GASTROENTEROLOGY

CLINICAL SCIENCE AND PRACTICE

GASTROENTEROLOGY
CLINICAL SCIENCE AND PRACTICE

Ian A. D. Bouchier
CBE, MD, FRCP, FRCP(Edin), HonFCP(SA), FFPHM, FRSA, FIBiol, FRS(Edin),
Professor of Medicine, Department of Medicine (RIE), University of Edinburgh,
The Royal Infirmary, Edinburgh, UK

Robert N. Allan
MD, PhD, FRCP
Consultant Physician, Queen Elizabeth Hospital,
Edgbaston, Birmingham, UK

Humphrey J. F. Hodgson
DM, FRCP
Professor of Gastroenterology, Royal Postgraduate Medical School;
Consultant Physician, Hammersmith Hospital,
London, UK

Michael R. B. Keighley
Barling Professor and Head, Department of Surgery, Queen Elizabeth Hospital,
Edgbaston, Birmingham, UK

SECOND EDITION
VOLUME TWO

W.B. SAUNDERS COMPANY LTD
LONDON PHILADELPHIA TORONTO SYDNEY TOKYO

This book is printed on acid free paper

W.B. Saunders Company Ltd

24–28 Oval Road
London NW1 7DX

The Curtis Center
Independence Square West
Philadelphia, PA 19106–3399

55 Horner Avenue
Toronto, Ontario M8Z 4X6, Canada

Harcourt Brace & Company (Australia) Pty Ltd
30–52 Smidmore St
Marrickville, NSW 2204, Australia

Harcourt Brace (Japan) Inc.
Ichibancho Central Building, 22-1 Ichibancho
Chiyoda-ku, Tokyo 102, Japan

First published 1984
Second edition 1993

A catalogue record for this book is available from the British Library.

Volume 1 ISBN 0-7020-1803-1
Volume 2 ISBN 0-7020-1804-X
Set ISBN 0-7020-1500-8

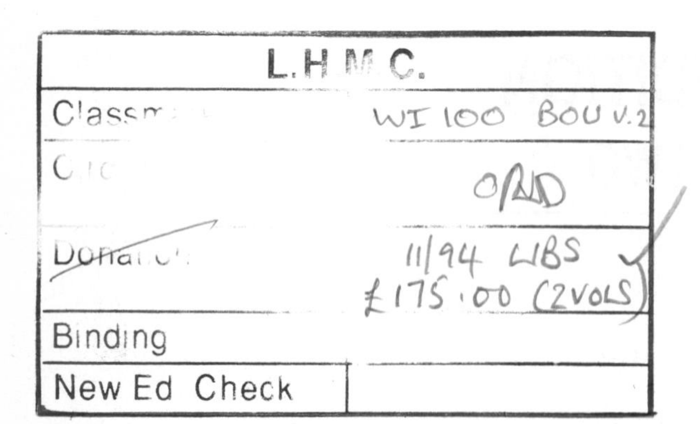

Typeset by Paston Press Ltd., Loddon, Norfolk
Printed and bound in Great Britain by The Bath Press

CONTENTS

VOLUME ONE

CHAPTER 5

GASTROINTESTINAL BLEEDING AND ISCHAEMIA

ACUTE UPPER GASTROINTESTINAL BLEEDING

A. Steger

INTRODUCTION

The management of bleeding from the gastrointestinal tract remains a major clinical problem, despite much work on diagnosis and treatment. Treatment is based on our increasing understanding of the relevant diseases and is becoming clearly defined with regard to both medical and surgical approaches. Despite this, there has been little change recently in the overall mortality from gastrointestinal bleeding; a 5–10% mortality being the range regarded as acceptable. It may be possible, however, to alter the outcome of gastrointestinal bleeding and reduce both rebleeding and mortality. This reflects specialist units for the management and monitoring of patients suffering from gastrointestinal haemorrhage, timing of endoscopy, a variety of endoscopic therapies, drug treatments and regimens and the timing of surgery and the operation performed. The mortality for upper gastrointestinal bleeds in specialist units has come down to 5% or lower[16] by these manoeuvres, but, recent changes in specialist practice are not yet generally applied. New approaches explored in the treatment of bleeding peptic ulcers and oesophageal varices should be extended to other causes of gastrointestinal bleeding.

There are about 30 000 admissions a year in England and Wales for gastrointestinal bleeding. To make further progress one priority is to reduce the number of patients in whom no cause of bleeding is found.[4,129] It is not possible to determine an exact breakdown and enumeration of the mortality of all diseases causing gastrointestinal bleeding from the information given in publications of the Office of Population Census and Surveys.[99,100] In 1988 there were 2125 deaths from bleeding peptic ulcers, just

Table 5.1 A total of 4431 cases of upper gastrointestinal haemorrhage giving causes and short-term outcome including rebleeding. (From OMGE International Upper GI Bleeding Survey, 1978–86[6] with permission of Scandinavian University Press)

Diagnosis	*n*	%	*Rebled (%)*	*Died (%)*
Peptic ulcer	1624	36.7	25.2	4.3
Varices	588	13.3	59.2	30.7
Erosions	298	6.7	15	7.1
Oesophagitis	183	4.1	7.7	3.6
Cancer	115	2.6	51.9	14.2
Mallory-Weiss	111	2.5	7	2
Other/multiple pathology	990	22.3	21.5	6.9
Normal endoscopy	229	6.7	2.6	0.4
No diagnosis made*	223	5	ND	ND

*No endoscopy, no diagnosis. ND = no data.

over half the total deaths from peptic ulceration. The OMGE Upper Gastrointestinal Bleeding Surveys[96] reported on over 4000 patients gathered over 8 years from the world and the causes of bleeding are shown in *Table 5.1*. Peptic ulcer disease and oesophageal varices accounted for about 50% of bleeding episodes; the overall mortality was 9.2% In the UK peptic ulceration accounts for nearer 50% of upper gastrointestinal bleeds and oesophageal varices 5–10%.[31] International comparisons are difficult because of different, and changing, disease patterns.

The acute bleeding peptic ulcer and its surgery is discussed in Chapter 2 (p. 306). As some therapies apply to non-ulcer haemorrhage and are described for 'upper gastrointestinal bleeding' in general rather than specific terms, there may be a small amount of overlap.

DIAGNOSIS

When a patient is seen with a suspected upper gastrointestinal haemorrhage a careful history and examination should be performed. Drugs and past medical and family history are relevant. Pulse and blood pressure measurement may indicate shock and further indication of a low circulating blood volume will be given by a low central venous pressure measurement or postural fall in blood pressure. Such observations indicate the severity of a bleed and have some prognostic value. Some cutaneous findings (spider naevi, telangiectasia, etc.) may be relevant to sources of blood loss.
Investigations include:

1. Haemoglobin
2. Platelet count
3. Haematocrit
4. Coagulation screen – especially if varices are suspected
5. Blood urea or blood urea nitrogen. This reflects a combination of dehydration, renal function and blood protein absorption from the gut. It is raised above the level expected from renal and circulatory considerations if blood has been lost into the upper gastrointestinal tract leading to absorption of broken-down blood and therefore may help distinguish between an upper and lower gastrointestinal bleed
6. Liver function tests
7. Calcium
8. Chest and abdominal radiographs for concomitant disease, which may alter diagnosis or management.

The main diagnostic investigation is fibreoptic endoscopy. The timing depends on the time of admission of the patient, the availability of endoscopic services and the patient's condition. All patients should be endoscoped within 24 hours of admission and ideally sooner. If a major bleed is suspected (tachycardia, systolic blood pressure under 100 mmHg, low central venous pressure, haemoglobin under 10 g/l) then endoscopy should be performed as soon as initial resuscitation has been adequately carried out.

Apart from the diagnostic role of endoscopy, therapeutic procedures may be performed to try and stop bleeding. Although early studies suggested endoscopy did not affect the outcome of upper gastrointestinal bleeding, this has changed with the recognition of differing endoscopic appearances of bleeding lesions, allowing better planning of treatment and rational endoscopic therapeutic intervention. This work relates predominantly to peptic ulcer haemorrhage, and is discussed on p. 308. The major stigmata of recent haemorrhage are a spurting (or bleeding) vessel or a visible vessel (in the base of an ulcer). These findings indicate a 50–80% chance of rebleeding. (The minor stigmata of haemorrhage include blood in the lumen, slight oozing and a flat red/black spot in the ulcer. These are associated with minimal risk of rebleeding and death.)[39] There is a need for similar criteria to be designed with respect to non-ulcer sources of bleeding. Diagnostic endoscopy in upper gastrointestinal bleeding is not just a question of looking. If a blood clot is seen obscuring the underlying mucosa and therefore any lesion, it must be washed away to allow full examination; this also applies to tissue slough and mucus. Endoscopy in upper gastrointestinal haemorrhage should be undertaken by the experienced endoscopist not the novice.

PRINCIPLES OF TREATMENT

MONITORING AND GENERAL CARE

Attention should be given to the clinical state of the patient, to the appearance of further bleeding and to the patient's pulse and blood pressure. Management is easier if these patients are monitored on a special unit attached to a gastroenterological ward, but of itself this is unlikely to reduce mortality. Patients with respiratory failure and those bleeding from oesophageal varices will often need the facilities of an intensive care unit. Urine output is particularly important and when this drops below 0.5 ml/kg per h, provided renal function was normal beforehand, it can be assumed that the patient has poor renal blood flow secondary to hypovolaemia. It may also be assumed that 20% of the blood volume has been lost and urgent resuscitation is necessary. Severe haemorrhagic shock occurs when more than 40% of the blood volume has been lost; in this situation there is inadequate perfusion of the heart and the brain. This seldom happens in modern hospitals but bleeding can be rapid in the elderly and in the patient with portal hypertension, and care must be taken to avoid irreversible circulatory damage. Changes in central venous pressure can be a useful guide to volume replacement.

The most important fluid for volume expansion is blood, but other fluids may be necessary, particularly at the moment of hospital admission. The fluid of choice on arrival at hospital is 0.9% sodium chloride or a balanced crystalloid solution. Care must be taken in transfusing saline, particularly in the elderly or in patients with heart disease, and it is contraindicated in patients with advanced liver disease. The expansion of blood volume is temporary but gives time for blood to be crossmatched, and the circulation is maintained adequately during this vital period. Colloids should be avoided at this stage, as leakage into the tissues provides problems for tissue lymphatics when the circulating blood volume has been re-established.

The place of transfusion in the patient with gastrointestinal haemorrhage has been questioned. In a small randomized trial, impedance clotting time was prolonged in those receiving a blood transfusion and those who were aggressively transfused had an increased rebleeding rate compared to those who were not transfused.[11] This work needs to be confirmed and most clinicians will require a lot of convincing that blood is not appropriate in the haemodynamically compromised patient.

BED REST

Bed rest has no therapeutic value per se and clearly depends on the clinical state of the patient. Once haemodynamic stability has been reached, bed rest has an adverse effect since thromboembolism is one of the most hazardous complications. Low dose heparin reduces the incidence of fatal pulmonary embolism after surgery but there is no reference to its use in non-operated patients with gastrointestinal bleeding.

SEDATION

Mild sedation is desirable in a restless patient, but care should be taken because the restlessness is frequently due to hypovolaemia. Diazepam is probably the best drug available but it should be used cautiously in hepatic disease.

ORAL INTAKE

Starvation was the traditional treatment until Meulengracht introduced early feeding and reported a reduced mortality. However, the reduced mortality was probably not due to feeding but to fluid replacement. Similar data were provided by Avery Jones but again the results were probably due to adequate transfusion. In the absence of definitive evidence on the effects of volume, acid and proteolysis in the stomach, no definite recommendations can be made for feeding. Management must therefore depend on the state of the patient and the likelihood of endoscopy or surgery.

NASOGASTRIC INTUBATION

The passage of a nasogastric tube is of much less importance since the introduction of endoscopy because one of its main functions was simply to detect whether there was free blood in the stomach. Opinion at the moment is rather against leaving such a tube in the stomach in view of its well recognized tendency to induce erosions. A nasogastric tube may play a role in the administration of drugs to the stomach, but otherwise its use should be discouraged.

TECHNIQUES OF THERAPEUTIC ENDOSCOPY

Endoscopy was initially claimed not to make any difference to the outcome of bleeding,[149] but this conclusion has to be modified with respect to the type of bleed (melaena, 'coffee grounds', massive haematemesis), the state of the patient (shocked or not), and the cause of the bleeding (erosions, ulcers or varices). Endoscopy allows diagnosis, some degree of prediction of further problems, and the potential for treatment as well. The value of the stigmata of recent haemorrhage in peptic ulceration is discussed in Chapter 2 (p. 308).

The methods used in the therapeutic endoscopic treatment of bleeding peptic ulcers (and varices) can be extended to treat haemorrhage from other causes. Technical drawbacks of surrounding tissue penetration, tissue damage and adherence of instrument to tissue (sticking) apply,[133] as does the principle of the use of the simplest, most effective technique available depending on the interest and experience of the operator. There are, in general, fewer published series of the results of these interventions in non-ulcer bleeding.

Endoscopy is generally well tolerated but hypoxia from respiratory depression due to sedative drugs such as midazolam can be a problem in the elderly.[8,9] Those undergoing endoscopy for upper gastrointestinal bleeding may require more sedation than normal and care should be taken that this is not excessive. To prevent hypoxia, oxygen can be given via nasal cannulas, and oxygen saturation (and pulse rate) monitored continuously with a laser Doppler pulse oximeter. Those at risk from developing endocarditis should receive prophylactic antibiotic cover for both diagnostic and therapeutic endoscopy.[107]

There is variation in the results of controlled trials as to the value of some methods (lasers) and factors to be taken into account include the experience of those doing the endoscopy.[73] There is great interest in a variety of physical methods to stop bleeding including thrombin, microwave probes and clips.

INJECTION

In treating oesophageal varices, injection works by causing intravariceal thrombosis followed by fibrosis. Experimentally sclerosants cause collagen formation for up to 30 days with variceal obliterations.[62] Transmural effects are seen which may explain the complications of fibrosis and strictures that can occur.

Injection is a simple, possibly underused method of stopping peptic ulcer bleeding;[79,125] in these reports, 78% of bleeding ulcers were stopped with a mixture of hypertonic saline and adrenaline in differing concentrations, the main one being 1:10 000. The effect of this is local pharmacological vasoconstriction together with the compressive effect of the volume (6–12 ml) injected.

There is increasing evidence of the effect of injection therapy in terms of reducing bleeding, the need for surgery and transfusion requirements. These findings apply whether an ulcer was bleeding, oozing or had stopped bleeding. Such work can be readily applied to other, non-ulcer causes of bleeding. In the past three years there has been increasing interest in injection techniques in the control of gastrointestinal bleeding for the simple reason that they are simple and cheap, the disposable part of one injection system costing about £40.

THERMAL

These methods all result in the deposition of energy around a bleeding point to cause tissue and vessel protein and collagen contraction and dehydration followed by thrombosis in the vessel that has bled. The technique is to place a ring of thermal energy around the bleeding point to intercept both entry and exit arms of the vessel that has bled.

Electrocoagulation

Experimental work has shown in an animal ulcer model that vessel compression is needed to ensure cessation of bleeding, a large Bicap probe being more effective than a non-contact laser beam.[3,64]

The bipolar electrode is possibly better than the monopolar with less sticking and more concentrated energy delivery as there is current between the closely applied points, rather than one between point and diathermy plate on the patient's surface. A probe with a film of liquid between a monopolar electrode and the tissue reduces adherence.[132] In endoscopic treatment it is, of course, the underlying vessel that is the target and inability to 'get' this may explain the failures.[63]

The multipolar electrocoagulator has been found in a small trial to be of value in treating bleeding from ulcers, Mallory-Weiss tears and vascular anomalies with a 90% haemostasis rate. Factors affected included repeat bleeding, transfusion requirements and further intervention.[76] One advantage electromechanical probes and injection methods may have over a laser light beam is that of mechanical compression at the time of delivering treatment.[118,134] There is perhaps a slightly greater chance of perforation with a monopolar than a bipolar electrocoagulator or heater probe as the last two stick less to tissue than the former.

Microwave thermal energy can also be used to treat bleeding points but is comparatively complex and costly.[75]

Laser

There has been some disparity between trials examining the use of different lasers in the treatment of bleeding ulcers. It is now established that because of its greater tissue penetration, the neomydium yttrium aluminium garnet (Nd-YAG) laser is more effective than the shorter wavelength argon laser. In trials studying bleeding peptic ulcers, with major stigmata of recent haemorrhage only under consideration, then a clear advantage was shown in association with laser treatment.[131,134] These trials were the first to show that therapeutic endoscopy had a place in the treatment of gastrointestinal bleeding. Other methods, however, may well produce as good results but without the need for the capital outlay for expensive equipment.

OTHER AGENTS

Butyl cyanoacrylate (butynate, a variety of 'superglue') is an effective haemostatic agent especially in conditions of mucosal bleeding such as gastric coagulopathy.

RADIOLOGY

Should an endoscopy service not be available, barium meal studies will show some lesions such as chronic peptic ulcers, cancers and varices (but without any treatment option) but they are not as useful as endoscopy at demonstrating erosions, gastritis or tears.[41,98]

Angiography can be of use when diagnosis is difficult but it is not a method for the occasional user and is best left to the expert enthusiast. The precise site of blood loss can be demonstrated by extravasation of contrast into the gut lumen but is rarely seen, so the demonstration of a potentially bleeding lesion is generally considered diagnostic. Bleeding rates of at least 0.5 ml/s are required for the direct demonstration of contrast leakage into the lumen.[91] Inter-arterial digital subtraction angiography can be of use in the detection of difficult bleeding lesions in the upper gastrointestinal tract before embolization.[113] Where the point of blood loss cannot be detected, the infusion of urokinase through carefully positioned catheters at selective visceral angiography can dissolve thrombus, restart bleeding and allow detection of the site of bleeding. This has its risks but may be necessary.[44] Techniques of angiography are discussed in greater detail later in this chapter.

99m Technetium sulphur colloid or pertechnetate-labelled red cell radionuclide scanning can detect blood loss at the lower rate of 0.1 ml/s and are mainly used in those with intermittent or chronic blood loss or those in whom there is doubt as to the site of blood loss.[59] These methods are simple to use and, if positive, indicate the area from which blood loss is coming and, for these reasons, the techniques are gaining popularity where available. Sulphur colloid scanning gives a rapid assessment of blood loss during the 20–40 minutes that the tracer is present in the circulation. Labelled red cells circulate for longer, but images obtained with this technique contain a persistent vascular background from circulating red cells which may make interpretation more difficult.

Angiography also can be used therapeutically with diffuse gastric bleeding or erosions or in patients thought unfit for surgery. The principle followed is that of arterial embolization of feeding blood vessels, or infusion of substances to cause vasoconstriction. Agents infused to stop bleeding include intra-arterial vasopressin and gelfoam. Although bleeding can be stopped in 75%, when rebleeding occurs there may be a 50% mortality rate, which is perhaps a reflection on the severity of such patients' illness to start with.[33] Vasopressin and embolization delivered by a selectively placed intra-arterial catheter in the treatment of upper gastrointestinal bleeding have been compared, with embolization being the more successful and preferred modality.[45]

Ultrasonography is useful in the detection of hepatosplenomegaly and can demonstrate the presence of intra-abdominal varices. Duplex Doppler (colour) sonographic studies can detect flow and its direction in the portal vein.

PHARMACOLOGICAL TREATMENT

Drug therapy in the context of acute gastrointestinal bleeding has a number of aims:

1. Enhancing the healing of mucosal ulcerative lesions, generally thought to be associated with hyperacidity.
2. Local control of the site of bleeding, generally by intra-arterial infusion.
3. Enhancement of clot formation and decrease in fibrinolysis.
4. Reduction in portal pressure.

Acid suppression in ulcer-associated bleeding

This is discussed in Chapter 2 (p. 310). The consensus from such studies is that it has been difficult to demonstrate that acid reduction improves mortality, or rebleeding within the acute episode, but most clinicians will begin such therapy with a view to starting the healing process. There are few studies that have addressed the effect of acid suppression in non-ulcer haemorrhages; in one study involving a variety of patients, including many on corticosteroids and non-steroidal anti-inflammatory drugs (NSAIDs), and largely, but not exclusively, bleeding from erosions, there was a reduction in blood loss in the group treated with acid suppression compared with the control group, with a reduction in rebleeding.[26,30] Pepsin inhibitors to reduce local proteolytic activity do not however, seem to be effective.[10]

Vasoconstrictors

Intra-arterial vasoconstrictors, such as vasopressin, are effective in controlling certain sorts of haemorrhage.[45] They may be particularly suitable for diffuse conditions such as widespread severe gastric erosions.[2] For more localized lesions, increasing use of therapeutic arterial embolization, particularly in the upper gastrointestinal tract where this can be performed relatively safely, has reduced enthusiasm for this procedure.[45]

There are other local approaches to stopping bleeding other than those of angiography or therapeutic endoscopy. Local cooling via a nasogastric tube with cold water (perhaps not generally considered a pharmacological approach) is widely practised in certain areas, although it has never been critically evaluated or proven.[10]

Blood coagulation

The increasing sophistication of transfusion services, and the availability of fresh frozen plasma, has made it easier to reverse clotting abnormalities, particularly in patients with liver disease. In the context of obstructive jaundice, vitamin K should be given to enhance coagulation factor synthesis. The antifibrinolytic drug tranexamic acid reduces transfusion requirements and the need for emergency surgery from benign gastric and duodenal lesions. Meta-analysis of the use of this drug in upper gastrointestinal bleeding suggests its use could lead to a 20% reduction in mortality, a 30% reduction in surgery and a 40% reduction in morbidity.[52] It is not clear whether the use of this drug can be extrapolated to non-ulcer associated bleeding and, despite the meta-analysis, the drug is not routinely used. Most studies were relatively small in number and a reporting bias may have crept in. The drug can be given intravenously, 1 g three times a day, with a reduced dose in renal impairment.

Splanchnic flow reduction

Drugs aimed at reducing splanchnic blood flow are most widely used in the context of portal hypertension. Somatostatin combines a reduction in splanchnic blood flow with a reduction in gastric acid secretion and in a controlled trial, a 72-hour infusion was reported to reduce the need for surgery, but not rebleeding or mortality;[83,84] but a somatostatin analogue was unhelpful in ulcer bleeding.[21]

CAUSES OF OESOPHAGEAL HAEMORRHAGE

MALLORY-WEISS TEAR

This is a tear in the mucosa at the level of the hiatus, a relatively common cause of upper gastrointestinal bleeding, accounting for about 5% of most published series. There is often a history of vomiting without blood in the vomitus before the haemorrhage, indicating that local pressure at the hiatus leads to a tear in the gastric or oesophageal mucosa.[85] The most common association is an acute alcoholic binge, which explains the peak incidence in males, aged from 20 to 50. Severe straining without vomiting, such as lifting or epilepsy, can also induce tears. If tears occur without obvious cause, however, bulimia is an association that may occur while self-induced vomiting is concealed.[152]

The tear can be in the gastric or oesophageal mucosa, and develops into a shallow ulcer which heals within a fortnight. More than one may be present. The diagnosis may be difficult to obtain with the endoscope. The tear may be seen either on the way into the stomach, or on retroverting the endoscope when the mucosal fold may hide the tear. There is often an associated hiatus hernia.

Most Mallory-Weiss tears stop bleeding spontaneously, but they can be injected. Surgery is only rarely required.[92] The use of a pressure tube such as a Sengstaken's tube is not recommended due to the possibility of causing extension or rupture.

INFECTIVE OESOPHAGITIS

Any infective oesophagitis may present as bleeding. Infection may be viral or fungal and it is uncommon for normal patients with no underlying cause such as malignancy, immunosuppression[130] or chemotherapy, to develop such infections.[6] The main organisms are viral: herpes simplex, cytomegalovirus, HIV 1, and fungal: *Candida*, moniliasis and aspergillus. Treatment of the relevant organism reduces the bleeding.[112]

Increasing numbers of drugs can cause oesophagitis, erosions and ulceration and possible bleeding; potassium chloride or quinidine are responsible in 60% of cases but other drugs include zidovidine, pivmecillinam, mexilitine and doxycycline.

PEPTIC AND STRESS-RELATED OESOPHAGITIS

The uncommon phenomenon of ectopic islands of gastric mucosa in the oesophagus (distinct from Barrett's oesophagus) may cause bleeding.[140] Barrett's oesophagus (discussed in Chapter 1) is found in up to 10% of patients with severe oesophagitis, and ulceration causing bleeding may be hard to treat in the columnar-lined Barrett's rather than the normal squamous-lined oesophageal epithelium. Omeprazole may have an advantage over H_2-antagonists here, as it has in the treatment of haemorrhagic reflux oesophagitis.[50,53,57,69] A very small percentage (up to 0.4%) of patients undergoing dilatation of a benign peptic oesophageal stricture bleed enough to need transfusion.[71] Operations on the oesophagus to control bleeding are rare unless portal hypertension is present.

Oesophageal bleeding in ventilated patients is prevented equally as well by sucralfate as by cimetidine.[19] It probably arises from acid reflux.

CARCINOMA OF THE OESOPHAGUS

Acute severe bleeding from oesophageal cancer is relatively uncommon and usually dysphagia and weight loss are present. Treatment is as appropriate for the stage of the disease, as discussed on p. 158. The Nd-YAG laser can be used to achieve haemostasis in bleeding oesophageal cancers,[87] and injection can also be attempted in emergencies.

OTHER CAUSES OF OESOPHAGEAL BLEEDING

Rare causes of oesophageal bleeding include aorto-oesophageal fistulas arising from aneurysms, oesophageal ulcers, foreign bodies, intrathoracic malignancies and intrathoracic vascular grafts. Pemphigus vulgaris, a rare disease, may lead to bullae and erosions in the oesophagus.

OESOPHAGEAL VARICES AND PORTAL HYPERTENSION

Survival after 5 years in those with cirrhosis and varices is 25%, with death or rebleeding most likely in the 2 weeks after bleeding.[27] Variceal size, portal pressure and a blue colour of the varices seen endoscopically seem to predict future bleeding.[123] Ultrasonographic measurement of the portal structures may correlate better with the occurrence of variceal bleeding than endoscopic assessment of variceal size.[90]

About 50% of those with varices bleed from them with a 30% risk of rebleeding at 6 weeks and 70% at a year. Mortality for each episode is up to 50%.

A study of the clinical history of varices in patients with primary biliary cirrhosis found that after varices developed, survival after 3 years was 59%. This was associated with haemorrhage in 41%, and survival after haemorrhage was 46%.[47]

Of those with a variceal bleed, 35–70% die depending on the hepatic reserve. Initial management is resuscitation with fluid and blood and correction of coagulopathy. After this comes the choice of vasopressin (with or without a vasodilator), injection sclerotherapy, balloon tamponade and surgery. All these options are not for the faint hearted or inexperienced. Of patients referred to the King's College liver unit with a Sengstaken–Blakemore tube in place, 50% of these had been incorrectly placed or managed.[147]

In the past 10 years, although there have been many detailed reports on the pharmacological management of variceal bleeding, there has been a trend towards the use of sclerotherapy as both the initial and definitive treatment for a bleeding episode.[136] This may give better results than balloon tamponade[104] as the initial treatment and does so in the longer term.[154] Although injection controls the bleeding episode in 90%,[38] it is repeated bleeds combined with the rate of failure of the diseased liver that determine the long-term outcome. The larger the varix and the higher the intravariceal pressure (over 12 mmHg) the more likely it is to bleed.[40,127]

MANAGEMENT OF VARICEAL BLEEDING

Management of variceal bleeding is complex, and may include mechanical, pharmacological, endoscopic, radiological and surgical manoeuvres. In addition these may be applied at the time of acute variceal haemorrhage, or after haemorrhage has occurred to prevent rebleeding. There are also some suggestions that medical treatment in particular may have a use prophylactically – before any bleeding has occurred.

For convenience, this section will discuss each particular mode of therapy in turn, outlining its use under each of these circumstances. Comparison between different approaches will be made as appropriate, and a final section provide a synthesis. Additional treatment appropriate to the chronic liver disease present in most patients with bleeding varices – prevention and treatment of encephalopathy, management of fluid balance including ascites, and correction of clotting abnormalities are relevant but fall outside the scope of this gastroenterological text. The discussion is also limited to the context of cirrhosis, and non-cirrhotic portal hypertension is not covered. Clinicians should, however, be alert to such possibilities, including varices secondary to splenic vein thrombosis, [80] the downhill varices of superior vena caval obstruction,[88] which require different approaches.

INJECTION SCLEROTHERAPY

Sclerotherapy for acute bleeding

Endoscopic therapy was first introduced in 1939[28] and has about a 90% success rate in the treatment of an episode of variceal bleeding. Sclerotherapy in the face of bleeding varices is a difficult task, not to be undertaken by the inexperienced. Anaesthetic assistance may be of great help in providing as stable a setting as possible for sclerotherapy to be performed. The use of an overtube to allow better and isolation of the bleeding point helps in the injection of acutely bleeding varices and should be available. There is probably little difference in outcome whether sclerosant is placed intravariceally or paravariceally, although the former is more popular and may help reduce mucosal complications. Manometry before injection can help increase the precision of intravariceal injection.[54] Providing obliteration results it does not really matter how it is done as long as the complication rate is low.[67] The timing of injections after the initial one has no effect on outcome.[153] Flexible endoscopic therapy has fewer complications than the use of a rigid endoscope.[12]

Injection therapy has complications, including bacteraemia in 50%, mild chest pain, pyrexia, aspiration, ulceration, strictures, oesophageal motor disorders and even brain and spinal cord infections. Sclerosant is detected in the pulmonary vasculature in 60% of those injected.[32]

One small trial showed that immediate injection stopped bleeding in 100% of cases and balloon tamponade in 90%, but both methods have their complications. After a week, fewer of those injected rebled.[95]

Agents used for injecting varices include 1.5% sodium tetradecyl sulfate, 5% ethanolamine oleate and absolute alcohol, but even if these are aimed into the variceal lumen, the area both within and around the varix is affected.[122] Ethanolamine as a sclerosant gives better control of postinjection bleeding and fewer injection ulcerations than sodium tetradecyl sulfate.[68] Five per cent ethanolamine oleate is a better sclerotherapy agent than 1% pilocanol.[66] Accessory agents used include disobutyl-2-cyanoacrylate 'superglue' and thrombin. Butylcyanoacrylate for control of acute variceal bleeding and treatment of fundal varices is claimed to be better than other agents.[126]

Laser therapy offers no advantage over injection sclerotherapy.

Long-term sclerotherapy

Following effective emergency sclerotherapy or indeed, successful conservative management by any means, most clinicians will enrol the surviving cirrhotic patient in a programme to obliterate varices. This approach has, in controlled trials, enhanced survival compared with controls without sclerotherapy.[70,154] Whether further enhancement of survival or, indeed, a greater reduction in the incidence of rebleeding, will follow combining sclerotherapy and β-blockade is currently unclear despite a number of trials.

Despite some logic in the approach, prophylactic sclerotherapy in the patient with cirrhosis who has never bled has not become widely practised and, indeed, in some controlled trials the prophylactic sclerotherapy was clearly deleterious.[49,124]

BALLOON TAMPONADE

Balloon tamponade in experienced hands can temporarily stop oesophageal variceal bleeding. The traditional approach of inserting a tube and decompressing next morning is usually followed by rebleeding, and aspiration (pneumonia in 10%) and oesophageal ulceration are notorious complications.[34,37,103] Its use is now being reduced as most will try early sclerotherapy in the acute phase; the approach may be useful to stabilize a patient to allow transfer to a specialist centre.

Important practical points are the use of a four-lumen tube (two balloons, gastric and upper oesophageal aspiration). Pressure necrosis should be avoided by intermittent decompression of the oesophageal balloon. Traction to increase the pressure of the gastric balloon at the oesophagogastric junction also predisposes to ulceration. Insertion of the balloon is easier if it is cold and therefore more rigid, and the oesophageal balloon pressure should be only 50–60 mmHg. The oesophagus should be regularly aspirated, and the whole episode kept to less than 24 hours.

In one small comparative trial (43 patients) more balloon tamponade treated patients rebled than did those treated with injections (19/23 to 9/20, $P < 0.05$). Other studies suggest that balloon compression is as good as injection sclerotherapy in stopping bleeding.[34,103]

DRUG THERAPY

Acute bleeding

The traditional drug therapy of acute variceal bleeding is vasopressin, which given intravenously can control bleeding in up to 60% of patients. Traditional bolus administration (20 units in 20 ml over 20 minutes) has given way to infusions (between 0.2 and 0.8 units per minute for 12–24 hours). This drug has a high cardiovascular complication rate, however, including myocardial infarction. The addition of an intravenous infusion of nitroglycerine can increase the effectiveness and reduce vasopressin related complications, and nitroglycerine patches have now been shown to be as effective and safer.[43] Glypressin is an alternative, synthetic formulation. In many studies in which vasopressin has been used, the overall hospital mortality has not been significantly greater than placebo, a reminder that it is the underlying degree of liver damage that is the main influence on the outcome of an episode of variceal bleeding.[58]

Intravenous somatostatin, infused at 250–500 μg per hour, has a similar or better effect than vasopressin with fewer side-effects. It is particularly expensive.[72,142]

Post-bleeding prophylaxis

Propranolol, given orally at a dose that reduces the pulse rate by 25%, has been shown to reduce rebleeding rates and improve mortality in a series of patients with alcoholic cirrhosis when given after an initial upper gastrointestinal bleed.[77] Improvement was seen in both variceal and diffuse gastric (erosive or portal hypertensive) haemorrhage. The precise effects of propranolol on the haemodynamics of the portal systemic circulation are poorly understood, but probably involves both splanchnic vasoconstriction and a reduction in cardiac output. These effects involve β_1- and β_2-receptors, so non-selective β-blockade is best.[155] There is probably a reduction in total hepatic blood flow, so liver function may deteriorate.

In the most successful therapeutic studies, β-blockade can reduce the incidence of recurrent variceal bleeding by up to 75%. So far physiological measurements have been unable to predict which patients on propranolol will rebleed.[146]

Prophylactic β-blockade

Meta-analysis of eight trials of non-selected β-blockade for the prophylaxis of bleeding in patients with cirrhosis who had never bled found that 45% of those treated bled compared with 66% in the control group ($P < 0.0001$). The differences in mortality were less striking: 22% in the β-blockade group and 28% in the control group. This improvement was not statistically significant.[24] As with comparative studies on the treatment of active variceal bleeding, it easier to improve bleeding rates than survival. In general, the better the initial liver function, the better the outcome.[48,102]

Other drug approaches

Drugs that increase the lower oesophageal pressure have been used to reduce oesophageal variceal bleeding in the short term. Metoclopramide reduces blood in flow to the area but whether there is a real clinical gain is unclear.[55]

SURGERY: ACUTE VARICEAL HAEMORRHAGE

General considerations

The direct surgical approach to acute variceal haemorrhage includes oesophageal transection, now generally performed with a 'gun stapler', with or without gastric vascularization, direct oversew of the bleeding vessel, or lowering of portal pressure by performance of a portacaval anastomosis. Among these, gun stapling has a slightly lower rate of controlling primary bleeding than portacaval shunting. On the other hand, shunting will predictably induce portal systemic encephalopathy. Emergency surgery inevitably has a higher mortality than elective surgery, but of the operations mentioned above, only portal–systemic shunting is considered for elective use, to prevent rebleeding; oversew and transection are limited in their use to stopping acute haemorrhage.

Direct oesophageal surgery

Although controlled trials have suggested that, as an initial approach in the bleeding cirrhotic, a greater proportion are controlled by transection than sclerotherapy,[56] most centres use this direct surgical approach when the logistically simpler and readily repeatable procedure of injection sclerotherapy has failed to achieve control.[105] The surgical operation perhaps surprisingly, does not increase mortality, probably reflecting its efficiency in stopping bleeding (usually 90% or more). Transection may give rise later to oesophageal strictures, but these are readily dilatable.

Portacaval decompression

Shunt operations have become less common, reflecting the growth of sclerotherapy, and the simpler surgical procedure of transection. In unselected series for acute bleeding the mortality may be 40–50%.[101] Selected patients – with good parenchymal liver function, perhaps non-cirrhotic livers, and selecting surgeons – may still be appropriate candidates after repeated serious bleeding. Early studies demonstrated that prophylactic surgery in patients who have never bled is inappropriate, as mortality is not improved, and encephalopathy enhanced.[25]

The precise type of shunt operation affects the development of postoperative encephalopathy and rebleeding. Rebleeding is less after portacaval shunting than the more distal shunts, whereas encephalopathy is more marked with the larger, proximal shunts.[51] Encephalopathy may be reduced further by distal splenorenal shunting rather than just splenorenal shunting.[150] Alternative approaches include the H-graft portacaval shunt, where a variation in the diameter of the shunt to below 10 mm leads to an improvement in encephalopathy and rebleeding rate.[121] The smaller the shunt the greater the risk of shunt thrombosis. The precise judgements in this area are difficult and often shaded by local expertise; the potential for liver transplantation, the morbidity and mortality of which is increased by previous shunt surgery, has also affected these decisions.[89,114]

Recently, interventional angiographic techniques allied with technical advances in stent formation have lead to the approach of transjugular intrahepatic portal systemic shunt: in effect railroading a wire mesh stent between the hepatic and the portal vein. The procedure offers the advantages of a surgical shunt without the surgical operation, and the size of the shunt can be modified to control encephalopathy. Its role is as yet undefined.[157]

OTHER APPROACHES

In acute bleeding, transhepatic obliteration of varices by interventional angiography can be achieved. The technique involves cannulation of the portal vein by passage of a guide-wire and catheter through the liver, and embolization of solid or irritant matter into the variceal run-off. The technique enjoyed a vogue in the 1970s and early 1980s. The high recurrence rate (for example 33% after 1 month) dampened enthusiasm for this lengthy procedure, whose complications included bleeding from the punctured liver and portal vein thrombosis.[135]

OVERALL TREATMENT APPROACH

There is a trend in the literature for the development of a policy where, if local treatment is unsuccessful with continued or early recurrent (24 hours) bleeding, then surgical decompression by either staple gun transection or portacaval shunting is the next step.[137] The patient should be as stable as possible; the results of surgery in the unstable patient are poor. It has been suggested that if two injection attempts fail then gun transection may prevent further continued rebleeding[18] but such a definition of injection sclerotherapy failure remains contentious. Whether recent approaches, such as the creation of a direct portal – systemic fistula by transhepatic or transjugular interventional radiology will alter this practice remains to be seen. After acute control, if established by sclerotherapy, most clinicians aim for long-term control with a course of sclerotherapy, and many now combine this with β-blockade.

GASTRIC BLEEDING ASSOCIATED WITH PORTAL HYPERTENSION

About 10% of variceal bleeds appear to come from gastric rather than oesophageal varices. These may be difficult to diagnose, becoming lost in folds of the stomach and requiring retroflexion of the endoscope. Their position also means that sclerotherapy is technically more difficult. Gastritis has also been found in 50% of patients with portal hypertension, and in some reports about 25% of the bleeds are attributed to gastritis rather than varices in this group of patients.[81,139] This portal hypertensive gastropathy consists of dilated tortuous submucosal veins and vascular ectasia. In some individuals this gives an appearance of diverging antral folds similar to the watermelon stomach.

The control of bleeding from gastric varices or portal hypertensive gastropathy may be more difficult than that of oesophageal variceal bleeding. Tamponade relying on the gastric balloon may be effective for strategically placed fundal lesions. Oesophageal transection is inappropriate, but a direct surgical approach with oversewing and a gastric devascularization may be attempted for emergency surgery. Decompressive surgery by formation of a portacaval shunt may be more logical in this group, and the transjugular, interventional, radiological approach to portal decompression may pay dividends in this group. Propranolol has been shown to be effective for prevention of re-bleeding from the portal hypertensive stomach.[77,139]

GASTRIC AND DUODENAL BLEEDING

The major role played by ulcers of the gastric and duodenal areas requires re-emphasis, as discussed in Chapter 2 (p. 306). Duodenitis, regarded by many as part of the spectrum of duodenal ulcer disease, may bleed and is not discussed in this section. In addition, any gastric tumour, or the rare gastric polyp, may bleed, but these are easily recognized and logically treated by injection, snaring or, commonly, surgery.

GASTRIC EROSIONS AND STRESS ULCERATION

Acute erosions of the gastric mucosa are common – seen in at least 10% of endoscopies. The constellation of minor abnormalities, of erythema, superficial haemorrhages and erosions, together constitute erosive gastritis. Erosions of more than 5 mm are generally dignified by the name of ulcers. Erosions are mainly associated with NSAIDs such as aspirin and indomethacin.[156] These are particularly prone to cause erosive gastritis on first use, within the first few days, and subsequent adaptation of the mucosa to the insult occurs. A substantial number of patients have continuing erosions, a disease entity which merges into NSAIDs-associated ulceration of the mucosa.[117] The erosions associated with NSAIDs are often linear, and characteristically appear in the antrum.

Alcohol is another common association of an acute erosive gastritis. Chronic erosive gastropathy is also common in renal failure, including chronic dialysis patients.[144] In the context of severe illness, as intensive care units, severe erosive gastritis and generalized acute stress ulceration throughout the stomach can occur and these can be particularly dangerous.[15]

Erosive gastritis predisposes to significant haemorrhage, even after apparently trivial intake of drugs such as aspirin. The superficial nature of the lesion on acute exposure to aspirin means that healing can take place rapidly, and most patients will respond to conservative treatment. Management can be difficult if haemorrhage persists, as bleeding may come from multiple sites, rendering endoscopic intervention difficult. Undersewing areas of diffuse erosion is seldom effective. Partial gastrectomy and vagotomy is probably the treatment of choice, although total gastrectomy may be required.[14]

Erosive gastritis is generally treated by transfusion if required, and either H_2-receptor antagonists, sucralfate, or a proton pump inhibitor. The evidence that these help stop bleeding is poor, but the role of these drugs in prevention of acute stress ulceration (see below) allows the logic of at least trying to prevent further ulceration.[60]

Prophylaxis against NSAIDs-induced gastric damage, and against blood loss, by the use of H_2-antagonists, or exogenous prostaglandins, is effective.[23] Prostaglandins are a logical approach to NSAIDs-induced erosions, as they replace the prostaglandin deficiency induced by the inhibitory activity of the NSAIDs against prostaglandin synthetase. Widespread prophylactic use of this class of drugs has been limited by side-effects such as diarrhoea, but use of the drugs is growing.

The erosive gastritis association with acute alcohol intake is well recognized but poorly documented, and its natural history is similar to that associated with acute NSAID-induced damage. In chronic alcoholics, portal gastropathy as discussed under gastric complications and portal hypertension may contribute to the picture.[81]

Acute bleeding from the upper gastrointestinal tract may complicate about 5% of admissions into intensive care units.[65] This is generally attributable to stress ulceration, the complex of severe confluent erosions from a combination of drug therapy, hypotension, renal failure, perhaps anxiety and other features. Considerable work has been done on the ability to prevent stress ulceration, with the endpoint of a trial generally being a reduction of measured blood loss rather than clinical episodes of significant gastrointestinal bleeding. High-dose antacids, sucralfate and H_2-antagonists are all effective, and proton pump inhibitors are likely to be.[60] The intravenously available preparations of H_2-antagonists have obvious advantages in this group of patients, although sucralfate can easily be delivered via a nasogastric tube.

Clinical bleeding can be severe and persistent, and associated with a high mortality. If conservative management fails, endoscopic control is worth trying but may be ineffective due to the widespread nature of the lesion.

Surgical procedures in patients bleeding from stress ulceration are associated with a mortality of between 33 and 50%, reflecting the group of patients who are severely ill, and the major surgical procedures required.[14] Intra-arterial pharmacological therapy with vasopressin at angiography has a high reported success rate, but an obvious reporting bias in its favour.[2] There seems no doubt that greater awareness of the problem, and the use of prophylaxis, is reducing the incidence of this complication.

ARTERIOVENOUS MALFORMATIONS

Angiodysplasia and arteriovenous malformations are now recognized to affect the whole of the gastrointestinal tract and not just the colon. They accounted for 4.4% of bleeding lesions in a series of 676 upper gastrointestinal endoscopies for haemorrhage.[22] The appearance varies, discrete, flat or raised but always red and varying in size from 2–10 mm. The shape may be pinpoint, stellate or web-like. There may be more than one lesion present in the upper gut and up to 50% may have colonic lesions.[35] Gastroduodenal arteriovenous malformations were found in 2% of all upper gastrointestinal bleeds and 3.7% of all major bleeds and, in this series, endoscopic therapy was noted to be useful.[111] Angiodysplasia bled in 23% of patients in whom it was seen at endoscopy (a total of 41 patients observed for 3 years), causing anaemia in 22%.[86]

The experience gained from the use of therapeutic endoscopy in treating bleeding ulcers has been extrapolated to other non-ulcer lesions although, as these are less common and less likely to be associated with major stigmata of recent haemorrhage, it is difficult to say how great a reduction in mortality this brings. Certainly if gastroduodenal angiodysplasias can be treated in this way, then repeated and difficult surgical resections may be avoided.[17]

Both the Nd-YAG and argon laser have been used to treat gastric and duodenal angiodysplasias and telangiectasias with better results being achieved with the former, a reflection of its greater tissue penetration.[17]

Diffuse vascular ectasia in the antrum can cause major blood loss and chronic anaemia. These are seen as red/blue linear streaks seeming to converge on the pylorus ('watermelon stomach'). These lesions consist of dilated ectactic vessels with a thickened gastric wall and fibrosis around the abnormal vessels.[74] Treatment can be local or resectional. In a small study, diffuse gastric vascular ectasia was found to be more common in females than males (7:1) and associated with cirrhosis and reduced gastrin levels and to cause chronic anaemia.[1] Such lesions are accessible to local endoscopic therapy[115] and surprisingly may respond to corticosteroid therapy, as well as to oestrogen–progesterone.[97]

Hereditary haemorrhagic telangiectasia has been found in a defined population to affect the stomach in 89% and the duodenum in 61%;[143] a few patients also had oesophageal or colonic lesions and the small intestine may also be involved. The mean age for the onset of bleeding was 55 years.

The more it is looked for, the more upper gastrointestinal tract angiodysplasia will be found. Repeated endoscopic therapy can reduce and, with time, stop bleeding from these lesions.[42] Alcohol injection reduced bleeding in gastroduodenal vascular abnormalities[115] and the heater probe was used to treat 22 patients with watermelon stomach and, although an average for four sessions were needed, antrectomy was avoided and in 8 out of 10, chronic bleeding was stopped.[108]

DIEULAFOY LESION

The Dieulafoy erosion occurs usually within 6 cm of the gastro-oesophageal junction and describes a discrete pinpoint ulceration over a branch of a gastric artery.[145] It is responsible for massive recurrent haemorrhage at any age. The mechanism of haemorrhage is thought to be superficial mucosal erosion penetrating this vessel. The Dieulafoy lesion is responsible for up to 1.5% of massive upper gastrointestinal bleeds.[36] Treatment can be by endoscopic therapy but the position of the bleeding point, often best viewed with a retroverted endoscope, may make this difficult and oversewing at laparotomy may be necessary.[106] Endoscopic treatment (injection, electrocoagulation) was performed successfully in 18 out of 22 patients.[13,110]

PANCREATITIS

Haemorrhage can complicate severe pancreatitis and be treated by arterial embolization but although control may be achieved, it may be at the cost of a high risk of development of septic complications needing debridement.[148] Similarly the spontaneous development of a fistula to the transverse colon is rare in pancreatitis but, when it occurs, may be associated with a 33% mortality due to sepsis or haemorrhage.[138] Bleeding is usually associated with pseudocyst formation after acute pancreatitis. In those with chronic pancreatic disease, splenic venous thrombosis can lead to extrahepatic portal hypertension and varices, curable by splenectomy.[80]

HAEMOBILIA

Haemobilia is a rare cause of upper gastrointestinal tract bleeding, which tends to be intermittent in nature so it is not always possible to see blood emerging from the ampulla. Angiography or pancreatography are usually required for diagnosis. Causes include pancreatitis *per se*, the development of an aneurysm of the gastroduodenal artery or one of its branches[128] (often after pancreatitis) and biliary–vascular fistulas. Increasing iatrogenic causes such as liver biopsy, endoscopic sphincterotomy, stenting, pancreatography and combined endoscopic radiological procedures are the main reasons for haemobilia developing and the temporal relationship to these events should indicate the cause.

Significant haemobilia complicates percutaneous transhepatic biliary drainage in up to approximately 5% of cases and may need to be stopped by arterial embolization.[93] Up to 10% of endoscopic sphincterotomies may be complicated by bleeding[46,78] and 2% may need surgery, these contributing to the mortality, albeit low, of the procedure. Indeed iatrogenic haemobilia has trebled in recent years and can be grouped as percutaneous, operative (including endoscopic) and from anticoagulation.[120] After a percutaneous procedure the placement of a nasobiliary catheter may allow the bleeding of haemobilia to settle without obstruction from blood clots.[5]

Percutaneous cholangioscopic lithotomy used in the management of common duct stones in association with strictures had minor bleeding in 14% and major bleeding requiring angiographic therapy in 10%.[61] Out of 1000 cholangiopancreatograms with sphincterotomies for common bile duct stones performed by the experienced group at the Middlesex Hospital, London, haemorrhage occurred as a complication in 3.9%[141] It must be appreciated that this type of figure represents the best in the range of complications after sphincterotomy. Severe bleeding may be managed angiographically with embolization.[29,119]

Haemobilia was also seen after balloon dilation of benign biliary strictures (20% in a controlled study comparing this treatment with surgery) and all needed arteriographic embolization to control the bleeding.[109] Expanding metallic stents used for biliary strictures had a high incidence of severe haemorrhage as a complication.[116]

OTHER CAUSES OF GASTRODUODENAL HAEMORRHAGE

Other miscellaneous causes of bleeding include aortoenteric fistulas (which should be considered in any patient presenting with gastrointestinal bleeding and a past history of aortic surgery), Wegener's granulomatosis, stomal ulceration, postgastrectomy biliary gastritis and polyps.

Aortoenteric fistulas may be spontaneous, but are commonly associated with Dacron grafts for aortic surgery. The site of predeliction is the fourth part of the duodenum, so endoscopic visualization is therefore difficult. A typical pattern is one or two brisk 'herald' bleeds preceding a catastrophic bleed and, in the setting of an aortic graft, early surgery is recommended. Aortography may be entirely unhelpful.

Of those patients with neurofibromatosis, 25% have gastrointestinal lesions and 60% present with bleeding.[151] Chemotherapy for lymphoma and gastrointestinal cancers has a high incidence of haemorrhage in those with ulcers and some recommend pretreatment ulcer surgery.[20] Duodenal diverticula may be linked with lesions which bleed such as erosions or polyps or ectopic gastric mucosa.

When surgery is inappropriate to treat haemorrhagic gastric cancer, interstitial laser hyperthermia can be used to cause a thermal shrinkage of the bleeding vessels and tumour.[7]

Other rare causes of bleeding include haemophilia with low factor VIII levels[94] and occult faecal bleeding of unknown origin in marathon runners.[82]

Some of these and other causes of gastrointestinal bleeding discussed above, even including peptic ulceration and varices, can be difficult to diagnose despite the ease of access to this area with an endoscope. For this reason they may be classified as chronic or obscure causes of gastrointestinal haemorrhage.

REFERENCES

1. Arendt, T., Barten, M., Lakner, V. *et al.* (1987) Diffuse antral vascular ectasia: cause of chronic gastrointestinal blood loss. *Endoscopy*, **19**, 218–220.
2. Athanasoulis, C.A., Baum, S., Waltman, A.C. *et al.* (1974) Control of acute mucosal haemorrhage by intra-arterial injection of posterior pituitary extractor. *New England Journal of Medicine*, **290**, 597–560.
3. Auth, D.C. (1986) Animal testing of endoscopic haemostasis with lasers and other devices. *Endoscopy*, **18** (2) 36–39.
4. Avery-Jones, F., Read, A.E. and Stubbe, J.L. (1959) Alimentary bleeding of obscure origin: follow up study and commentary. *British Medical Journal*, **1**, 1138–1142.
5. Baker, A.R., Corlett, S.K., Cookson, J.B. and Carr-Locke, D.L. (1987) Haemobilia treated by nasobiliary catheterization. *American Journal of Gastroenterology*, **82**, 783–785.
6. Barbare, J.C., Beaugrand, M., Galet, B. *et al.* (1984) Herpetic oesophagitis, a cause of post operative gastrointestinal bleeding (letter). *Gastroenterology, Clinical Biology*, **8**, 290–291.
7. Barr, H. and Krasner, N. (1989) Interstitial laser photocoagulation for treating bleeding gastric cancer. *British Medical Journal*, **299**, 659–660.
8. Bell, G.D., Bown, S., Morden, A., *et al.* (1987) Prevention of hypoxaemia during upper gastrointestinal endoscopy by means of oxygen via nasal cannulae. *The Lancet*, **1**, 1022–1024.
9. Bell, G.D., Spickett, G. P., Reeve, P.A. *et al.* (1987) Intravenous midazolam for upper gastrointestinal endoscopy: a study of 800 consecutive cases relating dose to age and sex of patient. *British Journal of Clinical Pharmacology*, **23**, 241–243.
10. Berstad, A. (1987) Antacids, pepsin inhibitors, and gastric cooling in the management of massive upper gastrointestinal haemorrhage. *Scandinavian Journal of Gastroenterology*, **22** (137), 33–38.
11. Blair, S.D., Janvrin, S.B., McCollum, C.N. and Greenhalgh, R.M. (1986) Effect of early blood transfusion on gastrointestinal haemorrhage. *British Journal of Surgery*, **73**, 783–785.
12. Bornman, P.C., Kahn, D., Terblanche, J. *et al.* (1988) Rigid versus fibreoptic endoscopic injection sclerotherapy: a prospective randomised controlled trial in patients with bleeding oesophageal varices. *Annals of Surgery*, **208**, 175–178.
13. Boron, B. and Mobarhan, S. (1987) Endoscopic treatment of Dieulafoy haemorrhages. *Journal of Clinical Gastroenterology*, **9**, 518–520.
14. Bowen, J. (1984) Surgical therapy in stress ulcerations. *Scandinavian Journal of Gastroenterology*, **19** (105) 97–100.
15. Bowen, J.C. and Rees, M. (1984) Acute stress ulcerations of the stomach: clinical correlates. *Scandinavian Journal of Gastroenterology*, **19** (105) 29–32.
16. Bown, S.G. (1991) Bleeding peptic ulcers. *British Medical Journal*, **302**, 1417–1418.
17. Bown, S.G., Swain, C.P., Storey, D.W. *et al.* (1985) Endoscopic laser therapy of vascular anomalies of the upper gastrointestinal tract. *Gut*, **26**, 1338–1348.
18. Burroughs, A.K., Hamilton, G., Philips, A. *et al.* (1989) A comparison of sclerotherapy with stapled transection of the oesophagus for emergency control of bleeding from oesophageal varices. *New England Journal of Medicine*, **321**, 857–862.
19. Cannon, L.A., Heiselman, D., Gardner, W. and Jones, J. (1987) Prophylaxis of upper gastrointestinal tract bleeding in mechanically ventilated patients – a randomized study comparing the efficacy of sucralfate, cimetidine and antacids. *Archives of Internal Medicine*, **147**, 2101–2106.
20. Chellingsworth, M.C. and Page, M.M. (1986) Fatal gastrointestinal haemorrhage (case report). *British Journal of Surgery*, **73**, 703.
21. Christiansen, J., Ottenjann, R. and von Arx, F. (1989) Placebo controlled trial with the somatostatin analogue SMS 201-995 in peptic ulcer bleeding. *Gastroenterology*, **97**, 568–574.
22. Clouse, R.E., Costigan, D.J., Mills, B.A. and Zuckerman, G.R. (1985) Angiodysplasia as a cause of upper gastrointestinal tract bleeding. *Archives of Internal Medicine*, **145**, 458–461.
23. Cohen, M.M., McReady, D.R., Clark, L. *et al.* (1985) Protection against aspirin induced antral and duodenal damage with enprostic. *Gastroenterology*, **88**, 382–387.
24. Conn, H.O. (1988) Prophylactic popranolol: the first big step. *Hepatology*, 167–170.
25. Conn, H.O. and Lindenmuth, W.W. (1968) Prophylactic portacaval anastomosis in cirrhotic patients with oesophageal varices: interim results with suggestions for subsequent investigations. *New England Journal of Medicine*, **279**, 725–732.
26. Coraggio, F., Scarpato, P., Spina, M. and Lombardi, S. (1984) Somatostatin and ranitidine in the control of iatrogenic haemorrhage of the upper gastrointestinal tract. *British Medical Journal*, **289**, 224.
27. Cortez. P.H., Abrantes, A., Esteves, A.V. *et al.* (1989) Long term prognosis of patients with cirrhosis of the liver and upper gastrointestinal

bleeding. *American Journal of Gastroenterology*, **84**, 1239–1243.
28. Crafoord, C. and Frenckner, P. (1939) New surgical treatment of varicose veins of the oesophagus. *Acta Otolaryngologica*, **27**, 422–429.
29. Czerniak, A., Thompson, J.N., Hemingway, A.P. *et al.* (1988) Haemobilia: a disease in evolution. *Archives of Surgery*, **123**, 718–721.
30. Daneshmend, T.K., Hawkey, C.J., Langman, M.J.S., Logan, R.F.A. *et al.* (1990) Omeprazole versus placebo for acute upper gastrointestinal bleeding: a randomised double-blind controlled trial in 1154 patients. *Gut*, **31**, A1206.
31. de Dombal, F.T., Clarke, J.R., Clamp, S.E. *et al.* (1986) Prognostic factors in upper G.I. bleeding. *Endoscopy*, **18** (2), 6–10.
32. DePuey, E.G., Richards, W.O., Millikan, W.J. and Henderson, J.M. (1988) Scintigraphic detection of pulmonary embolization of oesophageal variceal sclerosant. *Endoscopy*, **20**, 91–94.
33. Eckstein, M.R., Kelemouridis, V., Athanasoulis, C.A. *et al.* (1984) Gastric bleeding: therapy with intra-arterial vasopressin and transcatheter embolization. *Radiology*, **152**, 643–646.
34. Elewaut, A., De Man, M., De Vos, M. and Barbier, F. (1988) Endoscopic sclerotherapy: the value of balloon tamponade and the importance of disinfection. *Endoscopy*, **20**, 48–51.
35. Emanuel, R.B., Weiser, M.M., Shenoy, S.S. *et al.* (1985) Arteriovenous malformations as a cause of gastrointestinal bleeding: the importance of triple vessel angiographic studies in diagnosis and prevention of rebleeding. *Journal of Clinical Gastroenterology*, **7**, 237–246.
36. Farup, P.G., Tholfsen, J.K., Berner, A.A. *et al.* (1986) (Letter). Exulceration simplex dieulafoy – a report of 3 cases. *Endoscopy*, **18**, 252–253.
37. Feneyrou, B., Hanana, J., Daures, J.P. and Prioton, J.B. (1988) Initial control of bleeding from oesophageal varices with the Sangstaken – Blakemore tube. Experience in 82 patients. *American Journal of Surgery*, **155**, 509–511.
38. Fevery, J. (1986) Oesophageal varices. *Current Opinion in Gastroenterology*, **2** (4), 545–556.
39. Foster, D.N., Milorzewski, K.J.A. and Lowowski, M.S. (1974) Stigmata of recent haemorrhage in diagnosis and prognosis of upper gastrointestinal bleeding. *British Medical Journal*, **1**, 1173–1177.
40. Garcia, T.G., Groszmann, R.J., Fisher, R.L *et al.* (1985) Portal pressure, presence of gastroesophageal varices and variceal bleeding. *Hepatology*, **5**, 419–424.
41. Gelfand, D.W., Dale, W.J., Ott, D.J. *et al.* (1985) Duodenitis: endoscopic-radiological correlation in 272 patients. *Radiology*, **157**, 577–582.
42. Gilmore, P.R. (1988) Angiodysplasia of the upper gastrointestinal tract. *Journal of Clinical Gastroenterology*, **10**, 386–394.
43. Gimson, A.E.S., Westaby, D., Hegarty, J., Watson, A. and Williams, R. (1986) A randomised trial of vasopressin and vasopressin plus nitroglycerin in the control of acute variceal haemorrhage. *Hepatology*, **6**, 410–413.
44. Glickerman, D.J., Kowdley, K.V., Rosch, J. (1988) Urokinase in gastrointestinal bleeding. *Radiology*, **168**, 375–376.
45. Gomes, A.S., Lois, J.F. and McCoy, R.D. (1986) Angiographic treatment of gastrointestinal haemorrhage – comparison of vasopressin and embolization. *American Journal of Radiology*, **146**, 1031–1037.
46. Goodall, R.J.R. (1985) Bleeding after endoscopic sphincterotomy. *Annals of the Royal College of Surgeons of England*, **67**, 87–88.
47. Gores, G.J., Wiesner, R.H., Dickson, E.R. *et al.* (1989) Prospective evaluation of oesophageal varices in primary biliary cirrhosis: development, natural history and influence on survival. *Gastroenterology*, **96**, 1552–1559.
48. Grace, N.D. (1990) A hepatologists view of variceal bleeding. *American Journal of Surgery*, **160**, 26–31.
49. Gregory, P., Hartigan, P. *et al.* (1987) Prophylactic sclerotherapy for oesophageal varices in alcoholic liver disease: results of a VA co-operative randomised trial. *Gastroenterology*, **92**, 1414.
50. Hameeteman, W. and Tytgat, G.N. (1986) Healing of chronic Barrett's ulcers with omeprazole. *American Journal of Gastroenterology*, **81**, 764–766.
51. Harley, H.A.J., Morgan, T., Redeker, A.G. *et al.* (1986) Results of a randomised trial of end-to-side portacaval shunt and distal splenorenal shunt in alcoholic liver disease and variceal bleeding. *Gastroenterology*, **91**, 802–809.
52. Henry, D.A. and O'Connell, D.L. (1989) Effects of fibrinolytic inhibitors on mortality from upper gastrointestinal haemorrhage. *British Medical Journal*, **298**, 1142–1146.
53. Hetzel, D.J. and Bonnin, M. (1986) Long term management of haemorrhagic oesophagitis with cimetidine and omeprazole. *Australian and New Zealand Journal of Medicine*, **16**, 226–228.
54. Hosking, S.W., Robinson, P. and Johnson, A.G. (1987) Usefulness of manometric assessment of varices in maintenance sclerotherapy. A controlled trial. *Gastroenterology*, **93**, 846–851.
55. Hosking, S.W., Doss, W., El-Zeiny, H. *et al.* (1988) Pharmacological constriction of the lower oesophageal sphincter: a simple method of arresting variceal haemorrhage. *Gut*, **29**, 1098–1102.
56. Huizinga, W.K.J., Angora, I.B. and Baker, L.W. (1985) Oesophageal transection versus injection sclerotherapy in the management of bleeding esophageal varices in patients at high risk. **160**, 539–546.
57. Humphries, T.J. (1987) Effects of long term

medical treatment with cimetidine and bethanechol in patients with oesophagitis and Barrett's oesophagus. *Journal of Clinical Gastroenterology*, **9**, 28–32.

58. Hussey, K.P. (1985) Vasopressin therapy for upper gastrointestinal tract. Has its effectiveness been proved. *Archives of Internal Medicine*, **145**, 1263–1267.
59. Hyams, J.S., Leichtner, A.M. and Schwartz, A.N. (1985) Recent advances in diagnoses and treatment of gastrointestinal haemorrhage in infants and children. *Journal of Paediatrics*, **106**, 1–9.
60. Ivarsson, L. (1984) Antacids and H2 receptors antagonists in the prophylaxis and treatment of erosive gastritis: clinical aspects. *Scandinavian Journal of Gastroenterology*, **19** (105), 86–91.
61. Jeng, K., Chiang, H. and Shih, S. (1989) Limitations of percutaneous transhepatic cholangioscopy in the removal of complicated biliary calculi. *World Journal of Surgery*, **13**, 603–610.
62. Jensen, L.S., Lauberg, S., Juhl, C.O. and Andreassen, T.T. (1987) Oesophageal collagen content and mechanical strength after endoscopic sclerotherapy of oesophageal varices. An experimental study in rabbits. *Scandinavian Journal of Gastroenterology*, **22**, 743–749.
63. Johnston, J.H. (1984) The sentinel clot and invisible vessel: pathologic anatomy of bleeding peptic ulcer. *Gastrointestinal Endoscopy*, **30**, 313–314.
64. Johnson, J.H., Jensen, D.M. and Auth, D. (1987) Experimental comparison of endoscopic yttrium-aluminium-garnet laser, electrosurgery and heater probe for canine gut arterial coagulation. Importance of compression and avoidance of erosion. *Gastroenterology*, **92**, 1101–1108.
65. Kamade, T., Fusamoto, H., Karuano, S. *et al.* (1977) Acute gastro-duodenal haemorrhage in head injury. *American Journal of Gastroenterology*, **68**, 249–252.
66. Kitano, S., Iso, Y., Koyanagi, N. *et al.* (1987) Ethanolamine oleate is superior to polidocanol for endoscopic injection of oesophageal varices: a prospective randomised trial. *Hepatogastroenterology*, **34**, 19–23.
67. Kitano, S., Koyangi, N., Iso, Y., Higashi, H. and Sugimachi, K. (1987) Prevention of recurrence of oesophageal varices after endoscopic injection sclerotherapy with ethanolamine oleate. *Hepatology*, **7**, 810–815.
68. Kitano, S., Iso, Y., Yamaga, H. *et al.* (1988) Trial of sclerosing agents in patients with oesophageal varices. *British Journal of Surgery*, **75**, 751–753.
69. Klinkenburg-Knol, E.C., Jansen, J., Festen, H.P.M. *et al.* (1987) Double-blind multi-centre comparison of omeprazole and ranitidine in the treatment of reflux oesophagitis. *The Lancet*, **1**, 349–350.
70. Koch, H., Henning, H., Grimm, H. *et al.* (1986) Prophylactic sclerosing of oesophageal varices – results of a prospective controlled study. *Endoscopy*, **18**, 40–43.
71. Kozarek, R.A. (1986) Hydrostatic balloon dilation of gastrointestinal stenoses: a national survey. *Gastrointestinal Endoscopy*, **32**, 15–19.
72. Kravetz, D., Bosch, J., Teres, J. *et al.* (1984) Comparison of intravenous somatostatin and vasopressin in treatment of acute variceal haemorrhage. *Hepatology*, **4**, 442–446.
73. Krejs, G.J., Little, K.H., Westergaard, H. *et al.* (1987) Laser photocoagulation for the treatment of acute peptic ulcer bleeding: a randomised controlled clinical trial. *New England Journal of Medicine*, **316**, 1618–1621.
74. Kruger, R., Ryan, M.E., Dickson, K.B. and Nunez, J.F. (1987) Diffuse vascular ectasia of the gastric antrum. *American Journal of Gastroenterology*, **82**, 421–426.
75. Kuyama, Y., Yamamoto, N., Takashimizu, Y. *et al.* (1987) Endoscopic microwave treatment. *Gastrointestinal Endoscopy*, **33**, 229–232.
76. Laine, L. (1987) Multipolar electrocoagulation in the treatment of active upper gastrointestinal tract haemorrhage: a prospective controlled trial. *New England Journal of Medicine*, **316**, 1613–1617.
77. Lebrec, D., Poynard, T., Bernuau, J. *et al.* (1984) A randomised controlled study of popranolol for prevention of recurrent gastrointestinal bleeding in patients with cirrhosis: a final report. *Hepatology*, **4**, 355–358.
78. Leese, T., Neoptolomos, J.P. and Carr-Locke, D.L. (1985) Successes, failures, early complications and their management following endoscopic sphincterotomy: results in 394 consecutive patients from a single centre. *British Journal of Surgery*, **72**, 215–219.
79. Leung, J.W.C. and Chung, S.C.S. (1987) Endoscopic injection of adrenalin in bleeding peptic ulcers. *Gastrointestinal Endoscopy*, **33**, 73–75.
80. Little, A.G. and Moossa, A.R. (1981) Gastrointestinal haemorrhage from left-sided portal hypertension, an unappreciated complication of pancreatitis. *American Journal of Surgery*, **141**, 53–158.
81. McCormack, T.T., Sims, J., Eyre-Brook, I. *et al.* (1985) Gastric lesions in portal hypertension: inflammatory gastritis or congestive gastropathy? *Gut*, **26**, 1226–1232.
82. McMahon, L.F., Ryan, M.J., Larson, D. and Fisher, R.L. (1984) Occult gastrointestinal blood loss in marathon runners. *Annals of Internal Medicine*, **100**, 846–847.
83. Magnusson, I. (1987) Secretin and somatostatin in the treatment of upper gastrointestinal haemorrhage. *Scandinavian Journal of Gastroenterology*, **22** (137), 56–60.
84. Magnusson, I., Ihre, T., Johansson, C., Seligson, U., Törngren, S. and Urnäs-Moberg, K. (1985) Randomised double blind trial of somatostatin in

the treatment of massive upper gastrointestinal haemorrhage. *Gut*, **26**, 221–226.
85. Mallory, G.K. and Weiss, S. (1929) Haemorrhages from lacerations of the cardiac orifice of the stomach due to vomiting. *American Journal of Medical Science*, **178**, 506–509.
86. Marwick, T. and Kerlin, P. (1986) Angiodysplasia of the upper gastrointestinal tract: clinical spectrum in 41 cases. *Journal of Clinical Gastroenterology*, **8**, 404–407.
87. Mathus-Vliegen, E.M.H. and Tytgat, G.N.J. (1986) Laser photocoagulation in the palliative treatment of upper digestive tract tumours. *Cancer*, **57**, 396–399.
88. Maton, P.V., Allison, D.J. and Chadwick, V.S. (1980) Downhill esophageal varices and occlusion of superior and inferior vena cavas due to a systemic venulitus. *Journal of Clinical Gastroenterology*, **7**: 331–336.
89. Mazzaferro, V., Todo, S. and Tzakis, A.G. *et al.* (1990) Liver transplantation in patients with previous portasystemic shunt. *American Journal of Surgery*, **160**, 111–121.
90. Medhat, A., Iber, F.L., Dunne, M. and Baum, R. (1988) Ultrasonographic findings with bleeding and non-bleeding oesophageal varices. *American Journal of Gastroenterology*, **83**, 58–63.
91. Meyerovitz, M.F. and Fellows, K.E. (1984) Angiography in gastrointestinal bleeding in children. *American Journal of Gastroenterology*, **143**, 837–840.
92. Michel, L., Serrano, A. and Malt, R. (1980) Mallory-Weiss-Syndrome. Evolution of diagnostic and therapeutic patterns over two decades. *Annals of Surgery*, **192**, 716–720.
93. Mitchell, S.E., Shuman, L.S., Kaufman, S.L. *et al.* (1985) Biliary catheter drainage complicated by haemobilia: treatment by balloon embolotherapy. *Radiology*, **157**, 645–652.
94. Mittal, R., Spero, J.A., Lewis, J.H. *et al.* (1985) Patterns of gastrointestinal haemorrhage in haemophilia. *Gastroenterology*, **88**, 515–522.
95. Moreto, M., Zaballa, M., Bernal, A. *et al.* (1988) A randomized trail of tamponade or sclerotherapy as immediate treatment for bleeding oesophageal varices. *Surgery Gynaecology & Obstetrics*, **167**, 331–334.
96. Morgan, A.G. and Clamp, S.E. (1988) OMGE International upper gastrointestinal bleeding survey, 1978–86. *Scandinavian Journal of Gastroenterology*, **23** (144), 51–58.
97. Moss, S.F., Ghosh, P., Thomas, D.M., Jackson, J.E. and Calam, J. (1992), Antral vascular ectasia: maintenance treatment with oestrogen-progesterone. *Gut*, **33**, 715–717.
98. Munitz, H.A. Gelfand, D.W. and Ott, D.J. (1985) Upper gastrointestinal series: patient management and a study of 199 cases, 1985. *Gastrointestinal Radiology*, **10**, 227–281.
99. Office of Population Census and Surveys. Mortality surveillance, England and Wales, 1968–1985 (1988) London: HMSO.
100. Office of Population Census and Surveys. Mortality by cause, 1988, England and Wales (1990) London: HMSO.
101. Orloff, M.J., Beu, R.H., Hyde, P.V. and Stivolocki, W. (1980) Long term results of emergency portacaval shunt for bleeding oesophageal varices in unselected patients with alcoholic scirrhosis. *Annals of Surgery*, **192**, 325–337.
102. Pagliaro, L., Burroughs, A.K. and Sorensen, T.I.A. *et al.* (1990) β-blockers for preventing variceal bleeding (letter). *Lancet*, **336**, 1001–1002.
103. Panes, J., Teres, J., Bosch, J. and Rodes, J. (1988) Efficacy of balloon tamponade in treatment of bleeding gastric and oesophageal varices: results in 151 consecutive episodes. *Digestive Diseases and Sciences*, **33**, 454–459.
104. Paquet, K.J. and Feussner, H. (1985) Endoscopic sclerosis and oesophageal balloon tamponade in acute haemorrhage from oesophageal varices: a prospective controlled randomised trial. *Hepatology*, **5**, 580–583.
105. Paquet, K.J., Mercado, M.A. and Gad, H.A. (1990) Surgical procedures for bleeding oesophageal varices when sclerotherapy fails: a prospective study. *American Journal of Surgery*, **160**, 43–47.
106. Peitsch, W., Lange, W. and Schauer, A. (1987) Dieulafoy's disease – a rare but serious cause of acute upper gastrointestinal haemorrhage. *Deutsche Medicale Wochenschreibe*, **112**, 1940–1942.
107. Perucca, P.J. and Meyer, G.W. (1985) Who should have endocarditis prophylaxis for upper gastrointestinal procedures? *Gastrointestinal Endoscopy*, **31**, 285–287.
108. Petrini, J.L. and Johnson, J.H. (1898) Heat probe treatment for vascular ectasia. *Gastrointestinal Endoscopy*, **35**, 324–328.
109. Pitt, H.A., Kaufman, S.L., Coleman, J. *et al.* (1989) Benign post-operative biliary strictures. Operate or dilate? *Annals of Surgery*, **210**, 417–427.
110. Pointer, R., Schwab, G., Konigsrainer, A. and Dietze, O. (1988) Endoscopic treatment of Dieulafoy's disease. *Gastroenterology*, **94**, 563–566.
111. Quintero, E., Pique, J.M., Bombi, J.A. *et al.* (1986) Upper gastrointestinal bleeding caused by gastroduodenal vascular malformations; incidence, diagnosis and treatment. *Digestive Diseases and Sciences*, **31**, 897–905.
112. Rattner, H.M., Cooper, D.J. and Zaman, M.B. (1985) Severe bleeding from herpes oesophagitis. *American Journal of Gastroenterology*, **80**, 523–525.
113. Rees, C.R., Palmaz, J.C., Alvardo, R. *et al.* (1988) DSA in acute gastrointestinal haemorrhage. *Radiology*, **169**, 499–504.

114. Rocko, J.M., Howard, M.M. and Swan, K.G. (1986) Surgical management of bleeding oesophageal varices: results with 80 cases. *American Journal of Surgery*, **52**, 81–86.
115. Rose, J.D.R. (1987) Endoscopic injection of alcohol for bleeding from gastroduodenal vascular abnormalities. *British Medical Journal*, **295**, 93–94.
116. Rossi, P., Bezzi, M., Salvatori, F.M. *et al.* (1990) Percutaneous management of benign biliary strictures with balloon dilatation and self expanding metallic stents. *Cardiovascular Interventional Radiology*, **13**, 231–239.
117. Roth, S.H. and Bennett, R.E., (1987) Nonsteroidal anti-inflammatory drug gastropathy – recognition and response. *Archives of Internal Medicine*, **147**, 2093–2100.
118. Rutgeerts, P., Broeckaert, L., Coremans, G. *et al.* (1987) Randomized comparison of three haemostasis modalities for severely bleeding peptic ulcers: epinephrine 1% injection alone (1), epinephrine and polidocanol 1% injection (2), epinephrine injection followed by YAG laser (3), *Gastrointestinal Endoscopy*, **31**, 182(abst).
119. Saeed, M., Kadir, S., Kaufman, S.L. *et al.* (1989) Bleeding following endoscopic sphincterotomy: angiographic management by transcatheter embolization. *Gastrointestinal Endoscopy*, **35**, 300–303.
120. Sandblom, P. (1986) Iatrogenic haemobilia. *American Journal of Surgery*, **151**, 754–758.
121. Sarfeh, L.J., Rypins, E.B. and Mason, G.R. (1986) A systematic appraisal of portacaval H-graft diameters: clinical and haemodynamic perspectives. *Annals of Surgery*, **204**, 356–363.
122. Sarin, S.K., Mishra, S.P., Sachdev, G.K. *et al.* (1988) Ethanolamine oleate versus absolute alcohol as a variceal sclerosant: a prospective randomized controlled trial. *American Journal of Gastroenterology*, **83**, 526–530.
123. Sarin, S.K., Sundaram, K.R. and Ahuja, R.K. (1989) Predictors of variceal bleeding: an analysis of clinical, endoscopic and haemodynamic variables, with special references to intravariceal pressure. *Gut*, **30**, 1757–1764.
124. Sauerbruch, T., Wotzka, R., Kopcke, W. *et al.* (1988) Prophylactic sclerotherapy before the first episode of variceal haemorrhage in patients with cirrhosis. *New England Journal of Medicine*, **319**, 8–14.
125. Schuman, B.M. (1987) Endoscopic injection therapy for nonvariceal upper gastrointestinal haemorrhage – is it too good to be true? *Gastrointestinal Endoscopy*, **33**, 121–122.
126. Soehendra, N., Grimm, H., Nam, V. and Berger, D. (1987) N-butyl-2-cyanoacrylate: a supplement to endoscopic sclerotherapy. *Endoscopy*, **19**, 221–224.
127. Staritz, M., Poralla, T. *et al.* (1985) Intravascular oesophageal variceal pressure assessed by endoscopic fine needle puncture under basal conditions, Valsalva's manoeuvre and glyceryltrinitrate application. *Gut*, **26**, 525–530.
128. Steckman, M.L., Dooley, M.C., Jacques, P.F. and Powell, D.W. (1984) Major gastrointestinal haemorrhage from peripancreatic blood vessels in pancreatitis: treatment by embolization. *Digestive Disease and Sciences*, **29**, 486–497.
129. Steger, A.C. and Spencer, J. (1988) Obscure gastrointestinal bleeding. *British Medical Journal*, **296**, 3.
130. Steger, A.C., Timony, A.S.A., Griffen, S., Salem, R.R. and Williams, G. 1990. The influence of immunosuppression on peptic ulcer following renal transplantation and the role of endoscopy. *Nephrology Dialysis Transplantation*, **5**, 289–292.
131. Swain, C.P., Bown, S.G., Storey, D.W. *et al.* (1981) Controlled trial of argon laser photocoagulation in bleeding peptic ulcer. *The Lancet*, **2**, 1313–1316.
132. Swain, C.P., Mills T.N., Dark, J.M. *et al.* (1984) Comparative study of the safety and efficacy of liquid and dry monopolar electrocoagulation in experimental canine bleeding ulcers using computorized energy monitoring. *Gastroenterology*, **86**, 93–103.
133. Swain, C.P., Mills, T.N., Shemesh, E. *et al.* (1984) Which electrode? A comparison of four methods of electrocoagulation in experimental bleeding ulcers. *Gut*, **25**, 1424–1431.
134. Swain, C.P., Kirkham, J.S., Salmon, P.R., Bown, S.G. and Northfield, T.C. (1986) Controlled trial of Nd-YAG laser photocoagulation in bleeding peptic ulcers. *The Lancet*, **1**: 1113–1116.
135. Terabayashi, H., Ohnishi, K., Tsunoda, T. *et al.* (1987) Prospective controlled trial of elective endoscopic sclerotherapy in comparison with percutaneous transhepatic obliteration of oesophageal varices in patients with non-alcoholic cirrhosis. *Gastroenterology*, **93**, 1205–1209.
136. Terblanche, J. (1985) The long term management of patients after an oesophageal variceal bleed: the role of sclerotherapy. *British Journal of Surgery*, **72**, 88–90.
137. Terblanche, J., Burroughs, A.K. and Hobbs, K.E.F. (1989) Controversies in the management of bleeding oesophageal varices (two parts). *New England Journal of Medicine*, **320**, 1393–1398 & 1469–1475.
138. Thomas, C.T., Hinton, P.J. and Thomas, E. (1986) Spontaneous pancreatic duct-colon fistula. *Journal of Clinical Gastroenterology*, **8**, 69–73.
139. Triger, D.R. (1989) Natural history and treatment of portal hypertensive gastropathy. *Journal of Gastroenterology and Hepatology*, **1** suppl. 8–14.
140. Truong, L.D., Stroehlein, J.R. and McKenzie, J.C. (1986) Gastric heterotopia of the proximal oesophagus: a report of 4 cases detected by endoscopy and a review of the literature. *American Journal of Gastroenterology*, **81**, 1162–1166.
141. Vaira, D., Ainley, C., Williams, S. *et al.* (1989)

Endoscopic sphincterotomy in 1000 consecutive patients. *Lancet*, **1**, 431–433.
142. Valenzuela, J.E., Schubert, T., Fogel *et al.* (1989) A multicentre, randomized double blind trial of somatostatin in the management of acute haemorrhage from oesophageal varices. *Hepatology*, **10**, 958–961.
143. Vase, P. and Grove, O. (1986) Gastrointestinal lesions in hereditary haemorrhagic telangiectasia. *Gastroenterology*, **91**, 1079–1083.
144. Vaziri, N.D., Dure-Smith, B., Millar, R. *et al.* (1985) Pathology of gastrointestinal tract in chronic haemodialysis patients: an autopsy study in 78 cases. *American Journal of Gastroenterology*, **80**, 608–611.
145. Veldhuyzen, Z., Bartelsman, J.F.W.M., Schipper, M.E.I. and Tytgat, G.N.J. (1986) Recurrent massive haematemesis from Dieulafoy vascular malformations – a review of 101 cases. *Gut*, **27**, 213–222.
146. Villa, D., Jiron, M.I., Poynard, T. *et al.* Failure of haemodynamic measurements to predict recurrent gastrointestinal bleeding in cirrhotic patients receiving popranolol. *Journal of Hepatology*, **5**, 144–148.
147. Vlavianos, P., Gimson, A.E.S., Westaby, D. and Williams, R. (1989) Balloon tamponade in variceal bleeding: use and misuse. *British Medical Journal*, **298**, 1158.
148. Waltman, A.C., Luers, P.R. Athanasoulis, C.A. *et al.* (1986) Massive arterial haemorrhage in patients with pancreatitis. Complementary roles of surgery and transcatheter occlusive techniques. *Archives of Surgery*, **121**, 439–443.
149. Wara, P. and Stodkilde, H. (1985) Bleeding pattern before admission as a guideline for emergency endoscopy. *Scandinavian Journal of Gastroenterology*, **20**, 72–78.
150. Warren, W.D., Millikan, W.J., Henderson, J.M. *et al.* (1986) Splenopancreatic disconnection: improved selectivity of distal splenorenal shunt. *Annals of Surgery*, **204**, 346–355.
151. Waxman, B.P., Buzzard, A.J., Cox, J. and Stephens, M.J. (1986) Gastric and intestinal bleeding in multiple neurofibromatosis with cardiomyopathy. *Australian and New Zealand Journal of Surgery*, **56**, 171–173.
152. Weaver, D.H., Maxwell, J.G. and Castleton, K.B. (1969) Mallory-Weiss Syndrome. *American Journal of Surgery*, **118**: 887–889.
153. Westaby, D., Melia, W.M., MacDougall, B.R.D. *et al.* (1984) Injection sclerotherapy for oesophageal varices: a prospective randomised trial of different treatment schedules. *Gut*, **25**, 129–132.
154. Westaby, D., MacDougall, B.R.D. and Williams, R. (1985) Improved survival following injection sclerotherapy for oesophageal varices: final analysis of a controlled trial. *Hepatology*, **5**, 827–830.
155. Westaby, D., Melia, W.M., MacDougall, B.R.D. *et al.* (1985) $\beta 1$-selective adrenoreceptor blockade for the long term management of variceal bleeding. A prospective randomised trial to compare oral metoprolol with injection sclerotherapy in cirrhotics. *Gut*, **26**, 421–425.
156. Wyatt, J.I. and Dixon, M.F. (1988) Chronic gastritis – a pathogenetic approach. *Journal of Pathology*, **154**: 113–124.
157. Zemel, G., Karzen, B.T., Becker, G.J. *et al.* (1991) Percutaneous transjugular portal systemic shunt. *Journal of the American Medical Association*, **266**, 390–393.

ACUTE COLONIC AND OTHER LOWER GASTROINTESTINAL BLEEDING

J. Spencer

INTRODUCTION

Acute rectal blood loss is a fairly common cause of hospital admission. In the UK between 80 and 90% of admissions for alimentary bleeding will be due to proximal causes, predominantly peptic ulcer and oesophageal varices. A very small number present with 'obscure bleeding' mostly of small bowel origin. The remainder have lower intestinal bleeds, distal ileal bleeding – principally from a Meckel's diverticulum – being indistinguishable clinically from colonic.

Such rectal bleeding may present a considerable diagnostic and management problem. It may initially be difficult to distinguish upper from lower causes of haemorrhage, and within the colon, localization may be problematic. Mistaken diagnosis may lead to inappropriate surgery, and high risk of mortality. Modern diagnostic methods should, however, enable a correct diagnosis to be made in most patients. In the past, the difficulty of differentiating between right and left sided haemorrhage has led some surgeons to recommend total colectomy in order to save life.[19,47,56] This should not now be necessary.

AETIOLOGY AND CLINICAL FEATURES

Table 5.2 lists causes of lower gastrointestinal bleeding, based on a table from a study by Moncure *et al.* in 1989.[42] The bleeding patterns may vary with the age of the patient. Some are so characteristic as to be almost diagnostic; for example a young teenager with brisk red haemorrhage has a very high chance of having a bleeding Meckel's diverticulum.

In other cases there is much less certainty. Indeed, bleeding from caecal angiodysplasia can closely resemble melaena from the duodenum, so an attempt should always be made to exclude a more proximal cause.

Bleeding from polyps at any age may present acutely, but the haemorrhage is usually brief and rarely severe. The presence of mucus mixed with blood indicates inflammation, infarction (in ischaemic colitis) or neoplasia. Tumours occasionally erode a large vessel causing severe haemorrhage, but this is unusual.

All the lesions mentioned in *Table 5.2* can cause minor persistent or occult bleeding. In acute haemorrhage there is a major clinical difference between episodic bleeds, which may vary in intensity, and persistent unrelenting haemorrhage. The latter calls for early diagnosis and prompt treatment, which is usually surgical. Repeated bleeding, in episodes which often cease on admission to hospital, has its own diagnostic difficulty. The more severe persistent bleed may be easier to localize but, when this is not so, can lead easily to inappropriate surgery and carries a high mortality. A major cause of difficulty in the elderly is the differentiation between bleeding from diverticula and angiodysplasia.

Table 5.2 Causes of lower gastrointestinal bleeding. (From Moncure *et al*[4].)

Jejunum, ileum	*Colon, rectum*
Arteriovenous	*Angiodysplasia**
malformations	Arteriovenous
Angiodysplasia	malformations
Ulcers	*Ulcerations**
*Anastomotic**	*Diverticulosis**
Simple	*Cancer*
*Diverticula**	*Polyps*
Meckel's	*Haemorrhoids*
Acquired	Anal fissure
Crohn's disease	Stomal varices
Varices	Postoperative
Ischaemic ulcer	Postpolypectomy
Tuberculosis	Anastomotic
Arteritis	Trauma*
Blind loop	Ulcers
Angioma	Simple
Leiomyoma*	Stercoral
Cancer	Typhoid
Sarcoma	Amoebic
Polyps	
Uraemic ulcer	
Stomal varices	
Lymphoid hyperplasia	
*Trauma**	

*Lesions that usually bleed acutely, but may do so chronically. The most common lesions are italicized.

PROGNOSIS

MORTALITY

The mortality of acute lower gastrointestinal bleeding is reported as being of the order of 10–15%, although not many large series give accurate data.[37,52] This reflects the fact that heavy bleeding from the lower gut occurs principally in the elderly. Ten to twenty per cent of patients may require urgent surgery. The mortality from acute colonic surgery is high – up to 50% in some series, emphasizing the importance of proper diagnosis and management.[18]

REBLEEDING

The risk of rebleeding after initial treatment is clearly related to the primary cause. Single clearly defined causative lesions such as a Meckel's diverticulum or a cancer can be removed with a guaranteed outcome. Rebleeding usually occurs in one of four situations.

First, episodes of repeated bleeding occur if no localizing diagnosis can be made. Rarely, frequent repeated bleeds may suddenly cease, no clear diagnosis having been reached. It is most likely that in such cases thrombosis and healing has occurred in a vascular malformation, but this is pure conjecture.

Second, treatment may be successful initially, followed by recurrence. For example, caecal angiodysplasia treated endoscopically may behave in this way. It is possible that the vascular lesions have progressed meanwhile, but this again is conjectural because little is known of the natural history of such lesions.

Third, a causative lesion may be treated, perhaps by surgical removal, but at a later date a second lesion begins to bleed. This is particularly likely with angiodysplasia or other vascular lesions, which are often multiple.[55] Clearly in some cases the caecal lesion may have been identified, but was not the cause of bleeding, but this is not always the case. It would seem that caecal angiodysplasia is associated with an unusually high incidence of Meckel's diverticulum;[27] it is also associated with angiodysplasia of the stomach and jejunum in some cases.

Fourth, misdiagnosis may lead to inappropriate therapy, followed by rebleeding from the real undiagnosed cause. The classic error is the removal of sigmoid diverticular disease, because this was apparent on investigation or surgery, when bleeding arose from unrecognized angiodysplasia of the right colon.

INVESTIGATION

Before attempts are made at localization of the source of bleeding, initial assessment and resuscitation must be carried out. It is important to recognize that most episodes of acute rectal bleeding cease spontaneously. In the presence of severe bleeding, the use of a central venous line will help in the assessment of transfusion needs and continuing bleeding. A careful history and examination are required as for upper gastrointestinal bleeding. The description of blood lost may vary from the bright red blood of lower colonic bleeding, to maroon or near black stools from right-sided colonic haemorrhage or lower small intestinal blood loss. Rectal examination reveals the nature of the stool as well as detecting local lesions.

The choice of initial investigation must depend to some extent on the presentation and condition of the patient, and on any history of preceding events or episodes. It is important to leave investigative options open, so barium contrast studies should be avoided early on, as they preclude subsequent satisfactory angiographic studies. A suggested protocol is shown in *Table 5.3*. It is important to do a coagulation screen, particularly where there is a history of repeated haemorrhage. It must be remembered that a haemorrhagic tendency, for example, in von Willebrand's disease, may predispose to bleeding from a gut lesion, and it must not be assumed that the diathesis alone is the cause. This is particularly so if there is a sudden increase in bleeding after a history of lesser bleeds.

Endoscopy plays an important role. Usually an oesophagogastroduodenoscopy is necessary to be certain that bleeding is not from the upper gut. A recent previous endoscopy should not be relied on to exclude this step; vascular lesions may be intermittently visible and a previous negative examination does not exclude a source of bleeding in this area.

A rigid sigmoidoscopy is important. Local lesions can be identified, and clot and blood evacuated. After this a colonoscopy or flexible sigmoidoscopy may be attempted. This will often not succeed initially, though it may yield useful information about the site of bleeding without necessarily identifying the lesion. Early enthusiasm to use colonoscopy to diagnose the source of acute lower intestinal bleeding has passed. Acute lower gut bleeding stops spontaneously in between 75% and 90% of cases. A policy of colonoscopy after subsequent bowel cleansing either with tap-water enemas or oral agents such as polyethylene-glycol preparations is the most effective in diagnosis.[13] Even in unrelenting haemorrhage, however, colonoscopy is still safe and practical. If unsuccessful in the acute stage, repeated examination after spontaneous cessation is often helpful.[24] A large-channel instrument is essential for suction of blood, clot and residual stool if emergency colonoscopy is performed. Insertion must be cautious and visualization precede progress. It is suggested that overinflation may precipitate or aggravate bleeding.[15] Experienced endoscopists report that in 50% of such cases a bleeding site can be identified, although some, such as angiodysplasia,

Table 5.3 Steps in management of acute or massive lower intestinal haemorrhage

Diagnostic protocol
- Sigmoidoscopy
- Coagulation profile
- Blood urea nitrogen

Active bleeding	*Bleeding ceased*
Endoscopy	Colonoscopy/barium enema
Upper GI	Pertechnetate-99m scan
Colonoscopy	Selective angiography
Sulphur-colloid or RBC-scan (^{99m}Tc)	
Pertechnetate-99m scan	
Selective angiography	
Barium enema	
Upper GI small bowel series	

are easily obscured by bleeding. Bright, fresh blood issuing from a specific point is the most conclusive evidence of localization. Equally important, in 70% the region of colon from which bleeding originates can be estimated, thus permitting effective surgical treatment. Diffuse bleeding may be observed in conditions such as colitis. In addition, in a few cases, endoscopy may also be therapeutic, particularly if polyps amenable to snaring are responsible for haemorrhage.

RADIONUCLEIDE SCANS

These may be performed in two ways.[25,38] Sulphur colloid labelled with ^{99m}Tc given intravenously is cleared rapidly by the reticuloendothelial system and extravasation into the gut lumen may allow detection of extravasation of blood to bowel with bleeding rates as low as 0.5–1.0 ml per minute, but localization may still be difficult because of overlapping bowel. Distal passage of colloid within the gut lumen sometimes gives valuable information. The best that can be achieved, however, is a regional localization, for example, to 'upper small bowel' as a source of bleeding. The liver and spleen may mask the colonic flexures.

Alternatively, autologous red blood cells may be labelled in vitro with ^{99m}Tc and reinjected. Images are then obtained every 5 minutes for 30 minutes and then at greater intervals for up to 24 hours. In active bleeding the first images are most relevant. Red cell scanning is more reliable than colloid scanning but introduces a preparatory step that may delay use in an acute situation.

Pitfalls in the interpretation of scintiscans for bleeding include the misinterpretation of abnormalities produced by lesions such as abscesses, fibroids or radiation damage.

In a consecutive series of 49 patients with obscure bleeding, a site was located in 45% by red cell scanning. In most the site was proximal to the colon, reflecting the fact that colonic causes had usually been recognised previously either by endoscopy or radiology.[15]

A sodium pertechnetate isotope scan may be used to indicate the presence of a Meckel's diverticulum, as described later.[32,54,59] One use of isotope scans, rather than accurate localization of bleeding sites, is to indicate that bleeding is active, and angiography therefore more likely to be successful.

SELECTIVE ANGIOGRAPHY

Selective angiography has become an important tool in acute haemorrhage. When bleeding is active and persistent the site of haemorrhage has been identified in up to 80% of patients.[1,4,22,23,44,45] The procedure is technically demanding, however, and high quality studies are not universally available. This may in part explain the polarization of views in the literature. Angiography should be performed expeditiously and with full therapeutic support; it is easy for patients to become shocked during prolonged procedures leading to the view that the risks outweigh the benefits.[16] Proper monitoring should avoid such difficulties.

In acute bleeding, angiography may either reveal an anatomical abnormality representing the bleeding lesion, or may show extravasation of contrast into the gut. For the latter to occur, bleeding must be active, and occurring at a rate of at least 0.5 ml per minute. A three-vessel visceral angiogram is usually necessary but, in brisk bleeding, the vessel studied first must depend on the clinical impression as to the likely source of blood loss.

The usual sequence for abdominal angiography however, starts with the superior mesenteric artery. If the site of bleeding is not identified on either the regular or subtraction films, a magnification study of the right colon, caecum and distal small bowel with subtraction is performed. The magnification and subtraction films often show small angiodysplastic lesions with early venous drainage which may not be seen on the regular films (*Figures 5.1* and *5.2*). If this study is negative, a selective inferior mesenteric arteriogram should be performed. A negative superior and inferior mesenteric angiogram necessitates a selective injection into the coeliac trunk and its branches. The middle colic artery which supplies

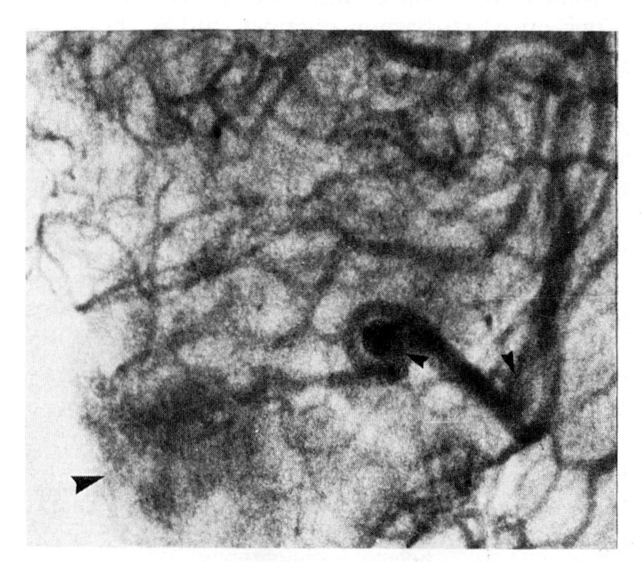

Figure 5.1 Angiodysplasia in the early capillary phase showing vascular tuft (large arrowhead) and early draining vein (small arrowhead).

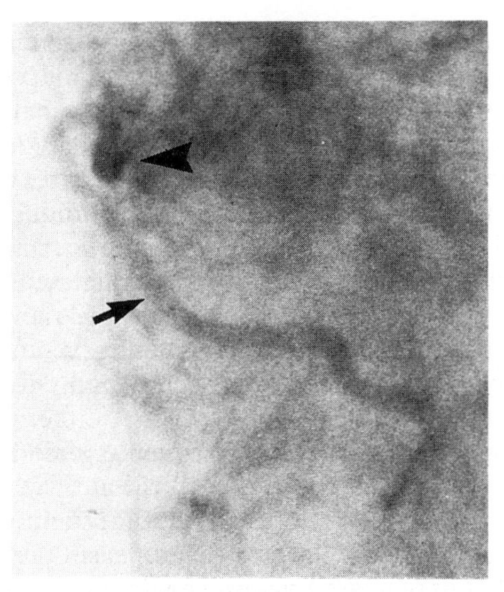

Figure 5.2 Angiodysplasia showing the vascular tuft (arrowhead) with the early draining vein (arrow).

part of the transverse colon may be an aberrant vessel and arise from the dorsal pancreatic artery. If this artery is not opacified, haemorrhage from this vessel will be missed. Also, a pancreatic tumour or abscess, or an aneurysm of the splenic artery, may erode into the transverse colon causing lower gastrointestinal haemorrhage. A coeliac axis injection will also ensure that a bleeding upper gastrointestinal lesion was not missed at earlier endoscopy.

The spectrum of findings when angiography is performed for acute colonic bleeding will vary according to the practice of the unit, whether colonoscopy has been performed and so on. Gostout reported 24 angiograms in acute bleeding, in which 12 revealed angiodysplasia.[26] This is the lesion most likely to be obscured at urgent colonoscopy, and one which early laparotomy, advocated instead of angiography by some, is most likely to miss.[16] There are not many full comparative studies. Jensen endoscoped 80 patients with acute bleeds and 74% had colonic lesions. In his series only 14% had been found on angiography, a yield which seems low considering that 30% of these lesions were arteriovenous malformations.[31]

Cussons *et al.* suggested that angiography gave a poor diagnostic yield and pointed out that laparotomy, which in their study was more effective diagnostically, should not be long delayed.[16] This study, however, included only nine angiograms for bleeding in an 18-month period; only one revealed a lesion, and the patient concerned became shocked during the radiological procedure. A second patient, in whom no angiographic diagnoses could be made, suffered a cardiac arrest during the procedure. In units with more extensive experience the yield is much higher. Koval *et al.* report angiograms in 63 patients with severe bleeding (with a mean transfusion requirement of over nine units). They found extravasation of contrast (46%), or a vascular anomaly (32%) in 78% of patients.[33] They pointed out that, unsurprisingly, extravasation of contrast into bowel was more likely to be seen with heavier bleeding, but they also used provocative manoeuvres such as heparin, tolazoline or streptokinase and, with these manoeuvres, the yield of extravasation doubled from 32% to 65%.[33]

If bleeding has stopped and a vascular tumour or angiodysplasia is suspected, the use of a vasodilator with magnification films enhances the early draining veins.

An occasional diagnostic technique in the angiographic setting is the injection of ^{99}m-technetium labelled sulphur colloid through a selectively sited catheter to localize slow bleeding. The potential for therapeutic use of angiography is discussed below.

BARIUM CONTRAST RADIOLOGY

A barium enema was once used commonly in the investigation of acute bleeding but, with the advent of colonoscopy and selective angiography, has been largely superceded. It is discouraged in the early stages because barium obscures the field for precise angiography. It was once believed that barium might even be therapeutic in diverticular bleeding, there being anecdotal reports of haemorrhage ceasing after such investigation. If the ileum is considered to be a possible source, then a small-bowel enema may be useful. The positive identification of a lesion on such an enema is very useful; however, a negative result must be treated with caution, as even gross lesions are occasionally missed due to overlapping of small bowel loops.

TREATMENT

ENDOSCOPIC TECHNIQUES

In colonic haemorrhage, endoscopic treatment falls into two main categories: namely colonoscopic removal of bleeding polypoid lesions; and other forms of ablative therapy.

Snare polypectomy is the appropriate treatment for those rare cases in which there has been massive bleeding from a polyp, and is occasionally used for bleeding from a fungating carcinoma. When there is active bleeding the procedure is facilitated by advancing beyond the lesion and snaring on withdrawal.

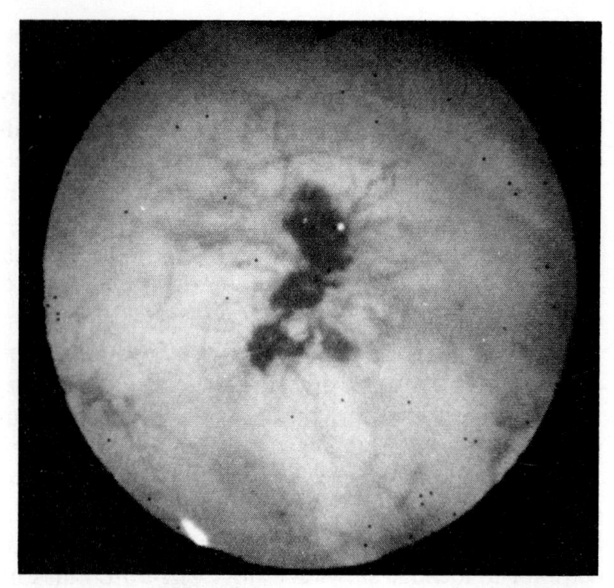

Figure 5.3 Angiodysplasia lesion seen at colonoscopy in the caecum of an elderly patient who presented with acute massive haemorrhage. The lesion is cherry red in colour and the dilated capillary network can be seen clearly.

Ablative therapy consists of coagulation or injection. Because of the thin-walled nature of the colon, there is always concern that coagulation, by whatever means, will lead to perforation. In one study of 115 patients, a comparison was made between the results of laser coagulation of lesions above and below the peritoneal reflection. Two thirds of these patients had presented with bleeding from tumours, arteriovenous malformations or radiation proctitis, and in half of these haemorrhage was acute. The procedures were considered successful in 83% in the rectum and in 87% in the colon. There was no difference in complication rates, even though 45% of the colonic lesions were in the particularly thin-walled caecum.[36] There was no laser-related morbidity. As in the duodenum, bleeding lesions may respond to injection with adrenaline, and this is rapidly becoming the first choice in non-polypoidal haemorrhage.[30]

Angiodysplasia (*Figure 5.3*) may, as already mentioned, be difficult to see in the acute stage, but elective colonoscopy after cessation of haemorrhage can permit electrocoagulation or laser therapy.[30] The lesions of angiodysplasia, Osler–Weber–Rendu and small angiomas are probably best managed by laser therapy.

THERAPEUTIC ANGIOGRAPHY

Once a site of bleeding has been identified by angiography, in selected cases treatment may be attempted by infusion of vasopressin. Bleeding within the inferior mesenteric territory such as a bleeding diverticulum (*Figure 5.4*) appears to respond well to peripheral intravenous infusion of

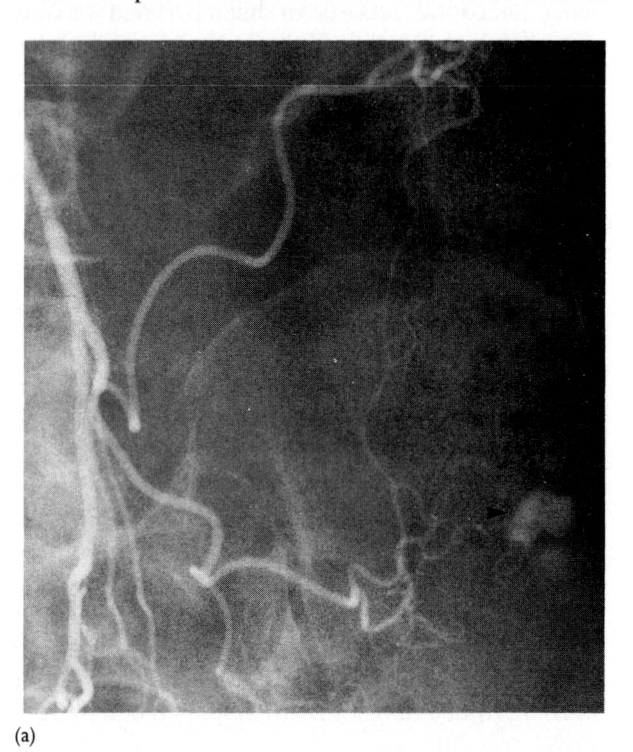

(a)

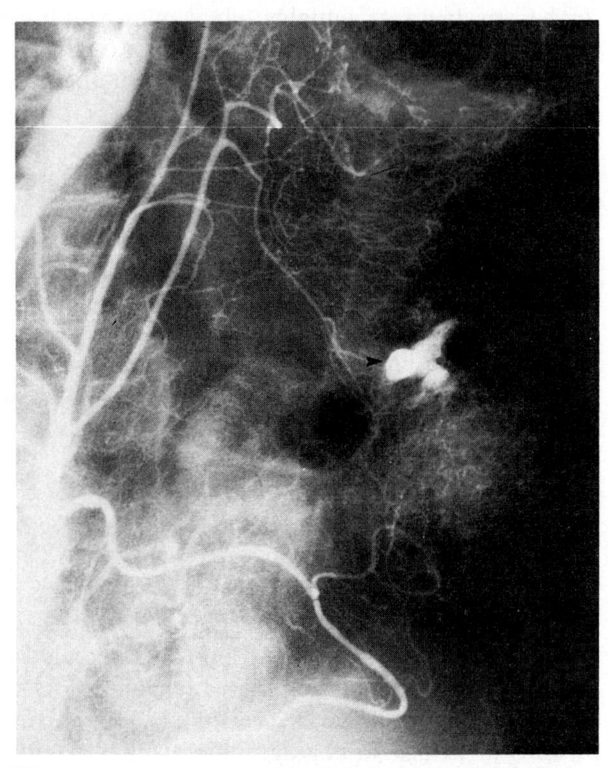

(b)

Figure 5.4 Bleeding diverticulum in the left colon seen at angiography with extravasation of contrast at the bleeding site (arrowhead).

vasopressin.[2,3,43] If there is no response to peripheral infusion a direct infusion into the mesenteric artery may be attempted. Bleeding within the superior mesenteric territory usually only responds to direct infusion into the major vessel.

Infusion therapy was initially used with some enthusiasm, but is now less widely employed. Its effect is temporary, and identification of a bleeding site should ideally be followed by direct assault – endoscopic or surgical in most cases – on the lesion. Continued bleeding, if not too severe, facilitates the identification of the lesion during direct exploration.

ARTERIOGRAPHIC EMBOLIZATION

This is occasionally a treatment option,[10] but has to be used with considerable caution because of the risks of bowel ischaemia,[48] causing infarction or perforation. It is therefore reserved for very pressing clinical situations (*Figure 5.5*). It has been used, for example, to arrest bleeding from an anastomotic site in a patient who had undergone several operations in rapid succession.[35] It is more useful higher in the gut where ischaemia is less likely than in the colon, and is the treatment of choice when mycotic aneurysms bleed in postoperative sepsis.

Disadvantages of this technique when compared with vasoconstriction are the lack of control and the fact that treatment is irreversible. Rebleeding may arise from sites with a dual blood supply and it is not always possible to place the catheter close to the bleeding lesion. Materials used for embolization currently include Gelfoam, Oxycel, Ivalon and cyanoacrylate. Gelfoam usually lyses within a few weeks to several months while Oxycel and Ivalon produce a longer occlusion. Ivalon frequently produces permanent occlusion as does cyanoacrylate but the latter is much more difficult to handle.

SURGERY

Ideally, the site of bleeding is localized before laparotomy and an appropriate resection is then indicated. In an acute situation this is not always achieved. In such cases a careful search for the bleeding source is made at laparotomy, which must include a careful examination of the small bowel. Meticulous palpation demands the emptying of each segment in turn by gentle 'stripping' movements, so that small lesions are not obscured by gut contents. On-table colonoscopy may be invaluable and if necessary colonic lavage can be carried out. A useful way of achieving this is to perform an appendicectomy and insert a catheter through a purse-string at its stump to irrigate the bowel.

The major problem at laparotomy, without prior localization, is to determine whether bleeding arises from the right or left colon, enabling an appropriate resection to be made. In the past, diverticular disease has been most problematic. Although diverticula are almost invariably more common on the left than on the right, experience with 'blind' resection of the left colon was frequently unsuccessful; indeed bleeding from the right colon seemed more common. In one series of 144 episodes of bleeding in 100 patients with diverticular disease, in 42 patients the bleeding was not red in colour, but black and tarry.[47] Such observations led to extensive bilateral resections in order to save life. It is very likely however that many of the right-sided bleeds may have been due to angiodysplasia, which often gives rise to tarry, melaena stools, though of course diverticula on the right do also bleed. Wrong surgical decisions have profound implications for the patient. With the use of angiography and on-table endoscopy, blind resections should rarely be necessary. In such an extreme situation it would be reasonable to resect

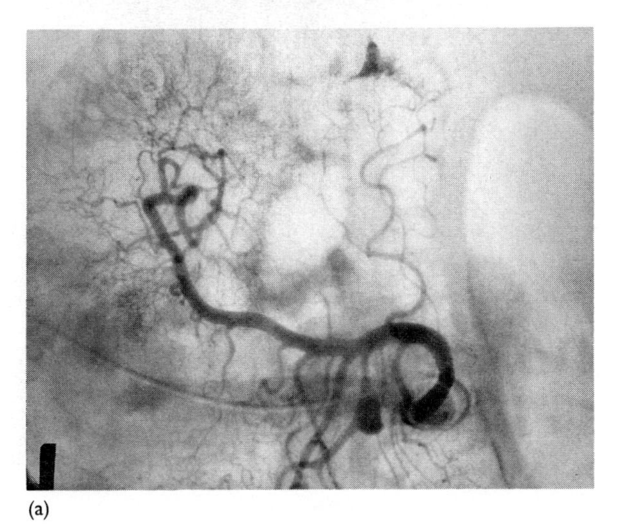

(a)

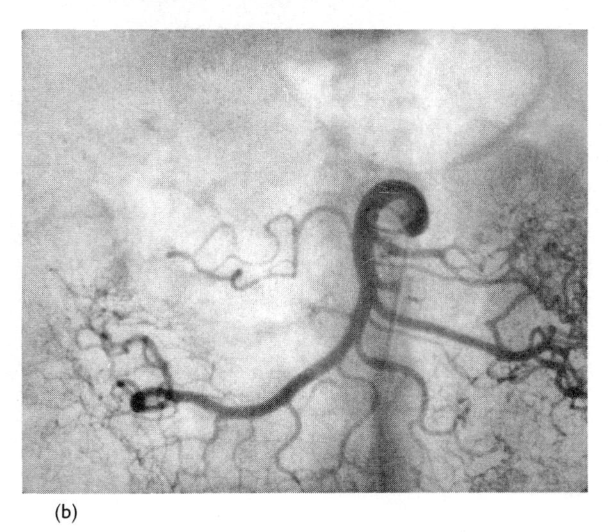

(b)

Figure 5.5 Embolization therapy. (a) Superior mesenteric arteriogram (arterial phase). (b) Superior mesenteric arteriogram following embolisation of the bleeding vessel with sterile absorbable gelatin sponge.

right or left according to the nature of the stool. When bleeding is particularly brisk, its origin may occasionally be identified by sectional cross-clamping of the bowel, and noting which segment fills with blood, but this is a rare situation. In the case of brisk but 'controllable' intermittent bleeding, there may still be a case for the formation of a transverse colostomy to identify the side which is bleeding, followed by resection later on. This rather desperate remedy, once quite commonly used, should rarely be necessary today.

AETIOLOGY

MECKEL'S DIVERTICULUM

Although not strictly a colonic condition, the clinical presentation is similar to that of right colonic bleeding lesions.

Such an ileal diverticulum occurs in about 2% of the population; although the incidence is equal in both sexes, symptoms are commoner in males. In infancy it usually lies about 30 cm proximal to the caecum, but this distance may be up to 90 cm in adults. The pouch represents the intestinal end of the vitellointestinal duct, and is of variable length and shape.

It is often lined with heterotopic gastric epithelium, occasionally associated with duodenal, pancreatic or colonic tissue. It is thought that between 10 and 20% of Meckel's diverticula are complicated by bleeding. Such haemorrhage arises as a result of peptic ulceration due to acid and pepsin secretion within the pouch, the ulcer being in the adjacent ileal mucosa, usually at the neck of the pouch. Such an ulcer may also perforate, and bleeding may be preceded by episodes of central abdominal pain. Although such bleeding can occur at any age, it is commonest in childhood, especially in the early 'teens'. Bleeding may be bright red or maroon in colour, and be either chronic, causing anaemia, acute, with severe bleeding, or recurrent, often with 'short, sharp' episodes of bleeding.

The presence of a diverticulum may be demonstrated on a small bowel enema, or on refluxed barium during a barium enema. It may also be demonstrated using a sodium pertechnetate isotope scan (*Figure 5.6*). It is important to realise that a negative technetium scan does not exlude the presence of a Meckel's; in some series the diagnosis rate has been high, but others have found that only 1 in 10 diverticula were detected. It is difficult to explain this wide variation in results. Selective superior mesenteric angiography may also be used to demonstrate a Meckel's; in the acute phase bleeding into the ileum may be seen, and in a quiescent phase the identification of a vitelline artery indicates the pres-

(a)

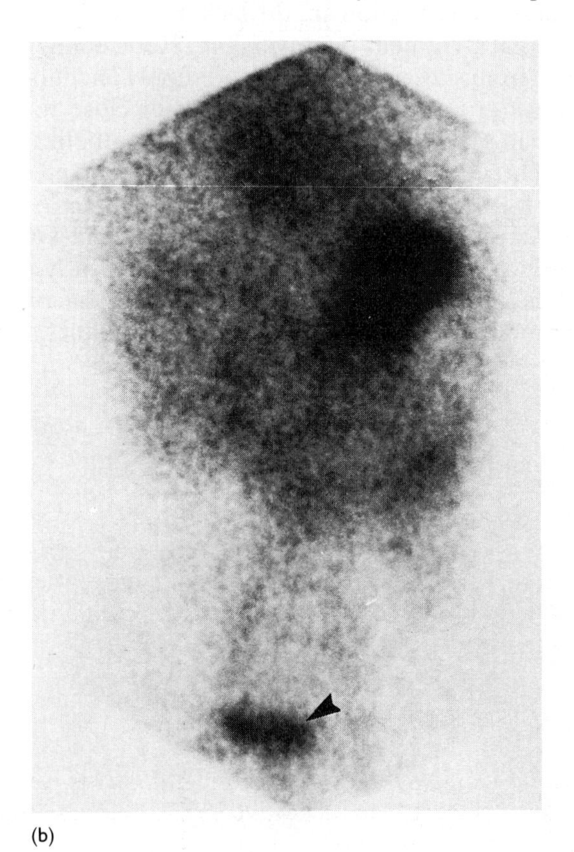

(b)

Figure 5.6 Meckel's diverticulum seen on a ^{99m}Tc pertechnetate scan showing the increased activity in the region of normal stomach and ectopic gastric mucosa (arrows). a) Anterior view; b) lateral view. (Courtesy of Dr G. Coates).

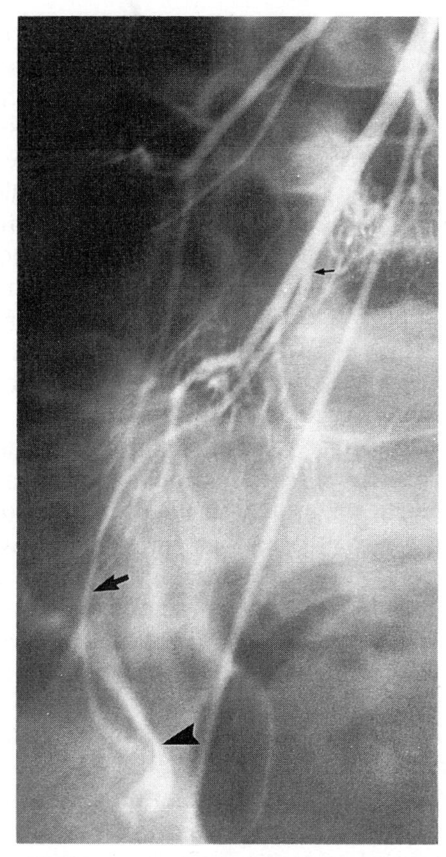

Figure 5.7 Bleeding Meckel's diverticulum seen at angiography in the arterial phase showing extravasation of contrast (arrowhead) and vitelline artery (large arrow) arising proximally (small arrow) from a major branch of the superior mesenteric artery (Courtesy of Dr R. J. Tuttle).

ence of a diverticulum, which must be the most likely (but not certain) source of haemorrhage (*Figure 5.7*).

Treatment is always surgical; resection of the diverticulum with either a wedge or length of adjacent ileum containing the ulcer is curative, except in those rare cases in which an incidental diverticulum is found in the presence of another bleeding lesion. It has been found, for example, that there is an unusually high incidence of diverticula in patients with angiographically demonstrated angiodysplasia, and in one series, in association with small bowel tumours.[17] Such associations are not as yet explained, or indeed substantiated from other sources.

INFLAMMATORY BOWEL DISEASE

Rectal bleeding is common in inflammatory bowel disease, especially in ulcerative colitis, and less frequently in Crohn's disease. If sigmoidoscopy is 'normal', up to 10% of patients who have persistent bleeding turn out eventually to have inflammatory bowel disease.[28] Massive bleeding, however, may be a presenting feature of localized Crohn's disease, especially in the young. In ulcerative colitis it usually occurs only in severe extensive disease.

In a review of 1526 patients with Crohn's disease seen at Mount Sinai Hospital, New York, 21 had severe acute bleeding, with 26 separate episodes. The incidence was 1.9% from large bowel lesions (17 of 929) and less, 0.7% from small bowel Crohn's (4 of 597 cases).[49] In a series of 913 patients in Aberdeen, 1.0% suffered life-threatening bleeding, with an age range of 21–63 years. In this series all bled from the colon.[34]

Mesleh and Lemons considered in 1983 that the ileum was the most common source of bleeding and that, in young subjects, Crohn's disease was the third commonest cause of bleeding after Meckelian ulceration and angiodysplasia.[39]

ANTIBIOTIC-ASSOCIATED COLITIS

This is an acute illness most often presenting as acute diarrhoea, usually with watery or mucoid stools. Gross bleeding may occasionally occur, but this is almost always in cases associated with the use of ampicillin. Sigmoidoscopy with biopsy is the most helpful diagnostic tool. Supportive measures, including transfusion in cases of haemorrhage, are important in therapy; more specific treatment is most often with vancomycin.

RADIATION-INDUCED COLITIS

Radiation-induced colitis is characterized principally by diarrhoea. In the initial stage of bowel damage an episode of bloody diarrhoea may occur. In the later chronic form of the disease there may be episodes of acute haemorrhage. This is almost always due to rectal or ileal ulceration, with bleeding from ectatic submucosal vessels.[57,60] Once episodes of bleeding occur, the progressive nature of this disease may demand surgical intervention to prevent crippling and life-threatening haemorrhage.[12] This is discussed further in Chapter 4.

TUMOURS

Benign polyps occasionally present with acute bleeding, though this is rarely severe. Juvenile polyps, though they typically have a short stalk, occasionally undergo torsion and auto-amputate. This is sometimes associated with massive bleeding.

Carcinomas of the colon may be associated with anaemia due to chronic bleeding, or bloody mucoid stools if left-sided. Acute brisk fresh haemorrhage may occur, but this is uncommon. Diagnosis by appropriate endoscopy or barium enema leads to surgical resection.

Bleeding from polyps may be controlled by snare excision, or by local electrocoagulation if bleeding is acute. The latter may be technically difficult, in which case surgical excision may be necessary.

VASCULAR ANOMALIES

Vascular anomalies, particularly angiodysplasia, are an important cause of bleeding which may be of an obscure nature. These are discussed as a whole below, in the section on obscure haemorrhage but, due to their frequency as a cause of acute bleeding, (as much as chronic), angiodysplasia of the colon is discussed here.

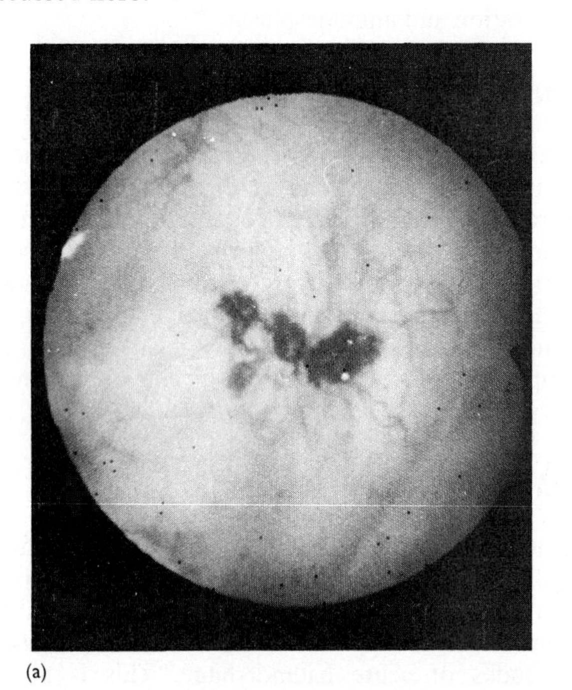

(a)

The lesions of angiodysplasia (*Figure 5.8*) are most commonly seen in the caecum and ascending colon but their frequency in the population is not known. Some workers believe that the lesions are unique to the right colon[8] although others have reported similar lesions elsewhere in the colon[9] and in the stomach and small bowel.[50] Baum *et al.*[5] suggest that angiodysplasia is an acquired lesion resulting from mucosal ischaemia, secondary to arteriovenous shunting in the mucosa which occurs with changes in intracolonic pressure.

Galloway *et al.*[51] who confirmed earlier reports of an association with aortic stenosis, believe that the lesions develop as a consequence of decreased perfusion pressure in the terminal branches of the superior mesenteric artery, secondary to a decreased ventricular output. A similar association with aortic valve disease and also chronic lung disease was noted by Rogers[50] whose patients were all diagnosed at colonoscopy. He has proposed that a lowered oxygen tension in the end-arterial vessels of the superior mesenteric artery results in capillary dilation and proliferation, eventually leading to a vascular abnormality.

Boley *et al.*[8,9] suggested that those lesions which occur in the right colon and caecum represent a separate and unique entity from other vascular lesions of the gastrointestinal tract. They base their conclusions on the evidence obtained from elegant injection techniques and painstaking study of the histopathology of the lesions. They explain the

Figure 5.8 (a) Angiodysplasia lesion in the caecum. The lesion is bright red and the dilated, irregular, superficial vessels can be seen clearly. (b) Gross specimen showing tortuous submucosal vessels communicating with two areas of mucosal angiodysplasia (upper right and upper left). A platelet thrombus plugs the site of haemorrhage (upper right).

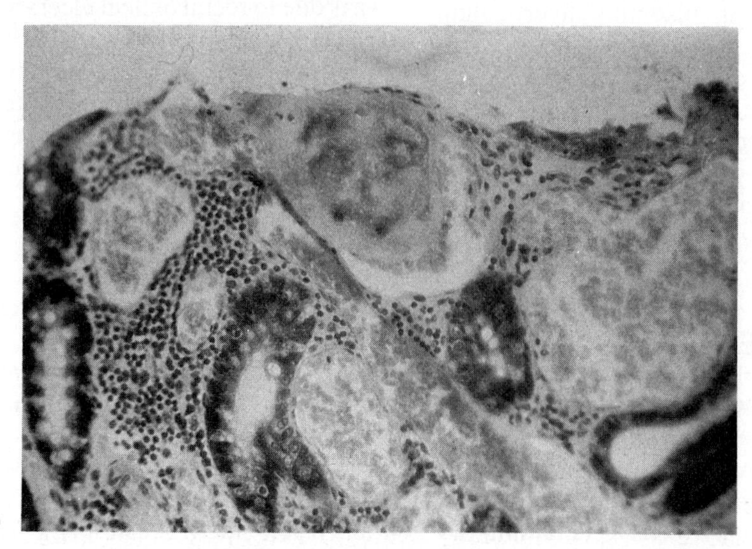

(b)

aetiology by a chronic intermittent partial obstruction of the submucosal veins at the point where they pass through the longitudinal and circular muscle layers of the bowel. This occlusion of the low pressure veins occurs over many years and does not affect the higher pressure arterial inflow. The resulting pressure differential causes capillary vessel and later capillary ring dilation with subsequent precapillary sphincter incompetence. Small arteriovenous malformations thus develop at the level of the mucosal capillaries. They attribute the frequency with which this lesion is now observed in the right colon to Laplace's law. When applied to the colon this states that the tension in the muscle of the bowel wall will be greater in that part of the colon with the greatest diameter, which is the caecum and right colon. From their extensive work Boley *et al.*[8] suggested that if angiodysplasia were due to ageing, lesions should be present in the colon of elderly patients who have not yet bled. They carried out injection and histopathological studies of the colon in a control group of 15 patients and identified mucosal ectasia in 27% and a large dilated submucosal vein in 53%.

The pathology of angiodysplasia of the right colon has been detailed by Mitsudo *et al.*[41] who have shown a spectrum from small early focal lesions to multiple large lesions. Superficial mucosal capillaries may or may not be dilated and mildly compress the lamina propria and communicate with a tortuous dilated submucosal vein. In more advanced cases, submucosal changes are more apparent and there is marked ectasia of mucosal vessels and the submucosal veins become increasingly tortuous and dilated while the arteries remain normal. The submucosal veins communicate with mucosal capillaries which are continuous with large or small groups of dilated vessels compressing the surrounding crypts. In severe cases, the capillary wall and attenuated epithelium are all that separate the capillary lumen from the colonic lumen (*Figure 5.8b*). It is clear from these observations how easily the wall may rupture and result in severe colonic bleeding.

The angiodysplastic appearances may be characteristic, with prominent ectatic vessels on the anti mesenteric border of the caecum, and an early-draining vein (see *Figures 5.1* and *5.2*). Appearances may be less convincing sometimes, and lesions seen at colonoscopy and angiography do not always correspond.

There is controversy over the preferred form of therapy. Colonoscopy with laser or heat coagulation is often effective, but has a high frequency of rebleeding, while surgery is more effective but obviously of greater risk.[30] A particular problem with angiodysplasia is whether angiographically identified areas of angiodysplasia are in fact the source of blood loss, particularly as evidence for multiple sites of angiodysplasia emerges.

ISCHAEMIC COLITIS

Acute infarction of the left colon is described on p. 1022. It is characterized by bloody diarrhoea and loin pain, and usually recovers spontaneously. Severe bleeding is very uncommon, and differentiation from other lesions depends on barium studies and colonoscopy. Massive bleeding, when it does occur, usually requires surgical resection.[14] Ischaemia should always be considered a likely cause of bleeding after aortic reconstruction.[53]

SOLITARY ULCER

Solitary ulcer of the rectum is discussed on p. 912; it may present with intermittent rectal bleeding. Although this is severe enough to cause anaemia, acute severe haemorrhage is very rare, and because of accessibility of the lesion, diagnosis is not difficult.

DIVERTICULAR DISEASE

Diverticular disease may cause chronic blood loss giving rise to anaemia, but may also give rise to major difficulty in assessing the location of the source of bleeding, which may be in the caecal area. For some reason yet unascertained, indigenous Japanese have a particular tendency to develop right-sided diverticula. Operation for bleeding is necessary only if bleeding does not stop on conservative management, or if it recurs during treatment.

Diverticular bleeding tends to be severe because it is arterial. It occurs from ruptured vasa recti at the neck of the diverticulum, or occasionally from the apex of the pouch when a vessel there is eroded by a faecolith (see *Figure 5.4*).

Bleeding ceases spontaneously in 80–90% of patients, and rebleeding occurs in about 25%.[20,21]

OTHER CAUSES

Other minor causes of lower gastrointestinal bleeding include haemorrhoids, colonic varices, trauma (including self-induced) and infections such as bacterial or amoebic colitis. Endoscopic investigation is the mainstay of these diagnoses.

SUMMARY

Acute colonic haemorrhage may be difficult to differentiate from ileal bleeding. It is often due to diverticular disease or angiodysplasia, but many other causes exist. Lesser bleeding of a chronic nature, and the difficulty of diagnosis in more obscure cases, are discussed in the next two sections.

REFERENCES

1. Allison, D.J., Hemingway, A.P. and Cunningham, D.A. (1982) Angiography in gastrointestinal bleeding. *Lancet*, **i**, 30–33.
2. Athanasoulis, C.A. (1982) Lower gastrointestinal bleeding. In *Interventional Radiology* (Eds) Athanasoulis, C.A., Pfister, R.C., Green, R.E. and Robertson, G.H. Philadelphia: W.B. Saunders.
3. Baum, S. (1982) Angiography and the gastrointestinal bleeder. *Radiology*, **142**, 569–572.
4. Baum, S., Athanasoulis, C.A. and Watman, A.C. (1974) Angiographic diagnosis and control of large bowel bleeding. *Diseases of the Colon and Rectum*, **17**, 447–453.
5. Baum, S., Athanasoulis, C.A., Waltman, A.C. *et al.* (1977) Angiodysplasia of the right colon: a cause of gastrointestinal bleeding. *American Journal of Roentgenology*, **29**, 789–794.
6. Behringer, S.E. and Albright, N.L. (1973) Diverticular disease of the colon. A frequent cause of bleeding. *American Journal of Surgery*, **125**, 419–423.
7. Boley, S.J. and Brandt, L.J. (1986) Vascular ectasias of the colon. *Digestive Diseases and Sciences*, **31**, 26S–42S.
8. Boley, S.J., Sammartano, R., Adamas, A. *et al.* (1977) On the nature and aetiology of vascular ectasias of the colon: degenerative lesions of aging. *Gastroenterology*, **72**, 650–660.
9. Boley, S.J., Sprayregan, S., Sammartano, R.J. *et al.* (1977) The pathophysiologic basis for the angiographic signs of vascular ectasias of the colon. *Diagnostic Radiology*, **125**, 615–621.
10. Bookestein, J.J. (1982) Angiographic diagnosis and transcatheter therapy of lower gastrointestinal bleeding. In *Interventional Radiology* pp. 55–89 (Eds) Athanasoulis, C.A., Pfister, R.C., Green, R.E. and Robertson, G.H. Philadelphia: W.B. Saunders.
11. Bourdette, D. and Greenberg, B. (1979) Twelve year history of gastrointestinal bleeding in a patient with calcific aortic stenosis and haemorrhagic telangiectasia. *Digestive Disease and Sciences,* **24**, 77–82.
12. Browning, G.G.P., Varma, J.S., Smith, A.N., Small, W.P. and Duncan, W. (1987) Late results of mucosal protectomy and colo-anal sleeve anastomosis for chronic irradiation rectal injury. *British Journal of Surgery*, **74**, 31–34.
13. Caos, A., Benner, K.G., Manier, J. *et al.* (1986) Colonoscopy after Golytely preparation in acute rectal bleeding. *Journal of Clinical Gastroenterology*, **8**, 46–49.
14. Chou, Y.H., Hse, S.C., Wang, C.Y., Chen, C.L. and How, S.W. (1989) Ischemic colitis as a cause of massive gastrointestinal bleeding and peritonitis: report of five cases. *Diseases of the Colon and Rectum*, **32**, 1065–1070.
15. Colachio, T.A., Forde, K.A., Patsos, T.J. and Nunez, D. (1982) Impact of modern diagnostic methods on the management of active rectal bleeding: Ten year experience. *American Journal of Surgery*, **143**, 607–610.
16. Cussons, P.D. and Berry, A.R. (1989) Comparison of the value of emergency mesenteric angiography and intraoperative colonoscopy with antegrade colonic irrigation in massive rectal haemorrhage. *Journal of the Royal College of Surgeons of Edinburgh*, **34**, 91–93.
17. Desa, L.A.J., Bridges, J., Grace, P.A., Krausz, T. and Spencer, J. (1991) Primary jejunoileal tumours: a review of 45 cases. *World Journal of Surgery*, **15**, 81–87.
18. Eaton, A.C. (1981) Emergency surgery for acute colonic haemorrhage: a retrospective study. *British Journal of Surgery*, **68**, 109–112.
19. Drapanas, T., Pennington, D.G., Kappelman, M. and Lindsay, E.S. (1973) Emergency subtotal colectomy – preferred approach to the management of massively bleeding diverticular disease. *Annals of Surgery*, **177**, 519–526.
20. Farrands, P.A. and Taylor, I. (1989) Management of acute lower gastrointestinal bleeding. Haemorrhage in a surgical unit over a 4 year period. *Journal of the Royal Society of Medicine*, **80**, 79–82.
21. Forde, K.A. (1989) Causes, diagnosis, and management of colonic bleeding. *Comprehensive Therapy*, **15**, 45–48.
22. Frey, C.F., Reuter, S.R. and Bookstein, J.J. (1970) Localisation of gastrointestinal haemhorrhage by selective angiography. *Surgery, Gynecology and Obstetrics*, **67**, 549–553.
23. Galloway, S.J., Casarella, W.J. and Shipkin, P.M. (1974) Vascular malformations of the right colon as a cause of bleeding in patients with aortic stenosis. *Radiology*, **113**, 11–15.
24. Gilbert, D.A. and Silverstein, F.E. (1987) Endoscopy in gastrointestinal bleeding. In *Gastroenterologic Endoscopy* (Ed) Sivak, M.V. p. 10. Philadelphia: W.B. Saunders.
25. Goergen, T.G. (1983) Serendipity in scintigraphic gastrointestinal bleeding studies. *Clinical Nuclear Medicine*, **8**, 396–399.
26. Gostout, C.J., Bowyer, B.A., Alquist, D.A., Viggiano, T.R. and Balm, R.K. (1988) Mucosal vascular malformations of the gastrointestinal tract: clinical observations and results of endoscopic neomydium: yttrium-aluminium-garnet laser therapy. *Mayo Clinic Proceedings*, **63**, 993–1003.
27. Hemingway, A. and Allison, D.J. (1982)

Angiodysplasia and Meckel's diverticulum: a congenital association? *British Journal of Surgery*, **69**, 493–496.

28. Hunt, R.H. (1978) Rectal bleeding. *Clinical Gastroenterology*, **7**, 719–740.
29. Hunt, R.M. (1984) Angiodysplasia of the colon. In *Advances in Gastrointestinal Endoscopy* (Ed.) Salmon, P.R. pp. 97–114. London: Chapman and Hall.
30. Hutcheson, D.F., Kaselin, J., Burnley, G.B. and Smith, G.W. (1987) Effect of therapy on bleeding rates in gastrointestinal angiodysplasia. *American Surgeons*, **53**, 6–12.
31. Jensen, D-.M. and Machicado, G.A. (1988) Diagnosis and treatment of severe hematochezia. The role of urgent colonoscopy after purge. *Gastroenterology,* **95**, 248–253.
32. Jewett, T.C., Duszniski, D.O. and Allen, J.F. (1970) The visualisation of Meckel's diverticulum with ^{99m}Tc pertechnetate. *Surgery*, **68**, 567–570.
33. Koval, G., Bennar, K.G., Rosch, J. and Kozak, B.E. (1989) Aggressive angiographic diagnosis in acute lower gastrointestinal haemorrhage. *Digestive Diseases and Sciences*, **32**, 248–253.
34. Kyle, J. (1991) Rarer complications of Crohn's (Dalziel's) disease. *Australian and New Zealand Journal of Surgery,* **61**, 489–492.
35. Lawler, G., Bircher, M., Spencer, J., Hemingway, A.P. and Allison, D.J. (1985) Embolisation in colonic bleeding. *British Journal of Radiology*, **58**, 83–84.
36. Low, D.E., Kozarek, R.A., Ball, T.J., Patterson, D.J. and Hill, L.D. (1989) Colorectal neomydium – YAG photoablative therapy. Comparing applications and complications on both sides of the peritoneal reflection. *Archives of Surgery*, **124**, 684–688.
37. Lyon, D.T. and Mantia, A.G. (1984) Large bowel haemangiomas. *Diseases of the Colon and Rectum*, **27**, 404–414.
38. McKusick, K.A., Frohlich, J., Callaghan, R.J. *et al.* (1981) ^{99m}Tc red blood cells for the detection of gastrointestinal bleeding: experience with 80 patients. *American Journal of Roentgenology*, **137**, 1113–1118.
39. Mesleh, G. and Lemons, J. (1983) Massive lower gastrointestinal haemorrhage in Crohn's disease. *Archives of Surgery*, **164**, 182–185.
40. Meyers, M. A., Alonso, D. R., Gray, G. F. and Baer, J. W. (1976) Pathogenesis of bleeding colonic diverticulosis, *Gastroenterology*, **71**, 577–583.
41. Mitsudo, S.M., Boley, S.J., Brandt, L.J. *et al.* (1979) Vascular ectasias of the right colon in the elderly: a district pathological entity. *Human Pathology*, **10**(5), 585–600.
42. Moncure, A.C., Tompkins, R.G., Athanasoulis, C.A. *et al.* (1989) Occult gastrointestinal bleeding: Newer techniques of diagnosis and therapy. *Advances in Surgery*, **22**, 141–177.
43. Naderi, M.J. and Bookestein, J.J. (1978) Rectal bleeding secondary to fecal impaction: angiographic diagnosis and treatment. *Radiology*, **126**, 387–389.
44. Nusbaum, M. and Baum, S. (1963) Radiographic demonstration of unknown sites of gastrointestinal bleeding. *Surgical Forum*, **14**, 374–375.
45. Nusbaum, M., Baum, S. and Blackmore, W.S. (1969) Clinical experience with the diagnosis and management of gastrointestinal haemorrhage by selective mesenteric catheterisation. *Annals of Surgery*, **170**, 506–514.
46. Ohri, S.K., Desa, L.A., Lee, H., Patel, T., Jackson, J., Lavender, J.P. and Spencer, J. (1992) The value of scintigraphic localisation of obscure gastrointestinal bleeding. *Journal of the Royal College of Surgeons of Edinburgh*, **37**, 328–332.
47. Ramanath, H.K. and Hinshaw, J.R. (1971) Management and mismanagement of bleeding colonic diverticula. *Archives of Surgery*, **103**, 311–314.
48. Resenkrantz, H., Bookestein, J.J., Bosen, R.J., Goff, W.B. and Healy, J.F. (1982) Colonic infarction after transcatheter embolisation for colonic haemorrhage. *Radiology*, **142**, 47–57.
49. Robert, J.R., Sachar, D.B. and Greenstein, A.J. (1991) Severe gastrointestinal haemorrhage in Crohn's disease. *Annals of Surgery*, **213**, 207–211.
50. Rogers, B.H.G. (1980) Endoscopic diagnosis and therapy of mucosal vascular abnormality of the gastrointestinal tract occurring in elderly patients and associated with cardiac, vascular and pulmonary disease. *Gastrointestinal Endoscopy*, **26**, 134–138.
51. Salem, R.R., Wood, C.B., Rees, H.C., Kheshavarzian, A., Hemingway, A.P. and Allison, D.J. (1985) A comparison of colonoscopy and selective visceral angiography in diagnosis of colonic angiodysplasia *Annals of the Royal College of Surgeons of England*, **67**, 225–226.
52. Schrock, T.R. (1988) Large intestine. In *Current Surgical Diagnosis and Treatment*, 8th edition, p. 586 (Ed.) Way, L.W. San Mateo: Appleton and Lange.
53. Schroeder, T., Christoffersen, J.D. and Anderson, J. (1985) Ischemic colitis complicating reconstruction of the abdominal aorta. *Surgery, Gynecology and Obstetrics*, **160**, 299–303.
54. Sfakianakis, G.N. and Conway, J.J. (1981) Detection of ectopic gastric mucosa in Meckel's diverticulum and other observations by scintigraphy. II Indications and methods – a ten year experience. *Journal of Nuclear Medicine*, **22**, 732–738.
55. Steger, A.C., Galland, R.B., Hemingway, A.P., Wood, C.B. and Spencer, J. (1987) Gastrointestinal haemorrhage from a second cause in patients with colonic angiodysplasia. *British Journal of Surgery,* **74**, 726–727.
56. Tagart, R.E.B. (1971) General peritonitis and haemorrhage complicating colonic diverticular disease. *Annals of the Royal College of Surgeons of England*, **55**, 175–183.

57. Taverner, D., Talbot, I.C., Carr-Locke, D.L. and Wicks, A.C.B. (1982) Massive bleeding from the ileum: a late complication of pelvic radiotherapy. *American Journal of Gastroenterology*, **77**, 29–31.
58. Thompson, J.N., Hemingway, A.P., McPherson, G.A.D., Rees, H.C., Allison, D.J. and Spencer, J. (1984) Obscure gastrointestinal haemorrhage of small bowel origin. *British Medical Journal*, **228**, 1663–1665.
59. Treves, S., Grand, R.J., Evalkis, A.J. (1978) Pentagastrin stimulation of Technetium-99m uptake by ectopic gastric mucosa in Meckel's diverticulum. *Radiology*, **128**, 711–712.
60. Warren, S. and Friedman, N.B. (1942) Pathology and pathologic diagnosis of radiation lesions in the gastrointenstinal tract. *American Journal of Pathology*, **18**, 499–513.

CHRONIC GASTROINTESTINAL HAEMORRHAGE

J. Spencer and M. Camilleri

Chronic haemorrhage may be overt or occult. Overt bleeding is defined as chronic if it is persistent but not severe enough to cause circulatory embarrassment. It may be seen in the form of melaena or red rectal bleeding. If occult, the clinical presentation is with anaemia, with evidence of occult bleeding on testing of the stools. In some patients chronic haemorrhage may be clinically interleaved with acute episodes.[68]

In some patients diagnosis is initially difficult. In early series in which endoscopy was not used, this was particularly the case. For example, Birke and Engstedt studied 1252 patients and could make no definitive diagnosis in 15%.[11] A similar proportion remained undiagnosed in another series in which endoscopy was employed.[23] With current investigation this percentage has fallen, with angiography having considerable impact. Chronic bleeding from the gut is always significant, and in particular it must be remembered that malignant tumours of the gut may be present, and curable. These include carcinomas of the stomach and caecum which are very common causes, and much rarer, small bowel tumours, which also often present in this way.[21]

The diagnostic problems are discussed in some detail later in this chapter, in the section on obscure haemorrhage.

AETIOLOGY

There are many causes of chronic blood loss, and these are listed in *Table 5.4*. Fuller descriptions of most entities appear in the appropriate sections of the book.

OESOPHAGEAL AND GASTRO-OESOPHAGEAL DISORDERS

These are more often associated with acute bleeding, although oesophagitis with ulceration may often present with chronic bleeding. Mallory-Weiss tears or varices may occasionally bleed chronically.

STOMACH DISORDERS

Gastritis, especially that associated with alcoholism, may cause chronic blood loss. The peculiar entity known as 'watermelon stomach' is particularly prone to bleed. In this condition inflamed and haemorrhagic streaks appear to radiate out from the pylorus into the antrum when seen endoscopically. These contrast with atrophic mucosa between them, giving rise to the appellation.[32] Cancers, leiomyomas (*Figure 5.9*) and other tumours often present with anaemia.

SMALL INTESTINE ABNORMALITIES

Peptic ulcers are more prone to acute bleeding but may present with anaemia. Jejunal or ileal ulceration may cause bleeding. Solitary 'non-specific' ulcers are included in this, as are those associated with potassium chloride ingestion. Chronic bleeding occurs in coeliac disease.

Small bowel tumours are uncommon, but always must be remembered in this context. Too often laparotomy is delayed and these tumours are advanced when first seen. Polyps, such as those in the Peutz-Jeghers syndrome, are important causes of chronic blood loss. They are associated with melanin pigmentation in the face and mouth (*Figure 5.10*).

Table 5.4 Classification of causes of chronic gastrointestinal haemorrhage

Oesophageal and gastro-oesophageal disorders
- Oesophageal ulceration and Barrett's syndrome
- Oesophagitis
- Hiatal hernia
- Tumours of oesophagus
- Oesophageal diverticula
- Mallory–Weiss syndrome
- Oesophageal and gastric varices

Disorders of the stomach
- Gastric ulcer
- Stomal ulcer
- Haemorrhagic gastritis and gastric erosions
- Tumours of stomach
  - Malignant tumours
  - Benign tumours and polyps
  - Adenoma, leiomyoma, haemangioma
- Gastric diverticula
- Watermelon stomach
- Dieulafoy disease

Disorders of the small intestine
- Duodenal ulcer
- Stomal ulcer
- Jejunal ulceration
- Tumours of small intestine
  - Lymphoma
  - Adenocarcinoma
  - Benign tumours
    - Leiomyoma, haemangioma, lipoma
    - Peutz–Jeghers syndrome
- Crohn's disease
- Tuberculosis
- Radiation damage
- Intussusception
- Small intestinal diverticula
  - Duodenal and jejunal diverticula
  - Meckel's diverticulum
- Enteric duplication cyst
- Small intestinal ischaemia

Disorders of the large intestine
- Ulcerative colitis
- Crohn's disease
- Rectal ulcer
- Anal fissure
- Haemorrhoids
- Tumours of large intestine
  - Malignant tumours
  - Benign tumours
    - Adenoma, haemangioma
    - Adenomatous and villous polyps
    - Familial polyposis of the colon
- Tuberculosis
- Radiation damage
- Diverticular disease of colon
- Ischaemic colitis
- Endometriosis
- Angiodysplasia (see vascular malformations)

Disorders of the liver and gallbladder
- Primary hepatic tumours
- Hepatic cirrhosis
- Viral hepatitis
- Hepatic abscess
- Hepatic cyst
- Aneurysm of hepatic artery
- Calculi
- Tumours of bile ducts or gallbladder
- Haemorrhagic cholecystitis

Disorder of the pancreas
- Acute pancreatitis
- Chronic pancreatitis
- Pancreatic pseudocyst
- Tumours of pancreas
- Splenic artery aneurysm

Vascular malformations
- Arteriovenous malformations
  - Angiodysplasia
  - Hereditary haemorrhagic telangiectasia (Osler–Weber–Rendu syndrome)
- Aneurysms and aorto-enteric fistulas
- Haemangiomas
  - Blue naevus bleb syndrome

Haematological disorders
- Haemophilia
- Christmas disease
- von Willebrand's disease
- Thrombocytopenia
- Purpuras
- Leukaemias
- Lymphoma
- Disseminated intravascular coagulation
- Polycythaemia rubra vera
- Haemolytic anaemias
- Aplastic anaemia
- Myelomatosis

Collagen disorders
- Systemic lupus erythematosus
- Polyarteritis nodosa
- Dermatomyositis
- Progressive systemic sclerosis
- Rheumatoid arthritis
- Henoch–Schönlein purpura

Inherited disorders of connective tissue
- Pseudoxanthoma elasticum (Groenblad–Strandberg syndrome)
- Ehlers–Danlos syndrome

Infections and infestations
- Amoebic colitis
- Bacillary dysenteric infection
- Pseudomembranous colitis
- Hookworm disease

(*Continued*)

Table 5.4 Classification of causes of chronic gastrointestinal haemorrhage (*continued*)

Drugs	*Drugs* (*continued*)
Acetylsalicylic acid	Anticoagulants
Indomethacin	Ethanol
Phenylbutazone	Ethacrynic acid
Oxyphenbutazone	Potassium chloride (Slow-K)
Benorylate	Emepronium bromide (Cetiprin)
Piroxicam	*Miscellaneous*
Naproxen	Primary amyloidosis
Ibuprofen	Uraemia
Aloxiprim	Renal carcinoma
Flufenamic acid	Aortic stenosis

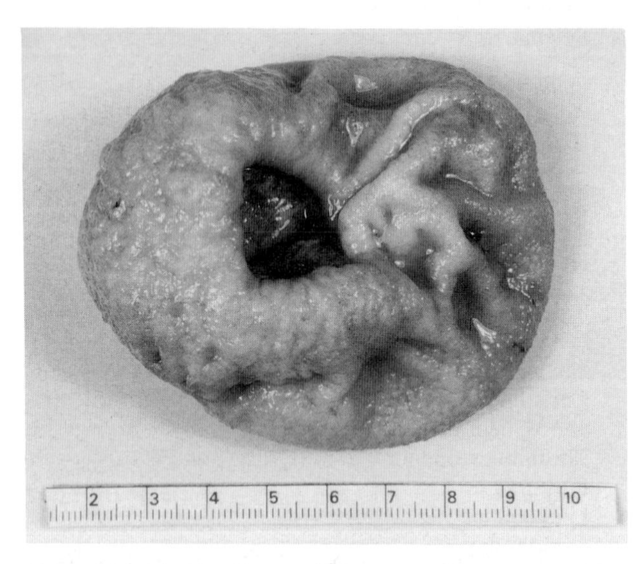

Figure 5.9 Leiomyosarcoma of the stomach which presented with haemorrhage. The cavitation of the tumour is typical of such stromal tumours.

Crohn's disease often features anaemia, in part due to blood loss. Jejunal diverticula are common, but rarely bleed. Meckel's diverticulum, in the ileum, does not often bleed chronically, but may do so. Enteric duplication cysts are also more likely to bleed acutely.

LARGE INTESTINE DISORDERS

All inflammatory diseases of the colon may bleed either acutely, or chronically. In the solitary rectal ulcer syndrome, chronic bleeding may occur, associated with mucus, rectal pain and altered bowel habit. Polyps and tumours, benign or malignant, may bleed chronically. Carcinomas of the right colon classically present with anaemia due to blood loss.

Diverticula may bleed acutely, but chronic bleeding is not at all common from these lesions. Endometriosis may present with bleeding. Most often the rectosigmoid is involved, though small bowel may be affected.

DISORDERS OF THE LIVER AND GALLBLADDER

These organs must not be forgotten as rare sites of chronic blood loss. Hepatoma, cirrhotic lesions, hepatitis, cysts or abscesses may all bleed. Abscesses associated with ascaris migration often bleed, though this is usually as acute episodes, and in children.

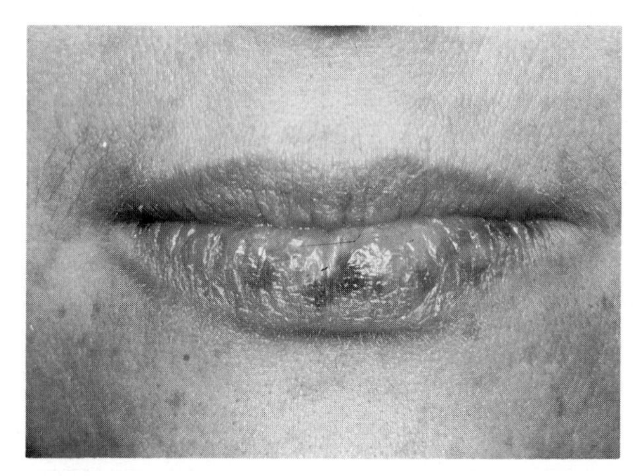

Figure 5.10 Peutz–Jeghers syndrome.

PANCREATIC DISORDERS

These occasionally bleed chronically, but that is extremely rare in pancreatitis. A splenic artery aneurysm may bleed down the pancreatic duct.

Other aneurysms may leak into the gut, although acute episodes of bleeding are much more common.[40]

VASCULAR MALFORMATIONS

Although these are rare in the gastrointestinal tract, with one large series suggesting an incidence of 1 in 14 000 individuals,[7] they rank high in importance as causes of obscure bleeding. They may be described according to the size and type of vessel affected, but it is useful, as suggested by Camilleri *et al.*[14] to classify them also with regard to the presence or absence of somatic or dermatological features (*Table 5.5*). This has the advantages of suggesting the likely clinical features, the preoperative investigations which will aid the diagnosis and localization of these lesions and hence their management. A classification by Richardson[69] aimed to differentiate those in whom surgical exploration was likely to be helpful. The classification was retrospective, however, and it does not seem possible prospectively to separate, as he suggests, between acquired lesions limited to the caecal area and those which are multiple, even though angiography sometimes permits this.

Arteriovenous malformations

The angiodysplastic lesions of the caecum have been discussed in the section on acute haemorrhage. Briefly they consist of irregularly shaped clusters of arteriolar, venular and capillary vessels located in the mucosa and submucosa of the intestine, most often in the right colon of elderly patients. Less commonly, lesions occur in the jejunum and stomach, and there have been several reports of such lesions causing gastrointestinal haemorrhage in younger patients, including adolescents.

They may present with obvious dark red bleeding in acute episodes, or with iron deficiency. In chronic haemorrhage, it seems reasonable to try the approach of local colonoscopic control by laser or heat ablation first. In difficult circumstances with extensive lesions, oestrogen therapy has been used with a reduction in transfusion requirements, being effective when 0.05 mg ethinyl oestradiol and 1 mg norethisterone were given daily in a controlled trial.[79]

Multiple phlebectasia

The term 'phlebectasia' refers to venous varicosities found in the gastrointestinal tract. There is some confusion in the literature of the first half of this century as this term was used to identify a small type of cavernous haemangioma.[28,49] The modern use of the term phlebectasia implies a non-neoplastic venous varicosity with abnormal endothelial lining, and this would appear to be indistinguishable from Gentry's[28] phlebectasia type of cavernous haemangioma.

Phlebectasias are not uncommon in the oesophagus and rectum and may also be found infrequently in the small intestine. There are at least seven well described cases of multiple intestinal phlebectasia reported in the recent literature[65] and to these one must add the large number reported in the earlier literature[28] in which they accounted for a third of all benign vascular lesions of the intestine. In all cases, the greatest density of lesions occurred in the mid-small bowel with a fall off in distribution

Table 5.5 A classification of intestinal vascular anomalies. (After Camilleri, Chadwick and Hodgson[8])

I Arteriovenous malformations (andiodysplasia, vascular ectasia)
II Multiple phlebectasia
III Telangiectasia
  (a) Hereditary haemorrhagic telangiectasia (Osler-Weber-Rendu)
  (b) Turner's syndrome
  (c) Calcinosis–Raynaud's–sclerodactyly-telangiectasia (CRST) syndrome and systemic sclerosis
IV Haemangioma
  (a) Capillary
  (b) Cavernous – single or diffuse
  (c) Mixed capillary – cavernous
  (d) Peutz-Jeghers syndrome
  (e) Blue rubber bleb naevus syndrome
  (f) Klippel-Trenaunay-Weber syndrome
V Disorders of connective tissue affecting blood vessels
  (a) Pseudoxanthoma elasticum
  (b) Ehlers-Danlos syndrome

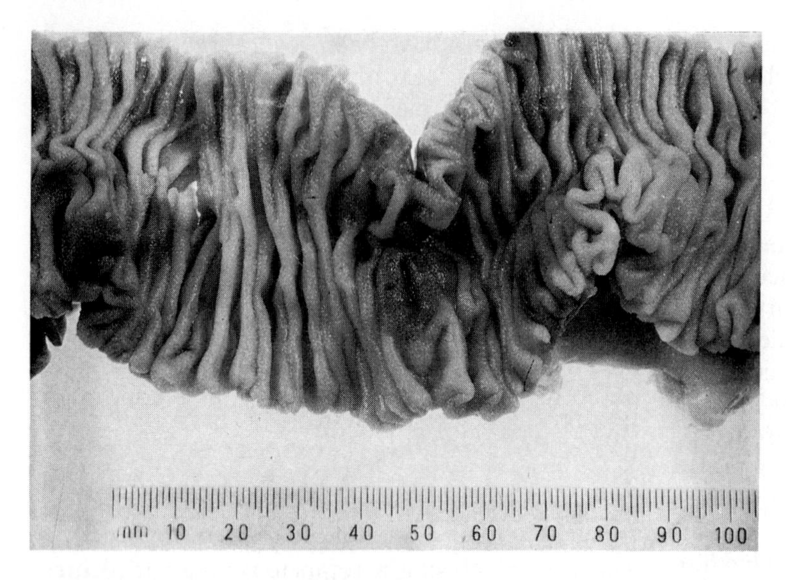

(a)

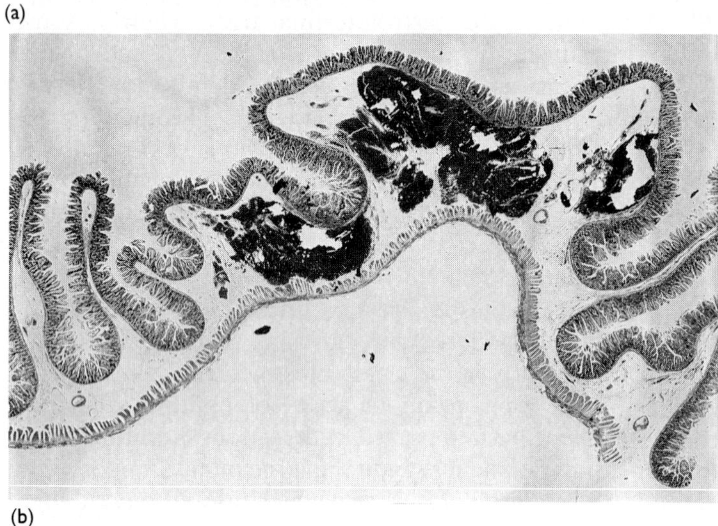

(b)

Figure 5.11 (a) Macroscopic appearance of the mucosal surface of resected jejunum showing multiple phlebactasia. (b) Whole-mount, low-power microscopy of lesion seen in (a). (Courtesy of Professor Hodgson).

proximally and distally. The lesions vary from a few millimetres to several centimetres in diameter. Grossly, they appear as dark, bluish-red nodules which are soft and compressible. The lesions are located in the submucosa and have abnormal endothelial lining. *Figure 5.11* shows the macroscopic and low-power microscopic appearances of this lesion. The mucosa overlying these lesions may be extremely thin. Similar varicose vessels may be seen entering the intestine at its mesenteric attachment.[74]

PRESENTATION AND DIAGNOSIS

In most cases, the diagnosis is made around the fifth or sixth decades, and the usual clinical presentations are occult bleeding or anaemia with alteration of stool colour. Although it has been stated that life-threatening haemorrhage does not occur in this condition,[12,65] the authors have seen this lesion presenting as massive gastrointestinal bleeding necessitating emergency laparotomy. It is striking that, although all preoperative diagnostic procedures have proved unsuccessful in the cases reported, in this patient, abdominal scanning after intravenous injection of Tc^{m} correctly localized bleeding to the jejunum.

TREATMENT

It is not surprising that reduction of the number of lesions by surgical excision of the mid-small bowel has not always been successful in stopping haemorrhage in every case. If surgical excision of all the lesions is not possible, intermittent blood transfusion and oral iron therapy are the mainstays of treatment.

Telangiectasia

Hereditary haemorrhagic telangiectasia (Osler–Weber–Rendu disease)

Up to 1977, this disorder had been reported in around 1500 members of 300 families. It is inherited as an autosomal dominant trait. Telangiectasia occur in the skin, mucous membranes and internal organs, resulting in recurrent haemorrhage. These

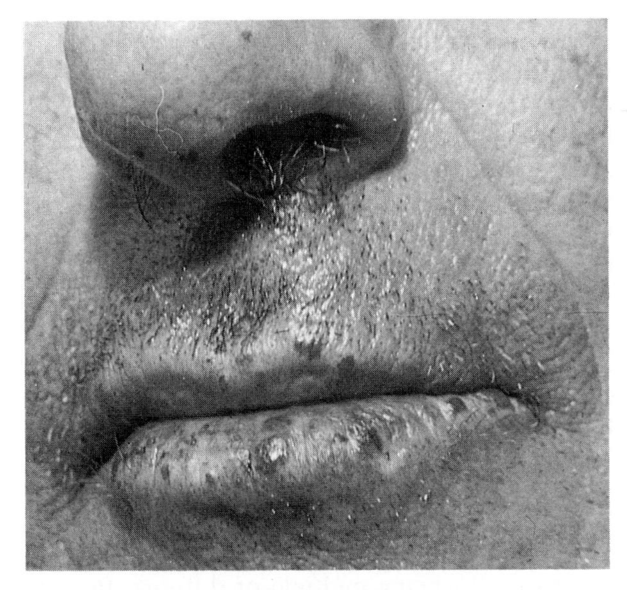

Figure 5.12 Hereditary haemorrhagic telangiectasia.

lesions arise from simple dilatation of normal vascular structures. Congenital thinning of the arterial muscle coat[24,75] and absent elastin in arteriolar walls may be responsible for the dilatation.

The telangiectasia are punctate, red to purple in colour, non-compressible and may be stellate or nodular.[24,75] Their size ranges from 1 to 4 mm and they occur on the face (*Figure 5.12*) and hands as well as the labial, buccal and nasal mucosae, and the conjunctiva. These mucocutaneous lesions usually appear in the second and third decades; the earliest haemorrhagic presentation is with repeated epistaxis in childhood. Bleeding from the gastrointestinal tract usually becomes manifest in the fourth decade[38,58] and occurs in about 15% of patients with this disorder. Vascular abnormalities also occur in the lung, liver, uterus, kidney, bladder, meninges, spinal cord and eye. One abnormality specific to the lung is the pulmonary arteriovenous fistula which may lead to cardiac failure and erythrocytosis.

The gastrointestinal presentation is usually with chronic blood loss. Gastroscopy may reveal multiple punctate lesions in the stomach[52,63] and colonoscopy may also show typical lesions.[47,76] Selective mesenteric arteriography may be necessary to localize the precise bleeding site, and some cases have required peroperative enteroscopy to detect the bleeding lesion.[33,34,50] Although about 40% of patients require blood transfusions, death due to excessive blood loss rarely occurs.

A number of gastrointestinal vascular anomalies have been reported in association with congenital or acquired von Willebrand's disease. These include diffuse gastrointestinal telangiectasia[1,51,33,34,50] similar to those of Osler–Weber–Rendu disease, and angiodysplasia consisting of masses of small tortuous, thin-walled blood vessels. The inheritance of the coagulopathy was linked to that of the telangiectasia in three generations of one family studied by Conlon *et al.*[17,18] These authors suggested that an endothelial defect was responsible for both disorders, resulting in inadequate synthesis of factor VIII and defective capillary structure. Ahr *et al.*[1] in a review of the literature on hereditary haemorrhagic telangiectasia, found some cases where a second haemostatic defect was present, often demonstrated only by prolonged bleeding times particularly after ingestion of aspirin. In the acquired variety, an inhibitor to factor VIII (present in the IgG fraction of plasma and lacking precipitating properties) has been reported in some cases[50] The presence of an associated clotting defect, or of disseminated intravascular coagulation, obviously increases the difficulty of managing acutely bleeding telangiectasia.[10]

Treatment

The management of patients with hereditary haemorrhagic telangiectasia should be conservative in the first instance. If bleeding continues despite blood transfusion, a search should be undertaken for an associated haemostatic defect and, failing this, selective mesenteric arteriography during active bleeding is mandatory to ensure localization and surgical excision of the bleeding telangiectasia. The role of hormonal therapy is still controversial. Some reports suggest that oestrogens are capable of stabilizing the brittle walls of blood vessels and may thus reduce the tendency to bleed;[55] however, a double-blind controlled clinical trial failed to show any benefit in terms of the frequency or intensity of bleeding or in the haemoglobin levels of patients with Osler–Weber–Rendu disease.[80]

Therapeutic embolization of affected blood vessels has been considered, and is certainly valuable for stopping bleeding from the upper respiratory tract in this condition.[2] However, when embolizing bleeding telangiectasia in the gut, the risk of causing infarction must be considered.

Telangiectasia associated with Turner's syndrome

Turner's syndrome is characterized by a variety of external somatic features as well as congenital malformations of internal organs, found in association with ovarian agenesis and a characteristic 45XO chromosome karyotype. The somatic features include infantilism, cubitus valgus, a webbed neck and shield-like chest. The congenital malformations include coarctation of the aorta, renal artery stenosis, septal defects in the heart, and lymphoedema.[35]

Turner's syndrome is associated with gastrointestinal haemorrhage due to vascular lesions in the intestinal wall.[25,48] These vascular anomalies have been described as haemangiomas, telangiectasias or dilated veins, and at laparotomy may be found throughout most of the small and large bowel and the mesentery but with a predilection for the small intestine. The incidence of gastrointestinal bleeding in Turner's syndrome is unknown. It occurred in 4 out of 56 patients in one series[35] but was not recorded in another series of 48 cases.[25]

Haemorrhage from these lesions is usually intermittent and often self-limiting, and death by exsanguination has only rarely been reported.[25,48] There are at least two well-documented reports suggesting that the vascular anomalies may spontaneously regress with time.[27,73] Thus the clinical presentation of these patients is often with bleeding before 20 years of age; after 30 years of age bleeding tends to be intermittent and self-limited.[72] Preoperative demonstration of bleeding vascular anomalies is difficult. Rutlin *et al.*[72] have demonstrated telangiectatic lesions in the duodenal bulb, caecum and ascending colon by fibreoptic endoscopy, but in most of the previous reports, diagnosis was reached at laparotomy.

Treatment

Because of the strong impression, based on both clinical and pathological findings, that lesions undergo spontaneous regression after the age of 30, a conservative approach is warranted[72] with intestinal resection restricted to small segments that include the bleeding lesions. Mesenteric arteriography may permit preoperative localization of both small or large intestinal bleeding lesions. It is possible that in the future, laser (or other) photocoagulation of bleeding lesions during upper gastrointestinal endoscopy, or colonoscopic diathermy or hot biopsy coagulation of colonic telangiectasia in patients with chronic anaemia may control haemorrhage in these patients as it has in those with caecal angiodysplasia.

Haemangiomas

For the sake of accuracy, it must be stated that the lesions discussed in this section are better classified as hamartomas since they are congenital or appear soon after birth, they cannot be easily distinguished on histopathological grounds from other acknowledged vascular malformations, and they do not grow disproportionately or indefinitely as true neoplasms do; they grow *pari passu* with the surrounding tissues without involving a greater area than that originally affected.[81] The term 'haemangioma' is retained for uniformity with the literature. These lesions may be classified according to the size of vessel affected – (i.e. capillary, cavernous or mixed) or according to their association with cutaneous or other somatic abnormalities (e.g. Peutz–Jeghers syndrome, Klippel–Trenaunay–Weber syndrome).

Intestinal haemangiomas are rare and usually non-hereditary. In a review of 1.4 million case records at the Mayo Clinic, Gentry *et al.*[28] found 106 vascular lesions of the intestine; 60 other cases were detected by reviewing 10 000 autopsy reports over 20 years at the same institution. Haemangiomas constituted 98% of the benign vascular tumours in this study.

Intestinal haemangiomas account for around 10% of all benign small intestinal tumours.[56] In River's review of 1399 cases in the literature,[71] it was shown that 5.4% of the tumours were solitary, localized lesions (3.7% being multiple or diffuse). In about half the cases, diagnosis was only reached at laparotomy. Wilson *et al.*[82] reviewed 1721 cases of benign small intestinal tumours from throughout the world and found 212 haemangiomas (the fifth commonest type of tumour). The distribution in the small intestine was predominantly in the jejunum (47%) and ileum (45%), with a minority in the duodenum (8%). Several authors stress the fact that most lesions are discrete, well circumscribed or encapsulated masses composed of blood vessels and are therefore hamartomas rather than true vascular neoplasms. The clinical presentations of 134 adequately documented small intestinal haemangiomas include haemorrhage (41%), abdominal pain (31%), and intussusception (13%). Rarely, abdominal masses are palpable (10%) and there may be evidence of weight loss.[82]

Clinical features

Capillary haemangiomas usually present with haemorrhage, and occasionally obstruction or perforation often associated with intramural bleeding. The larger cavernous and mixed lesions are more likely to result in ulceration or obstruction of the intestine, although gut haemorrhage remains a common clinical presentation. Of 18 cases of mixed haemangiomas reviewed by Gentry,[28] eight developed subacute intestinal obstruction, six had prominent gastrointestinal haemorrhage (which was fatal in three cases), and two were found incidentally at necropsy. Conversely, only 5% of cavernous haemangiomas are found incidentally at post mortem, the vast majority manifesting with haemorrhage (50%) or intestinal obstruction (35%).

Diffuse cavernous haemangiomas usually affect the colon and present with intermittent rectal bleeding (95%), often in childhood.

INVESTIGATIONS

Diagnosis of intestinal haemangiomas depends on a high index of suspicion in patients with haemorrhage particularly if associated with features that suggest subacute intestinal obstruction. Patients with cavernous haemangiomas may have calcified phleboliths in the region of the affected bowel on plain abdominal radiograph, a useful clue in children and young adults.[54] Mass lesions (single or multiple) may be visible on barium contrast examination by causing irregularity of the margins, stenosis or dilatations of intestinal loops.[61] Arteriography usually reveals the site of the vascular malformations by the appearance of contrast medium in vascular spaces in the bowel wall, often associated with slowing of the venous return from such lesions (in contrast to the early filling vein observed with angiodysplasia) (*Figure 5.12*). Rarely, cavernous haemangiomas may be detected endoscopically in the duodenum. The diagnosis of intestinal haemangiomas is often made at laparotomy in patients with intestinal obstruction or gut haemorrhage of unknown origin.

Capillary haemangiomas

These consist of small, closely packed blood vessels with a well differentiated hyperplastic endothelium which may obliterate the vascular space. They usually appear as single, discrete, encapsulated lesions, arising from the submucosal vascular plexus and enlarging towards the lumen of a hollow viscus. The lesions in the small intestine tend to be small plaques (around 1 cm^2) and constitute around 6% of vascular tumours in this organ.[28,49] Surgical resection is possible in most cases. There are a few reports of multiple intestinal capillary haemangiomatosis.

Cavernous haemangiomas

Cavernous haemangiomas consist of large blood-filled spaces or sinuses lined by single or multiple layers of endothelial cells. These spaces are supported by scant connective tissue septa that may contain smooth muscle fibres. Coagulation of blood within these spaces may occur and is followed by organization of the thrombus, hyalinization and eventually calcification. This process accounts for the distinctive radiological features of these lesions. Cavernous haemangiomas may be single or diffuse.

The single lesions, which account for 18% of all benign vascular lesions of the intestine[28,49] are usually polypoid and associated with the submucosal vascular plexus. They may enlarge and prolapse into the lumen of the viscus, resulting in ulceration, haemorrhage or intestinal obstruction; these manifestations occur in about 80% of patients with such lesions. The remainder are found incidentally at post mortem. The radiological features of these lesions are described above (*Figure 5.13*). Surgical excision was possible in about half the cases reviewed by Gentry.[28]

The multiple small simple cavernous haemangiomas described in the earlier literature are here classified as multiple phlebectasia.

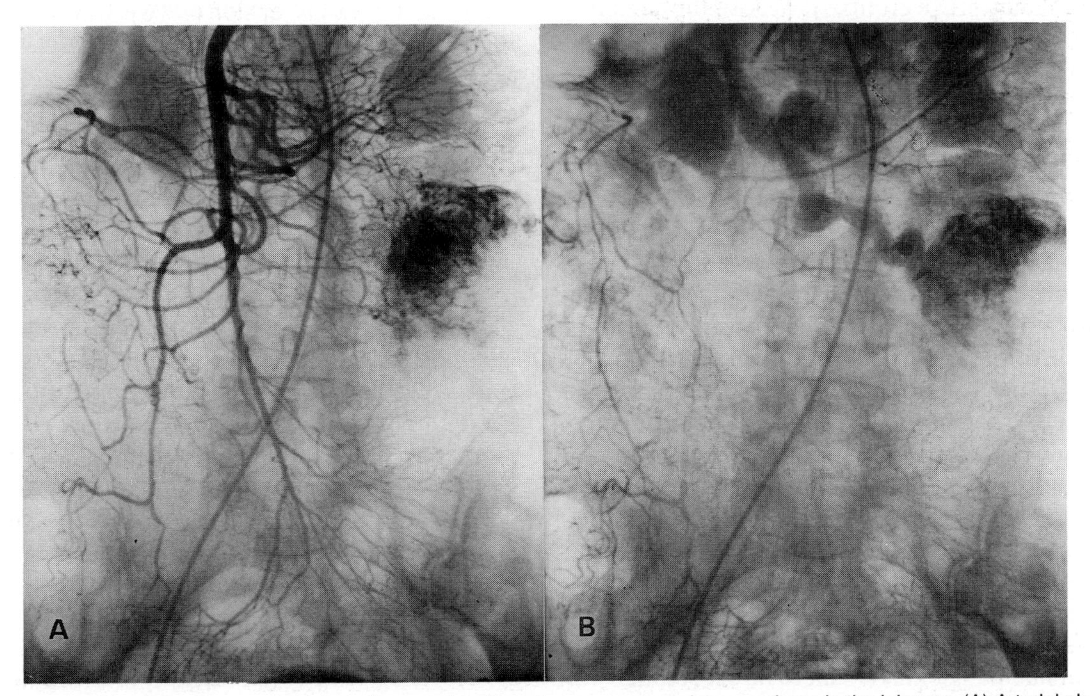

Figure 5.13 Selective superior mesenteric arteriogram showing a large cavernous haemangioma in the jejunum. (A) Arterial phase. (B) Venous phase. (Courtesy of Professor Allison).

Diffuse cavernous haemangiomas are characterized by great variation in size, shape and effect on the viscus in which they are located. Such lesions may involve 20–30 cm of one continuous segment of intestine, or there may be multiple lesions of this kind involving different segments of the gastrointestinal tract and surrounding viscera such as the urinary bladder. Diffuse cavernous haemangiomas account for 20% of all benign vascular lesions of the intestine. Their distribution appears to be equal for small intestine and colon. Their gross appearance on the luminal surface of the viscus is of a soft compressible, nodular, dark purple elevation under the mucosa. Microscopically they have the typical appearance of a cavernous haemangioma in most areas of the lesion; the periphery reveals numerous dilated tortuous vessels and an abundance of smooth muscle and connective tissue.

Overall this group has a very high mortality (about 30%) and morbidity, with continuing massive or chronic haemorrhage necessitating repeated transfusions of blood. Occasionally these diffuse lesions may spread to involve the urinary bladder and patients may present with haematuria.[8,28,77] There have been isolated reports of diffuse cavernous haemangiomas associated with lymphangiomatosis[77] as well as a protein-losing enteropathy which responded to surgical resection of a large segment of jejunum containing a diffuse lesion.[43] Extension of the haemangioma into the mesentery or retroperitoneum may result in haemorrhage at these sites. In a review of 47 cases of haemangiomas in the paediatric age group, 30 were of the cavernous variety (simple or diffuse) and the average duration of symptoms before diagnosis was 16 years.[60]

Radical surgery, where possible, appears to offer the only hope for cure in cases of diffuse cavernous haemangiomatosis of the intestine. Radiotherapy and sclerosing injections have been unsuccessful in controlling haemorrhage. Although high dose corticosteroids have been used successfully for large cutaneous angiomas there is no experience of this therapy for intestinal haemangiomas.

Selective arterial embolization of lesions shown to be bleeding at arteriography may be considered, particularly if multiple areas of diffuse haemangiomas are demonstrated. The therapeutic plan must be tailored to the individual patient after considering the severity of bleeding, response to conventional resuscitation, and disease extent.

The prognosis of patients with diffuse cavernous haemangiomas therefore depends on the extent of residual diseased intestine. Malignant transformation of haemangiomas is said to be exceedingly rare and most malignant haemangio-endotheliomas are thought to arise *de novo*.[81] There is one report of a patient with multiple simple capillary haemangiomas of the small and large bowel who died of gastrointestinal haemorrhage and was found at post mortem to have multiple malignant tumours in the gut and one in the bladder, all apparently arising in pre-existing haemangiomas.[59]

Mixed capillary and cavernous haemangiomas

These lesions account for 6–12% of all vascular malformations in the intestine.[37] They consist of solid areas of hyperplastic endothelial cells, partially obliterated vascular spaces and large blood-filled sinuses lined by a single endothelial cell layer. There is a variable amount of elastic and muscle tissue supporting these sinuses. The entire lesions tend to be encapsulated, and arise from submucosal vessels and enlarge towards the lumen of the viscus. They may eventually become pedunculated or ulcerate through the overlying epithelium. Since many of the mixed haemangiomas tend to be single (usually polypoid, occasionally diffuse in a single segment of bowel), surgical excision is frequently possible.

Peutz–Jeghers syndrome

There have been at least three papers which record the presence of mucocutaneous pigmentation with intestinal haemangiomas in the absence of polyposis, in the setting of a hereditary, dominantly-transmitted disease.

Jeghers *et al.*[44] described one patient with characteristic pigmentation and gastrointestinal bleeding without evidence of polyposis. Dormandy,[22] in a detailed study of five families (with 21 cases), found that four of the patients had pigmentation associated with gastrointestinal bleeding or abdominal pain but no evidence of polyposis. Bandler[5] reported a patient with mucocutaneous pigmentation and cavernous haemangiomas of the entire small intestine but no polyps. Two first-degree relatives of this patient also had haemangiomas of the intestine but no pigmentation.

Blue rubber bleb naevus syndrome

This disorder is inherited as an autosomal dominant trait,[9] although many reported cases appear to be sporadic.[30] It is characterized by cavernous haemangiomas of the skin, gastrointestinal tract and other viscera, including the liver, lung, spleen and joints. The skin lesions vary in number, may occur at any site including the palms and soles, and are present at birth but increase in number with age. They are typically blue, often tender, range in size from 1 mm to 2 cm across and have a wrinkled surface (*Figure 5.14*). They empty on digital pressure leaving a wrinkled blue sac that slowly refills over several minutes. Histologically, the skin haemangiomas

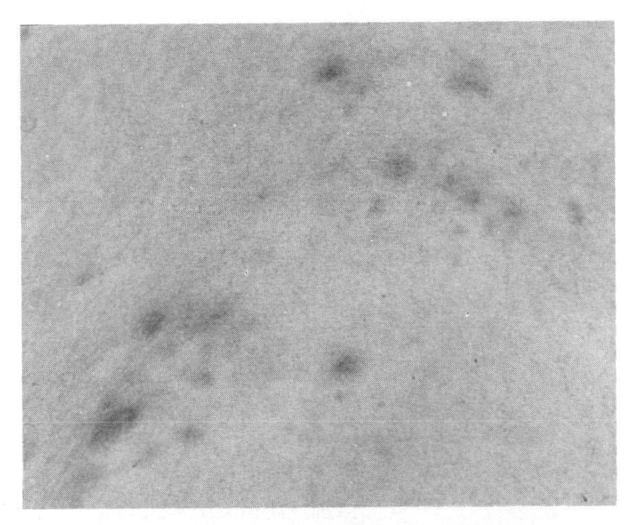

Figure 5.14 Blue rubber bleb naevus syndrome.

consist of clusters of dilated capillary spaces lined by cuboidal or flattened epithelium with a variable amount of connective tissue stroma.[4] Some reports also describe other elements present with the vascular lesions, such as smooth muscle cells and sweat glands.

The gastrointestinal tract lesions are usually multiple, but may be solitary. The onset of gastrointestinal bleeding may be at any time from early childhood to middle age. The small intestine is affected more frequently than the stomach and colon, and the lesions may be picked up on barium contrast examination as multiple mass lesions that may be mistaken for polyps. Angiography demonstrates arteriovenous malformations and may help to identify the site of bleeding, which is essential for surgical management of patients whose bleeding cannot be controlled medically.[4]

Klippel–Trenaunay–Weber syndrome

In 1990, Klippel and Trenaunay described a nonhereditary, sporadic disorder of children and young adults characterized by soft tissue and bony hypertrophy, varicose veins and port-wine haemangiomas, which are usually unilateral, often sharply demarcated, and involve a lower extremity, but are occasionally bilateral and affect the upper extremities, face or trunk.[66] Enlargement of the soft tissues may be gradual and may involve the whole limb, a portion of it, or selected digits. An underlying vascular abnormality consisting of atresia, hypoplasia, or obstruction of the deep venous system was noted in the 300 cases reported.[66] Parkes-Weber[64] described patients who, in association with the kind of abnormalities reported by Klippel and Tranaunay, also had arteriovenous fistulas with bruits over affected parts.

Other less frequent features of this syndrome include intermittent claudication, varicose ulcers, gangrene of an extremity, thrombophlebitis, varicose pulmonary veins, diffuse hair loss, dyskeratosis, altered sweating, lymphoedema, cutaneous lymphangiomas, dislocation of joints and gait abnormalities due to lower limb inequality, congestive cardiac failure, and bleeding from the urinary and gastrointestinal tracts.

The earliest report of gastrointestinal bleeding in association with limb hemihypertrophy is that of Hulke.[41] The affected patients were young boys (aged 7 and 5 years respectively) who had unilateral limb hypertrophy, cutaneous naevi, and gastrointestinal bleeding. One patient was found to have abnormal vessels on the serosal surface of the small and large intestine, as well as in the mesentery. The bowel vascular malformations may be mixed or cavernous haemangiomas.

Plain abdominal radiographs reveal phleboliths in the anatomical location of the colon and these increase in number and density with the patient's age. At colonoscopy, the bowel lumen is narrowed by multiple polypoid vascular masses that collapse on pressure and should only be biopsied with caution.[29] Similar irregularity of the bowel and prominent folds (resembling colonic varices) may be seen on barium enema. Arteriography shows slow venous drainage with contrast retained in vascular spaces in the colonic submucosa[29,66] and similar changes are visible in studies of the femoral artery. Arterial embolization has been considered by some authors but may lead to colonic infarction, especially as most lesions appear to affect the left side of the colon and rectum. Treatment necessitates primary resection of the affected intestinal segment with a permanent colostomy or 'pull-through' sphincter-saving procedure. This necessitates adequate delineation of the extent of bowel involvement with preoperative arteriography. Temporary relief may be obtained by ligation of the vessels supplying the colonic haemangioma.

Intestinal bleeding may be enhanced and postoperative haemostasis impaired when there is an associated consumptive coagulopathy resulting from intravascular clotting within the venous sinusoids of the cutaneous and visceral haemangiomas.

DISORDERS OF CONNECTIVE TISSUE AFFECTING BLOOD VESSELS

Pseudoxanthoma elasticum

This disorder demonstrates genetic heterogeneity in that both recessive and dominant modes of inheritance occur, and clinical variability is the rule.[20] Most cases are inherited as autosomal recessive.[31] No primary biochemical defect has been identified, although it is known that elastin metabolism is deranged.[15,78] The disorder affects the skin, mucous membranes and eyes, and the blood vessels of the gastrointestinal tract, heart and kidneys.[3,6] Prevalence figures are from 1/160 000 to 1/70 000, although these figures may be underestimating the true prevalence since they are based only on the number of reported cases.[20]

The skin changes are usually recognized in the second decade and usually affect regions of dermal stress, such as the neck, axillae and groin. These areas develop a characteristic yellowish, wrinkled appearance that simulates the skin of a plucked chicken (*Figure 5.15*). The skin eventually becomes lax and inelastic. Histologically there is a pathognomonic picture of clumping, fragmentation and calcification of elastic fibres in the mid- and deep dermis.

In most patients, alteration of elastic fibres on the retina, with rupture of the unsupported Bruch's membrane, results in the formation of angioid streaks. Other ocular problems are epithelial retinal pigment disturbances, atypical drusen, and neovascularization. Visual acuity often progressively worsens, especially when the macula becomes involved.

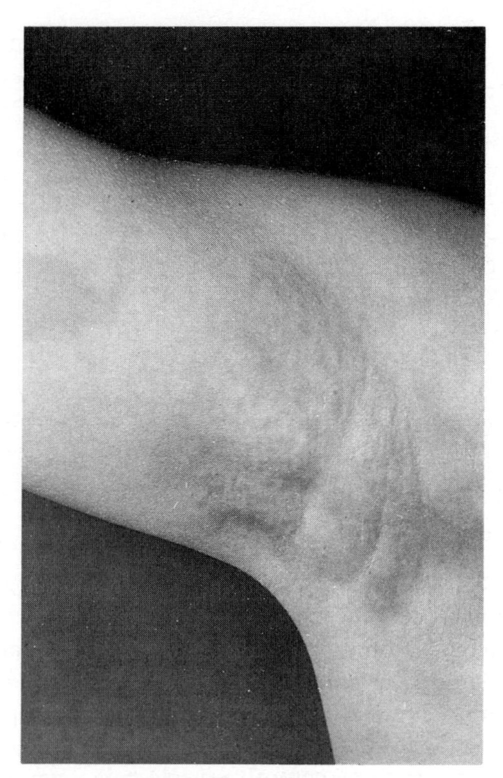

Figure 5.15 Pseudoxanthoma elasticum affecting axillary skin. (Courtesy of Dr Vickers.)

Medium-sized arteries degenerate and calcify in this disorder; such changes may result in weak peripheral pulses, intermittent claudication, angina, or strokes, and may be detected using plain radiography. Peripheral arterial occlusion, often unsuspected, and usually affecting radial, ulnar or posterior tibial arteries, occurred in a significant number of patients in one series.[31]

Haemorrhage is the most common presentation of gut involvement, and has been reported to occur as early as five years of age. There does appear to be a predilection for haemorrhage from the stomach.[20] Bleeding is thought to result from spontaneous vascular rupture and failure of calcified vessels to contract normally after injury, with resulting mucosal congestion and eventual erosion of the surface. Reports of the endoscopic appearance of the stomach describe a characteristic yellow, cobblestoned mucosa with a friable, oozing, eroded surface.[15,20,78] Proctoscopic examination also shows marked redundancy of rectal mucosa that becomes folded upon itself, and yellowish plaques similar to those seen in the stomach.[31] Barium contrast studies fail to reveal any abnormality; arteriography is reported to show abnormal, tortuous, narrowed mesenteric vessels as well as vascular malformations within the gastrointestinal tract.[3,6] This latter investigation may be necessary to demonstrate the site of bleeding if operative intervention is considered essential because of persistent haemorrhage. There has not, as yet, been a report of this technique during active bleeding. Fibreoptic endoscopy should be undertaken first, especially in view of the predilection for gastric bleeding. Resected specimens of stomach show that gastric submucosal arteries are calcified and the internal elastic lamina is deficient.[26] There is no evidence that anastomotic or incisional healing is impaired. Some authors have suggested that selective arterial embolization may be used to stop bleeding in these patients. Operative treatment is mandatory if haemorrhage cannot be controlled by such conservative means.

There is one report in the literature of coexistence of polyposis coli and pseudoxanthoma elasticum in one family.[62] Lesions such as peptic ulcer or hiatal hernia with oesophagitis may be more likely to bleed because of the underlying vascular abnormality in these patients. The significance of the former association is uncertain, but it highlights the importance of considering other treatable conditions when patients who suffer from pseudoxanthoma elasticum present with gut haemorrhage.

Ehlers–Danlos syndrome

This syndrome comprises a group of at least eight disorders.[45] It demonstrates genetic heterogeneity with documented kindreds showing autosomal dominant, autosomal recessive and sex-linked recessive patterns of inheritance. The spectrum of severity varies markedly from near normal to a life-threatening condition. The underlying aetiology is a defect in collagen synthesis, and the precise biochemical disorders are known for certain subgroups of the syndrome. There is a reduced content of type III collagen in subgroup IV, a deficiency of lysyl hydroxylase resulting in hydroxylysine deficiency in tissue collagen in subgroup VI, and deficiencies of lysyl oxidase and procollagen peptidase account for the disorder in subgroups V and VII.[39,45,46] Such biochemical markers are useful in distinguishing the various subgroups and provide a method for antenatal diagnosis which facilitates genetic counselling.

The syndrome is characterized by joint hyperextensibility (occasionally causing hip dislocation and clubfoot), bruising, skin elasticity and fragility, and formation of paper-thin scars. Redundant chordae tendineae may result in cardiac valve cusp prolapse or valvular incompetence. The more severe forms may be complicated by spontaneous arterial or even visceral rupture, the latter being seen almost exclusively in subgroup IV.[7] Massive dilatation of the oesophagus, stomach, or the small or large bowel have also been reported[36] and there is one well documented report of malabsorption due to bacterial overgrowth in a patient with the syndrome who had massive duodenal dilatation and multiple small intestinal diverticula.[37]

In a large series of 125 patients with this syndrome,[8] the gastrointestinal manifestations were haematemesis and melaena (6), jejunal intramural haemorrhage (1), colonic diverticular bleeding (2), colonic perforation (1), external piles (8) and skin splitting at the anal margin (5). Haematemesis and melaena were attributed to peptic ulceration in three, and a hiatal hernia in one patient, though no cause could be identified in two other patients. In view of the excessive tissue fragility, persistent haemorrhage and defective wound healing common in such patients, surgery should be avoided unless visceral rupture or uncontrollable haemorrhage supervene, and even angiography may be dangerous.

COLLAGEN–VASCULAR DISORDERS

Collagen disorders, such as systemic lupus erythematosus, polyarteritis nodosa, dermatomyositis and rheumatoid arthritis may be associated with visceral vasculitis which may cause chronic gut bleeding. They are discussed in Chapter 8.

HAEMATOLOGICAL DISORDERS

A wide range of haematological disorders may be associated with chronic gastrointestinal blood loss. These include clotting disorders, leukaemias, lymphomas, and haemolytic and aplastic anaemias. In polycythaemia rubra vera, chronic bleeding may result from thrombosis leading to local infarction of the gut with ulceration.

DRUGS

The possible drugs involved in chronic gastrointestinal bleeding are those already highlighted as potential causes of acute bleeding (and detailed in *Table 5.4*). It is generally rash to attribute chronic blood loss to anticoagulants, though they can exacerbate blood loss from many different lesions. Recently the role of non-steroidal anti-inflammatory drugs in causing a focal area of ulceration in the small intestine as well as the stomach has been highlighted.

Miscellaneous

Chronic gastrointestinal blood loss may occur in association with primary amyloidosis; localized ulceration may occur in the small intestine in this condition.

Chronic renal insufficiency and uraemia may cause bleeding from the duodenum or the colon, often in patients undergoing dialysis. Recurrent duodenal haemorrhage has also been reported in patients with renal carcinoma. Chronic or occult bleeding may also occur in patients with aortic stenosis, which may be associated with angiodysplasia.[16] Solitary ulcer of the caecum is also a rare cause of acute or chronic intestinal bleeding.

Factitious blood loss is difficult to diagnose, and frustrating to treat. Particular pointers are a medical or paramedical background in the patient.

CLINICAL FEATURES

EVIDENCE OF HAEMORRHAGE

The patient with overt bleeding will usually feature haemorrhage as the initial complaint. When bleeding is occult the patient is unaware of its presence, and then presents with anaemia, or with the other features of a systemic disease if this is present.

EVIDENCE OF CHRONIC IRON DEFICIENCY ANAEMIA

The typical features of anaemia may be present: fatigue, malaise, pallor, tachycardia, dyspnoea on exertion and oedema. Very commonly in the elderly the anaemia precipitates angina, which disappears with appropriate correction of the haemoglobin level.

UNDERLYING DISEASE

Underlying disease may give rise to the presenting symptoms, which, because of the wide range of possible diagnoses, are very varied. Any upper or lower bowel symptoms may be experienced.

INVESTIGATIONS

The major investigations used in the search for the cause of chronic bleeding have been discussed in the context of acute bleeding and the approach is summarized in the next section on obscure bleeding. A history of previous episodes, or of haemorrhage from multiple sites, or a family history of bleeding, suggest the possibility of one of the rarer hereditary conditions. A detailed history of drug ingestion is very important.

Characteristic physical features may suggest particular syndromes, as described separately. The presence of spider naevi, palmar erythema or jaundice suggest hepatic disease, and abdominal examination may reveal evidence of hepatomegaly, splenomegaly or masses suggesting neoplasia. A rectal examination is essential. The stools may be examined for parasites or ova.

LABORATORY TESTS

Standard haematological and biochemical tests should be performed and may provide a guide to the diagnosis. A complete blood count and blood film will determine if blood loss has been sufficient to cause anaemia and if the blood film suggests iron deficiency, confirmation will be obtained by determining the amount of stainable iron in the bone marrow or from serum ferritin determination. Serum iron levels are less reliable as the carrier protein, transferrin, is increased in iron deficiency but decreased in chronic disease. Platelet count, prothrombin time, bleeding time and partial thromboplastin time will detect clinically significant clotting defects in more than 90% of patients. An increased white cell count, if persistent, may suggest a neoplastic lesion or infection complicating colonic diverticula. Eosinophilia may point to hookworm disease, and thrombocythaemia suggests polycythemia rubra vera.

Routine biochemical tests, such as blood urea, electrolytes, sugar, albumin, globulin, calcium, magnesium, alkaline phosphatase, bilirubin and transaminases, may provide evidence of hepatic disease, inflammatory bowel disease or uraemia.

FAECAL STUDIES

Confirmation of faecal blood loss

Blood loss in the faeces may be obvious, depending upon the amount present or the site of blood loss. Thus, a distal source of chronic blood loss is more likely to give red blood in the stools than a proximal site, although this is not always the case. The presence of occult blood may be confirmed by a number of chemical tests which depend on the oxidation of a phenolic compound to a quinone structure by hydrogen peroxide catalysed by the peroxidase activity of haemoglobin.[42] Tests for faecal occult blood tend to be either highly sensitive (such as the formerly widely used benzidine and orthotolidine tests) or relatively insensitive (guaiac test). The highly sensitive tests tend to be positive after the shedding of 0.5–1.9 ml of blood in the gastrointestinal tract and a large number (over 70%) of false-positive reactions occur on an unrestricted diet. The relatively insensitive tests provide a positive result after passing 2–15 ml of blood and provide false-positive results in less than 25% of patients on a normal diet, but may give a false-negative reaction in up to 50% of patients. The interpretation of faecal occult blood tests is thus complicated by the loss of 'normal' small amounts of blood in the gastrointestinal tract, variations in the sensitivity of the chemical tests available, and the possibility that substances other than haemoglobin may be capable of producing a positive reaction, particularly with the 'sensitive' tests. False-positive results may occur with dietary meat or haemoglobin in poorly cooked meat and drugs containing bromide, iodide, potassium permanganate but not iron.

The present slide tests available, using either Haemoccult (guaiac) and Haemastix (orthotolidine), have been compared as screening procedures for occult gastrointestinal haemorrhage.[7] In a study of 438 patients, a false-positive rate of 22.9% was found with Haemastix, compared with 3.4% with Haemoccult. It was considered that the false-positive rate with Haemastix made this method unacceptable as a screening test, particularly in outpatients, although a test of greater sensitivity than Haemoccult may be needed in the investigation of hospital patients. Haemoccult may be too insensitive to detect lesions, particularly in the colon, which may be bleeding slowly or intermittently, but may be useful as a screening test in outpatients. In all patients suspected of chronic or occult gastrointestinal haemorrhage, repeated faecal occult blood tests may be necessary before occasional positive tests may provide confirmation of bleeding.

The test which is most commonly used at present is the relatively insensitive Haemoccult test which is less liable to provide false-positive results, may not routinely need dietary restriction before being applied but, if positive, provides valuable confirmation of gastrointestinal bleeding.

Quantitation of faecal blood loss

The amount of blood lost in the stools can be determined quantitatively by labelling the patient's circulating red blood cells with radioactive chromium (^{51}Cr), collecting the faeces and measuring the amount of faecal radioactivity.[68,69] Venous blood (20 ml) is drawn and, after labelling, is injected intravenously into the patient. The stools are collected for 5 days and, after preparation, the amount of radioactivity is determined by means of a scintillation counter. Using this method an average daily blood loss of 0.3–1.3 ml has been found in normal subjects. The value of the technique is to confirm abnormal faecal blood loss in patients suspected of having gastrointestinal bleeding but in whom faecal occult blood tests have been negative or equivocal, and to determine the amount of blood loss. The technique can also be used to calculate red cell survival.

REFERENCES

1. Ahr, D.J., Rickes, F.R., Hoyer, L.W. *et al.* (1977) Von Willebrand's disease and hemorrhagic telangiectasia: association of two complex disorders of hemostasis resulting in life threatening hemorrhage. *American Journal of Medicine*, **62**, 452–458.
2. Allison, D.J. (1982) Therapeutic embolisation. *Spectrum International*, **25**, 22–25.
3. Altman, L.K., Fialkow, P.J. and Parkor, F. (1974) Pseudoxanthoma elasticum. An underdiagnosed genetically heterogenous disorder with protean manifestations. *Archives of Internal Medicine*, **134**, 1048–1054.
4. Baker, A.L., Kahn, P.C., Binder, S.C. and Patterson, J.F. (1971) Gastrointestinal bleeding due to blue rubber bleb naevus syndrome. A case diagnosed by angiography. *Gastroenterology*, **61**, 530–533.
5. Bandler, M. (1960) Hemangiomas of the small intestine associated with mucocutaneous pigmentation. *Gastroenterology*, **38**, 643–645.
6. Bardsley, J.L. and Koehler, P.R. (1969) Pseudoxanthoma elasticum: angiographic manifestations in abdominal vessels. *Radiology*, **93**, 559–562.
7. Barrison, J.A., Primavesi, J., Gilmore, I.T. *et al.* (1981) Screening for occult gastrointestinal bleeding in hospital patients. *Journal of the Royal Society of Medicine*, **74**, 41–43.
8. Beighton, P.H., Murdoch, J.L. and Votteler, T. (1969) Gastrointestinal complications of the Ehlers–Danlos syndrome. *Gut*, **10**, 1004–1008.
9. Berlyne, G.M. and Berlyne, N. (1960) Anaemia due to 'Blue-Rubber-Bleb' naevus disease. *Lancet*, **ii**, 1275–1277.
10. Bick, R.L. (1971) Hereditary haemorrhage telangiectasia and disseminated intravascular coagulation: a new clinical syndrome. *Annals of the New York Academy of Sciences*, **370**, 851–854.
11. Birke, G., Engstedt, L. (1956) Melaena and haematemesis – a follow-up investigation with special reference to bleeding of unknown origin. *Gastroenterologia*, **85**, 97–115.
12. Cabal, E. and Holt, S. (1977) Polyarteritis as a cause of intestinal haemorrhage. *Gastroenterology*, **61**, 99–105.
13. Cameron, A.D. (1960) Gastrointestinal blood loss measured by radioactive chromium. *Gut*, 177–182.
14. Camilleri, M., Chadwick, V.S. and Hodgson, H.J.F. (1984) Vascular anomalies of the gastrointestinal tract. *Hepatogastroenterology*, **31**, 149–153.
15. Cocco, A.E., Grayer, D.I., Walker, B.A. and Martyn, L.J. (1969) The stomach in pseudoxanthoma elasticum. *Journal of the American Medical Association*, **210**, 2381–2382.
16. Cody, M.C., O'Donovan, T.P.B. and Hughes, R.W. (1974) Idiopathic gastrointestinal bleeding and aortic stenosis. *American Journal of Digestive Diseases*, **19**, 393–398.
17. Conlon, C.L., Weinger, R.S., Cimo, P.L. *et al.* (1978) Telangiectasia and von Willebrand's disease in two families. *Annals of Internal Medicine*, **89**, 921–924.
18. Conn, H.O. and Blitzer, B.L. (1976) Non association of adrenocorticosteroid therapy and peptic ulcer. *New England Journal of Medicine*, **294**, 473–479.
19. Cream, J.J., Gumpel, J.M. and Peachey, R.D.G. (1970) Schonlein-Henoch purpura in the adult: a study of 77 patients with anaphylactoid or Schonlein-Henoch purpura. *Quarterly Journal of Medicine*, **39**, 461–484.
20. Cunningham, J.R., Lippman, S.M., Renie, W.A. *et al.* (1980) Pseudoxanthoma elasticum: treatment of gastrointestinal haemorrhage by arterial embolisation and observations on autosomal dominant inheritance. *Johns Hopkins Medical Journal*, **147**, 168–173.
21. Desa, L.A.J., Bridger, J., Grace, P.A., Krausz, T. and Spencer, J. (1991) Primary jejunoileal tumours:

a review of 45 cases. *World Journal of Surgery*, **15**, 81–87.
22. Dormandy, T.L. (1957) Gastrointestinal polyposis with mucocutaneous pigmentation (Peutz–Jeghers syndrome). *New England Journal of Medicine*, **256**, 1093–1102.
23. Douvres, P.A. and Glass, G.B.J. (1970) Cryptogenic gastrointestinal haemorrhage. In *Progress in Gastroenterology, 2* (Ed.) Glass, G.B.J. New York and London: Grune and Stratton.
24. Edward, H. (1958) Haematemesis due to pseudoxanthoma elasticum. *Gastroenterology (Basel)*, **89**, 345–346.
25. Engel, E. and Forbes, A.P. (1965) Cytogenetic and clinical findings in 48 patients with congenitally defective or absent ovaries. *Medicine (Baltimore)*, **44**, 135–164.
26. Flatley, F.J., Atwell, M.E. and McEvoy, R.K. (1963) Pseudoxanthoma elasticum with gastric hemorrhage. *Archives of Internal Medicine*, **112**, 352–356.
27. Frame, B., Dhanwada, S.R., Ohorodnik, J.M. and Kwa, D.M. (1977) Gastrointestinal haemorrhage in Turner's syndrome. *Archives of Internal Medicine*, **137**, 691–692.
28. Gentry, R., Dockerty, M.B. and Clagett, O.T. (1949) Vascular malformations and vascular tumours of the gastrointestinal tract. *International Abstracts of Surgery*, **88**, 281–323.
29. Ghahremani, G.G., Kangarloo, H., Volberg, F. and Meyers, M.A. (1976) Diffuse cavernous haemangioma of the colon in the Klippel–Trenaunay syndrome. *Radiology*, **118**, 673–678.
30. Golitz, L.E. (1980) Heritable cutaneous disorders that affect the gastrointestinal tract. *Medical Clinics of North America*, **64**, 829–846.
31. Goodman, R.M., Smith, E.W., Paton, D. *et al.* (1963) Pseudoxanthoma elasticum. A clinical and histopathological study. *Medicine (Baltimore)*, **42**, 297–334.
32. Gouldesbrough, D.R. and Pell, A.C.H. (1991) Gastric antral vascular ectasia: a problem of recognition and diagnosis. *Gut*, **32**, 954–955.
33. Graham, D.Y., Agrawal, N.M. and Roth, S.H. (1988) Prevention of NSAID-induced gastric ulcer with misoprostol: multicentre, double-blind, placebo-controlled trial. *Lancet*, **ii**, 1277–1280.
34. Greenberg, G.R., Phillips, M.J., Tovee, E.B. and Jeejeebhoy, K.N. (1976) Fibreoptic endoscopy during laparotomy in the diagnosis of small intestinal bleeding. *Gastroenterology*, **71**, 133–135.
35. Haddad, H.M. and Wilkins, L. (1959) Congenital anomalies associated with gonadal aplasia. Review of 55 cases. *Pediatrics*, **23**, 885–902.
36. Harris, R.D. (1974) Small bowel dilatation in Ehlers Danlos syndrome: an unreported gastrointestinal manifestation. *British Journal of Radiology*, **47**, 623–627.
37. Hines, C.Jr and Davis, W.D. (1973) Ehlers Danlos syndrome with megaduodenum and malabsorption syndrome secondary to bacterial overgrowth: a report of the first case. *American Journal of Medicine*, **54**, 539–543.
38. Hodgson, C.H., Burchell, H.B., Good, C.A. and Clagett, O.T. (1959) Hereditary haemorrhagic telangiectasia and pulmonary arteriovenous fistula survey of a large family. *New England Journal of Medicine*, **261**, 625–636.
39. Hollister, D.W. (1978) Heritable disorders of connective tissue: Ehlers–Danlos syndrome. *Pediatric Clinics of North America*, **25**, 575–591.
40. Hong G.S., Wong, C.Y. and Nambiar, R. (1992) Massive lower gastrointestinal haemorrhage from a splenic artery pseudoaneurysm. *British Journal of Surgery*, **79**, 174.
41. Hulke, J.W. (1876) *Lancet*, **ii**, 857. Referred to by Shepherd, J.A. (1953) *British Journal of Surgery*, **40**, 409–421.
42. Irons, G.V. and Kirsner, J.B. (1965) Routine chemical tests of the stool for occult blood: an evaluation. *American Journal of Medical Science*, **249**, 247–260.
43. Jackson, A.E. and Peterson, C. (1967) Haemangioma of the small intestine causing protein-losing enteropathy. *Annals of Internal Medicine*, **66**, 1190–1196.
44. Jeghers, H., McKusick, V.A. and Katz, K.H. (1949) Generalised intestinal polyposis and melanin spots of oral mucosa, lips and digits: syndrome of diagnostic significance. *New England Journal of Medicine*, **241**, 993.
45. Krane, S.M. (1980) Understanding genetic disorders of collagen. *New England Journal of Medicine*, **303**, 101–102.
46. Krieg, T. (1981) Molecular defects of collagen metabolism in the Ehlers Danlos syndrome. *International Journal of Dermatology*, **20**, 415–425.
47. Kurata, J.H., Elashoff, J.D. and Grossman, M.I. (1982) Inadequacy of the literature on the relationship between drugs, ulcers and gastrointestinal bleeding. *Gastroenterology*, **82**, 373–382.
48. Lisser, H., Curtis, L.E., Escamilla, R.F. *et al.* (1947) The syndrome of congenital aplastic ovaries with sexual infantilism, high urinary gonadotrophins, short stature and other congenital abnormalities. *Journal of Clinical Endocrinology*, **7**, 665–687.
49. Lyon, D.T. and Mantia, A.G. (1984) Large bowel haemangiomas. *Diseases of the Colon and Rectum*, **27**, 404–414.
50. McGrath, K.M., Johnson, C.A. and Stuart, J.J. (1979) Acquired von Willebrand disease associated with an inhibitor to factor VIII antigen and gastrointestinal telangiectasia. *American Journal of Medicine*, **67**, 693–696.
51. McKusick, V.A. (1972) Pseudoxanthoma elasticum. In *Heritable Disorders of Connective Tissue, 4th Edition*, pp. 475–520. St Louis: CV Mosby.
52. McKusick, V.A. (1972) The Ehlers–Danlos syndrome. In *Heritable Disorders of Connective*

Tissue, 4th Edition, pp. 292–371. St Louis: CV Mosby.
53. McKusick, V.A. (1974) Multiple forms of the Ehlers–Danlos syndrome. *Archives of Surgery*, **109**, 475–476.
54. Marine, R. and Lattomus, W.W. (1958) Cavernous haemangioma of the gastrointestinal tract. *Radiology*, **70**, 860–863.
55. Menefee, M.G., Flessa, H.C., Glueck, H.I. and Hogg, S.P. (1975) Hereditary haemorrhagic telangiectasia (Osler–Rendu–Weber disease): An electron microscopic study of the vascular lesions before and after therapy with hormones. *Archives of Otolaryngology*, **101**, 246–251.
56. Miles, R.M., Crawford, D. and Duras, S. (1979) The small bowel tumour problem. An assessment based on a 20 year experience with 116 cases. *American Surgeon*, **189**, 732.
57. Mollison, P.L. and Veall, N. (1955) The use of the isotope ^{51}Cr as a label for red cells. *British Journal of Haematology*, **1**, 62–74.
58. Morgan, A.A. (1982) Recurrent gastrointestinal hemorrhage: an unusual cause. *American Journal of Gastroenterology*, **77**, 925–928.
59. Murray-Lyon, I.M., Doyle, D., Philpott, R.M. and Porter, N.H. (1971) Haemangiomatosis of the small and large bowel with histological malignant change. *Journal of Pathology*, **105**, 295–297.
60. Nader, P.R. and Margolin, F. (1966) Haemangioma causing gastrointestinal bleeding. *American Journal of Diseases of Children*, **111**, 215–222.
61. Nys, A. and Buyssens, N. (1963) Diffuse cavernous haemangiomatosis of the small intestine. *Gastroenterology*, **45**, 663–666.
62. O'Helleran, M. and Merrell, R.C. (1981) Pseudoxanthoma elasticum and polyposis coli: a novel co-mutation. *Archives of Surgery*, **116**, 476–477.
63. Ona, F.V. and Ahluwalia, M. (1980) Endoscopic appearance of gastric angiodysplasia in hereditary haemorrhagic telangiectasia. *American Journal of Gastroenterology*, **73**, 148–149.
64. Parkes-Weber, F. (1918) Haemangiectatic hypertrophy of limbs: congenital phlebarteriectasis and so-called congenital varicose veins. *British Journal of Childrens Disease*, **15**, 13.
65. Peoples, J.B., Kartha, R. and Sharif, S. (1981) Multiple phlebectasia of the small intestine. *American Surgeon*, **47**, 373–376.
66. Phillips, G.N., Gordon, D.H., Martin, E.C. *et al.* (1978) The Klippel–Trenaunay syndrome: clinical and radiological aspects. *Radiology*, **128**, 429–434.
67. Raiford, T.S. (1932) Tumours of the small intestine. *Archives of Surgery*, **25**, 122–177, 321–325.
68. Reuter, S.R. and Redman, H.C. (1977) Gastrointestinal bleeding. In *Gastrointestinal Angiography, 2nd Edition*, pp. 218–268. London, New York: W.B. Saunders.
69. Richardson, J.D. (1991) Vascular lesions of the intestines. *American Journal of Surgery*, **161**, 284–293.
70. Rissier, H.L. Jr (1959) Hemangiomatosis of the intestine. *Gastroenterologia*, **93**, 357–385.
71. River, L., Silverstein, J. and Tope, J.W. (1956) Benign neoplasms of the small intestine: a critical comprehensive review with reports of 20 new cases. *International Abstracts of Surgery*, **102**, 1–38.
72. Rutlin, E., Wisløff, E., Myren, J. and Serck-Hanssen, A. (1981) Intestinal telangiectasia in Turner's syndrome. *Endoscopy*, **13**, 86–87.
73. Scott, T. (1968) Turner's syndrome and vermiform phlebectasia of the bowel. *Transactions American Clinical Climatological Association*, **79**, 45–50.
74. Shandalow, S.L. (1956) Fatal massive gastrointestinal haemorrhage due to multiple phlebectasia of the small intestine. *Journal of the International College of Surgeons*, **24**, 445–447.
75. Shepherd, J.A. (1953) Angiomatous conditions of the gastrointestinal tract. *American Journal of Surgery*, **40**, 409–421.
76. Sogge, M.R. (1980) Detection of typical lesions of hereditary haemorrhagic telangiectasia by colonoscopy. *Gastroenterological Endoscopy*, **26**, 52–53.
77. Taylor, T.V. and Torrance, H.B. (1974) Haemangioma of the gastrointestinal tract. *British Journal of Surgery*, **61**, 236–238.
78. Uitto, J. (1979) Biochemistry of the elastic fibres in normal connective tissues and its alterations in diseases. *Journal of Investigative Dermatology*, **72**, 1–8.
79. Van Cutsem, E., Rutgeerts, P. and Van Trappen, G. (1990) Treatment of bleeding gastrointestinal vascular malformations with oestrogen-progesterone. *The Lancet*, **335**, 953–955.
80. Vase, P. (1981) Estrogen treatment of hereditary hemorrhagic telangiectasia: a double-blind controlled clinical trial. *Acta Medica Scandinavica*, **209**, 393–396.
81. Willis, R.A. (1962) Hamartomas and hamartomatous syndromes. In *The Borderland of Embryology and Pathology* 2nd edn (Ed.) Willis, B.A. pp. 351–392. London: Butterworth.
82. Wilson, J.M., Melvin, D.B., Gray, G. and Thorbjarnarson, B. (1975) Benign small bowel tumour. *American Surgeon*, **181**, 247–250.

NECROTIZING ENTEROCOLITIS

Caroline Doig

The main reason for gastrointestinal perforation in the neonate involving the large or small bowel is necrotizing enterocolitis.[45] About 10–20% of admissions to a neonatal surgical unit will be because of necrotizing enterocolitis or its complications. The incidence has increased to 24 per 1000 births with improved neonatal care, especially of the very small premature.[37] It can occur in the full term or older baby child[44,49] or after surgery.[31] If occurring in multiple births, not all babies will be involved.[38]

AETIOLOGY

The precise aetiology is probably multifactorial in a susceptible host infant with an anoxic episode, either at or after birth, leading to a reduction in the microcirculation with cell damage and ischaemia.[20] Changes in haemodynamics, as seen in exchange transfusions or with a patent ductus arteriosus,[36] can also lead to ischaemic bowel. Whether from anoxia or direct damage to the vessels even of a temporary nature,[47] such bowel has no defence to infection coming probably from the bowel lumen itself. In the full blown case, a mucosal ulcer allows gas from the lumen to enter the wall of the bowel giving the classical appearance of pneumocystis intestinalis. Less severe cases only exhibit a functional obstruction. As well as prematurity, stress of a traumatic birth, e.g. the cord around the neck or respiratory problems, lead to an increased incidence.[50]

The bowel at surgery is paper-thin with necrotic patches and inflammatory exudate or areas of perforation. The lumen will be filled with haemorrhagic debris while the mucosa may slough. Considering the complex intestinal flora pattern, it is not surprising that numerous organisms are grown, e.g. anaerobes, especially *Clostridia*[46] or *Escherichia coli*[4] and coagulase negative staphylococci[32] but no one organism can be implicated, although those in whom clostridia are implicated seem to have a more fulminating disease.[25]

Although it has been suggested that delaying feeding reduces the chance of necrotizing enterocolitis,[30] the disease may be evident within days of birth before feeding has started.[27] Different feeding regimens may allow different colonization of the bowel and so may be implicated. Breast milk, by producing immunological factors,[2] may reduce the incidence, although the disease is not a result of an immature immune mechanism.[12] Other factors may be increased intraluminal pressure and decreased pH.[15]

CLINICAL FEATURES

The baby may have only a functional obstruction with vomiting, abdominal distension and delay in the passage of meconium. Most babies will have abdominal distension with the passage of blood through the rectum. If complicated by septicaemia, disseminated intravascular coagulation will lead to bleeding problems and eventual death. The area and extent of bowel varies but the terminal ileum is frequently affected.

INVESTIGATIONS

An abdominal radiograph may show only gaseous distension with separation of loops of bowel by intraperitoneal fluid. In the established case, intramural gas as well as intraluminal gas gives an appearance of a target (*Figure 5.16*). A poor prognostic

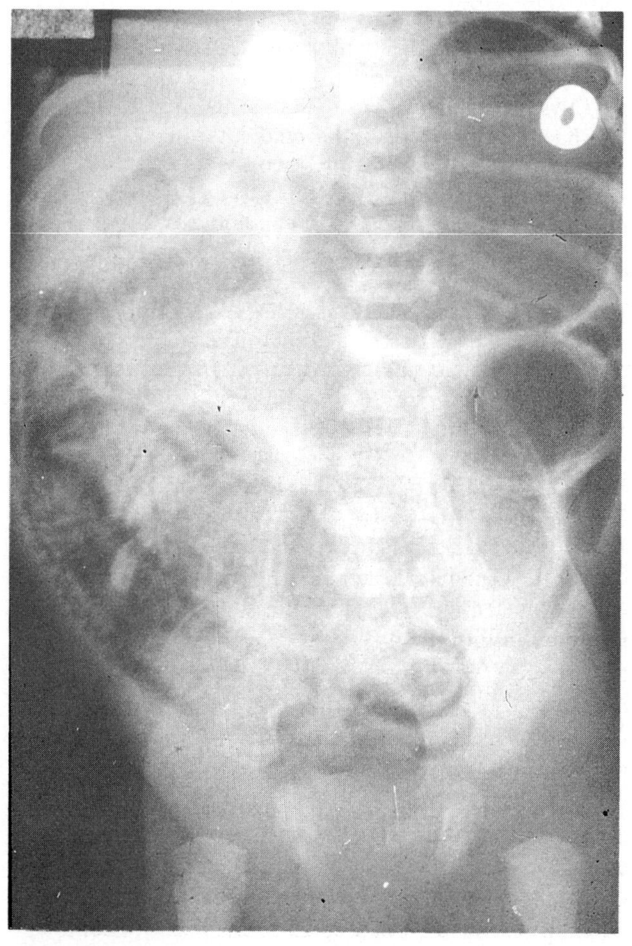

Figure 5.16 Plain abdominal radiograph with numerous areas of intramural gas.

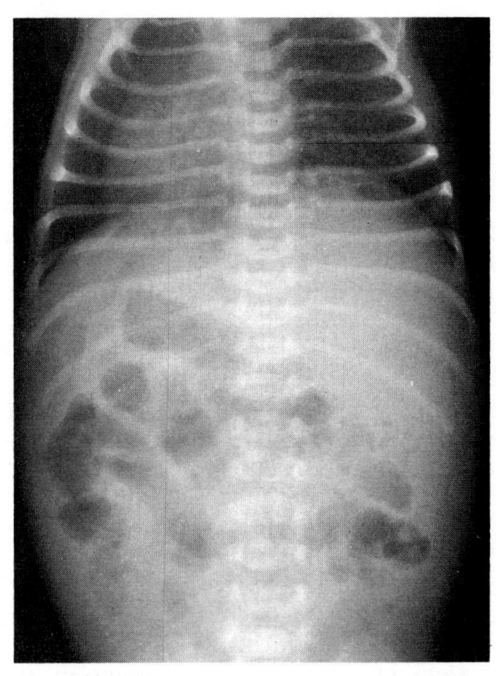

Figure 5.17 Free gas under diaphragm on abdominal X-ray. (Courtesy of Salford Health Authority.)

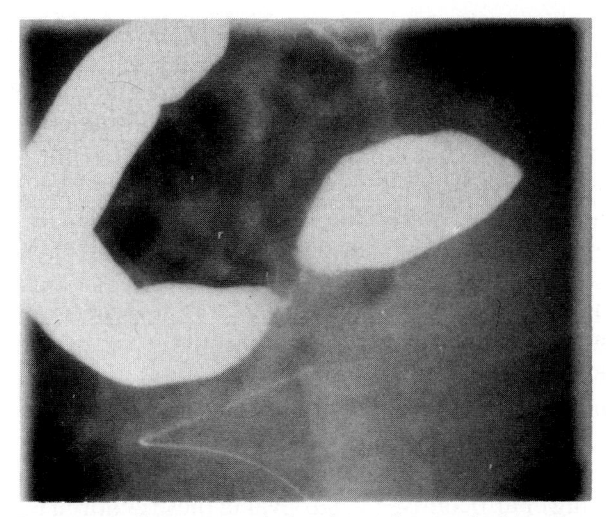

Figure 5.18 Transverse colonic stricture shown on barium enema.

sign, seen either on abdominal radiograph or ultrasound,[26] is gas, albeit transitory, in the portal venous system.[10,17]

If perforation has occurred, free gas is seen (*Figure 5.17*) although this can be missed initially. Even on the supine radiograph a haziness over the liver or odd-shaped gas shadow suggests gas outside the bowel. Bilious vomiting should alert one to the possibility of volvulus which can give a similar picture.[6]

TREATMENT

Diagnosis of necrotizing enterocolitis is often on suspicion alone, and therefore treatment should be started empirically. If uncomplicated, it is better to treat the baby conservatively without surgery by resting the bowel and treating the infection. Intravenous feeding for 2–3 weeks and appropriate antibiotics to treat the Gram negative and, more importantly, the anaerobic organisms (e.g. gentamycin and metronidazole) gives good results in most cases. In the very ill child, fresh frozen plasma or steroids may be indicated to treat the septicaemia and shock. Many of the very small babies with enterocolitis die with or without surgery but frequent radiographs,[3] even 6-hourly, will determine when perforation occurs, as it may be difficult in these very ill babies to know when this has occurred. Perforation occurs in about half of the cases.[29]

The disease process may resolve or lead on to late stricture formation. Problems with the introduction of feeding, bleeding[33] or recurrent abdominal distension necessitates a delayed barium study[5,21] to delineate strictures in the large or small bowel. Such strictures occur in a quarter of successful medically treated cases,[40] usually in the colon[24,42] (*Figure 5.18*) but not exclusively so. Resection and re-anastomosis gives good results, although balloon dilatation has been attempted.[1]

Even with aggressive medical treatment, surgery may be necessary, more especially for the complications of septicaemia, perforation and fistulas. Monitoring with platelet counts and abdominal radiographs help determine the timing of surgery.[34] Aggressive early surgery[28] does not give good results and surgery, usually resection with stomas, is reserved for the complications of peritonitis or abscess formation. If these occur, surgery is the only hope of saving these very ill and premature babies. If the child is too ill to undergo laparotomy, a drain inserted into the abdomen may improve the condition[7] until surgery can be performed. However in most of these babies die before definitive surgery can be carried out.

When surgery is performed it may be necessary to resect large areas of bowel, either colon or small bowel, leaving the child with less than adequate length of bowel. The decision is whether to bring out stomas,[35] which may be high in the small bowel or perform a primary anastomosis.[9,18,19] By anastomosing the bowel, problems with fluid losses and malabsorption can be avoided but problems with ischaemic anastomoses and breakdown are more likely. If stomas are performed – and this is the preferred choice[39] – these can be closed early[13,16] without problems.

As not all newborns with necrotizing enterocolitis will be sent to specialized medical or surgical units, it is not possible to gauge the true incidence of the disease or those requiring surgical intervention. All babies do not have the full blown picture and so will not be included in any statistics. Other problems of prematurity, e.g. respiratory problems, or intracranial haemorrhage, have a bearing on the eventual prognosis as do other congenital defects. Low platelet counts and pH[11] may help estimate the outcome. Although survival rates have improved[14] so that mortality rates are now less than 40%,[23] long-term sequelae, due perhaps more to the prematurity than the poor condition of the child, are not uncommon.[8,43]

Localized single perforations can occur through the gastrointestinal tract, unassociated with necrotizing enterocolitis.[48,51] Survival in these children is, in contrast, 80% with few sequelae.

FUNCTIONAL OBSTRUCTION

Mention has already been made of a possible lesser degree of necrotizing enterocolitis presenting as a functional obstruction. Failure to pass meconium associated with abdominal distension and vomiting are common presentations to a neonatal surgical unit.[22] Some will proceed to a full blown condition especially if there are associated factors of prematurity and respiratory distress. Others will settle after a few days of intravenous fluids and nasogastric suction. In all infants, Hirschsprung's disease, meconium ileus and sepsis should be excluded by suction biopsy, sweat test and an infection screen respectively. Other causes include hypothyroidism and hypoglycaemia associated with a diabetic mother. In such a child, barium enema appearances can mimic Hirschsprung's disease giving a 'hypoplastic left colon'. Functional obstruction can also complicate malrotation and in those children with short gut for whatever reason.[41]

REFERENCES

1. Ball, W.S., Kosloske, A.M., Jewell, P.F., Seigel, R.S. and Bartow, S.A. (1985) Balloon catheter dilatation of focal intestinal strictures following necrotizing enterocolitis. *Journal of Pediatric Surgery*, **20**, 637–641.
2. Barlow, B., Santulli, T.V., Heird, W.C., Pitt, J., Blanc, W.A. and Schullinger, J.N. (1974) An experimental study of acute neonatal enterocolitis: the importance of breast milk. *Journal of Pediatric Surgery*, **9**, 587–592.
3. Beasley, S.W., Auldist, A.W., Ramanujan, T.M. and Campnell, N.T. (1986) The surgical management of neonatal necrotizing enterocolitis, 1975–1984. *Pediatric Surgery*, **1**, 210–214.
4. Bell, M.J., Shackelford, P., Feigin, R.D., Ternberg, J.L. and Brotherton, T. (1979) Epidemiologic and bacteriologic evaluation of neonatal necrotizing enterocolitis. *Journal of Pediatric Surgery*, **14**, 1–9.
5. Born, M., Holgersen, L.O., Shahrivar, F., Stanley-Brown, E. and Hilfer, C. (1985) Routine contrast enemas for diagnosing and managing strictures following nonoperative treatment of necrotizing enterocolitis. *Journal of Pediatric Surgery*, **20**, 461–464.
6. Boulton, J.E., Ein, S.H., Reilly, B.J., Smith, B.T. and Pape, K.E. (1989) Necrotizing enterocolitis and volvulus in the premature neonate. *Journal of Pediatric Surgery*, **24**, 901–904.
7. Cheu, H.W., Sukarochana, K. and Lloyd, D.A. (1988) Peritoneal drainage for necrotizing enterocolitis. *Journal of Pediatric Surgery*, **23**, 557–580.
8. Cirkit, D., West, K.W., Schreiner, R. and Grosfeld, J.L. (1986) Long-term follow-up after surgical management of necrotizing enterocolitis: sixty-three cases. *Journal of Pediatric Surgery*, **21**, 533–537.
9. Cooper, A., Ross, A.J., O'Neill, J.A. and Schnaufer, L. (1988) Resection with primary anastomosis for necrotizing enterocolitis: a contrasting view. *Journal of Pediatric Surgery*, **23**, 64–67.
10. Donoghue, V. and Kelman, C.G. (1982) Transient portal venous gas in necrotizing enterocolitis. *British Journal of Radiology*, **55**, 681–682.
11. Dykes, E.H., Gilmour, W.H. and Azmy, A.F. (1985) Prediction of outcome following necrotizing enterocolitis in a neonatal surgical unit. *Journal of Pediatric Surgery*, **20**, 3–4.
12. Dykes, E.H., Liddell, R.H.A., Galloway, E. and Azmy, A.F. (1986) Immune competence in necrotizing enterocolitis. *Journal of Pediatric Surgery*, **21**, 211–214.
13. Festen, C., Severijnen, R.S.V.M. and Staak, F.H.J. vd. (1987) Early closure of enterostomy after exteriorization of small intestine for abdominal catastrophies. *Journal of Pediatric Surgery*, **22**, 144–146.
14. Freeman, R.B., Lloyd, D.J., Miller, S.S. and Duffy, P. (1988) Surgical treatment of necrotizing enterocolitis: a population-based study in the Grampian region, Scotland. *Journal of Pediatric Surgery*, **23**, 942–946.
15. Garstin, W.I.H., Kenny, B.D., McAneaney, D.S., Patterson, C.C. and Boston, V. E. (1987) The role of intraluminal tension and pH in the development of necrotizing enterocolitis: an animal model. *Journal of Pediatric Surgery*, **22**, 205–210.
16. Gertler, J.P., Seashore, J.H. and Touloukian, R.J. (1987) Early ileostomy closure in necrotizing enterocolitis. *Journal of Pediatric Surgery*, **22**, 140–143.

17. Griffiths, D.M. and Gough, M.H. (1986) Gas in the hepatic portal veins. *British Journal of Surgery*, **73**, 172–175.
18. Griffiths, D.M., Forbes, D.A., Pemberton, P.J. and Penn, I.A. (1989) Primary anastomosis for necrotizing enterocolitis: a 12-year experience. *Journal of Pediatric Surgery*, **24**, 515–517.
19. Harberg, F.J., McGill, C.W., Saleem, M.M., Halbert, R. and Anastassiou, P. (1983) Resection with primary anastomosis for necrotizing enterocolitis. *Journal of Pediatric Surgery*, **18**, 743–746.
20. Harrison, M.W., Connell, R.S., Campbell, J.R. and Webb, M.C. (1975) Microcirculatory changes in the gastrointestinal tract of the hypoxic puppy: an electron microscope study. *Journal of Pediatric Surgery*, **10**, 599–604.
21. Hartman, G.E., Drugas, G.T. and Shochat, S.J. (1988) Post-necrotizing enterocolitis strictures presenting with sepsis or perforation: risk of clinical observation. *Journal of Pediatric Surgery*, **23**, 562–567.
22. Howat, J.M. and Wilkinson, A.W.W. (1970) Functional intestinal obstruction in the neonate. *Archives of Disease in Childhood*, **45**, 800–808.
23. Jackman, S., Brerton, R.J. and Wright, V.M. (1990) Results of surgical treatment of neonatal necrotizing enterocolitis. *British Journal of Surgery*, **77**, 146–147.
24. Keily, E. and Eckstein, H.B. (1984) Colonic stricture and enterocolic fistulae following necrotizing enterocolitis. *British Journal of Surgery*, **71**, 613–619.
25. Kosloske, A.M. and Ulrich, J.A. (1980) A bacteriologic basis for the clinical presentations of necrotizing enterocolitis. *Journal of Pediatric Surgery*, **15**, 558–559.
26. Lindley, S., Mollitt, D., Seibert, J.J. and Golladay, E.S. (1986) Portal vein ultrasonography in the early diagnosis of necrotizing enterocolitis. *Journal of Pediatric Surgery*, **21**, 530–536.
27. Marchildon, M.B., Buck, B.E. and Abdenour, G. (1982) Necrotizing enterocolitis in the unfed infant. *Journal of Pediatric Surgery*, **17**, 620–623.
28. Martin, L.W. and Neblett, W.W. (1981) Early operation with intestinal diversion for necrotizing enterocolitis. *Journal of Pediatric Surgery*, **16**, 252–257.
29. Mazzoni, G., Doig, C.M., Bianchi, A. and Gough, D.C.S. (1987) Neonatal necrotizing enterocolitis: the surgical complications. *International Journal of Pediatric Surgery*, **1**, 13–17.
30. McCormack, C.J., Emmens, R.W. and Putman, T.C. (1987) Evaluation of factors in high risk neonatal necrotizing enterocolitis. *Journal of Pediatric Surgery*, **22**, 488–492.
31. Mollitt, D.L. and Golladay, E.S. (1982) Postoperative neonatal necrotizing enterocolitis. *Journal of Pediatric Surgery*, **17**, 757–759.
32. Mollitt, D.L., Tapas, J.J. and Talbert, J.L. (1988) The role of coagulase-negative staphylococcus in neonatal necrotizing enterocolitis. *Journal of Pediatric Surgery*, **23**, 60–64.
33. Nanjundiah, P., Lifschitz, C.H., Gopalakrishna, G.S., Cochran, W.J. and Klish, W.J. (1989) Intestinal strictures presenting with gastrointestinal blood loss. *Journal of Pediatric Surgery*, **24**, 174–178.
34. O'Neill, J.A., Stahlman, M.T. and Meng, H.C. (1975) Necrotizing enterocolitis in the newborn: operative indications. *Annals of Surgery*, **182**, 274–276.
35. O'Neill, J.A. and Holcomb, G.W. (1979) Surgical experience with neonatal necrotizing enterocolitis. *Annals of Surgery*, **189**, 612–617.
36. Palder, S.B., Schwartz, M.Z., Tyson, K.R.T. and Marr, C.C. (1988) Association of closure of patent ductus arteriosus and development of necrotizing enterocolitis. *Journal of Pediatric Surgery*, **23**, 422–427.
37. Pokorny, W.J., Garcia-Prats, J.A. and Barry, Y.N. (1986) Necrotizing enterocolitis: incidence, operative care and outcome. *Journal of Pediatric Surgery*, **21**, 1149–1154.
38. Powell, R.W., Dyess, D.L., Luterman, A., Simon N.P. and Ramenofsky, M.L. (1990) Necrotizing enterocolitis in multiple-birth infants. *Journal of Pediatric Surgery*, **25**, 319–324.
39. Ross, M.N., Wayne, E.R., Janik, J.S., Hanson, J.B., Burrington, J.D. and Chang, J.H.T. (1989) A standard of comparison for acute surgical necrotizing enterocolitis. *Journal of Pediatric Surgery*, **24**, 999–1006.
40. Schwartz, M.Z., Hayden, C.K., Richardson, C.J., Tyson, K.R.T. and Lobe, T.E. (1982) A prospective evaluation of intestinal stenosis following necrotizing enterocolitis. *Journal of Pediatric Surgery*, **17**, 764–766.
41. Shawis, R.N., Rangecroft, I., Cook, R.C.M. and Gough, D.C.S. (1984) Functional obstruction associated with malrotation and short small-bowel. *Journal of Pediatric Surgery*, **19**, 172–174.
42. Stein, H., Kavin, I. and Faerber, E.N. (1975) Colonic strictures following nonoperative management of necrotizing enterocolitis. *Journal of Pediatric Surgery*, **10**, 943–945.
43. Stevenson, D.K., Kernr, J.A., Malechowski, N. and Sunshine, P. (1981) Late morbidity among survivors of necrotizing enterocolitis. *Pediatrics*, **66**, 925–926.
44. Takayanagi, K. and Kapila, L. (1981) Necrotizing enterocolitis in older infants. *Archives of Disease in Childhood*, **56**, 468–469.
45. Tan, C.E.L., Keily, E.M., Agrawal, M., Brereton, R.J. and Spitz, L. (1989) Neonatal gastrointestinal perforations. *Journal of Pediatric Surgery*, **24**, 88–89.
46. Thomas, D.F.M. (1982) Pathogenesis of neonatal necrotizing enterocolitis. *Journal of the Royal Society of Medicine*, **75**, 838.
47. Tibboel, D., van Nie, C.J. and Molenaar, J.C.

(1980) The effects of temporary general hypoxia and local ischaemia on the development of the intestines: an experimental study. *Journal of Pediatric Surgery*, **15**, 57–59.
48. Weinberg, G., Kleinhaus, S. and Boley, S.J. (1989) Idiopathic intestinal perforations in the newborn: an increasingly common entity. *Journal of Pediatric Surgery*, **24**, 1007–1009.
49. West, K.W., Rescorla, F.J., Grosfeld, J.L. and Vane, D.W. (1989) Pneumatosis intestinalis in children beyond the neonatal period. *Journal of Pediatric Surgery*, **24**, 819–824.
50. Wijesinha, S.S. (1982) Neonatal necrotizing enterocolitis: new thoughts for the 'eighties. *Annals of the Royal College of Surgeons of England*, **64**, 506–509.
51. Zamir, O., Goldberg, M., Udassin, R., Peleg, O., Nissan, S. and Eyal, F. (1988) Idiopathic gastrointestinal perforation in the neonate. *Journal of Pediatric Surgery*, **23**, 335–339.

OBSCURE GASTROINTESTINAL BLEEDING

J. Spencer

DEFINITION

This term was coined to describe gastrointestinal bleeding, the source of which could not be determined by conventional standard investigations such as barium studies and endoscopy. It is a useful but somewhat vague concept and, as new investigations are used more routinely, less bleeding is 'obscure' in origin. For example, bleeding from caecal angiodysplasia has only been recognized relatively recently, and contributes very significantly to this group of patients; with the increasing use of colonoscopy and angiography it is more readily diagnosed and only the more subtle of such cases remain 'obscure'.

Chronic bleeding may be obscure in origin, and this has been discussed earlier. Other patients present with recurrent acute bleeds, sometimes widely spaced in time. Occasionally sequential bleeds end in a more severe and prolonged haemorrhage. This often represents deeper ulceration into a vascular mucosal lesion.

Though a rather indeterminate group, of the 25–30 000 people admitted to hospitals in the UK each year with gastrointestinal blood loss, about 5% are initially difficult to diagnose. This represents over 1200 patients.

Obscure bleeding falls into three categories. In the first the cause is common but has been unusually difficult to diagnose. Peptic ulcer, haemorrhoids, oesophageal varices and hiatus hernia may all be overlooked in this way, although all are accessible to readily available routine investigations.

The second category consists of multisystem disease (uncommon or not) with gastrointestinal lesions such as leukaemia, and Peutz–Jegher or Ehlers–Danlos syndrome, or coagulation disorders.

The third category is focal lesions that are not readily diagnosed either because they are very small, such as angiodysplasia, or because they are anatomically inaccessible, such as small bowel tumours.

Most of these have already been discussed in the previous sections on acute upper and lower gastrointestinal bleeding, and this section will concentrate on the diagnostic approach in this group of patients.

DIAGNOSTIC DILEMMAS

Although imaging techniques have advanced greatly, they may still be inadequate to confirm the origin of bleeding.

The greatest single problem relates to the relative inaccessibility of the small bowel. Barium studies are much less precise in that area, with much overlapping of gut and lack of a suitable double-contrast technique. Although small lesions may be demonstrated, occasionally gross abnormalities are overlooked. Radionucleotide scanning may be very helpful, but anatomical localization is rarely precise.

Vascular lesions may be very small, and most importantly may be *multiple*. The significance of vascular lesions seen at endoscopy or laparotomy may be difficult to assess. Small lesions may occasionally mysteriously appear and disappear, presumably as a result of circulatory shunting, increasing the difficulty of localization.

Endoscopic access to the small bowel is minimal and even with newer jejunoscopes gives imprecise localization and incomplete visualization of the source of bleeding.

At laparotomy the duodenum is particularly difficult to examine. Inexperienced operators may miss small lesions elsewhere in the small bowel, and may be misled by the ease with which the jejunum so readily empties its contents into the ileum, suggesting more distal bleeding. Gastric erosions may be either the cause or the result of haemorrhage.

Gut angiography is becoming increasingly sophisticated and useful but is not widely available. An inadequate angiogram giving a negative result can be very misleading.

AETIOLOGY

The lesions that caused obscure haemorrhage in a recent published series are listed, in *Table 5.6.*[23] Obviously any of the lesions discussed earlier in the context of chronic haemorrhage can cause obscure blood loss. 'Obscurity' results from inaccessibility using conventional diagnostic methods. It follows therefore that lesions in the liver, pancreas and small bowel are most likely to be 'obscure', but bleeding lesions of the liver and pancreas are relatively uncommon. Although angiodysplasia of the caecum and colon may be seen endoscopically, this is not always the case, and in many cases this diagnosis can only be made by arteriography. Most cases with obscure bleeding turn out to have angiodysplasia or small bowel lesions. A significant number of lesions remain undiscovered, although more sophisticated enteroscopy, either before or during surgery, is reducing this number.

INVESTIGATIONS

It is very important that there is no reluctance to repeat investigations in these patients where diagnosis is difficult. This applies particularly to endoscopy; vascular lesions are easily overlooked and may be visible only intermittently. If there is clear evidence of high bleeding, usually from a history of haematemesis, then concentration on the upper gut is pertinent. This must include pancreatography and hepatic angiography if no gastroduodenal lesion is found.

Interpretation of endoscopic findings may also vary: notably gastric antral vascular ectasia ('water melon stomach') is easily passed off by the inexperienced observer as antritis and its significance as a source of bleeding overlooked.[13]

In the acute situation, barium studies are best avoided as they preclude accurate angiographic assessment. They are best carried out in the interludes which usually occur between bleeds in such cases, and should then include a small-bowel enema, and a barium enema if colonoscopy has been incomplete.

Table 5.6 Causes of obscure bleeding in a series of 131 patients (From Thompson *et al.*,[23] with permission.)

Lesion	*n*
Colonic angiodysplasia	52
Arteriovascular malformations	
small bowel	16
gastric	4
Meckel's diverticulum	9
Small bowel tumours	7
Chronic pancreatitis	3
Colonic diverticular disease	3
Miscellaneous	16
No cause found	21
Table	131

COLONOSCOPY

Colonoscopy is of particular importance, as obscure bleeding very frequently arises from angiodysplasia of the caecum or ascending colon. In one series angiodysplasia was the cause of bleeding in 40% of 131 patients[23] and it may be responsible for nearly 4% of all gastrointestinal bleeding.[4] Most colonic sources can be identified if the whole colon is examined to the caecum. As the right colon is so frequently the source of bleeding, if the colonoscope will not pass the hepatic flexure easily – a common occurrence – then repeated attempts are to be encouraged.

ULTRASOUND AND COMPUTED TOMOGRAPHY (CT)

Ultrasound and CT, with contrast studies, are particularly useful in identifying hepatic and pancreatic lesions. Although these are unusual sources of haemorrhage, multiple haemangiomas of the liver can be confidently diagnosed and may be associated with similar lesions in the gut, for example in the Osler–Weber—Rendu disease. Chronic pancreatitis may be associated with bleeding into the gut, especially if acute episodes occur, and may be well documented on scanning.

RADIONUCLEOTIDE SCANNING

Radionucleotide scanning is of use during acute bleeding episodes, as discussed earlier but otherwise is of less value except in the quantification of blood loss. It may be, however, occasionally of value.[12]

FLUORESCEIN STRING TESTS

These tests were once much used in the search for occult sources of bleeding[14] and, although some found them useful, they have many inherent problems. Positioning in the gut at an appropriate time may be very difficult, but more importantly, interpretation of the findings has been found to be even more troublesome. Strong positive reactions at the cardia and pylorus, due to trauma, tend to obscure more relevant findings. With the advent of skilled angiography this test has largely been abandoned. In countries where such radiology is not available, the more sophisticated form of string test described by Pittman may still have a place.[19]

INTUBATION METHODS

Intubation methods have also fallen into disuse, but may have a place in patients who cannot be diagnosed by other means. A long intestinal tube is passed, with stepwise aspiration of contents for examination, perhaps including assessment of radioactivity after the intravenous injection of red cells labelled with ^{51}Cr.[18]

ENTEROSCOPY

This procedure is in its infancy. The current 'Endosonde' instrument may be passed transnasally into the stomach and on into much of the small bowel, forward transmission being by peristaltic action on an inflated balloon at its tip. Because of its small diameter, no flexion facility or biopsy or therapeutic channel is available. When the instrument has been passed to its full extent the small bowel is examined during gradual withdrawal. Views may be enhanced by manual palpation of the abdomen, but complete visualization is not possible. Nevertheless bleeding lesions have been seen in cases reported by Morris *et al.*[17]

In the absence of biopsy and coagulation channels such instruments will be of limited value. In many cases either a positive or negative investigation will need to be followed by a laparotomy, at which stage more precise enteroscopy and therapy can be pursued.

An alternative to 'Endosonde' enteroscopy is the use of 'push' instruments. These are larger in diameter, and progress is by the conventional endoscopic means of pushing the instrument. Some current instruments have the advantage of a channel for biopsy or coagulation, and progress down small bowel may be aided by use of an 'overtube' which prevents looping in the stomach. Considerable success has been reported using such instruments in the management of telangiectasia involving the upper small bowel.[16]

SELECTIVE VISCERAL ANGIOGRAPHY

This technique has become the most important specialist investigation, and should include a three-vessel study in every case.[1] It may be helpful in four ways.

Firstly, if bleeding is occurring during arteriography, contrast may be seen entering the gut, thus identifying the site of the lesion. For this to occur, bleeding must be at a minimum rate of 0.5 ml per minute.[3] If angiography is performed during a persistent bleed, the rate at which the origin is found is much higher.

Secondly, angiography may demonstrate anatomical features which give clues as to a possible cause. In particular, the presence of a vitelline branch from the superior mesenteric artery is almost certain evidence of the presence of a Meckel's diverticulum, which is very likely (but not certain) to be the source of haemorrhage (see *Figure 5.7*, p. 983).

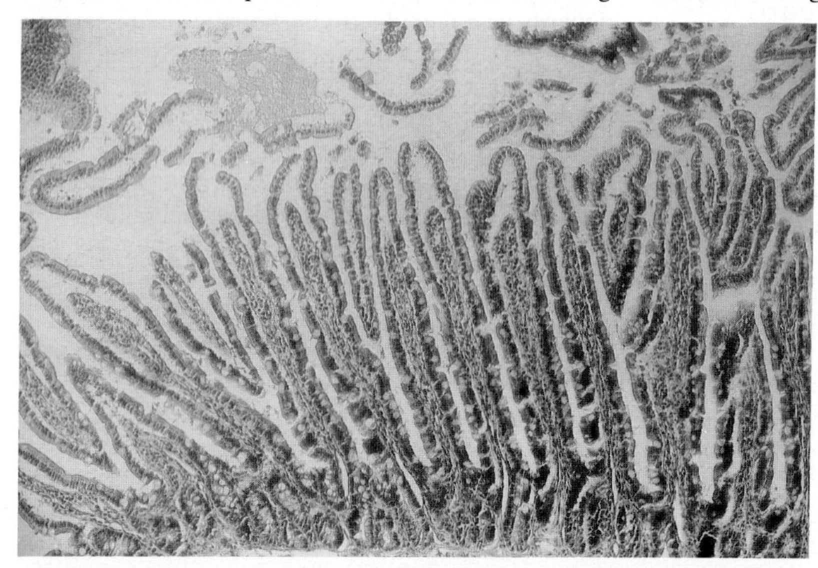

Figure 5.19 Ileum stained yellow (dark in this picture) by the injection of fluorescein into an artery supplying the arteriographically localized vascular lesion. (Courtesy of James Jackson.)

Thirdly, radiology may demonstrate a pathological lesion, even though it is not bleeding. Thus arteriovenous malformations or vascular tumours may be seen, even between episodes of bleeding.

Fourthly, angiography may aid in locating lesions invisible at laparotomy. Small vascular lesions may be visible radiologically and, by superselective techniques, a catheter may be introduced into feeding vessels. During operation, injection of fluorescein into the catheter highlights in yellow the section of bowel containing the invisible lesion, so that an appropriate resection can be performed. *Figure 5.19* illustrates a specimen identified by this method, in which post-operative injection of diluted barium demonstrates the lesion seen on preoperative angiography.

Alternatively, angiography during surgery with appropriate markers on the displayed bowel, will demonstrate the vascular pattern sufficiently well to recognize the loop containing the lesion seen on previous radiography.

SMALL-BOWEL ENEMA

If the ileum is considered to be a possible source, then a small-bowel enema may be useful. The positive identification of a lesion by this means is very useful; however, a negative result may be treated with caution, as even gross lesions are occasionally missed due to overlapping of small-bowel loops.

TREATMENT

In cases of obscure haemorrhage, it is essential to make a diagnosis whenever possible, even if this entails a laparotomy. It is better to subject a patient to a negative laparotomy than to allow a small-bowel tumour to progress dangerously. Many patients with obscure bleeding are elderly, however, and recurrent anaemia may often be managed by supportive therapy, including haematinics and occasional transfusion.

If vascular malformations are confidently diagnosed, and are multiple and not amenable to endoscopic therapy, then hormonal therapy should be considered. The most useful treatment is a combination of 0.05 mg ethinyloestradiol and 1.00 mg of norethisterone. This appears to have a rapid effect, and the benefit persists for several months after cessation of treatment. Because of this, intermittent therapy may be rational and may reduce adverse events. Current trials in this area are very promising (P. Rutgeerts, personal communication).[24,25]

Angiodysplasia may be treated endoscopically, which is an attractive proposition in the elderly. Coagulation may be by heat-probe, bipolar electrode or laser[6,7,15] with up to 70% of patients symptom free at a mean of 29 months after one treatment. The mortality of resection may be high – in one series as high as 18%,[21] particularly as patients coming to laparotomy may be bleeding acutely, with endoscopic treatment having already failed.

LAPAROTOMY

If judicious use of investigative methods has not revealed a site of bleeding, laparotomy is indicated. It will be necessary, in any case, for treatment of many lesions.

The value of laparotomy was reviewed by Retzloff, Hagedorn and Bartholomew[20] some years before many of the more modern investigations were possible. In their study 100 patients underwent surgical exploration but only 30% showed a definite site of haemorrhage and in 17% a possible site was considered. In 53% no lesion was found. This was, however, before angiodysplasia of the caecum, perhaps the commonest cause of obscure significant bleeding, was fully recognized.

In more recent studies, the importance of early laparotomy has been emphasized. In Birmingham, 14 of a series of 37 patients underwent laparotomy, and a causative lesion was found in nine.[8] These workers felt that the high mortality (16%) in their series was due to failure to make an earlier diagnosis, and they made a plea for earlier laparotomy. Small-bowel lesions are particularly likely to be missed without laparotomy, and obscure bleeding together with pain should prompt early laparotomy. Annular small-bowel ulceration[2] and tumours[9] are readily diagnosed, and the growth of tumours stopped by operation. Others still question the value of laparotomy[22] but it must be remembered that most lesions in the small bowel, a very common site for obscure lesions that bleed, will need a laparotomy for therapeutic reasons. In one series, 27 patients underwent laparotomy when radiography had failed to reveal a cause of obscure haemorrhage – in 21 a cause was found at operation and in most it was a small-bowel lesion.[23]

The technique of small-bowel examination at laparotomy is important, as small-bowel lesions are readily missed. Each section of gut must be emptied by careful 'stripping' movements, and palpated from different angles to avoid missing small lesions in the folds at the mesenteric or antimesenteric borders. Finding small anteriovascular malformations noticed at previous angiography is facilitated if superselective catheterization precedes laparotomy. With the feeding vessel cannulated, the area to be resected can be highlighted by the injection of intra-arterial fluorescein.

The value of laparotomy rests not only on careful examination technique but is, to some degree, related to age. Older patients are much more likely to be bleeding from lesions invisible to the surgeon than are younger ones (42% versus 8%),[23] making preoperative angiography particularly valuable in those over 45 years of age. This distinction, however, is mainly a reflection of the fact that the young are much more likely to be bleeding from a Meckel's diverticulum, and the old to be bleeding from angiodysplasia. If these two major diagnoses were excluded, it may be that laparotomy would carry a similar yield in all age groups.

INTRAOPERATIVE ENTEROSCOPY

This is a valuable procedure. It is best performed using a colonoscope passed through the mouth, the surgeon easing the endoscope around into the jejunum. The bowel is examined in segments, defined by gentle cross-clamping. This eliminates general inflation of the bowel, which prevents progress. With this technique, the distal ileum, and often the caecum, can be reached. The examination is both internal, by the endoscopist, and external, the surgeon viewing the transilluminated bowel wall. The presence of fresh blood within the lumen together with a vascular abnormality on transillumination is typical of small bleeding vascular lesions.[10]

Enteroscopy may also be performed by means of an enterotomy, or by retrograde passage after entry through the caecum. If caecal entry is employed, it is usual to remove the appendix and insert the endoscope through a purse-string suture at the caecal pole.

Bowden *et al.*[5] found intraoperative endoscopy to be useful in 28 of 30 patients, their series including colonoscopy during surgery.

REFERENCES

1. Allison, D.J., Hemingway, A.P. and Cunningham, D.A. (1982) Angiography in gastrointestinal bleeding. *The Lancet*, **ii**, 30–33.
2. Ballantyne, K.C., Morris, D.L., Hawkey, C.J. and Hardcastle, J.D. (1986) Haemorrhage from idiopathic annular ulcers of the small intestine. *Annals of the Royal College of Surgeons of England*, **68**, 245–248.
3. Baum, S. (1982) Angiography and the gastrointestinal bleeder. *Radiology*, **143**, 569–572.
4. Boley, S.J. and Brandt, L.J. (1986) Vascular ectasias of the colon. *Digestive Diseases and Sciences*, **31**, 26–42.
5. Bowden, T.A., Hooks, V.H., Teeslink, C.R., Parrish, R.A. and Mansberger, A.R. (1980) Occult gastrointestinal bleeding: locating the cause. *American Surgeon*, **46**, 80–87.
6. Bowers, J.H. and Dixon, J.A. (1982) Argon laser photocoagulation of vascular malformations in the GI tract: short term results. *Gastrointestinal Endoscopy*, **28**, 126.
7. Bown, S.G., Swain, C.P., Storey, D.W. *et al.* (1985) Endoscopic laser treatment of vascular abnormalities of the upper gastrointestinal tract. *Gut*, **26**, 1338.
8. Brearley, S., Hawker, P.C., Dorricott, N.J. *et al.* (1986) The importance of laparotomy in the diagnosis and management of intestinal bleeding of obscure origin. *Annals of the Royal College of Surgeons of England*, **68**, 245–248.
9. Desa, L.A.J., Bridger, J., Grace, P.A., Krausz, T. and Spencer, J. (1991) Primary jejunoileal tumours: a review of 45 cases. *World Journal of Surgery*, **15**, 81–87.
10. Desa, L.A., Ohri, S.K., Hutton, K.A.R., Lee, H. and Spencer, J. (1991) Role of intraoperative enteroscopy in obscure bleeding of small bowel origin. *British Journal of Surgery*, **78**, 192–195.
11. Fazio, V.W., Zelas, P. and Weakley, F.L. (1980) Intraoperative angiography and the localization of bleeding from the small intestine. *Surgery, Gynecology and Obstetrics*, **151**, 637–640.
12. Gordon, I. (1980) Gastrointestinal haemorrhage unrelated to gastric mucosa diagnosed on $^{99}Tc^{m}$ pertechnetate scans. *British Journal of Radiology*, **53**, 322–324.
13. Gouldesbrough, D.R. and Pell, A.C.H. (1991) Gastric antral vascular ectasia: a problem of recognition and diagnosis. *Gut*, **32**, 954–955.
14. Haynes, W.F., Pittman, F.E. and Christakis, G. (1960) Location of site of upper gastrointestinal tract haemorrhage by the fluorescein string test. *Surgery*, **48**, 821–827.
15. Jensen, D.M., Machicado, G.A. and Silpa, M.L. (1984) Treatment of GI angioma with argon laser, heater probe or bipolar electrocoagulation. *Gastrointestinal Endoscopy*, **30**, 184.
16. Lewis, B. and Waye, J. (1991) The nature of small intestinal angiodysplasia. *Gastroenterology*, **100**, A225.
17. Morris, A.J., Wasson, L., Park, R.H.R. and McKenzie, J.S. (1991) Small bowel enteroscopy with water insufflation – the first 80 cases. *Gut*, **32**, A1226.
18. Pillow, R.P., Hill, L.D., Ragen, P.A. *et al.* (1969) Newer methods for localisation of obscure small bowel bleeding. *Journal of the American Medical Association*, **207**, 1477–1480.
19. Pittman, F.E. (1964) The fluorescein string test. An analysis of its use and relationship to barium studies of the upper gastrointestinal tract in 122 cases of gastrointestinal tract haemorrhage. *Annals of Internal Medicine*, **60**, 418–429.
20. Retzloff, J.A., Hagedorn, A.B. and Bartholomew, L.G. (1961) Abdominal exploration for gastrointestinal bleeding of obscure origin. *Journal of the American Medical Association*, **177**, 104–107.

21. Salem, R.R., Thompson, J.N., Hemingway, A.P., Rees, H.C., Wood, C.B. and Alison, D.J. (1985) Outcome of surgery in colonic angiodysplasia. *Gut*, **26**, 1154–1155.
22. Spechler, S.J. and Schimmel, E.M. (1982) Gastrointestinal bleeding of unknown origin. *Archives of Internal Medicine*, **142**, 236–240.
23. Thompson, J.N., Salem, R.R., Hemingway, A.P. *et al.* (1987) Specialist investigation of obscure GI bleeding. *Gut*, **28**, 47–51.
24. van Cutsem, E., Rutgeerts, P., Geboes, K., van Gompel, F. and Vantrappen, G. (1988) Estrogen–progesterone treatment of Osler–Weber–Rendu disease. *Journal of Clinical Gastroenterology*, **10**, 676–679.
25. van Cutsem, E., Rutgeerts, P. and Vantrappen, G. (1990) Clinical practice. Treatment of bleeding gastro-intestinal vascular malformations with oestrogen-progesterone. *The Lancet*, **335**, 953–955.

THE SPLANCHNIC CIRCULATION IN SHOCK

U. Haglund

The splanchnic circulation has long been considered to play an important role in shock states. ‘An intestinal factor in shock’ was discussed by Lillehei in a series of experiments in which he could demonstrate much improved survival by cross perfusion of the gut during a period of severe haemorrhagic shock. Cross perfusion of other areas of the body had no similar effect.[14] The mechanism by which the splanchnic area has a role in shock has been a matter of some controversy. It was thought initially that gross circulatory changes within the splanchnic vasculature, leading to stagnation and pooling of blood and fluid in this vascular bed, were the most important factor. This has not been verified, however, and the modern concept is that the development of a distinct intestinal mucosal injury is the most important event, permitting release of toxic material to the general circulation.

SPLANCHNIC BLOOD FLOW CHANGES

Blood flow to the splanchnic area is reduced in most forms of shock. In certain forms, such as cardiac tamponade, the reduction in splanchnic blood flow is disproportionally great, whereas in others, such as sepsis, blood flow changes in parallel with cardiac index. The renin–angiotensin axis seems to be important in those situations with a disproportionate splanchnic vasoconstriction.[2] The distribution of blood flow within the gastrointestinal tract to the various layers of the gut changes during ischaemia and sepsis in such a way that a larger proportion of flow is directed to the mucosa.[5] Nonetheless, shock of various forms, as well as regional ischaemia from other causes, leads to the development of a characteristic injury of the villous layer of the mucosa (*Figure 5.20*, *Table 5.7*).[11,12]

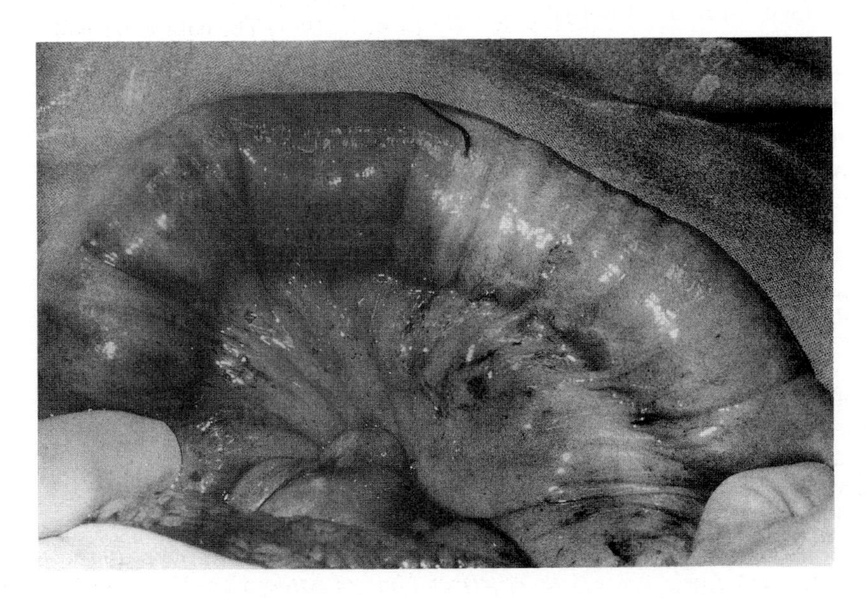

Figure 5.20 Intermediate grade of mucosal injury representative of what could be expected after a few hours of sepsis or shock or less than one hour of total warm ischaemia. Note the lifting of the epithelial lining and the obvious breakdown of the barrier between the lumen and the interior of the body.

Table 5.7 Regional consequences of partial or total warm intestinal ischaemia of various durations. (Data from Haglund, Bulkley and Grainger[12] and Park *et al.*[17])

Degree of ischaemia	*Duration (hours)*	*Type and extent of ischaemic injury*	*Re-perfusion injury*
Partial			
Flow >50%	Up to 6	None	
10–30%	Up to 1	Increased mucosal permeability	*
	2–3	Injury of the villi	*
Total	<20 min.	Increased mucosal permeability	
	20–60 min.	Injury of the villi	*
	1–2	Mucosal infarction	
	>8	Transmural infarction	

*Exacerbation of the ischaemic injury at re-perfusion.

It has been repeatedly demonstrated that the characteristic mucosal injury can be prevented if the superficial mucosa is supplied with oxygen during ischaemia or shock by intralumenal perfusion with oxygenated saline or similar measures.[5,13]

Reduced oxygen delivery therefore offers an obvious explanation for the development of mucosal injury. Reduced oxygen delivery is an obvious consequence of those conditions with disproportionate splanchnic vasoconstriction. In situations with mush less reduced blood flow, such as in sepsis, the development of hypoxic mucosal injury is harder to understand. A likely explanation is in the villous vascular anatomy. This consists of a central arterial vessel branching at the tip into a subepithelial network of capillaries and venules, creating the anatomical background for a countercurrent exchanger. The distance between the two sets of vessels is less than 20 micrometers which allows equilibrium for easily diffusible substances such as oxygen. A short circuiting of oxygen at the base of the villi is supported experimentally (see[13] for a review) and would be likely to become much more effective during hypotensive states where blood flow velocity is reduced. Short circuiting of oxygen in the villous countercurrent exchanger could well explain the paradox of hypoxic injury despite an almost unchanged volume of blood flow.[5]

SPLANCHNIC OXYGEN CONSUMPTION

A third mechanism contributing to the development of small intestinal hypoxic injury has recently been demonstrated.[1,3] The splanchnic area including the gut normally has an oxygen delivery that is much higher than the oxygen demand, and blood flow can be reduced by approximately 50% before oxygen consumption becomes dependent on delivery. In normal resting states, the oxygen extraction by the gut is therefore fairly low. In sepsis, however, where oxygen delivery to the splanchnic area falls in parallel with cardiac output, oxygen consumption is also rapidly increased by approximately 100%. Oxygen extraction by the gut then has to be increased and the oxygen content of the portal venous blood becomes much reduced. Despite these efforts there is a risk of flow-dependent hypoxia in the gut during sepsis.

There are thus three mechanisms:

1. Reduced oxygen delivery to the gut by vasoconstriction.
2. Reduced oxygen delivery to the tip of the villi due to increased efficacy of the villous countercurrent exchanger.
3. Increased demand of oxygen in sepsis.

They constitute possible explanations for the development of hypoxic mucosal injury during ischaemia and hypotension.

RE-PERFUSION INJURY

To further complicate the situation, intestinal mucosal injury may occur not only during ischaemia but also at re-perfusion, as initially demonstrated by Granger *et al.*[9] Re-perfusion injury in the gut may be very important for explaining functional changes and superficial morphological mucosal injury, whereas deeper (transmucosal or transmural) infarction does not seem to be influenced to any detectable degree by a re-perfusion component (see *Table 5.7*).[12] The re-perfusion injury that follows a period of partial intestinal ischaemia has been demonstrated to be secondary to the generation of oxygen-derived free radicals during re-perfusion. Free radicals are generated at this time following the conversion of xanthine dehydrogenase to xanthine oxidase during ischaemia.[9] Furthermore, adenosine triphosphate is catabolized to hypoxanthine but further breakdown to uric acid is oxygen dependent and cannot take place.

A substrate is thus accumulated, and an enzyme that generates free radicals is established. At re-perfusion, when oxygen is available in high amounts, a rapid conversion of hypoxanthine to uric acid may generate more oxygen-free radicals than the defence mechanisms of the body can tolerate. The endothelial cells probably are damaged initially by this process, which may later lead to microcirculatory disturbances, accumulation of activated polymorphonuclear leucocytes and further tissue damage.

IMPLICATIONS OF INJURY TO THE SMALL-INTESTINAL MUCOSA

Injury to the mucosa of the small intestine, regardless of whether it is functional (leading to increased permeability) or morphological, indicates a loss of the normal barrier between the intestinal lumen and the interior of the body. The loss of this barrier function has been associated with two fundamental processes which, either alone or combined, can explain the important role of the splanchnic area in shock, the release of cardiotoxic material, and bacterial translocation.

RELEASE OF CARDIOTOXIC MATERIAL

Cardiotoxic material has been demonstrated in intestinal venous blood, as well as in the lymphatic vessels draining the pancreas, in various forms of shock (see[10] for a review). The cardiotoxic material released[10,13] and the myocardial depressant factor from the pancreas[15] have several characteristics in common. Both seem to be water soluble with a molecular weight of about 500–1000 daltons, although they have not been fully identified chemically. Both factors probably consist of a number of small, related molecules which act in concert, and the very low concentration of each individual molecule makes chemical identification extremely cumbersome. The most striking difference between cardiotoxic material from the small intestine compared with that from the pancreas is that the latter is transported from the pancreas by the lymph whereas the former is found in the intestinal venous blood. Furthermore, the myocardial depressant factor is formed in the pancreas as a consequence of activated zymogenic and lysosomal proteases, whereas the mechanisms leading to the formation of cardiotoxic material in the gut is less clear.

BACTERIAL TRANSLOCATION

Bacteria and bacterial products constitute the other main type of substance released from the splanchnic area during shock. Even in normal conditions with a functionally intact intestinal mucosa, some degree of passage of bacteria and bacterial endotoxins does occur across the barrier, so-called translocation.[18] The amount is much increased during ischaemia, handling of the gut, bile duct obstruction and endotoxinaemia.[4,18] During ischaemia, and following re-perfusion, increased mucosal permeability perhaps later followed by frank morphological damage to the superficial part of the villi markedly enhances the leakage of bacteria and bacterial endotoxin from the gut lumen to the portal blood.

During the 1950s[8] such a mechanism was proposed as the basis of so-called irreversibility in shock but this concept, as a general phenomenon explaining all forms of severe shock, was at that time considered an oversimplification and was rejected. With increased insights into the process of translocation, and increased knowledge of the pathophysiology of multiple system organ failure, leakage of bacteria and bacterial products from the gut is now recognized as one possible mechanism for the development of chronic septicaemia and multiple organ failure.[16]

The proposed chain of events is that increased portal bacteremia, if not effectively handled by the reticuloendothelial cells of the liver, leads to generalized septicaemia. It should be noted in this context that the oxygen needs of the liver are also much increased during sepsis. At the same time, oxygen delivery is reduced as a function of decreased cardiac output and increased oxygen extraction of the gut,[1] so it is likely that the liver becomes hypoxic early during sepsis, and such a situation will greatly impair the efficacy of the liver defence system.

MULTIPLE ORGAN DYSFUNCTION AND INTESTINAL CIRCULATION

In addition to the above mechanisms, other organs in the splanchnic area may lead to a perpetuation of shock by their involvement in the multiple organ dysfunction (failure) syndrome, often complicating sepsis and shock in critically ill patients (*Table 5.8*). Events in the different splanchnic organs are considered to reflect similar pathophysiological

Table 5.8 Splanchnic involvement in multiple systems organ failure

Stomach	Gastric stress ulcerations
Small intestine	Mucosal injury
Colon	Ischaemic colitis
Gall bladder	Acalculous cholecystitis
Liver	Centrilobular liver necrosis

changes, outlined above for the small intestine, by combined ischaemia–re-perfusion injury. Consequently, aggressive resuscitation ensuring adequate oxygen delivery to meet the needs of the various tissues is the main prophylactic measure against splanchnic involvement in multiple organ failure.

MONITORING INTESTINAL CIRCULATION

It is obvious, therefore, that one important goal in the care of the critically ill and/or shocked patients is to maintain adequate splanchnic oxygenation. One problem in achieving this is the difficulty in monitoring the splanchnic circulation. Furthermore, even when techniques are available, such as measurement of superior mesenteric artery blood flow, it still remains difficult to determine what level of blood flow is adequate.

Recently, Fiddian-Green and co-workers described a tonometric technique that allows determination of oxygenation of the gastrointestinal mucosa.[6,7] This technique is an indirect way of measuring the superficial mucosal pH of part of the gastrointestinal tract. A catheter with a saline-filled silastic balloon is introduced into the gastric lumen by a nasogastric tube, or to the sigmoid colon by means of a sigmoidoscope. The PCO_2 in the gut lumen equilibrates over the silastic membrane with the PCO_2 in the saline, and reflects the PCO_2 of the superficial mucosa. Assuming that arterial bicarbonate equals that of the superficial mucosa, the arterial bicarbonate and saline PCO_2 levels allow calculation of mucosal pH using the Henderson–Hasselbalch formula.[6] A normal gastrointestinal mucosal pH is only possible with adequate oxygen delivery and adequate extraction and utilization of the delivered oxygen.

Experimental studies have demonstrated that periods of low gastrointestinal pH correspond to increased gastrointestinal permeability. In clinical series, it has been demonstrated that prolonged periods of low gastrointestinal mucosal pH are associated with increased mortality and morbidity following cardiac and vascular surgery, and also with an increased risk of extra abdominal infection following such surgery.[6] In principle, the ability to monitor mucosal pH should allow assessment of techniques aimed at maintaining or enhancing mucosal oxygenation.

REFERENCES

1. Arvidsson, D., Rasmussen, I., Almqvist, P., Niklasson, F. and Haglund, U. (1993) Splanchnic oxygen consumption in septic and hemorrhagic shock. *Surgery*, **109**, 190–197.
2. Bailey, R.W., Bulkley, G.B., Hamilton, S.R., Morris, J.B. and Haglund, U.H. (1987) Protection of the small intestine from nonocclusive mesenteric ischemic injury due to cardiogenic shock. *American Journal of Surgery*, **153**, 108–116.
3. Dahn, M.S., Lange, P., Lobdell, K., Hans, B., Jacobs, L.A. and Mitchell, R.A. (1987) Splanchnic and total body oxygen consumption differences in septic and injured patients. *Surgery*, **101**, 69–80.
4. Deitch, E.A., Berg, R. and Specian, R. (1987) Endotoxin promotes the translocation of bacteria from the gut. *Archives of Surgery*, **122**, 185–190.
5. Falk, A., Redfors, S., Myrvold, H. and Haglund, U. (1985) Small intestinal mucosal lesions in feline septic shock: a study on the pathogenesis. *Circulatory Shock*, **17**, 327–337.
6. Fiddian-Green, R. (1989) Studies in splanchnic ischemia and multiple organ failure. In *Splanchnic Ischemia and Multiple Organ Failure* (Eds) Marston, A., Bulkley, G.B., Fiddian-Green, R.G. and Haglund, U.H., pp. 349–363. London: Edward Arnold.
7. Fiddian-Green, R.G., McGough, E., Pittenger, G. and Rothman, E. (1983) Predictive value of intramural pH and other risk factors for massive bleeding from stress ulceration. *Gastroenterology*, **85**, 613–620.
8. Fine, J., Frank, H., Schweinburg, F., Jacob, S. and Gordon, T. (1952) The bacterial factor in traumatic shock. *Annals of the New York Academy of Sciences*, **55**, 429–437.
9. Granger, D.N., Rutili, G. and McCord, J. (1981) Superoxide radicals in feline intestinal ischemia. *Gastroenterology*, **81**, 22–29.
10. Haglund, U. (1989) Myocardial depressant factors. In *Splanchnic Ischemia and Multiple Organ Failure* (Eds) Marston, A., Bulkley, G.B., Fiddian-Green, R.G. and Haglund, U.H., pp. 349–363. London: Edward Arnold.
11. Haglund, U., Hultén, L., Lundgren, O. and Åhrén, C. (1975) Mucosal lesions in the human small intestine in shock. *Gut*, **16**, 979–984.
12. Haglund, U., Bulkley, G.B. and Granger, D.N. (1987) On the pathophysiology of intestinal ischemic injury. Clinical review. *Acta Chirurgica Scandinavica*, **153**, 321–324.
13. Haglund, U., Jodal, M. and Lundgren, O. (1984) The small bowel in arterial hypotension and shock. In *Physiology of the Intestinal Circulation* (Eds)

Shepherd, A.P. and Granger, D.N. pp. 305–319. New York: Raven Press.
14. Lillehei, R. (1957) The intestinal factor in irreversible hemorrhagic shock. *Surgery*, **42**, 1043–1054.
15. Lefer, A.M. (1978) Properties of cardioinhibitory factors produced in shock. *Federation Proceedings*, **37**, 2734–2740.
16. Meakins, J.L. and Marshall, J.C. (1989) The gut as the motor of multiple system organ failure. In *Splanchnic Ischemia and Multiple Organ Failure* (Eds) Marston, A., Bulkley, G.B., Fiddian-Green, R.G. and Haglund, U.H. pp. 349–363. London: Edward Arnold.
17. Park, P.O., Haglund, U., Bulkley, G.B. and Fält, K. (1990) The sequence of development of intestinal tissue injury following strangulation ischemia and reperfusion. *Surgery*, **107**, 574–580.
18. Wells, C.L., Maddaus, M.A. and Simmons, R.L. (1989) Bacterial translocation. In *Splanchnic Ischemia and Multiple Organ Failure* (Eds) Marston, A., Bulkley, G.B., Fiddian-Green, R.G. and Haglund, U.H. pp. 349–363. London: Edward Arnold.

ACUTE AND CHRONIC ISCHAEMIA OF THE GUT

L.W. Ottinger

The cellular and structural response of the gut to ischaemia is the same whatever the underlying cause. However, the clinical presentation and management of individual cases do not share this uniformity. Rather, they reflect aetiology as well as the factors of magnitude, extent and duration of circulatory deprivation. In this section, general elements common to all cases of gut ischaemia will be examined and then the major aetiological categories discussed. If one includes only cases of acute infarction suspected or diagnosed in premortem patients, about half will have a non-occlusive origin, there being no occlusion of major arteries or veins. Acute occlusion of the superior mesenteric artery or its branches, occlusion of the inferior mesenteric artery, venous thromboses and small vessel thromboses are the important other causes.[3,21] Finally, chronic ischaemia, a relatively rare clinical entity which takes the form of recurrent episodes of ischaemia without infarction, will be discussed.

ACUTE ISCHAEMIA

Anatomical factors

Three major arteries supply the abdominal part of the gastrointestinal tract. The *coeliac axis*, through the left and right gastric, short gastric and right gastroepiploic arteries, provides a relatively rich blood supply to the stomach. The anterior and posterior superior pancreaticoduodenal arteries provide a dual blood supply to the duodenum, being continuous with the inferior pancreaticoduodenal vessels from the superior mesenteric artery or its proximal branches. Additional collateral circulation occurs between the branches of the coeliac and the superior mesenteric arteries supplying the pancreas. The *superior mesenteric artery* supplies the jejunum, the ileum and the colon to the splenic flexure. Arcades connect its branches, the most peripheral of these constituting the marginal artery. The marginal artery gives rise to short end-arteries to the intestinal wall known as the vasa recti. The *inferior mesenteric artery*, a much smaller vessel, supplies the left and sigmoid colon, and most of the rectum. It anastomoses with the superior mesenteric artery through a common marginal artery, and with the middle and inferior haemorrhoidal arteries, which are branches of the hypogastrics. The relatively short length of intestine supplied by the coeliac axis, its rich collateral connections and the dual nature of its end branches makes ischaemic lesions of the stomach and duodenum very rare. The first two factors also apply to the inferior mesenteric artery, and there is, again, a relatively low incidence of occlusive lesions in its distribution.

The venous drainage parallels the arteries, except that the four major channels – the coronary, splenic, superior mesenteric and inferior mesenteric veins – combine in a single trunk, the portal vein. Collateral channels between the veins, and to the somatic venous system, are so numerous that infarction from thrombosis is rare unless the peripheral veins are involved.

Physiological factors

The normal arterial flow to the gut is about 10% of the cardiac output. It varies under conditions of both exercise and digestion, and the regulation of flow is complex. Not only is there control of flow at the arteriolar level by vasoconstriction and vasodilatation, but there is also autoregulation at the level of the vasculature in the villi. Extramucosal shunting is a third important factor in the control of circulation at the mucosal level.[15]

Flow is shown to increase in the presence of nutrients in the intestinal lumen. Endogenous hormones such as secretin, gastrin and cholecystokinin perhaps mediate this response. The influence of the autonomic nervous system on flow has also been demonstrated, but is complex and variable.

Flow can decrease in response to muscular activity or an increase in intraluminal pressure. Catecholamines and angiotensin II are potent reducers of blood flow. Cardiac glycosides also cause a decrease in flow due to a direct action at the arteriolar level. Under some circumstances of diminished cardiac output, flow may become severely reduced. Arteriolar constriction and extramucosal shunting may play an important role in promoting mucosal ischaemia, and their pharmacological reversal sometimes offers a useful avenue of therapy.

Pathophysiology

The first response to a degree of ischaemia sufficient to cause cell damage is noted in the mucosal layers. The earliest evidence of injury is in the submucosa and may be observed by electron microscopy after a period of ischaemia as short as 10 minutes.[7] By 30 minutes, light microscopy also reveals changes. These take the form of submucosal oedema and then haemorrhage. Plain radiographs and barium studies at this stage show mounds of fullness, often termed 'thumb-printing'. Mucosal slough follows, leading to ulceration and the release of blood into the lumen. With restoration of an adequate circulation, these changes are reversible and mucosal regeneration follows. This may be a prolonged process with recurrent bleeding and a transient period of impaired absorption. The muscular layers are more resistant to ischaemic injury. Initially muscle spasm occurs, but with the passage of time an atonic state develops. With moderate degrees of injury, fibrous strictures sometimes form, which usually become apparent 2–6 weeks later. More profound injuries lead to loss of integrity for the entire bowel wall. A characteristic foul, bloody transudate occurs in the early stages and frank perforation follows. The process may be hastened by the presence of digestive enzymes in the small bowel and by an inflammatory component in the colon. Serosal injury, especially in the colon, may lead to adhesive adhesions preventing general soilage for a time. Details of the pathophysiological process and its investigational background may be found in the review articles by Williams[27] and by Boley *et al.*[3]

The severity of intestinal injury reflects both the degree and the duration of the interruption of vascular flow. Extramucosal shunting and intraluminal pressure may worsen the injury. However, collateral flow in the arcades or marginal vessels distal to a site of arterial or venous occlusion and in intramural vessels may protect the peripheral portions of the bowel segment involved from injury. Both arterial spasm and a fall in cardiac output may contribute to the fall in perfusion; infarction may be precipitated by this means after a period of symptomatic ischaemia, even in the absence of worsening of the initial lesion. This is a major factor in producing the variety of clinical presentations so characteristic of mesenteric infarction.

Ischaemia may also cause abnormalities of motility and absorption, and intraluminal bleeding. With extensive tissue necrosis, metabolic acidosis and the systemic results of the release of vasoactive substances are sometimes observed.

Clinical features

Cases of acute intestinal injury, despite their varied aetiologies, are similar in clinical presentation. Though in many ways non-specific, this presentation is characteristic, and will almost always suggest the diagnosis. The single most striking element is abdominal pain. In some cases this is the result of muscle spasm or perforation with peritonitis. In the majority of patients, however, the pain is visceral and caused specifically by the ischaemia. Such pain is dull rather than sharp, constant rather than colicky, and is rather poorly localized, though the region of referral bears some relationship to the site of the injury. It may range from mild to remarkably severe.

Ischaemic pain does not necessarily imply tissue necrosis. The pain observed in syndromes of chronic ischaemia supports this fact. Furthermore, some cases of mesenteric infarction are preceded by hours or even days of such pain before an actual ischaemic injury is sustained. Nevertheless, pain is the most reliable and, at times, the only symptom marking the onset of infarction.

Ischaemia may influence intestinal motility, resulting in nausea, vomiting, bloating or diarrhoea. These features are so unspecific as to be of little diagnostic value.

Finally, intestinal bleeding is a usual result of mucosal infarction, leading to gross or occult blood in the gastric and rectal contents in most patients.

The combination of these non-specific elements will in most patients suggest the diagnosis of mesenteric infarction. However, the diagnosis is sometimes elusive in the early stages, particularly in the presence of symptoms and signs of related or unrelated disorders. Later, with the appearance of peritonitis, the diagnosis is more obvious, but by then irreversible injuries are to be expected, and the likelihood of survival declines accordingly.

Investigations

Laboratory determinations have little value in establishing the diagnosis in mesenteric ischaemia or infarction. The white cell count may be elevated, the extent to some degree reflecting the volume of infarcted tissue. Thus counts in excess of 20×10^9/l are frequently recorded, but in other cases of extensive infarction the count is normal. The serum amylase is elevated in about one half of patients, but seldom exceeds twice normal and rarely reaches the level expected in acute pancreatitis. Thus laboratory determinations are useful mainly in eliminating other causes of acute abdominal pain.

Plain radiographs of the abdomen are also seldom diagnostic.[26] In rare cases, spasm of the small bowel leads to a striking lack of bowel gas. The portal venous system may be filled with gas in late cases of extensive infarction. In the majority of cases, though, only dilatation of the bowel in a non-specific pattern of ileus is observed. With acute superior mesenteric artery occlusion there may be dilatation of the small and proximal large bowel, suggesting obstruction of the transverse colon. On the whole, just as with laboratory tests, plain films are mainly useful for excluding other causes of abdominal pain.

Conversely, angiography offers a specific diagnosis in many cases. A lateral aortogram may demonstrate obstruction of the origin of the mesenteric vessels. Selective studies show more peripheral arterial blocks. Less specific findings may be noted in cases of venous occlusion and non-occlusive infarction. Angiograms are, therefore, perhaps most useful in the patient with appropriate symptoms and a suspected diagnosis of mesenteric occlusion. In cases where the diagnosis seems more certain and the study would impose more than a slight delay, a laparotomy is a better diagnostic measure. If peritonitis is already present, delay is never acceptable.

An additional potential value of angiograms in superior mesenteric artery occlusion is the provision of anatomical information that will aid the surgeon in selecting the best type of reconstruction.[20] Angiographic techniques also provide a potent means of relieving mesenteric spasm through the direct infusion of antispasmodic drugs. Under the proper circumstances this may restore sufficient arterial flow to limit or prevent infarction. The clinical application is in practice sometimes limited by difficulty in patient selection and in integrating perfusion with surgical intervention.[3,4]

NON-OCCLUSIVE INFARCTION

The place of non-occlusive infarction in the general spectrum of mesenteric infarction is not readily defined. On the one hand, in large series upwards of one half of the patients investigated will have no macro-vascular occlusion;[3,21] on the other hand, the finding of mucosal infarction after death from whatever cause is frequent. If these latter cases are eliminated, however, and only those patients included in whom infarction made a substantial contribution to the clinical illness, non-occlusive infarction still remains the most common cause of ischaemic bowel necrosis. The cases are far from uniform, with many causes, presentations and associated medical problems; the classification 'non-occlusive infarction' represents more a grouping than a specific aetiology. The common factor is the development of bowel infarction in the absence of a demonstrable major vascular occlusion. Infarction may be superficial or deep, patchy or extensive, and involve the small or large bowel and even other visceral structures including the stomach. Because of the underlying causes, rather than the extent or irreversibility of the mesenteric injury, mortality is very high.

Aetiology

Non-occlusive infarction is the end result of a factor or factors that decrease blood flow to the bowel wall. In about a quarter of cases these factors are not identifiable. Known factors include a diminished cardiac output, as in coronary or valvular heart disease or arrhythmias, and insufficient peripheral perfusion, as in hypovolaemic or septic shock. A second factor in many older patients is the presence of stenotic lesions due to atherosclerotic occlusive disease in the central or peripheral portions of the mesenteric vessels. These lesions cause a further decrease in flow, sometimes to the critical level that will lead to infarction. Thus some patients with chronic intestinal ischaemia will develop non-occlusive infarction with or without another factor such as heart failure. Finaly, splanchnic artery spasm and shunting have an important role. These changes may reflect normal physiological shunting away from the splanchnic bed or a pathological degree of spasm. The latter may be in response to exogenous stimuli such as digitalis preparations or α-adrenergic agonists.

Clinical features

The clinical presentation differs from that in the general description only in that coexisting medical problems may tend to obscure the signs and symptoms. Abdominal pain and evidence of mucosal bleeding are present in the same proportion of patients, but may be overlooked in patients who are otherwise seriously ill. However, perforation with peritonitis is not missed so easily.

In a few patients a prior history of postprandial pain and weight loss will suggest a chronic ischaemic condition. The most helpful clinical symptom is abdominal pain. In a setting suggestive of ischaemia, this should lead to the presumptive diagnosis. Of course, pain from ischaemic bowel is probably relatively common in patients in intensive care settings and many do not develop infarction. The severity and persistence of the pain, as well as the presence of gastrointestinal bleeding and peritoneal signs, help to single out the patient with infarction.

Investigations

The clinical setting and symptoms will provide sufficient diagnostic evidence on which to base the practical elements of management. There are no direct measurements that are of value since there are no useful techniques for measuring in vivo mucosal blood flow. An increasing role for angiography in selected patients is advocated by some, their enthusiasm also reflecting the therapeutic value of angiographic techniques.[4] Given that the demands of proper management of associated and underlying conditions may preclude angiographic studies in many patients, indirect observation of splanchnic artery spasm and mural vascular changes may give clues to the diagnosis in an undertermined but substantial number of patients with non-occlusive infarction.[25] In practical terms, the presence of mesenteric emboli and the determination of the extent and location of atherosclerotic lesions will separate out those patients with an occlusive cause or contributing stenotic lesion from those with normal vessels.

Treatment

Measures to improve perfusion by treatment of the underlying central causes of decreased flow are essential. In many instances these measures will terminate symptoms of ischaemia or improve mural perfusion and limit infarction to the mucosal layers. The systemic use of drugs that may lead to splanchnic spasm may be unavoidable, but they should be eliminated when possible.

The development of peritoneal signs may dictate abdominal exploration, both to rule out some other cause such as cholecystitis or perforation of a peptic ulcer, and to resect segments of infarcted bowel. However, the latter does not greatly improve the chances of survival. The outcome is usually dictated by the underlying cause and, when this leads to bowel infarction, recovery is rare. The added burden of laparotomy may worsen the prognosis in some cases.

The use of local vasodilator drugs infused into the superior mesenteric artery through a percutaneously placed catheter will, in selected cases, lead to a marked increase in splanchnic perfusion. Papaverine is the drug frequently used for this purpose. Advocates of the technique point to a high incidence of survival compared with that observed in patients undergoing laparotomy. Although patient selection and treatment of patients who might have recovered without treatment cloud the evaluation of this approach, there is no question of its effectiveness in improving local perfusion.[4]

In patients in whom infarction has developed on a background of chronically compromised mesenteric arterial flow, restoration of flow will sometimes lead to patient survival.[23] This presupposes satisfactory reversal of any central cause of diminished circulation. The surgial considerations then do not differ from those of acute mesenteric thrombosis. In the absence of full thickness infarction, stenotic lesions may sometimes be managed by percutaneous transarterial dilatation. If satisfactory flow is restored, laparotomy may not be necessary or may be required in order to resect segments of non-viable intestine.

ACUTE SUPERIOR MESENTERIC ARTERY OCCLUSION

From a third to a half of all cases of mesenteric infarction are due to acute occlusion of the superior mesenteric artery or its branches. In many, perhaps the majority, the cause is an embolus. As with other peripheral emboli, most originate from the heart, either from a postinfarction mural thrombus or in association with atrial fibrillation. A few are of mycotic origin, usually from valvular vegetations. Trauma to the inner surface of the aorta, either from the placement of clamps during operations or the passage of a catheter for diagnostic studies of the heart or aorta and its branches, is a rare iatrogenic cause of emboli. The resultant emboli of atheromatous material may be large enough to behave like other emboli. However, in some cases they are small and numerous. They may then cause not only infarction of the intestine, but also other visceral organs. Death in such patients usually results from renal failure due to renal emboli.[14,20]

Large emboli typically lodge at or distal to the origin of the middle colic artery. With acute occlusion at this site, or more distally but within the main trunk, the area most severely affected is usually the terminal ileum. Insufficiency of collateral flow may modify this and, in many cases, infarction may develop in the entire area supplied by the vessel. When emboli pass into a major branch, ischaemic injury in the corresponding segment may develop or the collateral circulation may be sufficient to prevent actual infarction.

The other frequent cause of superior mesenteric artery occlusion is thrombosis. It tends to occur in any older group and to involve almost exclusively the proximal few centimetres of the vessel. This infarction due to thrombosis also tends to be more extensive. The site of predilection reflects the pattern of visceral atherosclerotic narrowing, which usually affects the proximal portion of the major vessels.[22] More peripheral lesions are seen but seldom lead to infarction, even when acute thrombosis occurs.

A third and rare cause is dissection of the aorta. Most such dissections originate in the thoracic aorta and are associated with transient occlusion of other aortic branches.

Clinical features

Infarction due to superior mesenteric occlusion tends to present a less difficult diagnostic problem than that due to other causes. This reflects the usual relatively abrupt onset of symptoms with characteristically severe, early pain in the absence of other acute medical problems.

The collateral circulation in most instances is, theoretically, adequate to avoid infarction. Thus a period of ischaemic pain without infarction is seen in many patients. This may last for several hours to days with fluctuation in severity or even disappearance of the pain. Direct observation of the circulation at laparotomy during this stage may be deceptive in that viable intestine and even faint peripheral pulses may suggest some other cause for pain, and a favourable opportunity for timely restoration of arterial flow may thus be forfeited. Angiography during this pre-infarction stage is especially useful. Later infarction ensues in response to extension of the thrombus, arterial spasm, bowel distension, or a fall in perfusing pressure.

Investigations

In the early stages the diagnosis is relatively obscure; later with infarction and perforation it becomes obvious. Severe abdominal pain in the absence of abdominal findings on examination, and without other explanation, should suggest mesenteric ischaemia. The finding of occult blood in the gastric and rectal contents, a history of emboli, and a marked leukocytosis are all helpful; plain abdominal films usually are not.

Angiography is of considerable use in the management of selected patients. Not only can it suggest the diagnosis but, by localizing the site of occlusion, it may also point to the specific cause and aid the surgeon in planning a reconstruction. Whether it should be used in all cases in which evidence of peritonitis is absent, and where the diagnosis of mesenteric infarction is under serious consideration, is an unanswered question. The anticipated delay, the general condition of the patient and the probability of some other diagnosis all influence the urgency of laparotomy and the advisability of angiography.[13]

Treatment

Except in a few cases of peripheral emboli without peritoneal signs and in cases of aortic dissection, immediate laparotomy is the preferred approach in all cases of acute mesenteric artery occlusion unless the patient is moribund. The surgeon should be prepared not only to resect infarcted bowel, but also to restore the arterial circulation.

With peripheral emboli and infarction, resection alone produces excellent rates of survival. With more central sites of occlusion, however, even extensive resection is, by itself, seldom successful. Either the patient will have insufficient remaining small intestine for survival or the unresected segments may undergo infarction in the early postoperative period.[2,20] Parenteral alimentation is a useful adjunct to management but cannot be used to maintain older patients after extensive small bowel resection.[11]

With central occlusion either from thrombosis or emboli, extensive areas of salvageable intestine will be found in about one half of patients requiring surgical exploration. Either an embolectomy for emboli, or a bypass for proximal thrombosis, may be performed. Embolectomy is almost always not only possible but also successful in restoring flow.[20,24] Thromboendarterectomy usually fails, is technically difficult, and, in most instances, is inferior to an aortic or iliac to mesenteric bypass.[6,20] Reconstruction is combined with resection when indicated. If segments of intestine are of questionable viability at the end of the operation, an elective laparotomy for further possible resection is advisable 12 to 24 hours later. The determination of viability intraoperatively may be aided by the use of fluorescein and observation of pulsatile mural blood vessels using a Doppler probe.[8] Postoperative complications of arterial reconstruction include thrombosis or re-embolization, bleeding from the arterial suture line, and bleeding from segments of bowel due to mucosal slough. Overall survival in cases of acute superior mesenteric artery occlusion remains poor, but is quite substantial in those cases successfully submitted to embolectomy.

VENOUS THROMBOSIS

Venous thrombosis, once regarded as a frequent cause of mesenteric infarction, is now thought to be responsible for 5–10% of cases.[12,21] The clinical presentation of venous thrombosis does not differ from that of other causes of intestinal ischaemia. It is reported that a period of ischaemic symptoms, which may last several days, often precedes infarction. Patients are sometimes febrile during this prodromal stage and have vague abdominal pain and a disturbance of bowel function.

Aetiology

When an underlying cause is discovered, it will most commonly be cirrhosis, a hepatic tumour or some other cause of acute portal vein thrombosis. Occlusion of the portal vein alone usually does not cause infarction; where infarction has occurred, propagation of the thrombus into the mesenteric vein is found. Other cases are associated with hypercoagulability states, compression by tumours, sepsis, trauma, and the use of oral contraceptives. In over half the cases, no underlying cause is found, though there may be evidence of venous thrombosis in other areas such as the extremities.

Investigations

Only the presence of bloodstained peritoneal fluid distinguishes mesenteric venous thrombosis from arterial infarction. It is not known how often the diagnosis may be suspected from angiographic studies but, in some cases, indirect findings are noted. These include arterial spasm, delayed clearing of small arteries and failure to opacify the portal system. The uncertainty of the findings and the non-specific signs and symptoms make preoperative diagnosis unusual. Recently, the use of Doppler ultrasound and dynamic CT imaging offer non-invasive means of suspecting the diagnosis.

Treatment

Thrombectomy seems to have little clinical application. This is because in most cases of infarction the thrombosis extends out to the edge of the bowel. It is this finding that gives rise to the rationale for a specific intraoperative diagnostic manoeuvre: when the mesentery of involved segments of bowel is incised, worm-like thrombus is extruded from the veins. Resection is the only successful approach to management.[21] The affected segment, usually the middle part of the small bowel, must be removed. A margin of normal bowel must be included, since infarction of the anastomosis is a common postoperative complication. Second-look operations 12 to 24 hours after initial resection are probably indicated in most patients. Postoperative anticoagulation, though unproven, is a logical step in the prevention of further thromboses and infarction but anticoagulants in the early postoperative period increase the risk of intra-abdominal bleeding.

ISCHAEMIC COLITIS

Ischaemic lesions of the left colon deserve separate consideration because several aspects of their presentation and management are different to those of infarction at more proximal levels of the intestinal tract. By contrast, lesions of the right and transverse colon (usually the result of superior mesenteric artery occlusion, but sometimes non-occlusive in origin) are covered by the principles already related earlier in this section. The term ischaemic colitis will be used to designate the more distal colonic lesions. They may be the result of inferior mesenteric artery occlusion or be non-occlusive in aetiology. They tend to be of limited extent, to involve a single segment, to be reversible, and to present a distinctive clinical picture. Their management does not include arterial reconstruction, and delayed rather than early surgical intervention is the rule, if necessary at all.

Aetiology

Occlusion of the inferior mesenteric artery due to atheroma is common in older patients but mesenteric infarction is rare. This reflects the small size of the interior mesenteric artery and the competence of the collateral supply to its distribution. In fact, many of the cases that are seen in clinical practice are the

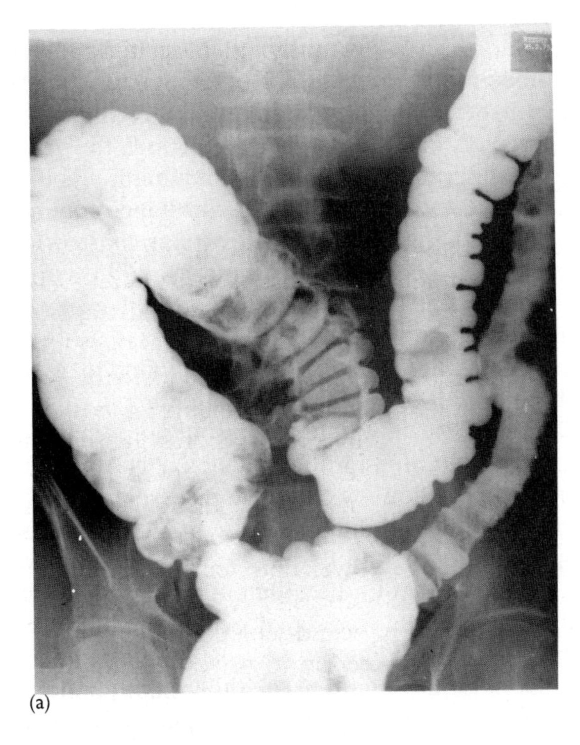

(a)

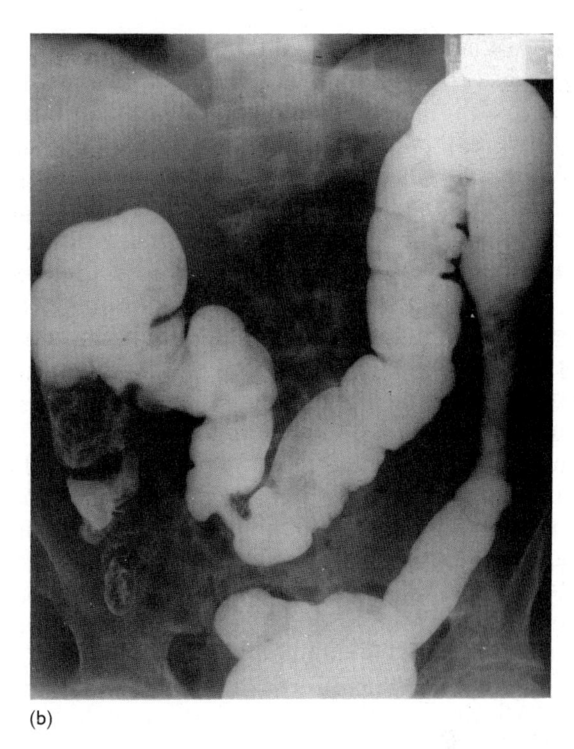

(b)

Figure 5.21 (a) An 'instant' barium enema from a patient with acute left-sided abdominal tenderness and bloody diarrhoea due to ischaemic colitis. Narrowing, 'thumb-printing' and oedema are seen in the descending colon. (b) Repeat barium enema from the same patient 10 weeks later. An ischaemic stricture of the descending colon is seen.

result of surgical ligation of the vessels in the course of colon resections or operations on the aorta. In the latter instance, a mucosal infarct that is centered in the distal sigmoid colon and extends from the descending colon to the rectum is produced. Although mucosal injuries are frequent, actual full thickness infarction is observed in only a small percentage of cases of ligation.

The more common cause is undefined non-occlusive infarction. Though underlying hypotension, cardiac failure, digitalis toxicity or a hypercoagulability state, including that observed in users of oral contraceptives, is seen in a few cases, in most, no such causative factor is apparent. Occlusion of small arteries and veins in the wall of the affected bowel is frequently seen but is thought to be a secondary manifestation.[5] The splenic flexure and the descending colon tend to be most commonly involved, though other segments may be affected. It is rare for more than a single isolated segment to be involved.[16,17]

Clinical course

Whether the cause is non-occlusive infarction or inferior mesenteric artery occlusion, the presentation is similar. Onset is acute with bloody diarrhoea, and early signs of peritoneal irritation over the affected segment. Bacterial invasion following loss of mucosal integrity is an important element. Spontaneous recovery is seen in most patients, though this may take several weeks. Rarely, a stricture develops. In patients with stricture, continued diarrhoea is observed, though the stricture is often not demonstrated until several weeks have elapsed. In a few patients, full thickness infarction or bacterial invasion may lead to perforation. Typically, this is delayed for a few days up to 3 weeks after the onset of symptoms. Continued evidence of inflammation occurs during this interval.

The general presentation of ischaemic colitis leads to a clinical picture that must be differentiated from that of other acute forms of colitis, obstruction, and from perforated diverticular disease. Barium enema studies, sometimes repeated, are very helpful in this regard. Submucosal oedema and haemorrhage in an evolving pattern are characteristic of ischaemic colitis.

Treatment

The diagnosis should be confirmed by radiography, except when a preceding surgical ligation of the inferior mesenteric artery makes the diagnosis obvious. Submucosal oedema and haemorrhage causing 'thumb-printing' may be diagnostic (*Figure 5.21*). If not, barium contrast studies should be performed. Without these findings, another diagnosis must be sought. When changes extend down into the rectum, sigmoidoscopy will show ischaemia and mucosal slough with ulceration. In most cases of non-occlusive infarction this will not be found.

When the diagnosis is sufficiently certain, management consists of close observation, intravenous fluids, restricting oral intake, and the use of parenteral antibiotics. Surgical intervention is reserved for cases in which perforation is suspected. Even when occlusion has occurred, inferior mesenteric artery reconstruction is not useful and is usually not possible. Worsening signs of sepsis and the development of palpable mass are common indications for laparotomy. Free perforation with soilage of the peritoneal cavity is rare. Resection with a proximal colostomy is the preferred operation. If the rectum is not severely involved, and this is usually so, later restoration of the colon's continuity may be anticipated. When operation is not performed, follow-up radiographic studies should be obtained to ensure that mucosal abnormalities have resolved, and that a neoplasm or more chronic form of colitis has not been overlooked.[2]

CHRONIC GUT ISCHAEMIA

In clinical practice, chronic intestinal ischaemia takes the form of recurrent transient episodes of ischaemia without structural damage to the gut itself. It is the intestine in the distribution of the superior mesenteric artery rather than the coeliac axis or inferior mesenteric artery that is affected. This reflects the large magnitude of variation of flow in the superior mesenteric artery with the various phases of digestion. In contrast, flow in the other vessels remains rather constant. Thus, chronic ischaemia is a disease of the small intestine rather than the stomach or colon.

In the hours following ingestion of a meal there is normally up to an eight-fold increase in superior mesenteric artery flow. When the flow is adequate during the resting state but, because of restriction of inflow, cannot meet these increased needs of the small intestine, periods of ischaemia ensue. These cause pain, the hallmark of gut ischaemia. This pain is felt in the mid and anterior abdomen but is of visceral type and likely to be characterized in vague terms with respect to nature, occurrence and location.

AETIOLOGY

Whatever the dominant systemic pattern may be, atherosclerotic occlusive disease seldom spares the visceral arteries. When advanced, mesenteric vascular lesions are seldom diffuse but characteristically occur in the origin or proximal 2 cm of the three major vessels.[10] Collateral inflow through the great peripheral arcades will suffice to maintain viability and, except under unusual circumstances, avoid symptoms as long as a period of slow narrowing precedes total occlusion. For this reason, the symptoms of chronic ischaemia are seldom if ever the result of disease involving a single vessel. Rather, severe narrowing or occlusion will be found to affect all three vessels in symptomatic patients.

The transient, flow-related episodes of ischaemia are the result of a probable imbalance between restriction of inflow by occlusive disease and restoration of flow through collaterals. In most patients, progression to occlusion is at a pace that does not exceed the capacity of the collaterals even at times of high demand. The finding of occlusion of two or even all three of the major vessels in asymptomatic patients is not unusual. On the other hand, patients with symptomatic chronic ischaemia will likely eventually experience infarction due to further progression of occlusive disease or other factors that reduce inflow. This tends to be extensive and is almost invariably fatal.

CLINICAL FEATURES

Episodes of ischaemia are the only specific symptoms of chronic mesenteric insufficiency. Vague and poorly characterized by the patient, they may be temporarily related to eating, coming on an hour or two after a meal. But many patients are old, inexact in their observations and irregular in their habits, and no pattern may emerge from the history. Still, without pain, the diagnosis may be confidently discarded. Conversely, the possibility of an ischaemic aetiology should be considered in any older patient with abdominal pain and no other apparent cause.

A second frequent element is weight loss. Though gradual, it may be profound. It has not been shown to be caused by a loss of absorptive capacity. Rather, it is the result of a conscious or unconscious aversion to eating because of the resulting pain.

There is also a non-specific change in bowel function. This is the result of alterations in motility or of changes in eating patterns. Patients may report early satiety, bloating, flatulence, diarrhoea or constipation. These symptoms obviously are not going to suggest the diagnosis, but they do lead the patient to repeatedly seek medical advice.

Also non-specific, but observed in most patients, is the presence of the symptoms and signs of advanced atherosclerotic disease in other systems, especially to the lower extremities. A history of smoking is surprisingly frequent, especially in younger women with a premature onset of atherosclerosis.

Finally, some patients will be noted to have or have had gastroduodenal ulcer disease of an unusual type.[1,9] This is characterized by shallow antral and proximal duodenal ulcers that are resistant to therapy. They are associated with usual peptic ulcer symptoms. These ulcers are thought to be a manifestation of advanced disease in the coeliac and superior mesenteric arteries and resultant ischaemia in the distribution of the pancreaticoduodenal arcades. Healing with revascularization has been reported.[9]

INVESTIGATIONS

The diagnosis rests in the demonstration of an advanced degree of impairment of circulation in the presence of an appropriate clinical history. Because of the protean nature of the symptoms and the low incidence of the condition even in the elderly, the diagnosis will be much more often advanced than confirmed.[18] And, for the same reasons, it is unsuspected in many patients until infarction makes it obvious. Patients usually have symptoms for months or even years before a diagnosis is established.

Doppler flow studies can be used for screening, but angiography is the standard method for determining the extent and severity of mesenteric vascular disease. Lateral aortography best demonstrates the origin and proximal segments of the coeliac and superior mesenteric arteries. Selective injections will give further details of peripheral and collateral flow but may precipitate infarction in the presence of severe ischaemia.

TREATMENT

Chronic pain and weight loss serve as an adequate reason for surgical repair in all but the high risk patient. Furthermore, most untreated cases eventually terminate in massive infarction. Non-surgical management has little value with one exception. Angiodilatation has been reported to successfully eliminate symptoms.[19] The low initial risk must be measured against an unknown but probably high incidence of recurrence with the further chance of infarction.

Surgical correction involves restoration of flow into either the coeliac or superior mesenteric arteries or both. This can be done by a number of operations which include thromboendarterectomy, re-implantation and bypass grafting. Revascularization of one vessel will eliminate symptoms, but doing both may offer some protection against subsequent failure due to progression of atherosclerotic disease. Surgical risk primarily reflects concurrent disease, especially coronary and renovascular occlusive lesions, rather than the operation itself. After successful revascularization, pain is eliminated but recovery of intestinal function usually takes many months. Some patients never regain lost weight.

REFERENCES

1. Allende, H.D. and Ona, F.V. (1982) Celiac artery and superior mesenteric artery insufficiency. Unusual cause of erosive gastroduodenitis. *Gastroenterology*, **82**, 763–766.
2. Bergan, J.J., Dean, R.H., Conn, J., Jr and Yao, J.S.T. (1975) Revascularization in treatment of mesenteric infarction. *Annals of Surgery*, **182**, 430–438.
3. Boley, S.J., Brandt, S.J. and Veith, F.J. (1978) Ischaemic disorders of the intestine. *Current Problems in Surgery*, **15**, 1–85.
4. Boley, S.J., Sprayregan, S., Siegelman, S.S. and Veith, F.J. (1977) Initial results from an aggressive roentgenological and surgical approach to acute mesenteric ischemia. *Surgery*, **82**, 848–855.
5. Brandt, L.J., Gomery, P., Mitsudo, S.M. *et al.* (1976) Disseminated intravascular coagulation in non-occlusive mesenteric ischemia: the lack of specificity of fibrin thrombi in intestinal infarction. *Gastroenterology*, **71**, 954–957.
6. Brittain, R.S. and Early, T.R. (1963) Emergency thrombo-endarterectomy of the superior mesenteric artery. *Annals of Surgery*, **158**, 138–143.
7. Brown, R.A., Chu-Jeng, C., Scott, H.J. and Gurd, F.N. (1970) Ultrastructural changes in the canine ileal mucosal cell after mesenteric arterial occlusion. *Archives of Surgery*, **101**, 290–297.
8. Bulkley, G.B., Zuidema, G.D., Hamilton, S.R. *et al.* (1981) Intraoperative determination of small intestinal viability following ischemic injury. *Annals of Surgery*, **193**, 628–637.
9. Cherry, R.D., Jabbari, J.M., Gorestky, C.A., Herba, M., Reich, D. and Blundel, P.E. (1986) Chronic mesenteric vascular insufficiency with gastric ulceration. *Gastroenterology*, **91**, 1548–1552.
10. Dick, A.P., Graff, R., Gregg, D.M., Peters, N. and Sarner, M. (1967) An arteriographic study of mesenteric arterial disease. I. Large vessel changes. *Gut*, **8**, 206–220.
11. Gusberg, R. and Gump, F.E. (1974) Combined surgical and nutritional management of patients with acute mesenteric vascular occlusion. *Annals of Surgery*, **179**, 358–361.
12. Hildebrand, H.D. and Zierler, R.E. (1980) Mesenteric vascular disease. *American Journal of Surgery*, **139**, 188–192.
13. Kaufman, S.L., Harrington, D.P. and Siegelman,

S.S. (1977) Superior mesenteric artery embolization: an angiographic emergency. *Radiology*, **124**, 625–630.
14. Kealy, W.F. (1978) Atheroembolism. *Journal of Clinical Pathology*, **31**, 984–989.
15. Lanciault, G. and Jacobson, E.D. (1976) Gastrointestinal circulation. Progress in gastroenterology. *Gastroenterology*, **71**, 851–873.
16. Marcuson, R.W. (1972) Ischaemic colitis. *Clinics in Gastroenterology*, **1**, 745–763.
17. Marston, A., Pheils, M.T., Thomas, M.L. and Morson, B.C. (1966) Ischemic colitis. *Gut*, **7**, 1–15.
18. Marston, A., Clarke, J.M., Garcia-Garcia, J. and Miller, A.L. (1985) Intestinal function and intestinal blood supply. *Gut*, **26**, 656–666.
19. Odurny, A., Sniderman, K.W. and Colapinto, R.F. (1988) Intestinal angina: Percutaneous transluminal angioplasty of the celiac and superior mesenteric arteries. *Radiology*, **167**, 56–62.
20. Ottinger, L.W. (1978) The surgical management of acute occlusion of the superior mesenteric artery. *Annals of Surgery*, **188**, 721–731.
21. Ottinger, L.W. and Austen, W.G. (1967) A study of 136 patients with mesenteric infarction. *Surgery, Gynecology and Obstetrics*, **124**, 251–261.
22. Reiner, L., Jimenez, F.A. and Rodriguez, F.L. (1963) Atherosclerosis in the mesenteric circulation: observations and correlations with aortic and coronary atherosclerosis. *American Heart Journal*, **66**, 200–210.
23. Russ, J.E., Haid, S.P., Yao, J.S.T. and Bergan, J.J. (1977) Surgical treatment of non-occlusive mesenteric infarction. *American Journal of Surgery*, **134**, 638–642.
24. Shaw, R.S. and Rutledge, R.H. (1957) Superior mesenteric artery embolectomy in the treatment of massive mesenteric infarction. *New England Journal of Medicine*, **257**, 595–598.
25. Siegelman, S.S., Sprayregan, S. and Boley, S.J. (1974) Angiographic diagnosis of mesenteric arterial vasoconstriction. *Radiology*, **112**, 533–542.
26. Tomchik, F.S., Wittenberg, J. and Ottinger, L.W. (1970) The roentgenographic spectrum of bowel infarction. *Radiology*, **96**, 249–260.
27. Williams, L.F. (1971) Vascular insufficiency of the intestines. Progress in gastroenterology. *Gastroenterology*, **61**, 757–777.

COELIAC AXIS COMPRESSION SYNDROME

W.C. Watson

DEFINITION

The coeliac axis compression syndrome describes abdominal pain or discomfort caused by complete or partial occlusion of the coeliac artery by the median arcuate ligament of the diaphragm, by the coeliac ganglia, or by a combination of these. Not all clinicians accept the existence of this entity, but well-documented cases have been reported.

ANATOMY

The coeliac artery rises from the ventral surface of the aorta at the level of the twelfth thoracic and first lumbar vertebrae, distal to the median arcuate ligament of the diaphragm. After a short anterior course (about 1.5 cm) between the right and left coeliac ganglia and above the upper border of the pancreas, it divides into the left gastric, hepatic and splenic arteries. Although this arrangement is fairly constant, variations are not uncommon and usually involve an alternative origin for one of the main branches. Important anastomotic channels connect the coeliac artery to the superior mesenteric artery, in particular the gastroduodenal artery and its pancreaticoduodenal branches.

PATHOLOGY

The main cause of the syndrome is compression of the coeliac axis by the median arcuate ligament of the diaphragm, either because of a higher than normal take-off of the artery, or because the ligament is in a lower position than normal. This causes a V-shaped indentation in the superior surface of the artery. Less frequently, occlusion occurs due to lateral or circumferential compression of the vessel by the coeliac ganglion[16,28] and periarterial fibrous tissue.[10] Mixed patterns also occur, and histology of the constricting tissue may show ganglion cells and ligamentous fibres.

Intrinsic occlusion of the coeliac artery by atherosclerosis, thrombosis, embolism, fibromuscular dysplasia and other pathologies may also be responsible for compression syndromes.

CLINICAL FEATURES

Diverse views are held as to whether or not coeliac axis compression is clinically significant. Some deny its existence[11,13,24,29] and some large radiological series[2,7] have shown a high frequency of coeliac axis compression in apparently normal subjects. In these two studies, however, 36 out of 74 (49%) and 7 out of 17 (41%) of the subjects with compression had unexplained abdominal pain, and five of the seven in Cornell's series[7] who had surgery for the compression improved. The presence of typical angiographic findings in asymptomatic subjects does not necessarily invalidate the syndrome,[6] as complete occlusion may occur without symptoms,[27] and occasionally patients may be asymptomatic even after occlusion of all three splanchnic vessels.[5,27]

Other authors accept it as a real entity and, since the last edition of this book, there have been significant additions to the literature corroborating this opinion[9,14,15,17,19,20,21,23,25,27,30,32] while there have been none denying it.

Most patients are women and the average age is in the late 30s and early 50s, but patients as young as 13 and as old as 80 have been reported.

The main presenting symptom is abdominal pain, which may be restricted to the epigastrium or radiate to the right or left upper quadrants or to the back. The pain is variously described as stabbing, cramping or a dull ache. In most patients it is intermittent, but in some it is constant. It may be associated with eating (usually a large meal), but is not relieved by antacids or antispasmodics. Some patients complain of vague upper abdominal distension. Diarrhoea may occur in some patients and weight loss is not uncommon. Nausea and vomiting are infrequent.

It is clear that these symptoms are not diagnostically different from many other gastrointestinal disorders. Patients in whom the diagnosis of coeliac axis compression syndrome is ultimately made have usually had numerous negative routine investigations and have not responded to a variety of treatments which may have included psychiatric therapy; in other words, they fall into the category of unexplained abdominal pain.

The only diagnostic physical sign is an abdominal bruit, best heard in the epigastrium. Epigastric bruits are not uncommon, however, and have been variously reported as occurring in 6.5%,[13] 15.9%[18] and 31%[31] of normal or asymptomatic individuals. In coeliac axis compression, however, the murmur has certain characteristic features.[31] It is best heard in the mid-epigastrium, or slightly to the left or just above this point.

It begins in early or mid-systole and has an ejection type of configuration. It is usually loud (grade 2 or 3 out of 3) and extends into early diastole. The diastolic component is much softer and must be listened for carefully. The murmur is best heard with the bell of the stethoscope (which needs to be directed at the acoustic axis of the murmur), varies with respiration (being loudest in expiration), and is very localized, becoming inaudible not more than 2 cm from the point of maximum intensity.

Occasionally patients with coeliac axis compression may have no murmur or the murmur may be faint because the artery is completely or almost completely occluded. In these patients, only a high index of clinical suspicion will lead to the definitive investigation of aortography.

INVESTIGATIONS

Routine investigations of abdominal pain, such as gallbladder and gastrointestinal radiology and endoscopy, are invariably negative. If they are not, an alternative diagnosis is made which should determine management until such time as it comes into question.

The definitive investigation is aortography using the Seldinger technique via the femoral artery. Views should be taken in expiration and inspiration, and in anteroposterior and lateral positions, and whenever possible selective catheterization of the coeliac and superior mesenteric arteries should be attempted. If the coeliac axis stenosis is severe and close to the root of the vessel, selective catheterization may not be possible. The author's centre has recently used the procedure of digital intravenous angiography which avoids arterial cannulation but requires more sophisticated equipment.

The purpose of radiology is threefold: firstly, to demonstrate the presence of coeliac artery compression; secondly, to determine the severity of the compression; and thirdly, to discover whether other major vessels (especially the superior mesenteric artery) are involved. The severity of the occlusion is assessed partly by the degree of compression (a percentage of the regular calibre of the vessel), the degree of post-stenotic dilatation, and the extent of the collateral filling (if any) from the superior mesenteric artery. *Figure 5.22* shows a typical example of severe coeliac axis compression with retrograde filling from the superior mesenteric artery.

Pancreatic dysfunction sometimes occurs in patients with coeliac compression syndrome. Incidences of 5 out of 22,[30] 1 out of 6,[4] and 2 out of 15,[22] have been reported. Pancreatic function tests are not diagnostic for the syndrome.

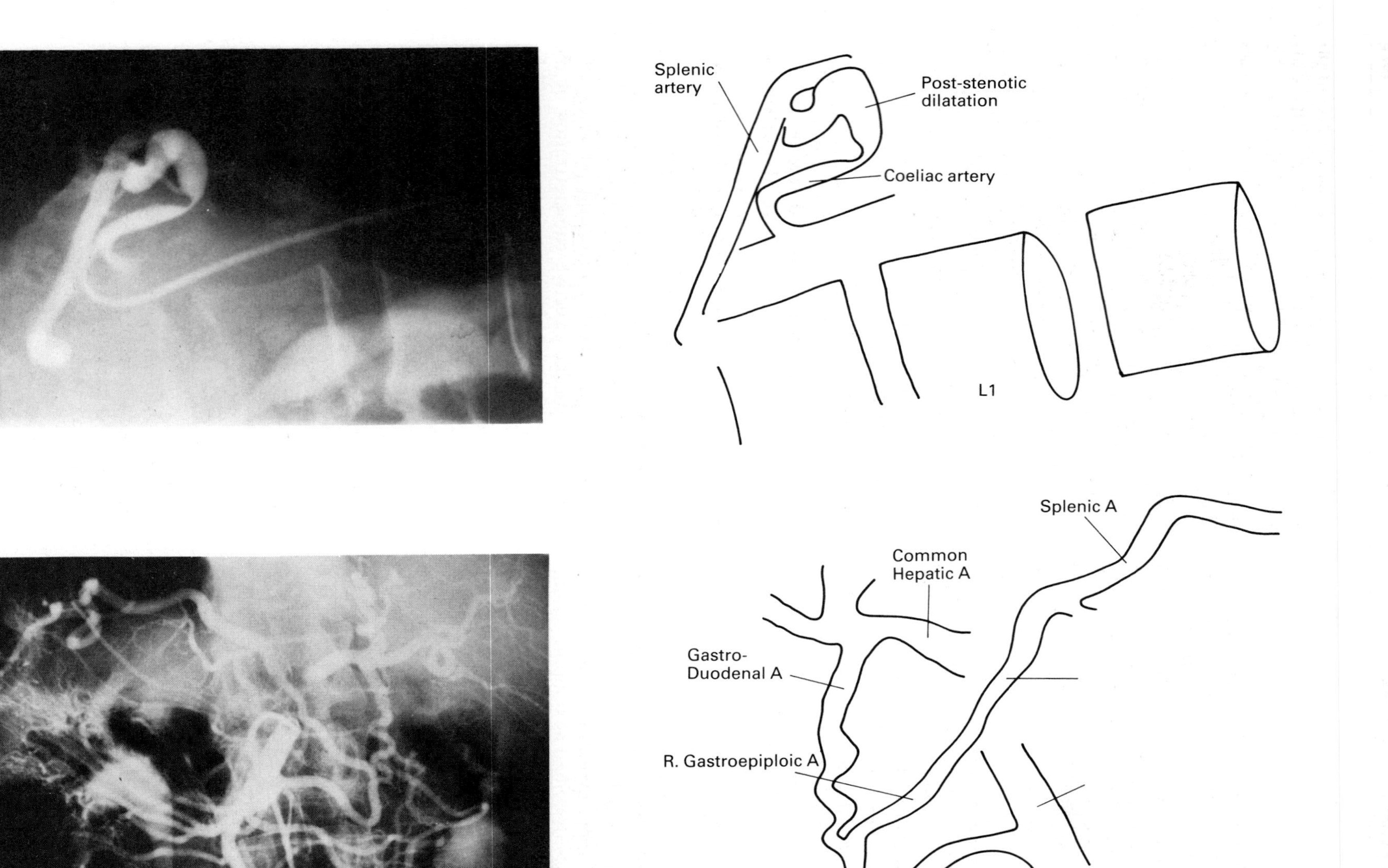

Figure 5.22 (a) Very tight compression of the coeliac artery by the median arcuate ligament of the diaphragm in an unusually distal location. (b) Retrograde collateral filling of the hepatic and splenic arteries from the superior mesenteric artery. The prominent anastomosis between the right gastroepiploic and dorsal pancreatic arteries is also unusual. (These films are from a 45 year old male with a 25 year history of undiagnosed persistent epigastric pain and progressive weight loss.)

TREATMENT

Whether patients are treated for the syndrome will depend on the personal opinion of the managing physician as to whether it is a real organic entity or not. If not, management continues as for any patient with chronic, undiagnosed abdominal pain.

Surgical relief of the arterial compression is safe and simple. It can be achieved in most patients by division of the median arcuate ligament, by dissection or excision of the encircling cuff of coeliac ganglia, or by a combination of both. If this approach is taken and the vessel does not pulsate, it may be dilated by a Fogarty catheter balloon inserted through an arteriotomy in the coeliac axis or one of its branches. A frequent consequence of this form of surgery is a periarterial sympathectomy.

Other surgical methods may be employed. Good results have been obtained by surgical bypass without correction of the compression. Lord, Stoney and Wylie[20] found that in 8 of their 12 patients, the coeliac artery remained narrow after division of the compressing bands and they proceeded to arterial reconstruction. Curl, Thompson and Stanley[8] advise inserting a graft or a bypass if a pressure gradient persists after the decompression. Others have resected the stenosed segment and reimplanted the artery elsewhere on the aorta.

RESULTS OF SURGERY

Reported results of operation have ranged from good to poor, but in recent years the balance of opinion has swung in favour of recognizing the entity. Part of the reason for this may be the stricter criteria for selection of patients for surgery[9,17,25,32] and validation of a good outcome by longer follow-up.[19,25]

THE PAIN MECHANISM

If coeliac artery compression causes pain, the reason for it doing so is not clear. The pain is not necessarily ischaemic; angiograms usually show adequate collateral filling of the coeliac artery and its main branches. If the pain is ischaemic it may be due to a 'steal' from the superior mesenteric artery to the coeliac bed.[12,26] If not, it may be due to neurogenic stimuli produced by throbbing of the compressed artery against the coeliac ganglion.[3,23] Whatever causes the pain, its relief has been attributed either to restoration of normal coeliac blood flow or to extirpation or transection of the coeliac ganglia.

Coeliac axis compression is, in the author's opinion, a real anatomical and pathological entity. This opinion is re-enforced by recent additions to the literature, but it is not universally recognized as being clinically significant. Even so, it seems reasonable to consider surgical decompression of the vessel in the small number of patients who are emotionally stable, who have distressing abdominal pain not explained by customary diagnoses and standard investigations, and who have not been helped by routine management including other kinds of surgery. The case is strengthened by such clinical features as weight loss, and pain which is aggravated by food, and not relieved by antacids or antispasmodics. This opinion is essentially similar to that of Brandt and Boley[1] which is based on a comprehensive review of the earlier literature.

REFERENCES

1. Brandt, L.J. and Boley, S.J. (1978) Celiac axis compression syndrome. A critical review. *Digestive Diseases*, **23**, 633–640.
2. Bron, K.M. and Redman, H.C. (1969) Splanchnic artery stenosis and occlusion. Incidence; arteriographic and clinical manifestations. *Radiology*, **92**, 323–328.
3. Carey, J.P., Stemmer, E.A. and Connolly, J.E. (1969) Median arcuate ligament syndrome. Experimental and clinical observations. *Archives of Surgery*, **99**, 441–446.
4. Charrette, E.P., Iyengar, S.R.K., Lynn, R.B., Paloschi, G.B. and West, R.O. (1971) Abdominal pain associated with celiac artery compression. *Surgery, Gynecology and Obstetrics*, **132**, 1009–1014.
5. Chiene, J. (1869) Complete obliteration of the coeliac and mesenteric arteries: the viscera receiving their blood-supply through the extra-peritoneal system of vessels. *Journal of Anatomy*, **3**, 65–72.
6. Colapinto, R.F., McLoughlin, M.J. and Weisbrod, G.L. (1972) The routine lateral aortogram and the celiac axis compression syndrome. *Radiology*, **103**, 557–563.
7. Cornell, S.H. (1971) Severe stenosis of the celiac artery. Analysis of patients with and without symptoms. *Radiology*, **99**, 311–316.
8. Curl, J.H., Thompson, N.W. and Stanley, J.C. (1971) Median arcuate ligament compression of the celiac and superior mesenteric arteries. *Annals of Surgery*, **173**, 314–420.
9. Daskalakis, M.K. (1982) Celiac axis compression syndrome, *International Surgery*, **67**, 442–444.
10. De Marino, V., Tournigand, P., Adhote, B. and Mercier, C. (1972) À propos des compressions éxtrinsèques de tronc coeliaque. *Journal de Chirurgie*, **104**, 289–306.
11. Drapanos, T. and Bron, K.M. (1966) Stenosis of

the celiac artery (editorial). *Annals of Surgery*, **164**, 1085–1088.
12. Dunbar, J.D., Molnar, W., Beman, F.M. and Marable, S.A. (1965) Compression of the celiac trunk and abdominal angina. Preliminary report of 15 cases. *American Journal of Roentgenology*, **95**, 731–744.
13. Edwards, A.J., Hamilton, J.D., Nichol, W.D., Taylor, G.W. and Dawson, A.M. (1970) Experience with coeliac axis compression syndrome. *British Medical Journal*, **1**, 342–345.
14. Ghosn, P.B., Rabbat, A.G., Trudel, J. *et al.* (1982) Celiac compression syndrome. *Canadian Journal of Surgery*, **25**, 377–379.
15. Gutnick, L.M. (1984) Celiac artery compression syndrome. *American Journal of Medicine*, **76**, 334–336.
16. Harjola, P.T. (1963) A rare obstruction of the celiac artery. *Annales Chirurgiae et Gynaecologiae Fenniae*, **52**, 547–550.
17. Jamieson, C.W. (1986) Celiac axis compression syndrome. *British Medical Journal*, **293**, 159–160.
18. Julius, S. and Stewart, B.H. (1967) Diagnostic significance of abdominal murmurs. *New England Journal of Medicine*, **276**, 1175–1178.
19. Kernohan, R.M., Barros, D.A.A., Cranley, B.T., Johnston, H.M. (1985) Further evidence supporting the existence of the celiac artery compression syndrome. *Archives of Surgery*, **120**, 1072–1076.
20. Lord, R.S.A., Stoney, R.J. and Wylie, E.J. (1968) Coeliac-axis compression. *The Lancet*, **2**, 795–798.
21. Lord, R.S. and Tracy, G.D. (1980) Celiac artery compression. *British Journal of Surgery*, **67**, 590–593.
22. Marable, S.A., Molnar, W. and Beman, F.M. (1966) Abdominal pain secondary to celiac axis compression. *American Journal of Surgery*, **111**, 493–495.
23. Marable, S.A., Kaplan, M.F. and Beman, F.M. (1968) Celiac compression syndrome. *American Journal of Surgery*, **115**, 97–102.
24. Mihas, A.A., Laws, H.L. and Jander, P.H. (1977) Surgical treatment of the celiac compression syndrome. *American Journal of Surgery*, **133**, 688–691.
25. Reilly, L.M., Ammar, A.D., Stoney, R.J. and Ehrenfeld, W.K. (1985) Late results following operative repair for celiac artery compression syndrome. *Journal of Vascular Surgery*, **2**, 79–91.
26. Reuter, S.R. and Olin, T. (1965) Stenosis of the celiac artery. *Radiology*, **85**, 617–627.
27. Rob, C. (1966) Surgical diseases of the celiac and mesenteric arteries. *Archives of Surgery*, **93**, 21–32.
28. Snyder, M.A., Mahoney, E.B. and Rob, C.G. (1967) Symptomatic celiac artery stenosis due to constriction by the neurofibrous tissue of the celiac ganglion. *Surgery*, **61**, 372–376.
29. Szilagyi, D.E., Rian, R.L., Elliott, J.P. and Smith, R.F. (1972) The celiac artery compression syndrome: Does it exist? *Surgery*, **72**, 849–863.
30. Watson, W.C. and Sadikali, F. (1977) Celiac axis compression. Experience with 20 patients and a critical appraisal of the syndrome. *Annals of Internal Medicine*, **86**, 278–284.
31. Watson, W.C., Williams, P.B. and Duffy, G. (1973) Epigastric bruits in patients with and without celiac axis compression. A phonoarteriographic study. *Annals of Internal Medicine*, **79**, 211–215.
32. Williams, S., Gillespie, P. and Little, J.M. (1985) Celiac axis compression syndrome: factors predicting a favorable outcome. *Surgery*, **98**, 879–887.

AORTIC ANEURYSMS

D.J. Ballard and J.W. Hallett, Jr

Aortic aneurysms are usually arteriosclerotic in origin, with the associated risk factors of male gender, age, smoking and hyperlipidaemia. The origin of the aneurysm is usually below the renals, but the renal artery origin may be involved. In addition, aortic aneurysms may be associated with iliac aneurysms. Thoracic aneurysms may extend into the suprarenal aortic area. In addition to clot formation within the aneurysm, which may contribute to ischaemic arterial disease of the legs due to embolization, an inflammatory reaction may occur externally to the aorta. Occasionally fungal or bacterial infection may lead to aneurysm formation (mycotic aneurysms).

CLINICAL FEATURES

Rupture may present with back pain and signs of retroperitoneal bleeding (*Figure 5.23*). A stuttering presentation may occur with symptoms over some days before the diagnosis is manifest. Clinical signs may include abdominal discomfort and tenderness, and the pulsatile expansile mass of the aneurysm, usually associated with evidence of diffuse atheromatous disease. The potential complications of aortic aneurysms are many (*Table 5.9*).

Table 5.9 Complications of unoperated abdominal aortic aneurysms (AAA) as potential independent indications for surgery

Rupture or suspected rupture (signs and/or symptoms of rupture or impending rupture)
- Abdominal, flank back or groin pain
- Hypotension (systolic blood pressure <100 mmHg)
- Aortocaval fistula
- Aortogastrointestinal fistula
- Imaging evidence of rupture (CT, MRI)

Complications of unoperated abdominal aortic aneurysm
- Embolism
- Thrombosis
- Infection involving AAA
- Ureteral obstruction
- Gastrointestinal obstruction
- Bile duct compression
- Symptomatic venous compression
- Renal artery compression
- Inflammatory AAA

CT = computed tomography. MRI = magnetic resonance imaging.

INVESTIGATIONS

In the active phase, there may be leukocytosis. Plain abdominal radiography will show curvilinear calcification, although this is often not striking. Ultrasound is currently the most useful means of screening for, or confirming the presence of an aneurysm, and evidence of rupture can also be demonstrated in this way. Computed tomography provides similar information, although it is generally less available in an emergency situation.

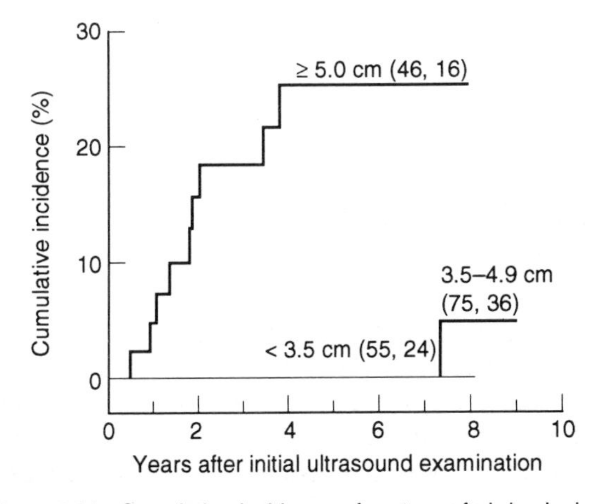

Figure 5.23 Cumulative incidence of rupture of abdominal aortic aneurysms, according to the diameter of the aneurysm at the initial ultrasound examination. (From Nevitt, Ballard and Hallett,[6] with permission.)

Table 5.10 The 30-day perioperative complications among 660 patients following surgery for non-ruptured abdominal aortic aneurysm in 1986 by members of the Canadian Society of Vascular Surgery. (Data from Johnston and Scobie.[5])

Event	%
Cardiac event	5.1
Prolongued ileus	11.0
Arrhythmia requiring treatment	10.5
Congestive heart failure	8.9
New arrhythmia	8.4
Respiratory failure	8.4
Diarrhoea with evidence of ischaemic colitis	7.1
Renal damage with increase in creatinine or BUN	5.4
Myocardial infarction	5.2
Intraoperative bleeding	4.8
Intraoperative limb ischaemia	3.5
Distal thromboembolism	3.3
Postoperative bleeding requiring transfusion	2.3
Superficial wound infection	1.5
Postoperative bleeding requiring repeat operation	1.4
Amputation	1.2
Coagulopathy	1.1
Graft thrombosis	0.9
Ischaemic colitis	0.6
Renal failure requiring dialysis	0.6
TIA or stroke	0.6
Deep infection	0.5
Graft infection	0.2
Paraplegia	0.2

BUN = blood urea nitrogen. TIA = transient ischaemic attack

TREATMENT

Once there is evidence of rupture, surgery is required, but the mortality is high, 30–60%. Symptoms of pain due to distension of the aneurysm suggest impeding rupture and necessitate early surgery.

The area of controversy is the asymptomatic aneurysm diagnosed incidentally. There are no controlled trials available, but a number of guidelines.[6] Evidence suggests that the risk of rupture of an aortic aneurysm of less than 5 cm in diameter is under 1% per year,[4] which should be compared with a 30-day perioperative mortality exceeding 4%[5] (*Table 5.10*), in a population among whom the 5-year survival following elective resection is approximately 60%.[7] Thus elective surgery is generally not indicated for aneurysms less than 5 cm. It is generally regarded as being appropriate for patients with aneurysms more than 6 cm. The optimal approach to the incidentally discovered 5–6 cm aneurysm is uncertain. Serial ultrasound observations[2,3] may help to identify patients who should be offered elective surgery.

REFERENCES

1. Ballard, D.J., Etchason, J.A., Hilborne, L.H. *et al.* (1992) Abdominal aortic aneurysm surgery: a literature review and rating of appropriateness and necessity. *RAND Publication JRA-04.*
2. Collin, J., Araujo, L. and Walton, J. (1989) How fast do very small abdominal aortic aneurysms grow? *European Journal of Vascular Surgery*, **3**, 15–17.
3. Cronenwett, J.L., Sargent, S.K., Wall, W.H. *et al.* (1990) Variables that affect the expansion rate and outcome of small abdominal aortic aneurysms. *Journal of Vascular Surgery*, **11**, 260–269.
4. Glimäker, H., Holmberg, L., Elvin, A. *et al.* (1991) Natural history of patients with abdominal aortic aneurysm. *European Journal of Vascular Surgery*, **5**, 125–130.
5. Johnston, K.W. and Scobie, T.K. (1988) Multicenter prospective study of nonruptured abdominal aortic aneurysms. I. Population and operative management. *Journal of Vascular Surgery*, **7**, 69–81.
6. Nevitt, M.P., Ballard, D.J. and Hallett, J.W., Jr (1989) Prognosis of abdominal aortic aneurysms: a population-based study. *New England Journal of Medicine*, **321**, 1009–1014.
7. Roger, V.L., Ballard, D.J., Hallet, J.W., Jr, Osmundson, P.J., Puetz, P.A. and Gersh, B.J. (1989) Influence of coronary artery disease on morbidity and mortality following abdominal aortic aneurysmectomy: a population-based study, 1971–87. *Journal of the American College of Cardiology*, **14**, 1245–1252.

CHAPTER 6

THE ACUTE ABDOMEN

OBSTRUCTION OF SMALL AND LARGE BOWEL AND ILEUS

D. Kumar

The small and large intestines perform important functions in maintaining homeostasis. Ingested food is broken down into simple carbohydrates, amino acids and fatty acids for absorption and transport to the liver. The upper intestine receives approximately 8 litres of fluid every day and extracts vitamins, electrolytes, water and trace elements so that 1–2 litres are subsequently delivered to the proximal colon where further water and electrolyte absorption takes place. This function is dependent upon an organized propagation of intestinal contents. This organized, propagated and propulsive activity is under neural, humoral and luminal control mechanisms. Intestinal obstruction can, therefore, lead to disruption of these important functions and result in changes in regional blood flow, whole body fluid and electrolyte imbalance, and impairment of host defence mechanisms. The interference of the normal aboral progression of intestinal contents results in intestinal obstruction. The term 'mechanical obstruction' is used when a physical barrier blocks the lumen, whereas failure of forward progression of bowel contents due to absent or disordered motility of bowel is called 'ileus'. When the blood supply of the intestines is compromised as a result of mechanical obstruction, gangrene occurs followed by perforation. Energetic resuscitation and surgical intervention is required at this stage to avoid a fatal outcome.

AETIOLOGY

Mechanical intestinal obstruction can be caused by a variety of factors. These can be broadly classified into luminal causes and extraluminal factors (*Table 6.1*). However, it has to be remembered that some of the factors listed in Table 6.1 produce mechanical obstruction by luminal as well as by extraluminal factors. For example, Crohn's disease may cause intestinal obstruction due to transmural inflammation, stricture formation or extrinsic compression due to abscess formation. Sometimes two separate mechanisms may account for an episode of obstruction as seen in cases where a loop of small bowel is adherent around an obstructing carcinoma. The age of the patient often gives important clues to the possible aetiological factors. Obvious examples are congenital anomalies in infants and children, and neoplastic disease in elderly patients. Obstructions due to hernias is seen in all age groups. In adults,

Table 6.1 Aetiology of intestinal obstruction

Luminal causes	*Extraluminal factors*
Atresia	Adhesions
Meckel's diverticulum	Hernias
Maltrotation	Volvulus
Hypertrophic pyloric stenosis	Carcinomatosis
Inflammatory bowel disease	Pancreatitis
(Crohn's, tuberculosis, diverticulitis)	Retroperitoneal haematoma
Strictures (Crohn's disease, tuberculosis, radiation, ischaemia)	Abscess/sepsis
Intussusception	Enteric neuropathy
Neoplasms	Aganglionosis
Medication	
Potassium chloride	
Non-steroidal anti-inflammatory drugs	
Constipation	
Gallstone ileus	
Enteroliths	
Foreign bodies	
Bezoars	

postoperative adhesions, neoplastic disease, strangulated hernias and inflammatory bowel disease are some of the important causes of intestinal obstruction. In the elderly population the causes of intestinal obstruction include postoperative adhesions, strangulated hernias, malignancy and mesenteric vascular insufficiency.

The incidence of adhesive obstruction appears to have risen over the last few decades whereas that of strangulated hernias has gradually fallen. This simply reflects the increased number of abdominal operations and elective repair of hernias before they develop complications such as strangulation. However, for all practical purposes adhesions, hernias and malignant disease still account for approximately 75% of all cases of intestinal obstruction.

PATHOPHYSIOLOGY

OBSTRUCTION

Simple obstruction implies mechanical obstruction of the intestine without occlusion of the blood supply. The bowel proximal to the obstruction distends. This distension is largely due to swallowed air.[46] The basic composition of small intestinal gas is that of air. The intraluminal pressures in the obstructed intestine are usually normal or slightly raised due to receptive relaxation of the smooth muscle of the intestinal wall in response to increased intraluminal pressure.[15] Vascular perfusion is maintained because transluminal pressures remain unchanged. Despite receptive relaxation, increases in the radius of the intestine result in increased wall tension and as a result there is an increased risk of perforation. This is particularly common in the caecum following distal bowel obstruction. With increasing distension and subsequent rises in pressure, the ability of the intestine to maintain perfusion is diminished.[37]

Fluid and electrolytes accumulate in the lumen and wall of the distended intestine proximal to the obstruction.[28,39] Intraluminal fluid accumulation may be due to either (1) translocation of fluid into the lumen because of increased osmolality resulting from enzymatic breakdown of intestinal contents[22] or (2) alterations in the blood supply to the small intestine. Some believe that the fluid is principally digestive secretions, whereas others believe that it results from the inability of the obstructed bowel to absorb water and electrolytes at the normal rate.

Prostaglandins may increase secretion and result in intraluminal fluid accumulation.[32] Failure of fluid and electrolyte absorption produces a progressive contraction of the extracellular fluid compartment and circulating volume, and vomiting accentuates the fluid depletion. The visceral vascular volume also increases which further reduces cardiac output.[10] These changes ultimately lead to hypovolaemic shock.

Acute obstruction is characterized by increased motor activity in the segment of bowel proximal to the occlusion[21,43] and cessation of nearly all motor activity in the bowel distal to the obstruction.[3] Following obstruction, the continuous peristaltic activity proximal to the obstruction changes to clustered contractions interspersed with motor quiescence. The periods of motor quiescence last for approximately 5 minutes in high obstruction and 10–15 minutes in low obstruction. Increased motor activity proximal to an obstruction appears to be mediated by cholinergic nerves. The distal inhibition may be partly mediated by non-cholinergic, non-adrenergic pathways.[33] The diminished intraluminal contents, distally, may also contribute to inhibition of motor activity in the distal segment.

Advanced mechanical obstruction results in luminal stasis and bacterial overgrowth. The Gram-negative and anaerobic organisms normally found in the colon begin to appear more proximally in the bowel.[37] Faeculent vomiting is, therefore, a feature of prolonged distal small bowel or colonic obstruction. Changes in luminal permeability allow absorption of endotoxins and bacteria. Although not so profound in human beings,[2] bacteraemia and endotoxiaemia do occur and potentiate the hypovolaemic shock; they may even precipitate renal failure.

STRANGULATION

The intestine has a remarkable capacity to withstand the effects of distension, increased secretion and decreased absorption. Interference with the mesenteric blood supply is the most serious complication of intestinal obstruction. This usually occurs secondary to a band adhesion, volvulus or hernia. However, if the vascular component is compromised then there is ischaemic disruption of intestinal mucosa. This disruption begins at the tips of the intestinal villi.[14] Extrinsic mechanical compression of the blood supply to the bowel results in vascular compromise, as normally encountered in an entrapped segment of bowel in a hernial sac or adhesion around a loop of bowel. Proximal and distal compression of the involved loop of bowel results in progressive oedema which further accentuates the vascular insufficiency. It is this progressive and sequential reduction in blood supply which characterizes strangulation. In small bowel volvulus there is obstruction to the venous outflow resulting in venous thrombosis. There is also associated mechanical obstruction of the lumen due to the twisting of bowel on its mesentry. As a result of this venous obstruction, blood starts to extravasate through disrupted capillaries into the bowel wall and the mesentry. As the integrity of the mucosa is breached, the luminal bacteria start to invade the submucosa. Bacterial toxins and bacteria cross the full thickness of the intestinal wall and enter the peritoneal cavity. The highly characteristic reddish-brown peritoneal fluid contains viable intestinal flora.[37] Endotoxins produced by Gram-negative bacteria are one of the most potent mediators of the systemic response to intestinal ischaemia. Kupffer's cells in the liver are responsible for the clearance of gut-derived endotoxins carried in the portal blood.[31] When there is an excess of endotoxin it spills over into the peripheral blood and exerts a systemic effect of which the most important is the release of interleukin-1 from macrophages.[11] This results in oedema, hypotension and acidosis.

TYPES OF OBSTRUCTION

ILEUS

Ileus is defined as the cessation of normal intestinal motility. It occurs with varying degrees of severity following surgery. This type of ileus is called 'postoperative ileus'. It is useful to differentiate postoperative ileus from other forms of ileus which may be secondary to the following:

1. Peritonitis
2. Intestinal ischaemia
3. Anaesthesia–general, spinal
4. Electrolyte disturbance
5. Trauma
6. Hypothyroidism
7. Spinal cord lesions
8. Drugs
9. Sympathectomy
10. Trace element deficiency–Mg^{++}, Ca^{++}.

Postoperative ileus

Postoperative ileus is the uncomplicated ileus following surgery which resolves spontaneously within 2–3 days. It involves the functional inhibition of propulsive bowel activity. During ileus there is no transit of bowel contents. Return of bowel sounds with subsequent passage of flatus or bowel movements indicates the end of ileus. In the small bowel, postoperative ileus is only transient,[4,45] whereas in the stomach it lasts for 24–48 hours and in the colon for 48–72 hours.[20,36,48] Occasionally the inhibition of propulsive activity lasts days to weeks. Postoperative ileus is probably due to the temporary inhibition of extrinsic control of motility. When prolonged, the intrinsic contractile systems may also be involved.[24] Breach of the peritoneum worsens ileus. However, inhibition of bowel motility is independent of the degree of bowel manipulation or the duration of surgery.[8,19] A number of factors including central and systemic factors, reflex systems and local factors have been implicated in the pathophysiology of ileus. Plasma catecholamines are elevated following surgery and high serum levels of catecholamines are associated with inhibition of motility.[1] Postoperative ileus is partially reversed by splanchnicectomy but not by adrenalectomy.[12] This highlights the importance of the sympathetic nervous system in mediating postoperative ileus. Parasympathetic stimulation increases motility, whereas stimulation of sympathic fibres inhibits motility. Sympathetic activation occurs due to stress and surgery and it thought to alter bowel motility during the postoperative period. The inhibitory reflex has a high and a low threshold component. The low threshold component is a spinal reflex which is abolished by division of the splanchnic nerves, anaesthesia and sectioning of the dorsal root fibres. The high threshold system is ganglionic and is abolished by excision of the prevertebral ganglia, although it is not affected by those manipulations that abolish the low threshold reflex.[16,23,51] An example of a low threshold reflex is intestino-intestinal reflex which has visceral afferent fibres originating in the bowel and cell bodies in the dorsal root ganglia. When activated these fibres activate inhibitory efferent sympathetic fibres which in turn results in inhibition of contractile activity.[18] In uncomplicated postoperative ileus, colonic motility is the worse affected segment. This is presumably due to α_2-receptor activation on cholinergic neurons which inhibits the release of acetylcholine and results in inhibition of colonic motility.[17] Patients with postoperative ileus treated with α-blockade combined with cholinergic stimulation resume colonic function earlier than non-treated patients.[29]

Anaesthetic agents inhibit motility.[25,50] They have the greatest effect on segments of the bowel most dependent on neural integration. In the colon, propagation of contraction is entirely dependent upon neuronal systems and, therefore, is more susceptible to the inhibitory effects of anaesthetic agents. Release of endogenous opiates has also been proposed as a cause of postoperative ileus. Small bowel myoelectrical activity and propulsion are inhibited by morphine.[47] However, treatment with naloxone does not reverse postoperative ileus, thereby suggesting that it may not be important in its pathogenesis.

The effect of laparotomy on migrating motor complex activity depends upon the extent of surgery. Division of abdominal muscles causes a transient inhibition of the migrating motor complex whereas its activity is completely abolished by opening the peritoneum. These inhibitory effects are blocked by splanchnicectomy.

Prolonged paralytic ileus

Hyponatraemia, hypokalaemia, hypocalcaemia and hypomagnesaemia all produce paralytic ileus. Intra-abdominal sepsis, retroperitoneal bleeding, peritonitis, excessive alcohol intake, opiates and phenothiazines have all been implicated in the causation of paralytic ileus. Similar to the postoperative ileus, over-activity of efferent sympathetic innervation is generally thought to be the cause of paralytic ileus. This may be mediated by both a direct effect of sympathetic fibres on intestinal ganglia and an indirect effect mediated by adrenaline and noradrenaline.

SMALL BOWEL OBSTRUCTION

Clinical features

Acute obstruction of the small intestine requires that the clinician make an accurate and early assessment of its cause. The causes of acute obstruction are as follows:

1. Small bowel obstruction:
   (a) congenital adhesions: malrotation
   (b) volvulus
   (c) adhesions
   (d) hernia: external and internal
   (e) Crohn's disease
   (f) endometriosis
   (g) radiation enteritis
   (h) tuberculosis
   (i) inflammatory mass: appendicitis, diverticular disease
   (j) talc
   (k) drugs.
2. Large bowel obstruction:
   (a) ischaemic stricture
   (b) intussusception
   (c) hernia
   (d) diverticular disease
   (e) endometriosis
   (f) Crohn's disease
   (g) volvulus: sigmoid, right colon, transverse colon
   (h) adenocarcinoma
   (i) tuberculosis
   (j) bilharzia.

As the narrowest part of the intestinal tract and, therefore, the most vulnerable to obstruction, the terminal ileum is the segment most likely to be involved in intussusception and adhesion formation. The symptom complex of acute small bowel obstruction is variable and depends on the site, degree and the duration of obstruction as well as the possible presence or absence of strangulation. There are four major symptoms that are characteristic of obstruction:

1. Abdominal pain
2. Vomiting
3. Abdominal distension
4. Constipation.

The pain is sudden, sharp and colicky in nature, and is often upper abdominal in high obstruction, periumbilical in low ileal obstruction and lower abdominal in colonic obstruction. If the obstruction is not relieved, the typical colicky pain may be replaced by a generalized abdominal discomfort. Between episodes of colic the patient feels relatively well and may be free of pain. In high intestinal obstruction there is an acute onset of colicky pain associated with profuse bilious vomiting. Abdominal distension may be slight or absent. Nausea and vomiting occur soon after the pain, and vomiting may relieve it. At first the vomitus contains bile, but with long-standing obstruction it changes to a yellow–brown colour and is faecal in odour. In distal small bowel obstruction the pain is mainly periumbilical or lower abdominal. This is often associated with moderate-to-severe distension of the abdomen. Inspection of the abdomen often shows previous incision scars, ventral or inguinal hernias or visible peristalsis. The combination of hyperactive bowel sounds and frequent abdominal cramps is highly suggestive of intestinal obstruction. Flatus or stool may be passed following the onset of pain. This is due to the presence of persistalsis distal to the obstruction. In incomplete obstruction the patient may complain of diarrhoea. Absolute constipation is a feature of complete obstruction. Patients with acute intestinal obstruction appear ill and anxious. Physical examination may reveal tachycardia, low-grade fever and dehydration. Marked distension of the abdomen may compromise respiratory function. Hypotension may occur due to fluid loss. The patient becomes restless as the frequency of colic increases. Rectal examination is often unhelpful. When strangulation occurs in the late stages the abdomen is often distended and silent. There is marked tachycardia with a low central venous pressure and possibly hypovolaemic shock. Signs of marked dehydration are often apparent. The pain becomes severe and persistent in nature and is often accompanied by guarding and rebound tenderness.

LARGE BOWEL OBSTRUCTION

Obstruction of the large intestine is often gradual in onset and occurs more commonly in patients over the age of 40 years. The most common presenting complaints are abdominal distension and constipation. Unlike small intestinal obstruction, pain is often absent or minimal unless peritonitis is present. The most common causes of large bowel obstruction are volvulus, acute diverticulitis and colorectal carcinomas. A history of progressive constipation over several months, associated with loss of appetite and/or weight, may provide important clues to the diagnosis. Nausea and vomiting are not features of early large bowel obstruction. It is only in late-stage obstruction that vomiting becomes a feature. The temperature and pulse are often within normal limits. The patient looks well and adequately hydrated. On examination the abdomen is distended but non-tender unless peritonitis supervenes. Unless the obstructing lesion is within reach of the examining finger rectal examination is often unhelpful.

Pseudo-obstruction

Pseudo-obstruction is a term coined to describe a patient with radiographic features of large bowel obstruction in whom no obstruction can be identified by contrast radiology or colonoscopy. The disorder must be identified because it is unnecessary and embarassing to operate on these patients.

Pseudo-obstruction may be a panenteric disorder and may be confused with ileus. There is a familial myopathy which presents early in life and it carries a poor prognosis which forms one aspect of the syndrome. The more familiar primary cause is a diffuse autonomic neuropathy of unknown aetiology which principally affects the colon, but which may also involve the oesophagus, stomach and small bowel. Secondary pseudo-obstruction may be due to intestinal ischaemia, a variety of drugs, collagen disorders, cardiac or renal disease, diabetes, and a range of metabolic and endocrine abnormalities.

INVESTIGATIONS

The main objective of laboratory and radiological investigations is: (1) to confirm the diagnosis of mechanical obstruction, and (2) to distinguish between simple obstruction and strangulation.

In most cases the diagnosis is made on clinical and surgical judgement. Haematological investigations may reveal an increase in haematocrit resulting from fluid loss from the intravascular space into the intestinal lumen and dehydration. The white cell count may be increased up to 20 000/mm^2. In the early stages, there is little change in plasma sodium, potassium and chloride concentrations; acid–base changes are also slight. In the untreated patient, there is gradual reduction in plasma sodium and chloride levels. There is metabolic acidosis due to the combined effects of dehydration, ketoacidosa and starvation. There may be superimposed respiratory acidosis due to restricted respiration as a result of an elevated diaphragm. A rising white cell count is often considered to be an indicator of bowel ischaemia. Very high white cell counts (40 000–

60 000/mm^2) suggest primary vascular occlusion in the mesentry.

The most important and accurate diagnostic tool is radiological examination of the abdomen with both erect and supine views. The supine film shows dilated loops of bowel whereas the erect film reveals air–fluid levels in dilated loops (*Figure 6.1*). Radiographs should be taken soon after admission to hospital, preferably within the first hour. A chest radiograph in the sitting position should also be included to exclude free gas under the diaphragm. The bowel distal to the obstruction shows little or no gas. This provides confirmatory evidence of the diagnosis. However, the predictive value of plain radiographs is probably around 85%.[13] Sometimes massively distended loops of small bowel can be mistaken for colonic obstruction. In the case of proximal intestinal obstruction, the segment of bowel above the obstruction is often decompressed by recent vomiting, hence no air–fluid levels are seen. In the case of distal obstruction a characteristic step-ladder pattern may be apparent. Radiological signs of ischaemia may also be present in the form of thumb printing, loss of mucosal pattern or thickening of the bowel wall. Free air in the peritoneal cavity suggests perforation complicating strangulation, although more than 50% of small and large bowel perforations do not cause pneumoperitoneum.[49] Visualization of both the inner and outer walls of the bowel suggests pneumoperitoneum. When loops of bowel are full of fluid, the dilatation may not be apparent on a plain radiograph (*Figure 6.2a*). In such cases ultrasonography or computed tomography (CT) may help in identifying the distended loops of bowel. Occasionally a contrast study may give further clues to the aetiology, site and degree of obstruction (*Figure 6.2b*).

In large bowel obstruction, laboratory findings reveal a normal haematocrit with a normal or elevated white cell count. Radiological examination may be helpful in defining the degree of obstruction and the level of obstruction. Supine and erect abdominal films show two distinct patterns of obstruction:

1. Closed loop obstruction with pronounced colonic and caecal dilatation (*Figure 6.3*).
2. Distension of the large and small intestines suggesting an incompetent iloecaecal valve (*Figure 6.4*).

Based just on plain radiographs, the site of obstruction is often unclear. Moreover, in the presence of small bowel distension, it is unsafe to assume that the ileocaecal valve is incompetent. Careful watch

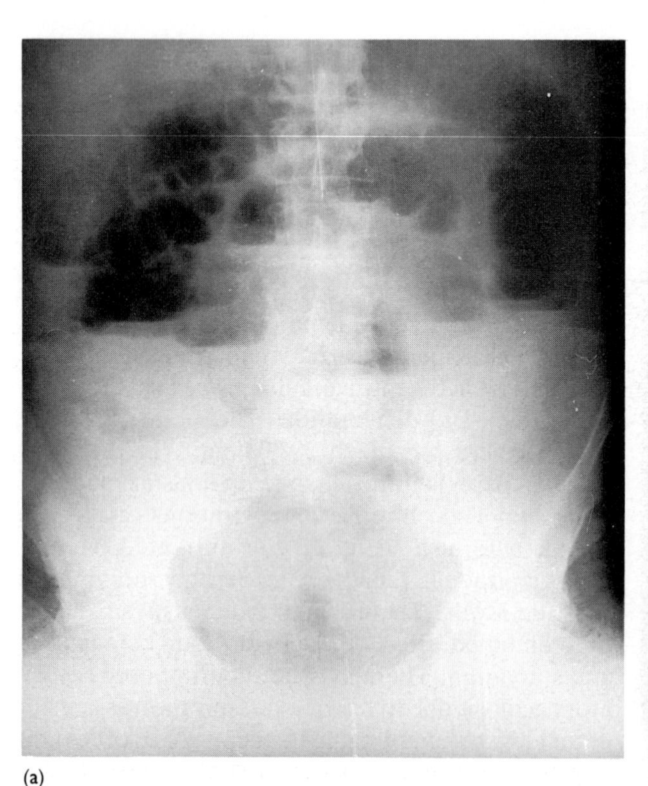

(a)

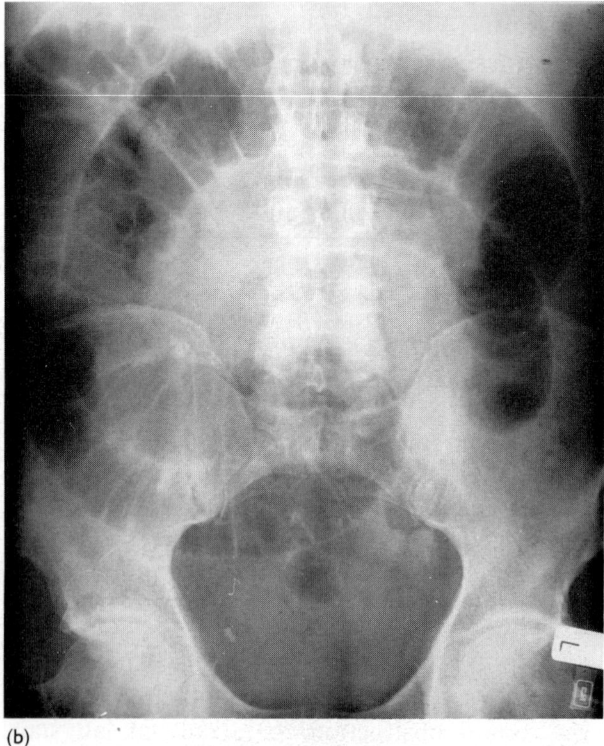

(b)

Figure 6.1 Erect (a) and supine (b) radiographs of the abdomen showing small bowel obstruction. Note the dilated loops of small bowel in the supine view and dilated loops with air–fluid levels in the erect film. (Courtesy of Dr J.R. Lee.)

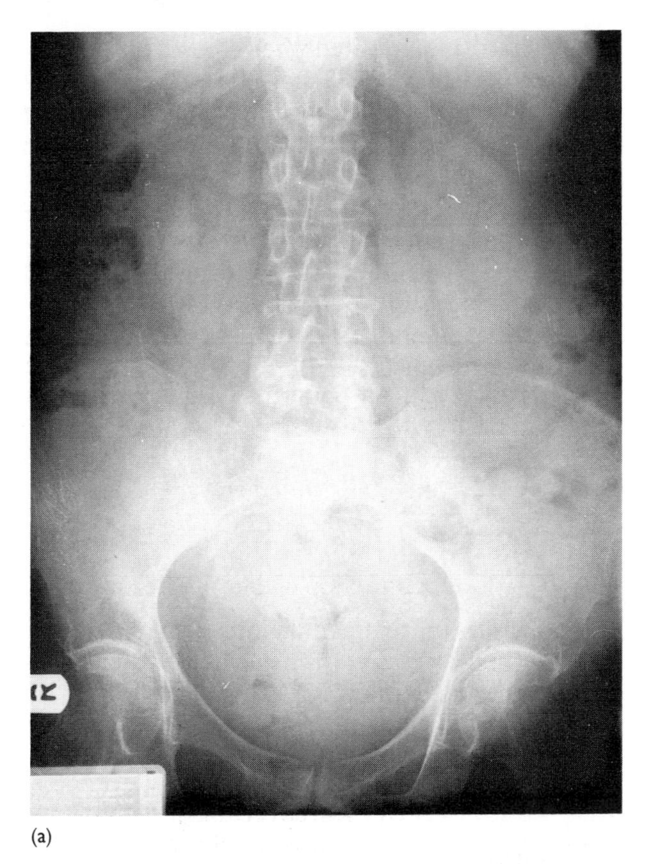
(a)

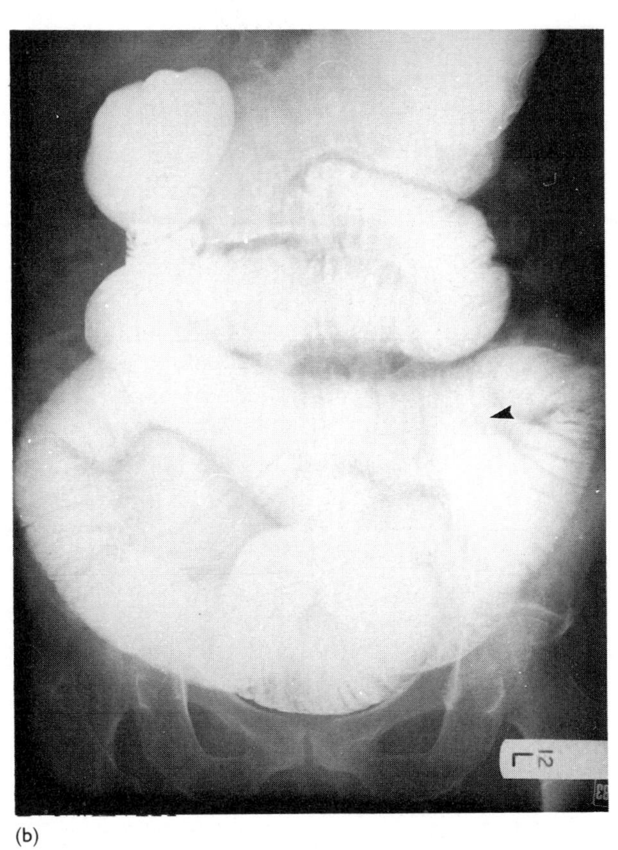
(b)

Figure 6.2 (a) Plain radiograph in a patient who was admitted with clinical signs of intestinal obstruction. Note the absence of air in the small bowel suggesting a fluid-filled obstruction. (b) Radiograph showing a contrast study in the same patient. Dilated loops of small intestine and the level of obstruction (arrow) are clearly seen. (Courtesy of Dr J.R. Lee.)

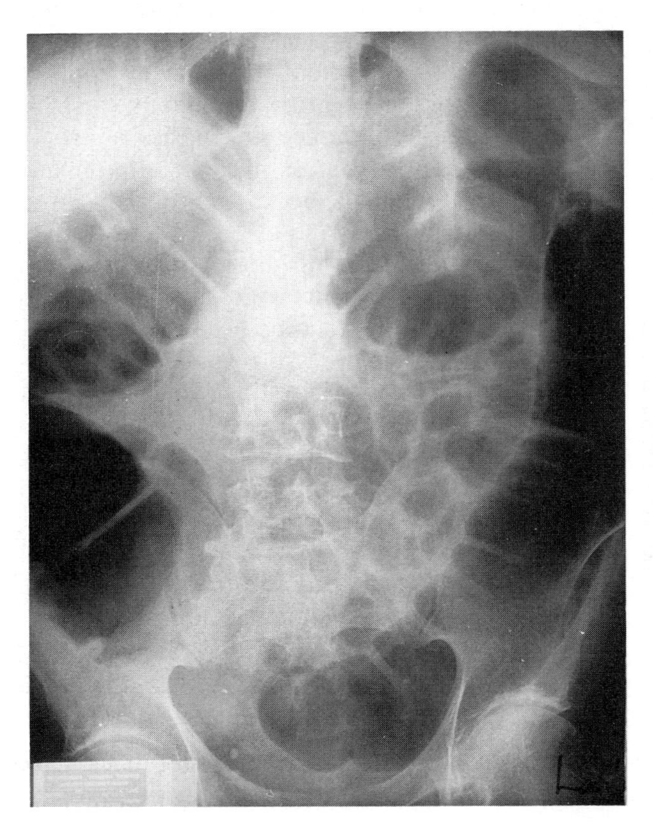

should be kept on caecal diameter because it is unsafe to allow the caecum to distend to a diameter beyond 10–12 cm. Further distension would initiate tears along the tenea and result in perforation. However, distension of the colon is not specific for mechanical obstruction of the large bowel. Therefore, contrast studies in the form of barium enema are often advised, particularly to exclude pseudo-obstruction. Occasionally, computed tomography is useful for the assessment of extraluminal pathologies such as diverticulitis.[26]

Proctosigmoidoscopy and flexible sigmoidoscopy may also be useful in establishing the site and nature of the obstruction. Care must be taken because air insufflation can worsen the colonic distension.

Contrast radiology is sometimes necessary. This includes barium enema, retrograde ileogram through an ileostomy and administration of contrast medium through a nasogastric tube or by mouth.

Figure 6.3 Radiograph showing marked colonic dilatation with no distension of the small bowel suggesting a competent ileocaecal valve. This is known as a 'closed loop' obstruction. (Courtesy of Dr J.R. Lee.)

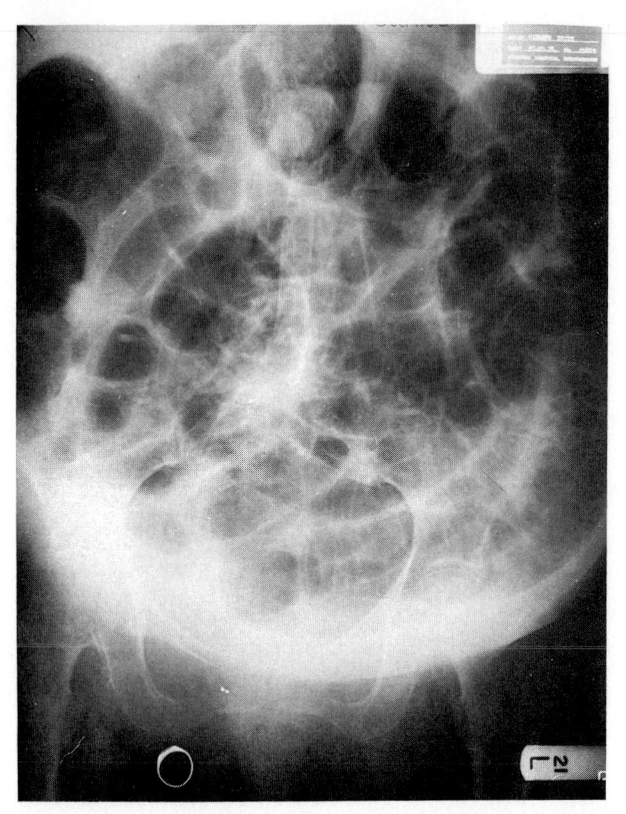

Figure 6.4 An example of an incompetent ileocaecal valve. Note the simultaneous distension of the colon and the small bowel. (Courtesy of Dr J.R. Lee.)

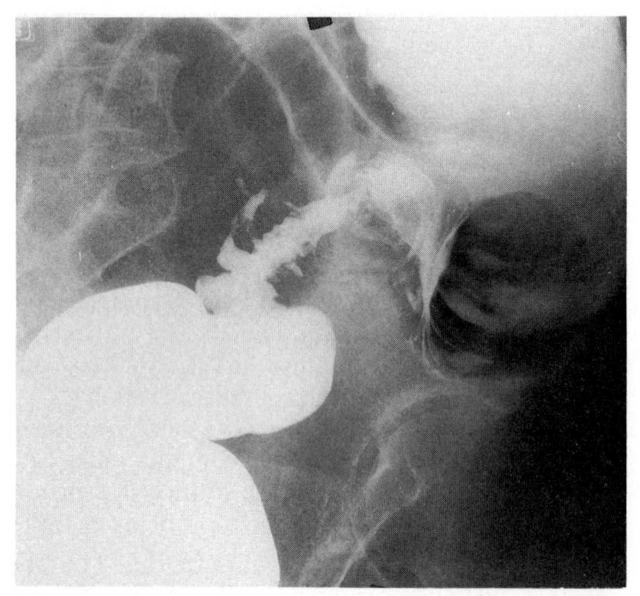

Figure 6.5 Barium enema in a patient who presented with colonic obstruction. The contrast study shows malignant obstruction of the distal sigmoid colon. Note distension of the colon proximal to the obstruction. (Courtesy of Dr J.R. Lee.)

Barium enema is indicated when colonic obstruction is suspected. This often reveals the type and level of obstruction (*Figure 6.5*). Barium enema may also be used to reduce a non-strangulated intussusception in children.

Care must be taken because introduction of barium in obstruction can cause perforation of inflammatory lesions and may also convert a partial obstruction into a complete obstruction.

The most common and most important indication for a contrast study is to differentiate between postoperative ileus and mechanical obstruction.

TREATMENT

The principles of treatment in intestinal obstruction are fluid and electrolyte replacement, decompression of bowel and timely intervention.

RESUSCITATION

This consists mainly of intestinal decompression using nasogastric suction and correction of fluid and electrolyte imbalance. Nearly all patients with intestinal obstruction are dehydrated. This is further accentuated by operation and the failure of the intestine to absorb fluid postoperatively. Severely dehydrated, shocked and elderly patients should also be catheterized, not only to obtain a sample of urine but to monitor the urine output in the first 24–48 hours. In the presence of sepsis, a broad-spectrum antibiotic such as a cephalosporin and metronidazole should be administered intravenously. The duration and extent of resuscitation depend upon whether a diagnosis of strangulation obstruction is suspected. Gastric decompression is carried out by nasogastric tubes such as the Miller–Abbot tube for decompression of the small intestine. Positioning of long intestinal tubes is difficult and the subsequent benefit controversial. Therefore, the routine use of such jejunal tubes has largely been abandoned. Sigmoid volvulus (*Figure 6.6*) can be decompressed using a rectal 'flatus' tube or by careful colonoscopy. Similarly, large bowel distension due to pseudo-obstruction may be decompressed with the help of a colonoscope.

SURGICAL POLICY

If the clinical and radiological features favour small bowel obstruction and there is no evidence of an

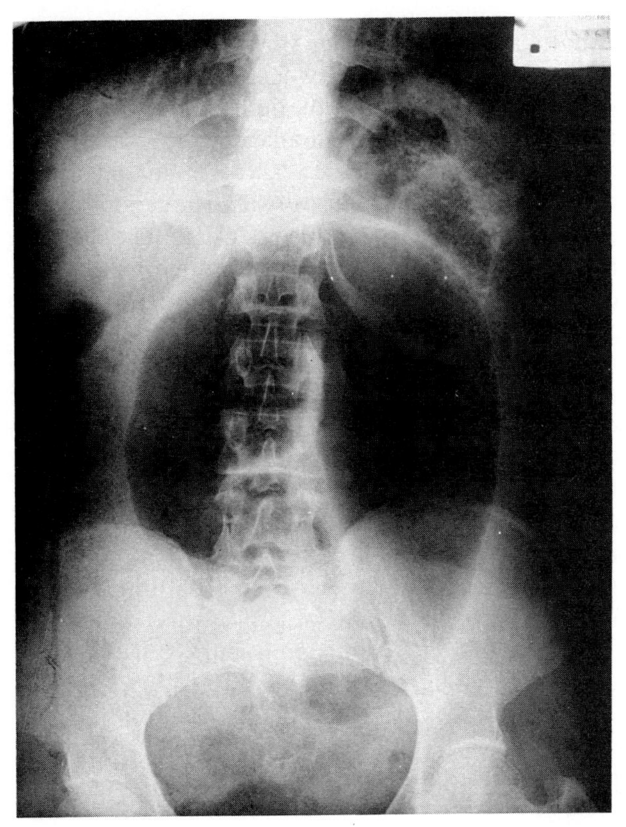

Figure 6.6 Radiographs showing an example of sigmoid volvulus. (Courtesy of Dr J.R. Lee.)

obstructed hernia or of intestinal infarction, the usual policy is to treat conservatively while carefully monitoring the patient's progress. Nasogastric decompression and intravenous fluids are continued in the hope that, particularly if the patient has had a previous laparotomy, the obstruction will resolve. If the patient has not had previous abdominal surgery, the possibility of obstruction around an inflammatory process or gallstones ileus should be considered. If there is no reduction in abdominal pain and distension, or if the bowel sounds become silent, there is a real fear of intestinal infarction and laparotomy should not be delayed.

If the clinical and radiological impression is of large bowel obstruction, the presence and site of large bowel occlusion should be identified by gentle, water-soluble contrast enema both to exclude pseudo-obstruction and to identify the site of occlusion. If an obstruction were identified in the large bowel, most patients would require surgery.

The management of adhesive obstruction, obstruction due to hernias, large bowel obstruction, and adynamic disorders of the small and large bowel will now be considered in greater detail.

Adhesions

Adhesions are one of the most common causes of intestinal obstruction and most laparotomies are followed by adhesion formation. It is controversial as to whether lysis of adhesions should be undertaken in cases with widespread dense adhesions involving multiple loops of small intestine. During such a procedure there is extensive denudation of the intestinal wall and the risk of multiple iatrogenic enterotomies. Several specialized procedures, including Noble's plication[30] and transmesenteric plication[6] have been advocated. However, neither of these procedures has met with long-term success. Most surgeons either perform lysis of adhesions alone with division of thick fibrous bands or use internal stenting with long intestinal tubes together with complete lysis of adhesions.

The ideal patient for tube decompression and intravenous fluid replacement therapy is one suspected of having adhesive small bowel obstruction secondary to a previous laparotomy without clinical signs of strangulation or gangrenous bowel. However, frequent evaluation of the efficacy of this treatment by an experienced surgeon is mandatory if serious complications such as strangulation and gangrene are to be avoided. If the diagnosis is in doubt, early diagnostic strategy rather than tube decompression should be followed. Marked leukocytosis with fever, tachycardia and localized abdominal tenderness, should lead to immediate laparotomy. Patients who do not respond to conservative measures by tube decompression in the first 48 hours should also be considered for surgery.

Hernias

When bowel becomes incarcerated in a hernia, it may be further complicated by strangulation. Under these circumstances the blood supply to the bowel is compromised in the neck of the sac, resulting in ischaemia and finally necrosis. Sometimes only the antimesenteric surface of the bowel is obstructed in a hernia, causing infarction of only a segment of the bowel wall. These are known as Richter's hernias. Approximately 10% of all inguinal hernias and 20% of all femoral hernias carry a risk of incarceration.[7] The small intestine is the most common organ found within the hernial sac of a strangulated hernia. The operation for a strangulated or incarcerated hernia involves adequate exposure of the hernial sac and careful dissection of the neck of the sac and the hernia contents. After the sac is opened the bowel must be carefully inspected to assess its viability. If the viability of the bowel is doubtful after wrapping it in a moist warm gauze for several minutes, then resection is the safest alternative. If the bowel is gangrenous then resection with end-to-end anastomosis is the operation of choice. The hernial sac is then resected and herniorraphy performed in the standard fashion.

Obstructed gangrenous femoral hernias are best exposed by the inguinal or the pre-peritoneal approach, the femoral or the combined approaches. The high approaches allow intestinal resection to be performed if necessary. A lower midline approach is sometimes used. This enables repair of both hernial orifices at the same time. Gangrene of the contents of the hernial sac should be suspected if dark-coloured fluid or a faeculent odour is present. If gangrene is suspected, special care must be taken to avoid reduction of the contents of the sac into the peritoneal cavity. If necrotic bowel is found then the necrotic tissue is resected followed by an end-to-end anastomosis and repair of the defect.

Incisional hernias are iatrogenic, and intestinal obstruction is common. Obstruction should be suspected in any patient with an incisional hernia who presents with colicky abdominal pain. The omentum and the small bowel are the most frequent contents of an incisional hernia. Usually, adhesions in the region of the hernial neck lead to intestinal obstruction. Umbilical hernias rarely cause obstruction but may do so when they are large. Internal hernias such as obturator hernia or paraduodenal hernias may occasionally lead to intestinal obstruction, but the diagnosis is often made at laparatomy.

Large bowel obstruction

Caecal or sigmoid volvulus may cause acute large bowel obstruction. Sigmoid volvulus is more common than caecal volvulus and occurs more frequently in patients resident in psychiatric hospitals. The patient usually presents with an acute onset of large bowel obstruction. Examination reveals a distended abdomen and the diagnosis is often established by erect and supine abdominal radiographs. Sigmoidoscopic or colonoscopic decompression of the twisted bowel is the procedure of choice. In patients with recurrent sigmoid volvulus, sigmoid colectomy may be necessary. At laparotomy the mesentery is thickened with a large redundant sigmoid colon. Resection of the sigmoid colon with an end-to-end colonic anastomosis is performed. Caecal volvulus usually occurs in patients of the middle and older age group with sudden onset of colicky right-sided pain associated with nausea and vomiting. The diagnosis is established by erect and supine abdominal radiographs. If the diagnosis is in doubt a barium enema will often confirm it. Resection of the twisted segment followed by an end-to-end primary anastomosis is the treatment of choice.

Malignant obstruction of the large bowel is another common cause of obstruction of the large intestine. Malignant large bowel obstruction often does not require emergency surgical treatment. The patients should be fully resuscitated with replacement of fluid and electrolytes, and urgent rather than emergency surgery carried out. If the patient is of a reasonable operative risk and has a left-sided obstruction, then the treatment of choice is a Hartman's procedure with an end colostomy and a mucous fistula. In right-sided colonic obstructions, resection and primary anastomosis are the treatment of choice. A method of intraoperative colonic irrigation has been advocated by some surgeons.[34] This technique has also been used by other investigators with good results. Advanced malignancy and peritonitis, however, are contraindications to primary anastomosis. Another option is to perform a primary anastomosis with a covering colostomy.

Postoperative ileus and pseudo-obstruction

The principal aim of treatment in patients with postoperative ileus and pseudo-obstruction is symptomatic relief and avoidance of surgical intervention. Nasogastric suction for bowel decompression remains the major form of therapy. A combination of nasointestinal intubation with intravenous hydration or total parenteral nutrition is the treatment of choice until the process resolves spontaneously. Parenteral nutrition should be started when there is pre-existing evidence of malnutrition in the form of weight loss and hypoalbuminaemia, and also when the ileus is expected to last for 7 days or longer. However, other forms of therapy have been tried and these include electrical stimulation, pharmacological agents and enteral feeding.

As a result of similarities between cardiac and intestinal smooth muscle oscillations, electrical stimulation of the bowel wall has been attempted for persistent ileus. This technique of electrical pacing, where electrical stimulation is applied directly to the bowel wall, has been achieved in dogs but not in humans.[35] Electrical stimulation of the bowel wall was reported initially to be successful but when compared to controls proved ineffective. Treatment of postoperative ileus with adrenergic inhibitors with or without cholinergic agonists has also been proposed.[40] α and β blockade with receptor antagonists, guanethidine, dihydroergotamine or adrenergic depletion with reserpine may improve postoperative ileus slightly but their use is limited by cardiovascular side effects.[5,41,44] Prostaglandins have also been used in the treatment of postoperative ileus. It has been suggested that they inhibit the release of noradrenaline and augment the release of acetylcholine from intramural neurons.[38] Prokinetic agents such as metaclopramide[9] and cisapride[42] have also been used for the treatment of postoperative ileus and pseudo-obstruction with varying degrees of success.

Recently, enteral feeding either by nasogastric intubation or needle jejunostomy has been advocated as a means of reducing the duration of postoperative ileus and/or for the treatment of pseudo-obstruction. Enteral feeding is said to stimulate the bowel mechanically, thereby reducing the duration of ileus.[27] However, a controlled randomized trial of postoperative treatment with nasoenteric tube against no specific therapy failed to reveal reduction of postoperative ileus by postoperative feeding.

Pseudo-obstruction may require repeated colonoscopic decompression, prolonged exposure to prokinetic drugs and even electrical pacing. In refractory cases, a loop ileostomy may have to be considered if small bowel motility is normal.

REFERENCES

1. Bernstein, A., Wright, A.C. and Spencer, D. (1967) Pheochromocytoma, as a cause of gastrointestinal distension. *Postgraduate Medical Journal*, **43**, 180–183.
2. Bounos, G., Hampson, L.G. and Gurd, F.N. (1964) Cellular nucleotides in hemorrhagic shock: relationship of intestinal metabolic changes to hemorrhagic enteritis and the barrier function of intestinal mucosa. *Annals of Surgery*, **160**, 650–668.
3. Carlson, R.S. and Wagensteen, O.H. (1930) Motor activity of the distal bowel in intestinal obstruction. *Proceedings of the Society of Experimental Biology and Medicine*, **27**, 676–681.
4. Carmichael, M.J., Weisbrodt, N.W. and Copeland, E.M. (1977) Effects of abdominal surgery on myoelectric activity in the dog. *American Journal of Surgery*, **133**, 34–38.
5. Catchpole, B.N. (1972) Treatment of ileus. *Surgery*, **71**, 313–314.
6. Childs, W.A. and Phillips, R.B. (1960) Experience with intestinal plication and a proposed modification. *Annals of Surgery*, **152**, 258–265.
7. Condon, R.E. and Nyhus, L.M. (1978) Complications of groin hernia. In: *Hernia*, 2nd edn, pp. 264–275 (Eds) Nyhus, L.M. and Condon, R.E. Philadelphia: J.B. Lippincot.
8. Condon, R.E., Cowles, V.E., Schulte, W.J., Frantzides, C.T., Mahoney, J.L. and Sarna, S.K. (1986) Resolution of postoperative ileus in humans. *Annals of Surgery*, **203**, 574–581.
9. Davidson, E.D., Hersh, T., Brinner, R.A., Barnett, S.M. and Boyle, L.P. (1979) The effects of metoclopramide on post operative ileus. A randomized double-blind study. *Annals of Surgery*, **190**: 27–30.
10. Derblom, H., Johansson, H. and Mylander, G. (1963) Vascular patterns of the intestinal villi in the obstructed small bowel of the rat. *Surgery*, **54**, 780–783.
11. Dinarello, C.A. (1984) Interleukin-1 and the pathogenesis of the acute phase response. *New England Journal of Medicine*, **311**, 1413–1418.
12. Dubois, A., Henry, D.P. and Kopin, I.J. (1975) Plasma catecholamines and postoperative gastric emptying and small bowel propulsion in the rat. *Gastroenterology*, **68**, 466–469.
13. Eisenberg, R.L. Heineken, P. and Hedgcock, M.W. (1983) Evaluation of plain abdominal radiographs in the diagnosis of abdominal pain. *Annals of Surgery*, **197**, 464–469.
14. Falk, A., Myrvold, H.E. and Lundgren, O. (1982) Mucosal lesions in the feline small intestine in septic shock. *Circulatory Shock*, **9**, 27–35.
15. Fondcaro, J.D. (1984) Intestinal blood flow and motility. In: *Physiology of the Intestinal Circulation*, pp. 107–120 (Eds) Shepherd, A.P. and Granger, D.N. New York: Raven Press.
16. Furness, J.B. and Costa, M. (1974) A dynamic ileus, its pathogenesis and treatment. *Medical Biology*, **52**, 82–89.
17. Gillis, R.A., Souza, J.D., Hicks, K.A. *et al.* (1987) Inhibitory control of proximal colonic motility by the sympathetic system. *American Journal of Physiology*, **253**, G531–539.
18. Glise, H., Lindahl, B.O. and Abrahamson, H. (1981) Reflex adrenergic inhibition of gastric motility by nociceptive intestinal stimulation and peritoneal irritation in the cat. *Scandinavian Journal of Gastroenterology*, **15**, 673–681.
19. Graber, J.N. Schulte, W.J. and Condon, R.E. (1980) The duration of postoperative ileus related to the extent and site of operative dissection. *Surgical Forum*, **21**, 141–144.
20. Harrower L.W. (1968) Postoperative ileus. *American Journal of Surgery*, **116**, 369–374.
21. Herrin, R.C. and Meek, W.J. (1933) Distension as a factor in intestinal obstruction. *Archives of Internal Medicine*, **55**, 152–168.
22. Johnson, L., Nordstrom, H. and Nylands, G. (1978) Experimental studies on fluid pathophysiology in small intestinal obstruction in the rat. Effects of intraluminal hypermotility. *Scandinavian Journal of Gastroenterology*, **13**, 49–56.
23. Kuntz, A. and Sacomanno, G. (1944) Reflex inhibition of intestinal motility through

decentralised prevertebral ganglia. *Journal of Neurophysiology*, **7**, 163–170.
24. Livingston, E.H. and Passaro, E.P. (1990) Postoperative ileus. *Digestive Disease and Sciences*, **35**, 121–132.
25. Marshall, F.N., Pittinger, C.B. and Long, J.P. (1961) Effects of halothane on gastrointestinal motility. *Anesthesiology*, **22**, 363–366.
26. Morris, J. Stellato, T.A. and Hagga, J.R. (1986) The role of computed tomography in colonic diverticulitis. *Annals of Surgery*, **204**, 128–132.
27. Moss, G. (1986) Discharge within twenty four hours of elective cholecystectomy. *Archives of Surgery*, **121**, 1159–1161.
28. Nadrowski, L.F. (1974) Pathophysiology and current treatment of intestinal obstruction. *Review of Surgery*, **31**, 381–402.
29. Neely, J. and Catchpole, B. (1971) The restoration of alimentary tract motility by pharmacological means. *British Journal of Surgery*, **58**, 21–28.
30. Noble, T.B. (1937) Plication of the small intestine as prophylaxis against adhesions. *American Journal of Surgery*, **35**, 41–44.
31. Nolan, J.P. (1981) Endotoxin, reticulodendothelial function and liver injury. *Hepatology*, **1**, 458–465.
32. Ohman V. (1984) The effects of luminal distension and obstruction on the intestinal circulation. In: *Physiology of the Intestinal Circulation*, pp. 321–334. (Eds) Shepherd, A.P. and Granger, D.N. New York: Raven Press.
33. Priholda, M. Flatt, A. and Summers, R.W. (1984) Mechanisms of motility changes during acute intestinal obstruction in the dog. *American Journal of Physiology*, **10**, G37–G42.
34. Radcliffe, A.G. and Dudley, H.A.F. (1983) Intraoperative antegrade irrigation of the large intestine. *Surgery, Gynecology and Obstetrics*, **156**, 721–723.
35. Richter, H.M. and Kelly, K.A. (1986) Effect of transection and pacing on human jejunal pacesetter potentials. *Gastroenterology*, **91**, 1380–1385.
36. Rothnie, N.G., Harper, R.A. and Catchpole, B.N. (1963) Early postoperative gastrointestinal activity. *The Lancet*, **2**, 64–67.
37. Russell, J.C. and Welsch, J.P. (1990) Pathophysiology of bowel obstruction. In: *Bowel Obstruction*, pp. 28–59. (Ed) Welch, J.P. Philadelphia: Saunders.
38. Ruwart, M.J., Klepper, M.S. and Rush, B.D. (1980) Mechanism of stimulation of gastrointestinal propulsion in postoperative ileus rates of 16,16-dimethyl PG32. *Advances in Prostaglandin Thromboxane Research*, **8**, 1609–1610.
39. Shin, C.S., Nimmannit, S. and Hoff, A. (1971) Body fluid compartment in patients with non strangulating obstruction of the small intestine. *Surgery, Gynecology and Obstetrics*, **132**, 980–984.
40. Smith, M.K., Kepson, R.P. and Catchpole B.N. (1965) Ileus: an experimental study. *British Journal of Surgery*, **52**, 381–386.
41. Smith, O., Stoicu, G. and Russo, I. (1979) Influence of alpha and beta blocking agents on recovery of intestinal transit and postoperative complications in aged patients. *Revista de Chirurgie, Oncologie, Radiologie, ORL, Oftalmologie, Stomatologie* **27**, 71–77.
42. Stacher, G., Steinringer, H., Schneider, C., Winklehner, S., Mittelbach, G. and Gaupmann, G. (1986) Effects of Cisapride on jejunal motor activity in fasting healthy humans. *Gastroenterology*, **90**, 1210–1226.
43. Summers, R.W., Yanda, R., Prihoda, M. and Flatt, A. (1983) Acute intestinal obstruction: an electromyographic study in dogs. *Gastroenterology*, **85**, 1301–1336.
44. Thorup, J., Wille Jorgensen, P., Jorgensen, T. and Kjaergaad, J. (1983) Dihydroergotamine in postoperative ileus. *Clinical Pharmacology and Therapeutics*, **34**, 54–55.
45. Tinckler, L.F. (1965) Surgery and intestinal motility. *British Journal of Surgery*, **52**, 140–150.
46. Wangensteen, O.H. and Rea, C.E. (1939) The distension factor in simple intestinal obstruction. An experimental study with exclusion of swallowed air by cervical oesophagostomy. *Surgery*, **5**, 327–339.
47. Weisbrodt, N.W., Sussman, S.E., Stewart, J.J. and Burks, T.F. (1980) Effect of morphine sulfate on intestinal transit and myoelectric activity of the small intestine of the rat. *Journal of Pharmacology and Experimental Therapeutics*. **214**, 333–338.
48. Wells, C., Rawlinson, K., Tinckler, L., Jones, H. and Saunders, J. (1961) Ileus and postoperative intestinal motility. *The Lancet*, **2**, 136–137.
49. Winek, T.G., Mosely, S. and Grout, G. (1988) Pneumoperitoneum and its association with ruptured abdominal viscus. *Archives of Surgery*, **123**, 709–712.
50. Wright, J.W., Healey, T.E.J., Balfour, T.W. and Hardcastle, J.D. (1982) Effects of inhalational anaesthetic agents on the electrical and mechanical activity of the rat duodenum. *British Journal of Anaesthesia*, **54**, 1223–1229.
51. Youmans, W.B. (1968) Innervation of gastrointestinal tract. In *Handbook of Physiology*, Vol. 4 (Ed.) Code, C.F. Washington DC: American Physiology Society.

PERITONITIS AND PERFORATION

N.S. Ambrose and J. Stewart

PATHOGENESIS

Peritonitis is a primary or secondary inflammation of the peritoneum. The aetiology may be aseptic and chemical, or septic in which case it may be viral or bacterial in origin. If it is bacterial, it may be specific from a single organism, such as the pneumococcus or mycobacteria, or non-specific from intestinal bacterial flora. The course of the peritonitis may be acute or chronic, localizing or non-localizing.

The peritoneum is a single layer of mesothelial cells, which lines the abdominal cavity and most of the viscera. The peritoneum forms a number of anatomical spaces as it covers the abdominal viscera, notably the greater and lesser sac, the para-ileal and para-duodenal fossa, the subphrenic and subhepatic spaces and the pelvis. It contains about 50–100 ml of straw-coloured fluid containing lymphocytes (50%) and macrophages (40%). The peritoneal fluid is in a constant state of flux as it circulates throughout the abdominal cavity, and as it is secreted and absorbed. The peritoneal mesothelium response to irritant stimuli is by increasing in volume, for instance following trauma there may be a rapid fluid shift into the peritoneum (300–500 ml/h).[5] The peritoneum has a number of defence mechanisms by which bacterial invasion may be overcome (*Figure 6.7*).

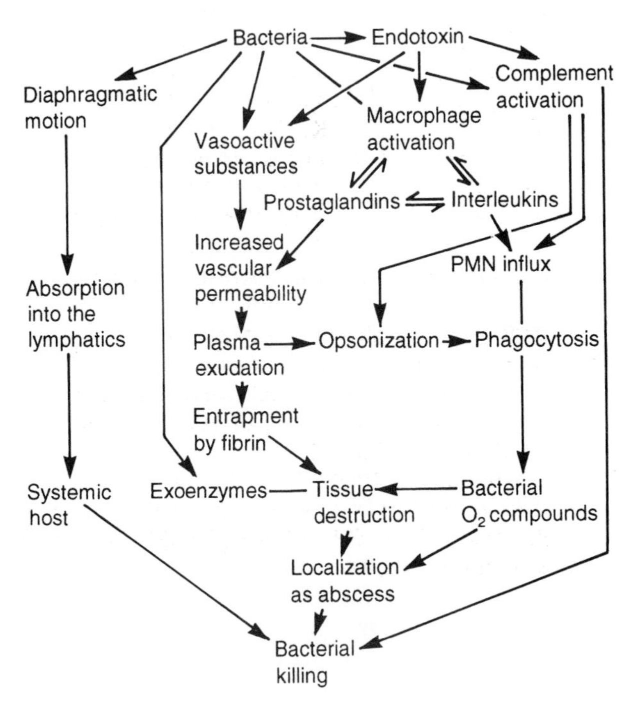

Figure 6.7 Diagrammatic representation of peritoneal defence mechanisms. (From Hau, T. (1990) *World Journal of Surgery*, **14**, 167–175.)

The prime function of the mesothelial peritoneal cells is to eliminate bacteria as they reach the peritoneal cavity. Phagocytosed bacteria quickly reach the lymphatics within a few minutes of their introduction onto the peritoneum.[2] Particulate matter is also phagocytosed and removed by the cephalad circulation of peritoneal fluid to the subdiaphragmatic lymphatics. This flow is maintained by pressure changes due to respiratory excursions as well as the valves within the lymphatics which prevent reverse flows.[1]

A second phase of defence against bacterial invasion of the peritoneum is the ability of the reticuloendothelial system, macrophages and lymphocytes to activate cellular and humoral immunological mechanisms in response to bacterial product, endotoxin and damaged cell walls.[3] A third and unique property of the peritoneum is the ability to isolate infection. It does so by the rapid production of fibrin precursors from the subbasement membrane venules in response to vasoactive substances. Fibrin traps bacteria and is not itself destroyed unless bacterial products are capable of fibrinolysis. Usually therefore fibrin forms an impermeable envelope.[4] The contained bacteria may not die but the surrounding polymorphs and lymphocytes do and in so doing bactericidal compounds form a minute abscess.

PRIMARY PERITONITIS

Primary peritonitis occurs in the absence of an overt intra-abdominal intestinal source. Patients with ascites are more prone to this condition particularly when an exogenous source is introduced by diagnostic aspiration. Spontaneous bacterial peritonitis is an uncommon but important complication of hepatic cirrhosis with or without ascites (page 1823). Commonly the bacteria found in primary peritonitis are haemolytic streptococci or pneumococci. It is thought they may gain entry to the peritoneum via the female genital tract accounting for the slight preponderance of females. Upper respiratory tract infection may be a predisposing cause. Often the diagnosis is made at laparotomy when despite a thorough search no breach is found in the gastrointestinal tract wall. Peritoneal aspiration may reveal Gram-negative organisms which makes the diagnosis of primary peritonitis more difficult to accept. At laparotomy the peritoneum is reddened and there is a milky-white, odourless exudate.

ASEPTIC PERITONITIS

Aseptic peritonitis is associated with either a chemical or foreign body irritation. Chemical peritonitis may be caused by irritation from bile, gastric or duodenal contents or meconium. The early reaction of the peritoneum to a perforated duodenal ulcer or gastric ulcer is a good example of this. The peritoneum is erythematous and there is considerable exudate of fibrin and lymph. The peritoneum may become secondarily infected after 12–24 hours. Foreign bodies may also provoke a reaction, probably the most important of which is starch peritonitis. Washing starch from gloves preoperatively or using powderless (starchless) gloves has reduced this condition effectively.

SECONDARY PERITONITIS

Most patients presenting with peritonitis have secondary peritonitis implying bacterial contamination from the gastrointestinal tract. A few patients may present with penetrating abdominal injuries or with exogenous derived infection. Perforation of a previously formed abscess into the peritoneal cavity causes acute bacterial peritonitis. The causes of secondary peritonitis are myriad but a systematic approach to classification is provided for ease of diagnosis (*Table 6.2*). Reference should be made to the text for an account of specific diseases.

Table 6.2 Causes of acute peritonitis and the differentiation from non-surgical causes of acute abdominal pain

Surgical	*Non-surgical*
Gastrointestinal	Cardiac
Perforated peptic ulcer	Pericarditis
Acute cholecystitis	Myocardial infarction
Acute pancreatitis	Pulmonary
Acute appendicitis	Pneumonia
Meckel's diverticulitis	Pulmonary infarction
Acute diverticulitis	Gastrointestinal
Small bowel obstruction	Hepatitis
Large bowel obstruction	Gastroenteritis
Traumatic ruptured viscus	Endocrine
Gynaecological	Diabetic ketoacidosis
Salpingitis	Adrenal insufficiency
Complicated ovarian cyst	Metabolic
Ectopic pregnancy	Acute intermittent porphyria
Vascular	Lead poisoning
Aneurysm	Familial Mediterranean fever
Ischaemia	Hyperlipidaemia
	Muscoloskeletal
	Rectus sheath haematoma
	CNS
	Tabes dorsalis
	Nerve root compression
	Renal
	Pyelonephritis
	Haematological
	Sickle-cell crisis

CLINICAL FEATURES

The history will in many cases provide an accurate guide to the pathology. The mode of onset of the pain, its character and its quality must be sought. Examination of the patient begins with an overall assessment from the end of the bed. The demeanor of the patient, rigidity and impaired abdominal wall movement and his or her conscious state will be noted immediately on inspection. Rapid, shallow respirations with dehydration, sunken eyes and cold clammy extremities suggest advanced peritonitis.

Symptoms and signs depend on the aetiology and particularly the duration of the process. Fever and tachycardia indicate a progressive illness often with hypotension, oliguria and hyperventilation. As the disease progresses the patient becomes less able to respond and may become hypothermic. Vomiting may be related to pain rather than to obstruction.

Abdominal pain of peritonitis may provide a useful clue to the diagnosis. When the inflammatory process starts, the visceral peritoneum, which is poorly innervated, allows only poor localization with diffuse cramp-like pain. The visceral peritoneum responds mostly to distension, pressure and traction and the biliary tract is better innervated than the rest of the intestines, thus allowing more accurate localization in this area. Parietal peritoneum with both somatic and visceral nerves is more likely to realize sensory stimuli from a local process, hence the finding of both local tenderness on palpation and rebound tenderness. Guarding of the anterior abdominal wall suggests local irritation. Onset of pain may give a clue to the aetiology. Sudden onset after a dull ache may suggest a perforated viscus. Shifting visceral pain or referred pain must be distinguished by a careful history. It is common to find shoulder tip pain in the presence of peritonitis as the parietal peritoneum of the diaphragm is irritated. In the presence of a perforation, pain may be felt among the track of the fluid that escapes. This is seen well after perforated duodenal ulcer with pain in the right lower quadrant and pelvic irritation in perforated appendicitis or diverticular disease.

In peritonitis the abdomen is usually distended with bowel sounds that are either hypoactive or absent. It is unusual to be able to feel a mass, but under anaesthesia prior to laparotomy a mass may be obvious giving further clues to its aetiology.

Rectal examination is mandatory, but may be difficult to interpret in the presence of severe pain.

INVESTIGATIONS

Only a few laboratory tests are useful in peritonitis. Blood should be taken for a full blood count and cross-matching, and a serum analyse should be requested. Serum should be kept for estimation of liver function tests if necessary at a later date. Urinalysis should be performed. Serum electrolytes are useful in the later management of the patient by parenteral fluid replacement. A peritoneal tap may be useful particularly in the presence of trauma, but there is always a small risk of introducing exogenous bacteria into the peritoneum.

RADIOLOGY

Good quality radiographs are essential for the accurate preoperative diagnosis of a patient with peritonitis. The radiographs should be reviewed by the clinician in charge and the radiologist prior to any decision to operate. Many patients clearly do not require radiological investigations such as those with appendicitis and those with ruptured aortic aneurysm. It is usual to request a chest radiograph, and erect and supine (or lateral decubitus depending on local expertise) abdominal radiographs. It is important to exclude bony fractures on all the radiographs seen. Calcification in organs, particularly the pancreas (*Figure 6.8*), or in calculi may indicate the site of the pathology.

An erect chest radiograph should exclude intrathoracic causes of abdominal pain and may reveal intra-abdominal free gas, gas in the mediastinum or subcutaneous emphysema. If an erect radiograph cannot be performed for technical reasons, then the lateral decubitus abdominal radiograph must be performed.

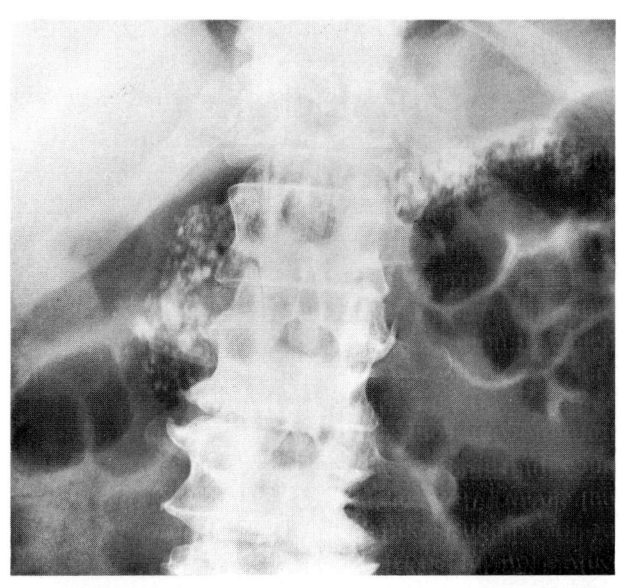

(a)

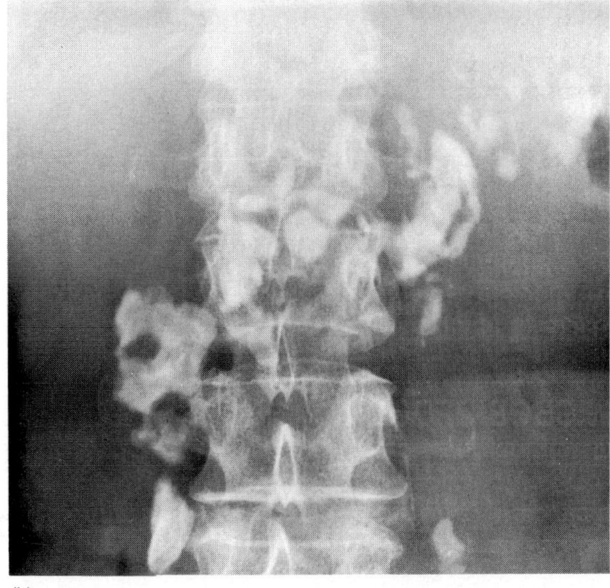

(b)

Figure 6.8 Plain abdominal radiographs: (a) microcalcification within the pancreas, indicative of acute-on-chronic pancreatitis – it is important to rule this out as a cause of peritonitis; (b) macrocalcification within the pancreas and associated lymph nodes.

Free intraperitoneal gas seen on any radiograph indicates a perforated viscus, provided that the patient has not had a laparoscopy or laparotomy within 10 days, although it is possible for mediastinal gas to track down into the retroperitoneum and into the peritoneal cavity (*Figure 6.9*).

The real value of abdominal radiographs lies in the interpretation of the bowel gas shadows. Local peritonitis and generalized peritonitis may have

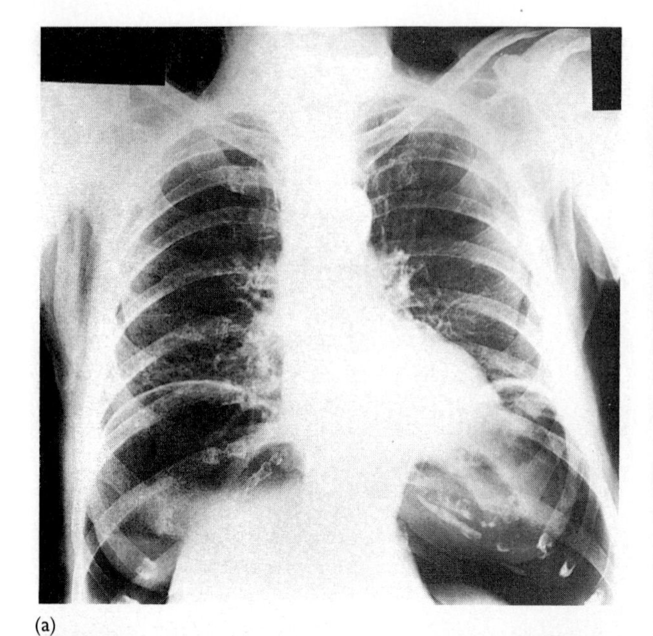

(a)

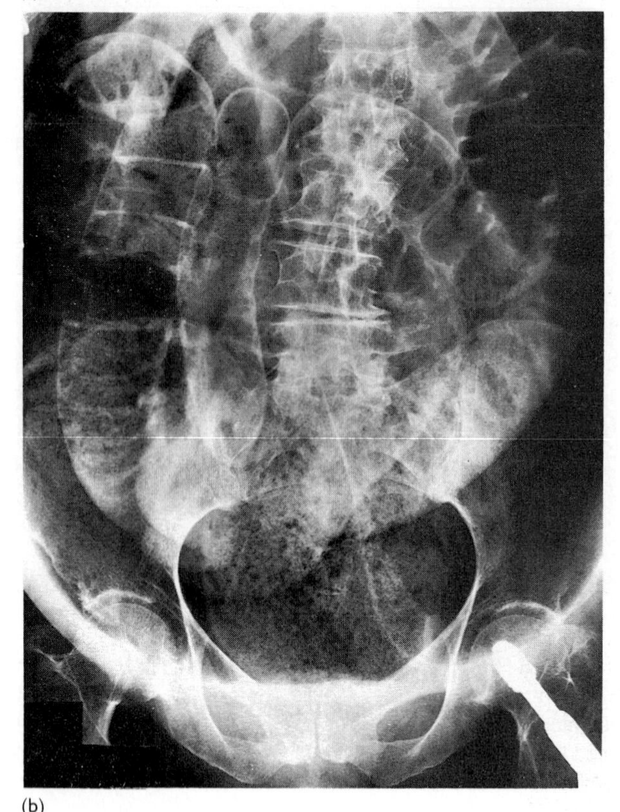

(b)

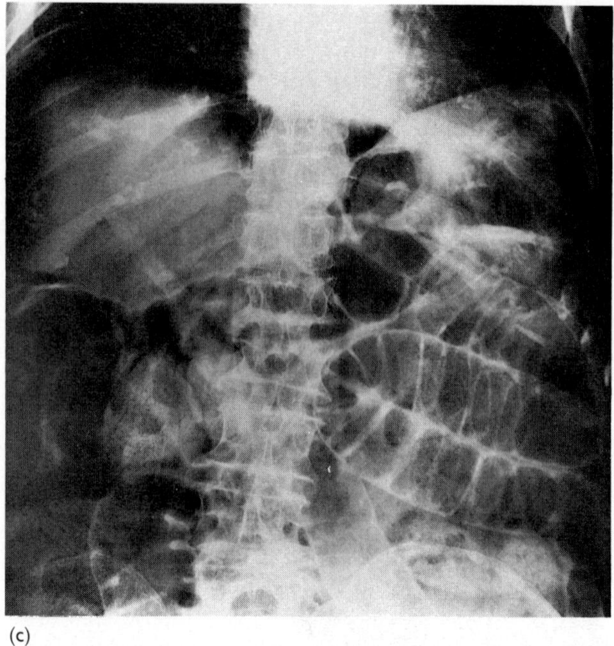

(c)

Figure 6.9 Gross pneumoperitoneum with air on both sides of the bowel wall. The falciform ligament is outlined, and the obliterated umbilical arteries can be seen on the supine radiograph. (a) Chest radiograph; (b) plain abdominal radiograph: supine; (c) plain erect abdominal radiograph.

characteristic radiological appearances. A sentinel loop may indicate a local area of irritation whilst a paucity of gas may reflect peritoneal fluid or high obstruction. The site of obstruction, whatever the cause, may be assumed from the characteristic bowel gas patterns in the jejunum, ileum and colon (*Figure 6.10*). The unusual must be recognized such as 'crack-packing' (*Figure 6.11*).

Air in places where it should not normally be present, such as the biliary tree, suggests a cholecyst or choledochoenteric fistula; if air is found in the bladder there may be an enterovesical fistula. These findings may indicate either sepsis or a fistula into a gas-filled viscus.

ULTRASOUND

Ultrasound has become a useful, quick, non-invasive investigation in patients with acute abdominal pain. It is particularly useful in those with acute biliary pain.

Contrast studies are not usually indicated unless more precise information is needed, as for instance in a possible perforated carcinoma of the colon (*Figure 6.12*) or in mesenteric ischaemia. Diagnosis of a perforated peptic ulcer may require a water-soluble contrast swallow and meal.

TREATMENT

Clearly the treatment of peritonitis must be directed at the primary cause which in most cases will require

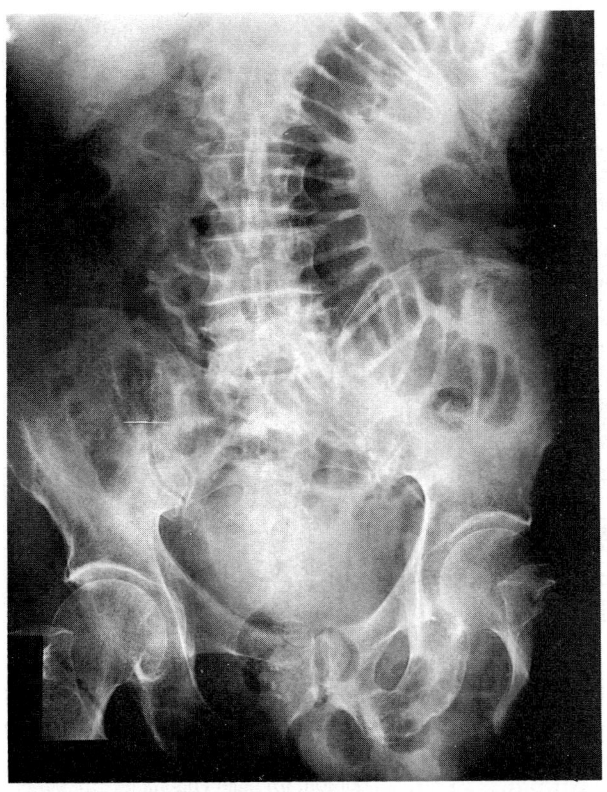

Figure 6.10 Small bowel obstruction due to a left inguinal hernia, with proximal dilatation and perforation.

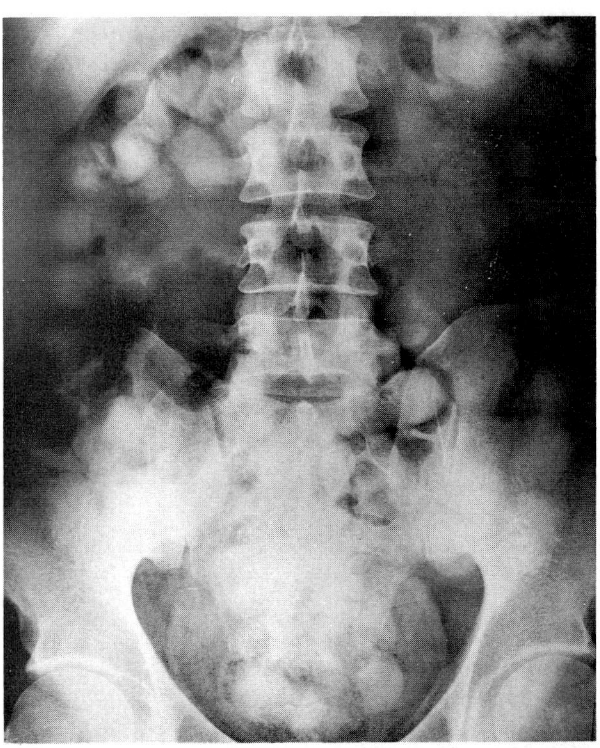

Figure 6.11 Plain abdominal radiograph showing multiple condoms containing cocaine within the bowel lumen.

surgical intervention. In resuscitating patients fluid needs to be replaced proportional to losses, and in attempting to do so accurate fluid balance must be achieved and a urine output re-established. This will require measurement of central venous pressure and hourly assessment of urine output. Therefore a urinary catheter must be passed. A broad-spectrum antibiotic must be prescribed and given intravenously – the spectrum must include the gut anaerobes but may be modified in the light of operative findings. Analgesia must be given to allow control of pain taking into account the respiratory function of the patient. In extreme cases it may be prudent to admit patients to the intensive care unit for preoper-

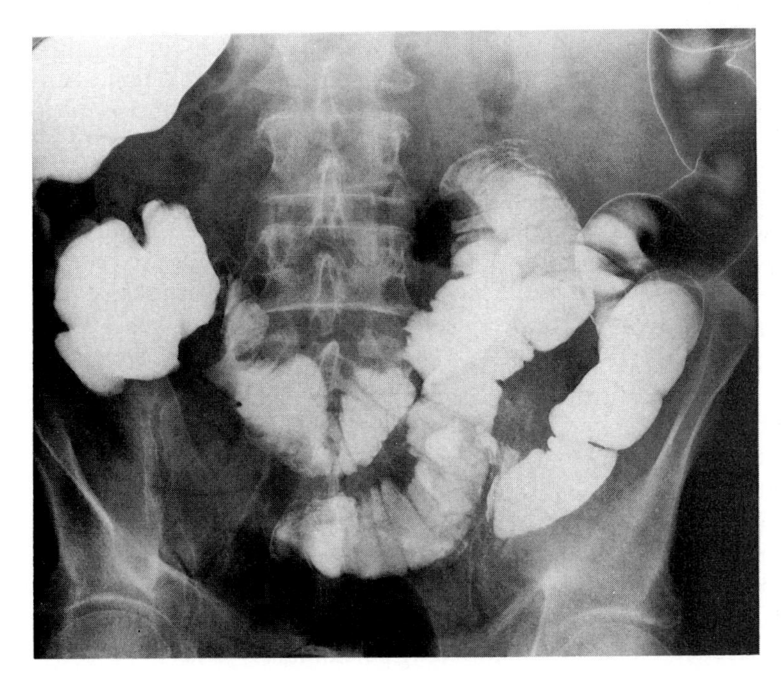

Figure 6.12 Contrast radiograph showing imprinting of the serosal surface of the bowel with peritoneal secondaries from a carcinoma of the colon.

ative monitoring and assessment. The primary cause of the peritonitis must be identified and the defect in the viscus is closed, exteriorized and resected.

REFERENCES

1. Allen, L. (1936) The peritoneal stomata. *Anatomical Record*, **67**, 89–103.
2. Hau, T., Hoffmann, R. and Simmons, R.L. (1978) Mechanisms of the adjuvant effect of haemoglobin in experimental peritonitis. 1. In vivo inhibition of peritoneal leukocytosis. *Surgery*, **83**, 223–229.
3. Largen, M.T. and Tannenbaum, C.S. (1986) LPS regulation of specific protein synthesis in murine peritoneal macrophages. *Journal of Immunology*, **136**, 988–993.
4. Majno, G. and Palade, G. E. (1961) Studies in inflammation. 1. The effect of histamine and serotonin on vascular permeability. An electron microscopic study. *Journal of Biophysical and Biochemical Cytology*, **11**, 571–605.
5. Samson, R. and Pasternak, B.M. (1979) Current state of surgery of the omentum. *Surgery, Gynecology and Obstetrics*, **149**, 437–442.

ABDOMINAL ABSCESSES

N.S. Ambrose and J. Stewart

Abscesses within the abdominal cavity usually comprise one of three major groups: intraperitoneal, retroperitoneal and visceral. Different types may occur depending on the underlying pathology. Commonly, abscesses may arise postoperatively or they may arise de novo from intestinal disease. The morbidity associated with intra-abdominal abscess is considerable. Accurate localization and early diagnosis may help to minimize this. The clinical course of an abscess may be insidious and diagnosis may not be considered for some time, hence therapy may be delayed.

MICROBIOLOGY

Bacteria reach the peritoneal cavity through perforations in the bowel or from primary infection of an abdominal organ.[4] Peritoneal contamination may also occur at operation on the gut.[3] Rarely bacteria may enter the abdominal cavity by extension of abscesses from adjacent organs such as the lung. Evidence also suggests that bacterial permeation through the bowel wall may lead to intra-abdominal abscesses in the absence of frank perforation.[8]

The intestinal bacterial population is extremely varied and the majority of bacteria isolated from abscesses derive from the gut flora. Fortunately, only a few intestinal bacteria are virulent enough to be found consistently causing sepsis in the abdominal cavity (*Table 6.3*). There is a qualitative difference in the bacteria isolated from abscesses in immunocompromised patients,[5] but little difference in the number and species from patients with free peritonitis and abscesses.[2] Clinical presentation may be modified by the early use of broad-spectrum antibiotics which may mask symptoms without eradicating the septic focus. Inadequate antibacterial therapy either in terms of its spectrum or its pharmacokinetics may allow an abscess to persist.

PATHOGENESIS

The pathogenic potential of bacteria within abscess cavities or those free within the peritoneal cavity is related to their ability to produce endotoxins, exoenzymes or by their direct action on the cell. Synergism between aerobic and anaerobic bacteria also plays an important role in pathogenic potential of abscesses.[1] The provision of growth factors, protection against host defences and creation of an environment suitable for growth are peculiar to different abscesses. The abscess wall acts as a physical barrier preventing the penetration of antibiotics which thus allows synergy between bacteria within the abscess.

Many substances may act as adjuvants which increase the pathogenicity of infections. Bile, gastric juice, necrotic material, blood, suture material and other foreign particles (such as bacterial polysaccharide) may inhibit phagocytosis, lower surface tension, reduce chemotaxis and activate macrophages. Thus contamination of the peritoneal cavity in the presence of substances may predispose to abscess or spreading peritonitis.

Table 6.3 Microbiology of intraperitoneal infections

	Peritonitis (*n* = 383)	*Subphrenic abscess* (*n* = 34)	*Immuno-suppressed patients* (*n* = 47)
Aerobic			
Staphylococci	29 (8%)	–	7 (15%)
Streptococci	108 (2%)	16 (47%)	20 (43%)
Escherichia coli	235 (61%)	23 (68%)	25 (53%)
Klebsiella/Enterobacter spp.	101 (26%)	5 (15%)	20 (43%)
Proteus sp.	87 (23%)	9 (26%)	5 (11%)
Pseudomonas sp.	30 (8%)	2 (6%)	9 (19%)
Serratia marcescapens	–	–	8 (8%)
Anaerobic			
Bacteroides sp.	288 (75%)	20 (59%)	11 (23%)
Anaerobic cocci	97 (25%)	12 (35%)	2 (4%)
Clostridia	67 (18%)	12 (35%)	4 (9%)
Fusobacteria	34 (9%)	9 (27%)	–
Eubacteria	94 (25%)	2 (6%)	–
Yeasts/fungi			
Candida spp.	6 (2%)	–	10 (21%)
Others	–	–	2 (4%)

Data from the literature.[3–5,7]

CLINICAL FEATURES

An abscess is associated with pain, swelling, tenderness, fever and general malaise. If superficial an abscess is both red and hot. Characteristically an abscess is associated with a high, swinging temperature. However, in patients who are immunocompromised these features may be absent altogether. Provided the patient is not neutropenic, polymorphonucleocytosis is generally found. The presence of an intra-abdominal abscess may be associated with abnormalities of liver function tests, particularly elevation of alkaline phosphatase. It is unusual for an abscess to cause obstruction unless it is extremely large but abscesses may be responsible for the failure of fistulas to resolve.

Abscesses in specific sites have well-recognized symptoms accompanying them. The types and origins of some common examples are given in *Table 6.4*.

INTRAPERITONEAL ABSCESSES

Primary perforation of the gut, secondary perforation associated with an anastamosis dehiscence, translocation of bacteria across bowel wall or a septic process anywhere in the peritoneal cavity may be responsible for intra-abdominal abscess. The abscess is usually walled by adjacent viscera, particularly the omentum, small bowel, peritoneum and the abdominal wall. Not uncommonly the process may produce more than one cavity in the same vicinity and is usually found in a dependent area (pelvis, paracolic gutters or subphrenic spaces).

Table 6.4 Sites and common sources of abscess

Site	*Source of abscess*
Visceral	Liver, spleen, pancreas, septicaemia
Subphrenic spaces	Ruptured viscus, postoperative
Subhepatic space	Gallbladder disease, postoperative
Lesser sac	Perforated gastric ulcer, pancreatitis
Interloop abscess	Any primary or secondary peritonitis
Retroperitoneal	Perforation of duodenum, ascending or descending colon, pancreatitis
Psoas	Disease of spine, kidneys or retroperitoneal gut
Pelvic	Appendicitis, diverticular disease, salpingitis, Crohn's disease, postoperative
Perianal	Pelvic sepsis or anorectal disease

Pelvic abscess

Pelvic abscess is a common sequel of intra-abdominal sepsis. It is characterized by urinary symptoms, tenesmus, passage of mucus per rectum and a palpable collection in the pelvis on rectal examination. It is seen in patients with appendicitis, diverticular disease and tubovarian abscess. It may follow peritonitis or pelvic surgery. Uncommonly a pelvic abscess is found following radiotherapy to the pelvis or in association with a pelvic tumour. Resolution of a pelvic abscess is uncommon and most require drainage. Undrained, most will discharge spontaneously through the rectum or vagina but uncommonly they may rupture into the peritoneal cavity causing peritonitis. It is usual to drain pelvic abscess through the rectum or the vagina depending on the location of the abscess when the patient is anaesthetized.

Subphrenic abscess

Subphrenic abscess is characterized by the surgical adage 'pus somewhere, pus nowhere, pus under the diaphragm'. It describes a collection of pus in contact with a diaphragmatic surface. As a consequence of the diversity of the peritoneal anatomy in this area, it is usual to describe several named collections such that accurate localization may be facilitated.[7] Right and left anterior and posterior subphrenic spaces are described as well as the subhepatic space (*Figure 6.13*) and in right and left extraperitoneal spaces. The most common collection around the liver is the right subhepatic space which may complicate peritonitis, upper gastrointestinal or pancreaticobiliary surgery, or biliary disease.

It is common to find no clinical signs in the abdomen but a chest radiograph may be grossly abnormal with effusion and consolidation. An elevated diaphragm may be visible on plain abdominal radiology and abnormal gas patterns may be visible.

RETROPERITONEAL ABSCESS

Psoas abscess is the most common of these. Whilst tuberculous psoas abscess from the lumbar or lower thoracic spine is now uncommon in Western practice, it is still seen in areas where the disease is endemic. Abscesses in this area are notoriously difficult to diagnose and may present below the inguinal ligament in the femoral triangle. Common causes include carcinoma of the colon and diverticular disease where perforation of the viscus occurs posteriorly. Retrocaecal or retroileal appendicitis may be complicated by a psoas abscess.

Ileal Crohn's disease may fistulate into the retroperitoneal space causing psoas abscess. Sepsis arising from either kidney or the lower dorsal and lumbar spine is an important cause of psoas abscess.

As many of these abscesses are associated with gas-forming bowel organisms they may be detected by plain radiographs. Abnormalities of hip movement, particularly a fixed flexion deformity associated with a limp, may misdirect the unwary clinician. It is vitally important that the underlying pathology be identified and treated because failure to do so could result in continuing sepsis or prolonged drainage due to fistula formation.

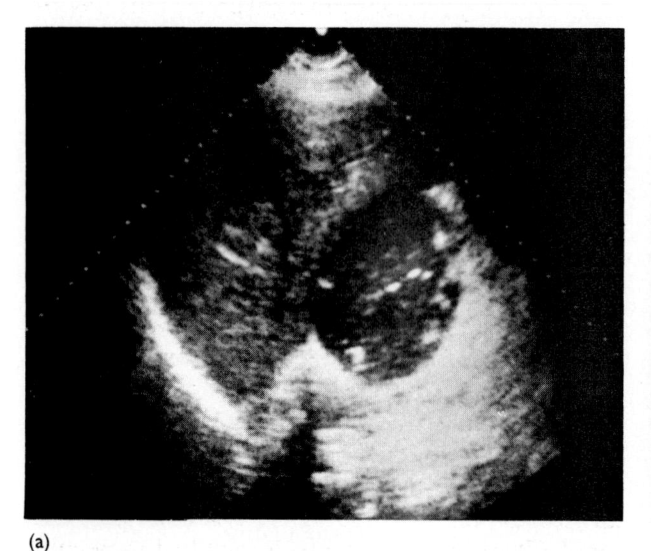

(a)

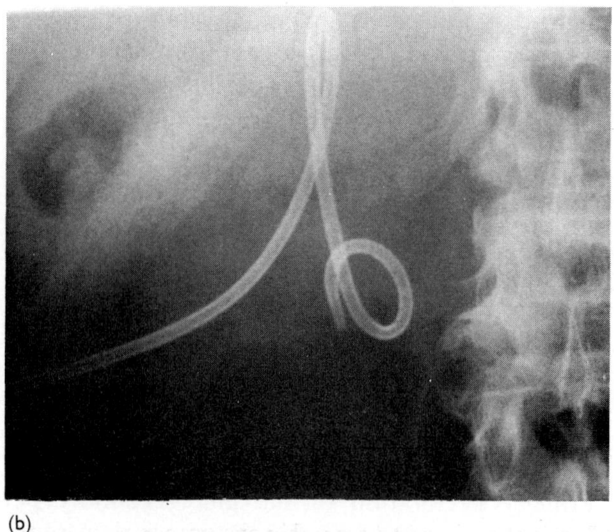

(b)

Figure 6.13 (a) Ultrasound of subhepatic abscess; (b) plain radiograph to show pigtail catheter within abscess cavity.

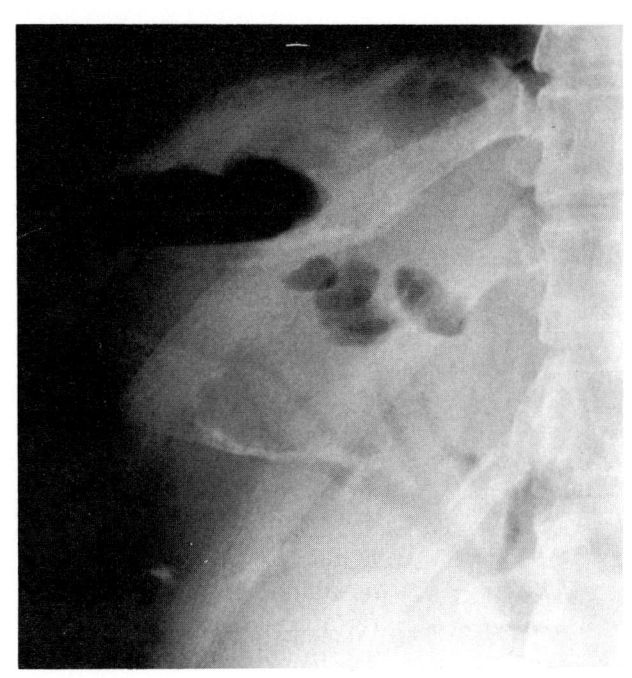

Figure 6.14 Plain radiograph showing gas-filled cavity within the liver and outlining biliary radicals.

VISCERAL ABSCESS

Across the world the most common visceral abscess is hepatic (*Figure 6.14*), but in the UK and USA hepatic abscess is uncommon. Splenic abscess is even more rare.

Most visceral abscesses are now of unknown aetiology. The decreasing incidence of portal pyaemia due to inflammatory disease of the gastrointestinal tract (appendicitis and diverticulitis particularly) and the increasing incidence of obstructed cholangitis in an increasingly elderly population has changed the pattern of hepatic abscess. Multiple abscesses in the liver caused by *Escherichia coli* or *Klebsiella* sp. are becoming more frequent and are usually secondary to biliary disease. Abscesses may be single or multiple. Multiple abscesses carry a high mortality which may be as high as 80%. Jaundice is a bad prognostic sign.

Clinically these patients are extremely ill with pain, chest signs, fever and night sweats. Hydatid and amoebic abscesses should be excluded by serology as treatable causes of intrahepatic cysts or abscesses.

INVESTIGATIONS

Clearly the overriding need in the presence of intra-abdominal pus is to achieve early drainage. Over the last 15 years, advances in visualization and localization of purulent collections within the peritoneal cavity have made enormous strides which have resulted in a progressive decrease in the morbidity and mortality of the condition. To reduce the mortality from its high level in untreated sepsis, early detection, accurate localization and early treatment are mandatory. Plain abdominal radiology, ultrasound, CT and radionuclide imaging are all important modalities of investigation. It is important that clinicians become familiar with all available techniques because they are complementary (*Table 6.5*).

Plain radiographs may be helpful by showing diagnostic extraluminal gas patterns, effusions, diaphragmatic displacement or a mass. Contrast radiology should be used sparingly because it will interfere with subsequent ultrasound or CT.

Ultrasound, although probably the most available non-invasive modality, has limitations. Tenderness may preclude good 'windows' for scanning. Bowel gas due to obstruction and ileus distorts the image. Bone and fat also make some windows impossible. The contents of the abscess may make different echo patterns difficult to interpret. As the origin of the abscess may be from a variety of organs the contents will be physically different (bile, lymph, urine, serum or blood). This may be particularly difficult in the pelvis where intraluminal ultrasound may be more efficient.

Computer-augmented tomography with contrast, particularly when faster scanners are utilized, achieves high resolution of many intravisceral and intraperitoneal collections where other modalities of imaging fail. Because of the cost and lack of availability of MRI scanning, CT will almost certainly remain the modality of choice for abscess detection in the next decade. Although drainage using CT presents many practical limitations (*Figure 6.15* and *Figure 6.16*), it may be very effective for deep abscesses.

Detection of abscesses and differentiation from inflammation may be achieved using radionuclide scanning, particularly using either gallium-67 or indium-111 as isotopes. Indium is usually preferred because it is more sensitive and can be chelated with EDTA (ethylenediamine tetraacetic acid) to leukocytes.

All of these imaging techniques offer different advantages and it is probable that more than one method will need to be used in most clinical situations. Whilst nuclide examination offers abscess localization and identification, it has the drawback that needle aspiration cannot be undertaken with the technique. By contrast, ultrasonography and rapid CT scanning provide a facility for needle-guided aspiration and percutaneous drainage.

Table 6.5 Advantages and disadvantages of imaging modalities

Imaging method	*Advantages*	*Disadvantages*
Plain radiograph	Available Quick	Inaccurate (50%)
Ultrasound	Available Drainage possible Sensitive (93%)	Limited by windows Ileus, fat, bone, pain, operator and equipment dependent
CT	Drainage possible Sensitive (95%) Extraperitoneal information	Timing (within 1 week) Multiple organ failure Size of cuts
MRI	Retroperitoneal image	Ferromagnetic incompatibility Scan time Uncooperative patients
Gallium-67	Inexpensive Sensitivity (80%)	Slow Tumour uptake Bowel excretion Acute infection missed
Indium-111	Specificity (93%) Infected prostheses	Labelling technique Leukocyte function Non-infected collections Stomas/incisions

TREATMENT

Once an abscess is detected it should be drained efficiently and quickly. Percutaneous drainage using ultrasound or CT has greatly reduced the morbidity from abscesses and is now the preferred method provided the abscess is not multilocular and provided it is accessible without the fear of damaging bile ducts, bowel, vascular structures or the urinary tract. Drainage depends on accurate localization. A number of rules need to be considered. It is unwise to penetrate solid organs, particularly the liver or spleen, or the pleural space to reach an abscess. Three or four separate abscesses may be effectively drained but more than this usually defies the ingenuity of most interventional radiologists. Staged percutaneous drainage followed by definitive surgery when the patient has been resuscitated should be considered where appropriate. The success of percutaneous drainage largely depends on patient selection, abscess location and localization, the type of abscess and the underlying pathology. The successes of percutaneous drainage is in the order of 80% and compares favourably with conventional surgical drainage.

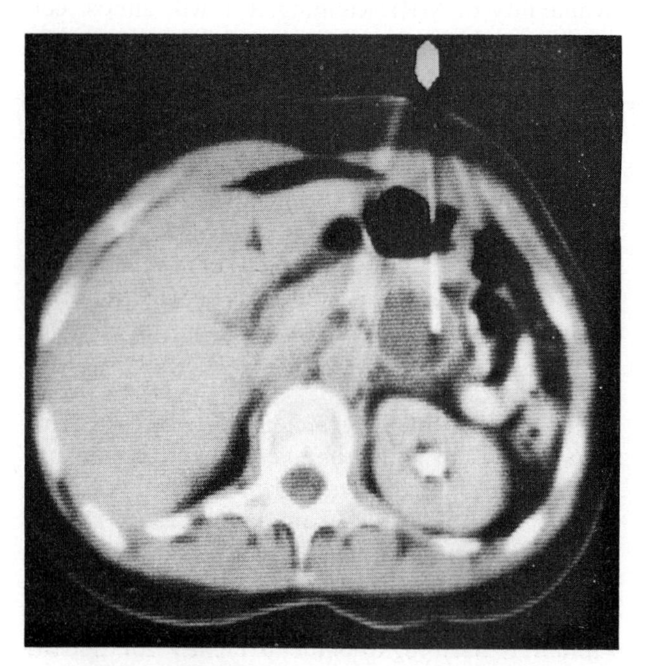

Figure 6.15 CT-guided drain into pancreatic abscess.

Mortality is dependent on the aetiology, the site, and the source of the abscess as well as a variety of host factors, and varies from 0% to 13%. Percutaneous drainage usually takes longer to drain completely than a surgically drained cavity. Complications of percutaneous drainage are similar to those of surgical drainage and include: septicaemia, vascular injury, visceral injury and fistula. Drainage of visceral abscesses within spleen, liver or pancreas using percutaneous techniques remain controversial.[6]

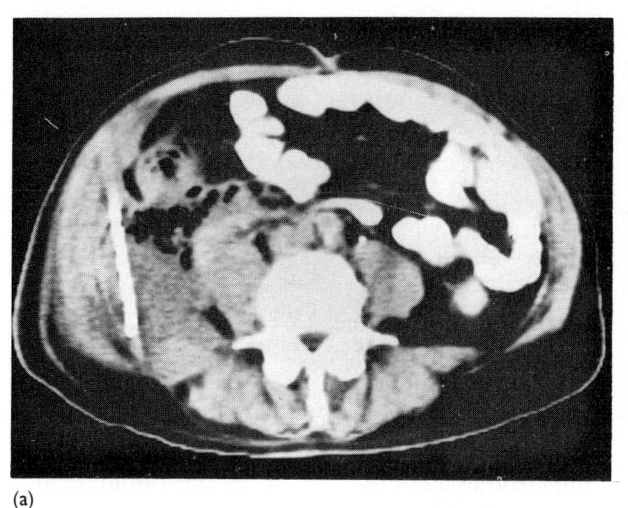

(a)

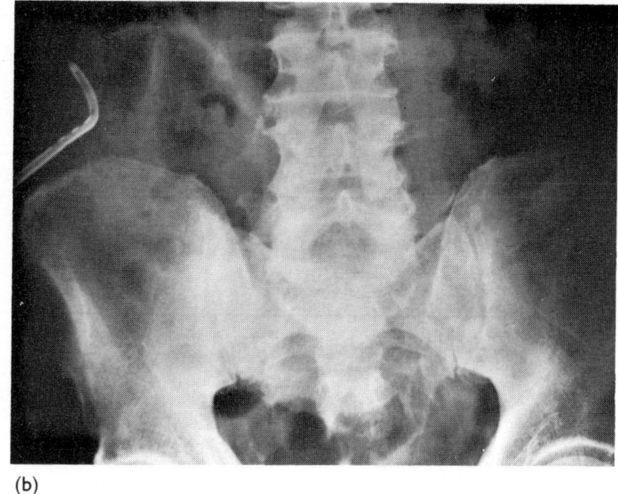

(b)

Figure 6.16 (a) Plain iliac fossa abscess drained under CT control; (b) plain radiograph to show position of pigtail catheter.

REFERENCES

1. Bjornson, H.S. (1982) Bacterial synergy, virulence factors and host defense mechanisms in the pathogenesis of intraabdominal infection. In: *Topics in Intraabdominal Surgical Infections* (Ed.) Simmons, R.L. pp. 65–78. Norwalk: Appleton-Century-Crofts.
2. Hau, T. (1990) Bacteria, toxins and the peritoneum. *World Journal of Surgery*. **14**, 167–175.
3. Hau, T., Ahrenholz, D.H. and Simmons, R.L. (1979) Secondary bacterial peritonitis: the biological basis of treatment. *Current Problems in Surgery*, **16**, 1.
4. Hau, T., Mozes, M.F. and Jonasson, O. (1975) Peritonitis nach Nierentransplantation. *Langenbecks Archiv für Chirurgie*, **353**, 269. 1975.
5. Hau, T., van Hook, E.J., Simmons, R.L. and Najarian, J.S. (1978) Prognostic factors of peritoneal infections in transplanted patients. *Surgery*, **84**, 403.
6. Pruett, T.L. and Simmons, R.L. (1988) Status of percutaneous catheter drainage of abscesses. *Surgical Clinics of North America*, **68**, 80–105.
7. Wang, S.M.S. and Wilson, S.E. (1977) Subphrenic abscess: the new epidemiology. *Archives of Surgery*, **112**, 934.
8. Wells, C.L., Rotstein, O.D., Pruett, T.L. and Simmons, R.L. (1986) Intestinal bacteria translocate into experimental abscesses. *Archives of Surgery*, **121**, 102–107.

ACUTE APPENDICITIS

D.J. Leaper

INTRODUCTION

The correct diagnosis of acute appendicitis is a great challenge, often best made by experienced middle-grade staff who manage the condition frequently, and the rewards of successful surgery are then achieved both quickly and in a satisfying way. Nevertheless, we should not become complacent: surgical intervention is still followed by an appreciable morbidity and mortality; wound infections and the number of perforated and gangrenous appendices can be lowered by active surveillance and audit of process; and controversies remain such as incidental appendicectomy, removal of normal appendices in young women, and the over-utilization of ultrasound and other imaging modalities which stimulate a large number of publications each year.

The first descriptions of the appendix have been attributed to Andreas Versalius (1543) and Vidii (1550) although it was seen earlier in the anatomical drawings of Leonardo da Vinci and Berengaria Da Carpi. Morgagni (1719) should be credited with the first accurate anatomical description. Appendicitis was described in autopsy studies by Lorenz Heister (1711) and John Hunter (1769). The first operation was successfully performed between these later two dates by Claudius Amyand (1735) who removed an inflamed appendix through a hernial sac. The most famous appendicectomy, and the drama which surrounded the event described so well by Ellis,[9] must be that performed by Treves on King Edward VII, thereby postponing his coronation.

Reginald Heber Fitz was one among many American and British surgeons who buried the controversy of 'typhlitis' and 'perityphlitis' and correctly advocated the advantages of early operation. Many of these surgeons did not publish their similar views but this background has been well summarized by Geroulanos[10] and Cooper.[5]

EPIDEMIOLOGY

In the developed Western countries appendicitis has been epidemic. Approximately 15% of people are subjected to appendicectomy, appendicitis being slightly more common in males than in females. Appendicitis can occur at any age, but the risk is maximal around the second decade of life with a 1% chance of developing the disease in each of the adolescent years.[25]

In the last 25 years admission rates have halved in England and Wales, although appendicectomy is still the most commonly performed abdominal operation.[29] This decline cannot be entirely attributed to the uptake of high-fibre diets because the decline began before this fashionable trend.[12] There are no clear racial or familial factors but this dietary link has become regarded as the most important factor.[4] It seems that in Western countries and those undergoing economic development there is widespread consumption of diets low in fibre and high in meat and sugar. This contrasts with Africa and Asia, particularly rural communities, where appendicitis is rare. When these communities migrate or are developed then appendicitis soon becomes as common as it is in the indigenous population of countries in which 'refined' diets are eaten.

PATHOLOGY

The true initiating factor of appendicitis remains hypothetical. There are two classic theories, one being of an obstructive cause and one catarrhal.[19] The obstructive cause is probably not disputed because many inflamed appendices are found to contain a faecalith (or other obstructing lesion such as a foreign body, mural lymphoid hyperplasia, worms, tumour or even a gallstone). The appendix has a good end-arterial blood supply and obstruction can lead to oedema and venous congestion, which in turn lead to arterial insufficiency and gangrene. Obstructing faecaliths are more likely to be associated with progression to gangrene and perforation. Obstruction can also be related to a distal obstructing pathology, usually inflammatory or neoplastic disease, which should not be forgotton, particularly in older patients.[13]

Infection may be an initiating factor in younger patients when specific or non-specific enteritis causes lymphoid hyperplasia. This was called catarrhal appendicitis and, because the blood supply to the appendix is not jeopardized so much, its progress tends to resolution. The epidemic of appendicitis in young adolescents may relate to the public health reforms which have been undertaken. It has been suggested that children are no longer exposed to the number and variety of pathogens as previously but if and when they are, in adolescence, they may develop appendicitis.[2,3] Once the appendicular mucosa is breached by infection, then inflammation and oedema leads to the pathological sequence that may result in peritonitis or gangrene.

The syndrome of chronic or recurrent appendicitis is still a thorny topic.[28] There is no doubt that many patients describe similar milder episodes of pain prior to the admission that ends in appendicectomy. Equally there are patients, with a history and findings on examination that are suggestive of early appendicitis, whose symptoms resolve with active observation. Who knows how many of these patients have chronic or recurrent appendicitis? Careful outpatient surveillance and audit have yet to give a clear answer.

The bacteria involved in appendicitis are essentially those that are present in the colon.[24] *Bacteroides* spp, coliforms (particularly *Escherichia coli*) and *Streptococcus faecalis* form the majority of harvested organisms with *Clostridium perfringens* and other streptococci and staphylococci forming the remainder, although the latter are rarely found in wound infections. The combination of anaerobe and aerobe acts in synergy and appropriate precautions at operation and with prophylactic antibiotics are mandatory.

CLINICAL FEATURES

The diagnosis of acute appendicitis is essentially clinical, but there is some pressure to avoid scars and adhesions (with a possible but unproven risk of infertility in women). There is a continuing diagnostic challenge[34] to reduce the number of negative appendicectomies (up to 20%), which are not performed without complications,[20] and are most common in young women. Consequently, there is a drive towards sophisticated investigations, however simple, but it was shown almost 20 years ago[7] that computer-aided diagnosis could improve diagnostic rates using clinical data alone.[22] Discriminant factors can be identified by multivariant analysis with scores[41] and aids [14] that reduce the negative appendicectomy rate without an increase in the incidence of gangrenous or perforated appendices. The simple act of form filling can improve diagnostic accuracy, and as acute appendicitis has such a variable history the active observation approach is justified when undertaken by experienced clinicians.

Classically acute appendicitis presents with visceral, ill-localized, mid-gut, periumbilical colic. There may be anorexia and vomiting, and constipation, but these are not useful discriminants. Within 12–24 hours the pain becomes parietal, well localised and constant in the right iliac fossa which is worsened by movement or coughing. The patient may be pyrexial (37–38°C) with facial flushing but fetor oris and a furred tongue are unhelpful. Tenderness is localized according to the anatomical position of the appendix. Tenderness with guarding and rebound over McBurney's point has been described for over a century.[26] This may be associated with psoas spasm, Rovsing's sign (tenderness in the right iliac fossa with pressure in the left iliac fossa) and Sherren's sign (hyperaesthesia in the right iliac fossa). In 15–20% of patients the appendix may be either retrocaecal (and cause confusion with cholecystitis or peptic ulceration) or retroileal (causing confusion with small bowel or ureteric obstruction). Pelvic appendicitis may cause diarrhoea or urinary frequency, and be confused with urinary tract infection or pelvic inflammatory disease in women.

The commonly seen diseases which may be confused with appendicitis are listed in Table 6.6. Non-specific abdominal pain is a widely used term for those patients who do not have a specific diagnosis made and who are sent home without further investigation; those patients who have a normal appendicectomy also belong to this category. This is a field requiring careful audit and surveillance. Only then can appropriate follow-up be instituted with feedback on negative appendicectomy rates or the later manifestation of other diseases.

Table 6.6 Differential diagnosis of acute appendicitis

Local disease	Non-specific abdominal pain Non-specific enteritis Mesenteric adenitis Specific enteritis (*Yersinia* spp., amoebiasis, tuberculosis, giardiasis, typhoid) Meckel's diverticulitis Solitary caecal diverticulum Sigmoid diverticulitis Inflammatory bowel disease (e.g. Crohn's) Neoplastic bowel disease (e.g. lymphoma) Irritable bowel syndrome Paracaecal hernia strangulation Torsion appendix epiploica
Pelvic disease (in women)	Ovarian twist or tumour Pelvic inflammatory disease salpingitis Ectopic pregnancy Ruptured ovarian cyst (includes Mittelschmirtz)
Upper abdomen and retroperitoneum	Peptic ulcer Cholelithiasis and pancreatitis Right ureteric colic Right pyelonephritis and urinary infection
Diaphragmatic musculoskeletal	Right pleurisy and pneumonia Spinal diseases Rectus sheath haematoma
Systemic and metabolic	Herpes zoster Syphilis Diabetes mellitus Acute intermittent porphyria Henoch–Schönlein disease

INVESTIGATIONS

Because the diagnosis is clinically based, investigations are usually ancillary or complementary.[36] Analysis may reveal infection or haematuria which may help to distinguish a urinary pathology. The white cell count is raised in most patients with acute appendicitis but is a poor discriminant. It is rarely necessary to utilize biochemical indices but, when there is doubt, an amylase estimation can exclude pancreatitis, the serum urea and electrolytes may be needed preoperatively in the elderly or those with generalized peritonitis, and C-reactive protein is non-specifically raised (although a surprising number of studies have investigated its value).

Plain abdominal radiographs are commonly, and wrongly, asked for on a routine basis but give poor discriminant help. The signs are many:[30] localized ileus with soft tissue density or caecal deformity; loss of psoas shadow; and faecaliths, foreign bodies or gas in the appendix; however, free peritoneal gas is rare.

The use of ultrasound with compression has been found to be discriminating and specifically useful in determining appendix abscess, mass or an alternative pathology.[32,35] Expertise is required: either the surgeon learns to use freely available ultrasound after hours or the radiologist must be reliable for an opinion when requested. Technetium scans, computed tomography (CT) and magnetic resonance imaging (MRI) are currently being investigated and many publications are being seen in the latest medical press. They are unlikely to have a significant part to play.

Laparoscopy is the clearest way forward to evaluate difficult patients' symptoms and signs, particularly young women where scars and adhesions need to be avoided.[8,31,43] As widespread expertise is obtained then laparoscopic appendicectomy may join the current trend towards minimally invasive surgery.

TREATMENT

The treatment of acute appendicitis, once diagnosed, is expeditious removal. Only in remote areas, or at sea, is there a place for conservatism. The operation is undertaken with general anaesthesia and antibiotic prophylaxis. The classic McBurney incision has been replaced by the more horizontal and cosmetic Lanz incision, which can be extended easily to allow more major procedures if necessary (such as right hemicolectomy or cholecystectomy.) The wound should be closed and a fresh incision made for a perforated duodenal or gastric ulcer. Too low an incision is to be deprecated as exposure can be limited. There is a case to be made for a laparotomy incision (lower midline) for elderly patients (over 60 years) because an initiating cause or other pathology may be found.[40] Retrograde removal of the appendix is best avoided but the whole structure must be excised with careful ligation and haemostasis. Stump inversion is not necessary but trials to prove or disprove this still continue.[39]

Antibiotic prophylaxis is mandatory and must be given preoperatively, ideally intravenously as a single dose at induction of anaesthesia.[18,23] To cover anaerobes and aerobes a combination of metronidazole and a second- or third-generation cephalosporin such as cefuroxime is ideal. There are differences in opinion regarding prophylaxis, however, because many reports have shown that a single intravenous dose of metronidazole, or a suppository given 1 hour preoperatively, is as good and much cheaper. There are others who recommend the use of broad-spectrum agents such as imipenem. Certainly, when spreading peritonitis is present a broad-spectrum cover is desirable and can be then continued as therapy for 3–5 days postoperatively.

Antibiotic treatment is advisable when the appendix has perforated. The rate of perforation is between 25% and 30% and occurs more commonly in the very young and elderly patients, but does not seem to be related to the length of history. Antibiotic lavage has been shown to be useful, but when peritonitis is localized it seems pointless to make it generalized by lavage ('peritoneal macrophages cannot swim and eat at the same time' was an expression coined by Richard Simmonds).[15] It is equally illogical to drain a patient's peritoneum after widespread peritonitis and it has been shown to offer no added protection after perforation.[11]

Traditional teaching has instructed that an *appendix mass* should be treated by conservative measures: the Ochsner–Sherren regimen.[37] Certainly, an appendix mass can resolve with bed rest, analgesia, intravenous fluids, antibiotics and bowel rest but it has been opined that an appendix mass, as well as an appendix abscess, can be operated on safely with appropriate skill and anaesthesia[17] thereby preventing the need for interval appendicectomy. This is a view also held by the author.

Appendix abscess may be managed conservatively but interventional radiology (ultrasound, or CT-guided percutaneous aspiration or drainage) or surgery is preferable. Surgery is mandatory if there are signs of spreading peritonitis or generalized sepsis.

If appendicitis is allowed to resolve, because there are no surgical facilities available or there is fear of damage in an operation for appendix mass, an interval appendicectomy is probably justified 1–2 months later. The operation is simple and avoids a 30% chance of further appendicitis; it also excludes other underlying disease which may be present, particularly in the elderly. The case for incidental appendicectomy during other procedures is still open to debate.[1,42] Even with appropriate prophylaxis there is an increased risk of wound infection. In fertile women the risk of adhesions and infertility following appendicectomy-related pelvic abscess does not justify coincidental appendicectomy, although the link is not proven. Certainly interval appendicectomy should be avoided in older patients where the future risk of developing acute appendicitis gives it no justification. The argument that interval appendicectomy occasionally reveals an appendix with coincidental pathology (such as a carcinoid) is a weak one.

ACUTE APPENDICITIS AT THE EXTREMES OF LIFE AND IN PREGNANCY

The overall mortality of appendicitis should be less than 1% of appendicectomies. This rises to 5% after perforation but deaths are mainly in very young and elderly patients. Mortality (and morbidity) continues to fall in relation to rapid diagnosis, appropriate treatment and good perioperative care and anaesthesia. Children suffer more perforations, particularly the youngest who have poor omental function and host defences.[33] Their increased mortality may also relate to parental delay and difficulties in history taking and atypical signs. The elderly suffer more perforations and the disease is often rapidly progressive, with the signs and symptoms being atypical and difficult to recognize.[16] The causes of death after appendicectomy are usually related to concurrent disease.[27]

In pregnancy there is poor localization of the signs of acute appendicitis because of the enlarging uterus, and the disease may be overlooked. The omentum may also be ineffective because of altered anatomical relationships.[38] The incidence of appendicitis is between 1 : 1500–6600 pregnancies and many other causes of abdominal pain should be assessed by the general surgeon and obstetrician together. The mortality following appendicectomy is virtually zero unless there is a perforation when maternal mortality may reach 17% and fetal mortality 43%.

COMPLICATIONS AFTER APPENDICECTOMY

Appendicitis may be followed by systemic complications common to all abdominal surgery and the local complications[6] are listed in Table 6.7. Wound complications of dehiscence or herniation are unusual, and an increased risk of right inguinal hernia is controversial, but infectious complications are relatively common. Appropriate prophylaxis and care during surgery results in a wound infection rate as low as 2–3% overall.[17] Delayed suture, favoured in North America after appendicectomy for perforation, has had few adherents in the United Kingdom where primary suture, even with continuous techniques, has not been found to be related to an increased incidence of wound infections. Pelvic collections are rarely seen and probably relate to inadequate peritoneal toilet in peritonitis, or to iatrogenic complications such as a haematoma which becomes infected. Subphrenic collections and certainly portal pyelophlebitis are historical.

Fistula related to appendiceal stump complications is uncommon and usually closes spontaneously provided a distal stenosing disease is not present. Obstruction following intussusception of the appendix stump is also a rarity.

Table 6.7 Local complications after appendicectomy

- Infection – wound
  – pelvis
- Dehiscence and hernia of wound
- Fistula } of appendix stump
- Intussusception } of appendix stump
- Adhesions and infertility

THE FUTURE

Laparoscopic appendicectomy is being widely practised and diagnostic laparoscopy is used to determine the cause of acute abdominal pain. It is likely that appendicitis will be managed in the future by minimally invasive surgery.[21]

REFERENCES

1. Andrew, M.H. and Roty, A.R. (1987) Incidental appendectomy with cholecystectomy: is the increased risk justified. *American Surgeon*, **53**, 553–557.
2. Baker, D. (1986) Epidemiology of appendicitis. In: *The Aetiology of Acute Appendicitis*, pp. 3–9. MRC Scientific Report No. 7. London: Medical Research Council.
3. Barker, D.J. and Morris, J. (1988) Acute appendicitis, bathrooms and diet in Britain and Ireland. *British Medical Journal*, **296**, 953–955.
4. Burkitt, D.P. (1971) The aetiology of appendicitis. *British Journal of Surgery*, **58**, 697–699.
5. Cooper, M.J. (1990) Manifestations of appendicitis. In: *Emergency Abdominal Surgery* (Eds) Williamson, R.C.N. and Cooper, M.J. Chap. 15, pp. 221–232. Edinburgh: Churchill Livingstone.
6. Cooperman, M. (1983) Complications of appendectomy. *Surgical Clinics of North America*. **63**, 1233–1247.
7. DeDombal, F.T., Leaper, D.J., Staniland, J.R., McCann, A.P. and Horrocks, J.C. (1972) Computer-aided diagnosis of acute abdominal pain. *British Medical Journal*, **2**, 9–13.
8. Deutsch, A.A., Zelikovsky, A. and Reiss, R. (1982) Laparoscopy in the prevention of

unnecessary appendectomies: a prospective study. *British Journal of Surgery*, **69**, 336–337.
9. Ellis, H. (1984) *Famous Operations*, Chap. 14, pp. 109–115. Pennsylvania: Harwal.
10. Geroulanos, S. and Largiader, F. (1988) Appendix-Appendizitis-Appendektomie. Ein Geschightlicher Uberblick. *Schweizerische Rundschau für Medizin Praxis (Bern)*, **77**, 867–875.
11. Greenall, M.J., Evans, M. and Pollock, A.V. (1978) Should you drain a perforated appendix? *British Journal of Surgery*, **65**, 880–882.
12. Heaton, K.W. (1987) Aetiology of acute appendicitis. *British Medical Journal*, **294**, 1632–1633.
13. Hill, J. and Leaper, D.J. (1986) Acute appendicitis and carcinoma of the colon. *Journal of the Royal Society of Medicine*, **79**, 678–680.
14. Hoffman, J. and Rasmussen, O.O. (1989) Aids in the diagnosis of acute appendicitis. *British Journal of Surgery*, **76**, 774–779.
15. Howard, R.J. and Simmonds, R.L. (1988) *Surgical Infectious Diseases*, 2nd Ed. Connecticut: Appleton and Lange.
16. Klein, S.R., Layden, L. Wright, J.F. and White, R.A. (1988) Appendicitis in the elderly. A diagnostic challenge. *Postgraduate Medicine*, **83**, 247–254.
17. Krukowski, Z.H. (1990) Appendicitis. **1**(86), 2044–2048.
18. Krukowski, Z.H., Irwin, S.T. Denholm, S. and Matheson, N.A. (1988) Preventing wound infection after appendicectomy. A review. *British Journal of Surgery*, **75**, 1023–1033.
19. Larner, A.J. (1988) The aetiology of appendicitis. *British Journal of Hospital Medicine*, **39**, 540–542.
20. Lau, W., Fan, S., Yiu, T., Chuk, W. and Wong, S.H. (1984) Negative findings at appendectomy. *American Journal of Surgery*, **148**, 375–378.
21. Leahy, P.F. (1989) Technique of laparoscopic appendicectomy. *British Journal of Surgery*, **76**, 616.
22. Leaper, D. J. (1990) New diagnostic techniques in the acute abdomen. Part I Computer aided diagnosis. In: Emergency Abdominal Surgery (Eds) Williamson, R.C.N. and Cooper, M.J. Chap. I pp. 1–5. Edinburgh: Churchill Livingstone.
23. Leaper, D.J. and Pritchett, C.J. (1989) Prophylactic antibiotics in general surgical practice. *Current Practice in Surgery*, **1**, 178–184.
24. Leigh, D.A. (1974) Bacterial flora of the appendix fossa and the incidence of wound infection. *Journal of Clinical Pathology*, **27**, 997–1000.
25. Ludbrook, J. and Spears, G.F.S. (1965) The risk of developing appendicitis. *British Journal of Surgery*, **52**, 856–858.
26. McBurney, C. (1989) Experience with early operative interference in cases of disease of the vermiform appendix. *New York Medical Journal*, **50**, 676–684.
27. McCallion, J. Canning, G.P., Knight, P.V. and McCallion, J.S. (1987) Acute appendicitis in the elderly: a 5 year retrospective study. *Age and Ageing*, **16**, 256–260.
28. Morson, B.C. and Dawson, I.M.P. (1979) Inflammatory disorders. In: *Gastrointestinal pathology*, pp. 455–465. London: Blackwell Scientific.
29. Noer, T. (1976) Decreasing incidence of acute appendicitis. *Acta Chirurgica Scandinavica*, **141**, 431–432.
30. Olutula, P.S. (1988) Plain film radiographic diagnosis of acute appendicitis: an evaluation of the signs. *Canadian Association of Radiologists' Journal*, **39**, 254–256.
31. Paterson-Brown, S., Thompson, J.N., Eckersley, J.R., Ponting, G.A. and Dudley, H.A.F. (1988) Which patients with suspected appendicitis should undergo laparoscopy? *British Medical Journal*, **286**, 1363–1364.
32. Pearson, R.H. (1988) Ultrasonography for diagnosing appendicitis. *British Medical Journal*, **297**, 309–310.
33. Pledger, H.G. Fahy, L.T. Van Mourik, G.A. and Bush, C.H. (1987) Deaths in children with a diagnosis of acute appendicitis in England and Wales. *British Medical Journal*, **295**, 1233–1235.
34. Bole, G.V. (1988) Appendicitis: The diagnostic challenge continues. *American Surgeon*, **54**, 609–612.
35. Puylaert, J.B., Rutgers, P.H., Lausang, R. *et al.* (1987) A prospective study of ultrasonography in the diagnosis of appendicitis. *New England Journal of Medicine*, **317**, 666–669.
36. Schwartz, S.I. (1987) Tempering the technological diagnosis of appendicitis. *New England Journal of Medicine*, **317**, 703–704.
37. Sherren, J. (1905) The causation and treatment of appendicitis. *The Practitioner*, **74**, 833–844.
38. Smoleniec, J. and James, D. (1990) General surgical problems in pregnancy. *British Journal of Surgery*, **77**, 1203–1204.
39. Street, D., Bodai, B.I., Owens, L.T. Moore, D.B., Walton, C.B. and Holcroft, J.W. (1988) Simple ligation vs stump inversion in appendectomy. *Archives of Surgery*, **123**, 689–690.
40. Sumpio, B.E., Ballantyne, G.H., Zdon, M.J. and Modlin, I.M. (1986) Perforated appendicitis and obstructing colonic carcinoma in the elderly. *Diseases of the Colon and Rectum*, **29**, 668–670.
41. Teicher, I., Landa, B., Cohen, M., Kabnick, L.S. and Wise, L. (1983) Scoring system to aid in diagnosis of appendicitis. *Annals of Surgery*, **198**, 753–759.
42. Voitk, A.J. and Lowry, J.B. (1988) Is interval appendicectomy a safe practice? *Canadian Journal of Surgery*, **31**, 448–451.
43. Whitworth, C.M., Whitworth, P.M., Sanfillipo, J. and Polk, H.C. (1988) Value of diagnostic laparoscopy in young women with possible appendicitis. *Surgical Gynecology and Obstetrics*, **167**, 187–190.

OTHER CAUSES OF ACUTE ABDOMEN

FOREIGN BODIES *(J. Temple)*

Foreign bodies may be introduced into the abdomen in one of three ways: (1) via the alimentary tract; (2) via the genitourinary tract; and (3) directly as a result of trauma.

Ingestion of foreign bodies is usually a problem in three groups of subjects: small children, elderly edentulous people, and psychiatric patients. The latter often deliberately ingest potentially dangerous objects such as pins, needles, nails and even razor blades. However, as these potentially dangerous objects are often found on radiograph to be lying in the stomach or small bowel in a patient who does not appear physically ill, the clinician should suspect that they have been well wrapped up in paper, tape or some other protective material. The best policy is to watch the progress of these objects by serial radiographs and operate only if the foreign body becomes obviously lodged or if there are signs of peritonitis or bleeding.

The variety of objects removed from the rectum is enormous. These may have been ingested orally or inserted anally, the latter usually as a result of deviant sexual practice. Removal of small foreign bodies can often be awaited naturally, but large objects may damage the rectum and require careful removal under general anaesthetic. If interperitoneal injury has occurred, a proximal colostomy is mandatory.

Foreign bodies may also be introduced into the abdomen by a penetrating injury. The missile itself or the structure through which it passed are carried along the track into the abdomen. Any penetrating injury in the abdomen should be explored for foreign bodies.

An acute abdomen occurs only when a foreign body penetrates either the gastrointestinal or genitourinary tract to produce a local abscess or generalised peritonitis. The aim of early exploration is to prevent these complications.

BLUNT ABDOMINAL TRAUMA

(J. Stewart)

The majority of civilian abdominal injuries are due to blunt trauma, usually resulting from automobile and industrial accidents.[16] By contrast, wartime injuries are usually penetrating in nature. Failure to manage abdominal injuries correctly accounts for a number of preventable deaths, a factor brought out in the recent Confidential Enquiry into Perioperative Deaths reported in the United Kingdom.[3] In the USA the failure to recognize and control intra-abdominal haemorrhage accounts for nearly 10% of traumatic deaths.[14]

Table 6.8 Pattern of injury found at laparotomy following blunt abdominal injury

Organ	*Relative incidence (%)*
Spleen	46
Liver	33
Mesentery	10
Urological	9
Pancreas	9
Small bowel	8
Colon	7
Duodenum	5
Vascular	4
Stomach	2

Adapted from McAnena *et al.*[16]

Due to the increase in the use of motorized transportation, the overall incidence of blunt abdominal trauma is increasing. Approximately 60% of civilian injuries of this type are due to automobile accidents.[6] The sudden rise in pressure to the abdomen is more likely to burst a solid organ than a hollow viscus, which may account for the greater incidence of solid organ injury (*Table 6.8*).

The abdomen represents a large part of the body, from the diaphragm superiorly to the infragluteal fold inferiorly. Blunt injuries to the back may also result in severe intra-abdominal trauma. The patient often suffers from multiple injuries and several specialities will be involved with appropriate management. The damage caused to intra-abdominal structures may be masked by other injuries or intoxicating agents. As many as one in three patients thought to have no serious injury at initial presentation will ultimately require a laparotomy.[17] Approximately 10% of civilian injuries that require a laparotomy are due to blunt abdominal trauma. In the stable patient the importance of repeated assessment by the same experienced surgeon is vital.

ANATOMY

For ease of evaluation the abdomen can be divided into four areas:

1. True abdomen

2. Intrathoracic abdomen
3. Pelvic abdomen
4. Retroperitoneal abdomen.

Apart from the true abdomen, the other areas are difficult to examine physically. The true abdomen contains the small and large bowel, the bladder when distended and the gravid uterus. The intrathoracic abdomen consists of the upper abdomen protected by the rib cage. It contains the stomach, spleen, liver, diaphragm and major blood vessels. The pelvic abdomen, surrounded by the bony pelvis, contains rectum, bladder, urethra, small bowel and, in the female, the uterus, tubes and ovaries.

The retroperitoneal abdomen contains the kidneys, pancreas, second and third portions of the duodenum, the major vessels, the aorta and inferior vena cava and the lymphatic channels.

PATHOPHYSIOLOGY

Injuries may be classified into high or low energy and several different types of process may occur.[10]

1. Compression of the abdominal viscera between the spinal column and the anterior abdominal wall causes a crush injury.
2. A sudden rise in intra-abdominal pressure may rupture a hollow viscus or burst a solid organ.
3. Sudden deceleration can cause severe shearing forces which may avulse organs or vascular pedicles.

The widespread introduction of seat belt devices and more recently inflation chambers have modified the basic types of injuries.[2] In some series there has been an increase in the number of mesenteric and visceral perforations over solid organ damage from seat belts. The spleen still remains the organ most frequently injured, followed by the liver, mesentery, kidneys and the pancreas.

History

Information as to the nature of the injury and the patient's initial condition and subsequent progress should be obtained from the emergency services.[14] Frontal, side and rear impact and rollover accidents have their own pattern of injury. The type of restraining device (if one was used) should be ascertained because lap belts are associated with different types of injuries from those associated with a lap and combined shoulder harness.[19] If the patient has rib fractures of the lower left chest, then there is a 20% chance that there will be an associated splenic injury. Similarly with rib fractures on the lower right side, there is a 10% chance of liver injury. The diaphragm is involved in about 4% of injuries and most commonly is affected on the left side. Following a compression injury with fractures of the upper limbs or spine, there is an associated risk of a major renal injury in 20% of cases. If possible a routine history with regard to other medical conditions, current and past drug therapy and allergies should also be obtained.

Physical examination

Examination should be performed with all of the patient's clothing removed. A thorough search should be made for any bruising, abrasions or puncture wounds as these may indicate intra-abdominal injuries. Similarly the marks left by tyres or seat belts are noted. The ribs are assessed for fractures. The initial shape and movement of the abdomen are noted as is the presence of any guarding, rebound or rigidity. In one series the presence of abdominal tenderness and guarding was associated with a 75% incidence of internal injuries. However, in up to 43% of cases there were no abdominal signs. Of these 44% were eventually subjected to a laparotomy and 77% of these had injuries requiring repair.[5]

The pelvis and hips should also be examined to exclude a major pelvic fracture. The perineum and urethral meatus are examined for bruising or fresh blood. Anal sphincter tone and the presence and position of the prostate are determined. A 'high riding prostate gland' indicates a post-membranous urethral distruption. The presence of thoracic trauma should always be considered particularly as the dome of the diaphragm may rise to the fourth intercostal space in full expiration.

The initial examination must be followed by repeated assessments as signs may well develop in an otherwise stable and asymptomatic patient.[15]

INVESTIGATIONS

Laboratory

Baseline haematological and biochemical investigations should be obtained. Although they are of limited use immediately following blunt abdominal trauma, alterations may indicate occult injury. A leukocytosis often occurs following trauma and is a non-specific finding. The serum amylase should be determined. A normal result does not exclude a pancreatic injury, although a grossly elevated isoenzyme may well indicate trauma to the pancreas.

Elevations of the serum amylase can occur with trauma to the proximal small bowel, parotid gland and the genitourinary tract. Baseline liver function tests should be obtained. The patient's blood group should be ascertained and appropriate volumes of blood products ordered and, if necessary, a coagulation screen performed. Blood should be available for rapid transfusion. In certain patients it will also be necessary to assess their hepatitis and HIV status. Urinalysis should be performed and again in certain patients analysis for drug metabolites may be required.

Radiology

Radiological investigations in the stable patient may provide useful information. The plain antero-posterior chest radiograph may reveal rib fractures or a ruptured diaphragm. Plain abdominal radiographs may show either free intra-abdominal gas following a visceral perforation or retroperitoneal gas. The ribs, spinous processes, vertebral bodies and pelvis should be examined for evidence of fractures. Some 500–800 ml free intraperitoneal blood is necessary for detection on a plain abdominal radiograph. Changes in the gas/air or fat interfaces may suggest collections around or displacement of organs. A variety of signs such as the loss of the flank-stripe, loss of the hepatic angle, or the accumulation of fluid over the bladder (the dog ear sign) have been described. A ruptured spleen may displace the stomach or colon causing changes in the usual gas patterns.[11]

The use of contrast radiological investigations is sometimes of value in the assessment of blunt injury to the duodenum. Duodenal injury following blunt trauma can occur as an isolated injury and may be difficult to diagnose early. Water-soluble contrast can be swallowed or introduced via a nasogastric tube.

Computed tomography of the abdomen

The use of computed tomography (CT) in the management of blunt abdominal trauma remains controversial. In the stable patient with the correct facilities available it may be of great value. In several studies the accuracy of abdominal CT in the management of blunt abdominal trauma has not been found to be as accurate as peritoneal lavage. CT scanning is not particularly accurate in the early assessment of pancreatic injury such as a blunt pancreatic fracture following a seat belt injury. It is also poor at detecting acute intestinal perforations. In pelvic fractures, however, CT scanning may be of value in assessing the fractures and the extent of the pelvic haematoma. In the assessment of liver and spleen injuries, such as burst fractures of the liver, contrast-enhanced CT scanning has been of value.[9]

Diagnostic abdominal ultrasound scanning

The improved new generation of real time and B-mode ultrasound machines has meant that diagnostic ultrasound is often used in the acute situation. The development of portable machines has increased availability in emergency departments. The use of ultrasound is of limited value in the diagnosis of a perforated viscus. It is of value in the assessment of liver or splenic damage and the detection of free intraperitoneal fluid. Gruessner, however, demonstrated that peritoneal lavage was superior in determining the need for a laparotomy to ultrasound. The use of abdominal ultrasound in assessing the abdomen must be regarded as a complementary study.[13]

Intravenous urography

The main indication for an intravenous urogram (IVU) is as a test of function. It will determine the presence of one or two functioning kidneys and the presence of a major renal parenchymal injury. The presence of gross haematuria is an indication for an intravenous urogram. However, there may be a vascular pedicle injury with only microscopic haematuria or no haematuria at all. At present an intravenous urogram is regarded as a screening investigation and may need to be complemented with a computed tomography scan or an arteriogram.

Abdominal peritoneal lavage

Abdominal peritoneal lavage has become a standard investigation in patients with blunt abdominal trauma, especially in the unconscious patient.[26] The technique was introduced by Root and colleagues in 1965.[25] Three main methods of introducing the lavage catheter are available: open, semi-open and closed. The lavage fluid consists of 1 litre warm physiological saline. If fresh blood is aspirated, the tap is positive. Fluid of doubtful significance is analysed for red and white cells, amylase and bile, and subjected to microscopy. In the presence of blunt abdominal trauma, visceral damage is present in more than 95% of patients in whom the red cell count is greater than 100 000/mm^3.[1,12] Diagnostic peritoneal lavage has an overall accuracy rate of 95% with a significant morbidity of less than 1%. Complications tend to occur with the closed method more frequently than other methods of introducing the cannula.[26]

THE CHILD WITH BLUNT ABDOMINAL TRAUMA

In children between the age of 1 and 14 years, trauma remains one of the major causes of death with blunt trauma accounting for 90% of these injuries.[7] Most injuries are as a result of automobile accidents, although many include other types of accidental trauma. The possibility of non-accidental injury due to child abuse must also be considered.

The abdomen in the small child tends not to have well-developed abdominal muscles compared to that of an adult, and has a relatively small antero-posterior diameter. The abdominal contents are therefore at greater risk of blunt injury. The initial assessment of the injured child is often difficult. This is due to a combination of fear, pain, other injuries including cerebral injury and hypoxia.

In the stable, cooperative child an abdominal CT may be of help in the assessment. The use of diagnostic peritoneal lavage has also been described as being of benefit particularly in those with multi-system injuries. The trend for splenic conservation, especially in children, has prompted a more conservative attitude to the child who is stable and suffering from a splenic injury.[8] The recognition of postsplenectomy sepsis due to pneumococci has provided further impetus for conservation of the spleen. It is now recognized that bleeding from minor splenic tears has often ceased by the time a laparotomy has been performed. This phenomenon has been ascribed to the presence of a greater capsule to parenchyma ratio than in the adult.[18] The use of double-contrast CT to monitor and follow patients who are stable is now accepted by most surgeons. The selective non-operative management of such cases, however, requires an experienced surgical and nursing staff.

BLUNT TRAUMA DURING PREGNANCY

The most common cause of blunt maternal injury are automobile accidents, domestic accidents and assault.[4,20] The management of blunt trauma involves some special considerations due to the altered maternal physiology and because the fetus may also be at risk.

The mother undergoes a series of physiological adaptations during pregnancy.[21] The maternal cardiac output increases by about 1 litre in the first 10 weeks of pregnancy. At about 20 weeks, the pregnant uterus can obstruct the maternal inferior vena cava when the mother is in the supine position.[27] The cardiac output may therefore be suddenly reduced. The maternal blood volume has also increased by as much as 45% at 28 weeks.[23] The risk of venous thrombosis is also increased and the release of thrombogenic mediators following trauma may initiate a disseminated intravascular coagulation. The intra-abdominal contents are displaced cephalad by the enlarging uterus. The larger the uterus, the greater the risk of injury. The blood flow to the uterus increases from 1 ml/second to 10 ml/second at term. There is therefore the risk of major haemorrhage if the uterus is sufficiently damaged.

The most common cause of death is due to haemorrhage and head injury. The bowel is reported to be less frequently injured. Uterine rupture is rare, occurring in only 0.6% of cases. In traumatic rupture of the uterus the fetal mortality is almost 100%, but maternal mortality is only about 10%.[22] The most common cause of fetal death after major trauma is abruptio placentae. After blunt abdominal trauma, abruptio placentae occurs in about 1–5% of minor injuries and 20–50% of major injuries. Direct fetal injury is not common as the amniotic fluid and soft tissues act to protect the fetus. Following blunt trauma, cranial injuries are the most common type of fetal injury. These occur especially when the fetal head is engaged in the third trimester and is at risk when the maternal pelvis is fractured.[25]

The risk of fetomaternal haemorrhage is four to five times greater in injured pregnant women than in non-injured pregnant women. It is more common if the placenta is sited anteriorly. The complications of fetomaternal haemorrhage include, cardiac dysrhythmias in the fetus, rhesus factor sensitization in the mother and death of the fetus from exsanguination.

REFERENCES

1. Alyono, D. and Perry, J.F. (1981) Value of quantitative cell count and amylase activity of peritoneal lavage fluid. *Journal of Traumas*, **21**, 345.
2. Arajarvi, E., Santavirto, S. and Tolonen, J. (1987) Abdominal injuries sustained in severe traffic accidents by seatbelt wearers. *Journal of Trauma*, **27**, 393.
3. Buck, N., Devlin, H.B. and Lunn, J.N. (1987) Confidential Enquiry into Perioperative Deaths. Nuffield Provincial Hospitals Trust and Kings Fund.
4. Crosby, W.M. and Costiloe, J.P. (1971) Safety of lap-restraint for pregnant victims of automobile collisions. *New England Journal of Medicine*, **284**, 632–636.
5. Davis, J.J., Cohn, I. and Nance, F.C. (1976) Diagnosis and management of blunt abdominal trauma. *Annals of Surgery*, **183**, 672.

6. DeVincenti, F.C., River, J.D., Laborde, E.J. *et al.* (1968) Blunt abdominal trauma. *Journal of Trauma*, **8**, 1004.
7. Eichelberger, M.R. and Randolph, J.G. (1985) Progress in paediatric trauma. *World Journal of Surgery*, **9**, 222.
8. Ein, S.H., Shandling, B., Simpson, J.S. *et al.* (1978) Non-operative management of traumatized spleen in children: How and why: *Journal of Pediatric Surgery*, **13**, 117.
9. Federle, M.P., Crass, R.A., Jefffrey, R.B. *et al.* (1982) Computed tomography in blunt abdominal trauma. *Archives of Surgery*, **117**, 645.
10. Feliciano, D.V. (1988) *Patterns of injury:* In: *Trauma.* (Eds) Mattox, K.L., Moore, E.E. and Feliciano, D.V. Norwalk, CT: Appleton & Lange.
11. Felson, B. and Klatte, E.C. (1975) Radiology of Abdominal Trauma. *Journal of the American Medical Association*, **231**, 1377.
12. Fischer, R.P., Beverlin, B.C., Engrav, L.H. *et al.* (1978) Diagnostic peritoneal lavage: Fourteen years and 2,586 patients later. *American Journal of Surgery*, **136**, 701.
13. Gruessner, R., Mentges, B., Duber, C. *et al.* (1989) Sonography vs peritoneal lavage in blunt abdominal trauma. *Journal of Trauma*, **29**, 242.
14. Hill, A.C., Schecter, W.P. and Trunkey, D.D. (1988) Abdominal trauma and indications for laparotomy. In: Trauma (Eds) Mattox, K.L., Moore, E.E. and Feliciano, D.V. Norwalk, CT: Appleton & Lange.
15. Hoyt, D.B. and Mackersie, R.C. (1988) *Abdominal Injuries: Essential Surgical Practice*. London: Butterworth Scientific.
16. McAnena, O.J., Moore, E.E. and Marx, J.A. (1990) Initial evaluation of the patient with blunt abdominal trauma. *Surgical Clinics of North America*, **70**, 3.
17. Moore, E.E. (1985) Resuscitation and evaluation of the injured patient. In: *Management of Trauma* (Eds) Zuidema, G.G., Ballinger, W. and Rutherford, R. Philadelphia: W.B. Saunders.
18. Moore, F.A., Moore, E.E., Moore, G.E. *et al.* (1984) Risk of splenic salvage after trauma: Analysis of 200 adults. *American Journal of Surgery*, 148.
19. Nygren, A. (1984) Injuries to car occupants – some aspects of the interior safety of cars. *Acta Otolologica Scandinavica*, **395**(suppl.).
20. Pearlman, M.D., Tintinalli, J.E. and Lorenz, R.P. (1990) A prospective controlled study of outcome after trauma during pregnancy. *American Journal of Obstetrics of Gynecology*, **162**, 1502–1510.
21. Pearlman, M.D., Tintinalli, J.E. and Lorenz, R.P. (1990) Blunt trauma during pregnancy. *New England Journal of Medicines*, **323**, 1609–1613.
22. Pepperell, R.J., Rubinstein, E. and MacIsaac, I.A. (1977) Motor-car accidents during pregnancy. *Medical Journal of Australia*, **1**, 203–205.
23. Pritchard, J.A. (1965) Changes in the blood volume during pregnancy and delivery. *Anesthesiology*, **26**, 393–399.
24. Root, H.D., Hauser, C.W., McKinley, C.R. *et al.* (1965) Diagnostic peritoneal lavage. *Surgery*, **57**, 633.
25. Rotthenberger, D., Quattlebaim, F.W., Perry, J.F., Zabel, J. and Fischer, R.P. (1978) Blunt maternal trauma: a review of 103 cases. *Journal of Trauma*, **18**, 173–179.
26. Thal, E.R. and Shires, G.T. (1973) Peritoneal lavage in blunt abdominal trauma. *American Journal of Surgery*, **125**, 64.
27. Ueland, K. and Hansen, J.M. (1969) Maternal cardiovascular dynamics. II. Posture and uterine contractions. *American Journal of Obstetrics and Gynecology*, **103**, 1–7.

CHAPTER 7

INFLAMMATORY BOWEL DISEASE

INCIDENCE, EPIDEMIOLOGY AND GENETICS

M.J.S. Langman

DESCRIPTIVE FEATURES

The incidence and prevalence of inflammatory bowel disease in the community can only be measured if all those who have the disease can be identified within a given population. Non-specific inflammatory bowel disease, in particular, poses a number of analytical problems.

DISEASE DEFINITION

The vast majority of cases of non-specific inflammatory bowel disease comprise either ulcerative colitis or Crohn's disease. Although individual features which are discussed elsewhere usually allow clinical distinction to be made between them, there are a minority of individuals in whom the distinction between ulcerative colitis and Crohn's disease cannot be made with certainty. Furthermore, the chance that any disease will be diagnosed depends upon access to sophisticated investigative methods which vary from place to place, especially from tropical under-developed areas to others with advanced Western patterns of industrialization. Thirdly, chronic non-specific inflammatory bowel disease is less likely to be recognised in areas where dysenteric illness is endemic. Even in places where infective dysenteric illness is uncommon, there will be a pool of cases of unknown and varying size which remain undiagnosed either through failure of presentation or through failure to recognize that the symptoms represent more than a simple disorder of bowel habit.

It is clear that incidence or prevalence data collected in different places or at different times can only be considered together provided these points are taken into account.

INDICES OF FREQUENCY

DEATH RATES

Few people die from Crohn's disease and ulcerative colitis; if they do it is usually from the complications of the disease or the complications of surgery. The chances of dying are also greater in older than in younger people. Fluctuations in death rates can therefore arise from variation in the age pattern of affected individuals, in the efficiency of treatment and in the clinical patterns of disease encountered, as well as from changes in patterns and fashions in death certification.

HOSPITAL ADMISSION RATES

Although most patients with Crohn's disease are likely to be admitted to hospital at some time or another, this is not true of ulcerative colitis, where the majority of individuals have mild disease limited to the distal large intestine. Outpatient treatment has probably become more common as medical treatment has improved, and this is likely to be true for both ulcerative colitis and Crohn's disease. It follows that disease frequency could be increasing even though hospital admission rates remain the same or even fall. Admission statistics also seldom allow repeated admissions of a single individual to be distinguished from single admissions of separate people.[35]

In general, there are more and more detailed data sets concerning disease frequency patterns which derive from countries with unitary medical care systems,[8,24,27,32,33,38,66,67,69] than from Western countries with other systems.[46–48]

Despite these difficulties, hospital admission rates probably form useful indices of Crohn's disease frequency but they are of little value in ulcerative colitis.

OUTPATIENTS AND OTHER DIAGNOSTIC REFERRAL RATES

Few sets of data are available. Even where they do exist the effects of changing diagnostic awareness, increasing diagnostic precision and greater general availability of diagnostic methods must be considered.

INCIDENCE AND PREVALENCE RATES

In general there are no striking differences in the age or sex incidence of colitis or Crohn's disease. Variations in sex incidence generally lie within the ratio of 1:5:1 for excesses of men, or women, with either disease, with no general consistency from one country, or study group, to another. Given environmental associations with smoking, and probably with oral contraceptive use, it is difficult to believe that examination of the sex ratios of the two diseases will yield significant clues to causes of disease frequency.

Examination of age-specific incidence rates tends to be hindered by uncertainty as to whether patients at set ages will necessarily present as disease symptoms manifest themselves. Recent data suggest a tendency for disease to be diagnosed rather later than earlier in life, but differences are small and there is no general consistency. Comparisons are hindered because disease may be sought more intensively in the elderly due to the perceived risk of cancer.

Table 7.1 Average annual incidence and prevalence rates for Crohn's disease per 100 000 population*

Place	Years	Incidence	Prevalence
England, Oxford[14]	1951–60	0.8	9.0
USA, Baltimore[53]	1960–63	1.8	–
Scotland, Aberdeen[32]	1955–68	2.0	32.5
England, North Tees[11]	1971–77	5.3	35.0
England, Nottingham[50]	1958–72	2.0	26.5
Norway, general survey[55]	1964–69	1.1	–
Switzerland, Basle[15]	1960–69	1.6	–
Denmark, Copenhagen[6]	1970–78	2.7	34.0
Sweden, Malmo[76]	1958–73	4.3	57.0
Sweden, Uppsala[13]	1965–83	6.1	–
Sweden, Stockholm[25]	1970–74	4.5	–
Wales, Cardiff[45]	1966–77	4.0	–
USA, Minnesota[19,63,71]	1943–47	0.8	–
	1973–77	6.8	–
	1978–82	4.3	91.0
New Zealand, Auckland[4,12]	1969–78	1.8	–

*Age-standardized and crude data are not separable in some of these data, and therefore no such distinctions have been attempted in compiling this table.

Table 7.2 Ulcerative colitis: average annual incidence rates (or first hospital admission rates), and prevalence rates per 100 000 population*

Place	Years	Incidence	Prevalence
Denmark, Copenhagen[6]	1961–67	7.3	44.1
	1962–78	8.1	117.7
England, North Tees[11]	1971–77	15.1	99.0
England, Oxford[14]	1951–60	6.5	79.9
Israel, Tel Aviv[18]	1961–70	3.6	37.4
New Zealand, Auckland[12]	1969–78	5.5	41.3
Norway, general survey[55]	1956–60	2.3	–
Scotland, NE[67,68]	1967–76	11.3	–
Sweden, Uppsala[13]	1965	7.0	–
	1983	11.0	–
USA, Baltimore[53]	1960–63	4.6	42.0
USA, Minnesota[71]	1935–64	9.7	–
	1960–79	13.6	212

*See footnote to *Table 7.1*.

The incidence and prevalence rates are given in *Tables 7.1* and *7.2* with data recorded predominantly in north-western Europe and North America. Data are available from these places for a number of reasons which include the high frequency of chronic non-specific inflammatory bowel disease, patterns of organization of medical care which ease the collection of data, and the ready availability of sophisticated diagnostic methods.

AREAS OF HIGH OR PROBABLE HIGH INCIDENCE OR PREVALENCE

Apart from the Scandinavian countries and the United Kingdom, disease frequency is certainly also high throughout North America, although the patterns of health care delivery there mitigate against the collection of coherent bodies of data. Details are available from Australia, New Zealand and White populations in South Africa. Reliable sets of data from elsewhere are sparse, but if the sizes of clinically reported series are reasonable indications, then those living elsewhere seem to be less frequently affected. Few sets of comparative data within countries exist, and even where they do interpretation is difficult given the wide confidence limits around point estimates of prevalence or incidence.[17]

AREAS OF LOW OR PROBABLE LOW INCIDENCE OR PREVALENCE

Series of clinical cases tend to be small and are reported infrequently from tropical areas, from Japan and Asia, from eastern and southern Europe, and from South America. To decide whether chronic non-specific inflammatory bowel disease is more or less common in these countries depends primarily upon inspired guesswork. The likelihood is that Crohn's disease and ulcerative colitis occur with reasonable if low frequency in southern Europe, but Crohn's disease tends to be under-reported in eastern Europe relative to ulcerative colitis, probably because it is relatively rare.

Moderate-sized sets of data have been reported from Czechoslovakia, Spain, Turkey, Japan and some parts of South America, but these probably represent investigator diligence rather than common disease frequency (for a general review see Lee[37]).

TIME TRENDS

The frequency with which Crohn's disease has been diagnosed rose steadily from the mid-1950s for about 20 years. Two possible reasons are increased diagnostic awareness and relabelling of ulcerative colitis as Crohn's disease, as well as a true increase in disease frequency. It is diffficult to gainsay the first, but there has been no general reduction in the apparent frequency of ulcerative colitis coinciding with the increase in Crohn's disease. Taken overall, it seems likely that the incidence of Crohn's disease has risen quite substantially (*Figure 7.1*). In the last 15 or 20 years it seems that disease frequency may have stabilized or fallen,[23,34] although the bases are unclear. The strongest environmental association has been with smoking, but a direct correlation with population smoking habits has not been observed.

The recorded frequency of ulcerative colitis has risen over the same time period, probably reflecting a rise in the frequency of ulcerative proctitis with little evidence of change in the incidence of extensive colitis. It is impossible to say whether this

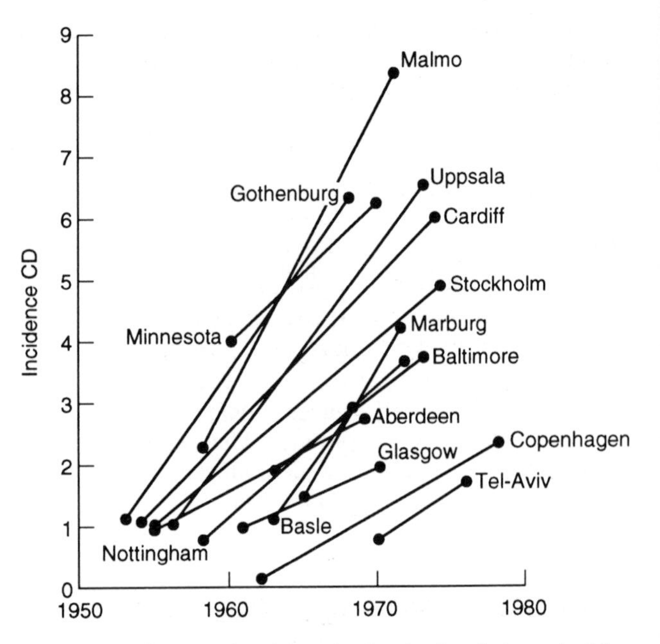

Figure 7.1 Comparative data sets showing trends towards rising incidence of Crohn's disease prior to 1980. (Figures are average rates per 100 000 of population per year.) [Reprinted with permission from Allan, R.N. *et al.* (1990). *Inflammatory Bowel Diseases.* Edinburgh: Churchill Livingstone.]

reflects a true increase in disease frequency or increased diagnostic awareness.

SOCIOECONOMIC PATTERNS

No particular occupational group seems to be at special risk of developing ulcerative colitis or Crohn's disease,[29] but there may be a general, if slight, tendency for both diseases to occur more often in people of higher socioeconomic grouping.

URBAN–RURAL DIFFERENCES

Differences between urban and rural incidence rates of inflammatory bowel disease have been detected by some[25,56] but not others. Overall the disease is rather less common in country dwellers. A reluctance of country dwellers to present with their symptoms could explain such differences as have been found.

ETHNIC VARIATION

Available information is limited because most studies of disease frequency have been conducted in places with White populations. In the USA the incidence of ulcerative colitis and Crohn's disease seems to be much lower in Black than in White people.[7] Maoris seem less likely to be affected by inflammatory bowel disease than White New Zealanders,[12,77] and Black (and to a lesser extent Indian) populations in South Africa than White populations.[37,64]

Jewish people seem to be more prone to inflammatory bowel disease than non-Jewish.[1] Within Israel itself both ulcerative colitis and Crohn's disease seem to be less common than in people living in northern Europe and North America.[18,54,61] Israeli-born and non-Ashkenazi Jews seem to be less susceptible than Jews born in Europe or North America. These differences suggest that environmental influences partly explain the increased susceptibility of individuals of Jewish extraction to inflammatory bowel disease.

PREDISPOSING FACTORS

ASSOCIATED DISEASE

An increased frequency of asthma, hay fever, allergic rhinitis and eczema has been detected in patients and their families.[21] As with other associated diseases, there is difficulty in distinguishing between hereditary and environmental effects.

DIET

The tendency for Crohn's disease and ulcerative colitis to occur in populations living in northern Europe and North America has inevitably suggested a causal association with dietary habits and particularly with a reduced dietary fibre and/or high refined sugar consumption. Suggestions that individual dietary habits might be important have not usually passed the test of time.[59]

SUGAR CONSUMPTION

In all studies (*Table 7.3*) Crohn's disease is associated with increased sugar consumption with approximately a doubling compared with matched controls. The increase does not seem to be explained by (1) increased sugar intake acting as a proxy for diminished fibre consumption, (2) altered taste perception in disease, (3) raised sugar consumption by smokers because smoking and sugar intake seem to be separate but interactive.[28]

Table 7.3 Sugar intake in Crohn's disease patients and in control individuals

	Average intake (g/day)		
Study	*Patients*	*Controls*	*No. of patients studied*
Martini and Brandes[44]	177	74	63
Miller *et al.*[49]	150	55	34
Thornton *et al.*[72]	122	65	30

INFECTION

The conflicting and generally disappointing results of experimental studies of the contagion hypothesis are discussed elsewhere. Epidemiological investigations suggest that patients are unable to transmit and to contract infection, but a limiting feature of these studies is that we do not understand what the appropriate timings might be.[50,51] The detection of lymphocytotoxic antibodies with increased frequency in the sera of family members of patients with inflammatory bowel disease could reflect common exposure to an infectious agent, although such findings are not necessarily specific for infection.[30,31] If the inverse correlation between the patterns of frequency of endemic dysenteries and of chronic non-specific inflammatory bowel disease is an epidemiological clue, then its nature eludes us.

If Crohn's disease and ulcerative colitis represent abnormal responses to infection from delayed exposure to causal agents which alter the pattern of host response, then the analogies of Hodgkin's disease[20,58] and paralytic poliomyelitis may be relevant.

CHILDHOOD FACTORS

As both Crohn's disease and ulcerative colitis reach their peak incidence in early adult life, it is natural to consider factors in childhood when seeking epidemiological clues.

Some data suggest that breast feeding exerts a protective influence[2,26] though, if true, it is unclear whether protection is in fact a direct consequence of breast feeding or arises for other associated factors.

SMOKING

There is a large and consistent body of evidence both in the UK,[2,42,70,73,74] and elsewhere, indicating that patients with colitis are particularly likely to be non-smokers, whereas those with Crohn's disease tend to be smokers. Relevant smoking habits seem to be those at the onset of disease, and the most persuasive explanation is that smoking habits determine the type of disease occurring. Differing risks of disease have been found with variations from approximately two- to fourfold increases or decreases (*Table 7.4*).

Table 7.4 Relative risks of inflammatory bowel disease for current smokers

Study	*Relative risk* *Crohn's disease*	*Ulcerative colitis*
Baltimore[9]	2.1	0.62
Bristol[73]	5.5	0.50
Liverpool[74]	3.2	0.18
Lund[3]	1.8	0.36
Milan[16]	2.9	0.61
N. Carolina[62]	1.9	0.80
Nottingham[42,70]	4.2	0.23
Orebro[41]	2.0	0.64

ORAL CONTRACEPTIVE USE

Most,[10,39,43,60,75] but not all,[36] evidence suggests that oral contraceptive use is associated with a modest increase in the risk of Crohn's disease. The basis is unclear but a vasculitic origin seems plausible. Another possibility is that any trend is explained by confounding, because oral contraceptive users also tend to be smokers. A similar trend has, however, been noted in ulcerative colitis[43] which, if real, would argue against the suggestion of confounding by association with smoking because colitics tend to be non-smokers.

GENETICS

Both Crohn's disease and ulcerative colitis occur more commonly than expected by chance within families.[13,40,57] In addition, where one of the diseases occurs in one family member, the same disease is more likely to manifest itself within the family than the other. This pattern could arise either from the play of common, predisposing, genetic factors within families, or from the play of common, predisposing, environmental influences.

Racial influences

Individuals of Jewish ancestry have been well known to be more liable to chronic inflammatory bowel disease, either Crohn's disease or colitis, than non-Jews. Again the difference could arise from genetic or environmental factors and distinction is difficult.

Genetic markers

Conclusive evidence of inherited liability to Crohn's disease or ulcerative colitis could come if it were possible to show that disease occurred more often than expected in those of, for example, a particular blood group. Although some studies of genetic markers have been disappointing, others have been supportive (*Table 7.5*).

Table 7.5 Prevalence of ulcerative colitis and Crohn's disease among first-degree relatives of patients

	Relatives			
	Percentage prevalence		*Risk ratio compared with general population*	
Patients	*Ulcerative colitis*	*Crohn's disease*	*Ulcerative colitis*	*Crohn's disease*
Ulcerative colitis	1.5	0.1	9.5	1.8
Crohn's disease	0.7	0.6	4.4	10.3

Table 7.6 HLA antigen meta-analysis of frequencies in patients with Crohn's disease and ulcerative colitis[4]

	Crohn's disease		*Ulcerative colitis*	
	Antigen	*Odds ratio*	*Antigen*	*Odds ratio*
Caucasian	A2	1.25	B27	1.81
	A11	0.62	Bw35	1.41
	B18	1.72		
Japanese	Not studied		B5	2.79

Negative studies have included a range of serological markers[5] as well as of ABO blood groups and secretor status. The nature of the inflammatory exudate, and the fact that class II antigens are expressed in the mucosa, make associations with the HLA antigens possible and even likely.

Individual studies have generally been too small to be convincing, and have been beset by the difficulty that random variations observed during multiple comparisons could be misinterpreted as real. By combining all results in a meta-analysis, it was possible to show small but significant trends, which differed for Crohn's disease and colitis, and for White and Japanese subjects (*Table 7.6*). No consistent patterns have been detected for a limited range of the D antigens.

The positive results obtained seem likely to be secondary to other, stronger, effects arising from linkage disequilibrium, which is strongly manifested within the HLA system. Thus coeliac disease is associated with HLA-B8 and -Dw3, the former arising through linkage disequilibrium with the latter (this being a phenomenon where in genetic rearrangements at meiotic division two genes tend to remain tied together).

REFERENCES

1. Acheson, E.D. (1960) The distribution of ulcerative colitis and regional enteritis in United States veterans with particular reference to the Jewish Religion. *Gut*, 1, 291–293.
2. Acheson, E.D. and Truelove, S.C. (1961) Early weaning in the aetiology of ulcerative colitis. *British Medical Journal*, **ii**, 929–933.
3. Benoni, C. and Nilsson, A. (1987) Smoking habits in patients with inflammatory bowel disease. A case control study. *Scandinavian Journal of Gastroenterology*, **22**, 1130–1136.
4. Biemond, I., Burnham, W.R., D'Amaro, J. and Langman, M.J.S. (1986) HLA-A and -B antigens in inflammatory bowel disease. *Gut*, **27**, 934–941.
5. Biemond, I., Weterman, I.T., Rood, J.J. *et al.* (1981) Search for genetic markers associated with Crohn's disease in the Netherlands. In *Recent Advances in Crohn's Disease* (Ed.) Pena, A.S., Weterman, I.T., Booth, C.C. and Strober, W. pp. 197–203. The Hague: Nijhoff.
6. Binder, V., Both, H., Hansen, P.K. *et al.* (1982) Incidence and prevalence of ulcerative colitis and Crohn's disease in the county of Copenhagen 1962–1978. *Gastroenterology*, **83**, 563–568.
7. Bonnevie, O. (1967) A socio-economic study of patients with ulcerative colitis. *Scandinavian Journal of Gastroenterology*, **2**, 129–136.
8. Bonnevie, O., Riis, P. and Anthonisen, P. (1968) An epidemiological study of ulcerative colitis in Copenhagen County. *Scandinavian Journal of Gastroenterology*, **3**, 432–438.
9. Calkins, B., Lilienfeld, A, Mendeloff, A., Garland, C., Monk, M. and Garland, F. (1984) Smoking factors in ulcerative colitis and Crohn's disease in Baltimore. *American Journal of Epidemiology*, **120**, 498.
10. Calkins, B.M., Mendeloff, A.I. and Garland, C. (1986) Inflammatory bowel disease in oral contraceptive users. *Gastroenterology*, **89**, 1046–1049.
11. Devlin, H.B., Datta, D. and Dellipiani, A.W. (1980) The incidence and prevalence of inflammatory bowel disease in North Tees Health District. *World Journal of Surgery*, **4**, 183–193.
12. Eason, R.J., Lee, S.P. and Jones, C.T. (1982) Inflammatory bowel disease in Auckland New Zealand. *Australasian and New Zealand Journal of Medicine*, **12**, 128–131.
13. Ekbom, A., Helmick, C., Zack, M. and Adami, H. (1991) The epidemiology of inflammatory bowel disease: a large population-based study in Sweden. *Gastroenterology*, **100**, 350–358.
14. Evans, J.G. and Acheson, E.C. (1965) An epidemiological study of ulcerative colitis and regional enteritis in the Oxford area. *Gut*, **6**, 311–324.
15. Fahrlander, H. and Baerlocher, C. (1970) Epidemiology of Crohn's disease in the Basle area. In *Regional Enteritis: Crohn's Disease* (Ed.) Engel, A. and Larssen, T. pp. 131–141. Fifth Skandia International Symposium. Stockholm: Nordisk Bokhandelus Forlag.
16. Franceschi, S., Panza, E., LaVecchia, C., Parazzini, P., Decarili, A. and Bianchi Porro, G. (1987) Non-specific inflammatory bowel disease and smoking. *American Journal of Epidemiology*, **125**, 445–452.
17. Garland, C.F., Lilienfeld, A.M., Mendeloff, A.I. *et al.* (1981) Incidence rates of ulcerative colitis and Crohn's disease in fifteen areas of the United States. *Gastroenterology*, **81**, 1115–1124.
18. Gilat, T., Ribak, J., Benaroya, Y. *et al.* (1974) Ulcerative colitis in the Jewish population of Tel-Aviv-Jafo. *Gastroenterology*, **66**, 335–342.
19. Gollop, J.H., Phillips, S.F., Melton, L.J. and Zinsmeister, A.R. (1988) Epidemiologic aspects of Crohn's disease: a population-based study in Olmsted County, Minnesota, 1943–82. *Gut*, **29**, 49–56.
20. Gutensohn, N. and Cole, P. (1981) Childhood social environment and Hodgkin's disease. *New England Journal of Medicine*, **304**, 135–140.
21. Hammer, B., Ashurst, P. and Naish, J. (1968) Diseases associated with ulcerative colitis and Crohn's disease. *Gut*, **9**, 17-21.
22. Harries, A.D., Baird, A. and Rhodes, J. (1982) Non-smoking. A feature of ulcerative colitis. *British Medical Journal*, **284**, 706.
23. Harries, A.D., Baird, A., Rhodes, J. and Mayberry, J.F. (1982) Has the rising incidence of Crohn's disease reached a plateau? *British Medical Journal*, **284**, 235.

24. Haug, K., Schrumpf, E., Barstad, S., Fluge, G. and Halvorsen, J.F. (1988) Epidemiology of ulcerative colitis in western Norway. *Scandinavian Journal of Gastroenterology*, **23**, 517–522.
25. Hellers, G. (1979) Crohn's disease in Stockholm County, 1955–1974. A study of epidemiology, results of surgical treatment and long-term prognosis. *Acta Chirurgica Scandinavia* (supplement 490), 1–84.
26. Hellers, G. (1981) Some epidemiological aspects of Crohn's disease in Stockholm County 1955–1979. In *Recent Advances in Crohn's Disease* (Ed.) Pena, A.S., Weterman, I.T., Booth, C.C. and Strober, W. pp. 158–162. The Hague: Nijhoff.
27. Hoj, L., Brix Jensen, P., Bonnevie, O. and Riis, P. (1973) An epidemiological study of regional enteritis and acute ileitis in Copenhagen County. *Scandinavian Journal of Gastroenterology*, **8**, 381–384.
28. Katschinski, B., Logan, R.F.A., Edmond, E.M. and Langman, M.J.S. (1988) Smoking and sugar consumption are separate but interactive risk factors in Crohn's disease. *Gut*, **303**, 261–263.
29. Keighley, A., Miller, D.S., Hughes, A.O. and Langman, M.J.S. (1976) The demographic and social characteristics of patients with Crohn's disease in the Nottingham area. *Scandinavian Journal of Gastroenterology*, **11**, 293–296.
30. Korsmeyer, S.J., Williams, R.C., Wilson, I.D. and Strickland, R.G. (1975) Lymphocytotoxic antibody in inflammatory bowel disease: a family study. *New England Journal of Medicine*, **293**, 1117–1120.
31. Kuiper, I., Weterman, I., Biemond, I. *et al.* (1981) Lymphocytotoxic antibody in patients with Crohn's disease and family members. In *Recent Advances in Crohn's Disease* (Ed.) Pena, A.G., Weterman, I.T., Booth, C.C. and Strober, W. pp. 341–347. The Hague: Nijhoff.
32. Kyle, J. (1971) An epidemiological study of Crohn's disease in North East Scotland. *Gastroenterology*, **61**, 826–833.
33. Kyle, J. (1972) *Crohn's Disease*. London: Heinemann Medical.
34. Kyle, J. and Stark, J. (1980) Fall in the incidence of Crohn's disease. *Gut*, **21**, 340–343.
35. Langman, M.J.S. (1979) *The Epidemiology of Chronic Digestive Disease*. London: Arnold.
36. Lashner, B.A., Kane, S.V. and Hanauer, S.B. (1989) Lack of association between oral contraceptive use and Crohn's disease: a community-based matched case-control study. *Gastroenterology*, **97**, 1442–1447.
37. Lee, E.C.G. (1981) *Crohn's Workshop: A Global Assessment of Crohn's Disease*. London: Heyden.
38. Lee, F.I. and Costello, F.T. (1985) Crohn's disease in Blackpool – incidence and prevalence 1968–80. *Gut*, **26**, 274–278.
39. Lesko, S.M., Kaufman, D.W., Rosenberg, L. *et al.* (1985) Evidence for an increased risk of Crohn's disease in oral contraceptive users. *Gastroenterology*, **89**, 1046–1049.
40. Lewkonia, R.M. and McConnell, R.B. (1976) Familial inflammatory bowel disease – heredity or environment? *Gut*, **17**, 235–243.
41. Lindberg, E., Tysk, C., Andersson, K. and Janerot, G. (1988) Smoking and inflammatory bowel disease. A case-control study. *Gut*, **29**, 352–357.
42. Logan, R.F.A., Edmond, M., Somerville, K.W. and Langman, M.J.S. (1984) Smoking and ulcerative colitis. *British Medical Journal*, **288**, 751–753.
43. Logan, R.F.A. and Kay, C.R. (1989) Oral contraception, smoking and inflammatory bowel disease – findings in the Royal College of General Practitioners Oral Contraceptive Study. *International Journal of Epidemiology*, **18**, 105–107.
44. Martini, G.A. and Brandes, J.W. (1976) Increased consumption of refined carbohydrates in patients with Crohn's disease. *Klinische Wochenschrift*, **54**, 357–371.
45. Mayberry, J., Rhodes, J. and Hughes, L.E. (1979) Incidence of Crohn's disease in Cardiff between 1934 and 1977. *Gut*, **120**, 602–608.
46. McDermott, F., Hughes, E.S.R. and Pihl, E. (1980) Mortality and morbidity of Crohn's disease and ulcerative colitis in Australia. *Medical Journal of Australia*, **1**, 534–536.
47. Mendeloff, A.I. and Dunn, J.P. (1971) *Digestive Diseases*. Cambridge, MA: Harvard University Press.
48. Mendeloff, A.I., Monk, M., Siegel, C.I. and Lilienfeld, A. (1966) Some epidemiological features of ulcerative colitis and regional enteritis – a preliminary report. *Gastroenterology*, **51**, 748–756.
49. Miller, B., Fervers, F., Rohbeck, R. and Strohmeyer, G. (1976) Zuckerkonsum bei patienten mit morbus Crohn. *Verhhandlungen de Deutschen Gesellschaft für Innere Medizin*, **82**, 922–924.
50. Miller, D.A., Keighley, A.C. and Langman, M.J.S. (1974) Changing patterns in epidemiology of Crohn's disease. *The Lancet*, **2**, 691–693.
51. Miller, D.S., Keighley, A., Smith, P.G. *et al.* (1975) Crohn's disease in Nottingham: a search for time-space clustering. *Gut*, **16**, 454–457.
52. Miller, D.S., Keighley, A., Smith, P.G. *et al.* (1976) A case control method for seeking evidence of contagion in Crohn's disease. *Gastroenterology*, **71**, 385–387.
53. Monk, M., Mendeloff, A.I., Siegel, C.I. and Lilienfeld, A. (1967) An epidemiological study of ulcerative colitis and regional enteritis among adults in Baltimore. I. Hospital incidence and prevalence, 1960–1963. *Gastroenterology*, **53**, 198–210.
54. Monk, M., Mendeloff, A.I., Siegel, C.I. and Lilienfeld, A. (1969) An epidemiological study of ulcerative colitis and regional enteritis among adults in Baltimore. II. Social and demographic factors. *Gastroenterology*, **56**, 847–857.
55. Myren, J., Gjone, E., Hertzberg, J.N. *et al.* (1971) Epidemiology of ulcerative colitis and regional enterocolitis (Crohn's disease) in Norway.

Scandinavian Journal of Gastroenterology, **5**, 511–514.
56. Norlen, B.J., Krause, U. and Bergman, L. (1970) An epidemiological study of Crohn's disease. *Scandinavian Journal of Gastroenterology*, **5**, 385–390.
57. Orholm, M., Monkholm, P., Langholz, E., Nielsen, O.H., Sorensen, T.I.A. and Binder, V. (1991) Familial occurrence of inflammatory bowel disease. *New England Journal of Medicine*, **324**, 84–88.
58. Paffenbarger, R.S., Wing, A.L. and Hyde, R.T. (1977) Characteristics in youth indicative of adult-onset Hodgkin's disease. *Journal of the National Cancer Institute*, **58**, 1489–1491.
59. Rawcliffe, P.M. and Truelove, S.C. (1978) Breakfast and Crohn's disease I. *British Medical Journal*, **2**, 539.
60. Rhodes, J.M., Cockel, R., Allan, R.N., Hawker, P.C., Dawson, J. and Elias, E. (1984) Colonic Crohn's disease and use of oral contraception. *British Medical Journal*, **288**, 595–596.
61. Rozen, O., Zonia, J., Yekutiel, P. and Gilat, T. (1979) Crohn's disease in the Jewish population of Tel-Aviv-Jafo. *Gastroenterology*, **76**, 25–30.
62. Sandler, R.S. and Holland, K.L. (1988) Smoking and infiammatory bowel disease. *Gastroenterology*, **94**, A398.
63. Sedlack, R.E., Nobrega, F.T., Kurland, L.T. and Sauer, W.G. (1972) Inflammatory colon disease in Rochester, Minnesota, 1935–1964. *Gastroenterology*, **62**, 935–941.
64. Segal, I., Tim, L.O., Hamilton, D.G. and Mannell, A. (1981) The Baragwanath experience of Crohn's disease and intestinal tuberculosis. In *A Global Assessment of Crohn's Disease* (Ed.) Lee, E.C.G. London: Heyden.
65. Shivananda, S., Pena, A.S., Nap, M. *et al.* (1987) Epidemiology of Crohn's disease in region Leiden, the Netherlands. *Gastroenterology*, **93**, 966–974.
66. Shivananda, S., Pena, A.S., Mayberry, J.F., Ruitenberg, E.J. and Hoedemaeker, P.J. (1987) Epidemiology of proctocolitis in the region of Leiden, the Netherlands. *Scandinavian Journal of Gastroenterology*, **22**, 993–1002.
67. Sinclair, T.S., Brunt, P.W., Ashley, N. and Mowat, G. (1983) Non specific proctitis in NE Scotland. A community study. *Gastroenterology*, **85**, 1–11.
68. Sinclair, T.S., Brunt, P.W. and Mowat, N.A.G. (1983) Non specific proctocolitis in north eastern Scotland: a community study. *Gastroenterology*, **81**, 1115–1124.
69. Smith, I.S., Young, S., Gillespie, G. *et al.* (1975) Epidemiological aspects of Crohn's disease in Clydesdale 1961–1970. *Gut*, **16**, 62–67.
70. Somerville, K.W., Logan, R.F.A., Edmond, E.M. and Langman, M.J.S. (1984) Smoking and Crohn's disease. *British Medical Journal*, **289**, 954–956.
71. Stonnington, C.M., Phillips, S.F., Melton, L.J. and Zinsmeister, A.R. (1987) Chronic ulcerative colitis: incidence and prevalence in a community. *Gut*, **28**, 402–409.
72. Thornton, J.R., Emmett, P.M. and Heaton, K.W. (1979) Diet and Crohn's disease: characteristics of the pre-illness diet. *British Medical Journal*, **2**, 762–764.
73. Thornton, J.R., Emmett, J.W. and Heaton, K.W. (1981). Smoking, sugar and inflammatory bowel disease. *British Medical Journal*, **290**, 1786–1787.
74. Tobin, M.W., Logan, R.F.A., Langman, M.J.S., McConnell, R.B. and Gilmore, I.T. (1987) Cigarette smoking and inflammatory bowel disease. *Gastroenterology*, **93**, 316–321.
75. Vessey, M.P., Jewell, D., Smith, A., Yeates, D. and McPherson, K. (1986) Chronic inflammatory bowel disease, cigarette smoking and use of oral contraceptives: findings in a large cohort study of women of child-bearing age. *British Medical Journal*, **292**, 1101–1103.
76. Wenckert, A., Henricksson, A. and Lindstrom, C. (1974) Incidence of Crohn's disease in the city of Malmo. *Scandinavian Journal of Gastroenterology*, **9** (supplement 27), 42.
77. Wigley, R.D. and MacLaurin, B.P. (1962) A study of ulcerative colitis in New Zealand, showing a low incidence in Maoris. *British Medical Journal*, **2**, 228–231.

AETIOLOGY AND PATHOGENESIS

J.M. Rhodes and H.H. Tsai

It is difficult both to define a disease whose aetiology is unknown and to determine the aetiology of a condition that cannot be clearly defined. This circular argument is particularly applicable to inflammatory bowel disease because there are many examples of conditions of widely differing aetiology which closely resemble ulcerative colitis or Crohn's disease. For example, bacterial dysentery, ischaemic colitis, irradiation colitis, intestinal tuberculosis, *Yersinia enterocolitica* enteritis and chronic granulomatous disease may all cause diagnostic confusion, presumably reflecting the limited range of inflammatory responses in response to a variety of stimuli.

ONE DISEASE OR TWO?

The first question that needs to be addressed is whether the conditions labelled as ulcerative colitis or Crohn's disease (regional enteritis) are separate diseases of different aetiology or whether they represent a continuous spectrum of inflammatory bowel disease with a common aetiology. The classic differences between the two conditions including the different histological features and their different anatomical distribution are weak arguments for considering them as different diseases when set against the wide variety of clinical and pathological manifestations that may result from infections such as tuberculosis, syphilis and leprosy. Epidemiological studies have provided better evidence for considering the two conditions as distinct entities. There is a striking difference in the smoking habits of patients with ulcerative colitis and Crohn's disease. Harries and colleagues in Cardiff showed that only 8% of 230 patients with ulcerative colitis were current smokers as compared with 44% of patients attending a fracture clinic.[82] This association between non-smoking and ulcerative colitis has since been confirmed in at least 12 other studies.[8,11,12,22,44,51,89,108,171,202,204,212] Patients with Crohn's disease smoke at least as much or more than age-matched controls.[44,83,100,191,202]

Dietary studies have also revealed differences between ulcerative colitis and Crohn's disease. Crohn's disease, unlike ulcerative colitis, is associated with a marked increase in the pre-illness consumption of refined sugar (see later) and there are many reports of impressive responses to dietary therapy in Crohn's disease which are not explicable on the basis of improved nutrition. There is little evidence in ulcerative colitis that alterations in diet alter the prognosis, and controlled trials of complete bowel rest combined with intravenous feeding have not shown any benefit.[52,125]

Family studies have shown some evidence of a link between ulcerative colitis and Crohn's disease. There is, for example, a 3.5-fold increase in risk for Crohn's disease in first-degree relatives of patients with ulcerative colitis.[132] Ulcerative colitis and Crohn's disease may therefore represent a spectrum of polygenic disease so that inheritance of only a few of the relevant genes might predispose to ulcerative colitis whilst inheritance of a more complete genotype would result in Crohn's disease.[124] Alternatively, a single inherited defect might result in different phenotypic expression depending on the presence of some environmental factor such as cigarette smoking.

The question of whether ulcerative colitis and Crohn's disease represent one disease or two will probably not be resolved until a convincing aetiology is discovered for one or both conditions.

ANIMAL MODELS

NATURALLY OCCURRING DISEASES

Primates

Primates in captivity are susceptible to a colitis which is strikingly similar to human ulcerative colitis. Colitis was reported in four Siamang gibbons in 1969[196] and in orang-utans in 1974[181] but recent attention has been focused on the colitis that affects the cotton-top tamarin, *Saguinus oedipus oedipus*. This primate quite predictably develops colitis when kept in captivity, the incidence rising from 18% of animals necropsied in the first year of captivity to 100% by the fourth year.[34] In addition 25–40% of the animals develop colonic cancer after 2–5 years in captivity.[34,35,104,115] histological features resemble human ulcerative colitis with crypt abscess formation and mucus depletion[42,118] and the disease responds to sulphasalazine.[118] As in human colitis, carcinomas begin as flat lesions rather than as adenomatous polyps.[34] In view of the report that in human ulcerative colitis the age-matched relative risk for cancer remains constant with time,[36] it is of interest that so far cancer predating the onset of colitis has not been reported in the monkeys, suggesting that in this animal model the colitis predisposes to cancer rather than being a co-inherited problem. It is curious that two other species of New World monkey, *Saguinus fuscicollis illigeri* and *Callithrix jacchus*, also develop colitis[15] in which there is no increased risk for cancer.[102] The cause of the colitis in monkeys is not clear but its apparent correlation with length of time in captivity lends some support to a possible link between colitis and psychological stress.

Dogs

Several breeds of dogs, boxers in particular, are prone to colitis. The boxer colitis usually has histological features resembling both Crohn's disease and Whipple's disease with granulomata and the presence of PAS-positive material (PAS = periodic acid–Schiff) within macrophages in the lamina propria.[210] Electron microscopic studies have demonstrated the presence of probable chlamydiae within phagocytic vacuoles[211] so the pathogenesis is probably different from human inflammatory bowel disease but interestingly there is usually a good response to sulphasalazine. There is a separate form of colitis in dogs which mimics ulcerative colitis and which may respond to corticosteroid therapy.[211]

TRANSMISSION OF DISEASE BETWEEN HUMANS AND ANIMALS

Dalziel first described the similarities between non-tuberculosis regional enteritis in humans and *Mycobacterium johnei* infection in goats[48] 19 years before Crohn's original report. Early trials of antituberculosis therapy in Crohn's disease were negative[186] but the agents used were probably not effective against *M. johnei*. There has been a resurgence of interest in this organism because of reports of its isolation from Crohn's disease tissue and the subsequent infection of goats inoculated with the isolate. The disease in ruminants is, however, invariably progressive and the response of human Crohn's disease to immunosuppressive therapy makes it unlikely that the two conditions are the same and *M. johnei* may just be one of many organisms causing secondary infection after penetrating areas of ulcerated intestinal mucosa.

Other examples of transmission of disease from humans to animals are less convincing. Granulomatous lesions have been induced in mice[129] and rabbits[33] by injection of filtered extracts of Crohn's disease tissue, but attempts to reproduce these results have not always been successful[199] so that some of the lesions may have been due to non-specific 'foreign body' reactions. More recently, Crohn's disease tissue extracts have induced lymphoma when injected into athymic nude mice[50] but it is not yet clear whether this response is specific for Crohn's disease tissue.[218]

EXPERIMENTAL MODELS

The wide variety of experimental models of inflammatory bowel disease is a reflection of the wide range of hypotheses for its aetiology. Microvascular ischaemia has been proposed as a mechanism for Crohn's disease and colonic artery ligation has been used as a model for colitis[18] as has occlusion of smaller end-arteries by intra-arterial injection of glass microspheres.[17] Lymphatic dilatation is a well-recognized histological feature of Crohn's disease and injection of sclerosant into subserosal and mesenteric lymphatics in experimental animals causes thickening of the terminal ileum but without ulceration or granuloma formation.[161] The disputed association between ulcerative colitis and stress has been studied by using pharmacological agents to alter the balance between sympathetic and parasympathetic activity. Experimental colitis has been induced by methacholine,[130] intraperitoneal adrenaline,[105] and prolonged administration of histamine[9] as well as by abdominal postganglionic sympathectomy.[9]

Several of the immunological hypotheses have been tested in animal models. These include the rectal instillation of antigens to which the animals have been previously sensitized[105] and the instillation of the potent sensitizer dinitrochlorobenzene.[157] A model has also been developed on the basis of the Auer modification of the Arthus phenomenon. Intravenously injected albumin–anti-albumin immune complexes are localized to the rectum by prior instillation of dilute formalin.[90] The formalin alone only produces mild hyperaemia whereas the injected immune complexes provoke a more severe inflammatory response with crypt abscess formation and mucus depletion. A chronic colitis results if the animal has previously been sensitized to the common enterobacterial (Kunin) antigen.[127]

The heightened interest in possible dietary aetiologies for Crohn's disease makes the carrageenan model worthy of careful consideration. Carrageenan is a sulphated polysaccharide, with a molecular weight of between 100 000 and 800 000, which is derived from red seaweeds and is widely used in the food industry as an emulsifier. In its undegraded form it is non-toxic,[21] but hydrolysis by dilute acid degrades it to a low-molecular-weight form (mol. wt of 30 000) which reproducibly provokes granuloma formation when injected subcutaneously into rats.[131] A series of studies has been performed to assess the effect of feeding the degraded carrageenan to animals. It has no effect on germ-free animals but in normally colonized animals (guinea-pigs) it provokes a colitis.[140] The development of colitis is dependent on the presence of particular strains of *Bacteroides vulgatus*.[139] Degraded carrageenan also promotes carcinogenesis when given to animals that have been fed a carcinogen.[215]

OVERLAP SYNDROMES

Sometimes the careful study of rare disorders may provide a clue to the aetiology of more common disorders. Chronic granulomatous disease is an inherited disorder of phagocyte function, usually X-linked, inducing an inability to cope with bacterial infection. It presents in childhood, typically with 'cold' abscesses, but one feature of the disease is granulomatous ulceration of the intestine which closely mimics Crohn's disease.[2] The molecular defect has been well characterized and is a cytochrome B abnormality resulting in an inability to kill phagocytosed bacteria because of a failure of free radical generation.[183]

There is a second phagocyte disorder, malakoplakia, which may also cause intestinal disease similar to Crohn's disease.[70] This is an acquired condition which is also due to a defect in the ability of phagocytes to kill phagocytosed bacteria and which can be corrected by high-dose vitamin C therapy.

Phagocyte function has been carefully studied in Crohn's disease without the demonstration of any convincing abnormality (see later) but there is still a strong suspicion that a reduced ability to cope with bacteria may explain some of the features of the disease.

SITE OF DISEASE AS A CLUE TO AETIOLOGY

Sir Samuel Wilks, who is usually credited with the first description of ulcerative colitis, must have encountered Crohn's disease as well for he was in no doubt that 'the end of the ileum and large intestine are the parts of the alimentary canal most liable to be affected from various causes for in them irritant substances lodge'.[225] Although Crohn's disease can affect any part of the intestine any hypothesis for its aetiology should take into account its predeliction for the terminal ileum and caecum. Possible explanations for this observation could include (1) increased permeability of the mucosa at this point (particularly overlying Peyer's patches); (2) the presence of large numbers of bacteria; and (3) stasis, as implied by Wilks.

Roles for stasis and/or bacteria in the pathogenesis of Crohn's disease are also implicated by the tendency for the disease to recur at or immediately proximal to the surgical anastomosis following resection. In one series reported from Birmingham, 57 out of 59 recurrences occurred at or immediately proximal to the anastomosis as opposed to only 7 out of 79 that were distal.[86]

Metastatic Crohn's disease is a rare but striking form of Crohn's disease which may provide further aetiological clues. Patients with Crohn's disease may develop granulomatous skin lesions remote from the intestine. Affected sites include the umbilicus[151], the thigh and forearm,[207] the penis[189] or the face.[14] The lesions may respond to treatment with metronidazole,[14] which suggests a defective capacity to respond to bacterial infection.

The tendency for ulcerative colitis to affect the distal colon more severely than the proximal colon must be a clue to its pathogenesis and suggests the importance of intraluminal factors. These factors, which might be bacterially secreted enzymes or peptides, would have to increase in concentration progressively from the proximal to the distal colon.

INFECTIOUS AGENTS

ULCERATIVE COLITIS

When medical microbiology was in its infancy it was difficult to distinguish idiopathic ulcerative colitis from bacillary dysentery; indeed, a standard medical textbook in 1904 stated that there was 'no need to regard idiopathic colitis and bacillary dysentery as different conditions'.[177] The hunt for an infective agent responsible for ulcerative colitis has contiued ever since. No specific organism has been identified which can reliably be detected in patients' faeces, but attacks of ulcerative colitis have been reported as a sequel to infection with a variety of pathogens including an unidentified diplococcus,[6] *Shigella* spp.,[1,5,66,67,93,117] *Salmonella* spp.,[54,113,200] *Campylobacter jejuni*,[134] *Clostridium difficile*,[20] *Aeromonas* spp.,[227] and *Giardia lamblia*.[73] It is uncertain whether the pathogenic organisms merely contribute to the relapse of colitis or actually provoke the development of chronic colitis.[198] Confusion is compounded by reports of corticosteroid-responsive 'ulcerative post-dysenteric colitis' following bacterial or amoebic dysentery.[155,158]

Faecal bacteria provide a rich source of foreign antigens and potentially toxic metabolites so they could have an important role in pathogenesis even if there is no specific pathogen. Seneca and Henderson[185] first suggested that the indigenous microbial flora might be involved in the pathogenesis of ulcerative colitis. The studies of carrageenan-induced colitis in guinea-pigs demonstrated the importance of the enteric flora[140,208] and showed that this experimental colitis could be prevented by concomitant administration of metronidazole.[141] The presence of *Bacteroides vulgatus* appears essential to the development of carrageenan-induced colitis[139,140] whereas *B. distasonis* and *Clostridium* spp. have been reported as essential in the development of a similar experimental colitis that is induced by synthetic dextran sulphate[138].

Using conventional microbiological techniques, exhaustive studies of the microflora in patients with inflammatory bowel disease have been inconclusive. Most studies[43,74] have shown little difference in the colonic flora of patients with ulcerative colitis when compared to controls. One study showed an increase in group D streptococci and a reduction in bifidobacteria compared to healthy controls.[209] Strains of these organisms isolated from patients with ulcerative colitis were more active in mucin degradation and lactate production.

Serotypes of *Escherichia coli* with specific adhesive properties to HeLa cells have been found more frequently in patients with acute colitis than in controls.[26,27,53] The adherence mechanism of this organism is mannose independent and its presence may indicate an increase in mucosal binding sites as a result of changes in carbohydrate expression secondary to the disease. An unusual strain of *E. coli*, serotype 0157 H7, has been associated with acute haemorrhage colitis but this does not develop into a chronic colitis.[217]

The search for viral agents in ulcerative colitis has been inconclusive. Riemann[168] reported electron microscopic findings of 'virus-like particles' in epithelial cells and macrophages in the mucosa of affected colons but others failed to confirm these findings.[57,224] Similarly there have been both positive[65,97,142,179] and negative reports[7,61,78,133,197] of serological testing for evidence of cytomegalovirus, Epstein–Barr virus or chlamydial infection in patients with ulcerative colitis.

CROHN'S DISEASE

Crohn, Ginsberg and Oppenheimer, in their classic description of the disease,[46] and Homans and Hass[91] carried out cultures on tissue from patients with regional enteritis but failed to demonstrate a transmissible agent. Patients have increased serum titres to the anaerobic organisms *Bacteroides fragilis*,[85,112] *Eubacterium* spp. and *Peptostreptococcus* spp.[223] but this does not necessarily imply a causative role for these organisms. Studies of the enteric flora of Crohn's disease patients have shown an increase in Gram-positive anaerobic coccoid rods when compared to healthy subjects.[222] The faecal content of cell wall-deficient bacteria is increased in both Crohn's disease and ulcerative colitis.[94] Although there is no convincing evidence for the involvement of any specific bacterial species in the aetiology of Crohn's disease, the effect of treatment with metronidazole[109,110] suggests that bacteria do have a role in the pathogenesis, perhaps by secondary infection of ulcerated tissue.

The similarities between Crohn's disease, human tuberculosis and Johne's disease of cattle[48] have understandably led to an intensive search for evidence of mycobacterial infection in Crohn's disease. That this search should still be actively pursued nearly 80 years later reflects the difficulty of excluding mycobacterial infection. The tuberculin skin test usually induces a normal or decreased response in Crohn's disease[12,76,201,226] and serum agglutinin reactions against *Mycobacterium paratuberculosis* and *M. avium intracellulare* do not differ from controls.[120] These findings do not rule out a mycobacterial aetiology. *Mycobacterium kansasii* has been isolated from the lymph node of a patient with Crohn's disease,[28] but this organism is ubiquitous and a common laboratory contaminant, and similar acid-fast bacteria have been found in tissue from patients with ulcerative colitis.[193] Considerable interest was aroused when Chiodini and colleagues[40] isolated a mycobacterium from Crohn's disease tissue that was later identified as *M. paratuberculosis* by DNA hybridization studies.[229] This organism was transmissible to goats and is the species responsible for Johne's disease of cattle. However, the isolation rates of this organism from Crohn's disease patients are low (2–15%) and, although a slow-growing strain of *M. chelonei* has also been isolated from Crohn's disease tissue,[72] extensive immunohistochemical studies searching for mycobacterial antigens in Crohn's disease tissue have proved negative,[106] as have studies using copy DNA probes to search for evidence of mycobacterial DNA.[29]

There have been several trials of antimycobacterial therapy in Crohn's disease with conflicting results. Several trials have been negative[60,92,186] but two studies have shown benefit with dapsone,[156,210] and several other studies of antimycobacterial therapy have produced promising results.[80,145,152,180,201,205,221] The significance of these trials is difficult to evaluate partly because *Mycobacterium johnei* is resistant to conventional antimycobacterial drugs but also because, in addition, some of the antimycobacterial drugs have immunosuppressive and anti-inflammatory effects. It seems unlikely that mycobacteria are the primary cause of Crohn's disease, in view of the beneficial effects of potent immunosuppressive agents such as corticosteroids, azathioprine and cyclosporine. Furthermore, the development of the acquired immune deficiency syndrome (AIDS), a condition in which atypical mycobacteria cause major problems, may result in the improvement of pre-existing Crohn's disease.[95]

Useful information has come from studies in which lymphocytes have been extracted from the mesenteric lymph nodes of patients with Crohn's disease or ulcerative colitis, fused with mouse myeloma cells and cultured so that they generate monoclonal antibodies, presumably with the same specificity as the antibodies that would have been produced by the mesenteric lymph nodes in the patient.[37] These antibodies have then been tested against a wide range of bacterial and dietary antigens. An increased proportion of cell lines generated from the lymph nodes of patients with Crohn's disease produced antibodies against pooled mycobacteria (30%) or against pooled miscellaneous organisms (36%) compared with those from ulcerative colitis (13% and 17%, respectively). Antibodies to food antigens (wheat, cabbage and milk) were rarely found. These results are compatible with the view that in Crohn's disease breaches in the mucosa allow access to a variety of bacteria, including some mycobacterial species. The secondary infection that results from the presence of these bacteria may well be important in pathogenesis but it seems unlikely that any single organism will prove responsible for the disease.

IMMUNOLOGY

Inflammation in the absence of any obvious pathogen has led many workers to seek immunological causes for ulcerative colitis and Crohn's disease. However, despite many hundreds of publications and the application of all available immunological techniques, no such cause has yet been found. It is difficult to formulate immunological hypotheses which adequately explain the site of the lesion in either disease. If there is an underlying immunological defect, why should the damage be almost entirely confined within the gastrointestinal tract and why should ulcerative colitis so typically affect the distal colon more than the proximal colon? Immunological studies have nevertheless been useful in highlighting several abnormalities which, although probably secondary to the disease, may have an important role in its perpetuation and because they provide insight into mechanisms of inflammation in the intestine and ways in which this might be modulated by drugs.

IMMUNOLOGICAL COMPETENCE

It has been suggested that patients with Crohn's disease are relatively anergic and unable to mount a normal cell-mediated immune response. Evidence for this comes from studies showing reduced Mantoux reactivity[150,226] but later studies which included carefully matched controls refuted this observation[19,69,178] and suggested that any anergy was either secondary to the disease itself or secondary to corticosteroid therapy.

It has been suggested that many patients with ulcerative colitis are atopic, but atopy is no more common in patients with ulcerative colitis than in controls.[126] Similarly the evidence for a role for food allergy in ulcerative colitis is scant. About one in five patients improve with elimination of cows' milk protein,[228] but the observation that complete bowel rest and intravenous feeding are of no benefit[53,125] rules out any very significant role for dietary antigens in this condition.

The similarity between Crohn's disease and the intestinal lesions of chronic granulomatous disease of childhood, an inherited phagocyte defect, has stimulated studies in all aspects of phagocyte function in Crohn's disease. Subtle defects in neutrophil polymorph phagocytosis have been shown,[135] but the ability of the phagocytes to generate an oxidative burst in order to kill phagocytosed bacteria is normal.[107,219] Considerable interest was stimulated by studies which showed reduced chemotaxis of patients' neutrophils in 'skin windows', i.e. serum-filled Perspex chambers placed over small areas of abraded skin.[184] When subsequent studies were performed on peripheral blood neutrophil polymorphs and monocytes they moved normally in vitro,[13,62,137,165] but there was evidence of the presence of inhibitors of chemotaxis in serum.[167] These studies can be summarized as showing evidence, not of a major underlying defect in phagocyte function, but of mild abnormalities, particularly in patients with active disease. This supports the clinical suspicion that some of the complications of Crohn's disease (perianal disease, fistula formation, metastatic disease) might be related to secondary defects in the ability to cope with bacterial infection.

Mild splenic hypofunction is a common feature of long-standing inflammatory bowel disease, whether Crohn's disease or ulcerative colitis, but it may be sufficiently marked to cause features of hyposplenism in the blood film and a marked diminution in splenic uptake on isotope scanning.[143] It is thought to be secondary to the continual bombardment of the reticuloendothelial system by antigenic material that has penetrated an inflamed or excessively permeable intestinal mucosa.

Numerous studies of lymphocyte function have been performed, both on peripheral blood lymphocytes and on lymphocytes extracted from mucosal samples. Many were performed while the methodology for assessing lymphocyte function was being developed and the results (particularly those for suppressor cell and natural killer cell activity) tend to be conflicting. The consensus now is that there is a general increase in lymphocytes within the mucosa but that the T-lymphocyte function is normal.[71,190] Mucosal B lymphocytes and plasma cells are both increased in ulcerative colitis and Crohn's disease, but in Crohn's disease there is a particular increase in immunocytes producing IgG_2 antibodies.[103,182] This subclass is typical of antibacterial antibodies which adds to the evidence that the mucosa in Crohn's disease is responding to some form of non-specific bacterial attack.

Circulating immune complexes have been sought because their presence would support the hypothesis that mucosal inflammation, particularly in ulcerative colitis, might represent an Auer reaction similar to the animal model of colitis that is based on this reaction. Confusion may have been caused in some of these studies by the method of serum storage because repeated freezing and thawing causes aggregation of immunoglobulin which has been shown to give rise to false-positive results in the tests used to detect immune complexes in serum.[191] The consensus now is that circulating complexes probably do not play a major role in pathogenesis, but may be responsible for some of the extra-intestinal manifestations of active disease such as arthritis, iritis and erythema nodosum.[87]

AUTOIMMUNITY

Many patients with ulcerative colitis or Crohn's disease have anti-colon antibodies detectable in the serum.[24,111] The antigen bound by these antibodies is located within goblet cells and probably a mucin, but the antibodies do not activate complement and do not have any cytotoxic effect. They are also found following gastroenteritis[32] which suggests that they are a secondary phenomenon. More recently a different autoantibody has been described in ulcerative colitis by Das and colleagues.[49] This is an IgG antibody which can be eluted from the colonic tissue of ulcerative colitis patients and which recognises a protein of molecular weight 40 000 present on the basolateral membrane of both normal and diseased colonic epithelial cells.

Peripheral blood lymphocytes which have an antibody-dependent cytotoxic effect on colonic epithial cells in vitro have been detected in the blood of patients with inflammatory bowel disease,[149,195] but the only cytotoxic lymphocytes that can be extracted from the mucosa are antibody independent.[173] In a study of over 1200 patients with inflammatory bowel disease, 6.6% of patients with ulcerative colitis had a recognized autoimmune disorder such as pernicious anaemia or thyroiditis compared with only 1.9% with Crohn's disease and 2.0% of controls.[190] There may be a subgroup of patients with ulcerative colitis in whom autoimmunity plays a part in the development of the disease phenotype. Sclerosing cholangitis, for example, is more common in HLA-DR3 individuals[39] whereas there is no HLA (histocompatibility locus antigen) association with ulcerative colitis in general. HLA-DR3 is associated with other autoimmune disorders and patients with sclerosing cholangitis can be shown to have antibodies in the serum which bind to an antigen in hepatic portal tracts.[38]

Studies of the microvasculature in the lesions of resected intestine from patients with Crohn's disease have shown abnormalities that would be consistent with a vasculitic pathogenesis[216] but such findings may be non-specific and control studies in disorders such as intestinal tuberculosis are needed to determine whether these changes are simply part of the inflammatory process.

There is a statistical association between oral contraceptive usage and colonic Crohn's disease[166] and possibly also with small bowel Crohn's disease.[31] There have also been anecdotal reports of colitis occurring shortly after oral contraceptives have been started and resolving when they are stopped. There is, however, no clear evidence for a direct causal relationship, although microvascular occlusion has been postulated as a possible mechanism.

Recently, antibodies to antigens in neutrophil cytoplasm (anti-neutrophil cytoplasmic antibodies, ANCA) have been found in the serum of patients with ulcerative colitis. Reported incidences range from 54%[30] to 85%.[56] Similar incidence of this antibody is detected in primary sclerosing cholangitis with or without colitis.[55] This is in contrast to Crohn's disease where only 10% of patients possess this antibody.[30] The pattern of staining is mainly perinuclear (p-ANCA) but cytoplasmic staining is also found.[30] The anti-neutrophil cytoplasmic antibodies found in ulcerative colitis are distinct from those found in Wegener's granulomatosis and their pathogenic role remains to be elucidated.

MECHANISMS OF INFLAMMATION AND THEIR MODULATION BY DRUGS

The presence of large numbers of inflammatory cells in the intestinal mucosa implies the presence of a high concentration of chemotactic factor. There are at least three likely contenders for this role:

1. Complement C5a
2. Leukotriene B_4
3. A bacterial chemotactic peptide such as formyl-methionyl-leucyl-phenylalanine (fMet Leu Phe).

There is some evidence of general complement activation in inflammatory bowel disease,[64,79] but in Crohn's disease a specific defect has been reported in the ability to generate C5a.[63] Leukotriene B_4 is an extremely potent chemotactic factor and is present in increased concentrations in the mucosa in inflammatory bowel disease.[187] fMet Leu Phe is produced by intestinal bacteria, and circulating neutrophils from patients with Crohn's disease (but not ulcerative colitis) have increased numbers of receptors for this peptide and an increased functional response,[3] perhaps reflecting frequent contact between neutrophils and intestinal bacteria in this disease. Platelet-activating factor (PAF), a species of phosphatidylcholine that is released by stimulated leukocytes, endothelial cells and platelets, may also have a key role in the development of inflammation. Colonic biopsies from patients with ulcerative colitis have a much greater potential to release platelet-activating factor than biopsies from controls or patients with Crohn's disease.[59] Platelet-activating factor is itself a powerful chemotactic factor but its synthesis is also closely linked to the synthesis of chemotactic leukotrienes.

Hopefully, the study of mechanisms of inflammation will lead to new forms of therapy, even if it does not lead directly to the cause of inflammatory bowel disease. Sulphasalazine and its active metabolite, 5-aminosalicylic acid, inhibit lipoxygenase,[194] the enzyme responsible for the generation of chemotactic leukotrienes from arachidonic acid, and it also inhibits the release of platelet-activating factor at concentrations that are probably achievable in the colonic mucosa.[59] Platelet-activating factor inhibition by other agents or antibodies seems to be a promising approach for the development of new therapies.

DIETARY FACTORS

Patients naturally assume that any chronic intestinal disease is likely to be related in some way to their diet. In ulcerative colitis, however, there is very little evidence for this concept. Approximately one in five patients benefit from exclusion of dairy products from the diet[228] but controlled trials have shown no benefit from total bowel rest and intravenous feeding[53,125] which would be expected if dietary factors were important, and there is no benefit from diversion ileostomy.[81] In Crohn's disease, there is clear evidence that dietary factors play a role in aetiology. Several trials have shown a therapeutic effect when patients with active disease are given intravenous feeding[68,114,213] or fed chemically defined formula diets[4,77,136,172,214] as their sole feed without any other form of therapy. It is unclear how these dietary therapies exert their effect. It does not seem necessary to avoid whole protein as good results have been reported with whole protein-based enteral feeds.[159] Although it has generally been assumed that dietary therapy works by excluding some harmful agent, some workers have reported beneficial results from supplementing a normal diet with an enteral feed,[84] which implies that part of the therapeutic effect may be due to improved nutrition. Epidemiological studies have also produced interesting information. Many studies have shown that patients with Crohn's disease have a high pre-illness intake of refined sugar.[23,75,96,99,119,121,122,123,144,188,203] These studies are difficult to interpret because they depend on the patients' recall of what their diets had been prior to their illness; furthermore there is no proof of a causal relationship between Crohn's disease and a high sugar intake. There is, for example, no evidence that it results in an altered microbial flora.[10]

ASSOCIATION WITH PSYCHOLOGICAL STRESS

Many patients with inflammatory bowel disease, particularly those with ulcerative colitis, comment that relapses of their disease tend to coincide with periods of psychological stress. This possible association has been difficult to prove or disprove as stress is difficult to quantify.[146,147,169,170] If the association is real there needs to be a biochemical explanation for the mucosal damage – possibly inhibition of mucus synthesis by catecholamines.

MUCOSAL PERMEABILITY

The evidence that lymphocytes in mesenteric lymph nodes of patients with Crohn's disease produce antibodies against a wide range of bacterial and dietary antigens fits well with the hypothesis that there might be an underlying increase in intestinal permeability in Crohn's disease. It is well recognized that patients with active disease have increased permeability, but this is probably secondary to the disease. Considerable interest has been attracted by the report that unaffected first-degree relatives of patients with Crohn's disease may have increased intestinal mucosal permeability. This story is still unclear because the permeability defect has so far only been demonstrated when Polyethylene glycol 400 has been used as the probe,[90] permeability to chromium-labelled EDTA (ethylenediaminetetra-acetic acid) and to sugar solutions having so far proved normal.[101]

MUCUS

In the colon there is a continual balance between mucus secretion and its breakdown by bacterial enzymes. About 1% of the normal human colonic flora are capable of using secreted mucus as their sole energy source.[128] A hypothesis for ulcerative colitis can be based on a postulated alteration in the relationship between mucus and bacteria.[163] If there was an inherited alteration in the colonic structure or synthesis of mucus which made the mucus unusually susceptible to bacterial enzymatic degradation, this might leave the mucosa relatively unprotected against attack by toxins or allergens. Because the mucus-degrading glycosidases are secreted by the colonic bacteria as exoenzymes, their concentration would be expected to rise progressively from the proximal to the distal colon, in keeping with the usual distribution of ulcerative colitis within the colon. Mucus is heavily glycosylated and one of the first steps in its breakdown is desialylation. Colonic mucin sialic acid is normally highly resistant to sialidase attack however because of *O*-acetyl substitution in the sialic molecule, but reduced *O*-acetylation of mucin sialic acids has been demonstrated histochemically in ulcerative colitis.[47,162] In ulcerative colitis a relative diminution of sulphomucins has also been found[58] and this would also tend to reduce the resistance of the mucus to bacterial breakdown. Studies of faecal mucus-degrading enzymes have shown increased concentrations of proteases,[45] and sulphatases,[206] and it is possible that fluctuations in the faecal concentrations of these enzymes, secondary to changes in the intestinal flora, may have a role in provoking relapse of disease.

Studies of mucus synthesis in ulcerative colitis have generally failed to show any striking abnormality,[116] but there is more evidence to suggest alterations in mucus structure. Although alterations in the chromatographic profile of purified mucins[153,154] are inconsistent,[160] the colonic mucins in ulcerative colitis have shortened oligosaccharide side chains[41] and alterations in lectin binding have been reported in both ulcerative colitis and Crohn's disease.[16,164] Although these are likely to be secondary phenomena they may still have important functional consequences.

MUCOSAL METABOLISM

Analysis of the nutritional requirement of the colonic mucosa has shown that over 70% of the energy supply of the colonic epithelium is derived from luminal short-chain fatty acids.[182] These fatty acids are derived from anaerobic bacterial metabolism.[174] Both in vitro and in vivo experiments have demonstrated a specific and selective failure of butyrate oxidation in colonic mucosa of active and quiescent colitis.[176] The inability of colonic mucosa to utilize its main energy source could explain the distribution of the disease in the large bowel, because the distal colon is more dependent on short-chain fatty acids than the proximal colon. The energy states of ATP, ADP and AMP in active colitis are also reduced.[98] It has been proposed that ulcerative colitis might result from a primary metabolic failure which is genetically determined.[175]

CONCLUSIONS

There is a natural tendency to be pessimistic about possible progress when diseases such as ulcerative colitis and Crohn's disease remain poorly understood many decades after their first recognition. Unfortunately, the lack of any clear pattern of inheritance has meant that so far new molecular biological techniques are relatively impotent in these conditions. Nevertheless, there are many clues available now and further careful study particularly, for example, of the mechanisms responsible for the beneficial effects of dietary therapy in Crohn's disease, are likely to produce valuable results.

REFERENCES

1. Acheson, E.D. and Nefzger, M.D. (1963) Ulcerative colitis in the United States Army in 1944. Epidemiology: comparison between patients and controls. *Gastroenterology*, **44**, 7–19.
2. Ament, M.E. and Ochs, H.D. (1973) Gastrointestinal manifestations of chronic granulomatous disease. *New England Journal of Medicine*, **288**, 382–387.
3. Anton, P.A., Targan, S.R. and Shanahan, F. (1989) Increased neutrophil receptors for and response to the proinflammatory bacterial peptide formyl-methionyl-leucyl-phenylalanine in Crohn's disease. *Gastroenterology*, **97**, 20–28.
4. Axelsson, C. and Jarnum, S. (1977) Assessment of the therapeutic value of an elemental diet in

chronic inflammatory bowel disease. *Scandinavian Journal of Gastroenterology*, **12**, 89–95.
5. Banks, B.M., Korelitz, B.I. and Zetzel, L. (1957) The cause of non-specific ulcerative colitis: review of twenty years' experience and late results. *Gastroenterology*, **32**, 983–1012.
6. Bargen, J.A. (1924) Experimental studies on the etiology of chronic ulcerative colitis. *Journal of the American Medical Association*, **83**, 332.
7. Beeken, W. (1979) Evidence of virus infection as a cause of Crohn's disease. *Zeitschrift für Gastroenterology*, **17**, 101–104.
8. Benoni, C. and Nilsson, A. (1984) Smoking habits in patients with inflammatory bowel disease. *Scandinavian Journal of Gastroenterology*, **19**, 824–827.
9. Berger, R.L. and Lium R. (1960) Abdominal postganglionic sympathectomy: a method for the production of an ulcerative colitis-like state in dogs. *Annals of Surgery*, **152**, 266–273.
10. Berghouse, L., Hori, S., Hill, M., Hudson, M., Lennard-Jones, J.E. and Rogers, E. (1984) Comparison between bacterial and oligosaccharide content of ileostomy effluent in subjects taking diets rich in refined and unrefined carbohydrates. *Gut*, **25**, 1071–1077.
11. Bianchi-Porro, G. (1987) Non-specific inflammatory bowel disease and smoking. *American Journal of Epidemiology*, **125**, 445–452.
12. Binder, H., Spiro, H. and Thayer, W. (1966) Delayed hypersensitivity in regional enteritis and ulcerative colitis. *American Journal Digestive Diseases*, **11**, 572–574.
13. Binder, V. and Riis, P. (1977) The leucocyte chemotactic function in patients with ulcerative colitis. *Scandinavian Journal of Gastroenterology*, **12**, 141–144.
14. Boerr, L.A., Bai, J.C., Olivares, L., Moran, C.E. and Kowalczuk, A. (1987) Cutaneous metastatic Crohn's disease: treatment with metronidazole. *American Journal of Gastroenterology*, **82**, 1326–1327.
15. Boland, C.R. and Clapp, N.K. (1987) Glycoconjugates in the colons of new world monkeys with spontaneous colitis. Association between inflammation and neoplasia. *Gastroenterology*, **92**, 625–634.
16. Boland, C.R., Lance, P., Levin, B., Riddell, R.H. and Kim, Y.S. (1984) Abnormal goblet cell glycoconjugates in rectal biopsies associated with an increased risk of neoplasia in patients with ulcerative colitis: early results of a prospective study, *Gut*, **25**, 1354–1371.
17. Boley, S.J., Krieger, H., Schultz, L. *et al.* (1965) Experimental aspects of peripheral vascular occlusion of the intestine. *Surgery, Gynecology and Obstetrics*, **121**, 789–794.
18. Boley, S.J., Schwartz, S., Lash, L. *et al.* (1963) Reversible peripheral vascular occlusion of the colon. *Surgery, Gynecology and Obstetrics*, **116**, 53–60.
19. Bolton, P.M., Jones, S.L., Newcombe, R.G., White, R.H. and Hughes, L.E. (1974) The immune competence of patients with inflammatory bowel disease. *Gut*, **15**, 213.
20. Bolton, R.P., Sherriff, R.J. and Read, A.E. (1980) *Clostridium difficile* associated diarrhoea: a role in inflammatory bowel disease? *The Lancet*, **1**, 383–384.
21. Bonfils, S. (1970) Carrageenan and the human gut. *The Lancet*, **2**, 414–415.
22. Boyko, E.J., Koepsell, T.D., Perera, D.R. and Inui, T.S. (1987) Risk of ulcerative colitis among former and current cigarette smokers. *New England Journal of Medicine*, **316**, 707–710.
23. Brauer, P.M., Gee, M.I., Grace, M. and Thompson, A.B.R. (1983) Diet of women with Crohn's and other gastrointestinal diseases. *Journal of the American Dietetic Association*, **82**, 659–664.
24. Broberger, O. and Perlmann, P. (1959) Autoantibodies in human ulcerative colitis. *Journal of Experimental Medicine*, **110**, 657–674.
25. Burke, D.A. and Axon, A.T. (1987) HeLa cell and buccal epithelial cell adhesion assays for detecting intestinal *Escherichia coli* with adhesive properties in ulcerative colitis. *Journal of Clinical Pathology*, **40**, 1402–1404.
26. Burke, D.A. and Axon, A.T. (1988) Hydrophobic adhesion of *E. Coli* in ulcerative colitis. *Gut*, **29**, 41–43.
27. Burke, D.A. and Axon, A.T. (1988) Ulcerative colitis and *E. coli* with adhesive properties. *Journal of Clinical Pathology*, **40**, 782–786.
28. Burnham, W.R., Lennard-Jones, J.E., Stanford, J.L. and Bird, R.G. (1978) Mycobacteria as a possible cause of inflammatory bowel disease. *The Lancet*, **2**, 693–696.
29. Butcher, P.D., McFadden, J.J. and Hermon-Taylor, J. (1988) Investigation of mycobacteria in Crohn's disease tissue by Southern blotting and DNA hybridization with cloned mycobacterial genomic DNA probes from a Crohn's disease isolated mycobacteria. *Gut*, **29**, 1222–1228.
30. Cambridge, G., Rampton, D.S., Stevens, T.K.J., McCarthy, D.A., Kamm, M. and Leaker, B. (1992) Anti-neutrophil cytoplasmic antibodies in inflammatory bowel disease. *Gut*, **33**, 668–674.
31. Camilleri, M., Schafler, K., Chadwick, V.S., Hodgson, H.J. and Weinbren, K. (1981) Periportal sinusoidal dilatation, inflammatory bowel disease, and the contraceptive pill. *Gastroenterology*, **80**, 810–815.
32. Carlsson, H.E., Lagercrantz, R. and Perlmann, P. (1977) Immunological studies in ulcerative colitis VIII. Antibodies to colon antigen in patients with ulcerative colitis, Crohn's disease and other diseases. *Scandinavian Journal of Gastroenterology*, **12**, 707–714.
33. Cave, D.R., Mitchell, D.N. and Brooke, B.N. (1976) Evidence of an agent transmissible from Crohn's disease tissue. *The Lancet*, **1**, 1311–1315.

34. Chalifoux, L.V. and Bronson, R.T. (1981) Colonic adenocarcinoma associated with chronic colitis in cotton top marmosets, *Saguinus oedipus*. *Gastroenterology*, **80**, 942–946.
35. Chalifoux, L.V., Bronson, R.T., Escajadillo, A. and McKenna, S. (1982) An analysis of the association of gastroenteric lesions with chronic wasting syndrome of marmosets. *Veterinary Pathology*, **19**, 141–162.
36. Chalmers, D.T., Murgatroyd, L.B. and Wadsworth, P.F. (1983) A survey of the pathology of marmosets (*Callithrix jacchus*) derived from a marmoset breeding unit. *Laboratory Animals*, **17**, 270–279.
37. Chao, L.P., Steele, J., Rodrigues, C., *et al.* (1988) Specificity of antibodies secreted by hybridomas generated from activated B cells in the mesenteric lymph nodes of patients with inflammatory bowel disease. *Gut*, **29**, 35–40.
38. Chapman, R.W., Cottone, M., Selby, W.S., Shepherd, H.A., Sherlock, S. and Jewell, D.P. (1986) Serum autoantibodies, ulcerative colitis and sclerosing cholangitis. *Gut*, **27**, 870–877.
39. Chapman, R.W., Varghese, Z., Gaul, R., Patel, G., Kokinon, N. and Sherlock, S. (1983) Association of primary sclerosing cholangitis with HLA B8. *Gut*, **24**, 38–41.
40. Chiodini, R.J., Van Kruiningen, H.J., Thayer, W.R., Merkel, R.S. and Coutu, J.A. (1984) Possible role of mycobacteria in inflammatory bowel disease. 1. An unclassified *Mycobacterium* species isolated from patients with Crohn's disease. *Digestive Diseases and Sciences*, **29**, 1073–1079.
41. Clamp, J.R., Fraser, G. and Read, A.E. (1981) Study of the carbohydrate content of mucus glycoproteins from normal and diseased colons. *Clinical Science*, **61**, 229–234.
42. Clapp, N.K., Henke, M.L., Lushbaug, C.C., Humason, G.L. and Gangaware, B.L. (1988) Effect of various biological factors on spontaneous marmoset and tamarin colitis. A retrospective histopathologic study. *Digestive Diseases and Sciences*, **33**, 1013–1019.
43. Cooke, E.M. (1967) A quantitative comparison of the faecal flora of patients with ulcerative colitis and that of normal persons. *Journal of Pathology and Bacteriology*, **94**, 439–444.
44. Cope, G.F., Heatley, R.V., Kelleher, J. and Lee, P.N. (1987) Cigarette smoking and inflammatory bowel disease: A review. *Human Toxicology*, **6**, 189–193.
45. Corfield, A.P., Williams, A.J.K., Clamp, J.R., Wagner, S.A. and Mountford, R.A. (1988) Degradation by bacterial enzymes of colonic mucus from normal subjects and patients with inflammatory bowel disease: the role of sialic acid metabolism and the detection of a novel *O*-acetyl sialic acid esterase. *Clinical Science*, **74**, 71–78.
46. Crohn, B.B., Ginsberg, L. and Oppenheimer, G. (1932) Regional ileitis: a pathologic and clinical entity. *Journal of the American Medical Association*, **99**, 1323–1329.
47. Culling, C.F.A., Reid, P.E. and Dunn, W.L. (1979) A histochemical comparison of the *O*-acylated sialic acids of the epithelial mucins in ulcerative colitis. Crohn's disease and normal controls. *Journal of Clinical Pathology*, **32**, 1272–1277.
48. Dalziel, T.K. (1913) Chronic interstitial enteritis. *British Medical Journal*, **2**, 1068–1070.
49. Das, K.M., Sakamaki, S. and Vecchi, M. (1989) Ulcerative colitis: specific antibodies against a colonic epithelial Mr 40,000 protein. *Immunology Investigations*, **18**, 459–472.
50. Das, K.M., Valenzuela, I., Williams, S.E., Soiero, R., Kadisch, A.S. and Baum, S.G. (1982) Studies of the etiology of Crohn's disease using athymic nude mice. *Gastroenterology*, **84**, 364–374.
51. de Castella, J. (1982) Letter (smoking). *British Medical Journal*, **284**, 1706.
52. Dickinson, R.J., Ashton, M.G., Axon, A.T.R., Smith, R.C., Yeung, C.K. and Hill, G.L. (1980) Controlled trial of intravenous hyperalimentation and total bowel rest as an adjunct to the routine therapy of acute colitis. *Gastroenterology*, **79**, 1199–2044.
53. Dickinson, R.J., Varian, S.A., Axon, A.T. and Cooke, E.M. (1980) Increased incidence of faecal coliforms with in vitro adhesive and invasive properties in patients with ulcerative colitis. *Gut*, **21**, 787–792.
54. Dronfield, M.W., Fletcher, J. and Langman, M.J.S. (1974) Coincident Salmonella infections and ulcerative colitis: problems of recognition and management. *British Medical Journal*, **1**, 99–100.
55. Duerr, R.H., Targan, S.R., Landers, C.J., LaRusso, N.F., Lindsay, K.L., Wiesner, R.H. and Shanahan, F. (1991) Neutrophil cytoplasmic antibodies: a link between primary sclerosing cholangitis and ulcerative colitis. *Gastroenterology*, **100**, 1385–1391.
56. Duerr, R.H., Targan, S.R., Landers, C.J., Sutherland, L.R. and Shanahan, F. (1991) Anti-neutrophil cytoplasmic antibodies in ulcerative colitis. *Gastroenterology*, **100**, 1590–1596.
57. Dvorak, A.M., Dickersin, G.R., Osage, J.E. and Monahan, R.A. (1978) Absence of virus structures in Crohn's disease tissues studied by electron microscopy. *The Lancet*, **1**, 328.
58. Ehsanullah, M., Filipe, M.I. and Gazzard, B. (1982) Mucin secretion in inflammatory bowel disease: correlation with disease activity and dysplasia. *Gut*, **23**, 484–489.
59. Eliakim, R., Karmeli, F., Razin, E. and Rachmilewitz, D. (1988) Role of platelet-activating factor in ulcerative colitis. Enhanced production during active disease and inhibition by sulfasalazine and prednisolone. *Gastroenterology*, **95**, 1167–1172.
60. Elliott, P.R., Burnham, W.R., Berghouse, L.M., Lennard-Jones, J.E. and Langman, M.J.S. (1982)

Sulphadoxime–pyrimethamine therapy in Crohn's disease. *Digestion*, **23**, 132–134.
61. Elliott, P.R., Forsey, T., Darougar, S., Treharne, J.D. and Lennard-Jones, J.E. (1981) Chlamydiae and inflammatory bowel disease. *Gut*, **22**, 25–27.
62. Elmgreen, J. (1984) Subnormal activation of phagocytes by complement in chronic inflammatory bowel disease? Neutrophil chemotaxis to complement split product C5a. *Gut*, **25**, 737–742.
63. Elmgreen, J., Berkowicz, A. and Sorensen, H. (1983) Defective release of C5a related chemo-attractant activity from complement in Crohn's disease. *Gut*, **24**, 525–531.
64. Elmgreen, J., Berkowicz, A. and Sorensen, H. (1983) Hypercatabolism of complement in Crohn's disease-assessment of circulating C3c. *Acta Medica Scandinavica*, **214**, 403–407.
65. Farmer, G.N.,Vincent, M.M., Fuccillo, D.A. *et al.* (1973) Viral investigations in ulcerative colitis and regional enteritis. *Gastroenterology*, **65**, 8–18.
66. Felsen, J. and Wolarsky, W. (1953) Acute and chronic bacillary dysentery and chronic ulcerative colitis. *Journal of the American Medical Association*, **153**, 1069–1072.
67. Felsen, J. (1936) The relationship of bacillary dysentery to distal ileitis, chronic ulcerative colitis and non-specific intestinal granuloma. *Annals of Internal Medicine*, **10**, 645–669.
68. Fischer, J.E., Foster, G.S., Abel, R.M., Abbott, W.M. and Ryan, J.A. (1973) Hyperalimentation as primary therapy for inflammatory bowel disease. *American Journal of Surgery,* **125**, 165–175.
69. Fletcher, J. and Hinton, J.M. (1967) Tuberculin sensitivity in Crohn's disease. *The Lancet*, **2**, 753.
70. Ganzales-Angulo, A., Corral, E., Garcia-Torres, R. and Quijano, M. (1965) Malakoplakia of the colon. *Gastroenterology*, **48**, 383–387.
71. Gibson, P.R., Van de Pol, E., Pullman, W. and Doe, W.F. (1988) Lysis of colonic epithelial cells by allogeneic mononuclear and lymphokine activated killer cells derived from peripheral blood and intestinal mucosa: evidence against a pathogenic role in IBD. *Gut*, **29**, 1076–1084.
72. Gitnick, G., Collins, J., Beaman, B. *et al.* (1989) Preliminary report on isolation of mycobacteria from patients with Crohn's disease. *Digestive Diseases and Science*, **34**, 925–932.
73. Goodman, M.J., Pearson, K.W., McGhie, D., Dutt, S. and Deodhar, S.G. (1980) *Campylobacter and Giardia lamblia* causing exacerbation of inflammatory bowel disease. *The Lancet*, **2**, 1247.
74. Gorbach, S., Nahas, L., Plant, A., Weinstein, L., Peterson, J. and Levitan, R. (1968) Studies of intestinal microflora. V. Fecal microbial ecology in ulcerative colitis and Crohn's disease: its relationship to severity of disease and chemotherapy. *Gastroenterology*, **54**, 575–587.
75. Graham, W.B., Torrance, B. and Taylor, T.V. (1978) Breakfast and Crohn's disease. *British Medical Journal*, **2**, 768.
76. Grange, J., Gibson, I. and Nasau, E. (1980) Enzyme-linked immunoabsorbent assay: a study of antibodies to *M. tuberculosis* in the IgG, IgA and IgM classes in tuberculosis, sarcoidosis and Crohn's disease. *Turbercle*, **61**, 145–152.
77. Greenberg, G.R., Fleming, C.R., Jeejeebhoy, K.N., Rosenberg, I.H., Sales, D. and Tremaine, W.J. (1988) Controlled trial of bowel rest and nutritional support in the management of Crohn's disease. *Gut*, **29**, 1309–1315.
78. Gump, D., Caul, E., Eade, O. *et al.* (1981) Lymphocytotoxic and microbial antibodies in Crohn's disease and matched controls. *Antonie van Leeunwenhoek*, **47**, 455–464.
79. Halstensen, T.S., Mollnes, T.E. and Brandtzaeg, P. (1989) Persistent complement activation in submucosal blood vessels of active inflammatory bowel disease: immunohistochemical evidence. *Gastroenterology*, **97**, 10–19.
80. Hampson, S., Parker, M., Saverymuttu, S., McFadden, J. and Herman-Taylor, J. (1988) Results of quadruple antimycobacterial chemotherapy in 17 Crohn's disease patients completing six months treatment. *Gastro-enterology*, **94**, A170.
81. Harper, P.H., Truelove, S.C., Lee, E.C.G., Kettlewell, M.G.W. and Jewell, D.P. (1983) Split ileostomy and ileocolostomy for Crohn's disease of the colon and ulcerative colitis: a 20 year survey. *Gut*, **24**, 106–113.
82. Harries, A.D., Baird, A. and Rhodes, J. (1982) Non-smoking: a feature of ulcerative colitis. *British Medical Journal*, **284**, 706.
83. Harries, A.D., Jones, L., Heatley, R.V. and Rhodes, J. (1982) Smoking habits and inflammatory bowel disease: effect on nutrition. *British Medical Journal*, **284**, 1161.
84. Harries, A.D., Jones, L.A., Danis, V., Fifield, R., Heatley, R.V. and Newcombe, R.G. (1983) Controlled trial of supplemental oral nutrition in Crohn's disease. *The Lancet*, **1**, 887–890.
85. Helphingstine, C.J., Hentges, D.J., Campbell, B.J., Butt, J. and Barrett, J. (1979) Antibodies detectable by counterimmunoelectrophoresis against Bacteroides antigens in serum of patients with inflammatory bowel disease. *Journal of Clinical Microbiology*, **9**, 373–378.
86. Higgens, C.S. and Allan, R.N. (1980) Crohn's disease of the distal ileum. *Gut*, **21**, 933–940.
87. Hodgson, H.J.F., Potter, B.J. and Jewell, D.P. (1977) Immune complexes in ulcerative colitis and Crohn's disease. *Clinical and Experimental Immunology*, **29**, 187–196.
88. Hodgson, H.J.F., Potter, B.J., Skinner, J. and Jewell, D.P. (1978) Immune-complex mediated colitis in rabbits. An experimental model. *Gut*, **19**, 225–232.
89. Holdstock, G., Savage, D., Harman, M. and Wright, P. (1984) Should patients with inflammatory bowel disease smoke? *British Medical Journal*, **288**, 362.
90. Hollander, D., Vadheim, C.M., Brettholtz, E.,

Petersen, G.M., Delahunty, T.J. and Rotter, J.I. (1986) Increased intestinal permeability in patients with Crohn's disease and their relatives. *Annals of Internal Medicine*, **105**, 883–885.
91. Homans, J. and Hass, G.M. (1933) Regional ileitis: a clinical, not a pathological entity. *New England Journal of Medicine*, **209**, 1315–1321.
92. Howell-Jones, J. and Lennard-Jones, J. (1966) Corticosteroids and corticotrophin in the treatment of Crohn's disease. *Gut*, **7**, 181–187.
93. Hurst, A.F. (1921) Ulcerative colitis. *Guy's Hospital Report*, **71**, 26.
94. Ibbotson, J.P., Pease, P.E. and Allan, R.N. (1987) Cell-wall deficient bacteria in inflammatory bowel disease. *European Journal of Clinical Microbiology*, **6**, 286–290.
95. James, S.P. (1988) Remission of Crohn's disease after human immunodeficiency virus infection. *Gastroenterology*, **95**, 1667–1669.
96. Jarnerot, G., Jarnmark, I. and Nilsson, K. (1983) Consumption of refined sugar in patients with Crohn's disease, ulcerative colitis, or irritable bowel syndrome. *Scandinavian Journal of Gastroenterology*, **18**, 999–1002.
97. Jarnerot, G. and Lantrop, K. (1972) Antibodies to EB virus in cases of patients with Crohn's disease. *New England Journal of Medicine*, **286**, 1215–1216.
98. Kameyama, J., Narui, H., Inui, M. and Sato, T. (1984) Energy levels in large intestinal mucosa in patients with ulcerative colitis. *Tohoku Journal of Experimental Medicine*, **143**, 253–254.
99. Kasper, H. and Sommer, H. (1979) Dietary fibre and nutrient intake in Crohn's disease. *American Journal of Clinical Nutrition*, **32**, 1898–1901.
100. Katschski, B., Logan, R.F.A., Edmond, M. and Langman, M.J.S. (1988) Smoking and sugar intake are separate but interactive risk factors in Crohn's disease. *Gut*, **29**, 1202–1206.
101. Katz, K.D., Hollander, D., Vadheim, C.M. *et al.* (1989) Intestinal permeability in patients with Crohn's disease and their healthy relatives. *Gastroenterology*, **97**, 927–931.
102. Kenedy, P.C. and Cello, R.M. (1966) Colitis of boxer dogs. *Gastroenterology*, **51**, 926–931.
103. Kett, K., Rognum, T.O. and Brandtzaeg, P. (1987) Mucosal subclass distribution of IgG-producing cells is different in ulcerative colitis and Crohn's disease of the colon. *Gastroenterology*, **93**, 919–924.
104. Kirkwood, J.K., Pearson, G.R. and Epstein, M.A. (1986) Adenocarcinoma of the large bowel and colitis in captive cotton-top tamarins (*Saguinus oedipus*). *Journal of Comparative Pathology*, **96**, 507–515.
105. Kirsner, J.B. (1961) Experimental 'colitis' with particular reference to hypersensitivity reactions in the colon. *Gastroenterology*, **40**, 307–312.
106. Kobayashi, K., Blaser, M.J. and Brown, W.R. (1989) Immunohistochemical examination for mycobacteria in intestinal tissues from patients with Crohn's disease. *Gastroenterology*, **96**, 1009–1015.
107. Koldkjaer, O., Klitgaard, N.A. and Schmidt, K.G. (1978) Cellular and humoral indices of disease activity in inflammatory bowel disease. *Digestion*, **17**, 387.
108. Kovacs, A. and Sawinsky, I. (1986) Smoking habits in inflammatory bowel disease. *Digestive Diseases and Science*, **31**, 844.
109. Krook, A., Danielsson, D., Kjellander, J. and Jarnerot, G. (1981) The effect of metronidazole and sulphasalazine on the faecal flora of patients with Crohn's disease. *Scandinavian Journal of Gastroenterology*, **16**, 183–192.
110. Krook, A., Kjellander, J. and Danielsson, D. (1982) Susceptibility of *Bacteroides* species to metronidazole during treatment of patients with Crohn's disease and healthy individuals. *Scandinavian Journal of Infectious Diseases*, **14**, 45–48.
111. Lagercrantz, R., Hammarstrom, S., Perlmann, P. and Gustafsson, B.E. (1966) Immunological studies in ulcerative colitis III. *Clinical and Experimental Immunology*, **1**, 263–276.
112. Lindberg, A.A., Weintraub, A. and Nord, C.E. (1979) The humoral antibody response to *Bacteroides fragilis* infections in humans. *Scandinavian Journal of Infectious Diseases*, suppl. 19, 46–51.
113. Lindeman, R.J., Weinstein, L., Levitan, R. and Patterson, J.F. (1967) Ulcerative colitis and intestinal salmonellosis. *American Journal of Medicine*, **254**, 855–861.
114. Lochs, H., Meryn, S., Marosi, L., Ferenci, P. and Hortnag, H. (1983) Has total bowel rest a beneficial effect in the treatment of Crohn's disease? *Clinical Nutrition*, **2**, 61-64.
115. Lushbaug, C.C., Humason, G.L., Swatzendruber, D.C., Richter, C.B. and Gengozian, N. (1978) Spontaneous colonic adenocarcinoma in marmosets. *Primates in Medicine*, **10**, 119–134.
116. MacDermott, R.P., Donaldson, R.M. and Trier, J.S. (1974) Glycoprotein synthesis and secretion by mucosal biopsies of rabbit colons and human rectum. *Journal of Clinical Investigation*, **54**, 545–554.
117. Mackie, T.T. (1932) Ulcerative colitis due to chronic infection with Flexner-bacillus. *Journal of the American Medical Academy*, **98**, 1706–1710.
118. Madara, J.L., Podolsky, D.K., King, N.W., Sehgal, P.K., Moore, R. and Winter, H.S. (1985) Characterisation of spontaneous colitis in cotton-top tamarins (*Saguinus oedipus*) and its response to sulfasalazine. *Gastroenterology*, **88**, 13–19.
119. Martini, G.A. and Brandes, J.W. (1976) Increased consumption of refined carbohydrates in patients with Crohn's disease. *Klinische Wochenschrift*, **54**, 367–371.
120. Matthews, N., Mayberry, J.F. and Rhodes, J. (1980) Agglutinins to bacteria in Crohn's disease. *Gut*, **21**, 376–380.
121. Mayberry, J.F., Rhodes, J., Allan, R. *et al.* (1981) Diet in Crohn's disease. Two studies of current

and previous habits in newly diagnosed patients. *Digestive Diseases and Science*, **26**, 444–448.
122. Mayberry, J.F., Rhodes, J. and Newcombe, R.G. (1978) Breakfast and dietary aspects of Crohn's disease. *British Medical Journal*, **2**, 1401.
123. Mayberry, J.F., Rhodes, J. and Newcombe, R.G. (1980) Increased sugar consumption in Crohn's disease. *Digestion*, **20**, 323–326.
124. McConnell, R.B. (1980) Inflammatory bowel disease: newer developments of genetic influence. In *Developments in Genetic Disease* (Ed.) Berk, J.E., Philadelphia: Lea & Febiger.
125. McIntyre, P.B., Powell-Tuck, J., Wood, S.R. *et al.* (1986) Controlled trial of bowel rest in the treatment of ulcerative colitis. *Gut*, **27**, 481–485.
126. Mee, A.S., Brown, D. and Jewell, D.P. (1979) Atopy in inflammatory bowel disease. *Scandinavian Journal of Gastroenterology*, **14**, 743–746.
127. Mee, A.S., McLaughlin, J.E., Hodgson, H.J.F., Potter, B.J. and Jewell, D.P. (1979) Chronic immune colitis in rabbits. *Gut*, **20**, 1–5.
128. Miller, R.S. and Hoskins, L.C. (1981) Mucin degradation in human colon ecosystems. Faecal population densities of mucin-degrading bacteria estimated by a "most probable number" method. *Gastroenterology*, **81**, 759–765.
129. Mitchell, D.N. and Rees, R.J.W. (1969) Agent transmissible from Crohn's disease tissue. *The Lancet*, **2**, 489–490.
130. Moeller, H.C. and Kirsner, J.B. (1954) The effect of drug-induced hypermotility on the gastrointestinal tract of dogs. *Gastroenterology*, **26**, 303–311.
131. Monis, B., Weinberg, T. and Spector, G.J. (1968) The carrageenan granuloma in the rat. *British Journal of Experimental Pathology*, **149**, 302–310.
132. Monsen, U., Brostrom, B., Nordenvall, B., Sorstad, J. and Hellers, G. (1987) Prevalence of inflammatory bowel disease among relatives of patients with ulcerative colitis. *Scandinavian Journal of Gastroenterology*, **22**, 214–218.
133. Munro, J., Mayberry, J., Matthews, N. and Rhodes, J. (1979) Chlamydia and Crohn's disease. *The Lancet*, **1**, 45–46.
134. Newman, A. and Lambert, J.R. (1980) Campylobacter causing flare-up in inflammatory bowel disease. *The Lancet*, **2**, 919.
135. Nielsen, O.H., Elmgreen, J., Thomson, B.S., Ahnfelt-Ronne, I. and Wilk, A. (1986) Release of leukotriene B4 and 5-hydroxyeicosotetraenoic acid during phagocytosis of artificial complexes by peripheral neutrophils in chronic inflammatory bowel disease. *Clinical and Experimental Immunology*, **65**, 465–471.
136. O'Morain, C., Segal, A.W. and Levi, A.J. (1980) Elemental diets in the treatment of acute Crohn's disease. *British Medical Journal*, **281**, 1173–1175.
137. O'Morain, C., Segal, A.W., Walker, D. and Levi, A.J. (1981) Abnormalities of neutrophil function do not cause the migration defect in Crohn's disease. *Gut*, **22**, 817–822.
138. Okayasu, I., Hatakeyama, S., Yamada, M., Ohkasu, T., Inagaki, Y. and Nakaya, R. (1990) A novel method in the induction of reliable experimental acute and chronic ulcerative colitis in mice. *Gastroenterology*, **98**, 694–702.
139. Onderdonk, A.B., Bronson, R. and Cisneros, R. (1987) Comparison of *Bacteroides vulgatus* strains in the enhancement of experimental ulcerative colitis. *Infection and Immunity*, **55**, 835–836.
140. Onderdonk, A.B., Franklin, M.L. and Cisneros, R.L. (1981) Production of experimental ulcerative colitis in gnotobiotic guinea pigs with a simplified microflora. *Infection and Immunity*, **32**, 225–231.
141. Onderdonk, A.B., Hermos, J.A., Dzink, J.L. and Bartlett, J.G. (1978) Protective effect of metronidazole in experimental ulcerative colitis. *Gastroenterology*, **74**, 521–526.
142. Orda, R., Samra, Z., Levy, Y., Shperber, Y. and Scapa, E. (1990) *Chlamydia trachomatis* and inflammatory bowel disease. *Journal of the Royal Society of Medicine*, **83**, 15–17.
143. Palmer, K.R., Sherriff, S.B., Holdsworth, C.D. *et al.* (1981) Further experience of hyposplenism in inflammatory bowel disease. *Quarterly Journal of Medicine*, **50**, 463.
144. Panza, W.J., Francheschi, S., LaVecchia *et al.* (1987) Dietary factors and the aetiology of inflammatory bowel disease. *Italian Journal of Gastroenterology*, **19**, 205–209.
145. Paris, J.C., Simon, V. and Paris, J. (1977) Etude critique des effets de la médication antituberculeuse. Dans une serie de 52 cas de formes severes de la maladie de Crohn. *Annals de Gastroenterologie et Hepatologie*, **13**, 427–433.
146. Paulley, J.W. (1990) Why do patients with ulcerative colitis relapse? (letter). *Gut*, **31**, 959.
147. Paulley, J.W. (1990) Why do patients with ulcerative colitis relapse? (letter). *Gut*, **31**, 1419.
148. Penny, W.J., Mayberry, J.F., Agget, P.J., Gilbert, J.O., Newcombe, R.G. and Rhodes, J. (1983) Relationship between trace elements, sugar consumption and taste in Crohn's disease. *Gut*, **24**, 288–292.
149. Perlmann, P. and Broberger, O. (1963) In vitro studies of ulcerative colitis. II Cytotoxic action of white blood cells from patients on human fetal colon cells. *Journal of Experimental Medicine*, **117**, 717–733.
150. Phear, D.N. (1958) The relation between regional ileitis and sarcoidosis. *The Lancet*, **2**, 1250–1251.
151. Phillips, R.K.S. and Glazer, G. (1981) Metastatic Crohn's disease of the umbilicus. *British Medical Journal*, **283**, 887.
152. Picciotto, A., Gesu, G.P., Schito, G.C., Testa, R., Varagone, G. and Celle, G. (1988) Antimycobacterial chemotherapy in two cases of inflammatory bowel disease. *The Lancet*, **1**, 536–537.
153. Podolsky, D.K. and Isselbacher, K.J. (1984)

Composition of human colonic mucin. Selective alteration in inflammatory bowel disease. *Journal of Clinical Investigation*, **72**, 142–153.
154. Podolsky, D.K. and Isselbacher, K.J. (1984) Glycoprotein composition of colonic mucosa. Specific alterations in ulcerative colitis. *Gastroenterology*, **87**, 991–998.
155. Powell, S.J. and Wilmot, A.J. (1966) Ulcerative post-dysenteric colitis. *Gut*, **7**, 438–443.
156. Prantera, C., Argentieri, R., Mangiarotti, R. and Levenstein, S. (1988) Dapsone and remission of Crohn's disease. *The Lancet*, **1**, 536.
157. Rabin, B.S. and Rogers, S.J. (1978) A cell-mediated immune model of inflammatory bowel disease in the rabbit. *Gastroenterology*, **75**, 29–33.
158. Rampton, D.S., Salmon, P.R. and Clark, C.G. (1983) Non-specific ulcerative colitis as a sequel to amoebic dysentery. *Journal of Clinical Gastroenterology*, **5**, 217–219.
159. Raouf, A.H., Hildrey, V., Daniel, J., Walker, R.J., Krasner, N., Elias, E. and Rhodes, J.M. (1991) Enteral feeding as sole therapy for Crohn's disease: a controlled trial of whole protein versus amino-acid based feed and a case study of dietary challenge. *Gut*, **32**, 702–707.
160. Raouf, A.H., Parker, N., Iddon, D. *et al.* (1991) Ion-exchange chromatography of purified colonic mucus glycoproteins in inflammatory bowel disease: absence of a selective subclass defect. *Gut*, **32**, 1139–1145.
161. Reichert, F.L. and Mathes, M.E. (1936) Experimental lymphedema of the intestinal tract and its relation to regional cicatrizing enteritis. *Annals of Surgery*, **104**, 601–616.
162. Reid, P.E., Culling, C.F.A., Dunn, W.L., Ramey, C.W. and Clay, M.G. (1984) Chemical and histochemical study of normal and diseased human gastroenterological tract. 1. A comparison between histologically normal colon, colonic tumours, ulcerative colitis and diverticular disease of the colon. *Histochemical Journal*, **16**, 235–251.
163. Rhodes, J.M., Black, R.R., Gallimore, R. and Savage, A. (1985) Histochemical demonstration of desialation and desulphation of normal and inflammatory bowel disease rectal mucus by faecal extracts. *Gut*, **26**, 1312–1318.
164. Rhodes, J.M., Black, R.R. and Savage, A. (1988) Altered lectin binding by colonic epithelial glycoconjugates in ulcerative colitis and Crohn's disease. *Digestive Diseases and Sciences*, **33**, 1359–1363.
165. Rhodes, J.M. and Jewell, D.P. (1983) Motility of neutrophils and monocytes in Crohn's disease and ulcerative colitis. *Gut*, **24**, 73–77.
166. Rhodes, J.M., Cockel, R., Allan, R.N., Hawker, P.C., Dawson, J. and Elias, E. (1984) Colonic Crohn's disease and use of oral contraception. *British Medical Journal*, **288**, 595–596.
167. Rhodes, J.M., Potter, B.J., Brown, D.J.C. and Jewell, D.P. (1982) Serum inhibitors of leucocyte chemotaxis in Crohn's disease and ulcerative colitis. *Gastroenterology*, **82**, 1327–1334.
168. Riemann, J.F. (1977) Further electron microscopic evidence of virus-like particles in Crohn's disease. *Acta Hepatogastroenterologica*, **24**, 116–118.
169. Riley, S.A., Mani, V., Goodman, M.J. and Lucas, S. (1990) Why do patients with ulcerative colitis relapse? *Gut*, **31**, 179–183.
170. Riley, S.A., Mani, V. and Goodman, M.J. (1990) Why do patients with ulcerative colitis relapse? Reply (letter). *Gut*, **31**, 959.
171. Roberts, C.J. and Diggle, R. (1982) Letter (smoking). *British Medical Journal*, **285**, 440.
172. Rocchio, M.A., Mocha, C., Haas, K.F. and Randall, H.T. (1974). Use of chemically defined diets in the management of patients with acute inflammatory bowel disease. *American Journal of Surgery*, **127**, 469–475.
173. Roche, J.K., Fiocchi, C. and Youngman, K. (1985) Sensitization to epithelial antigens in chronic mucosal inflammatory disease. Characterization of human intestinal mucosa-derived mononuclear cells reactive with purified epithelial cell associated components *in vitro*. *Journal of Clinical Investigation*, **75**, 522–530.
174. Roediger, W.E.W. (1980) The colonic epithelium in ulcerative colitis: an energy deficient disease? *The Lancet*, **2**, 712–715.
175. Roediger, W.E.W. (1988) What sequence of pathogenic events leads to acute ulcerative colitis? *Diseases of Colon and Rectum*, **31**, 482–487.
176. Roediger, W.E.W. (1982) Utilisation of nutrients by isolated epithelial cells of the rat colon. *Gastroenterology*, **83**, 424–429.
177. Rolleston, H.D. (1904) In *Diseases of the intestine and peritoneum* (Ed.) Nothnagel, D.H. pp. 254–255. Philadelphia: W.B. Saunders.
178. Ropke, C. (1972) Lymphocyte transformation and delayed hypersensitivity in Crohn's disease. *Scandinavian Journal of Gastroenterology*, **7**, 671.
179. Schuller, J.L., Piket-van Ulsen, J., Veeken, I.V.D., Michel, M.F. and Stolz, E. (1978) Antibodies against Chlamydia of the lymphogranuloma-venereum type in Crohn's disease. *The Lancet*, **1**, 19–20.
180. Schultz, M., Rieder, H., Hersh, T. and Riepe, S. (1987) Remission of Crohn's disease with antimycobacterial chemotherapy. *The Lancet*, **2**, 1391–1392.
181. Scott, G.B.D. and Keymer, I.F. (1974) Ulcerative colitis in apes: a comparison with the human disease. *Journal of Pathology*, **115**, 241–244.
182. Scott, M.G., Nahm, M.H., Nash, G.S., Bertovich, M.J. and MacDermott, R.P. (1986) Spontaneous secretion of IgG subclasses by intestinal mononuclear cells: differences between ulcerative colitis, Crohn's disease and controls. *Clinical and Experimental Immunology*, **66**, 209–215.
183. Segal, A.W. (1987) Absence of both cytochrome b245 subunits from neutrophils in X-linked chronic granulomatous disease. *Nature*, **326**, 88–90.

184. Segal, A.W. and Loewi, G. (1976) Neutrophil dysfunction in Crohn's disease. *The Lancet*, **2**, 219.
185. Seneca, H. and Henderson, E. (1950) Normal intestinal bacteria in ulcerative colitis. *Gastroenterology*, **15**, 34–39.
186. Shaffer, J., Hughes, S., Linaker, B., Baker, R. and Turnberg, L. (1984) Controlled trial of rifampicin and ethambutol in Crohn's disease. *Gut*, **25**, 203–205.
187. Sharon, P. and Stenson, W.F. (1984) Enhanced synthesis of leukotriene B4 by colonic mucosa in inflammatory bowel disease. *Gastroenterology*, **86**, 453–460.
188. Silkoff, K., Hallak, A., Yegana, L. *et al.* (1980) Consumption of refined carbohydrate by patients with Crohn's disease in Tel-Aviv-Yafo. *Postgraduate Medical Journal*, **56**, 842–846.
189. Slaney, G., Muller, S., Clay, J., Sumathipala, A.H.T., Hillenbrand, P. and Thompson, H. (1986) Crohn's disease involving the penis. *Gut*, **27**, 329–333.
190. Snook, J.A., de Silva, H.J. and Jewell, D.P. (1989) The association of autoimmune disorders with inflammatory bowel disease. *Quarterly Journal of Medicine*, **72**, 835–840.
191. Soltis, R.D., Hasz, D., Morris, M.J. and Wilson, I.D. (1979) Evidence against the presence of circulating immune complexes in chronic inflammatory bowel disease. *Gastroenterology*, **76**, 1380–1385.
192. Somerville, K.W., Logan, R.F.A., Edmond, M. and Langman, M.J.S. (1984) Smoking and Crohn's disease. *British Medical Journal*, **289**, 954–956.
193. Stanford, J. (1981) Acid-fast organisms in Crohn's disease and ulcerative colitis. In *Recent Advances in Crohn's Disease* (Ed.) Pena, A.S., Weterman, I.T., Booth, C.C. and Strober, W. pp. 274–277. The Hague: Martinus Nijhoff.
194. Stenson, W.F. and Lobos, E. (1982) Sulphasalazine inhibits the synthesis of chemotactic liquids by neutrophils. *Journal of Clinical Investigation*, **69**, 494–497.
195. Stobo, J.D., Tomasi, T.B., Huizenga, K.A., Spencer, R.J. and Shorter, R.G. (1976) In vitro studies of inflammatory bowel disease. Surface receptors of the mononuclear cell required to lyse allogenic colonic epithelial cells. *Gastroenterology*, **70**, 71–76.
196. Stout, C. and Snyder, R.L. (1969) Ulcerative-colitis-like lesion in Siamang gibbons. *Gastroenterology*, **57**, 256–260.
197. Swarbrick, E., Yungham, J., Price, H., Blackshaw, A. and Griffiths, P. (1979) *Chlamydia*, cytomegalovirus, and *Yersinia* in inflammatory bowel disease. *The Lancet*, **2**, 11–12.
198. Szilagyi, A., Gerson, M., Mendelson, J. and Yusuf, N. (1985) Salmonella infections complicating inflammatory bowel disease. *Journal of Clinical Gastroenterology*, **7**, 251–255.
199. Taub, R.N., Sachar, D., Siltzbach, L.E. and Janowitz, H. (1974) Transmission of ileitis and sarcoid granulomas to mice. *Transactions of the Association of American Physicians*, **87**, 219–224.
200. Taylor-Robinson, S., Miles, R., Whitehead, A. and Dickinson, R.J. (1989) Salmonella infection and ulcerative colitis. *The Lancet*, **1**, 1145.
201. Thayer, W.R., Coutu, J.A., Chiodini, R.J., Van Kruiningen, H.J. and Merkel, R.S. (1984) Possible role of mycobacteria in inflammatory bowel disease. II Mycobacterial antibodies in Crohn's disease. *Digestive Diseases and Science*, **29**, 1080–1085.
202. Thornton, J.R., Emmett, P.M. and Heaton, K.W. (1985) Smoking, sugar and inflammatory bowel disease. *British Medical Journal*, **290**, 1786–1787.
203. Thornton, J.R., Emmett, P.M. and Heaton, K.W. (1979) Diet and Crohn's disease: characteristics of the pre-illness diet. *British Medical Journal*, **2**, 762–764.
204. Tobin, M.V., Logan, R.F.A., Langman, M.J.S., McConnell, M.J.S. and Gilmore, I.T. (1987) Cigarette smoking and inflammatory bowel disease. *Gastroenterology*, **93**, 316–321.
205. Toulet, J., Rousselet, J. and Viteau, J.M. (1979) La rifampicine dans le traitment de la maladie de Crohn. *Gastroenterology and Clinical Biology*, **3**, 209–211.
206. Tsai, H.H., Sutherland, D., Gibson, G., Hart, C.A. and Rhodes, J.M. (1992) A novel fecal mucin sulfatase from human feces: its isolation, purification and characterization. *Clinical Science*, **82**, 447–454.
207. Tweedie, J.H. and McCann, B.G. (1984) Metastatic Crohn's disease of the thigh and forearm. *Gut*, **25**, 213–214.
208. van der Waaij, D., Cohen, B.J. and Anver, M.R. (1974) Mitigation of experimental inflammatory bowel disease in guinea pigs by selective elimination of the aerobic Gram-negative intestinal microflora. *Gastroenterology*, **67**, 460–472.
209. van der Weil-Korstanje, J.A.A. and Winkler, K. (1975) The fecal flora in ulcerative colitis. *Journal of Medical Microbiology*, **8**, 491–501.
210. Van Kruiningen, H.J. (1967) Granulomatous colitis of boxer dogs: comparative aspects. *Gastroenterology*, **53**, 114–122.
211. Van Kruiningen, H.J. (1972) Canine colitis comparable to regional enteritis and mucosal colitis of man. *Gastroenterology*, **62**, 1128–1142.
212. Vessey, M., Smith, A., Yeates, D., McPherson, K. and Jewell, D. (1986) Chronic inflammatory bowel disease, cigarette smoking, and the use of oral contraceptives: findings in a large cohort study of women of childbearing age. *British Medical Journal*, **292**, 1101–1103.
213. Vogel, C.M., Corwin, T.R. and Baue, A.E. (1974) Intravenous hyperalimentation in the treatment of inflammatory diseases of the bowel. *Archives of Surgery*, **108**, 460–467.
214. Voitk, A.J., Echave, V., Feller, J.H., Brown, R.A. and Gurd, F.N. (1973) Experience with elemental diet in the treatment of inflammatory

bowel disease. Is this primary therapy? *Archives of Surgery*, **107**, 329–333.
215. Wakabayashi, K., Inagaki, T., Fujimoto, Y. and Fukuka, Y. (1978) Induction by degraded carrageenan of colorectal tumors in rats. *Cancer Letters*, **4**, 171–176.
216. Wakefield, A.J., Sawyer, A.M., Dhillon, A.P., Pittilo, R.M., Rowles, P.M., Lewis, A.A.M. and Pounder, R.E. (1989) Pathogenesis of Crohn's disease: multifocal gastrointestinal infarction. *The Lancet*, **2**, 1057–1062.
217. Walker, C.W., Upson, R. and Warren, R.E. (1988) Haemorrhagic colitis: detection of a verotoxin producing *Escherichia coli* 0157 in a clinical microbiology laboratory. *Journal of Clinical Pathology*, **41**, 80–84.
218. Walvoort, H.C., Fazzi, G.E. and Pena, A.S. (1989) Seroreactivity of patients with Crohn's disease with lymph nodes of primed nude mice is independent of the tissue used for priming. *Gastroenterology*, **97**, 1097–1100.
219. Ward, M. and Eastwood, M.A. (1979) The nitroblue tetrazolium test in Crohn's disease and ulcerative colitis. *Digestion*, **14**, 179.
220. Ward, M. and McManus, J.P.A. (1975) Dapsone in Crohn's disease. *The Lancet*, **1**, 1236–1237.
221. Warren, J., Rees, H. and Cox, T. (1986) Remission of Crohn's disease with tuberculosis chemotherapy. *New England Journal of Medicine*, **314**, 182.
222. Wensink, F. and Custers-van Lieshaut (1981) The faecal flora of patients with Crohn's disease. *Journal of Hygiene*, **87**, 1–12.
223. Wensink, F. and van de Merwe, J.P. (1981) Serum agglutinins to *Eubacterium*, and *Peptostreptococcus* species in Crohn's and other diseases. *Journal of Hygiene*, **87**, 13–24.
224. Whorwell, P.J., Baldwin, R.C. and Wright, R. (1976) Ferritin in Crohn's disease tissue: detection by electron microscopy. *Gut*, **17**, 696–699.
225. Wilks, S. (1859) *Lectures on Pathological Anatomy*, p. 302. London: Longman.
226. Williams, W.J. (1965) A study of Crohn's syndrome using tissue extracts and the Kveim and Mantoux tests. *Gut*, **6**, 503.
227. Willoughby, J.M.T., Rahman, A.F.M.S. and Gregory, M.M. (1989) Chronic colitis after Aeromonas infection. *Gut*, **30**, 686–690.
228. Wright, R. and Truelove, S.C. (1965) A controlled therapeutic trial of various diets in ulcerative colitis. *British Medical Journal*, **251**, 138–141.
229. Yoshimura, H.H., Graham, D.Y., Estes, M.K. and Merkel, R.S. (1987) Investigation of association of mycobacteria with inflammatory bowel disease by nucleic acid hybridization. *Journal of Clinical Microbiology*, **25**, 45–51.

ULCERATIVE COLITIS

Ulcerative colitis is an inflammatory disease of the colon of unknown aetiology. It nearly always begins in the rectum and extends proximally to affect a variable extent of the colon. Although the first description of the disease is claimed by Wilks and Moxon in 1875, Samuel Wilks gave a very good description of the disease in 1859.[78,79] He distinguished ulcerative colitis from infective dysenteries, which were extremely common at the time, but it was not until the classic descriptions by Hurst in 1921[21] that the disease entity was fully accepted.

PATHOLOGY *(D.P. Jewell and S.P.L. Travis)*

MACROSCOPIC APPEARANCES

The disease may be confined to the rectum (usually termed 'haemorrhagic' or 'granular' proctitis) but it is uncertain whether this represents the same disease entity as ulcerative colitis. Proctitis remains confined to the rectum in about 60%, with only 30% extending to involve the sigmoid colon, and about 10% developing a universal colitis after 10 years.[56,61] The rectum is always involved, but occasionally there is relative sparing, especially in patients with severe extensive disease in a first attack, although microscopic abnormalities are always present on rectal biopsy.[64] Once the disease extends beyond the rectum, it may be manifest as a proctosigmoiditis, left-sided colitis, subtotal colitis or a universal (total) colitis. In patients with universal disease, there is frequently a mild inflammation of the terminal ileum (backwash ileitis).

In active disease the mucosal surface of the involved colon becomes uniformly haemorrhagic and granular. In severe disease there is ulceration (*Figure 7.2*) which may be extensive with stripping of large areas of mucous membrane. The ulceration may undermine adjacent mucosa with the formation of inflammatory polyps and mucosal bridges.

As the disease heals, the mucosa may either return to normal or become smooth and atrophic.

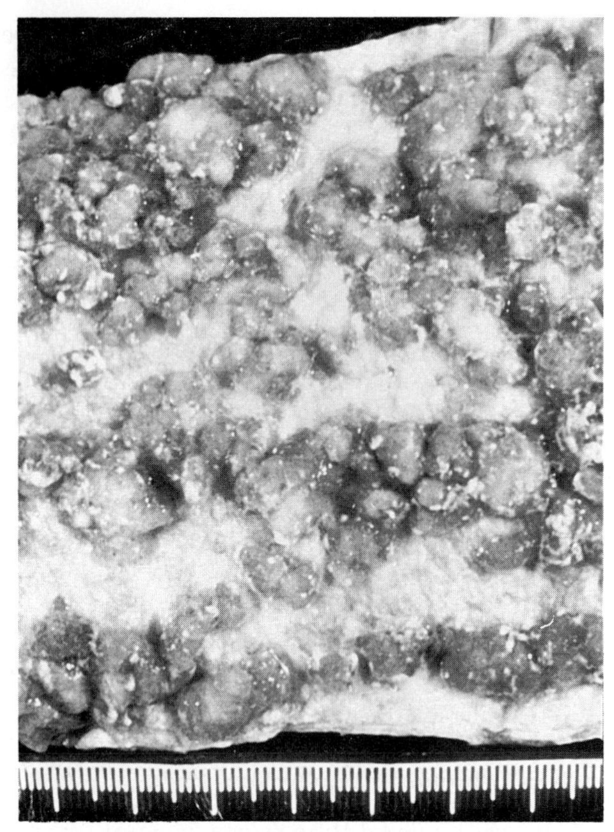

Figure 7.2 Resected bowel from a patient with severe ulcerative colitis. The mucosa is extensively ulcerated.

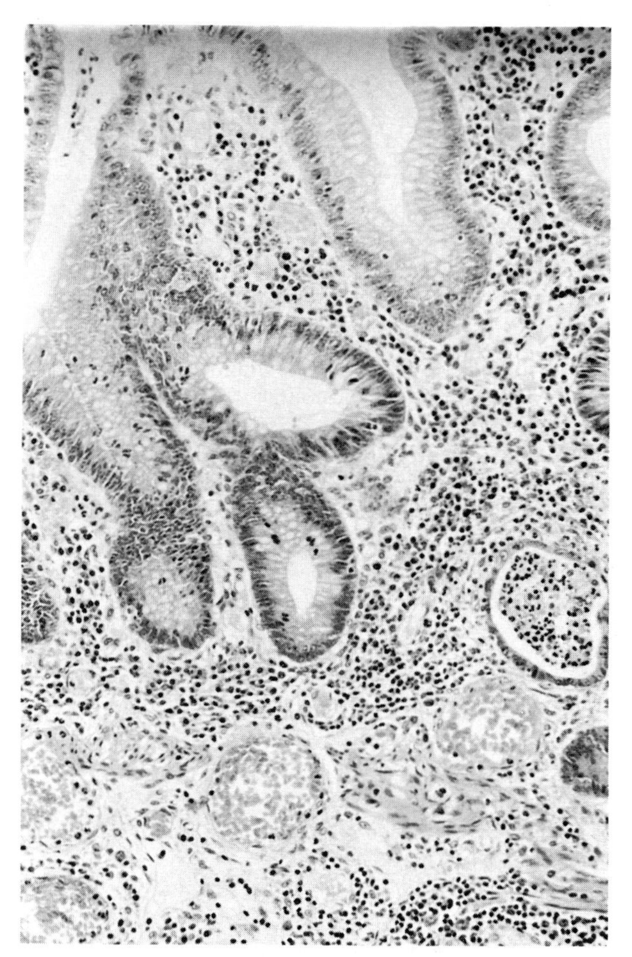

Figure 7.3 Moderatively active ulcerative colitis showing goblet cell depletion, cellular infiltration and increased vascularity. A crypt abscess is present.

Inflammatory polyps (pseudopolyps), formed by mucosal undermining and excessive granulation, become epithelialized and persist. Very large numbers of inflammatory polyps may be present. They are mainly found in the colon and are less pronounced in the rectum.

MICROSCOPIC APPEARANCES

The initial lesion is increasing vascularity and oedema of the mucosa, which becomes infiltrated with acute inflammatory cells – neutrophils, plasma cells and eosinophils – but lymphocytes and macrophages also accumulate. The neutrophils traverse between the epithelial cells into the crypts to form 'crypt abscesses'. This is characteristically accompanied by discharge of mucus from the goblet cells and this population of cells is therefore reduced in active disease (*Figure 7.3*). With increasing severity of disease, there is destruction of the glands and the surface epithelium (*Figure 7.4*). Although the inflammatory and ulcerating process may be severe, it is confined to the mucosa and does not extend appreciably into the deeper layers of the colonic wall, except in association with a perforation or an acute dilatation of the colon.

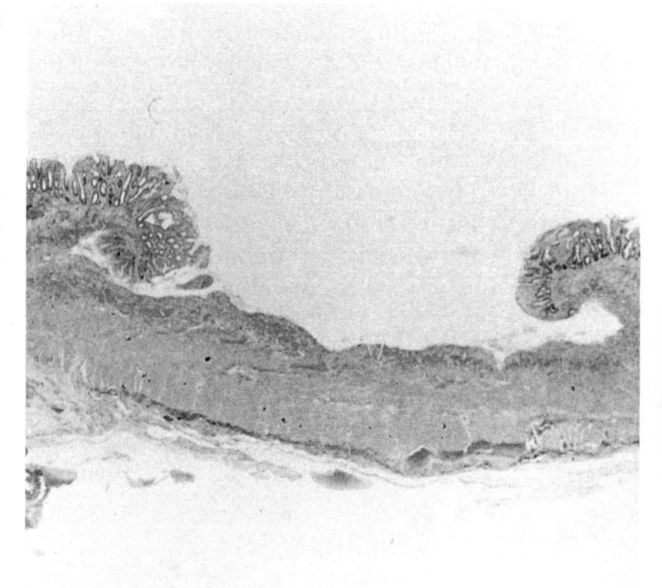

Figure 7.4 Section from the colon illustrated in Figure 7.2 to show the severe undermining ulceration. The mucosal islands that are shown radiologically in Figure 7.7 are well seen.

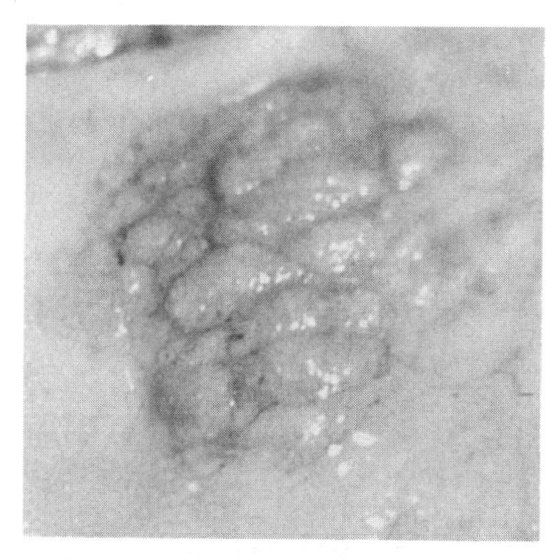

Figure 7.5 Macroscopic appearances of dysplasia in a patient with long-standing universal colitis.

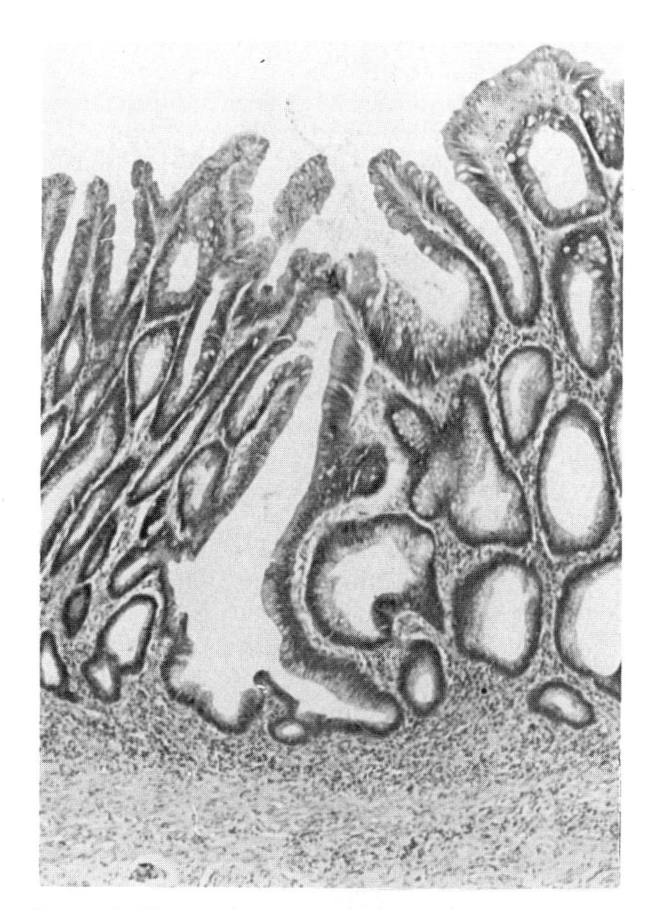

Figure 7.6 Histological appearance of the lesion shown in Figure 7.5. The hyperplastic epithelium is irregular and the mucosa is becoming polypoid. There is a pseudostratification and loss of goblet cells.

In remission the histological appearances of the mucosa may return to normal. However, there is usually some degree of mucosal atrophy. The colonic glands may be branched and reduced in number. They are often shorter than normal and do not extend down to the muscularis mucosae. In patients with long-standing disease, there may be hypertrophy of the muscularis and Paneth's cell hyperplasia at the base of the crypts.

Immunohistochemical stains show increased sialomucin production[17] and class II (HLA-DR) antigen expression[41] by colonic epithelial cells, as well as heterogeneity of the mononuclear cell infiltrate.[26,42] The consequences of these changes on mucosal protection,[53] or epithelial cell function,[18] may contribute to the distribution of disease.

In patients in whom the risk of developing colorectal cancer is increased, dysplastic lesions may occur which are considered to be precancerous.[35,77] They may occur anywhere in the colon and, in some cases, can be recognized macroscopically as rather irregular plaque-like lesions (*Figure 7.5*). The larger lesions can be identified radiologically or at colonoscopy. Histologically, there is irregularity of the tubules with crowding of epithelial cells and stratification of the nuclei which are pleomorphic (*Figure 7.6*). Mucus depletion is commonly present. These changes are present in the mucosa when there is no evidence of acute inflammation and, indeed, this is an important factor because an actively regenerating mucosa may resemble low-grade dysplasia.

CLINICAL PRESENTATION *(D.P. Jewell and S.P.L. Travis)*

The cardinal symptoms of ulcerative colitis are rectal bleeding, diarrhoea, the passage of mucus and abdominal pain.[10] The severity of the symptoms usually correlates with the severity of the disease, although it is not uncommon to find active disease at sigmoidoscopy in patients who are asymptomatic. Hence, endoscopic and histological assessment are necessary before an asymptomatic patient can be said to be in remission.

RECTAL BLEEDING

Patients with inflammation confined to the rectum (haemorrhagic proctitis) usually notice the passage of fresh blood either streaked on the outside of a normal stool or quite separate from faecal matter. The bleeding is frequently attributed to haemorrhoids by patients and even by their doctors. The passage or leakage of blood-stained mucus is a frequent symptom in these patients and should suggest a proctitis rather than haemorrhoids. With more extensive disease, the blood is mixed with the stool or there is a frank bloody diarrhoea. With severe disease, the stool becomes more like anchovy sauce as the blood is mixed with pus in addition to mucus and faecal material. Active ulcerative colitis without rectal bleeding is very unusual and either suggests a different diagnosis (such as Crohn's disease) or that the patient has not examined the stool.

DIARRHOEA

This is variable in degree. Patients with proctitis or proctosigmoiditis often complain of constipation and may never experience diarrhoea,[50] whereas if the whole colon is involved the diarrhoea can be severe and disabling. Most patients with active disease pass several liquid stoods daily and may have nocturnal diarrhoea. Urgency, and a feeling of incomplete evacuation, are common in association with active disease and patients may suffer distressing incontinence. Postprandial diarrhoea is also a common sympton. Mucus or frank pus is commonly mixed with the diarrhoea.

The pathophysiology of the diarrhoea is multifactorial. The principal change is failure to absorb salt and water,[59] due to reduced Na^+/K^+ ATPase pump activity, increased mucosal permeability, altered membrane phospholipids and increased concentrations of prostaglandins.[9] The loss of rectal reservoir capacity as a result of inflammation[52] and exudation of extracellular fluid from inflamed mucosa are contributory factors. Motility dysfunction results in slow small intestinal and proximal colonic transit[51] even in active disease, but rapid distal transit due to rectal irritability. Proximal constipation is commonly seen in distal colitis and is probably due to differences in motility between inflamed and non-inflamed areas.

ABDOMINAL PAIN

Pain is not a prominent symptom for most patients with ulcerative colitis. Mild colicky pain or lower abdominal discomfort relieved by defaecation may be present in some patients. However, severe pain may occur in those with fulminating attacks of the disease.

The cause of the pain is not known with certainty but is probably due to increased tension in the inflamed tissue caused by muscular contraction or distension.

OTHER SYMPTOMS

Patients with severe disease have usually lost weight and complain of malaise and lethargy. Symptoms of anaemia, such as shortness of breath, may also be present and patients may experience ankle swelling secondary to anaemia or hypoproteinaemia.

Weight loss is largely due to diminished food intake secondary to anorexia. Patients with fulminant disease are often nauseated or may even vomit, which further reduces intake. In addition, these patients are hypercatabolic and lose protein through the inflamed colon, both of which contribute to weight loss.

Patients may also present with symptoms referable to the extraintestinal manifestations of ulcerative colitis (see page 1200).

PHYSICAL SIGNS

Patients with mild disease have few, if any, abnormal physical signs. They are well nourished, not anaemic and show no evidence of having a chronic disease. Weight should, however, always be recorded and related to height on a centile chart in children or adolescents. On palpation of the abdomen, the colon is usually normal but minimal tenderness may show over the affected portion.

Patients with more severe disease usually look ill, with evidence of weight loss, and salt and water depletion. They are febrile and frequently anaemic with signs of iron deficiency. The skin may have the appearances associated with hypoproteinaemia and there may be dependent oedema. Oral candidiasis may be present. Beaking or frank clubbing of the nails often occurs in patients where the disease is chronic. Tachycardia is invariable, and postural hypotension may be present. Abdominal examination reveals marked tenderness along the length of the colon and rebound tenderness may be present. The abdomen may be distended and tympanitic, but is usually flat. Bowel sounds are often reduced. Minor perianal disease, such as a small fissure, may be present, but this is much less common than in patients with Crohn's disease. The signs of associated extraintestinal manifestations may also be present. Mouth ulcers are a common finding in patients with active disease.

DISEASE SEVERITY

It is useful to have a clinical guide to disease severity and the criteria of Truelove and Witts[70] are both simple and practical. *Severe disease* is defined as the passage of more than six stools daily with blood and associated with evidence of systemic disturbance such as fever, tachycardia, anaemia or an erythrocyte sedimentation rate (ESR) elevated to 30 mm/h or more. *Mild disease* consists of four or less stools per day with little or no blood and in the absence of systemic illness or an elevated ESR. *Moderate disease* is intermediate between mild and severe.

For all patients presenting with an acute attack of ulcerative colitis, 15% are severe, 25% moderate and 60% are mild.[15]

CLINICAL PRESENTATION

Patients with haemorrhagic proctitis usually present either with rectal bleeding associated with a normal bowel habit or they may actually complain of constipation. As the patient is not systemically ill, several weeks or even months may go by before a patient presents to a doctor.

The most common presentation of ulcerative colitis is the gradual onset of diarrhoea and rectal bleeding. In patients who start by passing blood as their only symptom, small quantities of blood are passed at the time of defaecation, although they may pass some blood and mucus separately; if this is allowed to persist, diarrhoea usually supervenes within a few weeks. Other patients begin with diarrhoea which, during the course of a few weeks or months, becomes frankly bloody.

Much less commonly, patients may present with an acute onset of bloody diarrhoea, anaemia, hypotension, fluid and electrolyte depletion, and may even become septicaemic. The local complications of acute dilatation of the colon, perforation or massive haemorrhage are sometimes present, and more commonly occur during the initial presenting attack.

EXTENT OF DISEASE AT PRESENTATION

In hospital-based series, about a third of patients have disease limited to the rectum, another third have more proximal disease, but not extending beyond the hepatic flexure, and the remainder have universal colitis.[76] In a population-based survey, 74% of patients had disease limited to the rectum or rectosigmoid colon.[61] The more extensive the disease, the more likely are systemic symptoms or local complications during an acute exacerbation, and the less good the outcome. Neither the extent of disease nor the severity of the first attack affects the frequency of relapse, but relapse is less frequent when colitis presents in the elderly.

COMPLICATIONS *(D.P. Jewell and S.P.L. Travis)*

The local complications of ulcerative colitis and their frequency are listed in *Table 7.7*. The extraintestinal complications, or manifestations, are discussed later in this chapter.

PERFORATION

This is the most dangerous of the local complications and is followed by faecal peritonitis. It only occurs in patients with severe disease, but the risk (0.3% of 1928 patients)[63] has fallen sharply in the last 20 years, probably as a result of early surgery for acute dilatation. It is still more common during the first attack,[16] perhaps because of the lack of fibrosis which is associated with earlier attacks and the absence of adhesions, which predispose to a free perforation. Perforation usually complicates acute dilatation, but may occur at other times, or as a complication of colonoscopy. Most perforations occur on the left side of the colon, especially in the sigmoid. There is no evidence that corticosteroid therapy predisposes to perforation – an assertion that has often been made.

The diagnosis may be difficult. The classic symptoms and signs of a colonic perforation, such as sudden onset of abdominal pain, distension, rebound tenderness and fever, are frequently absent. The minimal signs are largely due to faecal peritonitis in a patient already severely ill and their masking by large doses of corticosteroids. The more usual clinical picture is a sudden deterioration in the patient's general condition with a rise in pulse rate. Plain abdominal radiographs with decubitus views should be obtained immediately to demonstrate the presence of free air under the diaphragm.

The treatment is surgical with an emergency colectomy but is associated with a high morbidity.[16]

Table 7.7 Local complications of ulcerative colitis and their frequency

Complication	*Percentage of all patients*
Perforation	<1
Acute dilatation	2–10
Massive haemorrhage	<1
Perianal disease	<10
Strictures	<2
Carcinoma	3–5
Pseudopolyposis	15–30

ACUTE DILATATION

This is another uncommon but major complication usually associated with severe attacks of extensive ulcerative colitis. It is often termed 'toxic dilatation' and mainly affects the transverse colon. As for perforation, the only physical sign may be a sudden deterioration of the patient's general condition, although the abdomen is usually distended and it may be possible to visualize the contour of the colon. Bowel sounds are absent and there is a rapid pulse rate. Patients presenting with severe fulminating attacks should have abdominal girth monitored daily during the first few days of treatment and plain radiographs of the abdomen should be obtained at frequent intervals – even daily if there is a suspicion of impending dilatation. The plain radiographs demonstrate the dilated gas-filled colon without haustrations. In addition, 'mucosal islands' may be seen either as polypoid mucosal swellings along the edge of the colon, or *en face*. They represent small, inflamed and oedematous remnants of mucosa surrounded by severely ulcerated areas which have become denuded of most of their mucosa.

The risk of this complication is directly related to the severity of the attack and is mainly seen in patients with universal colitis, often during their first attack.[23] It rarely occurs in left-sided disease.[31] The pathogenesis of the complication is not known. Histologically, there is severe inflammation, which usually extends through the muscularis mucosae into the submocosa and muscle layers, together with thinning of the bowel wall.[40] It may be that the acute inflammatory reaction impairs the myenteric plexus but this is not yet proven. Possible risk factors include hypokalaemia or metabolic alkalosis, which impair colonic contractility, and hypoproteinaemia which leads to oedema of the bowel wall. Rapid correction of these disturbances with intravenous therapy may reverse the dilatation, at least in early cases.[68] Drugs which affect intestinal motility such as opiates, loperamide and anticholinergic agents may play a part. Generally these drugs should be avoided in patients with ulcerative colitis and are certainly contraindicated in acute attacks. A barium enema performed in patients with fulminant disease could perhaps precipitate acute dilatation but the evidence for this is weak. Finally, patients who have an associated infective diarrhoea (e.g. due to *Campylobacter* or *Salmonella* spp., or the toxin of *Clostridium difficile*) may be at particular risk of developing acute dilatation.

Treatment consists of rapid correction of fluid and electrolyte balance, and intravenous corticosteroids (see later). Nevertheless, most patients will require urgent colectomy once the initial medical treatment has corrected the major metabolic disturbances.

MASSIVE HAEMORRHAGE

This is a rare complication in patients with severe disease. The bleeding usually responds to transfusion and treatment of the disease, and rarely is an indication for an urgent colectomy.

PERIANAL DISEASE

Anal lesions, including haemorrhoids, rectal prolapse or perianal abscess, occur in a small proportion of patients with ulcerative colitis secondary to diarrhoea. More complex lesions, especially fistulas, suggest the possibility of Crohn's disease.

STRICTURES

Benign fibrous strictures are rare but may occur in patients with long-standing disease. Early series quoted a frequency of 11–12%, but this is almost certainly exaggerated by the inclusion of patients with Crohn's disease. The other major differential diagnosis is that of carcinoma. Colonoscopy with biopsy is helpful in making the correct diagnosis.

CARCINOMA

This is considered later (see page 1116).

PSEUDOPOLYPOSIS

Pseudopolyps are common in patients who have had recurrent attacks and occur mainly in the descending colon. They may occur singly or in clusters, and vary in shape and size from small, rounded, polypoid lesions to long, filiform lesions. They represent excessive granulation tissue (formed in response to the acute inflammation) which has become epithelialized. They may persist for years and occasionally become massive.[27] They can regress with time and have no malignant potential.[62]

DIAGNOSIS

The diagnosis of ulcerative colitis is based on the clinical picture, together with stool examination, sigmoidoscopic and radiological appearances, and the histological assessment of rectal and colonic biopsies.

STOOL EXAMINATION

Stool samples from patients with active ulceration contain large quantities of pus cells and frequently eosinophils. Stools should be cultured to exclude pathogens such as *Salmonella* spp. and *Shigella* spp., and special cultures should be set up to exclude *Campylobacter* spp. and *Clostridium difficile*. The presence of the toxin of *Clostridium difficile* should also be determined. To exclude amoebiasis, stools should be examined within a few minutes of obtaining the specimen.

SIGMOIDOSCOPY

This should be performed in all patients with a diarrhoeal illness and is best done in the unprepared patient. Minimal changes of early ulcerative colitis can thus be detected which can otherwise be masked by hyperaemia induced by preparative enemas. The earliest sigmoidoscopic sign of ulcerative colitis is loss of the normal vascular pattern and the mucosa appears hyperaemic and oedematous. The edges of the valves of Houston, which are normally sharp, become blunted. With more severe inflammation, the mucosa becomes granular and eventually friable so that touching or wiping of the mucosa results in small petechial haemorrhages. In patients with severe colitis, the mucosa bleeds spontaneously and becomes ulcerated. In these patients, the lumen usually contains large amounts of liquid reddish-brown stool (a combination of diarrhoea, pus and blood). In patients with long-standing disease, pseudopolyps may be seen on sigmoidoscopy. In remission, the sigmoidoscopic appearances may return to normal, but in patients who have had a long history of repeated attacks, the mucosa becomes pale and atrophic.

There is considerable observer variation in the interpretation of the mild changes, such as hyperaemia, granularity and oedema, but there is much greater uniformity concerning more severe changes such as friability, spontaneous bleeding and ulceration.[6]

RADIOLOGY

All patients with a severe attack should have a supine radiograph of the abdomen.[7] The interface between the mucosa and air within the colonic lumen is normally sharp. In the presence of severe disease, this becomes blurred and it is often possible to detect mucosal oedema or ulceration.[11] Thickening of the bowel wall may also be apparent. The plain radiograph is also useful in detecting the presence of faecal material. An inflamed segment of colon rarely contains faecal material and there are no faeces visible in patients with a severe universal colitis. The presence of faeces in the proximal colon is therefore a good indication that the disease is limited in extent. The radiograph demonstrates the width of the colon and an acute dilatation should be suspected if the diameter is greater than 5.5 cm. In severe cases, mucosal islands may be seen (*Figure 7.7*) and there may be distension of small bowel loops. Both these signs predict a high risk of failing medical therapy.[13,16] Plain radiographs also help to exclude a perforation.

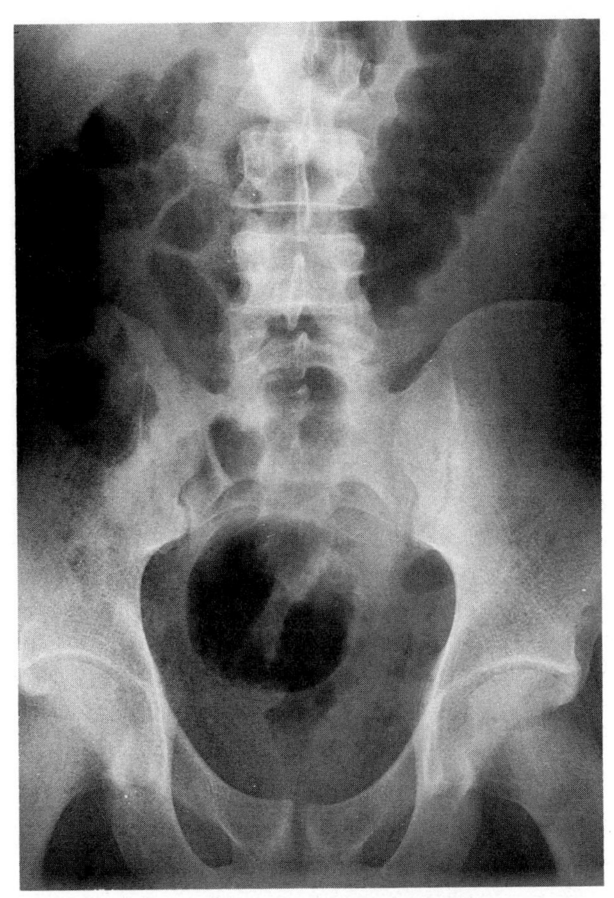

Figure 7.7 Plain radiograph of a patient with fulminating ulcerative colitis showing mucosal irregularity in the sigmoid and transverse colon. Mucosal islands in the transverse colon are clearly visible.

If the diagnosis is still in doubt, an 'instant' barium enema can be performed. A single contrast study without preparation is performed, allowing the barium to run in at low pressure without using a balloon catheter. However, barium studies are best avoided in these acutely ill patients and are contraindicated in patients with toxic megacolon.

Even in patients with less severe disease, care has to be taken if a barium enema is performed. Nevertheless, an air contrast procedure is safe, providing that (1) adequate preparation is obtained by gentle means, (2) the radiologist is aware that the disease is active, (3) the bowel is not over-distended with barium and air, and (4) the procedure is terminated if pain develops.

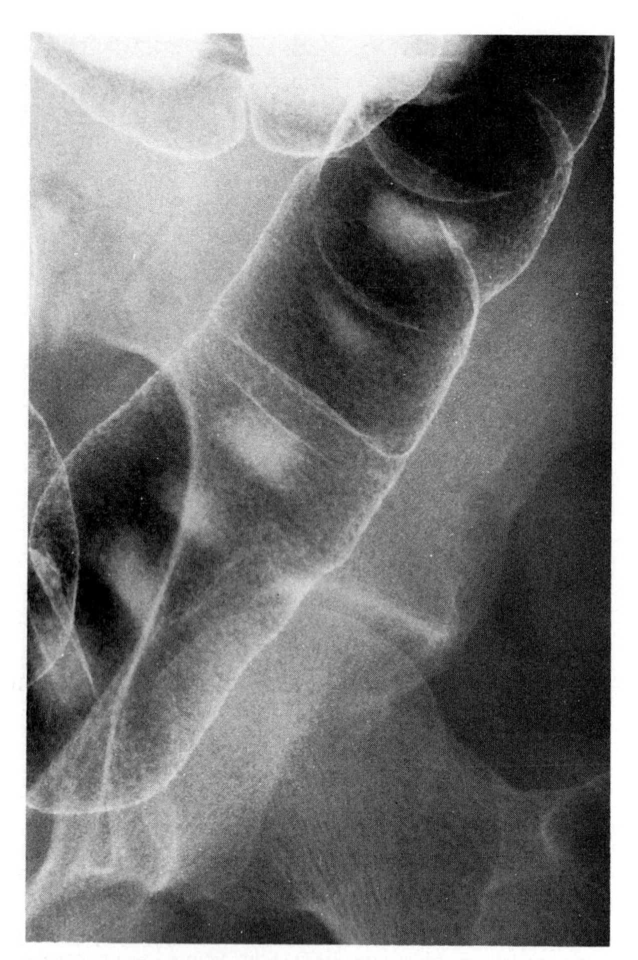

Figure 7.8 The fine granular appearances of mild ulcerative on a double-contrast barium enema.

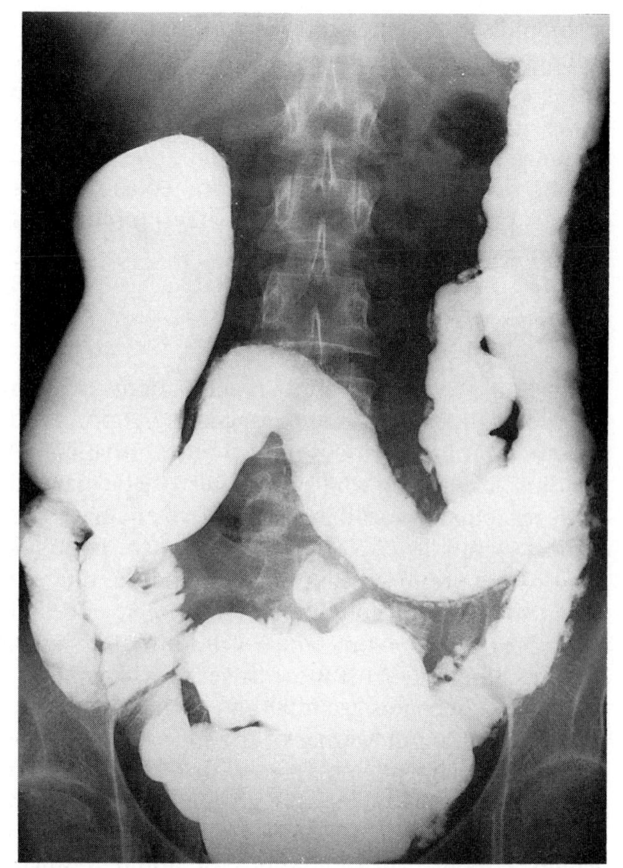

Figure 7.9 Single-contrast barium enema in a patient with severe ulcerative colitis showing deep ulceration.

In mildly active disease, the mucosa shows fine irregularities or serrations along the edge of the colon and appears granular when seen *en face* on an air contrast study (*Figure 7.8*). These abnormalities may be confined to the distal colon, but may be present throughout. With increasing severity of the disease, the ulcers become deeper and may appear as 'collar-stud' ulcers penetrating deep into the mucosa (*Figure 7.9*). As these deep ulcers undermine the epithelium, they may give rise to the radiological appearances of a 'double contour.' Loss of haustral pattern is a common sign and, in patients with long-standing disease, there may be shortening and narrowing of the colon. Pseudopolyps are often present in patients with long-standing disease. Widening of the presacral space seen on a lateral view of the pelvis is also commonly seen. This is probably another sign representing shortening and fibrosis of the rectum and it is not necessarily related to active disease or oedema of the pelvic tissues.

If there is doubt about whether the colonic disease is ulcerative colitis or Crohn's disease, a small bowel enema should be obtained to exclude ileal disease. However, for patients with ulcerative colitis, this examination should be normal, although the terminal ileum may appear featureless ('backwash ileitis') in those patients with severe universal disease.

COLONOSCOPY

This procedure is not usually necessary for diagnosis in most patients and is contraindicated in the presence of severe disease when the risk of perforation is high. If there are difficulties in the differential diagnosis, especially with respect to Crohn's disease, it can be useful because multiple biopsies can be obtained.[47] The principal uses of colonoscopy in patients with ulcerative colitis are in cancer surveillance and to determine the nature of a stricture or polyps shown radiologically. Colonoscopy is also helpful in defining the extent of disease in those patients whose symptoms are out of proportion to the radiological extent of disease. Commonly, the disease is much more extensive when assessed using multiple biopsies taken at endoscopy. Indeed, in one series up to 14% of the patients with a universal colitis on colonoscopy had a normal barium enema,[39] but prognostic factors, including the risk of cancer, are related to the extent of macroscopic disease.

RECTAL BIOPSY

A rectal biopsy should always be performed at the initial sigmoidoscopic examination. Once the diagnosis is established, some clinicians advise not taking further biopsy specimens. However, they are frequently useful, because there is incomplete agreement between the macroscopic appearances at sigmoidoscopy and the histological appearance.[6,75] Biopsy specimens should be carefully mounted on card or glass before fixation to ensure good orientation. Biopsies should be performed below 10 cm, i.e. below the peritoneal reflection, and preferably on the posterior wall. In this way, the risk of perforation becomes extremely small. The other complication is haemorrhage, which can be minimized by using small forceps and by ensuring haemostasis before the sigmoidoscope is removed.

Biopsy specimens taken at sigmoidoscopy or at endoscopy can be useful in the differential diagnosis of ulcerative colitis.[77] The characteristic appearances of Crohn's disease or ischaemic colitis may be present. Pseudomembranous colitis can often be diagnosed by biopsy specimens and a skilled histopathologist may distinguish an infective colitis from ulcerative colitis. Search for amoebae in suspected cases of amoebiasis is vital.

LABORATORY DATA

Many patients become iron deficient due to continued blood loss – 0.5 g elemental iron may be lost during a severe attack.[65] Hypochromic microcytic anaemia is therefore common in active disease, although anaemia is uncommon in patients with mild distal disease. Active inflammation is also associated with an eosinophilia, a monocytosis or thrombocytosis. The erythrocyte sedimentation rate is variably raised according to the severity of the disease.

Biochemical disturbance in patients with mild or moderate disease is uncommon, but severe attacks are associated with hypokalaemia, hypoalbuminaemia and a rise in α_2-globulins. Serum immunoglobulin concentrations usually increase but remain within the normal range, and fall again as the disease goes into remission. Serum orosomucoid and C-reactive protein concentrations behave as acute phase reactants and are useful in monitoring the inflammatory activity. Liver function tests may be abnormal in patients with fulminating attacks and show elevations of serum asparate transaminase or alkaline phosphatase. These are transitory changes and probably reflect a degree of fatty liver or non-specific changes in the liver secondary to toxaemia and under-nutrition. About 3% of patients will have persistently abnormal liver enzyme concentrations even when the disease is in remission, of which the most common is an elevated serum alkaline phosphatase.[60]

DIFFERENTIAL DIAGNOSIS

The more common diagnoses which must be considered in patients with suspected ulcerative colitis are listed in *Table 7.8*; they provide some practical points in differential diagnosis. For patients presenting with an acute onset of blood diarrhoea, an infective cause must be excluded. *Salmonella* spp., *Shigella* spp. or *Campylobacter jejuni* are the most common organisms causing self-limited colitis, but they may also provoke the first or subsequent attacks of ulcerative colitis. Pain is a prominent feature of *Campylobacter* infections. *Escherichia coli* serotype 0157: H7 may also cause haemorrhagic colitis, but the proximal colon is often more severely affected than the rectum.[19] The diagnosis is often missed, because serotyping of faecal *E. coli* is not routinely performed.

Sigmoidoscopic appearances of the infective colitides are similar to ulcerative colitis and it may also be difficult for the histopathologist to distinguish between them. Distorted crypt architecture, crypt atrophy, basal lymphoid aggregates and dense lymphocytic infiltrates have about an 80% probability of distinguishing inflammatory bowel disease from infective (self-limited colitis), but there may be substantial variations between histopathologists.[1] Pseudomembranous colitis is also diagnosed more frequently now that the toxin of *Clostridium difficile* can be detected. There is, of course, no reason why patients with ulcerative colitis should not contract an infective colitis, but it is then uncertain whether symptoms are solely due to the infection, or whether the infection triggers a relapse. Gonoccocal proctitis is easily overlooked in a gastroenterological clinic but, characteristically, it is associated with large quantities of purulent exudate. Chlamydial proctitis is much less common and appears macroscopically similar to ulcerative colitis. Opportunistic infections of the colon, such as herpes simplex and cytomegalovirus, may be seen in immunosuppressed patients and in AIDS sufferers. The ulcers are usually discrete and more likely to be confused with Crohn's disease than with ulcerative colitis. Histological appearances of a biopsy specimen usually provide the diagnosis.

Table 7.8 Differential diagnosis of ulcerative colitis

	Clinical	*Radiological*	*Histological*
Ulcerative colitis	Bloody diarrhoea	Extends proximally from rectum; fine mucosal inflammation	Acute inflammatory infiltrate; goblet cell depletion; distortion of crypts; crypt abscesses
Crohn's colitis	Anal lesions common	Segmental disease; rectal sparing; small bowel involvement; strictures, fissure ulcers and fistulas	Focal inflammation; submucosal involvement; granulomata; goblet cell preservation
Ischaemic colitis	Older age groups; vascular disease; sudden onset, often painful	Splenic flexure; 'thumb printing'; rectal involvement rare	Mucosal necrosis; ballooning of capillaries; red cell congestion; haemosiderin and fibrosis (chronic disease)
Infective colitis	Sudden onset usual; identifiable source with other cases (e.g. *Salmonella* spp.); pain may predominate (e.g. *Campylobacter* spp.); pathogens present in stool	Usually normal	Crypt architecture usually normal; neutrophil infiltrate
Pseudomembranous colitis	May be a history of antibiotics; 'membrane' may be seen on sigmoidoscopy; *Cl. difficile* toxin detectable in stools	Oedematous; shaggy outline	Similar to acute ischaemic colitis, but may show 'summit' lesions of fibropurulent exudate
Amoebic colitis	Travel in endemic area; amoebae in fresh stool	Discrete ulcers; amoeboma or strictures	Similar to ulcerative colitis; amoebae in lamina propria (chronic disease) or flask-shaped ulcers, readily shown by PAS stain
Collagenous colitis	Watery diarrhoea; rectal bleeding rare	Usually normal	>12 mm thick subepithelial collagen band
Microscopic colitis	Watery diarrhoea; often in older women; macroscopically normal colonic mucosa	Normal	Chronic inflammatory infiltrate; crypt distortion unusual

Collagenous colitis[29] and microscopic (also termed 'lymphocytic') colitis[28] are rare causes of recurrent diarrhoea, but without rectal bleeding. Older women are usually affected. Diagnosis is made by colonoscopy and serial biopsy, because the mucosa usually looks normal and the microscopic changes may be most prominent in the proximal colon.

TREATMENT

MEDICAL TREATMENT *(D.P. Jewell and S.P.L. Travis)*

All patients with ulcerative colitis must have the nature of the disease explained to them carefully and must appreciate that when symptoms recur they should report to their doctor early so that appropriate treatment can be given. Both patients and their close relatives often become upset by the symptoms, so that reassurance and moral support are vital in the overall management.

Active disease is generally treated with corticosteroids and, when the acute disease has settled, the remission maintained with compounds containing 5-aminosalicylic acid. The drugs that can be used will be discussed individually followed by guidelines for treating attacks according to severity.

Corticosteroids

The classic trials of Truelove and Witts[70,71] established the benefit of cortisone in the treatment of acute ulcerative colitis. Oral prednisolone is also effective and this is dose-related, although the higher doses (e.g. 60 mg daily) are associated with appreciable side effects. When prednisolone is given by mouth, it should be given as a single morning dose because this is as effective as a divided dose regimen but has fewer side effects.[34] Intramuscular ACTH may be marginally more effective than higher doses of cortisone, but is seldom needed. Topical corticosteroids, given as a retention enema, are also effective in healing active rectal disease and the combination of oral and topical steroids is more effective than either alone.[69] Absorption of steroid from the rectum is considerable if prednisolone phosphate enemas are used,[48] but this can be minimized either by using betamethasone enemas or, preferably, prednisolone *meta*-sulphobenzoate enemas.[33] The mechanism of action of steroids in ulcerative colitis remains uncertain, but inhibition of leukotriene synthesis, lysosomal membrane stabilization and reduced microvascular permeability[43] will decrease inflammation, whilst enhanced sodium and water transport[58] will decrease diarrhoea.

Corticosteroids should not be used as maintenance therapy because they are ineffective, at least in doses that are associated with an acceptable incidence of side effects. Neither cortisone in a dose of 37.5 mg daily,[71] nor prednisolone in a dose of 15 mg daily,[36] will maintain remission. An alternate-day regimen has been advocated as a way of minimizing side effects associated with higher doses.

Sulphasalazine

This drug consists of 5-aminosalicylic acid linked to sulphapyridine by a diazo bond. It is poorly absorbed in the small intestine and hence most of an orally administered dose is delivered to the colon. Colonic bacteria split the diazo bond and thereby release the two individual moieties. The active agent, at least for acute healing, is 5-aminosalicylic acid,[3,74] but the combination with sulphapyridine may still confer additional benefits. The mode of action of sulphasalazine is controversial.[22] In vitro studies have shown that it has a weak inhibitory effect on prostaglandin synthesis, but it may also reduce prostaglandin catabolism by inhibiting prostaglandin dehydrogenase. It inhibits polymorph and monocyte migration *in vitro* and this may be related to its ability to inhibit leukotriene synthesis, free radical and platelet-activating factor release. Sulphasalazine and 5-aminosalicylic acid may also inhibit lymphocyte function and prevent the induction of class II antigens on epithelial cells by interferon-γ. Sulphasalazine inhibits folate metabolism, but despite suggestions that folate supplements decrease the risk of dysplasia,[57] long-term use of sulphasalazine in distal colitis is not associated with an increased risk of colorectal cancer.

The dose-related side effects of sulphasalazine are largely caused by sulphapyridine and its metabolites, and include nausea, vomiting, diarrhoea and headache. Many of the non-dose-related side effects, such as erythema nodosum and other hypersensitivity rashes, may also be due to the sulphapyridine moiety. Rarely, agranulocytosis or a Heinz body haemolytic anaemia can occur, and sulphasalazine may cause male infertility. The drug mainly affects sperm motility but abnormal forms are often present and the total number of spermatozoa may be reduced. These changes are reversible once the drug is stopped.[67] The dose-related side effects of sulphasalazine can often be overcome by starting at a low dose (e.g. 0.5 g daily) and gradually working up to a full therapeutic dose, or using an enteric-coated preparation. For patients with hypersensitivity reactions, or continued intolerance, an alternative 5-aminosalicylic acid compound is recommended.

Sulphasalazine is more effective than a placebo in treating active disease, although it is not nearly as effective as corticosteroids.[72] Sulphasalazine enemas may be useful for active distal disease.[45] However, the major use of sulphasalazine is in long-term maintenance therapy because it reduces the frequency of recurrent attacks, an effect which operates over many years.[14] The optimum dose which gives maximal clinical effect with the fewest side effects is 2 g daily.[4]

Mesalazine and olsalazine

Mesalazine (1.2–2.4 g/day) or olsalazine (1 g/day) are indicated when there is sulphasalazine intolerance, hypersensitivity or male infertility, but not as initial treatment because they are appreciably more expensive than sulphasalazine which is usually well tolerated. Mesalazine (5-aminosalicylic acid) is available in slow-release preparations, either coated with an acrylic-based resin (Asacol),[55] or as microgranules coated with a semi-permeable ethyl cellulose membrane (Pentasa).[44] Olsalazine (Dipentum) consists of two molecules of 5-aminosalicylic acid joined by a diazo bond which is split by colonic bacteria.[25] Its pharmacodynamics are similar to those of sulphasalazine and it therefore delivers high concentrations of 5-aminosalicylic acid to the colonic lumen. All 5-aminosalicylic acid preparations have comparable efficacy to sulphasalazine[25,44,55] and are better tolerated, but side effects still occur in about 10% of patients. Enema preparations of mesalazine are effective in the treatment of distal colitis and may be especially useful when disease is refractory to steroids.[8]

Azathioprine

There is no evidence that azathioprine is of benefit for active disease. However, it may be of some value as long-term maintenance therapy in a dose of 1.5–2.0 mg/kg, especially for patients with established disease.[24] It should be reserved for those patients who frequently relapse once corticosteroids are tailed off. Azathioprine also has a steroid-sparing effect in those rare patients who appear to benefit from continuous therapy.[30] If a patient has a good response to azathioprine, the drug should be continued for 1–2 years. There may be risks of long-term therapy but these are probably small.[2,49]

Methotrexate

Preliminary reports on the use of methotrexate (15 mg/week by mouth) in refractory ulcerative colitis are encouraging,[32] but confirmation is needed.

Cyclosporin

The value of cyclosporin in active disease refractory to steroids is debatable,[5] and proper trials are required. Intravenous cyclosporin cannot yet be recommended as an alternative to surgery in severe attacks refractory to steroids, although some benefit has been reported.[38]

Cromoglycate

Despite promising results from early trials, all subsequent studies have shown no benefit, at least in doses up to 800 mg daily.

Antibiotics

Antibiotics have no place in the management of ulcerative colitis.[12]

TREATMENT OF ACUTE ATTACKS

MILD ATTACKS

Mild attacks are defined as the passage of no more than four motions daily, often with blood and mucus, by patients who are not systemically ill. These attacks are best treated with prednisolone in a dose of 20 mg daily in combination with sulphasalazine and steroid enema. Most patients are able to carry on their normal daily activities. This regimen rapidly renders the overwhelming majority of patients symptom-free. Oral steroids are maintained for at least 4 weeks before being tailed off. Rectal steroids are usually continued until oral steroids are stopped, and they can also be stopped if mucosal healing is apparent on sigmoidoscopy. Patients are maintained on sulphasalazine, mesalazine or olsalazine, as described above. If a good response is not obtained, the patient should be treated as for a moderate attack or may even require hospital admission.

MODERATE ATTACKS

These consist of passing more than four motions daily with blood, but in the absence of systemic illness. Prednisolone should be given in a dose of 40 mg daily for at least 1 week and then reduced over 2–3 weeks to 20 mg daily. The treatment schedule is otherwise similar to that outlined for mild attacks.

SEVERE ATTACKS

These are attacks in which there may be severe diarrhoea with bleeding in patients who may show any of the following: tachycardia, obvious salt and water deficiency, fever, anaemia and hypoalbuminaemia. All such patients must be admitted to hospital. Electrolyte, fluid and blood losses are corrected as quickly as possible and treatment should begin using intravenous fluids, nutrients and prednisolone 60 mg or hydrocortisone 400 mg daily. Intravenous antibiotics, such as tetracycline or metronidazole, have no role.[12] Hydrocortisone enemas should also be given, using 100 mg twice daily. These enemas are preferable to disposable enemas because they can be dripped into the inflamed colon at a slow rate, using a soft catheter and an intravenous infusion set, and are therefore more likely to be retained.

Patients in a severe attack should have careful monitoring of pulse rate, blood pressure, temperature and abdominal girth in order to detect the early signs of an acute dilatation or a perforation. Plain radiographs of the abdomen should be obtained to exclude these complications and are often repeated on a daily basis for the first few days.

About 70% of patients with severe attacks respond rapidly to this form of intravenous therapy in the first 5 days.[73] Experience has shown that patients not making a satisfactory response should be considered for urgent colectomy as few do well if medical therapy is continued. The factors which help to identify those patients who are likely to respond poorly and hence come to surgery, are a maximum temperature greater than 38°C, a maximum pulse rate of greater than 100/min, or a bowel frequency greater than 12 stools within the first 24 hours of hospital admission. A persistently low serum albumin (<30 g/l) during the first few days of treatment is another indicator of a poor prognosis.[37]

Patients who respond well to intravenous therapy should then receive oral corticosteroids (e.g. prednisolone 40 mg daily) and sulphasalazine. Hydrocortisone enemas should be continued or changed to a disposable enema (e.g. Predenema). A light diet is given.

There are a few patients who may have severe left-sided disease with proximal constipation. Exacerbations of the disease may not settle on intensive corticosteroid therapy unless the constipation is treated, perferably with a gentle osmotic purge.

MANAGEMENT OF PROCTITIS

Patients with symptomatic, haemorrhagic proctitis and normal colon are sometimes difficult to manage. Initially, topical steroids should be given in the form of a suppository or a foam, together with oral sulphasalazine. However, this regimen frequently fails to heal the inflammation. In these circumstances, oral corticosteroids or a sulphasalazine enema can be tried. If there is still no response, 5-aminosalicylic acid enemas (2 g/40 ml) can be tried, after treating any proximal constipation with an osmotic laxative (such as Picolax – sodium picosulphate – or lactulose).

THE ROLE OF DIET

In general, patients should be encouraged to eat a well-balanced high-fibre diet. Milk-free diets are not useful for most patients, although about 20% of patients appeared to benefit under the conditions of a controlled therapeutic trial.[80] Some of these patients probably had hypolactasia which may partly explain the benefit obtained. Patients with severe attacks of ulcerative colitis commonly have temporary hypolactasia.[46]

MAINTENANCE OF REMISSION

Once the patient is in remission, usually defined according to symptoms for the purposes of management, corticosteroids are tailed off as previously described. Sulphasalazine is continued in a dose of 2 g daily, on a long-term basis because this reduces the risk of a further relapse by about 75%, even after many years of treatment, Mesalazine 1.2 g/day or olsalazine 1 g/day are indicated for sulphasalazine intolerance.

COURSE AND PROGNOSIS

Most patients with ulcerative colitis suffer recurrent attacks of their disease,[15] but the reasons for relapse remain obscure.[54] The number of patients who have only one attack is very small and diminishes with increasing length of follow-up. In the few that never relapse, it may be that the initial attack represented an infection with *Campylobacter* spp. or *Clostridium difficile* at a time when modern diagnostic techniques were not available. About 8% of patients pursue a chronic continuous course and never have a prolonged remission.

The introduction of corticosteroids greatly reduced the overall mortality of ulcerative colitis but this is mainly in patients with mild or moderate attacks.[15] Severe attacks continue to be dangerous especially when they are of sudden onset and there is delay in making the diagnosis, when the patient is elderly, when universal colitis is present, or when a local complication intervenes. Nevertheless, developments in both medical and surgical treatment have reduced the mortality of severe attacks and, in the authors' hospital, mortality in this situation has fallen from about 33% in the pre-steroid era to less than 1% over the last 10 years.

The long-term prognosis has also probably improved with studies showing a survival curve which either does not differ appreciably from the expected survival curve,[56,66] or is only slightly decreased.[20] This improvement is probably due to the reduction in mortality during acute attacks, the reduction in operative mortality and the use of long-term sulphasalazine, which reduces the relapse rate to about one-quarter of that seen in patients who do not receive the drug.[14]

REFERENCES

1. Allison, M.C., Hamilton-Dutoit, S.J., Dhillon, A.P. *et al.* (1987) The value of rectal biopsy in distinguishing self-limited colitis from early inflammatory bowel disease. *Quarterly Journal of Medicine*, **65**, 985–996.
2. Alstead, E.M., Ritchie, J.K., Lennard-Jones, J.E. *et al.* (1990) Safety in azathioprine in pregnancy in inflammatory bowel disease. *Gastroenterology*, **99**, 443–446.
3. Azad Khan, A.K., Piris, J. and Truelove, S.C. (1977) An experiment to determine the active therapeutic moiety of sulphasalazine. *The Lancet*, **2**, 892–895.
4. Azad Khan, A.K., Howes, D.T., Piris, J. and Truelove, S.C. (1980) Optimum dose of sulphasalazine for maintenance treatment in ulcerative colitis. *Gut*, **21**, 232–240.
5. Baker, K. and Jewell, D.P. (1989) Cyclosporin A

for the treatment of severe colitis. *Alimentary Pharmacology and Therapeutics*, **3**, 143–149.

6. Baron, J.H., Connell, A.M. and Lennard-Jones, J.E. (1964) Variation between observers in describing mucosal appearances in proctocolitis. *British Medical Journal*, **1**, 89–92.
7. Bartram, C.I. (1976) Plain abdominal X-ray in acute colitis. *Proceedings of the Royal Society of Medicine*, **67**, 617–618.
8. Biddle, W.I. and Miner, P.B. (1990) Long term use of mesalamine enemas to induce remission in ulcerative colitis. *Gastroenterology*, **99**, 113–118.
9. Binder, H.J. and Sandle, G.I. (1987) Electrolyte absorption and secretion in the mammalian colon. In *Physiology of the Gastrointestinal Tract* (Ed.) Johnson, L.R. New York: Raven Press.
10. Both, H., Torp-Pedersen, K., Kriener, S. *et al.* (1983) Clinical manifestations of ulcerative colitis and Crohn's disease in a regional patient group. *Scandinavian Journal of Gastroenterology*, **18**, 987–991.
11. Buckell, N.A., Williams, G.I., Bartram, C.I. *et al.* (1980) Depth of ulceration in acute colitis. Correlation with outcome and clinical and radiologic features. *Gastroenterology*, **79**, 19–25.
12. Chapman, R.W.G., Selby, W.S. and Jewell, D.P. (1986) Controlled trial of metronidazole as an adjunct to corticosteroids in severe ulcerative colitis. *Gut*, **27**, 1210–1212.
13. Chew, C.N., Nolan, D.J. and Jewell, D.P. (1991) Small bowel gas in severe ulcerative colitis. *Gut*, **32**, 1535–1540.
14. Dissanayake, A.S. and Truelove, S.C. (1973) A controlled therapeutic trial of long-term maintenance treatment of ulcerative colitis with sulphasalazine. *Gut*, **14**, 923–926.
15. Edwards, F.C. and Truelove, S.C. (1963) The course and prognosis of ulcerative colitis. *Gut*, **4**, 299–315.
16. Edwards, F.C. and Truelove, S.C. (1964) The course and prognosis of ulcerative colitis. *Gut*, **5**, 1–22.
17. Ehsanullah, M., Filipe, M.I. and Gazard, B. (1982) Mucin secretion in inflammatory bowel disease: correlation with disease activity and dysplasia. *Gut*, **23**, 485–489.
18. Gibson, P.R., Van de Pol, E., Barratt, P.J. *et al.* (1988) Ulcerative colitis – a disease characterised by the abnormal epithelial cell. *Gut*, **29**, 516–521.
19. Griffin, P.M., Olmstead, L.C. and Petras, R.E. (1990) *Escherichia coli* 0157: H7-associated colitis. *Gastroenterology*, **99**, 142–149.
20. Gyde, S., Prior, P., Dow, M.J. *et al.* (1982) Mortality in ulcerative colitis. *Gastroenterology*, **83**, 36–43.
21. Hurst, A.F. (1921) Ulcerative colitis. *Guy's Hospital Report*, **71**, 24–41.
22. Ireland, A. and Jewell, D.P. (1990) Mechanism of action of 5-aminosalicylic acid and its derivatives. *Clinical Science*, **78**, 119–125.
23. Jalan, K.N., Sircus, W., Card, W.I. *et al.* (1969) An experience of ulcerative colitis. 1. Toxic dilatation in 55 cases. *Gastroenterology*, **57**, 68–82.
24. Jewell, D.P. and Truelove, S.C. (1974) Azathioprine in ulcerative colitis: final report on a controlled therapeutic trial. *British Medical Journal*, **2**, 627–630.
25. Jewell, D.P. and Truelove, S.C. (1988) Proceedings of the first international symposium on olsalazine in the treatment of ulcerative colitis. *Scandinavian Journal of Gastroenterology*, **23**, suppl. 148, 1–120.
26. Kaulfersch, W., Fiocchi, C. and Waldmann, T.A. (1988) Polyclonal nature of the intestinal mucosal lymphocyte populations in inflammatory bowel disease. *Gastroenterology*, **95**, 364–370.
27. Kelly, J.K., Langevin, J.M., Price, L.M. *et al.* (1986) Giant and symptomatic inflammatory polyps of the colon. *American Journal of Surgery and Pathology*, **10**, 420–428.
28. Kingham, J.G.C., Levison, D.A., Ball, J.A. *et al.* (1982) Microscopic colitis – a cause of watery diarrhoea. *British Medical Journal*, **285**, 1601–1604.
29. Kingham, J.G.C., Levison, D.A., Morson, B.C. *et al.* (1986) Collagenous colitis. *Gut*, **27**, 570–577.
30. Kirk, A.P. and Lennard-Jones, J.E. (1982) Controlled trial of azathioprine in chronic ulcerative colitis. *British Medical Journal*, **2**, 1291–1292.
31. Kisloff, B. and Adkins, J.C. (1981) Toxic megacolon developing in a patient with long standing distal ulcerative colitis. *American Journal of Gastroenterology*, **75**, 451–453.
32. Kozarek, R.A., Patterson, D.J., Bottoman, V.A. *et al.* (1990) Methotrexate: the long and the short of it. *Gastroenterology*, **98**, A183.
33. Lee, D.A.H., Taylor, M., James, V.H.T. and Walker, G. (1980) Rectally administered prednisolone – evidence for a predominantly local action. *Gut*, **21**, 215–218.
34. Lennard-Jones, J.E. (1983) Towards optimal use of corticosteroids in ulcerative colitis and Crohn's disease. *Gut*, **24**, 177–180.
35. Lennard-Jones, J.E., Melville, D.M., Morson, B.C. *et al.* (1990) Precancer and cancer in extensive ulcerative colitis: findings among 401 patients over 22 years. *Gut*, **31**, 800–806.
36. Lennard-Jones, J.E., Misiewicz, J.J., Connell, A.M. *et al.* (1965) Prednisone as maintenance treatment for ulcerative colitis in remission. *The Lancet*, **1**, 188–189.
37. Lennard-Jones, J.E., Ritchie, J.K., Hilder, W. and Spicer, C.C. (1975) Assessment of severity in colitis: a preliminary study. *Gut*, **16**, 579–584.
38. Lichtiger, S. and Present, D.H. (1990) Preliminary report: cyclosporin in treatment of severe ulcerative colitis. *The Lancet*, **336**, 16–19.
39. Loose, H. and Williams, C. (1974) Barium enema versus colonoscopy. *Proceedings of the Royal Society of Medicine*, **67**, 1033–1036.
40. Lumb, G., Protheroe, R.H.B. and Ramsay, G.S. (1955) Ulcerative colitis with dilatation of the colon. *British Journal of Surgery*, **43**, 182–188.
41. McDonald, G.B. and Jewell, D.P. (1987) Class II

antigen (HLA-DR) expression by intestinal epithelial cells in inflammatory diseases of the colon. *Journal of Clinical Pathology*, **40**, 312–317.
42. Mahida, Y.R., Patel, S., Gionchetti, P. *et al.* (1989) Macrophage subpopulations in lamina propria of normal and inflamed colon and terminal ileum. *Gut*, **30**, 826–834.
43. Meyers, S. and Janowitz, H.D. (1985) Systemic corticosteroid therapy of ulcerative colitis. *Gastroenterology*, **89**, 1189–1196.
44. Mulder, C.J.J., Tytgat, G.N.J., Weterman, I.T. *et al.* (1988) Double blind comparison of slow release 5-aminosalicylic and sulfasalazine in remission maintenance in ulcerative colitis. *Gastroenterology*, **95**, 1449–1453.
45. Palmer, K.R., Goepel, J.R. and Holdsworth, C.D. (1981) Sulphasalazine enemas in ulcerative colitis: a double-blind trial. *British Medical Journal*, **2**, 1571–1573.
46. Peña, A.S. and Truelove, S.C. (1973) Hypolactasia and ulcerative colitis. *Gastroenterology*, **64**, 400–404.
47. Peña, A., Bellando, P., Caldera, D. *et al.* (1987) Colonoscopy in inflammatory bowel disease. *Gastroenterology*, **92**, 181–185.
48. Powell-Tuck, J., Lennard-Jones, J.E., May, C.S. *et al.* (1976) Plasma prednisolone levels after administration of prednisolone-21-phosphate as a retention enema in colitis. *British Medical Journal*, **1**, 193–195.
49. Present, D.H., Meltzer, S.J., Krumholz, M.P. *et al.* (1989) 6-Mercaptopurine in the management of inflammatory bowel disease: short and long-term toxicity. *Annals of Internal Medicine*, **111**, 641–649.
50. Rao, S.C.C., Holdsworth, C.D. and Read, N.W. (1988) Symptoms and stool pattern in patients with ulcerative colitis. *Gut*, **29**, 342–345.
51. Rao, S.C.C., Read, N.W., Brown, C. *et al.* (1987) Studies on the mechanism of bowel disturbance in ulcerative colitis. *Gastroenterology*, **93**, 934–940.
52. Rao, S.C.C., Read, N.W., Davison, P.A. *et al.* (1987) Anorectal sensitivity and responses to rectal distension in patients with ulcerative colitis. *Gastroenterology*, **93**, 1270–1275.
53. Rhodes, J.M. (1989) Colonic mucus and mucosal glycoproteins: the key to colitis and cancer? *Gut*, **30**, 1660–1666.
54. Riley, S.A., Mani, V., Goodman, M.J. *et al.* (1990) Why do patients with ulcerative colitis relapse? *Gut*, **31**, 179–183.
55. Riley, S.A., Mani, V., Goodman, M.J. *et al.* (1988) Comparison of delayed release 5-aminosalicylic acid (mesalazine) and sulphasalazine in the treatment of ulcerative colitis relapse. *Gut*, **29**, 669–674.
56. Ritchie, J.K., Powell-Tuck, J. and Lennard-Jones, J.E. (1978) Clinical outcome of the first ten years of ulcerative colitis and proctitis. *Lancet*, **1**, 1140–1143.
57. Rosenberg, I.H. and Mason, J.B. (1989) Folate, dysplasia and cancer. *Gastroenterology*, **97**, 502–505.
58. Sandle, G.I., Hayslett, J.P. and Binder, H.J. (1986) Effect of glucocorticoids on rectal transport in normal subjects and patients with ulcerative colitis. *Gut*, **27**, 309–316.
59. Sandle, G.I., Higgs, N., Crowe, P. *et al.* (1990) Cellular basis for defective electrolyte transport in inflamed human colon. *Gastroenterology*, **99**, 99–105.
60. Shepherd, H.A., Selby, W.S., Chapman, R.W.G. *et al.* (1983) Ulcerative colitis and persistent liver dysfunction. *Quarterly Journal of Medicine*, **208**, 503–513.
61. Sinclair, T.S., Brunt, P.W. and Mowatt, N.A.G. (1983) Non-specific proctocolitis in Northeastern Scotland: a community study. *Gastroenterology*, **85**, 1–11.
62. Sloan, W.P., Bargen, J.A. and Baggenstoss, A.H. (1950) Local complications of chronic ulcerative colitis based on a study of 2000 cases. *Proceedings of Staff Meeting, Mayo Clinic*, **25**, 240–244.
63. Softley, A., Clamp, S.E., Bouchier, I.A.D. *et al.* (1988) Perforation of the intestine in inflammatory bowel disease: an OMGE survey. *Scandinavian Journal of Gastroenterology*, **23**, suppl. 144, 24–26.
64. Spiliadis, C.A. and Lennard-Jones, J.E. (1987) Ulcerative colitis with relative sparing of the rectum. *Diseases of Colon and Rectum*, **30**, 354–356.
65. Stack, B.H.R., Smith, T., Hywell Jones, J. and Fletcher, J. (1969) Measurement of blood and iron loss in colitis with a whole body counter. *Gut*, **10**, 769–773.
66. Stonnington, C.M., Phillips, S.F., Zinsmeister, A.R. *et al.* (1987) Prognosis of ulcerative colitis in a community. *Gut*, **28**, 1261–1266.
67. Toovey, S., Hudson, E., Hendry, W.F. and Levi, A.J. (1981) Sulphasalazine and male infertility – reversibility and possible mechanism. *Gut*. **22**, 445–451.
68. Torsoli, A. (1981) Toxic megacolon. Part II: prevention. *Clinics in Gastroenterology*, **10**, 117–121.
69. Truelove, S.C. (1960) Systemic and local corticosteroid therapy in ulcerative colitis. *British Medical Journal*, **1**, 464–467.
70. Truelove, S.C. and Witts, L.J. (1955) Cortisone in ulcerative colitis: final report on a therapeutic trial. *British Medical Journal*, **2**, 1041–1048.
71. Truelove, S.C. and Witts, L.J. (1959) Cortisone and corticotrophin in ulcerative colitis. *British Medical Journal*, **1**, 387–394.
72. Truelove, S.C., Watkinson, G. and Draper, G. (1962) Comparison of corticosteroids and sulphasalazine therapy in ulcerative colitis. *British Medical Journal*, **2**, 1708–1711.
73. Truelove, S.C., Willoughby, C.P., Lee, E.G. and Kettlewell, M.G.W. (1978) Further experience in the treatment of severe attacks of ulcerative colitis. *The Lancet*, **2**, 1086–1088.
74. Van Hees, P.A.M., Bakker, J.H. and van Tongeren, J.H.M. (1980) Effect of sulphapyridine,

5-aminosalicylic acid, and placebo in patients with idiopathic proctitis: a study to determine the active therapeutic moiety of sulphasalazine. *Gut*, **21**, 632–635.

75. Watts, J.M., Thomson, H. and Goligher, J.C. (1966) Sigmoidoscopy and cytology in the detection of microscopic disease of the rectal mucosa in ulcerative colitis. *Gut*, **7**, 288–294.
76. Watts, J.M., de Dombal, F.T., Watkinson, G. *et al.* (1966) Early course of ulcerative colitis. *Gut*, **7**, 16–31.
77. Whitehead, R. (1989) *Gastrointestinal and Oesophageal Pathology*. London: Churchill Livingstone.
78. Wilks, S. (1859) *Lectures of Pathological Anatomy*, 1st Ed. London: Langman & Roberts.
79. Wilks, S. (1859) Morbid appearances in the intestines of Miss Bankes. *Medical Times and Gazette*, **19**, 264–265.
80. Wright, R. and Truelove, S.C. (1965) A controlled therapeutic trial of various diets in ulcerative colitis. *British Medical Journal*, **2**, 138–141.

SURGICAL TREATMENT *(J.H. Pemberton)*

Chronic ulcerative colitis is primarily a medical problem, which if it becomes resistant to medical management may require surgical treatment. As experience with elective approaches to the management of chronic ulcerative colitis has broadened, prognosis has improved; more patients are referred earlier in the course of their disease, which, in turn, improves the results still further. Because patients are in relatively good health, surgeons can now consider performing alternatives to the classic operations described for ulcerative colitis. In patients with pancolitis, the standard approach in the USA historically has been proctocolectomy with abdominal ileostomy; the operation eliminates colonic disease effectively but of necessity results in a permanent stoma. The goal of alternative surgery is to gain *control* of enteric outflow.

The hypothesis is that if the quality of life is improved then patients would be more likely to accept an operation when indicated. Ideally, the operation should ensure that all disease is removed, and the pathway for defaecation is retained, thus minimizing the social and psychological impact of the operation.

The aims of this section are to consider established operations for chronic ulcerative colitis, describe alternatives, detail their rationale and goals, outline techniques briefly, assess results, and set forth the role of alternatives in the present-day management of patients with ulcerative colitis.

Table 7.9 Indications for operation in patients with chronic ulcerative colitis*

Intractable disease (on optimal medical management)
Growth retardation, inability to function socially or at work, complications of steroids
Severe dysplasia
Stricture
Cancer
Fulminating or toxic colitis
Haemorrhage (unremitting)
Perforation
Unremitting extraintestinal manifestations: arthritis, uveitis, pyoderma gangrenosum, erythema nodosum

*Modified from Glotzer, D.J. and Silen, W. (1980). Indications for operation in inflammatory bowel disease. In *Inflammatory Bowel Disease* (Ed.) Kirsner, J.B. and Shorter R.G. p. 499. Philadelphia: Lea & Febiger.

Indications for operation

Elective and emergency indications for surgery in patients with ulcerative colitis are listed in *Table 7.9*. The most common indication is persistent symptoms despite medical management. The *patient* must determine when symptoms are sufficiently troublesome to prompt surgical intervention. This decision, however, must be fully informed including the likely course of the disease, the surgical options available, their drawbacks and what life free of colitis would be like. In contrast, if dysplasia or other evidence of malignancy is found, the surgeon's hand is forced.

Proctocolectomy with Brooke ileostomy

The *aim* is to remove all diseased bowel and to establish a well-functioning stoma. The output of the stoma is managed effectively by an ileostomy appliance. The *rationale* for the operation is that proctocolectomy 'cures' the disease, the stoma is easy to manage, the rate of complications is low and the long-term functional results are quite good.

Patient selection

Patients of any body habitus and any age are candidates for this operation. An obese patient makes construction of the stoma more difficult. Moreover, obese patients tend to have more functional problems with their stomas than thinner patients do. Stryker *et al.* assessed the problem of elderly patients undergoing this procedure, and found that age alone was not a contraindication to Brooke ileostomy.[42]

Operation

The ileal branch of the ileocolic artery is sacrificed. The posterior dissection is performed close to the rectum, ensuring that the sympathetic nerves are protected at the sacral promontory and the hypogastric, and perirectal plexus are protected in the pelvis. An intersphincteric approach is used which excises only the internal sphincter and leaves the external anal sphincter, puborectalis muscle and levator plate intact.[25]

The site of the ileostomy in the right lower quadrant must be chosen preoperatively, preferably by a stoma therapist. The ileostomy is matured immediately in the manner used by Brooke.[9]

Complications

Overall mobidity ranges between 19% and 70%.[7] Septic complications occur in up to 30%,[8,40] and about a third of patients experience breakdown of the perineal wound after primary closure of the perineum. Small bowel obstruction requiring laparotomy occurs in 5–16% of patients,[25,39] which results in late mortality of about 1% per year.

Bladder paresis and sexual dysfunction do occur;[22,25] in the past, sexual dysfunction has been documented in 20–30% of men after proctectomy[10,16,47] and in 12% of women.

Complications related to the stoma itself have decreased in frequency since the mucosal eversion technique of Brooke was widely adopted.[9] Problems still occur, however, in 20–30% of patients.[37]

Clinical, functional and quality of life results

Rapid rehabilitation of patients with an ileostomy is the rule.[30] Recently, the author's group documented the clinical and functional results of a large group of Brooke ileostomy patients.[35] All patients who had a Brooke ileostomy constructed between 1966 and 1980 were sent a questionnaire. Of eligible patients, 675 responded (81%): 53% of the patients were men and the median age was 35 years. The mean follow-up was 8 years.

Delayed healing of the perineal wound was experienced by 33% of patients. Eighteen per cent required reoperation during the follow-up period; stomal revision alone was performed in 11%.

Most patients (93%) had no problems managing the stomas, but 11% had to care for the stoma at night. Occasional episodes of peristomal skin excoriation were reported by 40% of the patients.

Patients were asked to judge the manner in which their ileostomy affected seven 'activity status' categories (sexual function, sports, social activities, work at home, recreation, family relationships and travel). More patients noted restriction and fewer noted improvements in the more physically demanding categories compared with more socially oriented activities; fully 30% of patients indicated that their sexual activity had been restricted since their operation, whereas only 15% indicated it had improved. Overall, 75% of patients indicated that either the ileostomy had little effect or had improved their activity status.

In general, 95% of patients were satisfied with their ileostomies. However, 40% desired a change.

Although these results were quite acceptable, it was disturbing that in this most recent group of Brooke ileostomy patients, the quality of life seemed to differ little from that reported previously by Roy *et al*.[38] The drawbacks of the Brooke ileostomy remain, and justify the development of alternative procedures.

Ileostomy alternatives

Abdominal colectomy and ileal–rectal anastomosis

The *aim* of the ileal–rectal anastomosis operation (ileorectostomy) is to remove *most* of the diseased colon, thereby reducing the risks of haemorrhage, dilatation, perforation and malignant conditions, while retaining continence for stool and gas.

The *rationale* for ileorectal anastomosis is that the operation avoids a permanent stoma, greatly reduces the risks of pelvic nerve damage, is easy to perform, and other alternatives, should they be necessary, are not precluded.[2,15,19,48] The limitations of this approach are compelling: interval proctectomy is required in 6%–37% of patients; poor results occur in 50% of patients[1] and the risk of developing carcinoma in the retained rectum approaches 17% after 27 years.[13]

Patient selection

Patients are candidates for ileorectal anastomosis if there is minimal involvement of the rectum. Perhaps as important, patients must be willing to undergo frequent follow-up to screen for rectal cancer. Basically, patients of any age up to 70 years and of any body habitus may undergo ileorectal anastomosis.

The operation (*Figure 7.10*)

If in a preoperative proctoscopic examination the rectum dilates easily, performing an ileorectal anastomosis is reasonable. If not, an anastomosis should not be performed because the rectum will act as a non-distensible conduit for stool (i.e. a pipe) and incontinence usually results. A diverting ileostomy is not generally used because if the surgeon judges one is required, then the anastomosis should probably not be performed at all.

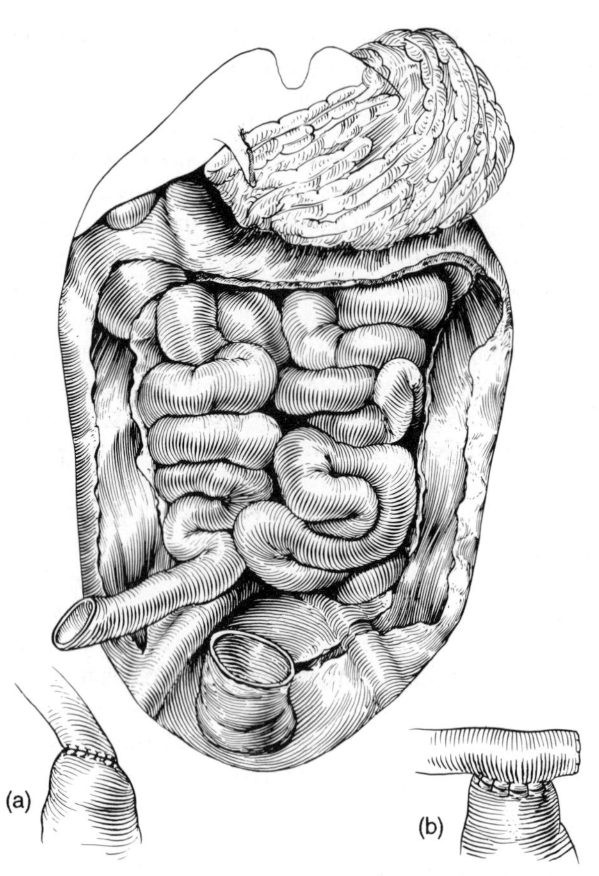

Figure 7.10 Ileorectal anastomosis: the abdominal colectomy has been completed, the specimen removed, and the ends of the bowel are ready for the anastomosis. Intestinal continuity is restored with either (a) an end-to-end or (b) an ileorectal anastomosis. [Reprinted with permission from Farnell, M.B. and Adson, M.A. (1985). Current results: The Mayo Clinic experience. In *Alternatives to Conventional Ileostomy* (Ed.) Dozois, R.R. pp. 81–99. Chicago: Year Book Medical.]

Complications

Surprisingly, operative mortality for elective ileorectal anastomosis varies between 2% and 8%.[6] Nearly all deaths result from anastomotic leakage,[3,32] which occurs relatively frequently (3–15%).[5,13] Small bowel obstruction occurred in 14–20% of patients.[4] Sexual function in men is usually preserved postoperatively, although up to 50% of women experience dyspareunia.[16]

Clinical outcome

Six months after ileorectal anastomosis, the mean stool frequency is about 5 in 24 hours.[32] Incontinence occurs in about 20% of patients,[31] and about 50% require bulking and/or constipating agents. Function improves steadily over the first 12–18 months and plateaus thereafter.

The best measure of a successful clinical outcome after ileorectal anastomosis is the rate of subsequent proctectomy. Such interval proctectomies are required for persistence or recurrent rectal disease or because rectal cancer supervenes. The late proctectomy rate for persistent or recurrent disease varies between 5%[2] and 58%;[23] it is 24% at the author's institution.[13] Moreover, the probabilities of patients achieving a good result after ileorectal anastomosis (i.e. requires no corticosteroids, is in good general health, has an acceptable stool frequency and no incontinence) are only 45% at the Mayo Clinic.[13] This is similar to the experience of others.[16,23]

The risk of cancer developing in the retained rectum is about 5% at 15 years after surgery; this increases to 15% at 30 years.[6,11,15,17,23] Unfortunately, these cancers are usually of advanced grade and stage compared with colorectal cancer in the general population.[6]

The quality of life after ileorectal anastomosis has been reported to be good;[29] the satisfaction is high and an active, productive lifestyle is usually preserved. Overall satisfaction is tempered, however, by the fact that patients often feel that they have not been cured because they must undergo frequent follow-up examinations.

Kock continent ileostomy

Since Kock first described the procedure of continent ileostomy in 1969, more than 1600 operations have been performed world wide.[14]

The *aims* of continent ileostomy are to remove the colon and rectum and to provide continence for faeces and gas while maintaining a cosmetically acceptable stoma. The *rationale* for the procedure is that colectomy and proctectomy 'cure' the disease, and the ileal pouch functions as a reservoir for gas and stool. Hopefully, by eliminating the necessity of wearing an external appliance, the quality of life would be improved.

Patient selection

Technically, patients are candidates for continent ileostomy if they do not have Crohn's disease, and if they are young (<55 years), thin and psychologically fit. At the Mayo Clinic, however, this operation is seldom offered to patients with chronic ulcerative colitis who have not yet had a proctocolectomy.

The operation

After completing the colectomy and proctectomy, the distal 45 cm of the ileum is used to construct the pouch, nipple valve and outflow tract. The stoma is sited at the hairline in the right lower quadrant. The outflow tract is short, and the stoma is flush with the skin.

Complications

At the author's institution, only 1 of 450 patients died after continent ileostomy,[12] Fazio and Church reported that complications included bowel obstruction (2–17%), haemorrhage (0.5–5%), sepsis (2–11%) and fistula (1–7%).[14] Delayed complications were valve extrusion, fistula and 'pouchitis'. Valve extrusion usually occurred during the first year after operation; surgery to revise the valve was required in 43% of the patients in the early operations and in 22% in those performed later.[12]

'Pouchitis' has occurred in 30% of continent ileostomy patients.[14] Excision of the pouch was required in less than 5% of patients over the longer term in the author's series.[12]

Clinical, functional and quality of life results

In the Mayo series[12] (mean follow-up 3.5 years), 75% of continent ileostomy patients were continent, 23% had occasional leakage and 3% wore an ileostomy bag. In the Cleveland series,[14] 91% of the patients were completely continent, and 5% occasionally leaked stool and gas. McLeod and Fazio reported that 93% of continent ileostomy patients felt that their expectations had been fully met and that all of them would undergo the operation again.[27] In contrast to these results, Valkamo found that only 37% of continent ileostomy patients were satisfied after the initial operation, but rates of satisfaction improved after surgical revision.[46]

In summary, the rate of complication and the rate of revisional surgery are quite high after continent ileostomy. Most patients, however, seem satisfied and achieve stomal continence *eventually*. The rate of late failure (>10 years) remains unknown.

Ileal pouch–anal anastomosis

The development of the ileal pouch–anal anastomosis operation (IPAA) has been described in detail.[33,41,50,51] Currently, at the Mayo Clinic, all patients undergoing ileoanal anastomosis actually undergo ileal *pouch*–anal anastomosis, usually using a 'J' design.[45]

The *aim* of the operation is to excise all diseased and potentially diseased colon and rectum while concomitantly restoring faecal continence and allowing defaecation to occur via the normal anatomical pathway. The *rationale* is that abdominal colectomy, proximal proctectomy *and distal rectal mucosal resection* remove all premalignant mucosa, but preserve the anal sphincter. The ileal pouch restores reservoir capacity. Because the distal rectal mucosal resection is performed endorectally, normal bladder and sexual function should be preserved. Finally a perineal wound is avoided.

Selection of patients

Under most circumstances, the operation should only be performed electively. Although no studies have documented the impact of severity of disease on outcome after ileal pouch–anal anastomosis, it seems obvious that the best results are achieved in patients who are not severely compromised. Conversely, in patients who require high-dose immunosuppressives (especially 6-mercaptopurine), have *uncontrolled* extraintestinal manifestations, or who are poorly nourished (low albumin), IPAA may not be indicated.

Certain patients are better candidates for IPAA than are others. Young, thin patients have a superior result compared to older, heavy patients.[28,34] Nearly all of the author's patients are on low or moderate doses of steroids so that this therapy is not a contraindication to surgery despite earlier reports to the contrary.[26] Finally, ideal candidates are intelligent, highly motivated, compliant and emotionally stable.

The operation (in brief)

The operation is performed in two stages. The abdominal colectomy, proximal proctectomy, distal endorectal mucosal resection, ileal 'J' pouch–anal anastomosis, and diverting loop ileostomy comprise the first stage. The protecting ileostomy is closed 8–12 weeks later at a second operation.

With the patient in the lithotomy position, a standard abdominal colectomy is performed except that the ileocolic vessels are preserved if possible. The ileal mesentery is mobilized to the level of the pancreas; this facilitates maximum mesenteric mobility.

Proctectomy

After elevating the rectum, the nerves at the sacral promontory are swept away from the superior haemorrhoidal vessels. The dissection is carried down to the level of the coccyx posteriorly, to the mid-vagina (or mid-prostate) anteriorly, and to the levators laterally.

J pouch

The mobility of the terminal ileum is ascertained; if a point on the antimesenteric aspect of ileum approximately 12–15 cm from the end reaches comfortably beyond the symphysis pubis, then the ileum will reach the anus without tension. The stapler is used to construct the pouch.

Endorectal mucosal resection

The laparotomy pad, placed earlier in the pelvis above the levators, is easily palpated and clearly visible within 3–5 cm of the dentate line posteriorly. The endorectal mucosal resection is started posteriorly at the dentate line. A submucosal plane is developed circumferentially. Neither residual rectal mucosa nor transitional epithelium remains in situ.

Ileal pouch–anal anastomosis

The apex of the pouch is delivered through the rectal muscular cuff to the dentate line. *Figure 7.11* is a diagram of the completed operation. An alternative method of performing this anastomosis is by the double staple technique.[49] At the Mayo Clinic, the ileoanal anastomosis is not stapled.

The final step is constructing a loop ileostomy in the right lower quadrant at a premarked site. In summary, the technical goals of the operation are to preserve the innervation of the bladder and genitalia, the anal sphincter and puborectalis muscles, and to construct a leak-proof pouch and tension-free anastomosis. If these goals are achieved, complications will be few, and the functional results are predictably good.

Ileal pouch–anal anastomosis has been performed in over 1100 patients at the Mayo Clinic between 1981 and 1991.

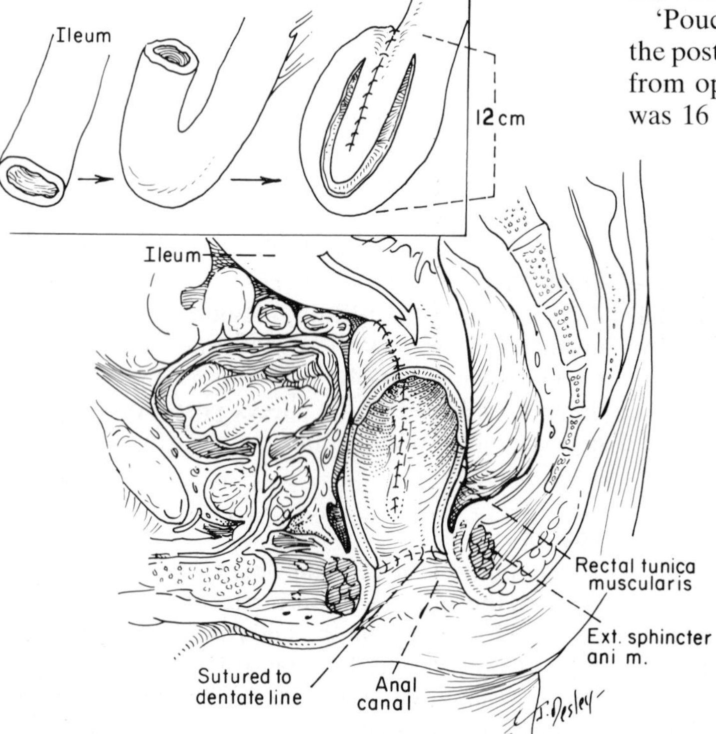

Figure 7.11 Diagram of the completed ileal pouch–anal anastomosis. [Reprinted with permission from Taylor, B.M., Beart, R.W. Jr, Dozois, R.R. *et al.* (1983). Straight ileo-anal anastomosis versus ileal pouch–anal anastomosis. *Archives of Surgery*, **118**, 696–701.]

Clinical results

The long-term results in 390 adults with chronic ulcerative colitis who had a 'J' pouch constructed and who were followed for a mean of 2.3 years (range 6 months to 5 years) were reported recently.[34]

Early results

One of the 390 patients (0.2%) died. Overall, 29% of patients had a postoperative complication. After the first operation, the most frequent complication was small bowel obstruction, which occurred in 22%; one-half required reoperation. Pelvic sepsis, which occurred in 5%, was manifest clinically as fever, leukocytosis and localized abdominal tenderness. One-third of the patients were treated successfully by antibiotic therapy alone, whereas the other two-thirds required operative drainage. Abdominal wound infections occurred in 3%. Urinary retention occurred transiently in 7% but required intermittent catheterization in less than 2%.

After closure of the ileostomy, 9% of patients had a small bowel obstruction for which operative correction was required in one-half. Anastomotic leakage at the site of ileostomy closure occurred in 2%.

Late results

The principal late complications were anastomotic stricture and 'pouchitis'. Most patients had web-like strictures at the anastomosis at the time of ileostomy closure; these were easily dilated and did not recur. Five per cent of the patients, however, had persistent strictures that required repeated dilatation.

'Pouchitis' occurred at variable times throughout the postoperative period. The mean (±s.d.) interval from operation to the first occurrence of pouchitis was 16 ± 14 months. Metronidazole (250 mg four

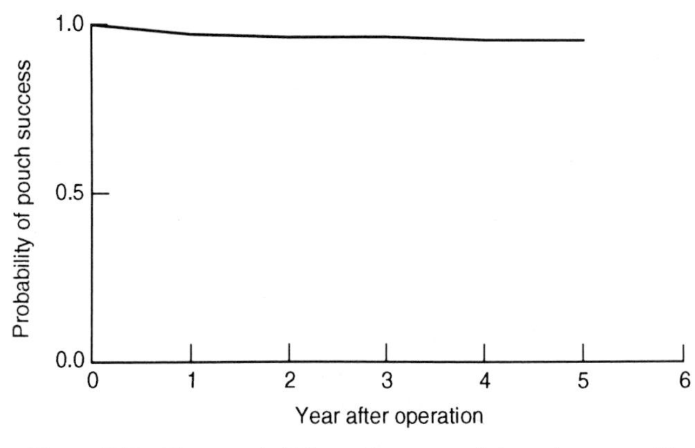

Figure 7.12 The probability of successful outcome with functioning pouch against year after operation. No patient failed after 3 years. [Reprinted with permission from Pemberton, J.H., Kelly, K.A., Beart, R.W. Jr, Wolff, B.G. and Ilstrup, D.M. (1987). Ileal pouch–anal anastomosis for chronic ulcerative colitis: long-term results. *Annals of Surgery*, **206**, 504–511.]

times daily) nearly always resulted in prompt resolution of symptoms. Several patients, however, have required continous low-dose metronidazole to prevent recurrence of 'pouchitis'.

Sexual dysfunction occurred in 11% of the men and 12% of the women; 1.5% of men were impotent and 4% complained of retrograde ejaculation. Dyspareunia occurred in 7% of the women and was the principal complaint.

Nearly all patients had a favourable outcome over 5 years (*Figure 7.12*); the operation only failed in 6%. The causes of failure were recurrent 'pouchitis', multiple stools, gross faecal incontinence and granulomatous ileitis.

Details of the stool frequency, patterns of continence, ability to discriminate gas from stool, and use of medication from 6 months to 5 years after ileal pouch–anal anastomosis are given in *Table 7.10* and *Figure 7.13*. The daytime and night-time stool frequency as well as the pattern of daytime continence did not change over time. In contrast, the incidence of nocturnal incontinence and dependency on medication declined.

Table 7.10 Functional results of ileal pouch–anal anastomosis from 6 months to 6 years postoperatively in 389 patients

	Follow-up at					
Parameter	*6 months*	*1 year*	*2 years*	*3 years*	*4 years*	*5 years*
No. of stools (mean ± s.d.)						
Day	5 ± 2	5 ± 3	6 ± 3	6 ± 2	6 ± 3	6 ± 2
Night	1 ± 1	1 ± 1	2 ± 2	2 ± 1	1 ± 1	2 ± 1
Able to discriminate gas from stool (% patients)	69	77	73	84	77	86
Diphenoxylate (Lomotil) (% patients)	26	19	17	25	6	4
Ispaghula (Metamucil) (% patients)	43	36	40	38	30	27

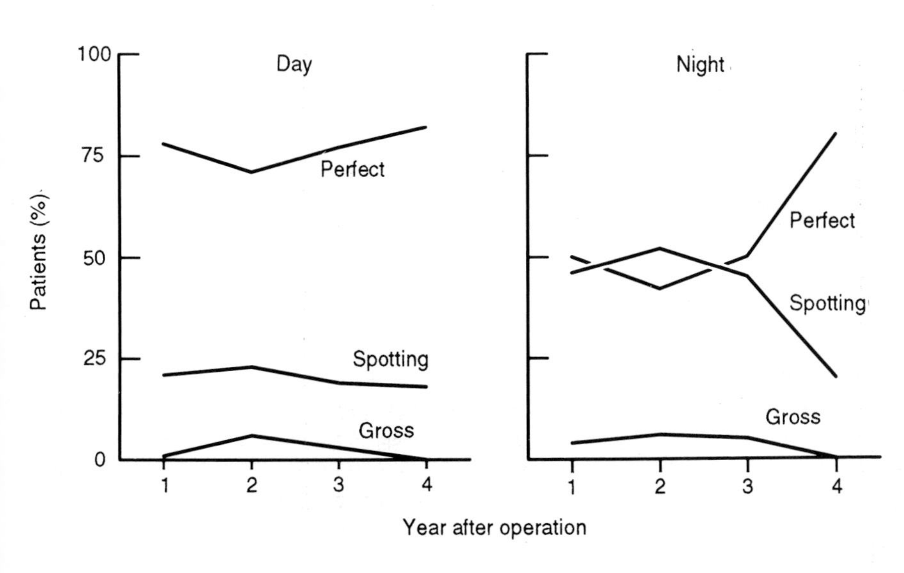

Figure 7.13 Daytime and night-time continence after ileal pouch–anal operation against the years after operation. Perfect = no faecal leakage. Spotting = faecal spotting of underclothes, 3 cm or less in diameter, two times or less per week. Gross = gross faecal incontinence more than two times per week. Data points are connected for illustrative purposes only. [Reprinted with permission from Pemberton, J.H., Kelly, K.A., Beart, R.W. Jr, Wolff, B.G. and Ilstrup, D.M. (1987). Ileal pouch–anal anastomosis for chronic ulcerative colitis: long-term results. *Annals of Surgery*, **206**, 504–511.]

Predictors of outcome

The older patients had more stools during the day than the younger patients did (≤50 years; 6 ± 3 stools/day; >50 years; 8 ± 4 stools/day; $P = 0.05$). Women and men had the same number of stools each day. Women, however, had more episodes of occasional incontinence than did men both during the day and at night. (Day: Women 33% vs men, 14%, $P < 0.001$; night: women 56% vs men 44%, $P < 0.02$.)

Patients who developed pelvic sepsis were no more likely to fail than those who did not, and they did not have any more sexual or urinary problems. The incidence of incontinence during follow-up was significantly affected by the *preoperative* stool frequency; the more stools before the operation, the more likely were patients to be incontinent after the operation ($P < 0.03$).

Quality of life

To determine whether there was any difference in the quality of life between patients with a ileal pouch–anal anastomosis and those with a Brooke ileostomy, the author's group surveyed 298 patients with the former (mean follow-up 47 months) and compared results to 406 Brooke ileostomy patients (mean follow-up 104 months) operated upon for chronic ulcerative colitis or familial adenomatous polyposis.[36] The mean age of the groups was similar (IPAA = 32 years; Brooke ileostomy = 38 years). The majority of both groups were satisfied with their operation (IPAA 95%; Brooke ileostomy 93%). After adjusting for age, diagnosis and reoperation rate, logistic regression analysis of performance scores in seven different categories was used to discriminate between operations. It was found that, in each performance category, the performance score discriminated between operations, with the probability of having had an ileal pouch–anal anastomosis operation increasing with improvement in performance scores ($P < 0.05$) (*Figure 7.14*). It was concluded that after IPAA, patients experienced significant advantages in performing daily activities compared to patients with Brooke ileostomy and thus experienced a better quality of life.

'Pouchitis'

At the Mayo Clinic, the incidence of 'pouchitis' has risen as follow-up has lengthened.[24] Among 734 patients in whom IPAA was performed between January 1981 and December 1988, the incidence of 'pouchitis' was 31% for patients with chronic ulcerative colitis and 6% for patients with familial adenomatous polyposis.[24] The mean time to first occurrence was 17 months. 'Pouchitis' *recurred* in 61% of patients at risk. Interestingly, patients with preoperative and postoperative extraintestinal manifestations (EIMS) of chronic ulcerative colitis had significantly higher rates of pouchitis than did patients without these manifestations (39% with preoperative EIMS vs 26% no EIMS; $p < 0.001$; 53% postoperative EIMS vs 25% no EIMS; $P < 0.001$). In 7 of 12 patients in whom extraintestinal manifestations disappeared after IPAA but then recurred, they recurred when 'pouchitis' occurred and abated when 'pouchitis' was treated. It was

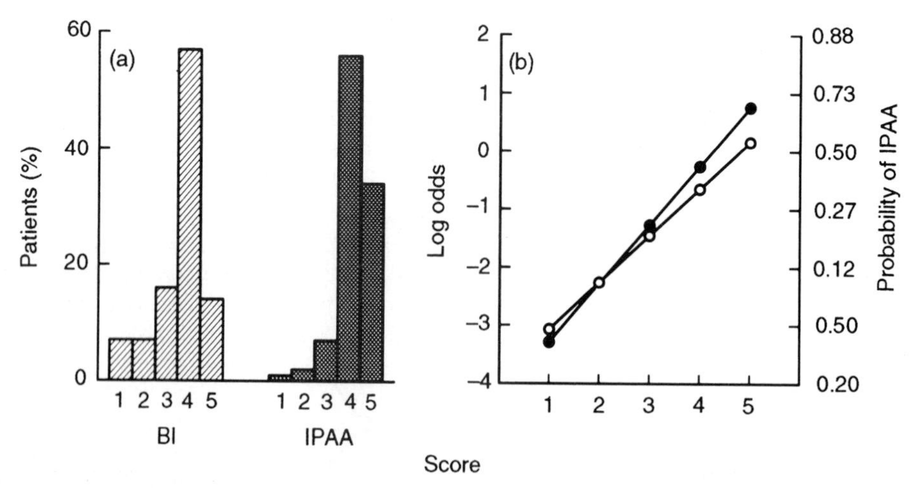

Figure 7.14 Comparison of performance status; category: sexual activity. (a) Overall distribution of patient performance scores for Brooke's ileostomy (BI) and ileal pouch–anal anastomosis (IPAA). The data indicate higher scores among IPAA patients. (b) Plots of estimated logarithm of probability of having had the IPAA operation in (●) 35- and 45-year-old patients with chronic ulcerative colitis, and no reoperation. The rising lines ([+] slopes) indicate that an improving performance score is associated with an increased probability of having had the IPAA operation in both age groups. Results in the other categories are similar. [Reprinted with permission from Pemberton, J.H., Phillips, S.F., Ready, R.R., Zinsmeister, A.R. and Beahrs, O.H. (1989). Quality of life after Brooke ileostomy and ileal pouch–anal anastomosis: comparison of performance status. *Annals of Surgery*, **209**, 620–628.]

concluded that 'pouchitis' occurred frequently after IPAA, that patients with extraintestinal manifestations of chronic ulcerative colitis were at higher risk of developing pouchitis than were patients who never had these manifestations, and that some patients experienced a temporal relationship between flares of extraintestinal manifestations and 'pouchitis'.

IPAA in patients with adenocarcinoma

Seventeen patients (13 with chronic ulcerative colitis, 4 with familial adenomatous polyposis) had a concomitant adenocarcinoma of the colon or rectum at the time of IPAA.[44] The stages of the tumours were: A – 5%; B1 – 32%; B2 – 18%; C1 and C2 – 45%. There were no operative deaths. The rate of pelvic sepsis was 18%, whilst it was 5% for all other IPAA patients. Both the cancer and non-cancer patients had the same daytime and night-time stool frequencies: six stools during the day/one stool during the night. The rate of daytime and night-time seepage was also the same: cancer 17% daytime/50% night-time incontinence; no cancer 23%/47%. It was concluded that IPAA is not contraindicated in patients with *resectable* colorectal cancer.

The anal transition zone

Johnston *et al.*[18] found improved sensation and better rates of perfect continence in patients in whom the anal transitional zone was spared. Keighley *et al.*[20] agreed that sensation was diminished after excision of the transition zone, but found no demonstrable improvement in continence in patients in whom the zone was retained. King and colleagues[21] found that 14 of 16 patients had mucosal inflammation consistent with chronic ulcerative colitis present in the sleeve of resected anal canal mucosa. Sugarman and colleagues who performed stapled ileal–anal anastomosis 2 cm above the dentate line reported that 19 of 20 patients had evidence of chronic ulcerative colitis at the margin of the staple line.[43] Whether sparing the anal transition zone results in improved function is unknown; all data presented to date are retrospective and/or not controlled. This issue is important; if a randomized prospective study supports improved results, then the secondary question of how to deal with retained rectal mucosa, which may present a risk for recurrent disease, dysplasia or malignant change, can be addressed.

Comparing the choices

Although the Brooke ileostomy is safe and reliable, it is not free of complications; up to 30% of patients have a septic complication, 20–25% require stomal revision, 15% have recurrent small bowel obstruction and stomal dysfunction occurs in up to 30%.

Ileal–rectal anastomosis

The primary *benefit* of ileorectal anastomosis is that the rectum is undisturbed by the operative dissection, defaecation mechanisms remain intact and the incidence of bladder or sexual problems is low. Moreover, there is no perineal wound. In many patients, the overall functional results are good. The major *problem* with ileorectal anastomosis is that diseased mucosa is left in situ. In a few patients, inflammatory changes will resolve, but in most, the disease process continues unabated. The sequelae of leaving disease behind include poor anastomotic healing, continued need for steroids, continued bleeding and mucus discharge, incontinence and high stool frequency if disease flares, and the possibility that cancer will occur. *Between 20% and 40% of these patients require proctocolectomy for one or several of these complications.*

Continent ileostomy

The major *benefit* is that although a stoma is constructed, discharge is controlled without using an external appliance. Moreover, all disease is removed. The principal *problem* is the impressively high rate of complications, nearly all of which require reoperation. A perineal wound accompanies this operation; the wound fails to heal promptly in about a third of the patients. Encouragingly, whereas the initial reoperation rate was more than 50%, it has now dropped into the 15–30% range.

Ileal pouch–anal anastomosis

The major *benefit* of ileal pouch–anal anastomosis is that it successfully restores faecal continence in most patients, but the major *problem* is that the complication rate is about 30%; complications such as pelvic infection, stricture, fistula, sinus tracts, pouch leakage, small bowel obstruction and 'pouchitis' continue to occur. Although occasional incontinence occurs in nearly all patients early after operation, particularly at night, this improves significantly over time. Moreover, major episodes of daytime incontinence occur in nearly 10% of patients but this incidence declines to zero by 4 years. Despite these problems, the benefits of ileal pouch–anal anastomosis are considerable: all disease is removed, the patients do not have a stoma, and anal defaecation is wilful and controlled.

Comment

The one alternative that fulfils the criteria for an ideal alternative to Brooke ileostomy is ileal pouch–anal anastomosis. Ileorectal anastomosis falls short because disease is left in situ, whereas the continent ileostomy operation necessitates an abdominal stoma.

This does not imply that ileorectal anastomosis and continent ileostomy are not useful. There are several specific instances in which ileo–rectal anastomosis may be the procedure of choice. One might be when a young person requires an operation, but he or she has yet to start a family or finish school. In these patients ileorectal anastomosis is an ideal choice to see them safely through adolescence without the problems of sexual or bladder dysfunction which might complicate ileal pouch–anal anastomosis. Moreover, patients of any age who are unwilling to accept *any* risk of sexual or bladder dysfunction should be offered ileol–rectal anastomosis. Of course, the rectum must be relatively free of disease if the operation is to be successful.

Also ileo–rectal anastomosis is an option for patients who are not candidates for ileal pouch–anal anastomosis because of age (>60 years) or body habitus (obesity). However, patients undergoing ileorectal anastomosis must be willing to undergo follow-up examinations at regular intervals and be amenable to proctectomy (and perhaps ileal pouch–anal anastomosis) where it is indicated.

Continent ileostomy plays a minor primary role in the management of patients with chronic ulcerative colitis; it is an option for patients who have already had a proctocolectomy and who desire control of the stoma.

Although no operation restores patients to normality, ileal pouch–anal anastomosis comes closest *without leaving disease in place*. Ileal pouch–anal anastomosis, therefore, is an important advance in the management of chronic ulcerative colitis. Although not applicable to all patients, ileal pouch–anal anastomosis should be considered the treatment of choice in nearly all young patients with chronic ulcerative colitis who face protocolectomy.

REFERENCES

1. Adson, M.A., Cooperman, A.M. and Farrow, G.M. (1972) Ileorectostomy for ulcerative disease of the colon. *Archives of Surgery*, **104**, 424–428.
2. Aylett, S.O. (1966) Three hundred cases of diffuse ulcerative colitis treated by total colectomy and ileo-rectal anastomosis. *British Medical Journal*, **1**, 1001–1005.
3. Aylett, S. (1963) Ulcerative colitis treated by total colectomy and ileorectal anastomosis: A ten-year review (Abridged). *Proceedings of the Royal Society of Medicine*, **56**, 183–190.
4. Aylett, S.O. (1960) Diffuse ulcerative colitis and its treatment by ileorectal anastomosis. *Annals of the Royal College of Surgery (England)*, **27**, 260–284.
5. Baker, W.N.W. (1970) The results of ileorectal anastomosis at St Mark's Hospital from 1952 to 1968. *Gut*, 235–239.
6. Baker, W.N.W., Glass, R.E., Ritchie, J.K. and Aylett, S.O. (1978) Cancer of the rectum following colectomy and ileorectal anastomosis for ulcerative colitis. *British Journal of Surgery*, **65**, 862–868.
7. Beauchamp, G., Beliveau, D. and Archambault, A. (1981) Death and complications after total colectomy for inflammatory bowel disease. *Canadian Journal of Surgery*, **24**, 463–466; 484.
8. Binder, S.C., Miller, H.H. and Deterling, R.A. Jr (1975) Emergency and urgent operations for ulcerative colitis: The procedure of choice. *Archives of Surgery*, **110**, 284–289.
9. Brooke, B.N. (1952) The management of ileostomy including its complications. *The Lancet*, **2**, 102–104.
10. Burnham, W.R., Lennard-Jones, J.E. and Brooke, B.N. (1977) Sexual problems among married ileostomists: Survey conducted by the Ileostomy Association of Great Britain and Ireland. *Gut*, **18**, 673–677.
11. Devroede, G. and Taylor, W.F. (1976) On calculating cancer risk and survival of ulcerative colitis patients with the life table method. *Gastroenterology*, **71**, 505–509.
12. Dozois, R.R., Kelly, K.A., Beart, R.W. Jr and Beahrs, O.H. (1985) Continent ileostomy: The Mayo Clinic experience. In *Alternatives to Conventional Ileostomy* (Ed.) Dozois, R.R. pp. 180–191. Chicago: Year Book Medical.
13. Farnell, M.B., Van Heerden, J.A., Beart, R.W. Jr and Weiland, L.H. (1980) Rectal preservation in nonspecific inflammatory disease of the colon. *Annals of Surgery*, **192**, 249–253.
14. Fazio, V.W. and Church, J.M. (1988) Complications and function of the continent ileostomy at the Cleveland Clinic. *World Journal of Surgery*, **12**, 148–154.
15. Grundfest, S.F., Fazio, V., Weiss, R.A. *et al.* (1981) The risk of cancer following colectomy and ileorectal anastomosis for extensive mucosal ulcerative colitis. *Annals of Surgery*, **193**, 9–14.
16. Grüner, O.-P.N., Naas, R., Fretheim, B. and Gjone, E. (1977) Marital status and sexual adjustment after colectomy: results in 178 patients operated on for ulcerative colitis. *Scandinavian Journal of Gastroenterology*, **12**, 193–197.
17. Johnson, W.R., McDermott, F.T., Hughes, E.S.R., Pihl, E.A. and Milne, B.J. (1983) The risk of rectal carcinoma following colectomy in ulcerative colitis. *Diseases of the Colon and Rectum*, **26**, 44–46.
18. Johnston, D., Holdsworth, P.J., Nasmyth, D.G. *et al.* (1987) Preservation of the entire anal canal in conservative proctocolectomy for ulcerative colitis: A pilot study comparing end-to-end ileo-anal anastomosis without mucosal resection with mucosal proctectomy and endo-anal anastomosis. *British Journal of Surgery*, **74**, 940–944.
19. Jones, P.F., Munro, A. and Ewen, S.W.B. (1977)

Colectomy and ileorectal anastomosis for colitis: Report on a personal series, with a critical review. *British Journal of Surgery*, **64**, 615–623.
20. Keighley, M.R.B., Winslet, M.C., Yoshoika, K. and Lightwood, R. (1987) Discrimination is not impaired by excision of the anal transition zone after restorative proctocolectomy. *British Journal of Surgery*, **74**, 1118–1121.
21. King, D.W., Lubowski, D.F. and Cook, T.A. (1987) Anal canal mucosa in restorative proctocolectomy for ulcerative colitis. *British Journal of Surgery*, **76**, 970–972.
22. Lee, E.C.G. and Dowling, B.L. (1972) Perimuscular excision of the rectum for Crohn's disease and ulcerative colitis: A conservation technique. *British Journal of Surgery*, **59**, 29–32.
23. Lindham, S. and Lagercrantz, R. (1980) Ulcerative colitis in childhood: Should the rectum be preserved at surgery? Long-term results in 50 patients. *Scandinavian Journal of Gastroenterology*, **15**, 123–127.
24. Lohmuller, J.L., Pemberton, J.H., Dozois, R.R., Ilstrup, D.M. and Van Heerden, J.A. (1990) Pouchitis and extraintestinal manifestations of inflammatory bowel disease after ileal pouch–anal anastomosis. *Annals of Surgery*, **211**, 622–629.
25. Lyttle, J.A. and Parks, A.G. (1977) Intersphincteric excision of the rectum. *British Journal of Surgery*, **64**, 413–416.
26. Martin, L.W., LeCoultre, C. and Schubert, W.K. (1977) Total colectomy and mucosal proctectomy with preservation of continence in ulcerative colitis. *Annals of Surgery*, **186**, 477–480.
27. McLeod, R.S. and Fazio, V.W. (1984) Quality of life with the continent ileostomy. *World Journal of Surgery*, **8**, 90–95.
28. Metcalf, A.M., Dozois, R.R., Kelly, K.A., Beart, R.W. Jr and Wolff, B.G. (1985) Ileal 'J' pouch–anal anastomosis: Clinical outcome. *Annals of Surgery*, **202**, 735–739.
29. Mignon, M. and Bonfils, S. (1985) Altered physiology in ulcerative colitis patients with ileorectal anastomosis. In *Alternatives to Conventional Ileostomy* (Ed.) Dozois, R.R. pp. 61–80. Chicago: Year Book Medical.
30. Morowitz, D.A. and Kirsner, J.B. (1981) Ileostomy in ulcerative colitis: A questionnaire study of 1,803 patients. *American Journal of Surgery*, **141**, 370–375.
31. Newton, C.R. and Baker, W.N.W. (1975) Comparison of bowel function after ileorectal anastomosis for ulcerative colitis and colonic polyposis. *Gut*, **16**, 785–791.
32. Parc, R., Levy, E., Frileux, P. and Loygue, J. (1985) Current results: Ileorectal anastomosis after total abdominal colectomy for ulcerative colitis. In *Alternatives to Conventional Ileostomy* (Ed.) Dozois, R.R. pp. 81–99. Chicago: Year Book Medical.
33. Pemberton, J.H., Heppell, J., Beart, R.W. Jr, Dozois, R.R. and Telander, R.L. (1982) Endorectal ileoanal anastomosis. *Surgery, Gynecology and Obstetrics*, **155**, 417–424.
34. Pemberton, J.H., Kelly, K.A., Beart, R.W. Jr, Wolff, B.G. and Ilstrup, D.M. (1987) Ileal pouch–anal anastomosis for chronic ulcerative colitis: Long-term results. *Annals of Surgery*, **206**, 504–513.
35. Pemberton, J.H., Phillips, S.F., Dozois, R.R. and Wendorf, L.J. (1985) Current clinical results. In *Alternatives to Conventional Ileostomy* (Ed.) Dozois, R.R. pp. 40–50. Chicago: Year Book Medical.
36. Pemberton, J.H., Phillips, S.F., Ready, R.R., Zinsmeister, A.R. and Beahrs, O.H. (1989) Quality of life after Brooke ileostomy and ileal pouch–anal anastomosis: Comparison of performance status. *Annals of Surgery*, **209**, 620–628.
37. Ritchie, J.K. (1971) Ileostomy and excisional surgery for chronic inflammatory disease of the colon: A survey of one hospital region. Part I. Results and complications of surgery. *Gut*, **12**, 528–536.
38. Roy, P.H., Sauer, W.G., Beahrs, O.H. and Farrow, G.M. (1970) Experience with ileostomies: Evaluation of long-term rehabilitation of 497 patients. *American Journal of Surgery*, **119**, 77–86.
39. Sirinek, K.R., Tetirick, C.E., Thomford, N.R. and Pace, W.G. (1977) Total proctocolectomy and ileostomy: Procedure of choice for acute toxic megacolon. *Archives of Surgery*, **112**, 518–522.
40. Steinberg, D.M., Allan, R.N., Brooke, B.N., Cooke, W.T. and Alexander-William, J. (1975) Sequelae of colectomy and ileostomy: Comparison between Crohn's colitis and ulcerative colitis. *Gastroenterology*, **68**, 33–39.
41. Stryker, S.J. and Dozois, R.R. (1985) The ileoanal anastomosis: Historical perspectives. In *Alternatives to Conventional Ileostomy*, (Ed.) Dozois, R.R. pp. 255–265. Chicago: Year Book Medical.
42. Stryker, S.J., Pemberton, J.H. and Zinsmeister, A.R. (1985) Long-term results of ileostomy in older patients. *Diseases of the Colon and Rectum*, **28**, 844–846.
43. Sugarman, H.J., Newsome, H.H., Decosta, G. and Zfass, A.M. (1992) Stapled ileoanal anastomosis for ulcerative colitis and familial polyposis without temporary diverting ileostomy. *Annals of Surgery*, in press.
44. Taylor, B.A., Wolff, B.G., Dozois, R.R., Kelly, K.A., Pemberton, J.H. and Beart, R.W. Jr (1988) Ileal pouch–anal anastomosis for chronic ulcerative colitis and familial polyposis coli complicated by adenocarcinoma. *Diseases of the Colon and Rectum*, **31**, 358–362.
45. Utsunomiya, J., Iwana, T., Imajo, M. *et al.* (1980) Total colectomy, mucosal proctectomy, and ileoanal anastomosis. *Diseases of the Colon and Rectum*, **23**, 459–466.
46. Valkamo, E. (1981) Ileostomy in ulcerative colitis: Academic dissection (thesis), Second Department of Surgery, University Central Hospital Helsinki Fairbairn.

47. Watts, J.Mc.K., de Dombal, F.T. and Goligher, J.C. (1966) Long-term complications and prognosis following major surgery for ulcerative colitis. *British Journal of Surgery*, **53**, 1014–1023.
48. Watts, J.Mc.K. and Hughes, S.R. (1977) Ulcerative colitis and Crohn's disease: Results after colectomy and ileorectal anastomosis. *British Journal of Surgery*, **64**, 77–83.
49. Williams, N.S. (1989) Stapling technique for pouch–anal anastomosis without the need for purse-string sutures. *British Journal of Surgery*, **76**, 348–349.
50. Williams, N.S. and Johnston, D. (1985) The current status of mucosal proctectomy and ileo-anal anastomosis in the surgical treatment of ulcerative colitis and adenomatous polyposis. *British Journal of Surgery*, **72**, 159–168.
51. Wong, W.D., Rothenberger, D.A. and Goldberg, S.M. (1985) Ileoanal pouch procedures. *Current Problems in Surgery*, **22**, (3), 1–78.

CANCER IN ULCERATIVE COLITIS

(S.N. Gyde)

Ulcerative colitis as a disease entity has been recognized for many years but the aetiology of this uncommon inflammation of the colon and rectum still remains obscure although genetic factors play a part.[51,52] The relationship between this inflammation of the bowel and the development of colorectal cancer remains equally obscure but there is no doubt that patients with ulcerative colitis who have long-standing extensive disease are at much greater risk of developing colorectal cancer than the general population. Patients with more limited disease (e.g. disease confined to the left side of the colon) have only a marginally increased risk and patients with

Table 7.11 Cancer incidence in ulcerative colitis: hospital series

			Cases		*Cancers*		*Results*
Authors and hospital series	*Year*	*Review period*	*Whole series*	*Extensive colitis*	*Whole series*	*Extensive colitis*	*Cumulative cancer incidence*
de Dombal *et al.*[14] General Infirmary, Leeds	1966	1952–1963	428	210	8	8	10 years 5% 20 years 21% 25 years 42%
McDougall[53] Gordon Hospital, London	1964	1947–1963	637	196	15	9	Extensive colitis Observed = 9, O/E = 30 Expected = 0.3
Edwards and Truelove[17] Radcliffe Infirmary, Oxford	1964	1938–1962	624	236	22	17	20 years Whole series 5.5% First attack (n = 250) 12.6%
Greenstein *et al.*[25] Mount Sinai Hospital, New York	1979	1960–1976	267	NS	26	21	Left-sided colitis O/E = 8.6 Extensive colitis O/E = 26.5
Lennard-Jones *et al.*[44] St Marks Hospital, London (Cancer surveillance in extensive colitis)	1983	1966–1980		303		13	
Prior *et al.*[64] Queen Elizabeth and General Hospitals, Birmingham	1982	1944–1976	676	462	35	35	Whole series (68% with extensive colitis) 25 years 8% 30 years 20%
Katza *et al.*[38] Private practice, New York	1983	1955–1980		106		4	Extensive colitis, patients all 10 years or more from onset, risk at 11 years 7.2%
Madjlessi *et al.*[49] Cleveland Clinic, Ohio, USA	1986	Cases to 1984	1248		82	74	Extensive colitis 20 years 11.9% 30 years 25.3% Left-sided colitis 20 years 1.8% 30 years 3.7%

O = observed; E = expected; NS = not stated.

inflammation confined to the rectum have no increased risk. However, if the rectum is left in situ in a patient who has had extensive disease, the retained rectum carries the risk of cancer in the patient with extensive disease (*Tables 7.11* and *7.12*).[2,14,17,18,25–28,30,32,38,39,47,53,63,64]

From available evidence, it is possible to discern patient groups at high, low and no excess risk of developing cancer and to document the increasing probability of developing cancer over time. It is also possible to examine how well ulcerative colitis patients survive once they have developed colorectal cancer and whether patients developing colorectal cancer in ulcerative colitis have a similar prognosis to patients developing colorectal cancer in the general population. It is possible to determine the stage needed to diagnose and treat cancer in ulcerative colitis in order to increase survival. The success (or lack of success) of methods currently used to 'screen' for cancer in ulcerative colitis in order to detect cancer at an early stage will be considered.

HISTORICAL PERSPECTIVE

Only a few years after ulcerative colitis was recognized as a disease entity, case reports were appearing of colorectal cancer complicating the disease.[3,36,79,80] Subsequently, there were many individual case reports in the literature, many reports from hospital series of patients relating to the cancer risk[14,17,23,26,38,44,47,53,59,64] and more recently prospective studies of incident cases in populations resident in defined geographical areas.[30,32,39]

Ulcerative colitis is an uncommon disease (incidence 5–10 per 100 000 population)[5,6,20,45,56,70,72,77] and it is only in hospitals specializing in the treatment of such patients that information can be gathered on relatively large groups of patients.

It is not surprising therefore that the great majority of studies concerning cancer incidence in ulcerative colitis have been based on information derived from hospital series of patients. Early reports from such series tended to express the cancer risk in terms of crude percentages, but by the mid-1960s most investigators were using actuarial methods to calculate the cumulative cancer risk over time.

Certain risk factors pertaining to the cancer incidence emerged from these early studies and have been confirmed by more recent reports. The most important risk factors can be summarized as follows.

Extent of disease

1. The increased cancer risk is mainly confined to patients with extensive or total colitis.

Table 7.12 Cancer incidence in ulcerative colitis: population-based series

			Cases		*Cancers*		*Results*
Authors and hospital series	*Year*	*Review period*	*Whole series*	*Extensive colitis*	*Whole series*	*Extensive colitis*	*Cumulative cancer incidence*
Hendriksen *et al.*[32] (Continuation of the Bonnevie study in Copenhagen County) All case of ulcerative colitis in Copenhagen County	1968/1985	1960–1978	783	124 (total colitis)	7	2 (total colitis)	Whole series 10 years 0.8% 15 years 1.1% 18 years 1.4% (CI 0.7–2.8) Median follow-up 6.7 years
Kewenter *et al.*[39] All cases in Goteburg City, Sweden diagnosed 'shortly' after onset of disease	1978	1952–1975	NS	234	NS	15	15 years 9.6% (CI 2.6–16.6) 20 years 24.2% (CI 11.0–37.4) Median follow-up 6.0 years Mean follow-up 8.5 years
Gyde *et al.*[30] Geographically defined cohorts from Stockholm County, Birmingham and Oxford	1988	1945–1986	823	486	35	29	Extensive colitis 20 years 7.2% (CI 3.6–10.8) 30 years 16.5% (CI 9.0–24)
Ekbom[18] Uppsala Health Care Region	1990	1965–1983	2509	741	36	NS	19 years 5.5%

CI = confidence intervals; NS = not stated.

2. Patients with left-sided colitis have been shown in some studies to have a small increase in risk.
3. Patients with proctitis have not shown any increased risk.

Duration of disease

Patients with long-standing disease are most at risk of developing cancer; the risk starts to increase 10 years from diagnosis, and continues to rise with time thereafter. No study has yet shown a levelling off of the cancer risk at any point in time once it has started to rise.

Age at onset of disease

The present evidence on this subject is conflicting. A recent report reinforces suggestions from other studies that young age at onset of disease is an independent risk factor separate from the effect of duration of disease.[17,18] Certainly childhood onset of the disease (below the age of 15 years) carries a particularly high risk of developing colorectal cancer at a young age.[15,25,55]

Age at diagnosis of cancer

In the general population the average age at diagnosis of colorectal cancer is around 60 years – in patients with ulcerative colitis it is around 50 years, some 10 years younger. In a large study from patients seen at St Mark's Hospital, London,[68] the average age at diagnosis of cancer was 63 years in the 4817 colorectal cancers from non-colitic patients, compared with an average age of 49 years in the 67 colorectal cancers occurring in ulcerative colitis patients seen over the same review period. In childhood-onset ulcerative colitis the average age at diagnosis of cancer is much earlier.[15,25,55]

In a large study of childhood-onset ulcerative colitis, from the Mayo Clinic, following 396 patients diagnosed at 14 years or younger, 52 of these children subsequently developed colorectal cancer. Calculating from the life tables it seems that at least 10 of the cancers were diagnosed before the age of 35 years and another 10 were diagnosed in the next decade before the age of 45 years.[15]

Distribution of cancer in ulcerative colitis

Langman[40] assembled data on colorectal cancer distribution in colitic and non-colitic patients (*Figure 7.15*). Colitic cancers tend to be more evenly distributed around the colon than non-colitic, which occur predominantly in the sigmoid colon and rec-

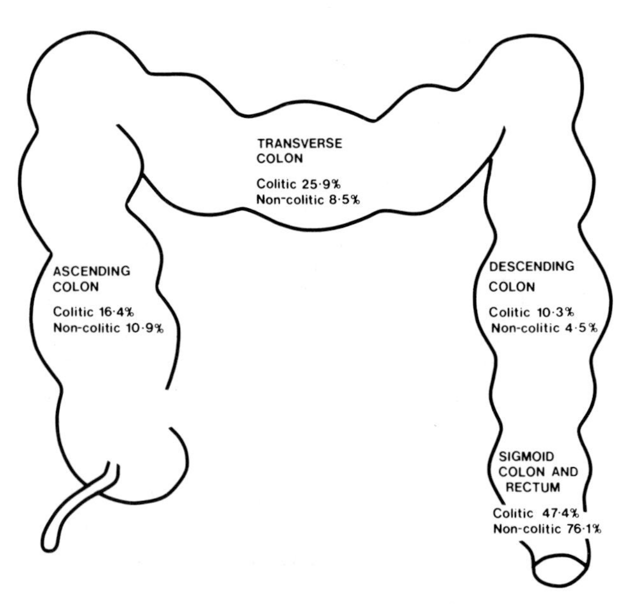

Figure 7.15 Distribution of colitic and non-colitic cancer. Colitic cancers: $n = 379$; non-colitic cancers: $n = 6277$.

tum. The different distribution of ulcerative colitis cancers might simply reflect a different distribution of cancers occurring in a younger age group. However, it has been shown that colorectal cancers in the general population, occurring below the age of 40 years, have a similar distribution to colorectal cancer occurring later in life, making this explanation unlikely. In clinical practice, fewer colitic cancers will be within the reach of the rigid sigmoidoscope (47.4%) when compared to the general population (76.1%), which has practical implications when investigating these patients.[8,40,48]

Survival from cancer in ulcerative colitis

Early reports suggested that ulcerative colitis patients developing colorectal cancer had a poor prognosis, considerably worse than the prognosis of patients with colorectal cancer in the general population.

More recently, analyses of survival (some series using the method of matched controls) suggest that the 5-year survival of colorectal cancer patients in ulcerative colitis is not significantly different from the general population. Results of these studies are summarized in *Table 7.13* and *Figure 7.16*. The crude 5-year survival in both colitic and non-colitic patients ranges from 33% to 55%.[31,33,35,41,68,73,76]

Multiple cancers and differentiation of cancers

All series show a higher incidence of multiple cancers in ulcerative colitis than in the control population, and these colitic cancers tend to be less well

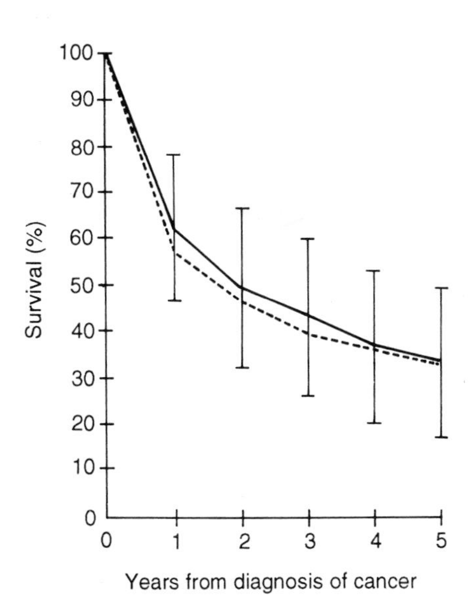

Figure 7.16 Pattern of survival of patients with colorectal cancer complicating ulcerative colitis. (—) Colorectal cancer patients; (- - -) general population. (From Gyde *et al.*[31])

differentiated. This increase in such cancers does not affect the virulence of the cancers in the colitic group, in that the 5-year survival of Dukes' A classification cancers (i.e. cancers in which survival was long enough for comparisons to be made) was independent of the degree of differentiation, and similar in both groups (*Table 7.13*).

A large proportion of the colitic patients presented with late cancer (*Table 7.13*). This must be due, in part, to the symptoms of cancer closely mimicking the symptoms of ulcerative colitis, which do not cause the alarm these symptoms might be expected to initiate in the general population prompting early investigation. Another factor may be that only 46% of cancers are within reach of the sigmoidoscope as opposed to 76% in the general population, making diagnosis more difficult (see *Figure 7.15*). There are also patients with apparently mild disease who do not require hospital referral until eventually they are referred to hospital presenting with late cancer complicating ulcerative colitis. Finally, there are some high-risk patients lost to follow-up who return after many years with symptomatic cancer.

ULCERATIVE COLITIS

Cumulative probability of developing cancer over time

The cancer incidence over time found in any given study on ulcerative colitis patients will depend upon the study 'sample' used. The aim of any study would be to produce results that would reflect the actual cancer incidence in the whole ulcerative colitis population, so that the results of any study might be generally applicable to any ulcerative colitis patient seen in any clinical setting.

Even having achieved this, the results will not necessarily reflect the cancer incidence in the disease itself, because in the general population there will be many patients who suffer from ulcerative colitis but in whom diagnosis has not been established. Of these undiagnosed patients some will die in their first attack, some will recover completely and some will have chronic persistent symptoms and may finally develop colorectal cancer. Those colorectal cancers occurring in undiagnosed patients will simply be recorded as colorectal cancer occurring in the general population. When considering the colorectal cancer incidence in ulcerative colitis referral is only being made to cases where the diagnosis has been made; and it would be reasonable to assume that most of such diagnoses are made by a hospital referral. The sample population for a cancer incidence study should be an unbiased sample of all ulcerative colitis patients diagnosed from the population.

If the study sample is biased the results will be biased and therefore not generally applicable.

Selection biases

Hospital series

Hospitals specializing in the treatment of ulcerative colitis tend to attract more severe and difficult cases which less specialized hospitals (where the original diagnosis may have been made) refer on.

Bias towards severity of disease

The most obvious bias is severity of disease with a high proportion of patients having extensive colitis. As these patients also have the highest risk for developing cancer, this bias will materially alter the risk found in the series as a whole. This bias can be overcome by separate analysis of the risk of the 'extensive colitis' group.

'Difficult cases' – bias towards cancer

Patients are often referred to specialist centres because of intractable symptoms that do not respond to normal therapy. Such patients may have cancer complicating their colitis, and such cancers, if included in an analysis, inflate the risk and this is not a true reflection of the risk in the series under review. This bias can be minimized by excluding any cancers diagnosed in the first year after referral.

Minimizing bias in hospital series

It is possible to use the valuable information collected in hospital series of patients, minimizing

Table 7.13 Survival of patients developing colorectal cancer complicating ulcerative colitis (UC)

Authors	*Year*	*Hospital series*	*Review period*	*Control group*	*Number of cancers**		*Patients with late cancer on referral*		*Number of cancers identified on histology of resected specimen for symptomatic colitis*	*Mean duration of symptoms to diagnosis of cancer*	*Mean 5-year survival (%)*	
							No.	*(%)*			*Cases*	*Controls*
Gyde *et al.*[31]	1983	Queen Elizabeth and General Hospitals, Birmingham Series of 676 UC patients	1944–1976	Colorectal cancers of the same median age as colitic cancers from West Midlands region	35	(4)	12	(34)	12	21 years	33.5	33
Van Heerden *et al.*[76]	1967	Mayo Clinic, USA Series of 726 patients undergoing surgery for UC	1961–1975	Non-colitic cancers matched for age, sex, Dukes classification and degree of differentiation (Broder's grade)	70	(16)	17	(24)	14	17.1 years (operable cases only)	41.7	47
Ritchie *et al.*[68]	1981	St Mark's, London Total series not -stated	1947–1980	4817 non-colitic cancers diagnosed at St Mark's over review period	67	(15)	19	(28)	NK	10 years in all but two cases	65.1 (in 57 operable cases)	47 (rectal cancers) 53 (colonic cancers)
Hughes *et al.*[33]	1978	University of Chicago hospitals and Clinics, USA Series of 1142 UC patients diagnosed in review period	1958–1976	Non-colitic cancers matched for age, sex, site and stage	29	(4)	–		NK	19.6 years	55.1	46.9

Lavery *et al.*[41]	1982	Cleveland Clinics, USA Total series not stated	1950–1979	Survival of UC cancers compared with group of non-colitic cancers diagnosed at Cleveland Clinic, 1950–1964	68 (3)	28 (41)	19	17 years	41	NK
Hulten *et al.*[36]	1979	Various Swedish hospitals over 10-year review period	10 years	Non-colitic cancers seen at Salgrens Hospital, Goteburg over review period, $n = 22$	25 (NK)	NK	NK	NK	12	25

NK = not known.
*Multiple cancers are indicated in parentheses.

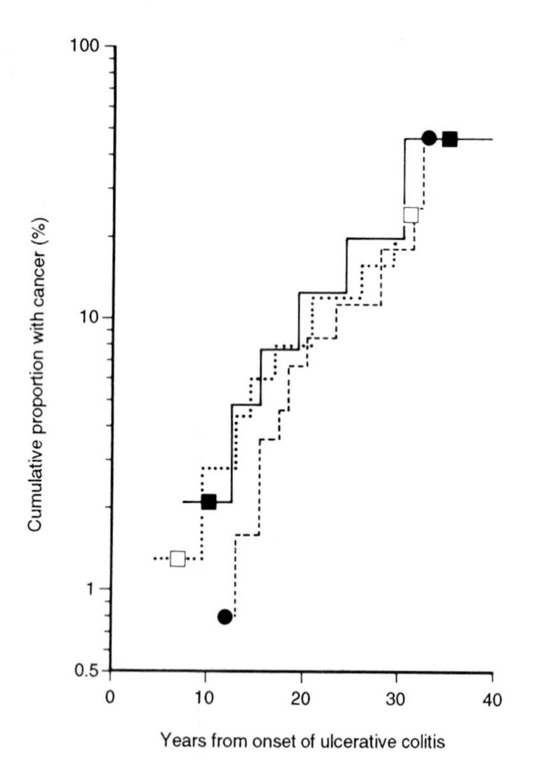

Figure 7.17 Colorectal cancer and extensive ulcerative colitis by centre: ■ Birmingham; □ Oxford; ● Sweden.

referral biases by basing studies on selected 'cohorts' of patients and discarding information on all other patients in the series.

The limitation of this method is that it requires good documentation on patients in hospital series for at least 20–30 years and this is often not available. This method was used successfully by Gyde *et al.*[30] in a recent report where patients were recruited from hospitals in three centres (Birmingham, Oxford and Stockholm). Patients were recruited from defined geographical areas and had been referred at or near onset of their disease, diagnosed between defined calendar years and aged 15 years or more at diagnosis (so excluding childhood-onset cases).

The remarkable similarity in this study for the cumulative cancer risk over time, analysed by the centres contributing patients (Birmingham, Oxford and Stockholm), suggests that the method of selecting 'cohorts' from the three hospital series did successfully eliminate the biases inherent in hospital series (*Figure 7.17*).

Population-based studies

In a population-based study, all incident cases of ulcerative colitis are recruited to the study from a defined population. A series of patients is accrued over time and the cancer incidence documented. This should be the most reliable method of determining the 'real' cancer incidence over time in the disease. Such studies are extremely time-consuming to carry out and will probably span more than the working lifetime of a single gastroenterology consultant. Because of the very low incidence of the disease, recruitment to any series is slow, and even then only a small proportion of patients (extensive colitis patients) are at high risk of developing cancer, with a latent period of at least 10 years from diagnosis in the high-risk group before the cancer risk becomes apparent.

These difficulties with prospective studies are illustrated by an excellent ongoing study in Copenhagen County (population 500 000). Over an 18-year period (1960–1978), 783 patients were recruited to the study, 124 with extensive disease. At the last report in 1985, with a median follow-up of 7 years, seven colorectal cancers had been observed. Although these are probably the best data we have concerning the cumulative cancer risk in ulcerative colitis, the numbers of cancers to date are small, giving wide confidence limits on estimates of the risk. Follow-up at present is short and would need to continue for many years to provide an accurate estimate of risk at 20–30 years from diagnosis.[5,32]

A recent report of a population-based study of cancer in ulcerative colitis (from Sweden) collected retrospective data on all cases of ulcerative colitis in six counties in central Sweden, and produced excellent data on 2509 cases of ulcerative colitis diagnosed between the years 1965 and 1983 ('incident cases') and followed up to 1984.[18] During the course of follow-up 36 cases of colorectal cancer were recorded. However, in the analysis of the cumulative cancer risk over time, these 36 cancers were combined with 55 cancers diagnosed in 635 patients who were diagnosed before 1965 ('prevalent' cases). As these 'prevalent' cases were a 'survivor' population (stated to be all alive on 1 January 1965) and as the date of diagnosis for the calculation of patient years at risk was not known, combining this group with the 'incident' cases to estimate the cumulative cancer risk over time biases the results from the incident cases, and makes the results of this potentially excellent study difficult to interpret. This reinforces the point made earlier that the 'sample' population is all important in any study.

Cumulative cancer incidence over time – results of studies

The cumulative cancer incidence over time in hospital-based studies and population studies is shown in *Tables 7.11* and *7.12*; *Table 7.14* documents the cancer risk in the retained rectum in ileorectal anastomosis. *Figures 7.17* and *7.18* are taken from the three-centre study[30] showing the

Table 7.14 Rectal cancer incidence in ileorectal anastomosis

Authors	Year	Hospital	Review period	No. of patients: Whole series	No. of patients: Extensive colitis	No. of rectal cancers: Whole series	No. of rectal cancers: Extensive colitis	No. of rectal cancers: Left-sided colitis	No. of cancers within 10 years of onset of disease	Cumulative cancer incidence (%)	Cumulative cancer incidence (years)	Dukes' classification of cancers at diagnosis: A	B	C	Distal metastasis
Baker *et al.*[2]	1978	Gordon Hospital, London	1952–1976	374	362	22	21	1	0	0 6 9 15	10 20 25 30	2	4	12	4
Grundfest *et al.*[28]	1981	Cleveland Clinic, USA	1957–1977	Nk	89	NK	4	NK	0	0 5 12.9	10 20 25	2	0	2	–
Oakley *et al.*[63]	1985	Cleveland Clinic, USA	1960–1982	145	NK	5	NK	NK	0	NK		3	0	1	1

NK = not known.

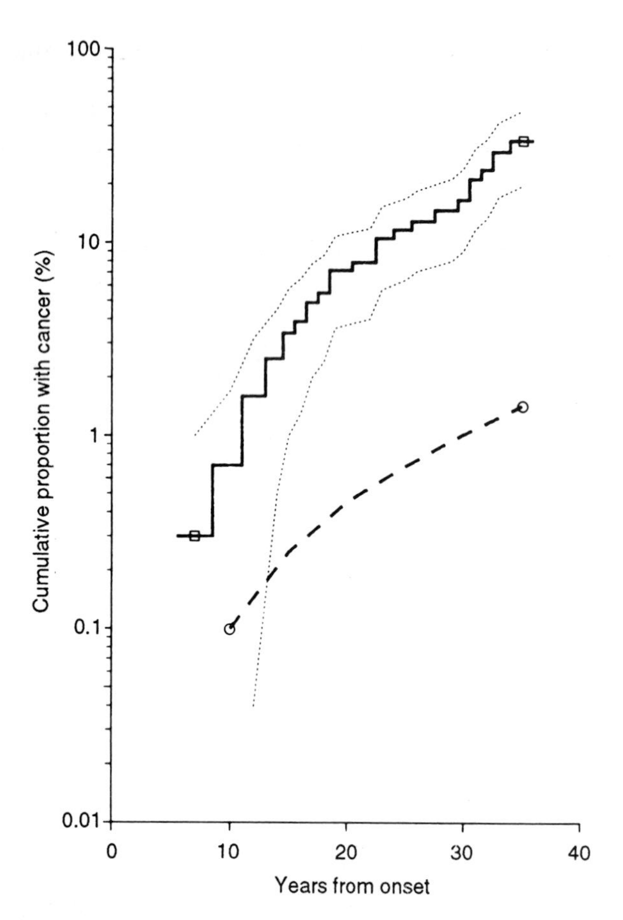

Figure 7.18 Cumulative risk with time of colorectal cancers in extensive colitis. (.......) 95% CI(+); (□—□) observed 95% CI(−); (○—○) expected.

cumulative probability of developing cancer over time.

Summarizing the results of these studies, it seems likely that the risk rises at around 0.5–1% per year after an interval of 10 years from diagnosis has elasped, giving a cumulative risk of developing cancer of 10–20% at 20 years from onset of disease and 20–30% at 30 years from onset.

The Copenhagen County population study has initially shown a very low risk in the overall series of 1.4% (confidence interval, CI 0.7–2.8). This low risk may be due, in part, to the policy of prophylactic panproctocolectomy at 10 years from onset of disease, as discussed in the early part of the study reported by Bonnevie *et al.* in 1968.[5,23]

Colorectal cancer in left sided colitis

Several studies have shown an increased risk of cancer in patients with left sided colitis, but a considerably lower risk than in patients with extensive colitis. This may be a real increase in risk. However, division of patients into extensive colitis and left sided colitis groups is a somewhat arbitrary procedure and is dependent on the diagnostic method used to make this distinction.

Initially a single contrast barium enema was the diagnostic method (and is still today in some centres). This was followed by double-contrast barium enema and more recently colonoscopy. Patients diagnosed as having left sided disease on single contrast barium enema might be considered to have extensive disease with more recent methods of double contrast barium enema or colonoscopy. The classification of some patients with extensive colitis into the left sided colitis group could significantly elevate the cancer risk found in that group.[18,25,30,48]

Cancer incidence in ileorectal anastomosis

The cancer incidence in two large series of patients with ileorectal anastomosis, carried out predominantly for extensive colitis, is shown in *Table 7.14.* Baker *et al.*[2] showed a cumulative cancer incidence of 9% 25 years from onset of disease, in close agreement with the results of Grundfest *et al.*[28] who reported a cumulative cancer incidence of 12.9% 25 years from onset of disease. No cancers occurred in either series in the first 10 years from onset of disease. Therefore, the retained rectum in patients with extensive colitis is at increased risk of developing cancer but this risk is less than in patients who have an intact colon with extensive colitis where cumulative cancer risk is between 20% and 30% 20 years from onset of disease (see *Tables 7.11* and *7.12*).[47,63]

Madjlessi and Farmer[47] recently reviewed the literature concerning cancer in the rectal stump following ileorectal anastomosis.

Bile duct cancer in ulcerative colitis

This is a rare complication associated with longstanding extensive disease and the only other site, except the large intestine, with a significantly increased cancer risk in ulcerative colitis.[1,12,49,67] The literature has been reviewed by Madjlessi *et al.*[49] including their own experience of 6 cases of bile duct carcinoma occurring in 1207 patients under review. In 25% of cases the diagnosis of bile duct carcinoma is only made at autopsy.

'Screening' for cancer: management of the high-risk group

Today, most patients with extensive colitis can be managed medically and remain in reasonably good health. However, cancer is a late complication and a significant cause of death in later years. Diagnosis of the cancer at an early stage followed by surgery can result in a complete cure. Prophylactic panproctocolectomy performed 10 years after diagnosis in these high-risk patients, to avoid cancer developing, was an approach recommended by some clinicians in the past, but in recent years has been superseded by 'screening' for cancer using dysplasia as a marker. This avoids major surgery, a pouch or life with a stoma, and the morbidity and occasional mortality associated with surgery for some patients. Ileorectal anastomosis with the rectal mucosa left in situ, although a more acceptable alternative to panproctocolectomy, leaves a rectum in place at risk of developing cancer. Some studies have shown that such patients are often lost to follow-up and only return many years later with advanced rectal cancer.

The use of dysplasia as a marker for cancer was suggested in a paper by Morson and Pang in 1967.[57] Many papers concerning the relationship between dysplasia and colorectal cancer in ulcerative colitis followed.[7,9,10,11,13,16,19,21,22,24,29,35,37,42–44,46,50,54,58,60–62,65,66,69,74,80]

These subsequent reports confirmed Morson and Pang's suggestion that dysplasia was a precursor of and a reliable 'marker' for cancerous change in the colon and rectum.

At this stage, having discovered a cancer 'marker' that could be used as a 'screening' test for cancer, it would have been appropriate to set up trials to establish the efficacy of the screening procedure. For example, rigorous clinical trials were set up prior to the introduction of breast cancer screening. These trials showed increased survival only in women over 50 years of age, diagnosed as having breast cancer in the group screened, compared with survival of women diagnosed as having breast cancer in the 'control' group. The positive benefits in survival shown by these trials have resulted in breast cancer screening being introduced on a population basis in England.[71]

Such trials have not been set up prior to screening for cancer in ulcerative colitis. Instead, observational studies were set up where screening was introduced in high-risk patients and the results observed, but with no comparative control group for comparison of survival.

'Screening' for cancer is now widely used in clinical practice for ulcerative colitis patients but with no clear idea of whether it is improving survival. The results of ongoing prospective studies vary considerably in the stage at which cancers are detected. In many instances the cancers have not been detected by the 'screen' but have been discovered because either the cancer has presented symptomatically or the cancer has been discovered coincidentally, often following surgery carried out for ill health due to the disease process itself.

The most successful prospective study so far was reported from Stockholm in a 15-year surveillance programme of 72 patients with total colitis. The two cancers identified were detected by the screening procedure itself (not coincidentally), both cancers being detected at an early stage (Dukes' stage A) where prospects for survival are good.[46]

In the last 6 years of the study, abnormal DNA patterns (aneuploidy) using flow cytometric analyses were included, and the study related these results to 'dysplasia' found at the time. This raises the possibility of a new 'marker' for cancer in these patients.

Problems in the use of 'dysplasia' as a marker for cancer

The numerous reports of surveillance programmes have highlighted many areas of concern in the use of 'dysplasia' as a marker. The major problems relate to the following:

1. Occurence of de novo cancers not associated with dysplastic change.
2. The patchy distribution of dysplasia.
3. Interobserver and intraobserver error relating to histopathological assessment of dysplastic change.
4. The natural history of dyplasia in the colon not being clearly established, also not establishing the proportion of cases with dysplastic change that will be followed by invasive carcinoma and at what time interval.

The problems relating to screening for cancer in ulcerative colitis have recently been reviewed.[11,29]

REFERENCES

1. Akwari, O., Van Heerden, J., Foulk, W. and Baggenstoss, A. (1975) Cancer of the bile ducts associated with ulcerative colitis. *Annals of Surgery*, **181**, 303–309.
2. Baker, W., Glass, R., Ritchie, J. and Aylett, S. (1978) Cancer of the rectum following colectomy and ileorectal anastomosis for ulcerative colitis. *British Journal of Surgery*, **65**, 862–868
3. Bargen, J.A. (1928) Chronic ulcerative colitis complicated by malignant neoplasia. *Archives of Surgery*, **17**, 561–576.
4. Blackstone, M., Riddell, R., Rogers, G. and Levin, B. (1981) Dysplasia-associated lesion or mass (DALM) detected by colonoscopy in longstanding ulcerative colitis: an indication for colectomy. *Gastroenterology*, **80**, 366–374.

5. Bonnevie, O., Riis, P. and Anthonisen, P. (1968) An epidemiological study of ulcerative colitis in Copenhagan County. *Scandinavian Journal of Gastroenterology*, **3**, 432–438.
6. Brostrom, O., Monsen, U., Nordenvall, B. *et al.* (1987) Prognosis and mortality of ulcerative colitis in Stockholm county, 1955–1979. *Scandinavian Journal of Gastroenterology*, **22**, 907–913.
7. Brostrom, O., Lofberg, R., Ost, A. and Reichard, H. (1986) Cancer surveillance of patients with longstanding ulcerative colitis: A clinical, endoscopical and histological study. *Gut*, **27**, 1408–1413.
8. Bulow, S. (1980) Colorectal cancer in patients less than 40 years of age in Denmark 1943–1967. *Diseases of the Colon and Rectum*, **23**, 327–336.
9. Butt, J.H., Lennard-Jones, J.E. and Ritchie, J.K. (1980) A practical approach to the risk of cancer in inflammatory bowel disease: Research, watch, or act? In *Inflammatory Bowel Disease*, (Ed) Winship, D.H., 64.6, pp 1203–1220, Philadelphia: WB Saunders.
10. Butt, J.H., Price, A. and Williams, C.B. (1983) Dysplasia and cancer in ulcerative colitis. In *Inflammatory Bowel Diseases*, 1st Edn (Ed.) Allan, R.N., Keighley, M.R.B., Alexander-Williams, J. and Hawkins, C.F. pp. 140–153. Edinburgh: Churchill Livingstone.
11. Collins, R.H., Feldman, M. and Fortran, J.S. (1987) Colon cancer, dysplasia and surveillance in patients with ulcerative colitis: a critical review. *New England Journal of Medicine*, **316**, 1654–1658.
12. Converse, C., Reagan, J. and Decosse, J. (1971) Ulcerative colitis and carcinoma of the bile ducts. *American Journal of Surgery*, **121**, 39–45.
13. Cook, M.G., Path, M.R.C. and Goligher, J.C. (1975) Carcinoma and epithelial dysplasia complicating ulcerative colitis. *Gastroenterology*, **68**, 1127–1136.
14. de Dombal, F.T., Watts, J., Watkinson, G. *et al.* (1966) Local complications of ulcerative colitis: Stricture, pseudopolyposis and carcinoma of the colon and rectum. *British Medical Journal*, **1**, 1442–1447.
15. Devroede, G.J., Taylor, W.F., Sauer, W.G. *et al.* (1971) Cancer risk and life expectancy of children with ulcerative colitis. *New England Journal of Medicine*, **285**, 17–21.
16. Dobbins, W.O. (1977) Current status of the pre-cancer lesions in ulcerative colitis. *Gastroenterology*, **73**, 1431–1433.
17. Edwards, F.C. and Truelove, S.C. (1964) The course and prognosis of ulcerative colitis. Part I, III, IV Carcinoma of the colon. *Gut*, **4**, 299–315.
18. Ekbom, A., Helmick, C., Zack, M. and Adami, H.O. (1990) Ulcerative colitis and colorectal cancer. A population based study. *New England Journal of Medicine*, 1228–1233.
19. Evans, D.J. and Pollack, D.J. (1972) In situ and invasive carcinoma of the colon patients with ulcerative colitis. *Gut*, **13**, 566–570.
20. Evans, J.G. and Acheson, E.D. (1965) An epidemiological study of ulcerative colitis and regional enteritis in the Oxford area. *Gut*, **6**, 311–324.
21. Fenoglio, C.M. and Pascal, R.R. (1973) Adenomatous epithelium, intraepithelial anaplasia, and invasive carcinoma in ulcerative colitis. *American Journal of Digestive Diseases*, **18**, 556–562.
22. Fozan, J.B.J. and Dixon, M.F. (1989) Colonoscopic surveillance in ulcerative colitis – dysplasia through the looking glass. *Gut*, **30**, 285–292.
23. Goldgraber, M.B. and Kirsner, J.B. (1964) Carcinoma of the colon in ulcerative colitis. *Cancer*, **17**, 657–665.
24. Granqvist, S., Gabrielson, N., Sundelin, P. and Thorgeirsson, T. (1980) Precancerous lesions in the mucosa in ulcerative colitis. *Scandinavian Journal of Gastroenterology*, **15**, 289–296.
25. Greenstein, A.J., Sachar, D.B. and Pucillo, A. (1979) Cancer in universal and left sided colitis: clinical and pathological features. *Mount Sinai Journal of Medicine*, **46**, 25.
26. Greenstein, A.J., Sachar, D.B., Smith, H. *et al.* (1979) Cancer risk in universal and left sided ulcerative colitis: factors determining risk. *Gastroenterology*, **77**, 290–294.
27. Greenstein, A.J., Sachar, D.B., Smith, H. *et al.* (1981) A comparison of the cancer risk in Crohn's Disease and ulcerative colitis. *Cancer*, **48**, 2742–2745.
28. Grundfest, S.F., Fazio, V., Weiss, R. *et al.* (1981) The cancer risk following colectomy and ileorectal anastomosis for extensive mucosal ulcerative colitis. *Annals of Surgery*, **193**, 9–14.
29. Gyde, S.N. (1990) Screening for colorectal cancer in ulcerative colitis: dubious benefits and high costs. *Gut*, **31**, 1089–1092.
30. Gyde, S.N., Prior, P., Allan, R.N. *et al.* (1988) Colorectal cancer in ulcerative colitis: A cohort study of primary referrals from three centres. *Gut*, **29**, 206–217.
31. Gyde, S.N., Prior, P., Thompson, H. *et al.* (1984) Survival of patients with colorectal cancer complicating ulcerative colitis. *Gut*, **25**, 228–231.
32. Hendriksen, C., Kreiner, S. and Binder, V. (1985) Long term prognosis in ulcerative colitis – based on results from a regional patient group from the County of Copenhagen. *Gut*, **26**, 158–163.
33. Hughes, R., Hall, T., Block, G. *et al.* (1978) The prognosis of carcinoma of the colon and rectum complicating ulcerative colitis. *Surgery*, Gynecology and Obstetrics, **146**, 46–48.
34. Hulten, L., Kewenter, J., Ahren, C. and Ojewkog, B. (1979) Clinical and morphological characteristics of colitis carcinoma and colorectal carcinoma in young people. *Scandinavian Journal of Gastroenterology*, **14**, 673–678.
35. Hulten, L., Kewenter, J. and Ahren, C. (1971) Precancer and carcinoma in chronic ulcerative colitis: a histopathological and clinical investigation.

Scandinavian Journal of Gastroenterology, **7**, 6634–6639.

36. Hurst, A.F. (1921) *Guy's Hospital Report*, **71**, 24–41.
37. Jones, H.W., Grogono, J. and Hoare, A.M. (1988) Surveillance in ulcerative colitis: Burdens and benefit. *Gut*, **29**, 325–331.
38. Katza, I., Brody, R., Morris, E. and Katz, S. (1983) Assessment of colorectal cancer risk in patients with ulcerative colitis. Experience from a private practice. *Gastroenterology*, **85**, 22–29.
39. Kewenter, J., Ahlman, H. and Hulten, L. (1978) Cancer risk in extensive colitis. *Annals of Surgery*, **188**, 824–827.
40. Langman, M.J. (1966) Epidemiology of cancer of the large intestine. *Proceedings of the Royal Society of Medicine*, **59**, 132–134.
41. Lavery, I., Chiulli, R., Jagelman, D. *et al.* (1982) Survival with carcinoma arising in mucosal ulcerative colitis. *Annals of Surgery*, **195**, 508–512.
42. Lennard-Jones, J., Morson, B., Ritchie, J. *et al.* (1977) Cancer in colitis: assessment of the individual risk by clinical and histological criteria. *Gastroenterology*, **73**, 1280–1289.
43. Lennard-Jones, J.E. (1985) Cancer risk in ulcerative colitis: surveillance or surgery. *British Journal of Surgery* (suppl.), 584–586.
44. Lennard-Jones, J.E., Morson, B.C., Ritchie, J.K. *et al.* (1983) Cancer surveillance in ulcerative colitis. Experience over 15 years. *The Lancet*, **2**, 149–152.
45. Linden, G. and Noller, C. (1971) Ulcerative colitis in Finland. II. One year incidence in all hospitals. *Diseases of the Colon and Rectum*, **14**, 264–266.
46. Lofberg, R., Bostrom, O., Karlen, P. *et al.* (1990) Colonoscopic surveillance in longstanding total ulcerative colitis – a 15-year follow-up study. *Gastroenterology*, **99**, 1021–1031.
47. Madjlessi, S.H. and Farmer, R.G. (1985) Squamous cell carcinoma of the rectal stump in a patient with ulcerative colitis. Report of a case and review of the literature. *Cleveland Clinic Quarterly*, **22**, 257–261.
48. Madjlessi, S.H., Farmer, R.G., Easley, K.A. and Beck, G.J. (1986) Colorectal and extracolonic malignancy in ulcerative colitis. *Cancer*, **58**, 1569–1574.
49. Madjlessi, S.H., Farmer, R.G. and Sivak, H.V. Jr (1987) Bile duct carcinoma in patients with ulcerative colitis. Relationship to sclerosing cholangitis: Report of six cases and review of the literature.
50. Manning, A.P., Bulgim, O.R., Dixon, M.F. and Axon, A.T.R. (1987) Screening by colonoscopy for colonic apithelial dysplasia in inflammatory bowel disease. *Gut*, **28**, 1489–1494.
51. Mayberry, J.F., Rhodes, J. and Newcombe, R.G. (1980) Familial presence of inflammatory bowel disease in relatives of patients with Crohn's disease. *British Medical Journal*, **1**, 84.
52. McConnell, R.B. (1980) Inflammatory bowel disease: newer views of genetic influences. In *Developments in Digestive Disease*, Volume 3 (Ed.) Berk, J.E. pp. 271–278. Philadelphia: Lea and Febiger.
53. McDougall, I. (1964) The cancer risk in ulcerative colitis. *The Lancet*, **2**, 655–659.
54. Melville, D.M., Jass, J.R., Shepherd, N.A. *et al.* (1988) Dysplasia and deoxyribonucleic acid aneuploidy in the assessment of precancerous changes in chronic ulcerative colitis. Observer variation and correlations. *Gastroenterology*, **95**, 668–675.
55. Michener, W.M., Farmer, R.G. and Mortimer, E.A. (1979) Long term prognosis of ulcerative colitis with onset in childhood or adolescence. *Journal of Clinical Gastroenterology*, **1**, 301.
56. Monk, M., Mendeloff, A.L., Siegel, C.I. and Lilienfield, A. (1967) An epidemiological study of ulcerative colitis and regional enteritis among adults in Baltimore. 1. Hospital incidence and prevalence 1960–1963. *Gastroenterology*, **53**, 198–210.
57. Morson, B. and Pang, L. (1967) Rectal biopsy as an aid to cancer control in ulcerative colitis. *Gut*, **8**, 423–434.
58. Myrvoid, H.E., Kock, N.G. and Ahren, C. (1974) Rectal biopsy and precancer in ulcerative colitis. *Gut*, **15**, 301–304.
59. Nefzger, M.D. and Acheson, E.D. (1963) Ulcerative colitis in the United States Army in 1944. *Gut*, **4**, 183–192.
60. Nugent, F.W. (1980) Surveillance of patients with ulcerative colitis: Lakey Clinic results. In *Colorectal Cancer: Prevention, Epidemiology, and Screening* (Ed.) Winawer, S.J., Schottenfield, D. and Sherlock, P. pp. 375–380. New York: Raven Press.
61. Nugent, F.W. and Haggitt, R.C. (1984) Results of a longterm prospective surveillance program for dysplasia in ulcerative colitis. *Gastroenterology*, **86**, 1197.
62. Nugent, F.W., Haggitt, R.C., Colcher, H. and Kutteruf, G.C. (1979) Malignant potential of chronic ulcerative colitis: preliminary report. *Gastroenterology*, **76**, 1–5.
63. Oakley, J.R., Jagelman, D.G., Fazio, V.W. *et al.* (1985) Complications and quality of life after ileorectal anastomosis for ulcerative colitis. *American Journal of Surgery*, **149**, 24–30.
64. Prior, P., Gyde, S.N., Macartney, J.C. *et al.* (1982) Cancer morbidity in ulcerative colitis. *Gut*, **23**, 490–497.
65. Ransohoff, D.F., Riddell, R.H. and Levin, B. (1985) Ulcerative colitis colonic cancer: problems in assessing the diagnostic usefulness of mucosal dysplasia. *Diseases of the Colon and Rectum*, **28**, 383–388.
66. Riddell, R.H., Goldman, H., Ransohoff, D.F. *et al.* (1985) Dysplasia in inflammatory bowel disease: standardized classification with provisional clinical applications. *Human Pathology*, **14**, 931–966.
67. Ritchie, J., Allan, R.N., Macartney, J. *et al.* (1974) Biliary tract carcinoma associated with ulcerative colitis. *Quarterly Journal of Medicine*, **170**, 263–279.

68. Ritchie, J., Hawley, P. and Lennard-Jones, J. (1981) Prognosis of carcinoma in ulcerative colitis. *Gut*, **22**, 752–755.
69. Rosenstock, E., Farmer, R.G., Petras, R. *et al.* (1985) Surveillance for colonic carcinoma in ulcerative colitis. *Gastroenterology*, **89**, 1342–1346.
70. Samuelsson, S.M. (1976) Ulcerative colitis in the County of Uppsala. Clinical, epidemiological and sociomedical aspects (dissertation). Acta Universitatis upsalienis.
71. Shapiro, S., Venet, W., Strax, P., Venet, L. and Roeser, R. (1982) Ten-fourteen year effect of breast cancer screening on mortality. *Journal of the National Cancer Institute*, **69**, 349–355.
72. Sinclair, T.S., Brunt, P.W., Ashley, N. and Mowat, G. (1983) Non-specific proctocolitis in North Eastern Scotland: A community study. *Gastroenterology*, **85**, 1–11.
73. Slaney, G. and Brooke, B.N. (1959) Cancer in ulcerative colitis. *The Lancet*, **2**, 694–698.
74. Stonnington, C.M., Philips, S.F., Zinsmeister, A.R. *et al.* (1987) Prognosis of chronic ulcerative colitis in a community. *Gut*, **28**, 1261–1266.
75. Teague, R.H. and Read, A.E. (1975) Polyposis in ulcerative colitis. *Gut*, **16**, 792–795.
76. Van Heerden, J.A., Judd, E.S. and Dockerty, M.B. (1967) Carcinoma of the extrahepatic bile ducts: a clinicopathologic study. *American Journal of Surgery*, **113**, 49–56.
77. Wigley, R.D. and MacLaurin, B.P. (1962) A study of ulcerative colitis in New Zealand showing a low incidence in Maoris. *British Medical Journal*, **2**, 228–231.
78. Wilks, S. (1859) *Lectures of Pathological Anatomy*, 1st Ed. London: Langman and Roberts.
79. Wilks, S. (1859) Mobid appearances in the intestines of Miss Banks. *Medical Times Gazette*, **19**, 264–265.
80. Yardley, J.H. and Keren, D.F. (1974) 'Precancer' lesions in ulcerative colitis: a retrospective study of rectal biopsy and colectomy specimens. *Cancer*, **34**, 835–844.

CROHN'S DISEASE

PATHOLOGY *(H. Thompson)*

Crohn's disease is a clinicopathological entity which can effect either the small intestine or the large intestine, and not infrequently both sites are involved at the time of clinical presentation or later during the course of this disorder.

The early stages of Crohn's disease are rarely observed and biopsy material may show non-specific inflammatory changes or occasionally granulomata. As the disease develops, ulceration appears in a focal segment of the gastrointestinal tract or throughout the colon. Endoscopic examination or double-contrast radiology may reveal aphthoid ulcers in the mucosa. Granulomata can be identified during this stage in biopsies of aphthoid ulcers or in biopsy material from the rectum, colon, perianal area, stomach, jejunum and ileocaecal lymph nodes. As this disease progresses more extensive ulceration associated with fissures develops in the diseased areas accompanied by hose pipe thickening of the bowel wall due to oedema and transmural inflammation. The mesenteric lymph nodes enlarge and show reactive changes with lymphoid hyperplasia, sinus catarrh and scattered granulomata. Jejunal biopsies may show convolutions, oedema and histological evidence of partial villous atrophy.

The gross and histological features of Crohn's disease will be discussed with reference to each anatomical zone.

INVOLVEMENT OF THE TERMINAL ILEUM (REGIONAL ILEITIS)

This is the most common and most familiar lesion in Crohn's disease which leads to ulceration (*Figures 7.19* and *7.20*) and hosepipe thickening (*Figure 7.21*) of a variable length of the distal ileum up to the ileocaecal valve. Only a few centimetres may be affected in some patients but more frequently the diseased segment measures 10–12 cm in length; it may extend to 30–40 cm in length with multiple affected segments or skip lesions. Foci of aphthoid ulceration are present in the early stages but in most resected specimens there is extensive ulceration or evidence of linear ulceration along the mesenteric attachment. The mucosa may show a cobblestone pattern or there may be oedema of the circular valvulae conniventes. Pseudopolyps may occur in a small proportion of cases and mucosal bridges are occasionally encountered. Stenosis and stricture formation are frequently observed radiologically and on gross examination of the specimen. Fissures, sinuses, fistulas and adhesions with kinking of small intestinal loops are found in patients with long-standing disease. Fruit pulp, tomato skins, fruit stones, a bolus of food debris and even coins have been discovered in the narrowed segment in patients with intestinal obstructions. Stercoliths resembling gallstones are occasionally found in association with single or multiple strictures. Disease extends into the adjacent caecum in 20% of cases, particularly

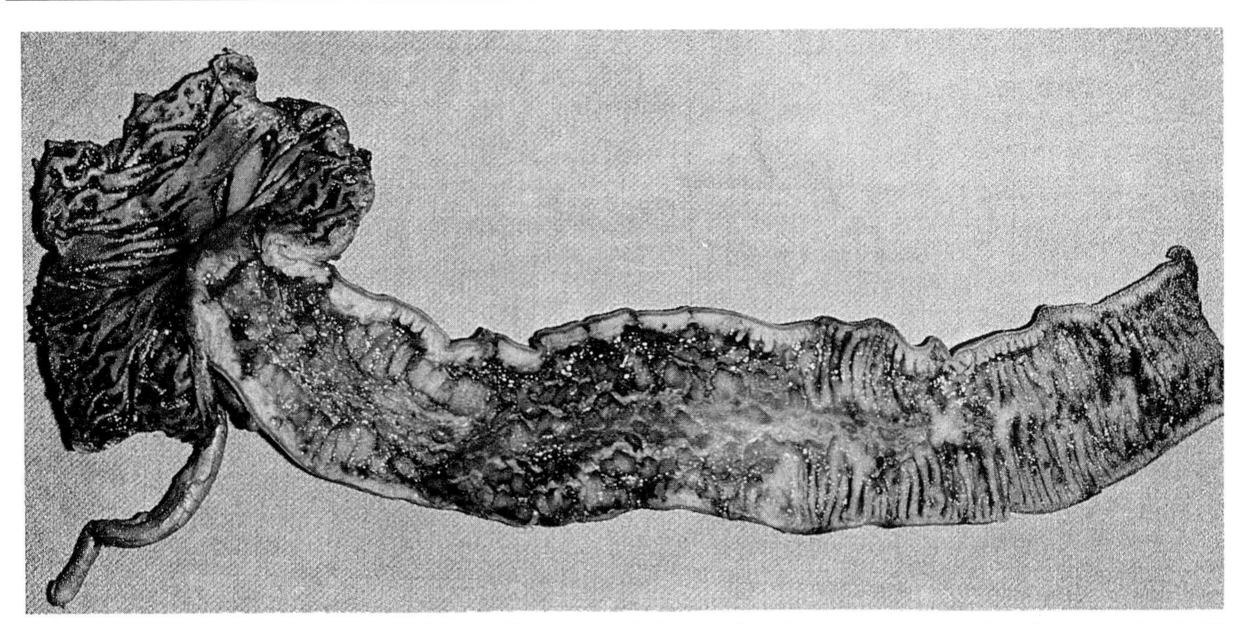

Figure 7.19 Regional ileitis involving terminal ileum with hosepipe thickening of the bowel wall and ulceration. The proximal part of the ileum shows ulceration on the mesenteric aspect.

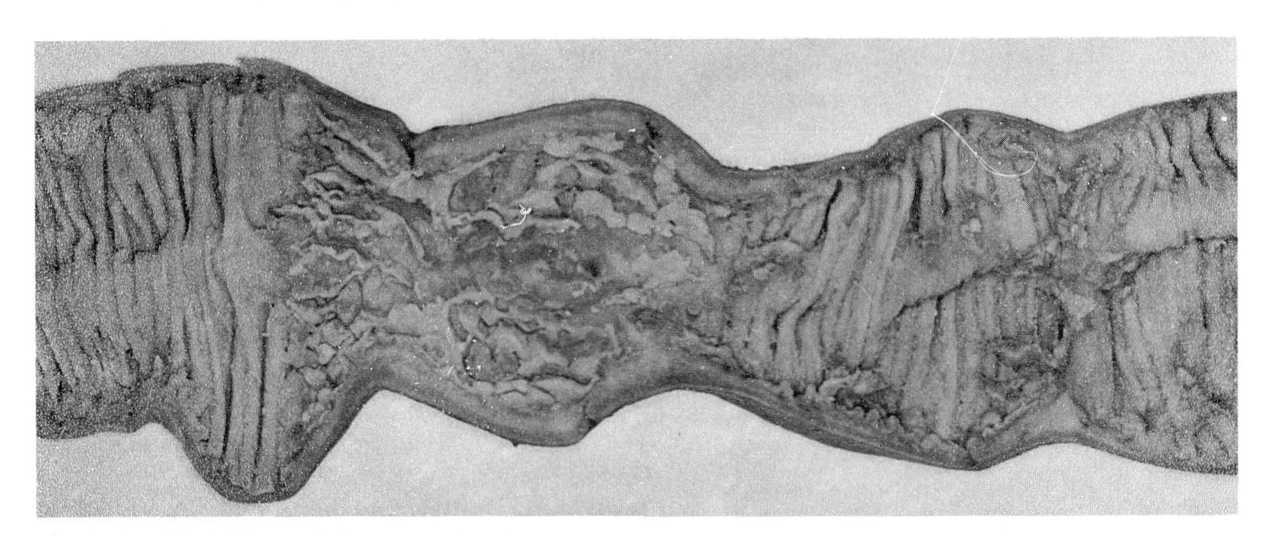

Figure 7.20 Crohn's disease of the small intestine with ulcerated strictures.

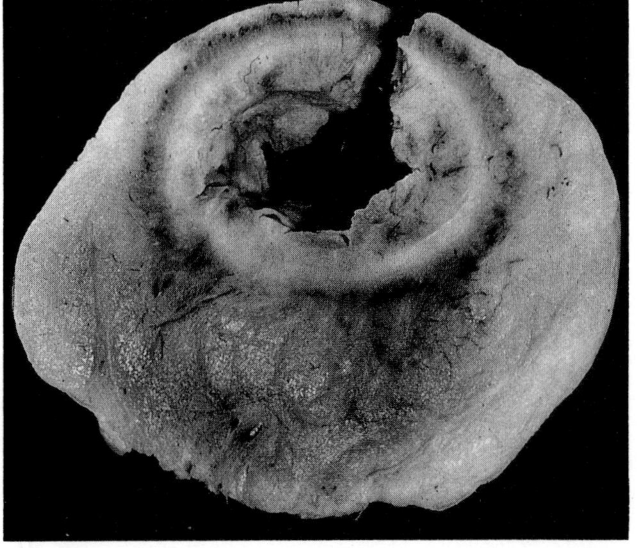

Figure 7.21 Hosepipe thickening in regional ileitis with oedema extending into mesenteric fat.

around the ileocaecal valve. The appendix may be thickened and involved, and Meckel's diverticulum is occasionally affected. Oedema extends into the mesenteric tissues. Abscesses loculate in the ileocaecal region in relation to loops of small bowel and ileocaecal lymph nodes. Recurrent ileal disease following hemicolectomy may be of the simple ulcerative type with no hosepipe thickening or strictures.

Histology

There is a wide spectrum of histological features which include ulceration, fissures (*Figure 7.22*), sinuses, oedema, lymphoid hyperplasia, granulomata, dilatation of lymphatic channels, thickening of the muscularis mucosae, fibrosis, microabscesses, chronic inflammatory cellular infiltration, neuromatous hyperplasia and angiitis. Non-caseating epithelioid cell follicles with Langhan's giant cells (*Figure 7.23)* are present in the bowel wall in 50–60% of cases and in the lymph nodes in about 25% of cases. Multiple sections must be examined for their detection and foreign body granulomata, which are frequently present, have to be carefully considered in differential diagnosis and excluded by polarizing microscopy. Endolymphatic granulomata may be prominent and microgranulomata are present in some cases. More diffuse granulomatous inflammation is found around fissures and sinuses. Eosinophilia is a prominent feature in some cases, to such an extent that a mistaken diagnosis of eosinophilic enteritis can be made. Epithelial regenerative changes are usually well developed and may simulate dysplasia. Crypt abscess formation is also seen *(Figure 7.24)*. Pseudopyloric gland metaplasia *(Figure 7.25)* is present in a high proportion of cases representing a regeneration phenomenon; parietal cells are occasionally identified in the metaplastic tubules. Angiitis is encountered in around 10% of specimens and may be inflammatory, necrotizing or

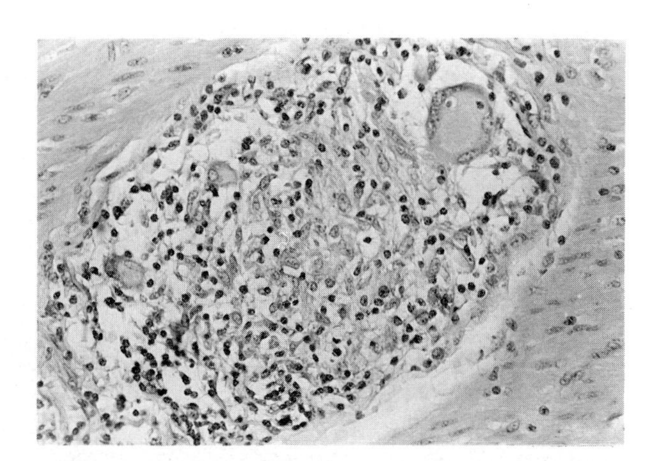

Figure 7.23 Non-caseating epithelioid cell follicle with Langhan's giant cell.

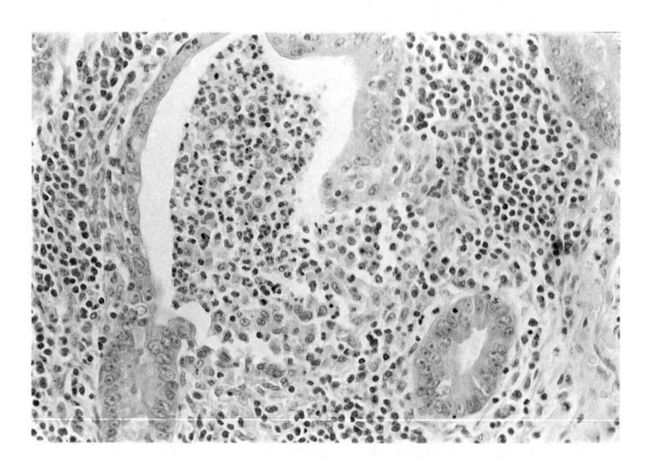

Figure 7.24 Crypt abscess in Crohn's disease.

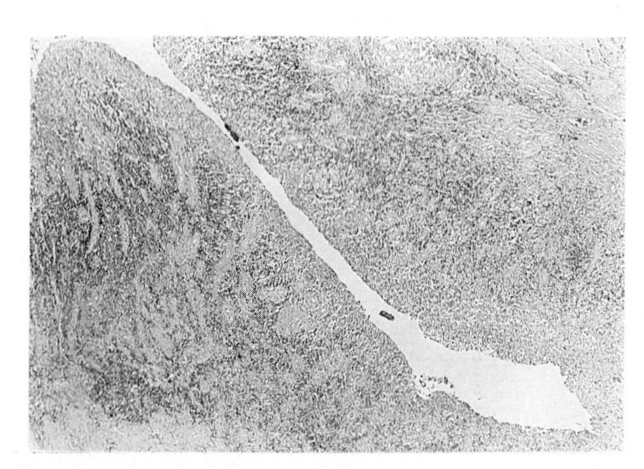

Figure 7.22 Fissure in ulcerated mucosa in regional ileitis.

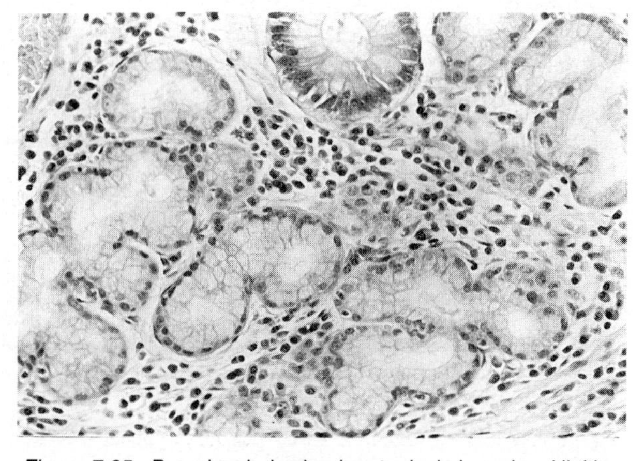

Figure 7.25 Pseudopyloric gland metaplasia in regional ileitis.

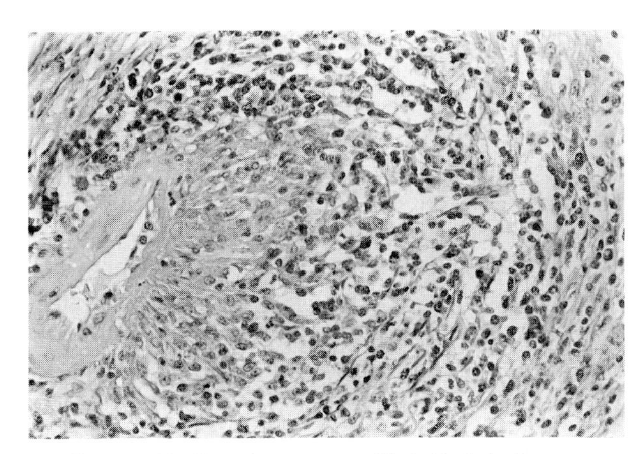

Figure 7.26 Granulomatous angiitis in Crohn's disease.

granulomatous *(Figure 7.26)* in type. Veins may also be involved. Endarteritis obliterans is frequently found and thrombosis is occasionally seen.

INVOLVEMENT OF THE COLON AND RECTUM

Discrete aphthoid ulcers which can be seen at endoscopy or demonstrated by double-contrast radiology represent the earliest lesions in Crohn's disease. This type of ulceration is not specific because it has been encountered in other infective disorders. Histological examination of aphthoid ulcers reveals focal superficial ulceration, lymphoid hyperplasia, occasional granulomata and even angiitis. As the disease progresses, linear ulceration *(Figure 7.27)*, discrete ulceration, cobblestone mucosa and, frequently, more florid ulceration develop. Fissures appear in the mucosa and may be associated with sinus, fistula or abscess formation particularly in the perianal region. Later in the disease, stenosis occurs either in hosepipe segments *(Figure 7.28)* or as short strictures. There is usually considerable thickening of the bowel wall as in regional ileitis due to oedema and transmural inflammation. Pseudopolyposis (see *Figure 7.27)* is a further feature of long-standing disease.

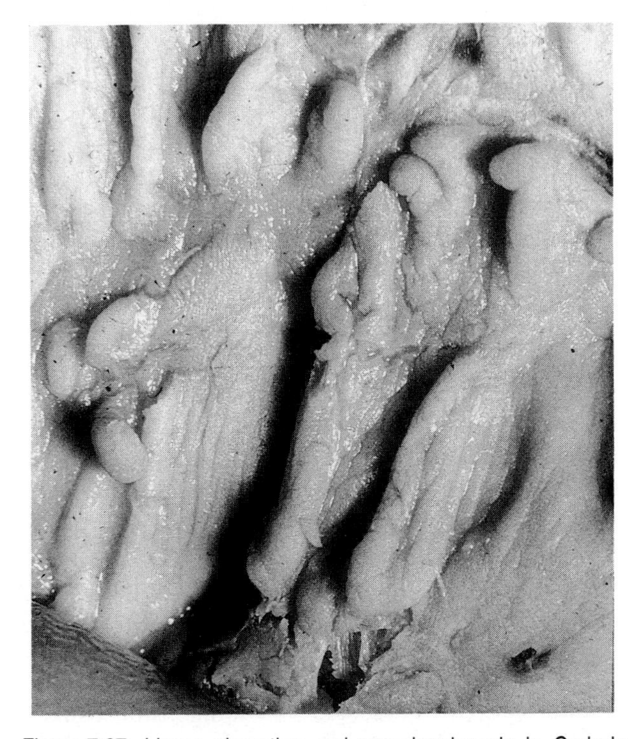

Figure 7.27 Linear ulceration and pseudopolyposis in Crohn's disease of the colon.

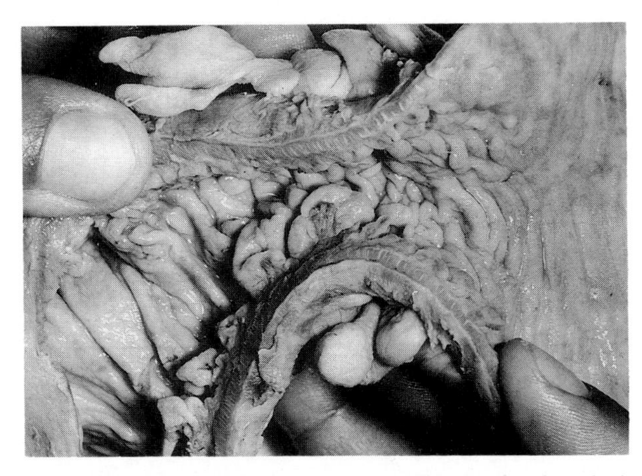

Figure 7.28 Short hosepipe segment with pseudopolyposis in Crohn's disease of the colon.

Segmental involvement of the colon and rectum is an interesting facet of the disease. Rectal sparing occurs in patients who have the features of segmental or right-sided colitis. The gross appearances are indistinguishable from ulcerative colitis in some cases and the diagnosis can only be established on histological criteria or where there is evidence of small bowel involvement. Local extension into the terminal ileum occurs in approximately 20% of cases of primary Crohn's disease of the colon.

Histology

The histological appearances are comparable with those found in regional ileitis with ulceration, fissures, lymphoid hyperplasia, oedema, fibrosis, thickening of the muscularis mucosae, neuromatous hyperplasia and non-caseating granulomata. The incidence of granulomata in Crohn's disease of the colon is around 70% and in rectal biopsy material 27.3% as recorded by Thompson and Bonser,[10] and 25% as recorded by Yardley and Hamilton.[12] Microgranulomata *(Figure 7.29)*, which represent subtle histological lesions with epithelioid cells and occasional Langhan's giant cells, raise a strong suspicion of Crohn's disease. Multiple endoscopic biopsies are more likely to be diagnostic than a single biopsy. In a stereomicroscopic and serial section

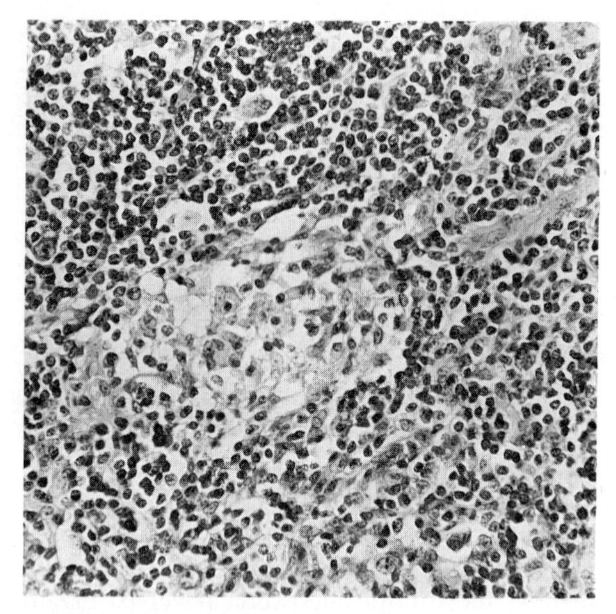

Figure 7.29 Microgranuloma in Crohn's disease of the colon.

study of rectal biopsies, Poulsen *et al.*[6] identified granulomata in 62% of rectal biopsies and an even higher incidence of 85% when two biopsies were examined from each patient. Confirmation of this study is awaited from other centres. Arteritis is a further feature; Thompson and Bonser[10] recorded an incidence of 1.5% in rectal biopsy material and around 10% in colectomy specimens. Epithelial regenerative changes occur but tend to be localized to ulcerated areas whilst the intervening mucosa appears normal. Absence of mucin depletion helps to distinguish Crohn's disease from ulcerative colitis. Focal non-specific inflammation as described by Yardley and Hamilton[12] and disproportionate inflammation are additional features. Granulomatous crypt abscesses are frequently present and granulomatous cryptitis is a further useful diagnostic feature.

INVOLVEMENT OF THE JEJUNUM

Primary localization can occur in the jejunum as well as secondary skip lesions complicating regional ileitis. The affected segment shows hosepipe thickening, narrowing and stenosis, occasionally amounting to stricture formation. Diaphragms are occasionally found as a coincidental congenital anomaly, although it is possible that Crohn's disease itself may lead to diaphragm formation. Diaphragms may also occur as a complication of non-steroidal anti-inflammatory drug abuse or as a complication of adult coeliac disease.

Histology

The histological appearances are typical and include ulceration, fissures, lymphoid hyperplasia and granulomata. Ulceration is usually most extensive along the mesenteric attachment. If granulomata are absent, then the diagnosis is much more difficult to sustain because the lesion has to be distinguished from polyarteritis nodosa, simple non-specific ulceration complicating adult coeliac disease, potassium-induced ulceration and ulcerative jejunitis.

INVOLVEMENT OF THE DUODENUM

The incidence of Crohn's disease of the duodenum complicating ileal or colonic disease is 4% in large clinical series. Stenosis is a common complication and a bypass operation may be necessary for persistent symptoms. The diagnosis can usually be established by endoscopy, radiology and biopsy. Granulomata are rarely encountered but they may be found in gastric biopsies taken from the same patient. Primary Crohn's disease of the duodenum is exceedingly rare. Duodenal ulcer disease is also a recognized complication of Crohn's disease and may be difficult to distinguish from granulomatous disease.

Perforation and haemorrhage represent additional complications of duodenal involvement. Clinical, radiological, endoscopic and pathological observations on Crohn's disease of the duodenum are documented by Fielding *et al.*[3] and by Thompson and Cockel.[11]

INVOLVEMENT OF THE STOMACH

This may be primary or secondary to Crohn's disease elsewhere in the gastrointestinal tract. Random gastric biopsies may show granulomata or an increased population of inflammatory cells. Significant disease is much less common and is associated with ulceration, fissures and thickening of the stomach wall. The pyloric region is most frequently affected but the lesion may be more extensive, involving the body mucosa. The gross appearances simulate linitis plastica or 'leather bottle stomach'. Patients with Crohn's disease of the duodenum may also have contiguous gastric disease. Non-caseating granulomata are nearly always present. Primary Crohn's disease of the stomach must be carefully differentiated from sarcoidosis, Wegener's granulomatosis, corrosive poisoning, tuberculosis, histoplasmosis and syphilis.

INVOLVEMENT OF OTHER SITES

Crohn's disease of the oesophagus is extremely rare but it has been well documented; the differential diagnosis includes peptic oesophagitis. Crohn's disease of the mouth and lips has been described, supported by historical changes. Crohn's disease of the appendix may be discovered during routine appendicectomy for appendicitis, but it should be emphasized that granulomatous disease of the appendix can occur without later development of Crohn's disease. Meckel's diverticulum can be involved by Crohn's disease in association with regional ileitis and it has also been described as a primary lesion. Primary Crohn's disease of the rectum and perianal region are uncommon, but well documented. Perianal disease is a familiar and extremely common feature of Crohn's disease. Fistulas and inflammatory changes in Crohn's disease can extend to involve the bladder, urinary tract, ovaries and tubes. More distant granulomatous lesions have also been described in the gallbladder, liver, synovial membranes of joints and the skin surface.

DYSPLASIA AND CANCER

There is a fourfold increased incidence of carcinoma of the colon and rectum in patients with long-standing Crohn's disease.[4] The author's group has encountered carcinoma of the small intestine[5] and cancer in fistulous tracts[1] complicating Crohn's disease. Cancer in the small intestine presents as the occult, diffusely infiltrating variety; colorectal malignant lesions may also be of this type. Dysplasia occurs as a complication of Crohn's disease in the small intestine, and also in the colon and rectum. Villous and tubular adenomas are also occasionally encountered. (See p. 1181.)

INVOLVEMENT OF THE LYMPH NODES

Adjacent lymph nodes are usually enlarged in association with gastrointestinal Crohn's disease. Abscess formation is a problem in the ileocaecal region in association with fissures and sinuses, and also between loops of involved small intestine. Sinus catarrh and reactive hyperplasia are prominent. Non-caseating granulomata with epithelioid cells and Langhan's giant cells are found in about 30% of cases. Foreign body giant cells are also occasionally found and coexistent caseating tuberculosis has been reported in the nodes. Reactive ileocaecal nodes not infrequently show old inactive calcified tuberculosis.

LYMPHOID HYPERPLASIA AND LYMPHOMA

Rarely, lymphoid hyperplasia and lymphocytic plasma cell infiltration are so well developed that they simulate lymphoma. Although malignant lymphoma has been reported in association with both regional ileitis and Crohn's disease of the colon, there is no statistical evidence of an increased incidence. Shepherd *et al.*[9] describe three cases of lymphoma complicating Crohn's disease and review the literature supporting an association between Crohn's disease and lymphoma.

HEPATIC DYSFUNCTION

A variety of complications occur in the liver[2] including fatty change, pericholangitis, granulomata, cirrhosis, amyloidosis and sclerosing cholangitis. There is an increased incidence of cholelithiasis and this can be complicated by suppurative cholangitis and multiple liver abscess formation.

BIOPSIES

The most important clue to the diagnosis of Crohn's disease lies in the identification of non-caseating granulomata or microgranulomata. Sections should be examined from at least three levels in the biopsy. Additional histological features are valuable in the assessment of rectal biopsies such as the presence of focal non-specific inflammation, disproportionate inflammation, distribution of neutrophils, absence of mucin depletion, and relatively normal crypt and surface epithelium. Multiple biopsies are more informative than a single biopsy. A recent claim[7] that an increased population of IgM cells in the lamina propria might be a helpful diagnostic feature of Crohn's disease has not yet been substantiated.

DIFFERENTIAL DIAGNOSIS

The location of the disease determines the differential diagnosis. In the small intestine, the principal entities include tuberculosis, non-steroidal anti-inflammatory drug abuse, adult coeliac disease with ulceration and strictures, ischaemic enteritis, eosinophilic enteritis and Behçet's syndrome. In the large intestine, the list includes ulcerative colitis, tuberculosis, diverticulitis, ischaemic colitis, schistosomiasis and Behçet's syndrome. In the perianal region tuberculosis, oleogranuloma and hidradenitis suppurativa must be considered.

REFERENCES

1. Buchmann, P., Allan, R.N., Thompson, H. and Alexander-Williams, J. (1980) Carcinoma in a rectovaginal fistula in a patient with Crohn's disease. *American Journal of Surgery*, **140**, 462–463.
2. Dew, M.J., Thompson H. and Allan, R.N. (1979) The spectrum of hepatic dysfunction in inflammatory bowel disease. *Quarterly Journal of Medicine* (*New Series*), **189**, 113–135.
3. Fielding, J.F., Toye, D.K.M., Beton, D.C. and Cooke, W.T. (1970) Crohn's disease of the stomach and duodenum. *Gut*, **11**, 1001–1006.
4. Gyde, S.N., Prior, P., Macartney, J.C. *et al.* (1980) Malignancy in Crohn's disease. *Gut*, **21**, 1024–1029.
5. Hawker, P.C., Gyde, S.N., Thompson, H. and Allan, R.N. (1981) Adenocarcinoma of the small intestine complicating Crohn's disease. *Gut*, **12**, 188–193.
6. Poulsen, S.S., Pedersen, W.T., Jarnum, S. (1984) 'Micro erosions' in rectal biopsies in Crohn's disease. *Scandinavian Journal of Gastroenterology*, **19**, 607–612.
7. Rosekrans, P.C.M., Maijer, C.J.L.M., van der Wal, A.M. *et al.* (1980) Immunoglobulin containing cells in inflammatory bowel disease. *Gut*, **21**, 941–947.
8. Scott, B.B., Goodall, A., Stephenson, P. and Jenkins, R. (1983) Rectal mucosal plasma cells in inflammatory bowel disease. *Gut*, **24**, 519–524.
9. Shepherd, W.A., Hall, P.A., Williams, G.T. *et al.* (1989) Primary malignant lymphoma of the large intestine complicating chronic inflammatory bowel disease. *Histopathology*, **15**, 325–337.
10. Thompson, H. and Bonser, R.S. (1981) Granuloma, arteritis and inflammatory cell counts in Crohn's disease. In *Recent Advances of Crohn's Disease* (Ed.) Pena, A.S., Weterman, I.T., Booth, C.C. and Stroler, W. pp. 80–83. The Hague: Martinus Nijhoff.
11. Thompson, H. and Cockel, R. (1982) Crohn's disease of the duodenum. *Schweizerische Rundschau für Medizin (Praxis)*, **71**, 374–377.
12. Yardley, J.H. and Hamilton, S.R. (1981) Focal nonspecific inflammation (FNI) in Crohn's disease. In *Recent Advances in Crohn's Disease* (Ed.) Pena, A.S., Weterman, I.T., Booth, C.C. and Stroler, W. pp. 62–66. The Hague: Martinus Nijhoff.

CLINICAL PRESENTATION *(R.N. Allan)*

Crohn's disease is an uncommon disorder so that the number of patients with Crohn's disease seen by any one doctor is usually small. Further, among the many patients referred to hospital, Crohn's disease is a rare explanation for abdominal symptoms. These features explain why the diagnosis is often delayed or overlooked.

The mean age at onset of symptoms is 30 years with an equal sex distribution. Persistent gastrointestinal symptoms in patients of this age group should alert the physician to the possibility of Crohn's disease. Crohn's disease may, however, occur at any age[37] and, to compound the difficulty, symptoms may be transient or intermittent, and patients are often asymptomatic at the time of the first consultation. Finally the term 'Crohn's disease' comprises a spectrum of disorders, the nature of whose presentation will vary according to the site and extent of the macroscopic involvement and whether any local complications have occurred.

History

General comments

A careful history from the symptomatic patient will usually elicit symptoms suggestive of organic disease which would warrant further investigation. The site of macroscopic disease can be readily identified radiologically but only after the investigation has been requested! Features such as persistent change in bowel habit, urgency, diarrhoea at night and rectal bleeding all point to an organic basis for symptoms. Careful assessment should be made of the frequency and severity of abdominal pain. Discussion with the family provides a new and helpful slant when the severity and importance of symptoms is uncertain. Clear evidence of a change in appetite and weight loss are also useful pointers. In children even severe abdominal symptoms may only be revealed by careful direct questioning.

Anorexia is sometimes confused with anorexia nervosa and the label 'irritable bowel syndrome' should not be applied lightly until organic disease has been carefully considered and excluded. Rarely patients with persistent symptoms but no abnormal physical signs in whom blood tests and good-quality radiological investigations are normal develop macroscopic or radiological evidence of Crohn's disease several years later. Those few patients with significant and positive symptoms can readily be kept under review to ensure that the correct diagnosis is established.

Physical examination

Physical examination usually reveals clear signs that suggest organic disease and points the way to further investigation, but of course a completely normal physical examination does not exclude Crohn's disease. The clinical features that suggest the diagnosis include the extraintestinal manifestation of finger clubbing, arthritis or erythema nodosum. There may be clear evidence of recent weight loss or a palpable mass or enterocutaneous fistula on abdominal examination. A simple perineal examination usually points to the diagnosis because most patients with Crohn's disease have perianal lesions. The presence of skin tags may be a helpful early pointer to the diagnosis.

The history and physical examination will not only suggest whether there are organic features worthy of further investigation, but will also help to determine the site of macroscopic disease and whether local complications are present.

Among a large series of patients with Crohn's disease referred to the General Hospital, Birmingham, the distribution of macroscopic disease at presentation was: distal ileum with or without involvement of the right colon (66%), extensive colonic involvement (14%), distal colonic involvement (5%), diffuse small bowel disease (5%), other sites (7%).[18,20] The specific features at presentation are determined by the site of macroscopic disease.

Distal ileal disease

The distal ileum, with or without involvement of the right colon, is the most common site of macroscopic disease. Symptoms usually arise from the macroscopic change in the distal ileum. Macroscopic disease of the right colon alone is rare.

Obstructive symptoms

With active mucosal disease

Recurrent bouts of subacute colicky abdominal pain, abdominal distension and rumbling are usually associated with systemic disturbance including malaise, fever, anorexia and weight loss.

The abdominal pain may be associated with diarrhoea, probably caused by increased sodium and water secretion from the small intestine proximal to the stenotic segment.

Inactive mucosal fibrous stricture

Distal ileal Crohn's disease has usually progressed to fibrous stricture formation by the time that the diagnosis is made. Stricture formation leads to intermittent obstructive symptoms which are usually short-lived and the patient is well and symptom-free between these episodes.

The pain may be vague, intermittent or atypical in site. Persistent or recurrent symptoms should prompt a request for a barium follow-through examination.[13] Some patients elude early diagnosis because an endoscopy and barium enema examination have been requested. The changes in the distal ileum are easily overlooked particularly if there is no retrograde filling of the distal ileum with contrast during the barium enema examination.

Abscess formation

Abscess formation results from either local perforation proximal to a stricture, perforation through a penetrating ulcer or inflammatory change in locally involved lymph nodes. This complication is associated with systemic disturbance anorexia, weight loss, fever and malaise. On examination, there is usually, but not invariably, either a tender mass in the right iliac fossa or psoas spasm.

Local sepsis, if undetected, can lead to severe malnutrition. Such a patient is illustrated in *Figure 7.30*. She had been treated by resection of the distal ileum some 5 years earlier. Her symptoms had recurred and she was advised to rest at home. Three months later at her first consultation she was wasted, anaemic, dehydrated and there was a palpable mass in the right iliac fossa. At laparotomy a large abscess was drained and recurrent Crohn's disease of the

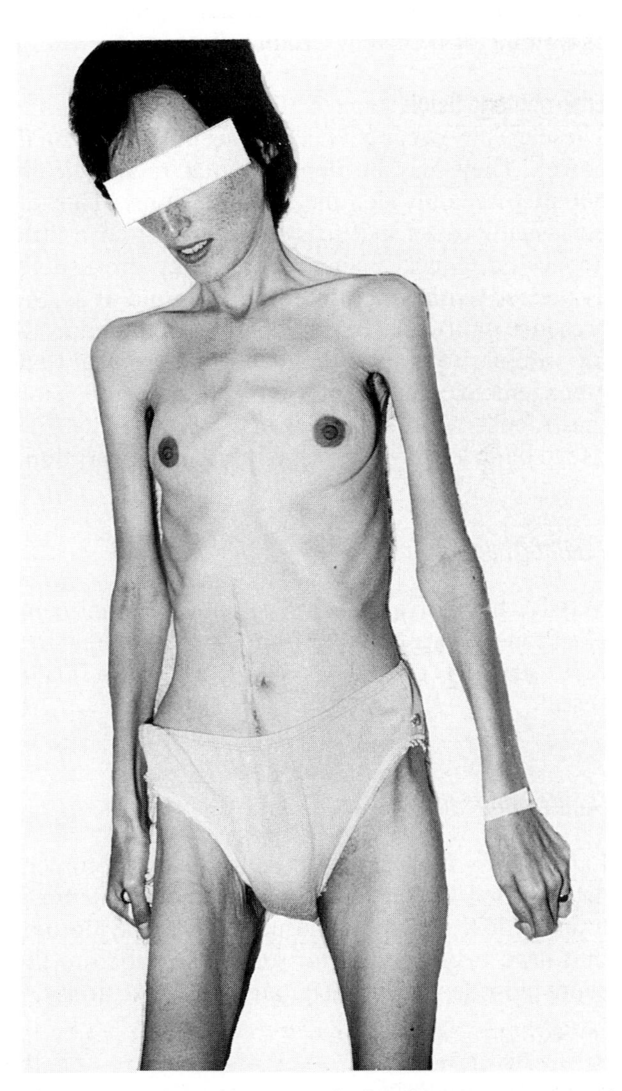

Figure 7.30 Abscess formation in Crohn's disease: appearance at presentation after resting at home for 3 months. Note scar of previous resection of distal ileum for Crohn's disease some 5 years previously.

ileum was resected. The stricture which had given rise to such severe complications was only 2 cm in length!

Fistula formation

Enterocutaneous fistula[19]

Enterocutaneous fistulas may follow laparotomy for suspected appendicitis. The fistula does not arise from the appendix stump but from adjacent loops of ileum damaged at surgery, or from the site of a local perforation which has been oversewn. Fistula formation commonly follows incision and drainage of a local abscess. Spontaneous enterocutaneous fistulas are rare but may be a presenting feature in recurrent Crohn's disease. They must be distinguished from post-operative enterocutaneous fistulas which follow an anastomotic leak where there is no evidence of residual or recurrent Crohn's disease.

Enteroenteric fistula[15]

These usually occur between adjacent loops of small bowel. They may be demonstrated radiologically but are often only identified at laparotomy. They do not usually cause specific symptoms and have little impact on clinical management. They are usually associated with stricture formation and it is the presence or absence of symptoms from the underlying stricture formation that determines appropriate management. Enteroenteric fistulas at other sites (gastrocolic or enterocolic) may occasionally give rise to blind loop syndromes or even malabsorption.

Haemorrhage

Massive haemorrhage is a rare but important complication.[39] It arises either from ulcers proximal to a tight stricture or follows infiltration of a major vessel.

'Acute appendix'

Laparotomy may be undertaken to exclude appendicitis when Crohn's disease of the distal ileum is found. Close questioning usually reveals symptoms that have been present for some weeks before the acute episode which precipitated the laparotomy.

Colonic involvement[2]

The most common symptoms of extensive colonic involvement are diarrhoea and general malaise, often associated with anorexia and weight loss. The onset is usually insidious. A few patients present with fulminating colitis. Obstructive symptoms are uncommon, although vague persistent abdominal discomfort is often a feature.

Left-sided disease

This is a common site in older patients and usually associated with diverticular disease. The symptoms may mimic the underlying diverticular disease with attacks of pain in the left lower quadrant and intermittent diarrhoea. The natural history is usually benign with little systemic disturbance except for a few patients who present acutely with colonic perforation either initially or unexpectedly during the course of follow-up.

Perianal disease[4]

More than two-thirds of patients have perianal disease which is usually painless and asymptomatic. The appearances often look distressing to the examiner's eye, but perianal disease is only painful when complicated by local abscess formation or active anal fissure. Such episodes readily alert the clinician to the possibility of Crohn's disease, but the diagnosis has usually been made before complications ensue.

Diffuse small bowel disease[7]

This is a rare site for Crohn's disease although rather more common in children than in adults. The diagnosis may be elusive because the symptoms can be subtle particularly when there is no change in bowel habit. Even when the radiological examination shows extensive changes the patient may be asymptomatic, except perhaps for some mild peripheral oedema due to low serum albumin levels.

More commonly the patients present with severe symptoms of malaise, anorexia, weight loss, peripheral oedema and a low serum albumin.

The pattern of presentation varies according to the interval between the onset of symptoms and diagnosis. With time the diffuse change may either revert to normal or heal leaving multiple short strictures which lead to recurrent episodes of intestinal obstruction.

Oesophageal disease

Oesophageal disease is rare. Dyer *et al.*[10] described two cases of Crohn's disease of the oesophagus but could find no other examples in more than 2000 reported cases of Crohn's disease in 12 large reported series. Huchzermyer *et al.*[25] identified 21 cases from the literature including 5 of their own. Thirty-one cases of proven or presumed oesophageal Crohn's disease from the literature have been reviewed by Weterman.[47]

The most common symptom is progressive dysphagia causing marked weight loss which can become severe within a few weeks. Examination is often unhelpful except to confirm the weight loss. Aphthous ulcers may be present in the mouth.[14] Confusion can arise with fungal infections such as candidiasis, especially in patients receiving corticosteroids or immunosuppressive therapy.

Gastric and duodenal disease

The first report of duodenal involvement was published by Gottlieb and Aloent in 1937.[17] At least 200 cases had been reported in the literature by 1977.[33] A recent review of 89 patients with duodenal Crohn's disease (some of whom were included in an earlier series[33]) suggests that medical treatment relieves symptoms in the majority and only a third require surgical treatment, usually for obstructive symptoms.[34] The duodenum is more commonly involved than the stomach. Gastroduodenal lesions are usually associated with macroscopic disease in other parts of the gastrointestinal tract.

Epigastric pain is the predominant symptom, which often mimics peptic ulcer, although the poor response to antacids and H_2-receptor blockers may arouse suspicion. The macroscopic lesions can progress to stricture formation which causes abdominal pain, anorexia, nausea, vomiting and weight loss. Bleeding is uncommon. Physical examination is usually unhelpful except to confirm weight loss, but occasionally a succussion splash is found. It is surprising how few symptoms may be associated with what appears radiologically to be a tight duodenal stricture.

Extraintestinal manifestations

In some patients extraintestinal manifestations predominate. These features include erythema nodosum, aphthous ulcers of the mouth, acute arthritis, ankylosing spondylitis, ocular lesions or even pyoderma gangrenosum. Growth retardation in children occasionally occurs as the only symptom. However, gastrointestinal symptoms can usually be elicited on careful enquiry.

Summary

The history and physical examination often suggest the presence of organic disease and may suggest the site of macroscopic disease and, in particular, whether or not local complications have supervened.

DIAGNOSIS *(R.N. Allan)*

The diagnosis of the symptomatic patient should follow a clear analytical pathway to determine the site of macroscopic disease, whether the disease is active or inactive, and the identification or exclusion of metabolic problems or local complications.

The clinical features alert the clinician to the possibility that the symptomatic patient has Crohn's disease. Certain uncommon presentations such as ankylosing spondylitis or growth retardation alone may delay the diagnosis, but these presentations are rare. In most patients a good quality barium follow-through or barium enema examination will identify the characteristic features and define the site of macroscopic disease. The quality of the films must be considered in interpreting the report because, for example, the terminal ileum may not have been displayed well and early lesions in the colon, particularly aphthous ulcers, may have been overlooked. In a few symptomatic patients good quality radiological studies may be entirely normal for several years before unequivocal radiological change develops. The patient who has undergone extensive investigation and acquired a label of functional bowel disorder may be referred later to a colleague. The demonstration of a total colitis on repeat barium enema examination undermines everyone's confidence, except those of the colleague!

Rigid or flexible sigmoidoscopy or colonoscopy may reveal characteristic perianal disease or patchy mucosal change and, rarely, the classic aphthous ulcers. Biopsy can be helpful and granulomata may be identified even in apparently normal uninvolved mucosa, although many of these changes are confined to the submucosa whereas biopsies are often limited to the mucosa.

Laboratory tests are helpful, particularly as a screening procedure at the first outpatient visit. The symptomatic patient with abdominal pain and diarrhoea can readily be screened by measuring the haemoglobin, packed cell volume, serum iron, total iron-binding capacity, serum albumin, serum globulin and acute phase proteins (orosomucoids or C-reative proteins). The erythrocyte sedimentation rate (ESR) is helpful if elevated but normal values do not exclude Crohn's disease, because in some patients the result may be normal in the presence of active macroscopic disease. Normal values for all these indices are uncommon in patients with Crohn's disease except where the symptoms are due to an inactive fibrous stricture, or where there are short segments of active disease; however, in both these situations the radiological features are usually characteristic of Crohn's disease.

The symptomatic patient with established Crohn's disease should be subject to regular critical clinical reanalysis. The site and extent of macroscopic disease should be reviewed. Contrast radiological examination should be undertaken as often as indicated by the clinical problem. In most patients, particularly those with inactive disease, many years may elapse between examinations. However, patients with severe symptoms may require re-evaluation after only a few weeks. Distal ileal mucosal inflammatory lesions may progress to fibrous stricture. Patients with aphthous ulceration of the colon who have unexpected or persistent symptoms may require repeat barium enema examination or colonoscopy because the changes can progress to extensive colonic involvement within a few weeks. Patients with diffuse small bowel disease may need reassessment because the changes may either resolve or strictures may develop during the healing phase. The strictures may be amenable to surgical intervention. Diffuse small bowel disease may occasionally be followed by the development of extensive colonic disease in previously normal large bowel.

The possibility of metabolic problems inducing symptoms must be considered, for example, the malaise associated with fluid and electrolyte depletion (particularly potassium loss). Anaemia is common and may explain the symptoms of malaise or tiredness. Muscle weakness may be due to calcium malabsorption and osteomalacia. Trace metal deficiency, usually magnesium and occasionally zinc, should be considered and corrected, especially in patients with persistent diarrhoea. Correction of these metabolic problems will relieve many symptoms previously ascribed to 'the Crohn's disease'.

The local complications which may cause symptoms include stricture, abscess and fistula formation. They should all be considered and identified or excluded.

In patients with abdominal pain the symptoms may be due to associated disorders which appear in Crohn's disease more commonly than expected in the general population such as peptic ulcer, gallstones and renal stones, rather than the underlying disease itself.

Radiology

Developments in radiology have been well reviewed by Goldberg and Jeffrey.[16] The role and value of air contrast studies of the gastrointestinal tract are now well established (see also page 1141).

The value of infusion techniques in Crohn's disease of the small intestine have been analysed by Nolan and Gourtsoyiannis.[32] A variety of changes has been identified including discrete, longitudinal and fissure ulcers and sinuses. The double-contrast technique may even demonstrate small bowel adhesions. The natural history of the radiological appearances of discrete mucosal 'aphthous' ulcers has been well documented in serial studies.[28] The radiological findings correlate well with the pathological appearances. Many of the characteristic features are missing using a single-contrast technique.[21]

Newer techniques including gallium scanning,[38] grey scale ultrasound[24] and angiography of the gut[44] may all contribute to diagnosis.

A number of papers have assessed the use of isotope-labelled granulocytes in the assessment of inflammatory bowel disease. Patients prefer this technique but the sensitivity is not as good as conventional techniques and cannot be recommended for routine use, although it may well be of value in patients where there are real diagnostic dilemmas.[9]

Endoscopy

The role of colonoscopy in inflammatory bowel disease has been summarized in two good reviews.[23,48] Pera and his colleagues have evaluated a large number of endoscopic signs at colonoscopy. They concluded that discontinuous involvement, anal lesions and cobblestone mucosa are still the best hallmarks for Crohn's disease.[35] Although most patients with inflammatory bowel disease do not require colonoscopy, it plays an important role where there are diagnostic doubts or difficulties; it is used to determine the extent or severity of disease, the nature of stricture formation, to take mucosal biopsies to detect dysplasia and for primary diagnosis in children (see also page 1212).

The magnifying colonoscope with dye spraying is an interesting technique for demonstrating minute mucosal structure and has been recommended for monitoring response to treatment, the early detection of recurrence and for the prediction of remission.[41]

Histopathology

The value of large bowel biopsy in the differential diagnosis of inflammatory bowel disease has been reviewed by Chambers and Morson.[6] Surawicz *et al.*[40] examined 243 rectal biopsies from 90 patients with Crohn's disease and showed that, even with multiple serial sectioning, epithelioid granulomata were found in only 25%. Granulomata appear to be more common in the rectum and anus than elsewhere in the gastrointestinal tract, although these studies did not correct for variations in mucosal volume.[22] Specific features have been identified by stereomicroscopic examination of rectal biopsies from patients with ulcerative colitis. They include changes in the mucosal pattern, irregular enlarged gland openings filled with exudate, and patchy localization of goblet cells.[36] Scanning electron microscopy studies can readily distinguish between ulcerative colitis and Crohn's disease. Image analysis based on measurements of mucosal dimension, architecture and cell counts in both the lamina propria and epithelium of rectal biopsies showed that the most powerful discriminant was increased lamina propria cellularity in distinguishing chronic colitis from non-specific colitis.[26] For further information on histopathology, see page 1128.

Laboratory indices and diagnosis

Interpretation of laboratory data requires critical analysis. The information it provides complements the clinical history, physical findings, and the results of radiological and sigmoidoscopic examinations.

In most symptomatic patients presenting for the first time, the laboratory indices will be abnormal. Unexplained anaemia, elevated ESR or acute phase proteins, such as C-reactive proteins or serum orosomucoids, and a low serum albumin all point to an organic basis in patients presenting with abdominal symptoms.

Serum albumin levels are useful as indices of activity. They reflect the degree of inflammatory activity in the gut because there is a close relationship between serum albumin levels and gastrointestinal protein loss in inflammatory bowel disease.[27]

The half-life of serum albumin is of the order of 20 days so that serum albumin levels do not alter rapidly but reflect the situation over a period of 1–2 weeks.

Acute phase proteins are also useful in determining disease activity. Seromucoids, a group of α_1-glycoproteins soluble in 0.6 mol/l perchloric acid, were first used by Cooke and his colleagues.[8] The predominant protein is orosomucoid (acid α_1-glycoprotein), for which a specific assay of α_1-glycoprotein is available.[43] The half-life of seromucoids is about 5 days, so the speed of response is much more rapid than serum albumin. A variety of other acute phase proteins have also been utilized.[46]

An elevated ESR is a useful index and reflects the increased secretion of α-globulin, fibrinogen and α-globulin by the liver. However, the ESR is sometimes normal in proteins with active inflammatory bowel disease. A normal ESR does not therefore exclude active disease.

Other useful laboratory indices include C-reactive protein which correlates well with clinical indices of activity.[11] These proteins have a short half-life and so are a sensitive index for rapid assessment of change in severity.

Problems in diagnosis

The distinction between ulcerative colitis and Crohn's disease is probably still best drawn by Kirsner[29] whilst the differential diagnosis of ulcerative colitis and Crohn's disease from other specific inflammatory bowel diseases has been the subject of an excellent review.[42] Tuberculosis of the gastrointestinal tract has to be considered seriously in the differential diagnosis, particularly in the immigrant population.[12] Campylobacter enterocolitis has recently been highlighted in the differential diagnosis.[30] Late-onset Crohn's disease is often found in association with diverticular disease.[3]

The diagnostic errors and reasons for delay in the diagnosis of Crohn's disease have been analysed in a large series of patients.[1] A group of 140 patients with Crohn's disease were grouped according to the site of macroscopic disease – small bowel (61), ileocolic (30), colon alone (40) and anorectal (9). In these patients, the mean interval between the onset of symptoms and referral to hospital was only 2.9 months so that the family practitioner is completely exonerated from blame for the delay in establishing the diagnosis.

The correst diagnosis was established in two-thirds of the patients within 2 years of the onset of symptoms. The diagnostic problems in 20% were confined to the distinction between ulcerative colitis and Crohn's disease, which had little effect on management.

Misdiagnosis was most common in small bowel disease. A diagnosis of acute appendicitis which proves to be Crohn's disease may dent the pride of the diagnostician, but has limited impact on management. On careful questioning, most patients with Crohn's disease of the distal ileum mimicking acute appendicitis reveal a history of abdominal symptoms for several months before the acute episode supervened. A label of psychiatric disorder was common. Other patients presenting with abdominal pain had diagnostic labels of peptic ulcer or gallstones attached to them.

The most common misdiagnosis in ileocolonic and colonic disease was to attach a psychiatric label to abdominal symptoms which subsequently were shown to have an organic basis. Overall an incorrect diagnosis of psychiatric disorders was made in 19% of the patients.

Simple screening tests for organic disease were helpful but not diagnostic because only half the patients were anaemic and two-thirds had an elevated ESR. The diagnostic confusion commonly arose because of the non-specific nature of the initial symptoms which led the patients to be referred to a number of different specialists.

Diagnostic tests to avoid such pitfalls have always been an attractive proposition. Walker[45] demonstrated that normal buccal mucosa from patients with Crohn's disease incubated with their own serum and then stained with deposited antibody by fluorescent techniques showed a positive reaction not observed in mucosa from normal subjects or patients with ulcerative colitis. Further work suggests that the tests may not be sufficiently specific to be used in differential diagnosis.[31]

REFERENCES

1. Admans, H., Whorwell, P.J. and Wright, R. (1980) Diagnosis of Crohn's disease. *Digestive Diseases and Science*, **25**, 911–915.
2. Allan, R.N., Steinberg, D.M., Alexander-Williams, J. and Cooke, W.T. (1977) Crohn's disease involving the colon: an audit of clinical management. *Gastroenterology*, **73**, 723–732.
3. Berman, I.R., Corman, M.L., Collier, J.A. and Veidenheimer, M.C. (1979) Late onset Crohn's disease in patients with colonic diverticulitis. *Diseases of the Colon and Rectum*, **22**, 524–529.
4. Buchmann, P., Keighley, M.R.B., Alexander-Williams, J. and Allan, R.N. (1980) The natural history of perianal Crohn's disease. *American Journal of Surgery*, **140**, 642–644.
5. Chambers, T.J. and Morson, B.C. (1977) The granuloma in Crohn's disease. *Gut*, **20**, 269–274.
6. Chambers, T.J. and Morson, B.C. (1980) Large bowel biopsy in the differential diagnosis of inflammatory bowel disease. *Investigative Cell Pathology*, **3**, 159–173.
7. Cooke, W.T. and Swan, C.J.H. (1974) Diffuse jejuno ileitis. *Quarterly Journal of Medicine*, **43**, 583.
8. Cooke, W.T., Fowler, D.C. and Cox, E.V. (1958) The clinical significance of seromucoids in regional ileitis and ulcerative colitis. *Gastroenterology*, **34**, 910–919.
9. Crama-Bohbouth, G.E., Arndt, J.W., Pena, A.S. *et al.* (1988) Value of indium-III granulocyte scintigraphy in the assessment of Crohn's disease of the small intestine—Prospective investigation. *Digestion*, **40**, 227–236.
10. Dyer, N.K., Cooke, P.I. and Kemp Harper, R.A. (1969) Oesophageal stricture associated with Crohn's disease. *Gut*, **10**, 549–554.
11. Fagan, E.A., Dyck, R.F., Maton, P.N. *et al.* (1982) Serum levels of C-reactive protein in Crohn's disease and ulcerative colitis. *European Journal of Clinical Investigation*, **12**, 351–359.
12. Findlay, J.M. (1979) Tuberculosis of the gastrointestinal tract in Bradford 1967–1977. *Journal of the Royal Society of Medicine*, **72**, 587–590.
13. Fraser, G.M. and Adam, R.D. (1988) Modification to the gas enhanced small bowel barium follow through examination using gastrograffin and compression. *Clinical Radiology*, **39**, 537–541.
14. Geboes, K., Janssens, J., Rutgeerts, P. and Vantrappen, G. (1986) Crohn's disease of the oesophagus. *Journal of Clinical Gastroenterology*, **84**, 249–254.
15. Givel, J.C., Hawker, P.C., Allan, R.N. and Alexander-Williams, J. (1983) Entero-enteric fistula complicating Crohn's disease. *Journal of Clinical Gastroenterology*, **5**, 321–323.
16. Goldberg, H.I. and Jeffrey, R.B. (1980) Recent advances in the radiographic evaluation of inflammatory bowel disease. *Medical Clinics of North America*, **64**, 1059–1081.
17. Gottlieb, C.H. and Aloent, S. (1937) Regional jejunitis. *American Journal of Roentgenology*, **38**, 881–883.
18. Gyde, S.N., Prior, P., Macartney, J.C. *et al.* (1980) Malignancy in Crohn's disease. *Gut*, **21**, 1024–1029.
19. Hawker, P.C., Givel, J.C., Keighley, M.R.B. *et al.* (1983) Management of enterocutaneous fistulae in Crohn's disease. *Gut*, **24**, 284–287.
20. Higgens, C.S. and Allan, R.N. (1980) Crohn's disease of the distal ileum. *Gut*, **21**, 933–940.
21. Hildell, J., Lindstrom, C. and Wenckert, A. (1979) Radiographic appearances in Crohn's disease. 1. Accuracy of radiographic methods. *Acta Radiologica (Diagnosis)*, **20**, 609–625.
22. Hill, R.M., Kent, T.H. and Hansen, R.N. (1979) Clinical usefulness of rectal biopsy in Crohn's disease. *Gastroenterology*, **77**, 938–944.
23. Hogan, W.J., Hensley, G.T. and Greenen, J.E. (1980) Endoscopic evaluation of inflammatory bowel disease. *Medical Clinics of North America*, **64**, 1083–1102.
24. Holt, S. and Samuel, E. (1979) Grey scale ultrasound in Crohn's disease. *Gut*, **20**, 590–595.
25. Huchzermyer, G., Paul, F., Seifert, E. *et al.* (1976) Endoscopic results in five patients with Crohn's disease of the oesophagus. *Endoscopy*, **8**, 75–81.
26. Jenkins, D., Goodall, A., Drew, K. and Scott, B.B. (1988) What is colitis? Statistical approach to distinguishing clinically important inflammatory change in rectal biopsy specimens. *Journal of Clinical Pathology*, **41**, 72–79.
27. Jensen, K.B., Jarnum, S., Koudhal, G. and Kristensen, M. (1976) Serum orosomucoid in ulcerative colitis. Its relation to clinical activity, protein loss and turnover of albumin, IgG. *Scandinavian Journal of Gastroenterology*, **11**, 177–183.
28. Joffe, N. (1980) Radiographic appearances and course of discrete mucosal ulcers in Crohn's disease of the colon. *Gastrointestinal Radiology*, **5**, 371–378.
29. Kirsner, J.B. (1975) Problems in the differentiation of ulcerative colitis and Crohn's disease: the need

for repeated diagnostic evaluation. *Gastroenterology*, **68**, 187–191.
30. Loss, R.W., Mangle, J.C. and Pereira, M. (1980) Campylobacter colitis presenting as inflammatory bowel disease with segmental colonic ulceration. *Gastroenterology*, **79**, 138–140.
31. Matthews, N., Tapper-Jones, L., Mayberry, J.F. and Rhodes, J. (1979) Buccal biopsy in diagnosis of Crohn's disease. *The Lancet*, **1**, 500–501.
32. Nolan, D.J. and Gourtsoyiannis, N.C. (1980) Crohn's disease of the small intestine: a review of the radiological appearances in 100 consecutive patients scanned by a barium infusion technique. *Clinical Radiology*, **31**, 597–603.
33. Nugent, F.W., Richmond, M. and Park, S.K. (1977) Crohn's disease of the duodenum. *Gut*, **18**, 115–120.
34. Nugent, F.W. and Roy, M.A. (1989) Duodenal Crohn's disease: an analysis of 89 cases. *American Journal of Gastroenterology*, **84**, 249–254.
35. Pera, A., Bellando, P., Caldera, D. *et al.* (1987) Colonoscopy in inflammatory bowel disease: Diagnostic accuracy and proposal of an endoscopic score. *Gastroenterology*, **92**, 181–185.
36. Poulsen, S.S., Christensen, K.C., Petri, M. and Jarnum, S. (1980) Stereomicroscopic examination of stained rectal biopsies in ulcerative colitis and Crohn's disease. *Scandinavian Journal of Gastroenterology*, **15**, 535–544.
37. Puntis, J., McNeish, A.S. and Allan, R.N. (1984) Long term prognosis of childhood onset of Crohn's disease. *Gut*, **25**, 329–336.
38. Rheingold, O.J., Tedesco, F.J., Block, F.E. *et al.* (1979) (^{67}Ga) Citrate scintiscanning in active inflammatory bowel disease. *Digestive Diseases and Science*, **24**, 363–368.
39. Rubin, M., Herrington, J.R. and Schneider, R. (1980) Regional enteritis with major gastrointestinal haemorrhage as the initial manifestation. *Archives of Internal Medicine*, **140**, 217–219.
40. Surawicz, C.M., Meisel, J.L., Ylvisaker, T. *et al.* (1981) Rectal biopsy in the diagnosis of Crohn's disease: value of multiple biopsies and serial sectioning. *Gastroenterology*, **80**, 60–71.
41. Tada, M., Misaki, F., Shimono, M. *et al.* (1978) Endoscopic studies on the microscopic structure of colonic mucosa in the follow-up observation of ulcerative colitis. *Gastroenterologica Japonica*, **13**, 72–76.
42. Tedesco, F.H. (1980) Differential diagnosis of ulcerative colitis and Crohn's ileo-colitis and other specific inflammatory disease of the bowel. *Medical Clinics of North America*, **64**, 1173–1183.
43. Thaw, P.A. and Allbutt, E.C. (1980) A critical evaluation of serum seromucoid assay and its replacement by a serum alpha-1-acid gylcoprotein assay. *Annals of Clinical Biochemistry*, **17**, 140–143.
44. Tsuchiya, M., Muira, S., Asakura, H. *et al.* (1980) Angiographic evaluation of vascular changes in ulcerative colitis. *Angiography*, **31**, 147–153.
45. Walker, J.E. (1978) Possible diagnostic test for Crohn's disease by use of buccal mucosa. *The Lancet*, **2**, 759–760.
46. Weeke, B. and Jarnum, S. (1971) Serum concentrations of 19 serum proteins in Crohn's disease and ulcerative colitis. *Gut*, **12**, 297–302.
47. Weterman, I. (1983) Oral, oesophageal and gastroduodenal Crohn's disease. In *Inflammatory Bowel Diseases* (Ed.) Allan, R.N., Keighley, M.R.B., Alexander-Williams, J. and Hawkins, C.F. Edinburgh: Churchill Livingstone.
48. Williams, C.B. and Wayne, J.C. (1978) Colonoscopy in inflammatory bowel disease. *Clinics in Gastroenterology*, **7**, 701–717.

RADIOLOGY AND ENDOSCOPY

(J.R. Lee)

The roles of endoscopy and radiology in Crohn's disease are complementary. Both are of value in the diagnosis and assessment of upper gastrointestinal and large bowel disease but radiology is superior for routine use in the small intestine. Endoscopy, in general, allows a more accurate close-up assessment of the gastrointestinal mucosa, but good quality double-contrast barium radiology also has a high accuracy, approaching, and occasionally superior to, endoscopy. Which of these methods is used depends a great deal upon the experience and availability of the radiologist and endoscopist. Not all patients with known or suspected Crohn's disease warrant endoscopy. A prime indication is to establish the presence and extent of the disease in patients with normal or doubtful radiological studies. The aim of both radiology and endoscopy is to demonstrate the essential pathological features of Crohn's disease – oedema, ulceration, fibrosis and fistulas. The hallmark of Crohn's disease is the asymmetry and discontinuous distribution of the disease process.

RADIOLOGY

Radiology is widely available and the greater use of double-contrast barium examinations using improved barium suspensions and pharmacological techniques has improved the visualization of fine mucosal detail. In general, barium studies are more comfortable for the patient and give a superior overall picture of the extent of the disease. The features and extent of extraluminal disease can only be detected and assessed by radiology. A permanent record of the examination is, of course, an integral part of the procedure.

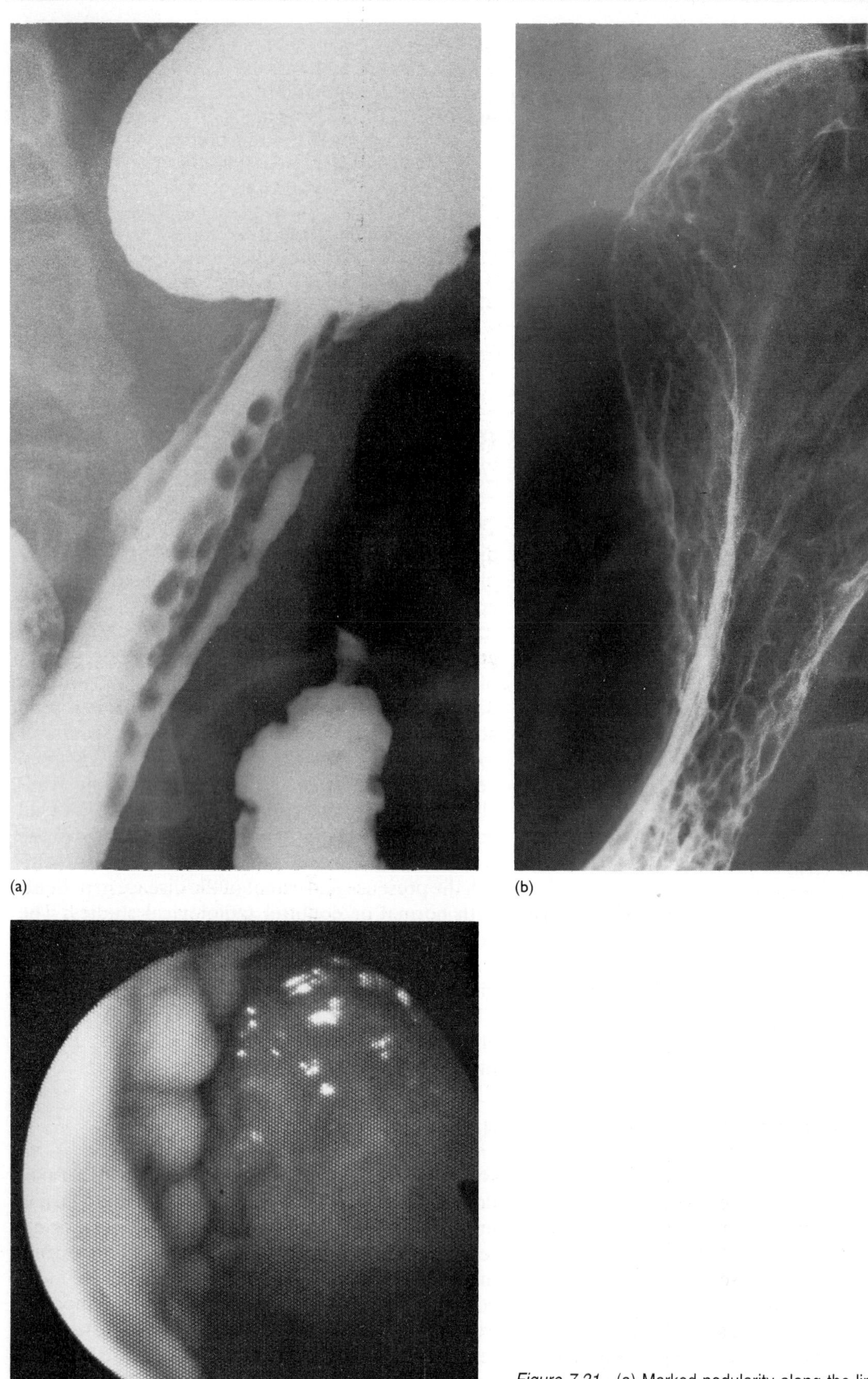

Figure 7.31 (a) Marked nodularity along the line of rugal folds in single-contrast barium-filled phase; (b) the same patient in double (air) contrast phase. (c) The endoscopic appearance. Note that there is no ulceration between the nodules.

ENDOSCOPY

Medical staff experienced in endoscopy are not so readily available and the examination can be uncomfortable for the patient. Endoscopic procedures require sedation of the patient and are more hazardous than a barium examination. However, in experienced hands, endoscopy gives a better evaluation of the mucosal appearance than radiology. The mucosa is seen in full colour and alteration of mucosal vascularity can be an indication of early disease. Aphthous ulceration is better seen than with radiology. The field of view through an endoscope is, however, small, and the extent of the disease may be difficult to record. Permanent documentation of the mucosal appearance is not a regular feature of endoscopic examinations, although this is more easily done with greater availability of video-endoscopy and the opinion and experience of the examiner are extremely important. A particular and important strength of endoscopy is the ability to obtain tissue for histological examination for an exact diagnosis. Tissue biopsies obtained via an endoscope are small, often involving only the surface of the mucosa. The presence of the diagnostic epithelioid granulomata can usually be found only in a relatively small number of biopsies, and the definite histological diagnosis can be made in less than 25% of patients.[22] It is important, therefore, to take numerous biopsies from several sites.[21] The most reliable site for a successful diagnostic biopsy is on the margin of the early lesion such as an aphthous ulcer.[16]

OEDEMA

In the early stages, the mucosa becomes swollen. Radiologically this can be seen as a coarsening of the fine mucosal detail. This is best seen in the colon on double-contrast barium enema. Endoscopically, the vascularity may be altered, either becoming more prominent with an overall reddening of the mucosa or the normal vascular pattern may be obscured by thickened, oedematous mucosa. In later stages, the mucosal folds become thickened, straightened and distorted and these may be seen both radiologically and through the endoscope. Mucosal nodules may be seen, and these are often discrete. Some nodularity is due to surrounding ulceration, leaving islands of normal mucosa. This is best seen endoscopically. Some nodularity, however, is due to mucosal thickening without associated ulceration (*Figure 7.31*). Gross oedema may affect the whole bowel wall thickness and give rise to 'hosepipe thickening' with swollen loops of intestine. Radiologically, this is best seen in the distal ileum where it is shown by separation of the barium-filled bowel (*Figure 7.32*). It is also seen well on computed tomography (CT) scans (*Figure 7.33*). Endoscopically, areas of hosepipe thickening will be shown as a narrowed lumen with a stiff non-pliable wall often associated with mucosal ulceration.

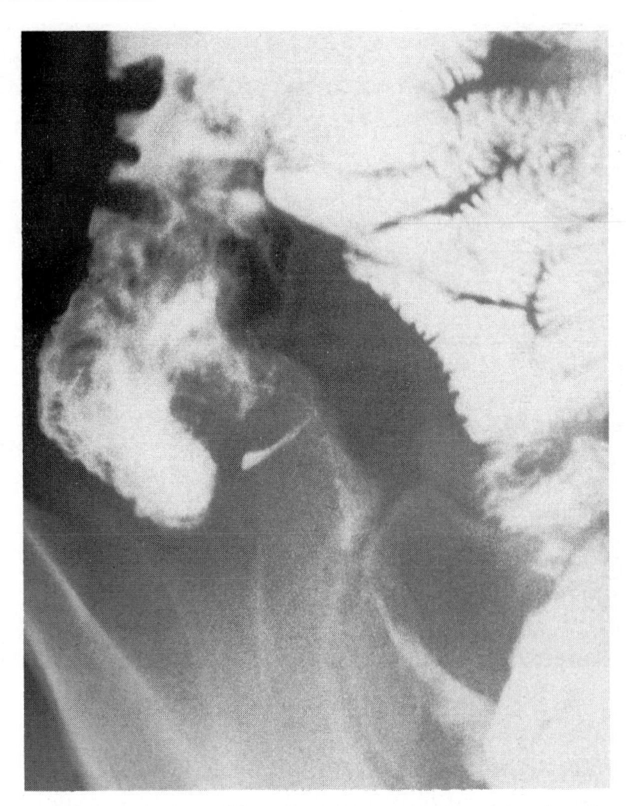

Figure 7.32 Barium follow-through examination showing the narrowed ulcerated terminal ileum separated from adjacent barium-filled bowel by grossly oedematous ileum. There is a deep sinus/fissure 2 cm from the ileocaecal valve.

ULCERATION

Shallow aphthous or aphthoid ulceration is probably the earliest stage of ulceration that can be shown macroscopically.[14] It is intramucosal and cannot be seen radiologically in profile projecting outside the bowel lumen. It is seen *en face* as a central speck of barium with a dark translucent surround of mucosal oedema.

Endoscopically, there is usually an erythematous area with a small central depression, and as the ulcer becomes larger the central area shows a white slough in the base. Aphthous ulcers may be entirely discrete with large areas of surrounding normal mucosa and both endoscopically and radiologically are best seen in the colon (*Figure 7.34*). Disease progression

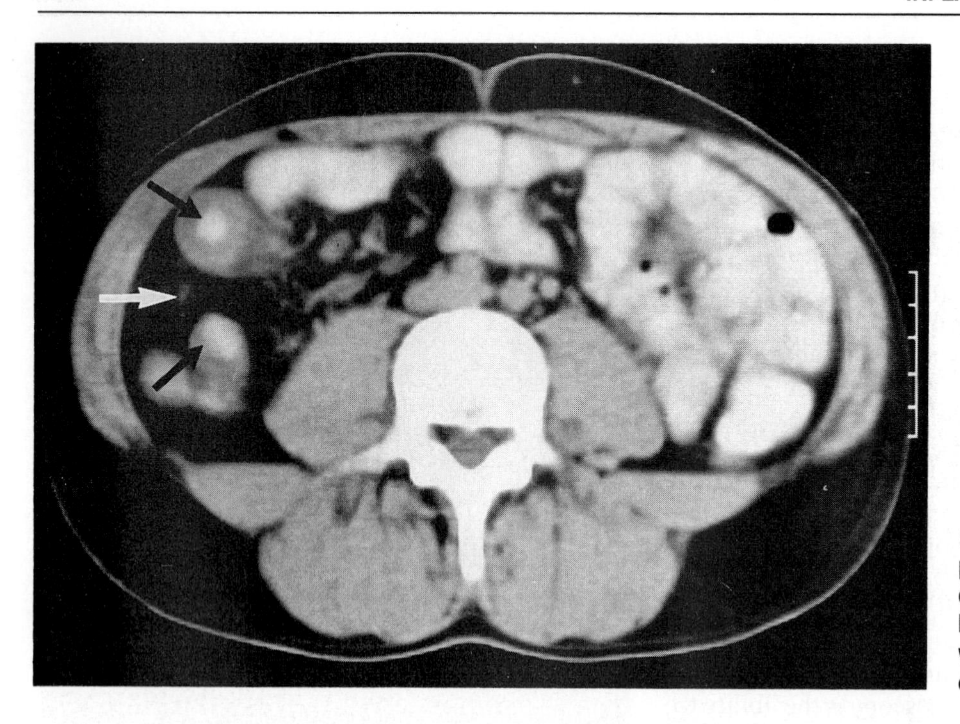

Figure 7.33 CT examination of a patient with terminal ileal Crohn's disease. Thickened loops of small bowel are shown (black arrows) with intervening increased mesenteric fat (white arrow).

leads to an increase in ulceration, both geographically and deep into the mucosa with ulcer coalescence. This gives rise to a varying pattern of ulceration which is often bizarre. Long linear ulcers may occur, which in the colon are along the line of the taenia coli (*Figure 7.35*). Large areas of mucosal ulceration lead to denuded patches. Linear and transverse ulceration together show as a 'cobblestone' pattern (*Figure 7.36*). Deep, penetrating ulcers are said to have a 'rosethorn' appearance radiologically but this is not pathognomonic of Crohn's disease.[18] In the author's experience use of double-contrast radiology stretches the bowel wall and obliterates some of the deep ulceration, especially in the colon. Intramucosal extension gives rise to a 'collar stud' lesion[11] which, if multiple, shows as a continuous track in the submucosa radiologically. Varying stages of ulceration may occur at the same time, and usually severe ulceration is surrounded at the margin by shallow ulcers.

FIBROSIS

Fibrosis develops as the disease heals. If it occurs in a circumferential manner then a stricture will result. Many apparent strictures are, however, due to spasm or oedema. Fluoroscopy or endoscopy, aided by an intravenous antispasmodic drug, will normally distinguish the two types. Shortening from fibrosis in the long axis of the bowel will often lead to pseudosacculation as the disease process is usually asymmetrical and the mesenteric border is frequently more affected.[13] Transmural fibrosis will lead to angulation and adherence of bowel loops which can give rise to intestinal obstruction.

FISTULAS

Fistulas are probably an extension of deep, transmural ulcerations which penetrate into adjacent structures. The most commonly found fistulas are enteroenteric, and the majority are short and within a few centimetres of the ileocaecal valve, giving rise to minimal short bowel circuit. Fistulas between terminal ileum and sigmoid colon give rise to more obvious clinical symptoms such as diarrhoea. Many fistulas are complex, with many pathways, and are the result of an abscess. Sinuses are the precursor of fistulas and often arise from the terminal ileum (see *Figure 7.32*) or the anal region. Most patients with perianal lesions in Crohn's disease, however, have a normal rectum radiologically. Although fistulas may be seen using CT this is not a reliable method of detection. Contrast radiology remains the method of choice.

EXTRALUMINAL DISEASE

Using cross-sectional methods of imaging such as ultrasound, computed tomography and magnetic resonance imaging, it is now appreciated that extraluminal manifestations, such as fatty infiltration of the mesentery, lymph node enlargement, bowel wall thickening and abscess formation, are more common than previously thought and more easily detected.[5]

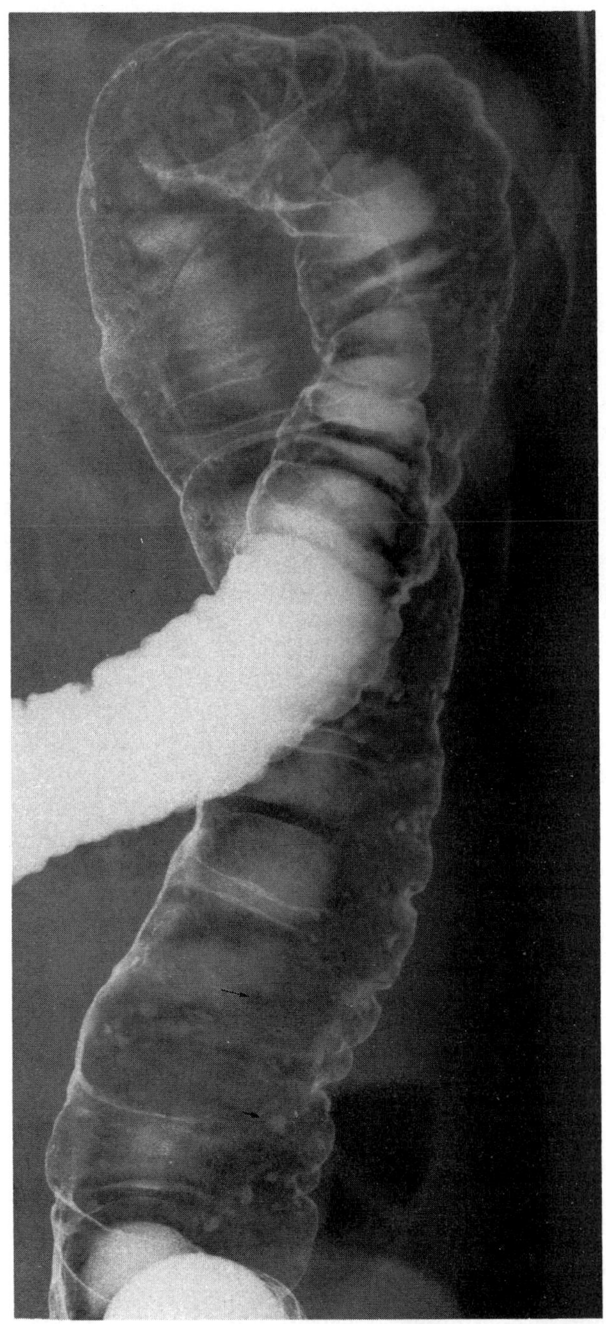

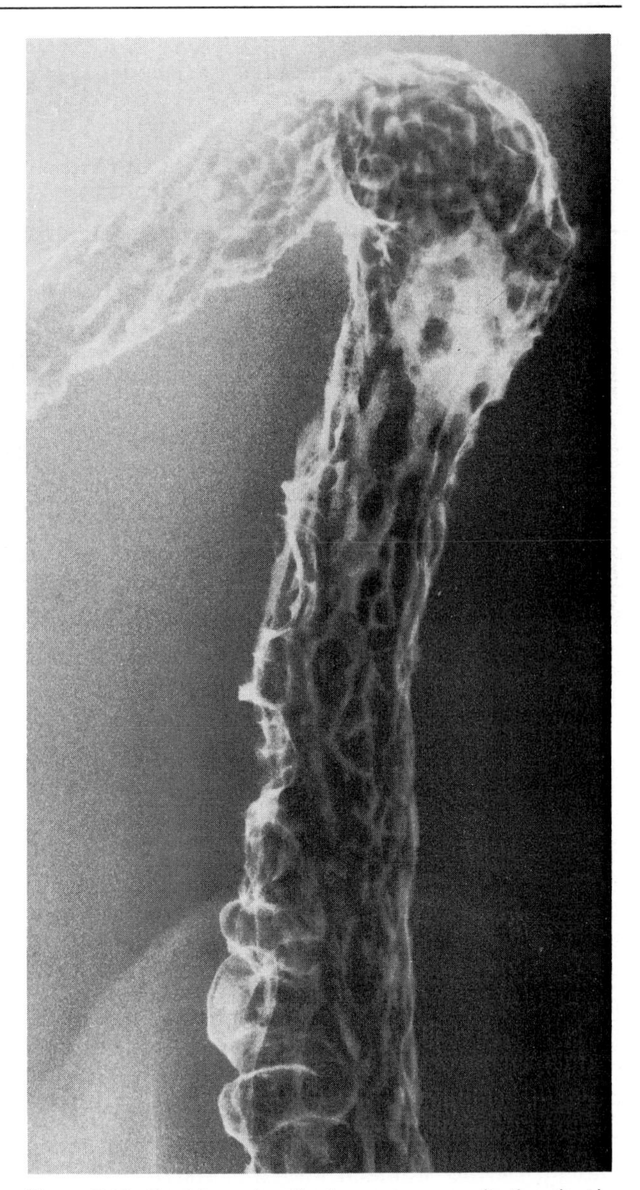

Figure 7.36 Double-contrast barium enema examination showing marked 'cobblestone' formation of the mucosa with longitudinal and transverse ulceration.

Figure 7.34 Double-contrast barium enema examination in a colon studded with discrete shallow aphthous ulcers of varying size. The white areas represent the shallow ulcer crater and the narrow dark halo represents surrounding oedema. In between the ulcers the colonic mucosa is normal.

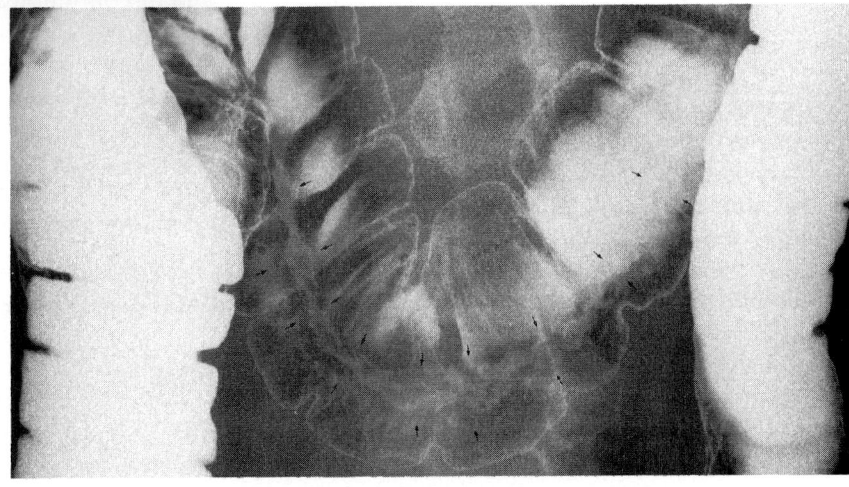

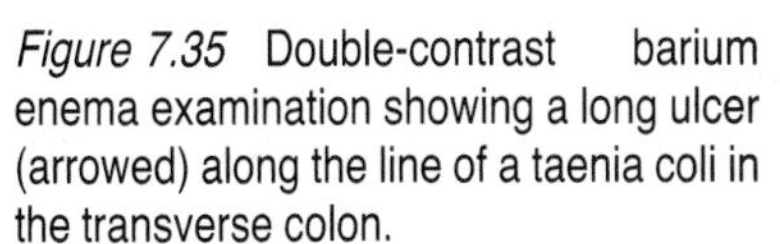

Figure 7.35 Double-contrast barium enema examination showing a long ulcer (arrowed) along the line of a taenia coli in the transverse colon.

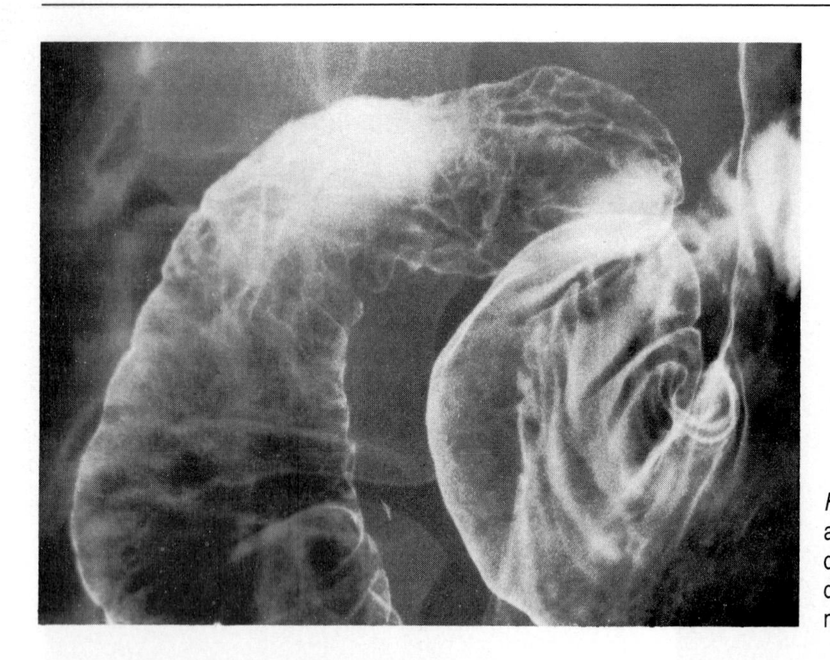

Figure 7.37 Double-contrast barium meal examination showing mosaic appearance of the duodenal cap and proximal part of the descending duodenum. There is an abrupt change to normal mucosa in the remaining parts of the duodenum.

FEATURES AT SPECIFIC SITES

Oesophagus, stomach and duodenum

These parts can be examined easily and accurately by endoscopy and double-contrast barium meal examination which has an accuracy approaching that of endoscopy.[6,9] Crohn's disease of the oesophagus is uncommon. Its features are mimicked by those of reflux oesophagitis, which is extremely common. Endoscopically, they are very similar and Crohn's disease of the oesophagus is rarely diagnosed radiologically. Oesophageal Crohn's disease can progress to stricture or fistula formation.[3] The granulomatous process more commonly affects the antrum of the stomach and the first part of the duodenum, usually in contiguity. In its severe form, it leads to narrowing of the gastric outlet, which may require surgical bypass for relief. Severe disease of the stomach is recorded in 1–4% of patients[4] and severe duodenal disease is found in 4–7% of patients with Crohn's disease elsewhere in the gastrointestinal tract. However, routine demonstration of the surface mucosa by double-contrast barium examinations has revealed lesser mucosal abnormalities of the stomach and duodenum in up to 40% of patients with Crohn's disease of the ileum or colon[10] and this has been the author's experience. Mucosal abnormalities are also seen endoscopically in either the oesophagus, stomach or duodenum in approximately 50% of patients with small or large bowel Crohn's disease.[8] Correlation between endoscopy, radiology and histology, however, is not exact. Minor histological abnormalities, some diagnostic of Crohn's disease, are found in patients who are radiologically and endoscopically normal. The minor changes of oedema and aphthous ulceration are usually indistinguishable, radiologically and endoscopically, from the gastroduodenal erosions seen in peptic ulcer disease. Mucosal irregularity along the line of rugal folds is sometimes seen in the stomach. This appearance is specific for Crohn's disease (see *Figure 7.31*). Radiologically, a mosaic pattern may be seen, either in the stomach or duodenum, which probably represents the end-stage of severe ulceration (*Figure 7.37*).

Differential diagnosis

The main differential diagnosis is peptic ulceration of the oesophagus, stomach and duodenum, in all its manifestations. Both Crohn's disease and peptic ulceration involve mucosal oedema, shallow aphthous ulceration, deeper ulceration, fibrosis and peptic perforation which may simulate fistula formation. Both disease processes may be asymmetrical and discontinuous. Ulceration in Crohn's disease is usually more extensive and severe than is normally seen in peptic ulcer disease (*Figure 7.38*).

Furthermore, Crohn's disease of the stomach and duodenum is rarely, if ever, seen without Crohn's disease elsewhere in the gastrointestinal tract. Differential diagnosis includes neoplasia, lymphoma, sarcoid and tuberculosis.

SMALL INTESTINE

Distal ileum

The distal ileum, although the most common site affected by Crohn's disease, is unfortunately also

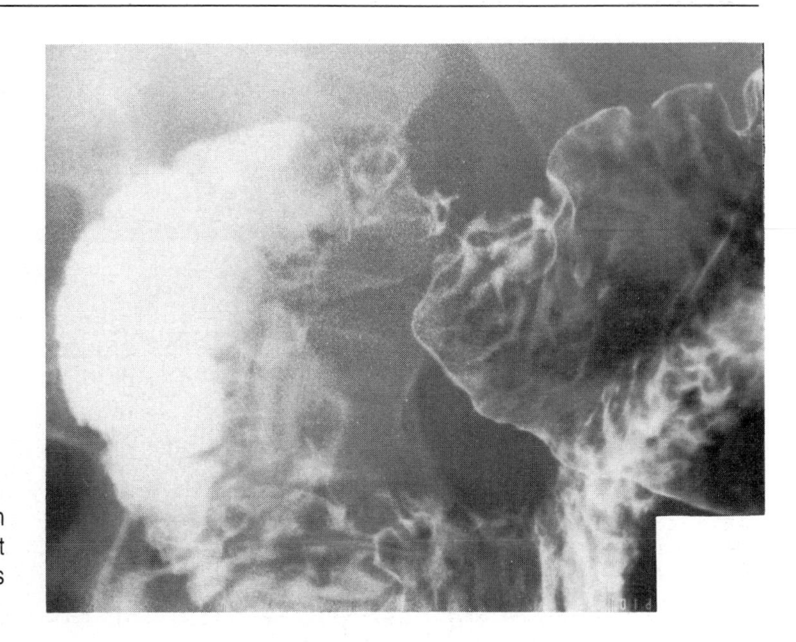

Figure 7.38 Marked narrowing of the gastric antrum and duodenal cap as shown by a double-contrast barium meal examination. The antrum reveals numerous aphthous ulcers.

the area most difficult to examine by radiology and endoscopy except where the patient has an ileostomy. The disease is therefore often well advanced before a diagnosis is established. The early radiological signs are spasm, irritability and mucosal swelling with nodularity. Shallow ulceration may be seen radiologically and endoscopically. Later, the bowel wall becomes thickened and shows radiologically as a separated loop of barium-filled bowel (see *Figure 7.32*). Thickened bowel is well demonstrated by the use of CT (see *Figure 7.33*). The disease may also present as a long, continuous symmetrical segment. If severe spasm and oedema are present the classic 'string signs' may be seen on radiographs, but this appearance is rarely due to permanent fibrosis. Thickened terminal ileum may induce an indentation of the medial wall of the caecum, causing a narrowed caecum on barium enema examination.

Jejunoileitis

Diffuse involvement of the proximal small bowel is much less common than disease of the distal ileum. It occurs more commonly in younger patients and radiologically shows as diffuse thickening and nodularity of the valvulae conniventes, with shallow ulceration at the apices of the mucosal folds. It is an area which thus far is rarely examined by an endoscope. More extensive ulceration may lead to large areas of effaced mucosa which later give rise to strictures (*Figure 7.39*).

Differential diagnosis

Early disease confined to the distal ileum may be confused with yersinia enterocolitis, although the latter condition is transient and never results in stricture or fistula formation.[20] Ileocaecal tuberculosis may be identical on radiology, but the presence of longitudinal ulceration is an important factor in differentiating Crohn's disease from tuberculosis.[19] Lymphoma may present a difficult problem in diagnosis. The presence of large focal ulceration is in favour of lymphoma. Carcinoid tumours with fibrosis occasionally simulate Crohn's disease.[2] Ischaemia rarely causes confusion with Crohn's disease in the small bowel. Its sudden onset and rapid resolution or perforation and death usually makes the distinction all too easy.

LARGE INTESTINE

The incidence of colonic Crohn's disease is increasing perhaps in part because earlier diagnosis has been achieved by improved radiology and endoscopy, aided by more effective large bowel cleansing. Most patients with colitis can safely undergo full bowel preparation without significant systemic disturbance. Only patients with toxic megacolon are exempt from this rule, but this complication is now rarely seen. Crohn's disease classically affects the proximal colon, usually with associated disease in the distal ileum.[15] The rectum is affected in about 50% of patients,[17] but this is much less than in ulcerative colitis where the rectum is invariably involved. A few patients have continuous total colonic involvement with Crohn's disease.[7] Shallow aphthous ulceration is seen in the early stages, usually surrounded by normal mucosa (see *Figure 7.34*). Progression of the ulceration leads to a 'cobblestone' or nodular appearance (see *Figure 7.36*) and occasionally geographically large ulcer-

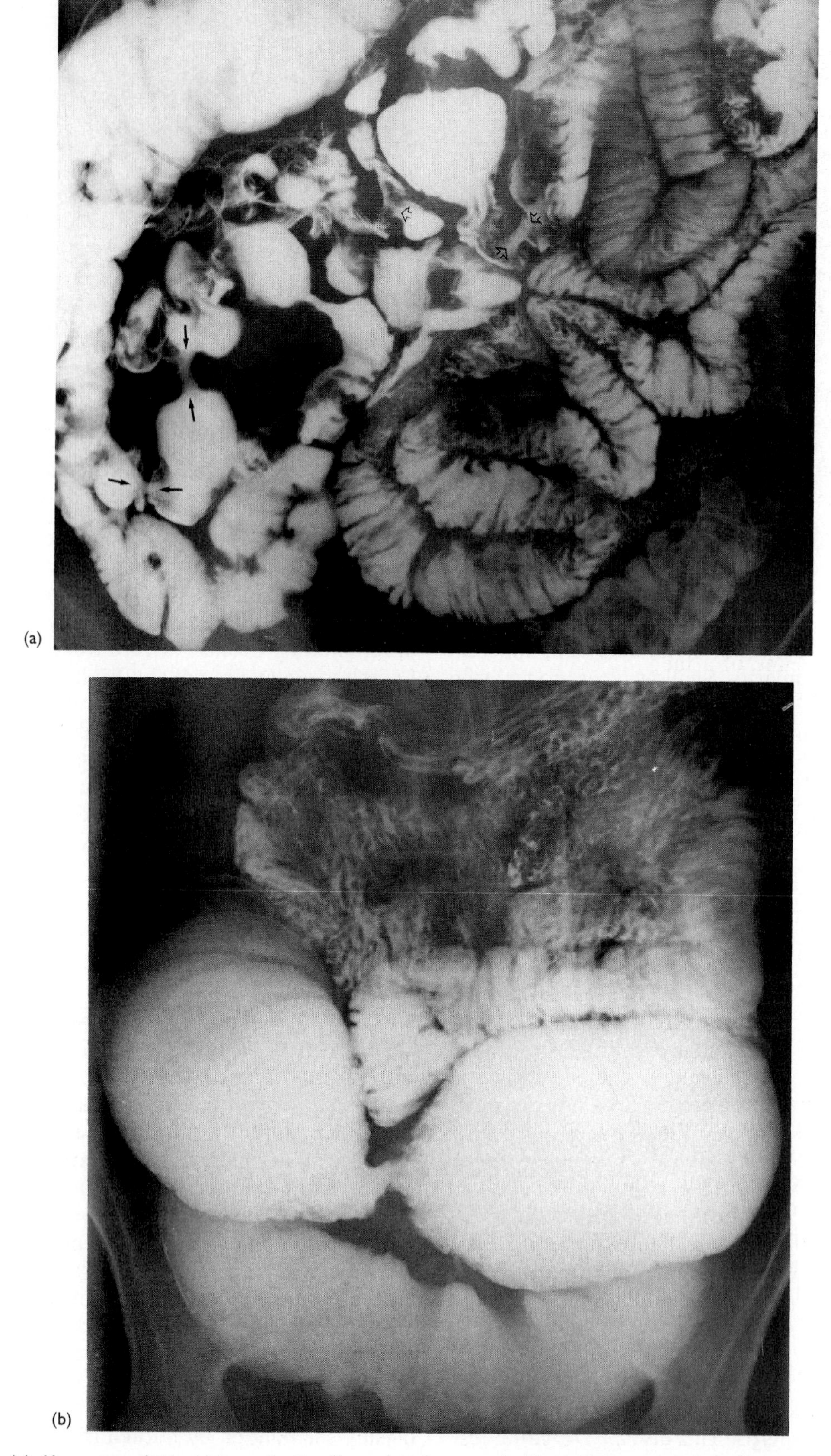

Figure 7.39 (a) Numerous short strictures in the ileum (single arrows). The strictures are typically asymmetrical leading to pseudosacculation (open arrows). (b) A single short stricture which has progressed to partial obstruction of the small bowel with gross dilatation.

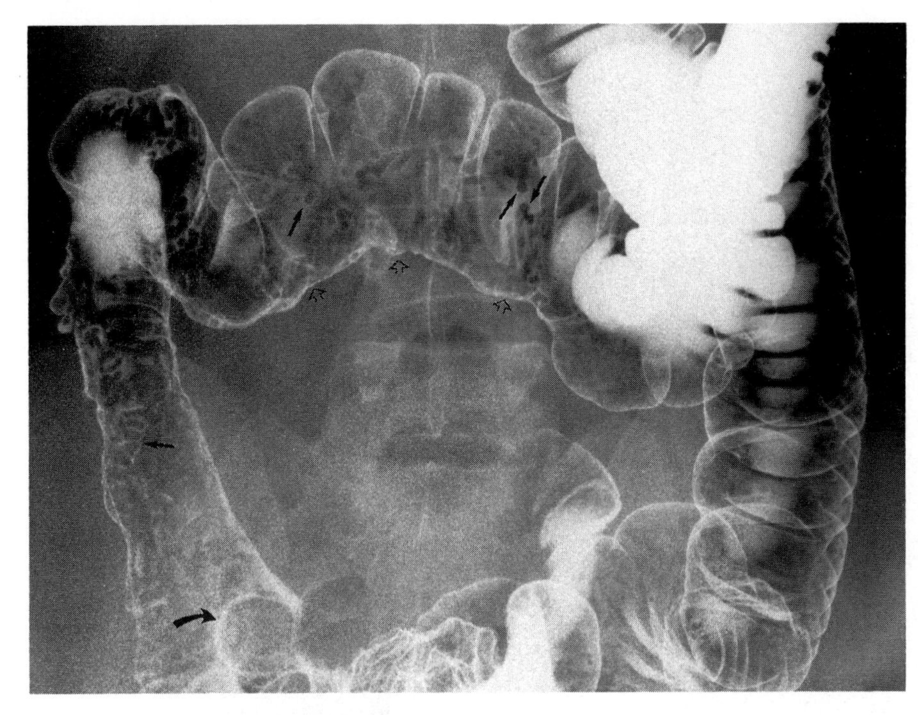

Figure 7.40 Double-contrast barium enema examination showing several features of Crohn's disease. Pseudopolyps are seen in the ascending and transverse colon (filled arrows). Asymmetrical involvement of the mesenteric border (open arrows) with normal mucosa on the opposite antimesenteric border. The ileocaecal valve is grossly oedematous (curved arrow).

ation may be seen. This sometimes occurs in a linear fashion along the line of a taenia coli (see *Figure 7.35*). The ulcerated areas usually show less severe ulceration at the margins, but occasionally the demarcation can be abrupt. Pseudopolyposis, due to inflammatory polyps in areas of quiescent disease, are increasingly seen both endoscopically and on radiograph, the latter due to improvement in barium techniques. The inflammatory polyps in Crohn's disease are asymmetrical and discontinuous (*Figure 7.40*), unlike those in ulcerative colitis, which occur continuously and distally. Occasionally the polyps may fuse, causing bridges across the intestinal lumen. These are visualized well endoscopically but rarely on a barium enema examination. Pseudopolyps may be focal and actually occlude the bowel lumen, which can be mistaken for a neoplasm.[1] Acute Crohn's colitis may progress to an acute toxic dilatation as in ulcerative colitis. This is a contraindication both to radiological examination and endoscopy. Fibrosis occurring in the circumferential axis will result in strictures that radiologically may be difficult to distinguish from neoplasia. Longitudinal fibrosis on the mesenteric border causes pseudosacculation.

Differential diagnosis

In Western societies the main differential diagnosis is from ulcerative colitis. This disease is continuous proximally from the rectum and symmetrical about the colonic circumference, but rarely Crohn's disease may also have both these features. Crohn's disease is more often distributed patchily in the proximal colon with normal intervening mucosa. There is a much higher tendency to form strictures and fistulas in Crohn's disease. It may be impossible to differentiate the two conditions radiologically. Endoscopy makes the distinction more readily in the early stages. The diffuse, reddened, granular mucosa of ulcerative colitis is more easily seen than on a radiograph. In severe disease, however, where the ulceration is more marked and extensive, the distinction on endoscopy may not be so easily made.[22] The underlying pathology may not be apparent for several months or years. In the author's experience, when it is difficult to distinguish between the two conditions, Crohn's disease is usually the final diagnosis. Ileocaecal tuberculosis is usually impossible to distinguish both radiologically and endoscopically (*Figure 7.41*). Tuberculosis may occasionally affect discontinuous isolated colonic segments and in Western countries the diagnosis may not be made until a histological examination has been performed. Crohn's strictures in the colon can be confused with neoplasia and occasionally ischaemia. Carcinomatous strictures usually have a shouldered margin with raised edges which are more easily seen endoscopically and can be confirmed by endoscopic biopsy. Demonstration of metastases on CT also makes the distinction easier. Strictures of Crohn's disease tend to be tapered, and the margins and transition to normal mucosa not so definite. Ischaemia may be extremely difficult to distinguish from Crohn's disease in the elderly. Both conditions in this age group tend to affect the sigmoid colon and

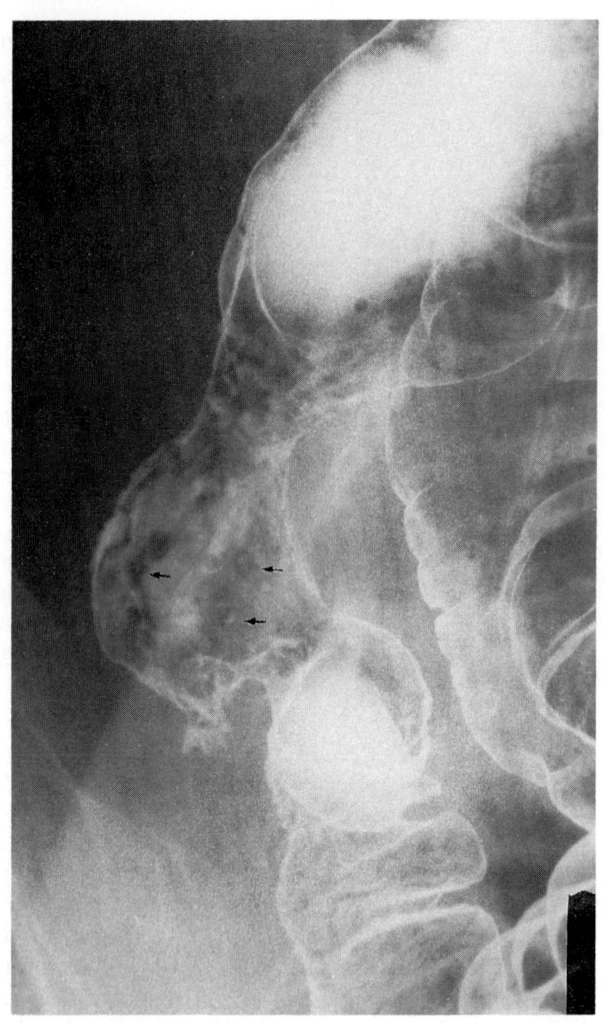

Figure 7.41 Contracted ulcerated caecum and proximal ascending colon affected by tuberculosis. There are several small aphthous ulcers (arrows). Appearances are indistinguishable from Crohn's disease.

diverticular disease is commonly a further complication, giving rise to a confusing appearance both on radiograph and through the endoscope. Ischaemia tends to settle within a few weeks or leads to perforation. Both severe diverticular disease, and Crohn's disease, may give rise to longitudinal submucosal or paracolic sinuses on a barium enema examination.[12] In the early stages of the disease, with mucosal oedema and shallow aphthous ulceration, Behçet's disease and amoebic colitis may be considered but in Western countries the demonstration of aphthous ulceration in the colon favours a diagnosis of Crohn's disease.[17]

RECURRENT DISEASE FOLLOWING SURGERY

This is not uncommon. It has the same features as the primary disease, but tends to occur in typical sites. After an ileocaecal resection with an ileocolic anastomosis, recurrent disease almost invariably occurs in the 'new' terminal ileum and this is true even if the colonic resection is more extensive with a distal ileocolic anastomosis. In gastroduodenal disease, with a bypass gastrojejunostomy, the disease process often extends into the jejunum adjacent to the anastomosis.

REFERENCES

1. Bernstein, J.R., Ghahremani, G.G., Paige, M.L. and Rosenberg, J.L. (1978) Localised giant pseudopolyposis of the colon in ulcerative and granulomatous colitis. *Gastrointestinal Radiology*, **3**, 431–435.
2. Chang, S.F., Burrell, M.I., Belleza, N.A. and Spiro, H.M. (1978) Borderlands with diagnosis of regional enteritis: trends in over diagnosis and value of a therapeutic trial. *Gastrointestinal Radiology*, **3**, 67–72.
3. Cynn, W.S., Chon, H., Gureghian, R.A. and Levin, B.L. (1975) Crohn's disease of the oesophagus. *American Journal of Roentgenology*, **125**, 359–364.
4. Fielding, J.F., Toye, D.K.M., Beton, D.C. and Cooke, W.T. (1970) Crohn's disease of the stomach and duodenum. *Gut*, **11**, 1001–1006.
5. Gore, R.M. (1987) Cross sectional imaging of inflammatory bowel disease. *Radiologic Clinics of North America*, **253**, 115–131.
6. Herlinger, H., Glanville, J.N. and Kreel, L. (1977) An evaluation of the double contrast barium meal against endoscopy. *Clinical Radiology*, **28**, 307–314.
7. Joffe, N. (1981) Diffuse mucosal granularity in double contrast studies of Crohn's disease of the colon. *Clinical Radiology*, **32**, 85–90.
8. Korelitz, B.I., Waye, J.S., Kreuning, J. *et al.* (1981) Crohn's disease in endoscopic biopsies of the gastric antrum and duodenum. *American Journal of Gastroenterology*, **76**, 103–109.
9. Laufer, I. (1976) Assessment of the accuracy of double contrast gastroduodenal radiology. *Gastroenterology*, **71**, 874–878.
10. Laufer, I. (1979) *Double Contrast Gastrointestinal Radiology with Endoscopic Correlation*, p. 168. Philadelphia: W.B. Saunders.
11. Lichtenstein, J.E., Madewell, J.E. and Feigin, D.S. (1979) The collar button ulcer. *Gastrointestinal Radiology*, **4**, 79–84.
12. Marshak, R.H. (1975) Granulomatous disease of the intestinal tract (Crohn's disease). *Radiology*, **114**, 3–22.
13. Meyers, M.A. (1976) Clinical involvement of mesenteric and antimesenteric borders of small bowel loops. Radiologic interpretation of pathologic alterations. *Gastrointestinal Radiology*, **1**, 49–58.
14. Morson, B.C. and Dawson, M.P. (Ed.) (1979) *Gastrointestinal Pathology*, 12th Ed. pp. 272–336. Oxford: Blackwell Scientific.

15. Nelson, J.A., Margulis, A.R., Goldberg, H.I. and Lawson, T.L. (1973) Granulomatous colitis: significance of involvement of the terminal ileum. *Gastroenterology*, **64**, 1071–1076.
16. Potzi, R., Walgram, M., Lochs, H. *et al.* (1989) Diagnostic significance of endoscopic biopsy in Crohn's disease. *Endoscopy* **21**, 60–62.
17. Simpkins, K.C. (1976) The barium enema in Crohn's colitis. In *The Management of Crohn's Disease*, (Ed.) Weterman, I.T., Pena, A.S. and Booth, C.C. pp. 62–67. Amsterdam: Excertpa Medica.
18. Stanley, P., Kelsey Fry, I., Dawson, A.M. and Dyer, N. (1971) Radiological signs of ulcerative colitis and Crohn's disease of the colon. *Clinical Radiology*, **22**, 434–442.
19. Tsukasa, S., Tokjdome, K., Irisa, T., Nishimata, Y., Hashimoto, S. and Shirakabe, H. (1978) Roentogenographic diagnosis of Crohn's disease of the small intestine. *Stomach and Intestine*, **13**, 335–349.
20. Vantrappen, G., Agg, H.O., Ponette, E., Geboes, K. and Bertrand, P.H. (1977) Yersinia enteritis and enterocolitis: gastroenterological aspects. *Gastroenterology*, **72**, 220–227.
21. Weterman, I.T. (1981) Colonoscopy in Crohn's disease. In *Crohn's Workshop* (Ed.) Lee, E.C.G. pp. 33–38. London: Heyden.
22. Williams, C.B. and Waye, J.D. (1978) Colonoscopy in inflammatory bowel disease. *Clinics in Gastroenterology*, **7**, 701–717.

TREATMENT

MEDICAL TREATMENT *(J.E. Lennard-Jones, revised by R.N. Allan)*

This section aims to provide guidance on the medical treatment of Crohn's disease. The best way of managing Crohn's disease is to analyse the current symptoms and base treatment on this. Controlled drug trials provide guidance for an overall strategy but the response in the individual is unpredictable. Drug therapy is only one aspect of treatment; dietary manipulation, replacement of nutritional deficits and surgical measures are all equally important and at all times must be combined together with encouragement and support of the patients and their families.

Drugs used in the treatment of Crohn's disease may be broadly grouped into anti-inflammatory compounds, drugs that may act by affecting immune responses, antibacterial drugs and symptomatic treatments. The results of controlled trials are summarized first followed by general conclusions about the likely circumstances in which each type of drug may be expected to provide benefit. Finally, suggestions are offered about the way in which drugs may be used in different types of Crohn's disease.

ANTI-INFLAMMATORY DRUGS

Sulphasalazine

Pharmacology and metabolism

Sulphasalazine – salicyl-azo-sulphapyridine – is split at the azo link by enteric bacteria to yield 5-aminosalicylic acid and sulphapyridine.

Therapeutic experiments in a small number of patients with colonic Crohn's disease, and in a larger number of patients with ulcerative colitis, suggest that sulphasalazine and 5-aminosalicylic acid applied directly to the inflamed colonic mucosa are therapeutically active, but sulphapyridine is not.[19] At present, there is no certainty as to the mode of action of this drug, but 5-aminosalicylic acid is the important constituent of the molecule and may be the active moiety.

Potential side effects

The potential side effects of sulphasalazine are dependent on the blood level of sulphapyridine and on individual hypersensitivity. The blood level of sulphapyridine depends not only on dose but also on the patient's genetic ability to acetylate the drug at a fast or slow rate. High levels of sulphapyridine may be associated with malaise, headache, nausea, dyspepsia and mild haemolysis. the most frequent idiosyncratic reaction is a skin rash; other reactions such as blood dyscrasias are rare. An important side effect is decreased fertility in men while they are taking sulphasalazine, an adverse effect almost certainly due to the sulphapyridine part of the molecule. There is a decrease in sperm count and motility with an increase in the proportion of abnormal forms. Fertility returns within 2 or 3 months of stopping the drug.[43]

Evidence for clinical effectiveness

The clinical effectiveness of sulphasalazine will be considered in active disease, in inactive disease and after resection.

ACTIVE DISEASE

In the American National Co-operative Crohn's Disease Study (NCCDS), sulphasalazine – 1 g/15 kg body weight (maximum 5 g) daily given over 4 months – proved no better than placebo in ileal disease, but was effective in ileocolic ($P = 0.027$) and colonic ($P = 0.006$) disease.[40] Reanalysis of data in another smaller trial[2] also showed no certain benefit in disease confined to the small bowel, but a therapeutic effect in ileocolic and colonic disease ($P < 0.05$). Another controlled trial[46] showed unequivocal benefit of the drug in a dose of 4–6 g daily over a period of 26 weeks; patients with small intestinal disease seemed to do as well as those with disease involving the colon but the number of patients was small. In the European Co-operative Crohn's Disease Study[24] treatment was with either 3 g/day sulphasalazine or placebo for 6 weeks. Sulphasalazine was superior to placebo for active colonic disease ($P < 0.05$) but not at other sites.

INACTIVE DISEASE

In the NCCDS trial, sulphasalazine in a dose of 0.5 g/15 kg body weight (maximum 2.5 g) daily failed to reduce the relapse rate among patients with inactive disease over 1–2 years. The European studies[24] confirmed that sulphasalazine 3 g/day was of no statistically significant benefit in quiescent disease.

AFTER RESECTION

Four trials have failed to show that sulphasalazine given over periods of up to 2 years reduces the relapse rate after resection.[3,22,40,49] The authors of one trial[49] calculated that between 110 and 130 patients would be needed in each treatment group to ensure a high probability of showing that the relapse rate is halved by treatment. So far, no trial has achieved this size, and until such a trial is completed the effect of sulphasalazine as a maintenance treatment remains uncertain. However, the results to date are not encouraging.

The role of sulphasalazine in treatment of Crohn's disease

The controlled trials confirm a clinical impression that sulphasalazine is often beneficial in the treatment of active ileocolonic or colonic Crohn's disease. The response is significantly better than placebo but not often dramatic. The drug seems to be most effective early in the course of disease and its effects are often disappointing in patients with a long history. There is little evidence from controlled trials to support the use of the drug in extensive small bowel disease, although clinical experience suggests that the drug can be effective. There is no evidence to support the use of long-term sulphasalazine therapy to reduce the rate of relapse in patients treated medically or the rate of recurrence in patients after resection, although individual patients are seen in whom long-term treatment does seem helpful.

Preparations of 5-aminosalicylic acid

As the sulphapyridine component of sulphasalazine is responsible for many of the side effects, considerable effort has been exerted to produce new modes of delivery of 5-aminosalicylic acid.

One analogue has been prepared in which two molecules of 5-aminosalicylic acid are joined by an azo link so that, on bacterial cleavage of the diazo bond, two molecules of 5-aminosalicylic acid are liberated. 5-aminosalicylate has also been prepared in an acrylic coating whose break-up is pH dependent, so that the drug is released in the mid-small intestine as the pH becomes more alkaline. Preparations are also available where the 5-aminosalicylate is in microgranular form and is a combination of these two preparations.

Another analogue has been prepared in which 5-aminosalicylic acid is linked to the harmless carrier benzoylalanine.

The concept is that higher doses of 5-aminosalicylate might be delivered with these new preparations and that the release site could be better targeted to either the small or the large intestine.

If 5-aminosalicylic acid is given by mouth it is likely to be absorbed in the upper small intestine and excreted in the urine. In theory different delayed release preparations can be prepared which liberate 5-aminosalicylic acid in either the small intestine or the proximal or distal colon.

5-Aminosalicylate in active disease

Preliminary results from a multicentre placebo-controlled variable dose study of oral mesalazine (Pentasa) for active Crohn's disease, 199 patients (of a planned 240) were randomized to receive either placebo or, mesalazine 1 g, 2 g or 4 g per day for 16 weeks. Preliminary results have suggested that mesalazine 4 g/day is effective as a single agent for the treatment of active Crohn's disease.[14]

In a 16-week controlled trial of 67 patients with active disease, there was no overall benefit in outcome but there was some benefit in patients with small bowel disease suggesting that clinical trials with larger doses of 5-aminosalicylates would be worth while.[32]

Solutions of 5-aminosalicylic acid tend to become discoloured due to oxidation of this unstable compound. Such solutions have given encouraging results when administered as a retention enema in ulcerative colitis, but no data are yet available on their use in Crohn's disease.

Corticosteroids

Pharmacology and metabolism

The corticosteroids most commonly used in the treatment of Crohn's disease are prednisone or prednisolone. Prednisone is hydroxylated to prednisolone in the body and both are lipid-soluble. For parenteral and topical administration, the water-soluble compound prednisolone-21-phosphate or 6-methylprednisolone may be preferable.

In the blood, cortisol or prednisolone is partially bound to an α-globulin – transcortin – and to albumin. Only the unbound steroid is metabolically active and the level of free corticosteroid rises if the serum albumin level falls, with an associated increase in drug side effects and perhaps therapeutic activity. The biological effects of these drugs on experimentally induced inflammation persist longer than would be predicted from the plasma level. Thus the plasma half-life of prednisolone after intravenous administration is around 3–4 hours, but the biological half-life is 18–36 hours.

When compared with a normal control group, absorption of prednisolone given by mouth was reduced in seven patients with Crohn's disease.[35] All but one of the patients had ileal disease of mild-to-moderate severity, but there was no steatorrhoea or excess protein loss from the gut. Other workers have not shown decreased absorption of prednisolone in Crohn's disease, but the results suggest that there may be differences in patients with small or large bowel involvement.[42]

Potential side effects

The possible side effects of corticosteroid therapy are well known and limit the therapeutic usefulness of these drugs. Depression of the hypothalamic–pituitary–adrenal axis may be prevented by dosage schedules designed to give intermittent rather than continuous high blood levels, particularly if the high therapeutic level coincides with the physiological peak cortisol level in the morning. It is also probable that intermittent high blood levels, with normal levels for much of the time, cause fewer metabolic side effects than persistently raised blood levels. Reduced prednisolone absorption in some patients with small intestinal Crohn's disease may lead to fewer side effects than in patients with normal absorption taking an equivalent dose.

It has been suggested that corticosteroids retard growth in children and that the use of corticotrophin minimizes this side effect. It is now apparent that growth retardation in Crohn's disease is generally due to poor food intake and the role of corticosteroids in this complication is difficult to assess.[17]

Evidence for therapeutic effectiveness

The clinical effectiveness will be considered in acute disease, active disease and quiescent disease or after resection.

Acute disease

The most serious acute form of the disease is severe Crohn's colitis. There has been no controlled trial restricted to Crohn's colitis, but at least one trial[15] has included patients with both Crohn's colitis and ulcerative colitis. This trial showed that corticotrophin 40 units daily gave equivalent results to hydrocortisone 300 mg daily (both drugs given intravenously). Side effects, especially oedema, tend to be more common with a hydrocortisone infusion than with prednisolone and most clinicians now use the equivalent dose of prednisolone 60 mg daily given as a trial of treatment for several days.

Active disease

The NCCDS trial showed that prednisone 0.25–0.75 mg/kg body weight (maximum 60 mg) daily given over 4 months, the dose being adjusted to the activity of the disease, was more effective than placebo ($P < 0.0006$). These results applied to patients with ileal ($P = 0.002$) and ileocolonic disease ($P = 0.008$), but the results in patients with colonic disease were not significant perhaps due to the small size of the group.[40]

In the European Co-operative Crohn's Disease Study a tapered 6-week course of oral 6-methylprednisolone (from 48 mg/day to 12 mg/day) was more effective than placebo overall ($P < 0.001$) and in ether small or large bowel disease alone ($P < 0.05$) and in small and large bowel disease together ($P < 0.05$).[24]

Quiescent disease or after resection

Three trials have failed to show benefit from low doses of corticosteroids in preventing relapse in patients with inactive disease or after resection. Prednisolone 7.5 mg daily for up to 3 years did not reduce the relapse rate nor did it affect recurrence or extension of disease among 33 patients when compared with 26 patients who received a control tablet.[39] Prednisone 0.25 mg/kg body weight (maximum 20 mg) daily was not apparently superior to placebo over 1–2 years in maintaining remission in the NCCDS trial. A course of prednisolone (with sulphasalazine 3 g daily), beginning with 15 mg and reducing to nil 33 weeks after resection, failed to reduce the recurrence rate over the first three post-operative years.[3]

The European Study identified a small subgroup of patients with active disease in whom continuous administration of low dose methylprednisolone (8 mg/day) after initial improvement with a higher dose was superior to placebo over a period of 2 years.[24] A small study has shown that patients with minimal symptoms but abnormal laboratory tests showing evidence of persistent inflammation developed a symptomatic relapse less frequently over the next 6 months if given methylprednisolone 0.25 mg/kg per day than if given placebo.[7]

The role of corticosteroids in Crohn's disease

The main role of corticosteroids in medical treatment is to suppress acute inflammation of the gut. Before starting treatment it is important to ensure, as far as possible, that the symptoms are due to inflammation of the intestine, rather than to an abscess or other infective episode. An initial dose of 20–40 mg prednisolone given by mouth, or in severe cases 60 mg prednisolone given intravenously, is advisable with the aim of controlling the symptoms as soon as possible. Thereafter, usually at the end of the first or second week of treatment, the dose can be progressively reduced as long as clinical improvement is maintained and the course of treatment is completed in 4–8 weeks. It is important that neither the patient nor the doctor should regard such treatment as curative; it is best thought of as a measure to control a temporary exacerbation.

Long-term corticosteroid treatment should not be given to a patient who is well in the hope of preventing trouble. However, occasional patients are seen in whom it proves difficult or impossible to withdraw corticosteroid treatment without an immediate recurrence of symptoms. Such patients appear to have 'active chronic' disease which can be suppressed by long-term corticosteroid treatment. In such patients, it may be necessary to continue corticosteroid treatment for a long period provided that the inflammation cannot be controlled by other drugs and that surgical treatment is inappropriate. This clinical experience was backed by the findings in the European study.[24] It is in such patients that the use of azathioprine or 6-mercaptopurine should be considered for its steroid-sparing effect.

Topical corticosteroids are a useful treatment for inflammation of the mouth, distal colon, anal canal or perianal skin.

Combination of a corticosteroid and sulphasalazine

As both these drugs are effective in the treatment of active Crohn's disease, it is reasonable to ask whether or not the beneficial effects are additive. A controlled trial of prednisone, with or without sulphasalazine, has failed to show that the addition of sulphasalazine increased the rate of remission in active disease or reduced the relapse rate in patients with inactive disease, or that sulphasalazine exerted a steroid-sparing effect.[38] The European study showed that a combination of 6-methylprednisolone and sulphasalazine was the more effective regimen when the disease was localized to the colon, and superior to other drugs used alone.[24]

DRUGS WITH A POSSIBLE EFFECT ON IMMUNITY

Azathioprine and 6-mercaptopurine

Pharmacology and metabolism

6-Mercaptopurine is a purine antagonist which interferes with nucleic acid synthesis. Azathioprine was derived from 6-mercaptopurine by conjugation of a free thiol group with the aim of decreasing toxicity without loss of effectiveness. Azathioprine is largely converted to 6-mercaptopurine in the body and the similar metabolic pathways suggest that both drugs can be expected to have similar clinical effects.

After oral administration, the drugs are absorbed to a variable extent, but there has been no work yet to correlate blood levels with clinical effectiveness in Crohn's disease. Breakdown of these drugs to the urinary metabolite, 6-thiouric acid, requires xanthine oxidase. If the xanthine oxidase inhibitor, allopurinol, is given, the rate of breakdown is reduced and toxic levels may result unless the dose of azathioprine or 6-mercaptopurine is reduced.

Both drugs have proven immunosuppressant action and could act in Crohn's disease by altering the immune response in an undefined way. The circulating K-cell activity and the plasma cell count in the lamina propria rise in patients with Crohn's disease when the drug is stopped.[10] Patients with Crohn's disease treated with azathioprine have a significantly lower K-cell activity than untreated patients.[11] Both drugs have a non-specific anti-inflammatory effect and there is some evidence that azathioprine has anti-bacterial activity against enteric anaerobes.

Potential side effects

In high doses, both drugs suppress the bone marrow and this danger sets an upper limit on the doses that can be used for an inflammatory disorder. The dose of azathioprine used in Crohn's disease is usually between 2 and 2.5 mg/kg body weight daily. In the NCCDS trial, 2 out of 59 patients developed severe and 7 moderate leukopenia while taking azathioprine at 2.5 mg/kg body weight daily for up to 4 months.[37] The only drug-related death among all reported controlled trials occurred from bone marrow failure after treatment with azathioprine in this dose range for 11 years.[28] The starting dose of 6-mercaptopurine used in the one controlled trial was 1.5 mg/kg body weight daily and on this dose most patients developed mild and two developed severe leukopenia.[30]

About 1 in 300 patients has congenital deficiency of the enzyme, 3-methyltransferase, concerned with the metabolism of these drugs.[21] Such patients develop toxic levels of a metabolite with consequent marrow suppression. This deficiency cannot be detected before treatment and manifests itself within 12 weeks of starting the drug. For this reason, blood counts are advisable every 2 weeks during the first 3 months of treatment and thereafter the author arranges monthly blood counts.

About one in ten patients is unable to take these drugs because of side effects. In the two largest controlled trials, one of which included 113 patients given azathioprine, and the other 68 patients given 6-mercaptopurine, the following complications caused treatment to be withdrawn; severe nausea (3), pancreatitis (6), fever (3), and leukopenia (6).[30,37] All these side effects resolved without long-term sequelae when the drug was stopped.

There has been concern that an increased frequency of malignant disease might occur among patients treated with immunosuppressive drugs. A prospective survey[16] among patients treated for a variety of disorders, but excluding transplants, included 280 patients with inflammatory bowel disease. Among the total series of 1349 patients, four developed non-Hodgkin's lymphoma (expected number = 0.34, $P < 0.001$), two squamous carcinoma of the skin (expected number = 0.38, $P = 0.06$) and 34 developed other tumours (expected number 21.74, $P < 0.01$). The increased incidence of malignant disease could be due to other factors, for example, some of the diseases treated could be associated with an increased incidence of malignant disease regardless of treatment. However, caution in the use of immunosuppressive drugs is clearly indicated especially as few patients have been followed after treatment for many years.

Evidence of therapeutic effectiveness

The clinical effectiveness will be considered in active disease, chronic active disease and quiescent disease.

Active disease

In the NCCDS trial no significant effect of azathioprine in active Crohn's disease was demonstrable, although the published results do show a trend in favour of the drug.[40] Two cross-over trials have also failed to show that azathioprine is helpful in active Crohn's disease.[18,33] These results must be accepted with caution because, in the NCCDS trial, corticosteroids were withdrawn from many patients just before azathioprine was started, and the part played by drug side effects in limiting the number of patients who completed the treatment period with azathioprine is difficult to assess. In the other two trials, there was a high proportion of patients with severe structural complications of the disease which would not be expected to respond to drug therapy.

Active chronic disease

A trial of 6-mercaptopurine was performed using 83 patients who were chronically ill, with a mean duration of continuous active symptoms of 4.3 years, and who were failures of therapy with sulphasalazine and steroids, but for whom surgery was not imminent.[30] Among 39 patients who received treatment with both 6-mercaptopurine and a control tablet during the 2-year cross-over design, 26 improved with 6-mercaptopurine and only 3 with placebo ($P < 0.0001$). Of all patients treated during the first year of the trial, 26 out of 36 who received 6-mercaptopurine improved compared with 5 out of 36 who received a control tablet ($P < 0.001$). In this trial, 60 out of 83 patients were taking prednisolone in a mean dose of 20 mg daily and 43 patients were taking sulphasalazine. Among the 44 prednisone-treated patients who received 6-mercaptopurine for at least 6 months, it was possible to withdraw the steroid in 24 patients and reduce the dose substantially in another 9. By contrast, during placebo treatment, steroids could be discontinued or reduced in only 14 out of 39 patients ($P < 0.001$).

In a trial of azathioprine, prednisolone was given with or without this drug in the treatment of acute disease.[51] It proved possible to withdraw the prednisolone from most of the patients given azathioprine and 10 of these 11 patients remained in remission and completed the trial, whereas 8 of 11 receiving placebo were withdrawn early because of relapse ($P < 0.01$). In another trial, 20 patients with Crohn's disease who had received at least 10 mg prednisone daily over 3 months were divided equally into two groups and given in addition either azathioprine or a placebo tablet respectively.[34] The mean reduction of 15.5 mg in the daily dose of prednisone among those receiving azathioprine was greater than the mean reduction of 6.1 mg in the placebo group ($P < 0.05$). In a long-term but uncontrolled study of 42 patients, from a series of 207 patients with Crohn's disease in Scandinavia, there was evidence that both azathioprine and 6-mercaptopurine could be of benefit and enable reduction or withdrawal of corticosteroid therapy.[27]

QUIESCENT DISEASE

A group of 51 patients who were in good health after treatment of their Crohn's disease with azathioprine, 2 mg/kg body weight daily for at least 6 months, was divided randomly and in double-blind fashion, either to a group in which azathioprine was continued or to one in which a control tablet was substituted.[28] The trial lasted 1 year unless relapse occurred earlier. The cumulative probability of relapse was nil at 6 months and 5% (±5 s.d.) at a year among those on azathioprine, compared with 25% (±9 s.d.) at 6 months and 41% (±11 s.d.) at a year among those in the control group ($P < 0.01$). The relapse rate did not correlate with the duration of pre-trial clinical remission or the duration of azathioprine treatment.

In the NCCDS trial azathioprine 1 mg/kg body weight daily was given for 1 or 2 years to patients who were well at the start of the trial.[40] Approximately 25% of patients in the trial experienced a relapse by the end of the first year and 40% by the end of the second year. Patients receiving azathioprine did not rank significantly better than placebo as judged by life table analysis.

The role of azathioprine or 6-mercaptopurine in Crohn's disease

These two drugs act slowly over several months and exert a steroid-sparing and anti-inflammatory effect in patients with chronic active Crohn's disease. In such patients given azathioprine or 6-mercaptopurine, it is often possible to reduce the dose of or withdraw prednisolone. The disease tends to relapse when azathioprine or 6-mercaptopurine is withdrawn and it is necessary to continue treatment for months or years, provided that the drug is well tolerated. At present, the optimal length of treatment cannot be defined. As these drugs are potentially dangerous they should be used only if simpler measures have failed, surgical treatment is inappropriate and the disease is causing ill health or disability. Azathioprine is best given in a dose of 2 mg/kg body weight and 6-mercaptopurine in an initial dose of 1.5 mg/kg body weight. Regular blood counts should be performed at intervals of 2 weeks for 3 months and thereafter monthly. Bone marrow depression is uncommon once the recommended dose has been given for 3 months with no adverse effects.

Present and his colleagues, who have treated nearly 400 inflammatory bowel disease patients with 6-mercaptopurine for a mean duration of 5 years, have reported the observed toxicity which includes pancreatitis (3.3%), bone marrow depression (2%), allergic reactions (2%) and drug hepatitis (0.3%). All complications were reversible and there was no mortality.[31]

OTHER DRUGS GIVEN WITH THE AIM OF AFFECTING IMMUNE RESPONSE

Cyclosporin is a potent immunosuppressive agent with specific effects on T-lymphocyte-mediated immunity. Its administration in the field of transplantation is well established and there are well-established side effects, particularly nephrotoxicity.

In a study of 73 patients who were intolerant or resistant to corticosteroids randomly assigned to receive either cyclosporin (5–7.5 mg/kg per day) for 3 months or placebo, improvement occurred in 59% of the treatment group and 32% of the placebo group ($P = 0.032$). Improvement occurred after 2 weeks of treatment. In the succeeding 3 months after the trial period had been completed when therapy was gradually withdrawn, improvement was maintained in 38% of the treatment group and 15% of the placebo group.[8] The benefit was not dramatic in most patients and the improvement was largely confined to a small subgroup of a few patients.

At present its use should be restricted to controlled trials. It remains to be seen whether it will prove possible to identify that small group of patients who might have substantial benefit because its widespread use will be precluded by the high incidence of nephrotoxicity.

Disodium cromoglycate is not absorbed from the gut and it was hoped that it would benefit inflammatory bowel disease by preventing liberation of histamine and other chemical mediators from mast cells, as it appears to do in asthma. Unfortunately, these hopes have not been fulfilled and a controlled trial has failed to show benefit in active or slightly active Crohn's disease.[4] Levamisole,[41,50] oral BCG[9] and transfer factor[47] have been tested in controlled trials without demonstrable benefit.

ANTIBACTERIAL DRUGS

Antibacterial drugs may reduce secondary infection or reduce the antigenic stimulus of enteric bacteria to diseased mucosa. An uncontrolled study has suggested that broad-spectrum antibiotics given continuously in various combinations over periods of up to 5 years can result in considerable benefit.[25] Few antibacterial drugs tested so far have been tested by controlled trial.

Metronidazole

Metronidazole has a marked antibacterial action against anaerobic organisms such as *Bacteroides* species. When given by mouth the proportion of anaerobes in the faecal bacterial flora falls and there is a corresponding increase in aerobes so that the total flora is unchanged.[20]

Clinical experience

In a small double-blind cross-over trial,[5] following 20 patients given metronidazole at 1 g daily for 2 months, in addition to other treatments, clinical and haematological improvements ($P < 0.01$) were noted among the 6 patients with colonic disease but in the group as a whole the only significant effects were a rise in haemoglobin level and a fall in sedimentation rate during the period of receiving the metronidazole.

In a larger, randomized, double-blind, cross-over trial over 4 months, metronidazole 0.4 g twice daily was compared with sulphasalazine 1.5 g twice daily in patients with an elevated clinical activity index and serum orosomucoid level.[45] About one-third of the patients had disease confined to the small bowel and the remainder had colonic disease with or without ileal involvement. The clinical disease activity index improved to the same extent with both drugs during the first 4 months, but the orosomucoid level fell and the haemoglobin level rose further in the metronidazole group. During the second 4 months after cross-over, those patients who had not responded to sulphasalazine responded to metronidazole, but there was no response to sulphasalazine after failure of metronidazole. The authors concluded that metronidazole is slightly more effective than sulphasalazine in the treatment of active Crohn's disease.

Uncontrolled observations have suggested that metronidazole 20 mg/kg body weight given over months, up to 3 years, benefited 26 patients with severe perineal Crohn's disease.[6] Deterioration of the perineal lesions occurred in about three-quarters of those in whom withdrawal of metronidazole was attempted.

Side effects

The major side effect of metronidazole is a peripheral neuropathy. In the group of patients treated with the drug at a dose of 20 mg/kg body weight daily, one-half developed paraesthesiae, usually of the feet, after a mean treatment period of 6.5 months. The neuropathy usually recovered over months when the drug was withdrawn (although it persisted for almost 2 years in one patient) and it disappeared in some patients when the dose was reduced. Other side effects can be a metallic taste, nausea, anorexia, headache and a furry tongue. It is said that metronidazole can react with alcohol to give a disulfiram-like effect and moderation in alcohol consumption is usually advised, though few, if any, patients complain of this side effect.

There has been concern that metronidazole might be carcinogenic but no evidence that this is so in humans has been forthcoming. Metronidazole did not induce an increased frequency of chromosomal aberrations at a daily dose of 800 mg for 4 months in a group of patients with Crohn's disease.[45] There is no conclusive evidence at present to suggest that the drug is teratogenic, but in the absence of data caution is needed in the use of metronidazole during pregnancy.

Anti-mycobacterial drugs

Sulphadoxine is a long-acting sulphonamide (half-life 4–8 days) and pyrimethamine (closely related to trimethoprim, but longer acting) acts in sequential blockade with sulphonamides on folic acid metabolism. Together these drugs are active against a wide range of organisms, including some mycobacteria. In a controlled trial among 51 patients with chronic active Crohn's disease, this drug combination given in one weekly dose was compared with a control tablet; no benefit was apparent from the combined drug.[12]

A combination of rifampicin and isoniazide was not shown to be effective by controlled trial.[36] Likewise, clofazimine was not shown to be beneficial in a controlled trial.[1] Quadruple therapy has been proposed and encouraging initial results have been reported[13] but the results of a controlled trial are awaited.

Dapsone apparently benefited six patients to whom it was given[48] but no further observations have been published.

SYMPTOMATIC DRUG THERAPY

Antidiarrhoeal drugs

Double-blind cross-over studies have shown that loperamide decreases stool frequency and weight, with a corresponding trend towards solid consistency, in Crohn's disease, after ileocolic resection, or after colectomy and ileorectal anastomosis.[23,29] In the first of these trials, loperamide in a mean dose of 6.9 mg daily was shown to be superior to diphenoxylate, at a mean dose of 17.7 mg daily, in terms of stool frequency and consistency ($P = 0.01$) and patients' preference ($P = 0.002$). Loperamide[44] and codeine phosphate[26] both reduce ileostomy output by about 20–25%; diphenoxylate appeared less effective.

When the terminal ileum is diseased or after ileal resection, bile salts entering the colon may induce secretion of water and electrolytes, and thus cause diarrhoea. Cholestyramine 4 g daily, or sometimes smaller doses with meals, can be helpful in this situation, but in practice this treatment is often either ineffective or unacceptable to the patient. In patients with ileal disease and diarrhoea, a trial of cholestyramine in full doses may be made. If there is no response the treatment should be abandoned; if there is a good response, the minimal dose of cholestyramine necessary to maintain improvement should be established by progressive reduction in the total daily dose.

Antispasmodic and analgesic drugs

Antispasmodics are of doubtful benefit but are sometimes used in patients with bolus colic when no other treatment is possible. Certain patients with chronic pain, unrelieved by measures already outlined, seem to need regular doses of non-addictive analgesic drugs.

WHICH ASPECTS OF THE DISEASE RESPOND TO DRUG THERAPY?

Drug treatment can reduce inflammation of the gut and to some extent reduce secondary infection. Drugs can affect the function of the intestine to reduce diarrhoea or malabsorption. Lastly, by improving the sense of well-being or reducing local or systemic symptoms, drugs can improve appetite and thus nutrition.

Clinical assessment should define the patients' complaints precisely. As Crohn's disease cannot be cured, treatment should be directed to the disability that it causes. Endoscopic and radiological investigations should be used to assess the detectable extent and structural complications of the disease. Appropriate measurements should be used to define any general or specific nutritional deficits.

Once this assessment is complete, drug therapy may be used, where appropriate, to try and relieve an inflammatory, infective, systemic or symptomatic component of the disorder. A limited goal should be set and simple observations recorded to establish whether or not the goal is achieved within a reasonable time. If no progress is made then a different treatment should be employed until a useful result is obtained. At every stage, all possible drug, nutritional and surgical therapies should be considered in deciding on a treatment policy.

DRUG TREATMENT OF DIFFERENT TYPES OF DISEASE

Crohn's disease of the lips and mouth

Crohn's disease may be associated with ulceration, and sometimes swelling of the lips, buccal mucosa, gingival sulcus or tongue. Topical corticosteroids are helpful. Preparations available are slowly dissolving hydrocortisone lozenges, each containing 2.5 mg hydrocortisone as the sodium succinate, which should be held between the gum and the cheek near an ulcer four times daily, or triamcinolone dental paste applied to the inflamed area several times daily. In very severe cases, prednisolone-21-phosphate (Prednesol) 5 mg in 30 ml water three or four times daily can be used as a mouth wash and gargle before being swallowed.

Extensive involvement of the small intestine

Patients with widespread small bowel disease, but without obstructive symptoms due to stricture formation, often respond well to drug therapy. Some remain well as long as sulphasalazine is continued with a tendency of relapse when it is stopped. Antibacterial drugs may be tried and may be particularly helpful if there is bacterial overgrowth in the small bowel. Corticosteroids by mouth generally help, but often have to be continued in a maintenance dose equivalent to prednisolone 10–15 mg daily over months or years. In such circumstances, azathioprine may be useful for its steroid-sparing and anti-inflammatory effect.

Ileocaecal disease

Disease limited to the ileocaecal region tends to present with obstructive symptoms or local pain and tenderness. Drug therapy can produce temporary relief but rarely leads to satisfactory control of the disease in the long term. Surgical treatment is indicated or often becomes needed for persistent local pain, bolus colic, general ill health or a local complication. Sulphasalazine or metronidazole are worth initial trial if there is no clear indication for surgery. Corticosteroid treatment may lead to symptomatic improvement but the drug is difficult to withdraw and local structural complications are liable to develop while treatment is continued.

Ileocolonic and colonic disease

Patients with predominantly colonic disease often respond well to drug therapy. Sulphasalazine or metronidazole is usually the first drug to try and, if successful, can be given over a prolonged period. Severe colitis with fever, anorexia, abdominal pain and tenderness, and diarrhoea often respond to a corticosteroid given intravenously. The usual regime is to give 20 mg 6-methylprednisolone as a bolus every 8 hours. Less severely ill patients often respond to prednisolone 30 or 40 mg daily by mouth, usually given in one morning dose, and continued for about 2 weeks before progressive reduction in dose over 6–8 weeks once improvement has been obtained; sometimes relapse of symptoms tends to occur when the dose is reduced to 10 mg daily or less. In these circumstances, azathioprine can be given if there is no contraindication and the disease severity warrants its use, to take advantage of its steroid-sparing and anti-inflammatory effect.

Anorectal disease

Crohn's disease limited to the rectum and sigmoid colon may respond to topical corticosteroid therapy using suppositories (Predsol), a foam (Colifoam) or retention enemas. Prednisolone as the water-soluble metasulphabenzoate (Predenema) is absorbed less from an enema than prednisolone-21-phosphate (Predsol).

Topical treatment with sulphasalazine or 5-aminosalicylic acid as an enema, or sulphasalazine as a suppository, may also be beneficial.

Anal pain due to chronic fissure or ulcer may respond to treatment with a steroid cream, such as betamethasone valerate (Betnovate 0.1%), applied by the patient on a rubber finger cot or anal dilator. This cream can also be applied to ulcers on the perineal skin or in the natal cleft or groins.

Perianal fistulas may cause surprisingly little disability, despite their appearance, as long as drainage of pus is free. Such fistulas may close, or become dry and indolent, if the intestinal disease is controlled as already described. Long-term metronidazole has been reported to give good results in a dose of 20 mg/kg body weight daily given over many months, though often results are disappointing. Most clinicians use a rather smaller dose as side effects are common with this large dose.

Unhealed perineal wounds

In some patients surgical wounds fail to heal after treatment of fistulas or removal of rectum. Widespread ulceration of the perineum with characteristic ulcers in the natal cleft and groins can develop.

Such patients are very difficult to treat. Surgical toilet and frequent cleansing of the area, avoiding maceration of healthy skin, are essential. Topical corticosteroids as a cream or applied as a solution of prednisolone-21-phosphate may help. In severe cases, if there is no response to local measures, systemic corticosteroids in a low dose, such as prednisolone 10–20 mg combined with azathioprine 2 mg/kg body weight daily, is a justifiable treatment and often appears to promote healing.

Crohn's disease with associated disorders

Intestinal disease associated with erythema nodosum, pyoderma or arthritis usually responds to systemic (oral or parenteral) corticosteroid therapy. Inflammation of the eye may occur without obvious activity of the intestinal disease and can often be treated by local measures. Sacroiliitis and ankylosing spondylitis tend to follow a course independent of the intestinal disease and require a non-steroidal anti-inflammatory drug for the relief of pain and stiffness.

Internal and external intestinal fistulas

Spontaneous fistulas between neighbouring loops of intestine generally require surgical treatment, though such fistulas can be an incidental finding in a symptomless patient. An enterovesical fistula is generally an indication for operation.

A spontaneous enterocutaneous fistula is generally the result of chronic intestinal perforation with subsequent rupture or drainage of the resulting abscess through the skin. Such fistulas do not usually close with drug therapy, unlike postoperative fistulas which tend to close spontaneously. Patients have been reported in whom closure of a spontaneous fistula has followed the use of azathioprine or 6-mercaptopurine, but this is not the general experience. Antibacterial drugs may reduce the output of pus, but rarely eliminate the abscess cavity.

Intra-abdominal and perianal abscesses

Almost all such abscesses require surgical drainage. As most are due to a chronic perforation of diseased intestine, the use of antibacterial drugs is unlikely to be successful. Similarly perianal abscesses rarely respond to antibacterial drugs.

Obstructive episodes

Most obstructive episodes in Crohn's disease are due to structural narrowing of the gut or an adhesion from previous surgery. Occasionally, a corticosteroid given by mouth, perhaps combined with antibacterial drugs, may lead to temporary relief if the obstruction is due to an exacerbation of Crohn's disease with oedema. Even so, elective surgery treatment is often needed for recurrent episodes. Drug treatment can be useful to obtain a temporary respite during which a patient's nutritional state can be improved before elective, rather then urgent, surgical treatment.

CONCLUSION

Drug treatment in Crohn's disease is only a part of the overall treatment which often includes dietary manipulation, nutritional replacement and surgical measures. Many patients never require any drug therapy, for example those who present with obstructive symptoms due to terminal ileal disease and who are successfully treated by resection of the diseased segment. At present drug treatment of Crohn's disease is non-specific, empirical and often disappointing. The physician looks forward to the day when a specific harmless remedy becomes available which can cure this distressing disorder or at least prevent recurrence after initial medical or surgical treatment.

REFERENCES

1. Afdhal, N.H., Long, A., Lennon, J., Crowe, J. and O'Donoghue, D.P. (1987) Controlled trial of clofazimine in Crohn's disease. *Gut*, **28**, A1391.
2. Anthonisen, P., Barany, F., Folkenborg, O. *et al.* (1974) The clinical effect of salazosulphapyridine (Salazopyrin) in Crohn's disease: a controlled double-blind study. *Scandinavian Journal of Gastroenterology*, **9**, 549–554.
3. Bergman, L. and Krause, U. (1976) Postoperative treatment with corticosteroids and salicylazosulphapyridine (Salazopyrin) after radical resection for Crohn's disease. *Scandinavian Journal of Gastroenterology*, **11**, 651–656.
4. Binder, V., Elsborg, L., Greibe, J. *et al.* (1991) Disodium cromoglycate in the treatment of ulcerative colitis and Crohn's disease. *Gut*, **22**, 55–60.
5. Blichfeldt, P., Blomhoff, J.P., Myhre, E. and Gjone, E. (1978) Metronidazole in Crohn's disease: a double blind cross-over clinical trial. *Scandinavian Journal of Gastroenterology*, **13**, 123–127.
6. Brandt, L.J., Bernstein, L.H., Boley, S.J. and Frank, M.S. (1982) Metronidazole therapy for perineal Crohn's disease: a follow-up study. *Gastroenterology*, **83**, 383–387.
7. Brignola, C., Campieri, M., Farrugia, P. *et al.* (1988) The possible utility of steroids in the prevention of relapses of Crohn's disease in remission. *Journal of Clinical Gastroenterology*, **10**, 31–34.
8. Brynskov, J., Freund, L., Rasmussen, S.N. *et al.* (1989) A placebo controlled double blind randomised trial of cyclosporin therapy in active Crohn's disease. *New England Journal of Medicine*, **321**, 845–850.
9. Burnham, W.R., Lennard-Jones, J.R., Hecketsweiler, P. *et al.* (1979) Oral BCG vaccine in Crohn's disease. *Gut*, **20**, 229–233.
10. Campbell, A.C., Skinner, J.M., Hersey, P. *et al.* (1974) Immunosuppression in the treatment of inflammatory bowel disease. I. Changes in lymphoid sub-populations in the blood and rectal mucosa following cessation of treatment with azathioprine. *Clinical and Experimental Immunology*, **16**, 521–533.
11. Eckhardt, R., Kloos, P., Dierich, M.P. and Meyer sum Buschenfelde, K.H. (1977) K-lymphocytes (Killer cells) in Crohn's disease and acute virus B-hepatitis. *Gut*, **18**, 1010–1016.
12. Elliott, P.R., Burnham, W.R., Berghouse, L.M. *et al.* (1982) Sulphadoxine–pyrimethamine therapy in Crohn's disease. *Digestion*, **23**, 132–134.
13. Hampson, S.J., Parker, M.C., Saverymuttu, S.H., Joseph, A.E., McFadden, J.-J.P. and Hermon-Taylor, J. (1989) Quadruple antimycobacterial chemotherapy in Crohn's disease: results at 9 months of a pilot study in 20 patients. *Alimentary Pharmacology and Therapeutics*, **3**, 343–352.
14. Hanauer, S.B., Belker, M.E., Gitnick, G. *et al.* (1990) Multi centre placebo controlled dose ranging study oral pentasa for active Crohn's disease. *Gastroenterology*, **98**, A173.
15. Kaplan, H.P., Portnoy, B., Binder, H.J. *et al.* (1975) A controlled evaluation of intravenous adrenocorticotrophic hormone and hydrocortisone in the treatment of acute colitis. *Gastroenterology*, **69**, 91–95.
16. Kinlen, L.J., Sheil, A.G.R., Peto, J. and Doll, R. (1979) Collaborative United Kingdom–Australasian study of cancer in patients treated with immunosuppressive drugs. *British Medical Journal*, **2**, 1461–1466.
17. Kirschner, B.S., Voinchet, O. and Rosenberg, I.H. (1978) Growth retardation in inflammatory bowel disease. *Gastroenterology*, **75**, 504–511.
18. Klein, M., Binder, H.J., Mitchell, M. *et al.* (1974) Treatment of Crohn's disease with azathioprine: a controlled evaluation. *Gastroenterology*, **66**, 916–922.
19. Klotz, U., Maier, K., Fischer, C. and Heinkel, K. (1980) Therapeutic efficacy of sulfasalazine and its metabolites in patients with ulcerative colitis and Crohn's disease. *New England Journal of Medicine*, **303**, 1499–1502.
20. Krook, A., Danielsson, D., Kjellander, J. and Jarnerot, G. (1981) The effect of metronidazole and sulfasalazine on the faecal flora in patients with

Crohn's disease. *Scandinavian Journal of Gastroenterology*, **16**, 183–192.

21. Lennard, L., Van Loon, J. and Weinshilboum, R.M. (1989) Pharmacogenetics of acute azathioprine toxicity: Relationship to thiopurine methyltransferase genetic polymorphism. *Clinical Pharmacology and Therapeutics*, **46**, 149–154.
22. Lennard-Jones, J.E. (1977) Sulphasalazine in asymptomatic Crohn's disease. *Gut*, **18**, 69–72.
23. Mainguet, P. and Fiasse, R. (1977) Double-blind placebo-controlled study of loperamide (Imodium) in chronic diarrhoea caused by ileocolic disease or resection. *Gut*, **18**, 575–579.
24. Malchow, H., Ewe, K., Brandes, J.W. *et al.* (1986) European Co-operative Crohn's Disease Study: results of drug treatment. *Gastroenterology*, **86**, 249–266.
25. Moss, A.A., Carbone, J.V. and Kressel, H.Y. (1978) Radiologic and clinical assessment of broad spectrum antibiotic therapy in Crohn's disease. *American Journal of Roentgenology*, **131**, 787–790.
26. Newton, C.R. (1978) Effect of codeine phosphate, Lomotil and Isogel on ileostomy function. *Gut*, **19**, 377–383.
27. Nyman, M., Hansson, I. and Eriksson, W. (1985) Long-term immunosuppressive treatment in Crohn's disease. *Scandinavian Journal of Gastroenterology*, **20**, 1197–1203.
28. O'Donoghue, D.P., Dawson, A.M., Powell-Tuck, J. *et al.* (1978) Double-blind withdrawal trial of azathioprine as maintenance treatment for Crohn's disease. *The Lancet*, **2**, 955–957.
29. Pelemans, W. and Vantrappen, G. (1976) A double-blind crossover comparison of loperamide with diphenoxylate in the symptomatic treatment of chronic diarrhoea. *Gastroenterology*, **70**, 1030–1034.
30. Present, D.H., Korelitz, B.I., Wisch, N. *et al.* (1980) Treatment of Crohn's disease with 6-mercaptopurine: a long-term randomized double blind study. *New England Journal of Medicine*, **302**, 981–987.
31. Present, D.H., Meltzer, S.J. Krumbolz, M.P. Wolke, A. and Korelitz, B.I. (1989) 6-Mercaptopurine in the management of inflammatory bowel disease: short and long-term toxicity. *Annals of Internal Medicine*, **111**, 641–649.
32. Rasmussen, S.N., Lauritsen, K., Tage-Jensen, U. *et al.* (1987) 5-Amino Salicylic acid in the treatment of Crohn's disease. A 16 week double blind placebo controlled multicentre study with Pentasa. *Scandinavian Journal of Gastroenterology*, **22**, 877–883.
33. Rhodes, J. Bainton, D., Beck, P. and Campbell, H. (1971) Controlled trial of azathioprine in Crohn's disease. *The Lancet*, **2**, 1273–1276.
34. Rosenberg, J.L., Levin, B., Wall, A.J. and Kirsner, J.B. (1975) A controlled trial of azathioprine in Crohn's disease. *Digestive Diseases*, **20**, 721–726.
35. Shaffer, J.L., Williams, S.E., Turnberg, L.A. *et al.* (1983) Absorption of prednisolone in patients with Crohn's disease. *Gut*, **24**, 182–186.
36. Shaffer, J.L., Hughes, S., Linaker, B.D., Baker, R.D. and Turnberg, L.A. (1984) Controlled trial of rifampicin and ethambutol in Crohn's disease. *Gut*, **25**, 203–205.
37. Singleton, J.W., Law, D.H., Kelley, M.L. Jr *et al.* (1979) National Co-operative Crohn's Disease Study: adverse reactions to study drugs. *Gastroenterology*, **77**, 870–882.
38. Singleton, J.W., Summers, R.W., Kern, F. Jr *et al.* (1979) A trial of sulfasalazine as adjunctive therapy in Crohn's disease. *Gastroenterology*, **77**, 887–897.
39. Smith, R.C., Rhodes, J., Heatley, R.V. *et al.* (1978) Low dose steroids and clinical relapse in Crohn's disease: a controlled trial. *Gut*, **19**, 606–610.
40. Summers, R.W., Switz, D.M., Sessions, J.T. Jr *et al.* (1979) National Co-operative Crohn's Disease Study: Results of drug treatment. *Gastroenterology*, **77**, 847–869.
41. Swarbrick, E.G. and O'Donoghue, D.P. (1979) Levamisole in Crohn's disease. *The Lancet*, **1**, 392.
42. Tanner, A.R., Halliday, J.W. and Powell, L.W. (1981) Serum prednisolone levels in Crohn's disease and coeliac disease following oral prednisolone administration. *Digestion*, **21**, 310–315.
43. Toovey, S., Hudson, E., Hendry, W.F. and Levi, A.J. (1981) Sulphasalazine and male infertility: reversibility and possible mechanism. *Gut*, **22**, 445–451.
44. Tytgat, G.N. and Huibregtse, K. (1975) Loperamide and ileostomy output: placebo-controlled double-blink crossover study. *British Medical Journal*, **2**, 667.
45. Ursing, B., Alm, T., Barany, F. *et al.* (1982) A comparative study of metronidazole and sulfasalazine for active Crohn's disease: the Co-operative Crohn's Disease Study in Sweden. *Gastroenterology*, **83**, 550–562.
46. Van Hees, P.A.M., Van Lier, H.J.J., Van Elteren, P.H. *et al.* (1981) Effect of sulphasalazine in patients with active Crohn's disease: a controlled double-blind study. *Gut*, **22**, 404–409.
47. Vicary, F.R., Chambers, J.D. and Dhillon, P. (1979) Double-blind trial of the use of transfer factor in the treatment of Crohn's disease. *Gut*, **20**, 408–413.
48. Ward, M. and McManus, J.P.A. (1975) Dapsone in Crohn's disease. *The Lancet*, **1**, 1236–1237.
49. Wenckert, A., Kristensen, M., Eklund, A.E. *et al.* (1978) The long-term prophylactic effect of salazosulphapyridine (Salazopyrin) in primarily resected patients with Crohn's disease. A controlled double-blind trial. *Scandinavian Journal of Gastroenterology*, **13**, 161–167.
50. Wesdorp, E., Schellekens, P.T.A., Weening, R. *et al.* (1977) Levamisole in Crohn's disease: a double-blind controlled trial. *Gut*, **18**, A971–A972.
51. Willoughby, J.M.T., Kumar, P.J., Beckett, J. and Dawson, A.M. (1971) Controlled trial of azathioprine in Crohn's disease. *The Lancet*, **2**, 944–947.

SURGICAL TREATMENT *(M.R.B. Keighley)*

Small bowel Crohn's disease

Over 80% of patients with ileal Crohn's disease will require surgical treatment. The likelihood of resection increases with duration of follow-up. A few patients have a short history with acute non-obstructing ileitis which may resolve completely.

The majority of patients develop obstruction, an abscess or fistula, and a few will require emergency surgery for perforation, bleeding, misdiagnosed apendicitis or malignancy. The risk of reoperation for recrudescence is about 50% at 10 years. Most patients have their first operation in the second decade, assuming that the life expectancy in Crohn's disease is little different from that in the non-Crohn's disease population; most patients are likely to need three or four resections in their lifetime. Provided the surgical policy is to conserve bowel length, serious morbidity should not occur even if four resections are needed.

Elective surgical treatment

First resection

Ileal Crohn's disease has a remarkably uniform pathology. Commonly 10–15 cm of terminal ileum is involved with a thickened wall and some fat wrapping. The ileal mesentery is thickened and contains enlarged lymph nodes. The caecum and right colon often appear to be remarkably normal at laparotomy. The ileum is sometimes adherent to the omentum, other loops of bowel or to the fallopian tubes. There may be proximal skip lesions, an abscess or a fistula to another loop of bowel or skin.

The indications for surgical intervention are usually obstruction, but in a few cases the main indication is an abscess or fistula.

PREFERRED SURGICAL TREATMENT

Resection is the preferred option. Without resection, the clinician cannot be absolutely certain of the diagnosis and bypass may not prevent the development of local sepsis. A long inflamed segment is not amenable to strictureplasty.

EXTENT OF RESECTION

The aim of resection is merely to remove the segment or segments which are causing complications. For first resections this generally entails removing 10–15 cm of terminal ileum and taking the lower pole of the caecum which includes the appendix and the ileum to a point where there is relatively healthy bowel of normal calibre without ulceration.

A wide excision may be responsible for long-term morbidity and Crohn's disease cannot be cured by resection because it is a panenteric disease.[124] It was argued at one time that a wide resection might reduce the risk of disease recurrence[49] and that the mesenteric lymph nodes formed an important focus of recurrent disease if they were not removed.[26]

Two Scandinavian papers report lower recurrence rates after radical resections. Bergman and Krause[20] reported recurrence rates at a mean 10-year follow-up of 29% after radical resection compared with 84% for the remainder. This difference persisted when the same patients were reviewed 8 years later.[80] Nygaard and Fausa[99] also demonstrated significantly lower recurrence rates during the first year after radical resection than after very localized excisions. Consequently, surgeons in the past have performed cancer-like operations for inflammatory disease in the belief that if nodes or residual disease were not removed recurrence was invariable.[131] Frozen section examination of the resection lines has been used to ensure that all the disease had been removed in order to minimize recurrence. Although frozen sections are difficult to interpret,[61] this practice continues at some centres.[102]

Karesen and others[72] reported crude recurrence rates of 66% where there was microscopic evidence of disease at the resection margin, compared with 14% in those that did not. Lindhagen and others[89] divided 110 patients into three groups based on histological examination of the resection margin: in 41 the margins were normal, 39 had minor inflammatory changes and 30 had macroscopic ulceration with crypt abscesses and ganulomata on microscopy. The cumulative recurrence rate at 10 years for patients with macroscopic changes was 73% compared with 44% in those with minor inflammation and 37% for normal margins. Further evidence to support the influence of microscopic disease at resection margins was reported by Wolff and colleagues[131] at the Mayo Clinic. The cumulative recurrence rate in 39 patients with disease at one or other margin was 90% at 8 years compared with 47% in the remainder.

Other authors have failed to demonstrate any association between microscopic changes at the resection margin and recurrence.[2,29,101,116] Pennington and others[102] studied 97 patients undergoing 103 resections: 52 specimens had normal resection margins but microscopic changes were present in the other 51 specimens. They found no difference in crude or cumulative recurrence rates between the groups based on clinical recurrence, suture line recurrence or reoperation rates.

There is good evidence, based upon microscopic evidence of granulomata or inflammatory cell infiltrates at resection margins, to demonstrate that resection margin involvement has no influence on the subsequent risk of recurrence.[40,66,89] Thus Cooper and Williams[33] reported crude recurrence rates of 38% where there was evidence of residual disease at resection margins, compared with 29% when the resection margins were apparently free of disease. Indeed Glass and Baker[50] even suggested that the presence of granulomata at resection margins might protect against a high recurrence rate.

Based on long-term observations on the natural history of Crohn's disease, it is now known that recurrence is invariable anyway; indeed the surgical procedure probably has little influence on recurrence rates.[127]

Length of diseased bowel

A wider resection may be necessary if there is an abscess or a fistula.[56] Nevertheless, the concept of *en bloc* excision should be avoided. If a large inflammatory mass is found with multiple enteroenteric fistulas and large cavitating mesenteric nodes, it is worth while isolating the segment from the rest of the peritoneal cavity and dissecting off all the loops from the diseased segment. Uninvolved loops can be preserved and small stenotic segments can be treated by strictureplasty,[7,85] leaving a relatively short primary diseased segment for resection and anastomosis.

Timing of surgical resection

Hultein[69] considers that the risk of extensive bowel resection is greater and the morbidity of surgical therapy much higher in patients with advanced disease. It is generally wiser to operate early before the onset of complications, because this carries a low morbidity and only very short bowel segments will have to be removed. Advanced disease is commonly associated with abscess or fistula at the time of resection, and is attended by a high incidence of postoperative complications, whereas early disease which was not associated with intra-abdominal sepsis carries a low incidence of complications (12%).

Recurrence after ileal resection

The cumulative 10-year recurrence rate is 35% irrespective of the number of previous resections, the duration of symptoms, the age at diagnosis or whether the disease is resected or bypassed.[66] Reoperation rates are naturally lower than recurrence rates. Reoperation rates at 5 and 10 years are reported as 25% and 33% respectively,[15] and are uninfluenced by duration of disease or the age of the patients[14] (*Figure 7.42*). Rutgeerts and others[108] performed an endoscopic survey in 114 patients who had already had an ileal resection

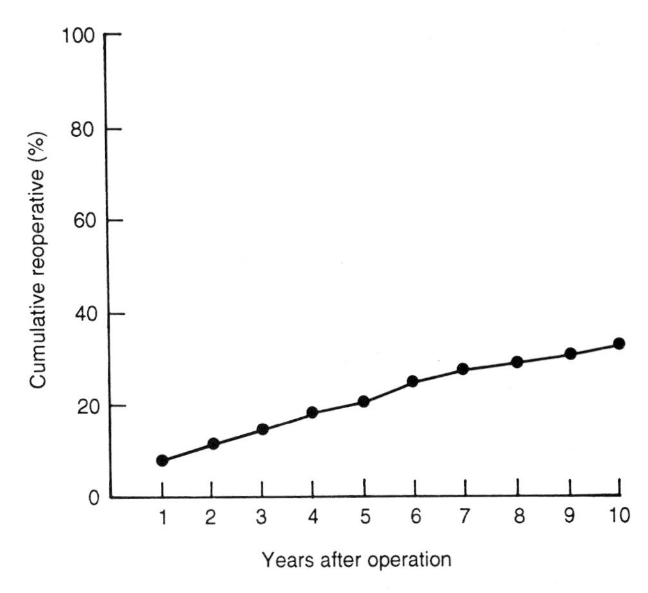

Figure 7.42 Cumulative reoperation rates after first resection for distal ileal Crohn's disease in years from time of the first operation. (Reproduced with permission from *Surgery of the Colon, Rectum, Anus* (1993) M.R.B. Keighley and N.S. Williams. London: WB Saunders.)

for Crohn's disease. Endoscopic evidence of recurrence was identified in 72% of these patients within a year of operation but few had symptoms of recurrence. Hence asymptomatic recurrence often occurs early and recurrence of disease is almost invariable.

Metabolic sequelae

After ileal resection patients usually complain of increased frequency of defaecation, loose stools and occasional urgency. Vitamin deficiency may also complicate ileal resection, the most specific deficiency after ileal resection being malabsorption of vitamin B_{12} with subsequent depletion of stores, necessitating parenteral replacement.[13,46] Disturbances in the enterohepatic circulation may be manifested by an increased incidence of cholelithiasis[12,74] as well as urolithiasis.[37]

Malabsorption is rare after a Crohn's disease resection, but it may be evident after bypass procedures and may be due to residual active disease. Serious malabsorption only becomes difficult to manage when patients have lost two-thirds or more of their ileum.[64]

Alternative surgical therapy: bypass

When Crohn and his colleagues described regional ileitis, resection was the preferred surgical option.[4] In the ensuing years resection was replaced by bypass operations because of the high mortality rates at that time after ileal resection.[49] As a consequence bypass became popular with a much lower

Table 7.15 Indications for reoperation: bypass compared with resection

	Side-to-side bypass (%)*	*Resections and end-to-end anastomosis† (%)*
Fistula	33	5
Abscess	29	5
Recurrence	24	42
Mean interval between initial operation and reoperation (years)	4.1	5.9

From Alexander-Williams *et al.*[6]
*$n = 21$.
†$n = 89$.

mortality.[48] The operation involved either a side-to-side anastomosis or an exclusion bypass by leaving the Crohn's disease segment out of circuit.

Schofield[113] reported an 89% recurrence rate at 5 years after bypass compared with an 18% 5-year recurrence rate after resection. Fielding and others[43] reported significantly higher recurrence rates after bypass (44%) compared with resection (26%). However, Banks and others[17] reported recurrence rates that were identical after resection or bypass. Alexander Williams and colleagues[6] found that the disease-free interval was shorter after bypass operations. Furthermore, there was a high incidence of complications, particularly enterocutaneous fistula (33%) or postoperative abscess (29%), after bypass compared with fistula in only 5%, and in abscess in only 5% after resection (*Table 7.15*).

Hence bypass surgery for Crohn's disease fell into disrepute with reports of serious metabolic sequelae and persistent sepsis. Occasional ileal malignancy complicating long-standing bypass procedures for ileal Crohn's disease is a further argument against bypass.[58]

Operations for recurrent Crohn's disease

Recurrence is inevitable after resection for Crohn's disease. Greenstein *et al.*[56] showed that penetrating disease (fistula and abscess) had a 73% reoperation rate compared with 29% in obstructing disease. Furthermore, disease which initially presented with an abscess and fistula tends to recur in this way (*Table 7.16*).

The aim of resection for recurrent small bowel Crohn's disease is to remove obstructing or pene-

Table 7.16 Natural history of Crohn's disease

Pattern of presentation	*Perforating (n = 375)*	*Non-perforating (n = 395)*
Fistula	240	–
Abscess	91	–
Free perforation	44	–
Obstruction		239
Intractability		132
Bleeding		15
Acute colitis		9
Recurrence		
Recurrence with fistula, abscess or free perforation (%)	73	29
Recurrence with obstruction, bleeding or colitis (%)	27	71

From Greenstein *et al.*[56]

trating disease while ensuring that as much small bowel as possible is preserved. Preserving bowel that can never function normally is a worthless exercise; however, leaving a patient with the short-gut syndrome is to inflict life-long morbidity.

Strictureplasty

The concept of non-resectional surgery started with bypass operations.[49] The prospect of alleviating obstruction by strictureplasty without creating a blind loop, with the risk of bacterial overgrowth, folate depletion and disturbed bile salt chemistry by enteroplasty, has been explored in many centres. Lee[85] pioneered the concept of treating Crohn's disease strictures by strictureplasty. He operated on patients with intestinal obstruction and malnutrition in whom excisional surgery was contraindicated either because there was diffuse disease or a 'short bowel' from previous resections. The Oxford group undertook what they described as 'minimal surgery'.

The author's group has used the principle of strictureplasty to treat enteric strictures in Crohn's disease since 1976. They have now performed 245 strictureplasties in 61 patients (*Table 7.17*). The indications for the 89 operations in this study were recurrent intestinal obstruction in 81 patients, enterocutaneous fistulas in 7 patients and ileostomy bleeding in 1. An associated resection was performed at 24 operations.

Dehn and others[35] reported the Oxford results. There was overall symptomatic improvement in more than 90% of their 24 cases with no leaks or fistulas. The St Marks' experience with strictureplasty was rather more disappointing. Kendall and others[75] reported the results of 95 patients treated by 458 strictureplasties: 6 developed recurrent symptoms between 2 and 6 months after operation, and a very high recurrence rate was observed in patients with active small bowel disease.

Fazio's report from the Cleveland Clinic is the largest North American experience.[41] Fifty patients had 225 strictureplasties; there was no operative mortality. Serious morbidity was reported in 16%, which included three enterocutaneous fistulas, two postoperative abscesses and two patients who had serious intra-abdominal haemorrhage. All patients were improved, and in particular, abdominal pain was invariably alleviated.

Twenty-four of 46 patients in Birmingham, followed up for more than 5 years, have since required further operations, usually for strictures elsewhere in the gastrointestinal tract. However, it may be difficult to determine whether these are strictureplasty recurrences or missed proximal skip lesions. Three patients who required reoperation were found to have small bowel carcinomas but it was uncertain whether these tumours developed at the site of a previous strictureplasty. Based on these findings, a full-thickness biopsy of the bowel wall is advised if strictureplasty is undertaken.

The complication rate for strictureplasties was remarkably low. Major complications developed in nine patients. Seven patients developed enterocutaneous fistulas due to either a missed distal stenosis malnutrition or sepsis.

The high rate of postoperative enterocutaneous fistula has been the subject of closer scrutiny. The incidence of pre-existing abscess or fistula was significantly greater in the patients who developed a postoperative leak. As a result of these findings, the author's group no longer advise the use of an unprotected strictureplasty for recurrent disease in the presence of a coexisting abscess or enterocutaneous fistula. Four of the leaks were from 37 Finney or J-pouch strictureplasties, compared with 3 from 208 Heineke-Micklicz strictureplasties. This argues against long strictureplasties for recurrent Crohn's disease.

A 6-month assessment after operation indicated that 36 (80%) of 45 patients became pain free, with improvement in their general well-being. Body weight and serum albumin improved significantly after strictureplasty with a mean weight gain of 3.4 kg over the first 6 months.

A high incidence of recurrence is now recognized after strictureplasty; one reason is that it tends to be used for patients with multifocal Crohn's disease and often in those who have had multiple previous resections. A higher incidence of recrudescence would therefore be expected than after a simple resection in which a single site of Crohn's disease is resected with an end-to-end anastomosis between normal bowel.

When resection and strictureplasty were compared in terms of the surgery-free interval, a much higher rate was observed after strictureplasty. The surgery-free interval was only 2.9 years after strictureplasty compared with 7.9 years after resec-

Table 7.17 Strictureplasty at the General Hospital, Birmingham

Number of patients	61
Total number of operations	89
Number of patients having previous resection	47
Total number of strictureplasties	245
Sites:	
Duodenum	7
Jejunum	89
Ileum	119
Ileocaecal	20
Ileorectal	10

Table 7.18 Comparison between resection and strictureplasty

	Resections (*n = 41*)	*Strictureplasty* (*n = 41*)
Number of operations	221	130
Duration of follow-up (years)	17.2	15.2
Surgery-free interval (years)	7.9	2.9

From Sayfan *et al.*[110]

tion (*Table 7.18*) despite careful intraoperative testing in the strictureplasty group to detect proximal or distal strictures. It is therefore felt that strictureplasty and miniresection should now be compared in a randomized trial.

Surgery in diffuse small bowel Crohn's disease

The entity of diffuse small bowel disease was first highlighted by Cooke and Swan[31] who reported 18 patients with diffuse disease (5% of the entire Crohn's disease practice), 13 of whom required an operation. A few patients have multiple foci of activity in the proximal ileum and jejunum which may be the site of perforation and bleeding. In multifocal disease it is often difficult to tell which of the multiple lesions is responsible for symptoms. The most common indication for operation is recurrent intestinal obstruction, usually provoked by solid food. Weight loss is common and often occurs due to anorexia or the fear that eating will cause abdominal colic.

Fazio and Galanduik[40] reviewed the Cleveland Clinic experience of diffuse disease. Recurrent partial small bowel obstruction was the symptom that principally required surgical treatment. Consequently, a number of patients underwent multiple strictureplasties to preserve small bowel, because many had had previous extensive resections. They reported weight gain, pain relief and rapid normalization of serum albumin in all patients after operation.

In 1989 we identified 42 patients with diffuse small bowel disease. The most striking surgical difference between localized and diffuse disease was the proportion having multiple strictureplasties in the diffuse small bowel disease. Possibly the most disturbing data relate to mortality. Nine of 27 patients with diffuse disease reported by Andrews and Allan[14] died: including 3 from small bowel carcinoma, 3 from sepsis, 1 from thromboembolism and 1 from metabolic causes.

The author believes that miniresection and strictureplasty have an important role in diffuse small bowel disease for the relief of symptoms, control of metabolic sequelae and improvement of nutrition. Major resections should be avoided but the long-term prognosis in some patients should be guarded.

Surgical treatment of gastroduodenal Crohn's disease

Gastroduodenal Crohn's disease nearly always occurs in association with disease elsewhere in the alimentary tract. The complications of gastroduodenal Crohn's disease which require surgical intervention are bleeding, stenosis or both.

As it is not advisable to resect the duodenum, this is the one area of the bowel in which bypass is still considered the preferred surgical treatment. The best results were said to follow gastro-jejunostomy[44] but the jejunum is particularly susceptible to acid/peptic digestion and, as some patients have gastric hypersecretion, vagotomy reduces the high risk of stomal ulceration. Selective vagotomy has theoretical advantages over truncal vagotomy in that it is less likely to provoke diarrhoea. With the advent of H_2-receptor antagonists and proton pump inhibitors duodenal strictureplasty alone is now preferred to gastrojejunal bypass and vagotomy.

Murray and colleagues[97] reported the surgical treatment of gastroduodenal Crohn's disease at the Lahey Clinic in 70 patients, 27 of whom (38%) underwent some form of surgical treatment. The mainstay of surgical treatment was some form of bypass either a gastrojejunostomy or a Roux-en-Y duodenojejunostomy in 14: surprisingly 8 patients underwent a localized resection. Vagotomy was used sparingly because of post-vagotomy diarrhoea, but five patients developed stomal ulcers despite vagotomy. Complications of surgical treatment were high: two patients developed duodenal fistulas after resection, one patient sustained a bile duct injury, four patients suffered from gastric outlet obstruction despite gastrojejunostomy and five developed stomal ulcers.

The surgical management of duodenal Crohn's disease is difficult and should not be undertaken lightly unless the patient has a fistula. Obstructive disease can now be managed by strictureplasty which carries a lower incidence of peptic ulceration and impaired gastric emptying than gastrojejunostomy. Vagotomy should be used sparingly.

Urgent surgical intervention for acute complications

Free perforation

The most common pathology is a free perforation of the ileum with small bowel contents in the peritoneal cavity.[1] The small bowel is nearly always obstructed.

Occasionally the perforation may arise from the jejunum or sigmoid colon. It has been suggested that the perforation may be secondary to ischaemia; steroids and non-steroidal anti-inflammatory medication have also been implicated. Perforation of bowel may occur without faecal peritonitis if this arises from a bypassed segment of ileum or right colon. Occasionally perforation may be due to a carcinoma complicating Crohn's disease.[58]

The results of simply oversewing a perforated segment of Crohn's disease are disastrous.[95] Nasr and others[98] reported 13 patients treated in this manner, 5 of whom died of continuing sepsis.

As all patients have chronic obstructive disease, the safest policy is to resect the obstructed and perforated segment of bowel. The dilemma then facing the surgeon is whether to perform a primary anastomosis or to opt for the safer policy of delivering both bowel ends to the surface as an end ileostomy and a mucous fistula. If the colon has perforated, an anastomosis is not advisable. If the faecal peritonitis is of long standing or the patient is compromised by being malnourished or having another system failure, it is not advisable to perform an anastomosis. If, as is more likely, the patient presents early and the perforation is in the ileum, a primary anastomosis can usually be undertaken safely.

Exanguinating haemorrhage

Profound, persistent or recurrent intestinal blood loss is a rare complication of Crohn's disease. Bleeding is usually from an ulcer on the mesenteric border of the small bowel. Occasionally massive blood loss may complicate a linear ulcer in the colon. The event is rare, and Barber and others[18] report only 3 cases among 257 with Crohn's disease.

Clinicians must exclude more common disorders which may coexist with Crohn's disease as a cause of intestinal blood loss. The most likely diagnosis is a bleeding peptic ulcer.

Most patients who continue to bleed require laparotomy in the Lloyd-Davies position to facilitate intraoperative panendoscopy. The site of bleeding will need resection. The author's group has encountered three such cases, all occurring in the small bowel when the site was localized by transillumination during intraoperative ileoscopy.

Acute appendicitis/acute ileitis

Acute appendicitis is uncommon in patients with Crohn's disease,[79] perhaps so rare that the argument for performing a prophylactic appendicectomy is difficult to justify.

The appendix, however, is commonly abnormal in Crohn's disease. Larsen and others[82] report that over half of all patients with Crohn's disease have granulomata in the appendix. So that appendicectomy has been advocated as a means of establishing a diagnosis in difficult cases.

Occasionally when a surgeon is operating for suspected appendicitis through a grid iron incision, he or she will be surprised to discover that the appendix is normal and that the terminal ileum is hyperaemic.

The ileitis may merely represent an acute infection from an organism such as *Yersinia enterocolitica*, a form of arteritis affecting the gut or acute Crohn's disease. More commonly the ileum is partially obstructed due to Crohn's disease.

The surgeon is faced with a dilemma if acute ileitis is discovered through a grid iron incision. Traditionally surgeons have been taught to take out the appendix because it is now known that fistulas virtually never complicate appendicectomy even in ileal Crohn's disease. Furthermore there may be confusion if the patient presents in a casualty department with right iliac fossa pain and a grid iron incision if the appendix has not been removed.[4]

Although fistulas from the appendix stump virtually never complicate appendicectomy the fact remains that enterocutaneous fistulas from the involved ileum commonly complicate an emergency exploration of the right iliac fossa if the ileum is left in situ (see *Table 7.19*). Therefore to leave the ileum and remove the appendix is hardly logical, particularly as the risk of appendicitis if it is not removed is low.[115]

If at laparotomy, irrespective of the type of incision used, the ileum is acutely inflamed, it should not be resected unless the appearances are typical of chronic ileal Crohn's disease. If the ileum is not removed it would be advisable to perform early radiology of the gut as well as cultures and serology to exclude specific intestinal pathogens. If the radiological appearances are typical of stenotic Crohn's disease and *Yersinia* spp. is excluded, early re-laparotomy and resection are advisable.

Table 7.19 Complications following laparotomy and appendicectomy in acute ileal Crohn's disease in 24 patients

Compilation	*Numbers*
Right iliac fossa mass	8
Enterocutaneous fistula	5
Enteroenteric fistula	2
Ileal perforation	1
Obstructed ileal disease	3
Duodenal Crohn's disease	1

From Simonwitz *et al.*[115]

If at laparotomy the appearances are typical of chronic Crohn's disease, it would be entirely reasonable in the author's view to perform an ileal resection and ileocolonic anastomosis, both to establish the diagnosis and to prevent further local complications.

Acute intestinal obstruction

Acute intestinal obstruction from small bowel Crohn's disease is exceedingly rare.[71] If a patient with Crohn's disease presents with abdominal distension, colicky pain, vomiting and has obstructive bowel sounds, the cause of the obstruction is likely to be some other pathology, such as an undisclosed femoral hernia. Acute-on-chronic obstruction in Crohn's disease may be due to the development of a carcinoma.[60] Occasionally acute obstruction may be due to undigested food particles acting as a ball valve between two Crohn's disease strictures.[4]

Untreated acute obstruction may result in small bowel infarction. To have to resect infarcted bowel in Crohn's disease is nothing short of a tragedy, because the lifelong morbidity from the short bowel syndrome might have been averted.

LARGE BOWEL CROHN'S DISEASE

The proportion of patients requiring surgical treatment for colonic Crohn's disease is only marginally less than for ileal disease, and approximately two-thirds of patients with colorectal Crohn's disease eventually require a resection. A small proportion of patients, usually no more than 5–10%, requires an emergency operation for fulminating colitis which may be complicated by toxic dilatation or even colonic perforation. The preferred surgical option for those patients with toxic dilatation or perforation is subtotal colectomy and an ileostomy.

Elective resection is usually advised because of progressive deterioration of health with anorexia, weight loss, malaise, diarrhoea and urgency. Sometimes complications such as abscess, fistula or malignancy are indications for surgery whereas in others severe perianal disease may be the main reason. The surgical options fall into three main categories: sphincter preservation with restoration of intestinal continuity (segmental or subtotal colectomy and anastomosis), construction of a stoma with sphincter preservation (colectomy and ileostomy or faecal diversion alone) or resection of the bowel and sphincters (proctocolectomy or rectal amputation alone).

Elective surgical treatment of colonic Crohn's disease

Indications

The main indications for surgical intervention are intractable diarrhoea and malaise, and severe perianal or rectal disease. In right-sided disease, the ileal component dominates the clinical picture and the majority of patients present with obstructive symptoms, intra-abdominal abscess and enterocutaneous fistula. In patients with sigmoid disease the presentation may mimic diverticular disease with localized obstruction, pericolic abscess or free perforation. If the left-sided disease is more extensive, surgical resection may be indicated if medical control of diarrhoea, urgency and general malaise is ineffective. The other indications for surgical intervention are severe anorectal disease complicated by stricture, chronic sepsis and a narrow, contracted, inflamed rectum.

Operation rates

Overall operation rates are remarkably similar, thus Goligher[53] reported that 250 of 352 patients (71%) with large bowel Crohn's disease eventually required a resection. This is almost identical to the author's own experience where 272 of 360 patients (75%) with large bowel Crohn's disease required an operation. Right-sided disease is usually associated with ileal disease causing obstructive symptoms; consequently the operation rate is high: 89%.[15] Left-sided disease tends to affect an older population particularly if confined to the sigmoid with a lower operation rate – 62% – but in extensive colonic disease, the operation rate is higher – 79%.

Despite the fact that over half of all patients with left-sided or extensive disease eventually require a permanent stoma, the quality of life is generally good. Over 70% of patients are completely well and are able to lead the same sort of life as they had enjoyed before the onset of their disease.[53]

Recurrence after operations for colonic Crohn's disease

Unlike ileal disease, in which the type of operation, and extent of resection, are unrelated to the risk of recurrence, recurrence after operations for colonic disease is closely related to the type of surgical procedure.

Ritchie[103] showed that the recurrence rate 10 years after proctocolectomy was only 9% compared with 50% after ileorectal anastomosis. Goligher[53] reported crude 8-year recurrence rates of 14% after proctocolectomy and 61% after ileorectal anastomosis. It was also found that ileal recurrence was significantly more common after ileorectal anastomosis than after proctocolectomy.[111]

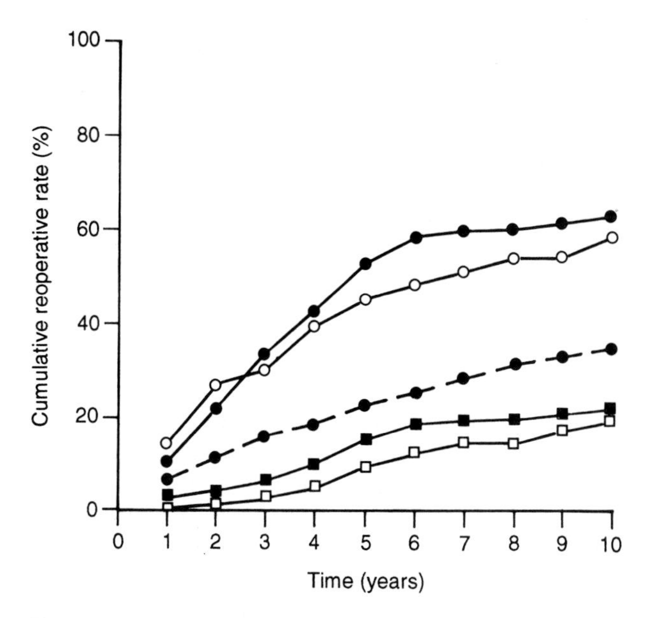

Figure 7.43 Cumulative reoperation rates for recurrent disease after colectomy and ileorectal anastomosis (●), after panproctocolectomy (□), after total colectomy and ileostomy (○), after segmental colectomy (■), compared with ileocaecal resection (×). (Reproduced with permission from *Surgery of the Colon, Rectum, Anus* (1993) M.R.B. Keighley and N.S. Williams. London: WB Saunders.)

The author's group compared reoperations in the first 10 years after operative treatment of colonic Crohn's disease with ileocaecal resection for ileal disease (*Figure 7.43*). Segmental colectomy and subtotal colectomy with ileorectal anastomosis had significantly higher recurrence rates compared with either total colectomy and ileostomy or proctocolectomy.

Ileal disease at the time of colectomy may influence ileal recurrence rates.[90] Thus at the Cleveland Clinic the recurrence rate 11 years after proctocolectomy or colectomy and ileostomy was 46% if there was ileal disease, compared with only 23% if the ileum appeared to be normal.

Recurrence rates are generally higher in patients who are young when they first present.[60,90] This is hardly surprising because the duration of observation in surviving patients is much greater in the young.

Morbidity and mortality

Abdominal wound sepsis after colonic resection occurs in 7–14%.[10,57] These postoperative infections are much more common in patients who have pre-existing infection before resection.[69]

Late complications include enterocutaneous fistula, abdominal sepsis, intestinal obstruction, ileostomy complications and perianal disease. The increased risk of gallstones occurring in up to 6% and urolithiasis reported in 35% have already been discussed.

The morbidity of the unhealed perineal wound is only relevant after rectal excision. Impaired perineal wound healing occurs in over 60% of patients and persistent perineal sinus is reported in 10% of patients.[60,105,112] This complication has lead to alternative surgical approaches being explored such as colectomy and ileostomy alone, conservative proctocolectomy or faecal diversion alone.[83]

Sexual problems may complicate rectal excision: impotence or impaired erection may occur in men and severe dyspareunia in women. The incidence of male dysfunction has been reduced by close perimuscular dissection of the rectum.[84,87] Dyspareunia may also be reduced by avoiding a perineal wound using the options proposed above. Some sexual morbidity is directly due to the presence of a stoma.

In Crohn's disease the incidence of ileostomy dysfunction is much higher than in ulcerative colitis.[117] Consequently there is a much higher rate of ileostomy revision and acute-or-chronic electrolyte disturbance.[122]

Most early deaths are due to sepsis and are usually the result of anastomotic dehiscence. Late deaths are either due to unrelated disease, recurrence or late sepsis.[15,58,60]

Surgical options

Sphincter preservation and restoration of intestinal continuity

This combination is the most attractive one to patients. There is no stoma and no perineal wound, there is negligible social or sexual morbidity, anal continence is preserved, and the functional outcome is generally good provided the rectum is spared. However, there is always a risk of anastomotic breakdown particularly in malnourished patients with coexisting sepsis. Furthermore, these operations carry the highest incidence of recurrent Crohn's disease.

Segmental colectomy

Localized strictures of the colon in the presence of a normal rectum is the most common indication for segmental colectomy.[67,109] Occasionally the localized strictured segment may be complicated by a pericolic abscess or an enteroenteric fistula.

One advantage of segmental colectomy is that the proximal colon can often be preserved with the functional benefit of improved sodium absorption.[107] The main disadvantage is the high incidence of recurrence both in the ileum and in the remaining large bowel. It is believed that segmental colectomy is a perfectly reasonable surgical option in selected patients with short skip lesions in the colon and with minimal disease elsewhere.

However, in the author's experience the recurrence rates are high after segmental colectomy both in the ileum, the residual colon and in the rectum.[8] Sanfey *et al.*[109] also found that repeat resection was needed in 7 of 16 patients 8 years after segmental colectomy. The author's group found that the reoperation rate was 66% at 10 years and that 10 of 36 patients had required a proctocolectomy for extensive colorectal recurrence.[8] Some might argue that recurrence is so common that this procedure should never be advised for colonic Crohn's disease and that all patients should be treated by subtotal colectomy. The reoperation rates after subtotal colectomy were therefore compared with segmental colectomy. Although reoperation rates at 10 years were lower after subtotal colectomy (53% vs 66%), the difference was not statistically significant and the disease-free interval tended to converge with time. We conclude therefore that segmental colectomy has a useful place in a few selected patients with localized colonic disease.

Subtotal colectomy and ileorectal or ileosigmoid anastomosis

A high proportion of patients have either continuous colonic Crohn's disease with rectal sparing or multiple strictures in the large bowel with a normal rectum. It was found that 80 of 272 patients requiring an operation for colonic Crohn's disease were suitable for treatment by ileorectal anastomosis.[15] The St Mark's group had an almost identical experience and reported that 81 of 250 patients were considered suitable for treatment by subtotal colectomy and primary anastomosis. This operation is contraindicated where there is active perianal disease or extensive small bowel involvement.[3,51,90]

The great advantage of subtotal colectomy and a primary anastomosis is that the source of the chronic protein-losing colitis or sepsis is eliminated without the imposition of a permanent stoma or a perineal wound. The social, sexual and marital advantages for young women with Crohn's colitis are considerable. They may complete their education, start a career or enjoy normal family life, have children and have a satisfactory sexual relationship with their partner while they are young, even though at least half will eventually require rectal excision.[11]

A satisfactory functional outcome and a low risk of early proctectomy are largely determined by the degree of rectal distensibility, compliance and absence of macroscopic proctitis.[123] Quite often the sigmoid colon is not obviously diseased; under these circumstances there are functional advantages in preserving the sigmoid colon and performing an ileosigmoid anastomosis.[39]

The most important source of morbidity is anastomotic dehiscence which has a reported incidence of 5–30%.[32,42,47,53] A covering loop ileostomy will reduce the sequelae of this complication and may even reduce its incidence. The risk of anastomotic dehiscence is closely related to the nutritional state of the patient, high-dose steroids and pre-existing abdominal sepsis. Under these circumstances some, including the author's group, would advise a subtotal colectomy and ileostomy, so that an anastomosis can be postponed until the sepsis has resolved.[32]

Many patients have a good functional result after ileorectal anastomosis, particularly if it is performed at the level of the rectosigmoid junction to maximize reservoir function of the rectum. The majority of patients will have less than six bowel actions per day and troublesome diarrhoea is unusual.[9]

There is no clear relationship between the severity of the proctocolitis and frequency of defaecation.[24] Even moderate perianal disease may be associated with reasonable functional results and a low recurrence rate.[11] Lefton and others[86] reported that the best results were in young patients with rectal and sigmoid sparing. Steroids have little influence on the eventual functional outcome.[67]

Between 59% and 65% patients will have a satisfactory result without further surgery after a mean follow-up period of approximately 10 years.[11,105] Flint *et al.*,[47] from combined data, reported a recurrence rate of 47% (32–66%) in 192 patients undergoing ileorectal anastomosis compared with 25% (2–52%) in a series of 345 patients undergoing proctocolectomy. The finding that the recurrence rate after ileorectal anastomosis is approximately twice that after proctocolectomy, in crude terms, has been confirmed by Allan *et al.*[86] and Goligher.[53]

Recurrence does not always imply a proctocolectomy and ileostomy because recurrence may often be dealt with by local ileal resection, if the recurrence is in the small bowel just proximal to the ileorectal anastomosis.[68] The proctectomy rate in the author's group is slightly less than half the overall reoperation rate and only a third of the patients in fact required a rectal excision 10 years after the original operation.

Sphincter preservation with a stoma

There are certain circumstances where a primary anastomosis after colonic resection is dangerous and where colectomy, rectal preservation and ileostomy are indicated. These include emergency colectomy for fulminating colitis and colectomy in the presence of severe rectal disease or abdominal sepsis. There are other patients in whom a sphincter ablative operation is indicated because of severe anorectal disease where the patient cannot accept a permanent stoma for religious, social or marital reasons. The options in these patients include: a proximal stoma alone without any resection, a stoma proximal to a resection and anastomosis or a colectomy and ileostomy.

Subtotal colectomy and ileostomy

Total colectomy and end-ileostomy with either a mucous fistula or an oversewn rectal stump has the advantage of safety, and ileal recurrence is low, being similar to that seen after proctocolectomy. The main indication for this operation is as an emergency procedure for severe colitis but the incidence of subsequently restoring intestinal continuity may be low.[96] Subtotal colectomy and ileostomy may also be used in patients with severe proctitis or in patients with severe perianal disease where a delay in perineal wound healing or even a persistent perineal sinus is anticipated. The major disadvantages of total colectomy with end-ileostomy are the retention of a rectal stump, which may be a source of residual or recurrent morbidity, and the problems inherent in the stoma. The presence of an ileostomy, even though theoretically temporary, may be associated with psychological, social and physical difficulties.[36] This may represent an unacceptable alternative to the potential complications and recurrence rates with ileorectal anastomosis for the young or poorly adjusted patient.

Total colectomy is associated with a mortality of between 2% and 8%.[15] The mortality is higher for emergency operation. Most patients are rapidly restored to health, and can discontinue long-term medical therapy, but approximately 50% of patients develop specific stoma complications within a year of ileostomy construction.

Recurrence rates in the ileum are essentially identical to those occurring after proctocolectomy.[53] One of the problems with colectomy and ileostomy is that the rectum is often ignored unless there is persistent disease or diversion proctitis. These patients often refuse sigmoidoscopy or, because they are so well, default from follow-up. The author's group has at least one patient who developed a late rectal adenocarcinoma complicating a defunctioned rectovaginal fistula. Others also report malignancy in the rectum after faecal diversion.[16]

Faecal diversion

Faecal diversion can be achieved by split or loop ileostomy. In 1975 Lee[83] suggested that beside disease recurrence, three factors had to be considered in the management of large bowel Crohn's disease: (1) the probability of a permanent stoma if the disease is diffuse or involves the rectum; (2) the hazards of a total colectomy in a malnourished patient; and (3) the high morbidity and mortality of intra-abdominal sepsis. Faecal diversion was advocated by the Oxford group as an alternative to conventional surgical resection in three instances: firstly to achieve colonic healing and allow intestinal continuity to be restored without resection where disease was diffuse but not severe enough to warrant proctocolectomy; secondly, to facilitate major resection in those with poor health; and thirdly to limit resection in patients with diffuse disease.

These indications have subsequently been expanded to include the avoidance of growth retardation in children with diffuse colitis requiring steroids, and to protect or avoid a primary anastomosis.[63] More recently faecal diversion has been advocated in the management of refractory perianal disease and as a means of delaying or even preventing proctocolectomy.[62] Faecal diversion has also been advocated to allow perianal and rectovaginal fistulas to heal spontaneously[132] or to facilitate repair of rectovaginal fistulas.[120] Others argue, however, that faecal diversion has no impact on perianal disease[104] and that faecal diversion may in fact exacerbate rectal disease by creating the iatrogenic disorder of diversion proctocolitis.[51,78,106]

Faecal diversion has an undeniable role in protecting an intestinal anastomosis after resection for Crohn's disease. It is useful where there are technical difficulties with the anastomosis, if the anastomosis has been constructed through existing Crohn's disease, if the patient is malnourished or if there is coexisting abdominal sepsis.[132] Faecal diversion may have a pivotal role in the management of postoperative enterocutaneous fistulas. Usually faecal diversion under these circumstances is performed by merely raising a loop ileostomy above a fistula, but if there is extensive sepsis complete defunction by exteriorizing both ends of the bowel may be safer.[83]

The main problem with faecal diversion is that some patients with a macroscopically normal rectum actually develop severe proctocolitis when the faecal stream is diverted.[51,78] This condition may be very difficult to distinguish from reactivation of Crohn's proctitis[27,79] but it improves when intestinal continuity is restored.[77]

A critical review of the outcome of faecal diversion has been reported from Cleveland, Oxford and Birmingham. In Cleveland, Zelas and Jagelman[132] used loop ileostomy to divert 79 patients who had failed to respond to medical therapy or who had severe perianal disease. They reported initial improvement in 72 patients (91%) but 24 patients

Table 7.20 Results of faecal diversion in Crohn's colitis

	*Stoma + resection (n = 51)**	*stoma alone (n = 44)**
Immediate remission	47 (92)	36 (82)
Sustained remission: 12 months	42 (82)	31 (70)
Steroids: before:after	16:2	30:9
Restoration of intestinal continuity	25 (50)	6 (14)
Remain defunctioned	10 (20)	21 (47)
Proctocolectomy	16 (31)	17 (39)

*Numbers in parentheses are the percentages.

(33%) subsequently relapsed. All patients in whom the stoma was closed without a resection relapsed.

In Oxford Lee[83] reported the outcome of 69 patients treated by split ileostomy: 22 (32%) eventually required a proctocolectomy, 9 (13%) were able to have a more limited resection, whereas 25 (36%) still remained defunctioned and only 18 (26%) were able to achieve restoration of intestinal continuity.

The results of the author's group of faecal diversion are summarized in *Table 7.20*. When a loop ileostomy was used alone, 82% achieved an immediate remission; this was sustained for a year in 70% but in only 14% of patients was it possible to restore intestinal continuity without resection. These results were quite different from those achieved when loop ileostomy was used with an intestinal resection.

Harper and others[62] reported the impact of split ileostomy in 19 patients with fistula-in-ano: 11 improved, 4 relapsed while diverted, 1 relapsed after ileostomy closure and only 3 patients were able to achieve restoration of intestinal continuity. The results in 12 women with rectovaginal fistulas were as follows: 5 improved but the fistula remained unhealed, 5 were successfully repaired, but all relapsed when the stoma was closed and only 2 healed in the long term.

Despite the risks of causing diversion proctocolitis it is believed that faecal diversion has a valuable role in the surgical treatment of Crohn's disease. Proximal diversion under certain circumstances increases the safety of resection and primary anastomosis. Faecal diversion may prove valuable in Crohn's disease complicated by abscess or fistulas. Use of a loop ileostomy may be essential to ensure successful reconstruction of the anal sphincter or the rectovaginal septum.

The place of faecal diversion alone is perhaps more controversial. There are many examples of patients, particularly with severe rectal and perianal disease, where construction of a loop ileostomy has rapidly restored health, allowed perirectal sepsis to resolve and enabled a patient to come to terms with an ileostomy. In many of these patients, their quality of life is such that they do not want any further operations. There is a slightly increased risk of malignancy in the defunctioned large bowel. Many patients with perirectal disease will eventually need a proctocolectomy.

Faecal diversion has occasionally been used in children with growth retardation in order to withdraw steroid administration so that growth spurts can be achieved. This strategy has been particularly valuable in children who show objective improvement with total parenteral nutrition.

Overall the number of patients in whom this form of management is indicated is limited. The advantage is that proximal loop ileostomy is a relatively minor procedure and diversion is associated with a high incidence of disease remission. In most patients loop ileostomy adequately defunctions the colon; furthermore management and closure are much easier than for patients with a split ileostomy. As the role of surgery is to control symptoms while preserving bowel, faecal diversion may provide an attractive alternative to conventional ablative surgery in selected cases.

Conservative proctocolectomy

The concept of removing the colon and rectum while preserving the anal canal and sphincters has been explored by a few groups recently.[119] This approach is more applicable to ulcerative colitis than to Crohn's disease. The rationale for this approach is that the morbidity of the unhealed perineal wound or persistent perineal sinus might be eliminated, while removing the diseased process. A further potential advantage might be to reduce the incidence of dyspareunia.

There are two forms of conservative proctectomy. The more usual procedure involves full rectal mobilization by the abdominal route to the level of the levator ani with closure either of the upper anal canal or the lower rectum by suture or staples with removal of the rectum. In the alternative technique, instead of closing the lower rectum or anal canal, the mucosa of the anorectum is excised to the dentate line, as in mucosal proctectomy.

The results of conservative proctocolectomy have been reported from St Mark's Hospital,[119] Oxford and Birmingham.[129] There is remarkable concordance in the findings from all three centres and the overall opinion is that conservative proctocolectomy is generally not a satisfactory alternative to conventional total rectal excision. Early complications are common and include bleeding, pelvic seromas and particularly pelvic sepsis. Sepsis is usually due to over-active sphincters which prevents drainage of purulent material collecting in the lower pelvis. In the author's own experience five of eight patients had persistent pelvic or perineal sepsis with intermittent offensive discharge and four patients required a proctectomy.[128]

This approach is often technically impossible in Crohn's disease patients due to scarring around the anal canal from intersphincteric sepsis, fistulas and chronic mucosal inflammation. Consequently, the author's group and others believe that this method of proctectomy has little place in the management of Crohn's disease.

Sphincter ablation and permanent stoma

Almost half of all patients requiring surgery for large bowel Crohn's disease will eventually require an operation to remove the rectum and a permanent stoma. Usually the inflammatory process involves the rectum, necessitating total proctocolectomy and ileostomy as the initial operation. In other patients a secondary proctectomy is performed for progressive rectal involvement or recurrence in the rectum after sphincter-conserving operations such as subtotal colectomy and ileostomy or ileorectal anastomosis, segmental colectomy or even proximal loop ileostomy used alone or to protect a distal anastomosis. In a few patients with severe rectal disease and an uninvolved colon, the best option may be rectal excision alone.[55,103]

The advantages of sphincter ablative surgery and a permanent ileostomy are that the operation restores patients to good health and alleviates socially incapacitating diarrhoea, urgency, incontinence, severe perianal sepsis with chronic discharging fistulas and mucorrhoea. If these patients will accept that, for them, life with an ileostomy is infinitely preferable to permanent sepsis and incontinence, this approach should be strongly recommended. Also there is no later risk of malignancy in chronic fistulas or in the defunctioned rectum. Furthermore, the risk of recurrent disease in the ileum after proctocolectomy is lower than after any other operation for Crohn's disease. Thus there are many advantages in these surgical options provided the patient will accept a permanent stoma.

Sadly for some patients, rectal excision and a stoma is in itself associated with morbidity. In 35% of patients, perineal wound healing is not achieved in 3 months and in 10% of patients there is a long-standing, persistent, perineal sinus.[112] There is also the potential sexual morbidity attending rectal excision with impaired erection or retrograde ejaculation in men and distressing dyspareunia from perineal scarring in women. Stoma complications and their sexual morbidity are also common in Crohn's disease. For all these reasons, the option of sphincter ablative surgery is probably being practised with less enthusiasm today than it was 20 years ago.

Abdominoperineal excision of the rectum

The rectum is involved alone in a small proportion of patients with Crohn's disease. These patients usually have extensive perianal and rectal disease. If such patients cannot be controlled by repeat dilatation or are not controlled with medical therapy, the rectum alone may be excised with the construction of an end-colostomy.

There are few reports on the outcome of rectal excision alone, because the majority of patients have coexisting ileal or colonic disease necessitating a proctocolectomy. Lockhart-Mummery[91] has the largest series which includes 24 patients. The cumulative probability of recurrence was remarkably low, being 6% at 5 years and 11% at 10 years. These authors conclude therefore that the operation has a place for a small group of patients with localized anorectal disease. Williams and Hughes[126] also support the use of this operation for anorectal Crohn's disease and have used it in nine patients. However, there were two operative deaths, one admittedly from malignancy but the other from sepsis. Perineal healing within 3 months of operation occurred in only one patient and three had a persistent perineal sinus. Problems with the colostomy were also reported in two patients. Nevertheless, the recurrence rate was very low and only one patient required a proctocolectomy. This option has only been used in four patients by the author's group; recurrences in the colon necessitated proctocolectomy in three and the stomatherapists found that most patients had difficulty managing a rather wet colostomy. Therefore they found that it was generally preferable to use a proctocolectomy even if the disease appears to be confined to the rectum, but accept that others have found rectal excision alone to be a perfectly acceptable procedure for anorectal disease.

Proctocolectomy and ileostomy

Proctocolectomy is indicated for extensive colonic disease involving the rectum with or without perianal disease. The operation may even be indicated for severe anorectal disease even in the presence of an apparently normal colon. The patient must understand that the operation necessitates a permanent end-ileostomy because any form of restorative procedure is contraindicated.[22,76]

Many patients eventually undergo what is sometimes termed 'completion proctocolectomy' as a consequence of rectal recurrence or progressive rectal disease after colectomy with ileostomy, ileorectal anastomosis or after faecal diversion, the usual indication being persistent discharge from the defunctioned rectum or active perianal disease.

Proctocolectomy has an operative mortality rate of 3–9%.[65,90,111] Goligher[54] reported a mortality of 8.9% after protocolectomy compared with 2.8% following colectomy and ileorectal anastomosis.

Hospital stay is often prolonged after proctocolectomy; this is largely attributed to patients having to learn to care for their stoma together with delay in perineal wound healing.

Complications in the author's own practice include abdominal wound sepsis in 8%, perineal wound sepsis in 22%, abdominal abscess in 9%, intra-abdominal bleeding in 7%, thromboembolism in 3% and septicaemia in 1%. Intestinal obstruction requiring repeat laparotomy was needed in 11 patients (14%).

Delayed or unhealed perineal wounds are associated with high fistula-in-ano, faecal contamination and postoperative perineal wound sepsis.[19,34,70] The incidence of ileostomy dysfunction is high[117] and may be associated with disease recurrence. The most common complications are retraction, prolapse, fistula formation and obstruction.[122] Most ileostomy complications can be managed by local revision. In the presence of recurrent Crohn's disease, however, laparotomy and resection are often necessary.

In the early days of surgery for Crohn's disease colitis it was not fully appreciated that recurrent ileal disease might occur later as it had done after ileocaecal resections. Goligher's observations in 1972 may seem unremarkable today, but he carefully described the pathological findings in seven patients who developed ileal recurrence following either colectomy and ileostomy or proctocolectomy.[52] In two cases, ulceration and cobblestoning of the mucosa was evident on the ileostomy itself, whilst in the remainder the recurrence was just inside the abdominal wall causing stenosis, bleeding, parastomal sepsis and fistula.

Recurrent Crohn's disease in the ileum developed in 20 of 182 patients who had been treated at St Mark's Hospital by proctocolectomy. The rate of recurrence both at that Institution and in the author's own was significantly less than after ileorectal anastomosis.[103] The cumulative recurrence rates after proctocolectomy being 7% at 5 years, 11% at 10 years and 22% at 20 years.

We must conclude therefore that, although proctocolectomy is associated with the morbidity of a perineal wound and the ileostomy, and even though the operative mortality is slightly higher than restorative resection, the long-term prognosis in these patients who come to terms with a permanent stoma are excellent. Proctocolectomy has the lowest incidence of recurrent disease following any operation for Crohn's disease. Furthermore, there are fewer late deaths from gastrointestinal malignancy or recurrent disease causing sepsis or repeated operations.

Emergency surgical treatment for colonic Crohn's disease

Emergency colectomy may be required for acute fulminating colitis or for a perforated paracolic abscess. The indications for colectomy are acute fulminating colitis and its complications such as toxic dilatation, colonic perforation, persisting acute colitis or colorectal haemorrhage.

Acute fulminating colitis

Approximately 20–30% of all patients presenting with acute fulminating colitis will eventually be found to have Crohn's disease and not ulcerative colitis.[38,45,94]

Severe disintegrating disease or toxic dilatation may be complicated by perforation which is accompanied by severe circulatory failure and a rigid silent abdomen. The complications of toxic dilatation or free perforation carry a mortality of 20–50%.[114,125]

At least 40% of patients with fulminating colitis who have underlying Crohn's disease will have some evidence of perianal disease.[73] Bleeding is often less prominent if the underlying diagnosis is Crohn's disease. More patients with Crohn's disease tend to give a history of previous intestinal symptoms, particularly diarrhoea, urgency and abdominal pain.[130]

Mortensen and others[96] described 18 patients presenting to St Mark's Hospital with acute fulminating colitis who had underlying Crohn's disease. In at least nine of these patients, a diagnosis of Crohn's disease was not suspected when they presented with acute colitis. Twelve patients developed toxic dilatation, two of whom were complicated by colonic perforation. Colonic perforation also developed without dilatation in three patients and only three had uncomplicated acute fulminating colitis.

Usually there are certain macroscopic features of Crohn's disease even in fulminating colitis. Perianal disease is evident in 50% of patients; there is often, although not invariably, some ileal involvement. There is usually some thickening in at least a part of the wall of the colon, linear ulceration with cobblestoning of the mucosa is often absent in acute fulminating colitis, but other tell-tale signs of Crohn's disease may be present such as deep fissures and penetrating ulcers with localized sepsis. Segmental involvement is often evident and there is evidence of rectal sparing in over half of the patients with acute Crohn's disease.

Toxic dilatation

Toxic dilatation is due to bacterial fermentation in the colon causing gaseous distension and impaired blood supply to the muscle coat of the colon.[121] There is mucosal ischaemia with sloughing of the colonic mucosa leaving denuded muscle and mucosal islands. This disintegrating process quickly progresses to perforation.[93]

Toxic dilatation complicating Crohn's colitis may be precipitated by barium enema examination or exacerbated by taking anticholinergics, opiates or antidiarrhoeal agents. The incidence of this event in Crohn's disease ranges from 4.4% to 6.3%. The diagnosis is made clinically when the diameter of the transverse colon exceeds 5.5 cm. The mortality of toxic dilatation exceeds 40% particularly if surgical intervention is delayed or the colon is allowed to perforate.[28] Brooke[23] reviewed 23 cases of toxic dilatation complicating Crohn's colitis, 9 of whom died. Grieco and others[59] reported 5 patients from 78 with Crohn's ileocolitis who developed toxic megacolon (6.3%). Occasionally colonic dilatation may occur secondary to a colonic stricture, but perforation is exceedingly rare.[118]

Free perforation

Free perforation is not necessarily a complication of toxic dilatation and may occur without any evidence of dilating disease. Free perforation of the colon with toxic dilatation occurs in up to 3% of patients with Crohn's disease.[25] Perforations usually occur in the descending colon or sigmoid but caecal perforation has been reported in Crohn's disease.[81] Perforations may complicate high-dose steroid therapy.

Free perforation may complicate disease in the sigmoid colon which either masquerades as or occurs in combination with diverticular disease.[21] Malignant or granulomatous diverticulitis may present with a pericolic abscess, or with purulent or faecal peritonitis.[92] There is a high incidence of local complications with fistulas, abscess and free perforation.[30] Rectal involvement is often progressive,[5] extraintestinal manifestations are common[88] and 76% have perianal disease.

Conservative management

Urgent considerations include rapid resuscitation with intravenous colloids and crystalloids to replace blood volume and electrolyte deficiencies. The author's group advises high-dose intravenous steroids, usually hydrocortisone 100 mg 6-hourly, and intravenous antibiotics.

Bedrest with graduated compression stockings to prevent thromboembolic complications is commenced on admission, but prophylactic subcutaneous heparin is not given because of the risks of exacerbating colonic bleeding. All patients are admitted to the gastrointestinal unit where they can be carefully monitored and kept under close scrutiny by the nursing staff. Perhaps the most important parameter is the daily monitoring of abdominal girth and plain radiograph. Radiological evidence of impending dilatation with a transverse diameter of the colon exceeding 5.5 cm, and plain radiographic evidence of mucosal islands, retroperitoneal gas or pneumoperitoneum, should be used as an absolute indication for laparotomy.

Surgical intervention

If a diagnosis of Crohn's colitis has been established which from our experience is the case in approximately half of all patients, then a rather more aggressive intervention is called for than in ulcerative colitis. The reason for this is that fewer patients with acute Crohn's colitis go into remission compared with acute ulcerative colitis. Furthermore, the morbidity of delayed surgical treatment is higher and the long-term prospect of retaining the colon is far less in Crohn's colitis.[15,96,130]

If a patient with acute Crohn's colitis shows no evidence of improvement in 72 hours, or if there is deterioration despite intravenous fluids, steroids and antibiotics during the first 72 hours, then a colectomy with ileostomy and mucous fistula is advised. If there are signs of toxic dilatation, impending or actual perforation, then a colectomy is performed immediately. If there is initial improvement which is not sustained or if there is later deterioration despite intensive steroid therapy and nutritional support, then a colectomy with oversewing of the rectal stump and an end-ileostomy or an ileorectal anastomosis is advised.

Subtotal colectomy and ileostomy

Subtotal colectomy and ileostomy is the operation most widely used for patients with acute fulminating colitis or its complications. The advantages are that the disintegrating colon is removed, so that any associated sepsis can resolve, there is no anastomosis hence the risk of sepsis from that source is eliminated, and the patient has an opportunity to experience an end-ileostomy. Furthermore, the option of a subtotal colectomy and ileostomy does not necessarily commit the patient to a permanent stoma, hence a period of adjustment can take place in the knowledge that surgery performed is only a temporary solution to a life-threatening situation. In other words it leaves all options open while removing the major source of disease. As the rectum is never initially involved in perforation or toxic dilatation, it may be safely preserved. Just occasionally severe bleeding may occur from the rectal stump necessitating early proctectomy, but in Crohn's disease this is rarely necessary.

There are two situations in which a mucous fistula would be preferred to closure of the rectal stump. The first is if the rectum is severely inflamed; a mucous fistula would then provide easier access to the rectum for the administration of topical steroids. The second is the risk that the rectal stump might leak after closure.[130] Only if the rectum is very severely diseased, if there is pre-existing pelvic sepsis, or if the patient is on high doses of steroids, would there be a high risk of leakage from a closed rectal stump. Usually therefore the rectum is closed by staples or sutures at the pelvic brim.

Restorative proctocolectomy and ileoanal anastomosis

At laparotomy fulminating ulcerative colitis may be indistinguishable from Crohn's colitis. Even in Crohn's colitis the appendix and terminal ileum may be normal. The eager surgeon wishing to prevent the stigma of a permanent stoma, and believing the disease to be ulcerative colitis, may be tempted to perform a restorative proctocolectomy and ileoanal anastomosis even without a covering ileostomy, on the basis that the patient has only been on steroids for a few days. The risks of leakage and pelvic sepsis under these circumstances are considerable and if the diagnosis proves to be Crohn's disease then it is likely that the patient will lose 50 cm of terminal ileum because of chronic pelvic sepsis or complications.

The option of an emergency restorative proctocolectomy should be resisted, however good the evidence for ulcerative colitis. The incidence of complications which could permanently wreck the function of a pouch are too high. Irrespective of the diagnosis, the preferred surgical option in acute colitis is subtotal colectomy and ileostomy.

Subtotal colectomy and ileorectal anastomosis

There are a few patients in whom this option might be worthy of serious consideration, but it is not advised for the treatment of fulminating colitis. If a patient is known to have Crohn's disease and previous investigations have shown that there is rectal sparing, there may be a place for subtotal colectomy and ileorectal anastomosis if such a patient develops an acute relapse of colitis necessitating emergency admission and early surgical intervention.

The advantage is that the patient has a single operation for the control of complicated colitis and the procedure is reported to be safe provided that there is no pre-existing sepsis.[47]

Proctocolectomy and ileostomy

The author's group argues against the use of proctocolectomy as an emergency operation. The rectum rarely, if ever, needs to be removed for acute Crohn's disease. There is a high morbidity from pelvic and perineal sepsis when the rectum is removed from the pelvis, particularly in the presence of toxic dilatation or colonic perforation, when contamination is inevitable. Finally the mortality of emergency proctocolectomy is still prohibitively high.[10,55,57]

Defunction

The concept of defunctioning the colon and diverting the faecal stream is an attractive approach in chronic disease,[63,83] but it clearly cannot be used for toxic dilatation or perforation and it is doubtful whether this is a safe option in acute fulminating colitis.[100]

Preferred surgical option

Subtotal colectomy and ileostomy with or without a mucous fistula is the preferred surgical option for almost all patients requiring an emergency colectomy for acute fulminating colitis, or its complications. This option removes the perforating or dilating disease, allows thorough histological scrutiny of the resection specimen, avoids anastomosis and keeps all therapeutic options open.

REFERENCES

1. Abascal, J., Diaz-Rojas, F., Jorge, J. *et al.* (1982) Free perforation of the small bowel in Crohn's disease. *World Journal of Surgery*, **6**, 216–220.
2. Adolff, M., Arnaud, J.P. and Ollier, J.C. (1987)

Does the histologic appearance at the margin of resection affect the postoperative recurrence rate in Crohn's disease. *Annals of Surgery*, **53**, 543–546.
3. Adson, M.A., Cooperman, A.M. and Farrow, G.M. (1972) Ileorectostomy for ulcerative diseases of the colon. *Archives of Surgery*, **104**, 424–428.
4. Alexander-Williams, J. (1971) The place of surgery in Crohn's disease. *Gut*, **12**, 739–749.
5. Alexander-Williams, J. (1976) Late onset Crohn's disease. In *The Management of Crohn's Disease* (Ed.) Weterman, I.T., Pena, A.S. and Booth, C.C. p.43. Amsterdam: Excerpta Medica.
6. Alexander-Williams, J., Fielding, J.F. and Cooke, W.T. (1972) A comparison of results of excision and bypass for ileal Crohn's disease. *Gut*, **13**, 973–975.
7. Alexander-Williams, J. and Fornaro, M. (1982) Strictureplasty beim morbus Crohn. *Der Chirug.*, **53**, 799–801.
8. Allan, A., Andrews, J., Hilton, C.J., Keighley, M.R.B., Allan, R.N. and Alexander-Williams, J. (1989) Segmental colonic resection is an appropriate operation for short skip lesions due to Crohn's disease in the colon. *World Journal of Surgery*, **13**, 611–616.
9. Allan, R., Steinberg, D.M., Alexander-Williams, J. and Cooke, W.T. (1977) Crohn's disease involving the colon: an audit of clinical management. *Gastroenterology*, **73**, 723–732.
10. Allsop, J.R. and Lee, E.C.G. (1978) Factors which influenced postoperative complications in patients with ulcerative colitis or Crohn's disease of the colon on corticosteroids. *Gut*, **19**, 729–734.
11. Ambrose, N.S., Keighley, M.R.B., Alexander-Williams, J. and Allan, R.N. (1984) Clinical impact of colectomy and ileorectal anastomosis in the management of Crohn's disease. *Gut*, **25**, 223–227.
12. Andersson, H., Bosaeus, I., Hellberg, R. and Hulten, L. (1982) Effect of a low-fat diet and antidiarrhoeal agents on bowel habits after excisional surgery for classical Crohn's disease. *Acta Chirurgica Scandinavica*, **148**, 285–290.
13. Andersson, H., Filipsson, S. and Hulten, L. (1978) An evaluation of the bile salt malabsorption before and after surgery in patients with Crohn's disease. *Scandinavian Journal of Gastroenterology*, **13**, 249.
14. Andrews, H.A. and Allan, R.N. (1990) Crohn's disease of the small intestine. In *Inflammatory Bowel Disease*, 2nd Ed. (Ed.) Allan, R.N., Keighley, M.R.B., Alexander-Williams, J. and Hawkins, C. pp. 329–337. Edinburgh: Churchill-Livingstone.
15. Andrews, H.A., Lewis, P. and Allan, R.N. (1989) Prognosis after surgery for colonic Crohn's disease. *British Journal of Surgery*, **76**, 1184–1190.
16. Ball, C.S., Wujanto, R., Harbourbi, N.Y. and Schofield, P.F. (1988) Carcinoma in anal Crohn's disease: discussion paper. *Journal of the Royal Society of Medicine*, **81**, 217–219.
17. Banks, B.M., Zetzel, L. and Richter, H.S. (1969) Morbidity and mortality in regional enteritis. *American Journal of Digestive Diseases*, **14**, 369–379.
18. Barber, K.W. Jr, Waugh, J.M., Beahrs, O.H. and Sauer, W.G. (1962) Indications for and the results of the surgical treatment of regional enteritis. *Annals of Surgery*, **156**, 472–482.
19. Bardot, P., Keighley, M.R.B. and Alexander-Williams, J. (1980) Perineal wound healing after proctectomy for carcinoma and inflammatory disease. *British Journal of Surgery*, **67**, 275–276.
20. Bergman, L. and Krause, U. (1977) Crohn's disease: a long-term study of the clinical course in 186 patients. *Scandinavian Journal of Gastroenterology*, **12**, 937–944.
21. Berman, I.R., Corman, M.L., Coller, J.A. and Veidenheimer, M.C. (1979) Late onset Crohn's disease in patients with colonic diverticulitis. *Disease of the Colon and Rectum*, **22**, 524–529.
22. Block, G.E. (1980) Surgical management of Crohn's colitis. *New England Journal of Medicine*, **302**, 1068–1070.
23. Brooke, B.N. (1972) Crohn's disease of the large bowel. *British Medical Journal*, **1**, 310–311.
24. Buchmann, P., Mogg, G.A.G., Alexander-Williams, J., Allan, R.N. and Keighley, M.R.B. (1980) Relationship of proctitis and rectal capacity in Crohn's disease. *Gut*, **21**, 137–140.
25. Bundred, N.J., Dixon, J.M., Lumsden, A.B., Gilmour, H.M. and Davies, G.C. (1985) Free perforation in Crohn's colitis: a ten year review. *Diseases of the Colon and Rectum*, **28**, 35–37.
26. Burman, J.H., Cooke, W.T. and Alexander-Williams, J. (1971) The fate of ileorectal anastomosis in Crohn's disease. *Gut*, **12**, 432–436.
27. Burman, J.H., Thompson, H., Cooke, W.T. and Williams, J.A. (1971) The effects of diversion of intestinal contents on the progress of Crohn's disease of the large bowel. *Gut*, **12**, 11–15.
28. Cello, J.P. and Meyer, J.H. (1978) Ulcerative colitis. In *Gastrointestinal Disease* (Ed.) Sleisenger, M.H. and Fordtran, J.S. p. 1597. Philadelphia, W.B. Saunders.
29. Chardavoyne, R., Flint, G.W., Pollack, S. and Wise, L. (1986) Factors affecting recurrence following resection for Crohn's disease. *Diseases of the Colon and Rectum*, **29**, 495–502.
30. Colcock, B.P. and Stahmann, F.D. (1972) Fistulas complicating diverticular disease of the sigmoid colon. *Annals of Surgery*, **175**, 838.
31. Cooke, W.T. and Swan, C.J.H. (1974) Diffuse jejuno-ileitis of Crohn's disease. *Quarterly Journal of Medicine*, **72**, 583–601.
32. Cooper, J.C., Jones, D. and Williams, N.S. (1986) Outcome of colectomy and ileorectal anastomosis in Crohn's disease. *Annals of the Royal College of Surgeons of England*, **68**, 279–282.
33. Cooper, J.C. and Williams, N.S. (1986) The influence of microscopic disease at the margin of resection on recurrence rates in Crohn's disease.

Annals of the Royal College of Surgeons of England, **68**, 23–26.

34. Corman, M.L., Veidenheimer, M.C., Coller, J.A. and Ross, V.H. (1978) Perineal wound healing after proctectomy after inflammatory bowel disease. *Diseases of the Colon and Rectum*, **21**, 155–159.
35. Dehn, T.C.B., Kettlewell, M.G.W., Mortensen, N.J.McC., Lee, E.C.G. and Jewell, D.P. (1989) Ten year experience of strictureplasty for obstructive Crohn's disease. *British Journal of Surgery*, **76**, 339–341.
36. Devlin, H.B., Plant, J.A. and Griffin, M. (1971) Aftermath of surgery for anorectal cancer. *British Medical Journal*, **3**, 413–418.
37. Ernest, D.L., Johnson, G., Williams, H.E. and Admirand, W.H. (1974) Hyperoxaluria in patients with ileal resection. *Gastroenterology*, **66**, 1114.
38. Farmer, R.G., Hawk, W.A. and Turnbull, R.B. (1968) Regional enteritis of the colon: a clinical and pathological comparison with ulcerative colitis. *American Journal of Digestive Diseases*, **13**, 501–514.
39. Farnell, M.B., Van Heerden, J.A., Beart, R.W. and Wiland, L.H. (1980) Rectal preservation in nonspecific inflammatory disease of the colon. *Annals of Surgery*, **192**, 249–253.
40. Fazio, V.W. and Galandiuk, S. (1985) Strictureplasty in diffuse Crohn's jejunoileitis. *Diseases of the Colon and Rectum*, **28**, 512–518.
41. Fazio, V.W., Galandiuk, S., Jagelman, M.D. and Lavery, I.C. (1989) Strictureplasty in Crohn's disease. *Annals of Surgery*, **210**, 621–625.
42. Fazio, V., Turnbull, R.B. and Goldsmith, M.G. (1975) Ileorectal anastomosis: A safe surgical technique. *Diseases of the Colon and Rectum*, **18**, 107–114.
43. Fielding, J.F. (1970) Crohn's disease. MD Thesis, University of Cork.
44. Fielding, J.F., Toye, D.K., Beton, D.C. and Cooke, W.T. (1970) Crohn's disease of the stomach and duodenum. *Gut*, **11**, 1101–1106.
45. Fielding, J.F. and Truelove, S.C. (1972) Crohn's disease of the large bowel. *British Medical Journal*, **1**, 310.
46. Filipsson, S., Hulten, L. and Lindstedt, G. (1978) Malabsorption of fat and vitamin B12 before and after resection for Crohn's disease. *Scandinavian Journal of Gastroenterology*, **13**, 529.
47. Flint, G., Strauss, R., Platt, N. and Wise, L. (1977) Ileorectal anastomosis in patients with Crohn's disease of the colon. *Gut*, **18**, 236–239.
48. Garlock, J.H. (1967) Surgery of the small intestine. In *Garlock's Surgery of the Alimentary Tract*, pp. 241–292. London: Butterworth.
49. Garlock, J.H. and Crohn, B.B. (1945) An appraisal of the results of surgery in treatment of regional ileitis. *Journal of the American Medical Association*, **127**, 205–208.
50. Glass, R.E. and Baker, W.N.W. (1976) Role of the granuloma in recurrent Crohn's disease. *Gut*, **17**, 75–77.
51. Glotzer, D.J., Glick, M.E. and Goldman, H. (1981) Proctitis and colitis following diversion of the fecal stream. *Gastroenterology*, **80**, 438–441.
52. Goligher, J.C. (1972) Ileal recurrence after ileostomy and excision of the large bowel for Crohn's disease. *British Journal of Surgery*, **59**, 253–259.
53. Goligher, J.C. (1979) The outcome of excisional operations for primary and recurrent Crohn's disease of the large intestine. *Surgical Gynecology and Obstetrics*, **148**, 1–8.
54. Goligher, J.C. (1985) The long-term results of excisional surgery for primary and recurrent Crohn's disease of the large intestine. *Diseases of the Colon and Rectum*, **28**, 51–55.
55. Goligher, J.C. (1988) Surgical treatment of Crohn's disease affecting mainly or entirely the large bowel. *World Journal of Surgery*, **12**, 186–190.
56. Greenstein, A.J., Lachman, P., Sachar, D.B. *et al.* (1988) Perforating and non-perforating indications for repeated operations in Crohn's disease: evidence for two clinical forms. *Gut*, **29**, 588–592.
57. Greenstein, A.J., Meyers, S., Sher, L., Heimann, T. and Aufses, A.H. (1981) Surgery and its sequelae in Crohn's colitis and ileocolitis. *Archives of Surgery*, **116**, 285–288.
58. Greenstein, A.J., Sachar, D., Pucillo, A. *et al.* (1978) Cancer in Crohn's disease after diversionary surgery. *American Journal of Surgery*, **135**, 86–90.
59. Grieco, M.B., Bordan, D.L., Geiss, A.C. and Beil, A.R. (1980) Toxic megacolon complicating Crohn's colitis. *Annals of Surgery*, **191**, 75–80.
60. Gyde, S.N., Prior, P., Macartney, J.C., Thompson, H., Waterhouse, J.A.H. and Allan, R.N. (1980) Malignancy in Crohn's disease. *Gut*, **21**, 1024–1029.
61. Hamilton, S.R., Reese, J., Pennington, L. *et al.* (1985) The role of resection margin frozen section in the surgical management of Crohn's disease. *Surgical Gynecology and Obstetrics*, **160**, 57–62.
62. Harper, P.H., Kettlewell, M.G.W. and Lee, E.C.G. (1982) The effect of split ileostomy on perianal Crohn's disease. *British Journal of Surgery*, **69**, 608–610.
63. Harper, P.H., Truelove, S.C., Lee, E.C.G., Kettlewell, M.G.W. and Jewell, D.P. (1983) Split ileostomy and ileocolostomy for Crohn's disease of the colon and ulcerative colitis: a 20 year survey. *Gut*, **24**, 106–113.
64. Hellberg, R., Hulten, L. and Bjorn-Rasmussen, E. (1982) The nutritional and haematological status before and after primary and subsequent resectional procedures for classical Crohn's disease and Crohn's colitis. *Acta Chirurgica Scandinavica*, **148**, 453–460.
65. Hellers, G. (1979) Crohn's disease in Stockholm County 1955–1974. *Acta Chirurgica Scandinavica*, (Suppl.) **490**, 1–84.

66. Higgens, C.S. and Allan, R.N. (1980) Crohn's disease of the distal ileum. *Gut*, **21**, 933–940.
67. Howel Jones, J., Lennard-Jones, J.E. and Lockhart-Mummery, H.E. (1966) Experience in the treatment of Crohn's disease of the large intestine. *Gut*, **7**, 448–452.
68. Hughes, E.S.R., McDermott, F.T. and Masterton, J.P. (1980) Ileorectal anastomosis for inflammatory bowel disease: 15 year follow up. *Diseases of the Colon and Rectum*, **23**, 399–400.
69. Hulten, L. (1988) Surgical treatment of Crohn's disease of the small bowel or ileocecum. *World Journal of Surgery*, **12**, 180–185.
70. Irvin, T.I. and Goligher, J.C. (1975) A controlled clinical trial of three different methods of perineal wound management following excision of the rectum. *British Journal of Surgery*, **62**, 287–291.
71. Javett, S.L. and Brooke, B.N. (1970) Acute dilatation of colon in Crohn's disease. *The Lancet*, **2**, 126–128.
72. Karesen, R., Serch-Hanssen, A., Thoresen, B.O. and Hertsberg, J. (1981) Crohn's disease: long-term results of surgical treatment. *Scandinavian Journal of Gastroenterology*, **16**, 57–64.
73. Keighley, M.R.B. and Allan, R.N. (1986) Current status and influence of operation on perianal Crohn's disease. *International Journal Colorectal Disease*, **1**, 104–107.
74. Kelly, T., Klein, R. and Woodford, J. (1972) Alteration in gallstone solubility following distal ileal resection. *Archives of Surgery*, **105**, 352.
75. Kendall, G.P., Hawley, P.R., Nicholls, R.J. and Lennard-Jones, J.E. (1986) Strictureplasty: a good operation for small bowel Crohn's disease? *Diseases of the Colon and Rectum*, **29**, 312–316.
76. Kock, N.G. (1969) Intra-abdominal reservoir in patients with permanent ileostomy. *Archives of Surgery*, **99**, 223–231.
77. Korelitz, B.I., Cheskin, L.J., Sohn, N. and Sommers, S.C. (1984) Proctitis after fecal diversion in Crohn's disease and its elimination with reanastomosis: implications for surgical management. Report of 4 cases. *Gastroenterology*, **87**, 710–714.
78. Korelitz, B.I. Cheskin, L.J., Sohn, N. and Sommers, S.C. (1985) The fate of the rectal segment after diversion of the fecal stream in Crohn's disease: its implications for surgical management. *Journal of Clinical Gastroenterology*, **7**, 37–43.
79. Korelitz, B.I. and Sommers, S.C. (1974) Differential diagnosis of ulcerative colitis and granulomatous colitis by sigmoidoscopy, rectal biopsy and cell counts of rectal mucosa. *American Journal of Gastroenterology*, **61**, 460–469.
80. Krause, U., Ejerblad, S. and Bergman, L. (1985) Crohn's disease: a long-term study of the clinical course in 1986 patients. *Scandinavian Journal of Gastroenterology*, **20**, 516–524.
81. Kyle, J., Caradis, T., Duncan, T. *et al.* (1968) Free perforation in regional enteritis. *American Journal of Digestive Diseases*, **13**, 275–283.
82. Larsen, E., Axelsson, C. and Johansen, A. (1970) The pathology of the appendix in morbus Crohn and ulcerative colitis. *Acta Pathologica Microbiologica Immunologica Scandinavica*, (Suppl.) **21**, 161–165.
83. Lee, E. (1975) Split ileostomy in the treatment of Crohn's disease of the colon. *Annals of the Royal College of Surgeons of England*, **56**, 94–102.
84. Lee, E.C.G. and Dowling, B.L. (1972) Perimuscular excision of the rectum for Crohn's disease and ulcerative colitis. A conservative technique. *British Journal of Surgery*, **59**, 29–32.
85. Lee, E.C.G. and Papaioannou, N. (1982) Minimal surgery for chronic obstruction in patients with extensive or universal Crohn's disease. *Annals of the Royal College of Surgeons of England*, **64**, 229.
86. Lefton, H.B., Farmer, R.G. and Fazio, V. (1975) Ileorectal anastomosis for Crohn's disease of the colon. *Gastroenterology*, **69**, 612–617.
87. Leicester, R.J., Ritchie, J.K., Wadsworth, J., Thompson, J.P. and Hawley, P.R. (1984) Sexual function and perineal wound healing after intersphincteric excision of the rectum for inflammatory bowel disease. *Diseases of the Colon and Rectum*, **27**, 244–248.
88. Lennard-Jones, J.E. (1972) Differentiation between Crohn's disease, ulcerative colitis and diverticulitis. *Clinical Gastroenterology*, **1**, 367.
89. Lindhagen, T., Ekelund, G., Leandoer, L., Hildell, J., Lindstrom, C. and Wenckert, A. (1983) Crohn's disease in a defined population course and results of surgical treatment. I Small bowel disease. *Acta Chirurgica Scandinavica*, **149**, 407–413.
90. Locke, M.R., Fazio, V.W., Farmer, R.G., Jagelman, D.G., Lavery, I.C. and Weakley, F.L. (1981) Proximal recurrence and the fate of the rectum following excisional surgery for Crohn's disease of the large bowel. *Annals of Surgery*, **194**, 754–760.
91. Lockhart-Mummery, H.E. (1975) Symposium: Crohn's disease: anal lesions. *Diseases of the Colon and Rectum*, **18**, 200–202.
92. Marshak, R.H., Janowitz, H.D. and Present, D.H. (1970) Granulomatous colitis in association with diverticula. *New England Journal of Medicine*, **283**, 1080.
93. Marshak, R.H., Lester, L.J. and Friedman, A.I. (1950) Megacolon, a complication of ulcerative colitis. *Gastroenterology*, **16**, 768.
94. McGovern, V.J. and Goulston, S.J.M. (1968) Crohn's disease of the colon. *Gut*, **9**, 164–176.
95. Menguy, R. (1972) Surgical management of free perforation of the small intestine complicating regional enteritis. *Annals of Surgery*, **175**, 178.
96. Mortensen, N.J.McC., Ritchie, J.K., Hawley,

P.R., Tood, I.P. and Lennard-Jones, J.E. (1984) Surgery for acute Crohn's colitis: results and long term follow up. *British Journal of Surgery*, **71**, 783–784.

97. Murray, J.J., Schoetz, D.J., Nugent, F.W., Coller, J.A. and Veidenheimer, M.C. (1984) Surgical management of Crohn's disease involving the duodenum. *American Journal of Surgery*, **147**, 58–65.
98. Nasr, K., Morowitz, D.A., Anderson, J.G. *et al.* (1968) Free perforation in regional enteritis. *American Journal of Digestive Diseases*, **13**, 275–283.
99. Nygaard, K. and Fausa, O. (1977) Crohn's disease: recurrence after surgical treatment. *Scandinavian Journal of Gastroenterology*, **12**, 577–584.
100. Oberhelman, H.A. (1976) Inflammatory disease of the bowel: indications for surgery. *Diseases of the Colon and Rectum*, **19**, 582–583.
101. Papaioannou, N., Piris, J., Lee, E.C.G. and Kettlewell, M.G.W. (1979) The relationship between histological inflammation in the cut ends after resection of Crohn's disease and recurrence. *Gut*, **20**, A916.
102. Pennington, L., Hamilton, S.R., Bayless, T.M. and Cameron, J.L. (1980) Surgical management of Crohn's disease. *Annals of Surgery*, **192**, 311–317.
103. Ritchie, J.K. (1990) The results of surgery for large bowel Crohn's disease. *Annals of the Royal College of Surgeons of England*, **72**, 155–157.
104. Ritchie, J.K. and Lennard-Jones, J.E. (1976) Crohn's disease of the distal large bowel. *Scandinavian Journal of Gastroenterology*, **11**, 433–436.
105. Ritchie, J.K. and Lockhart-Mummery, H.E. (1973) Non-restorative surgery in the treatment of Crohn's disease of the large bowel. *Gut*, **14**, 263–269.
106. Roediger, W.E.W. (1990) The starved colon – diminished mucosal nutrition, diminished absorption and colitis. *Diseases of the Colon and Rectum*, **33**, 858–862.
107. Roediger, W.E.W., Rigol, G. and Rae, D. (1984) Sodium absorption with bacterial fatty acids and bile salts in the proximal and distal colon as a guide to colonic resection. *Diseases of the Colon and Rectum*, **27**, 1–5.
108. Rutgeerts, P., Geboes, K., Vantrappen, G., Kerremans, R., Coenegrachts, J.L. and Coremans, G. (1984) Natural history of recurrent Crohn's disease at the ileocolonic anastomosis after curative surgery. *Gut*, **25**, 665–672.
109. Sanfey, H., Bayless, T.M. and Cameron, J.L. (1984) Crohn's disease of the colon. Is there a role for limited resection? *American Journal of Surgery*, **147**, 38–42.
110. Sayfan, J., Wilson, G.A.L., Allan, A., Andrews, H. and Alexander-Williams, J. (1989) Recurrence after strictureplasty or resection for Crohn's disease. *British Journal of Surgery*, **76**, 335–338.
111. Scammell, B., Ambrose, N.S., Alexander-Williams, J., Allan, R.N. and Keighley, M.R.B. (1985) Recurrent small bowel Crohn's disease is more frequent after subtotal colectomy and ileorectal anastomosis than proctocolectomy. *Disease of the Colon and Rectum*, **28**, 770–771.
112. Scammell, B.E. and Keighley, M.R.B. (1986) Delayed perineal wound healing after proctectomy for Crohn's colitis. *British Journal of Surgery*, **73**, 150–152.
113. Schofield, P.F. (1965) The natural history and treatment of Crohn's disease. *Annals of the Royal College of Surgeons of England,* **36**, 258–279.
114. Schofield, P.J. (1983) Toxic dilatation and perforation in inflammatory bowel disease. *Annals of the Royal College of Surgeons of England*, **64**, 318–320.
115. Simonowitz, D.A., Rusch, V.W. and Stevenson, J.K. (1982) Natural history of incidental appendectomy in patients with Crohn's disease who required subsequent bowel resection. *American Journal of Surgery*, **143**, 171–173.
116. Speranza, V., Simi, M., Leardi, S. and Del Papa, M. (1986) Recurrence of Crohn's disease: are there any risk factors? *Journal of Clinical Gastroenterology*, **8**, 640–646.
117. Steinberg, D.M., Allan, R.N., Brooke, B.N., Cooke, W.T. and Alexander-Williams, J. (1975) Sequelae of colectomy and ileostomy: comparison between Crohn's colitis and ulcerative colitis. *Gastroenterology*, **68**, 33–39.
118. Svanes, S., Thunold, S., Skaar, R. *et al.* (1976) Dilatation of the colon with free perforation due to mechanical obstruction in Crohn's disease. *Acta Chirurgica Scandinavica*, **142**, 181–185.
119. Talbot, R.W., Ritchie, J.K. and Northover, J.M.A. (1989) Conservative proctocolectomy: A dubious option in ulcerative colitis. *British Journal of Surgery*, **76**, 738–739.
120. Tuxen, P.A. and Castro, A.J. (1979) Rectovaginal fistula in Crohn's disease. *Diseases of the Colon and Rectum*, **22**, 58–62.
121. Wakefield, A.J., Sawyer, A.M., Dhillon, A.P. *et al.* (1989) Pathogenesis of Crohn's disease: multifocal gastrointestinal infarction. *The Lancet*, **2**, 1057–1062.
122. Weaver, R.M., Alexander-Williams, J. and Keighley, M.R.B. (1988) Indications and outcome of reoperation for ileostomy complications in inflammatory bowel disease. *International Journal of Colorectal Diseases*, **3**, 38–42.
123. Weaver, R.M. and Keighley, M.R.B. (1986) Measurement of rectal capacity in the assessment of patients for colectomy and ileorectal anastomosis in Crohn's colitis. *Diseases of the Colon and Rectum*, **29**, 443–445.
124. Weterman, I.T. (1976) Course and long-term

prognosis of Crohn's disease. MD thesis, Leiden, Delft: W.D. Meinimar.
125. Whorwell, P.J. and Isaacson, P. (1981) Toxic dilatation of colon in Crohn's disease. *The Lancet*, **2**, 1334–1337.
126. Williams, J.G. and Hughes, L.E. (1989) Effect of perioperative blood transfusion on recurrence of Crohn's disease. *The Lancet*, **2**, 131–132.
127. Williams, J.G., Wong, W.D., Rothenberger, D.A. and Goldberg, S.M. (1991) Recurrence of Crohn's disease after resection. *British Journal of Surgery*, **78**, 10–19.
128. Winslet, M.C., Alexander-Williams, J. and Keighley, M.R.B. (1990) Conservative proctocolectomy with low transection of the anorectum is a poor alternative to conventional proctocolectomy in inflammatory bowel disease. *International Journal of Colorectal Diseases*, **5**, 117–119.
129. Winslet, M.C. and Keighley, M.R.B. (1988) Defunctioned proctitis: a diagnostic dilemma. *Gut*, **29**, A1454.
130. Winslet, M.C. and Keighley, M.R.B. (1990) Surgery for Crohn's disease of the colon. In *Inflammatory Bowel Diseases*, 2nd Ed. (ed.) Allan, R.N., Keighley, M.R.B., Alexander-Williams, J. and Hawkins, C. pp. 473–482. Edinburgh: Churchill Livingstone.
131. Wolff, B.G., Beart, R.J. Jr, Frydenberg, H.B., Weiland, L.H., Agrez, M.V. and Ilstrup, D.M. (1983) The importance of disease-free margins in resections for Crohn's disease. *Diseases of the Colon and Rectum*, **26**, 239–243.
132. Zelas, P. and Jagelman, D.G. (1980) Loop ileostomy in the management of Crohn's colitis in the debilitated patient. *Annals of Surgery*, **191**, 164–168.

CANCER IN CROHN'S DISEASE

(S.N. Gyde)

Crohn's disease and ulcerative colitis are classified under the broad heading of 'inflammatory bowel disease', although superficially they appear to be very different diseases. However, genetic studies leave little doubt that these two apparently disparate conditions are linked by some common inheritance.[36,40] In ulcerative colitis, the disease process is confined to the colon and rectum, and the inflammation limited to the mucosa. Crohn's disease can affect the whole gastrointestinal tract and the inflammatory process affects the full thickness of the bowel wall leading to complications such as stricture, chronic abscess and fistula formation.

In a recent report of a study of the families of a single series of Crohn's disease patients in New York ($n = 353$), over 20% ($n = 72$) of patients had relatives with either Crohn's disease or ulcerative colitis.[36] Given this common predisposition, an increased cancer risk in one of these diseases might be associated with an increased cancer risk in the other.

The enormous body of literature concerning the cancer risk in ulcerative colitis demonstrates that this disease carries a considerably increased risk of developing colorectal cancer above that in the general population. In comparison there are few studies in the literature concerning the cancer risk in Crohn's disease.

This suggests that cancer complicating Crohn's disease is uncommon and does not pose a particular clinical problem.

Reviewing the world literature Hawker *et al.*[33] detailed 61 cases of small bowel cancer and Zinkin *et al.*[52] detailed 44 cases of large bowel cancer.

Considering Dr Crohn and his colleagues first described 'regional iteitis' as a disease entity in 1932[14] which was closely followed by reports in the literature of the first cases of cancer complicating the disease, in 1948, of colonic cancer[50] and, in 1956, of small bowel cancer,[23] the number of cases reported in the world literature is small.

FACTORS AFFECTING THE NUMBER OF CANCERS SEEN

Surgical resection

In contrast to ulcerative colitis, where effective medical therapy is available. Crohn's disease surgical resection of the diseased bowel is often the most effective treatment. Severely diseased bowel in Crohn's disease is, therefore, usually resected well before the long latent period necessary for cancer to develop.

Bypass procedure and strictureplasty

Bypass procedures were common in the early years of surgical treatment of Crohn's disease patients. Such procedures allowed diseased bowel to remain in situ for many years, and many of the reported cancers have developed in bypassed loops.[27,33]

Misclassification

Prior to 1960, patients with colonic Crohn's disease, without small bowel involvement, were classified as having ulcerative colitis. In 1960, Lockhart-Mummery and Morson[39] described the histopathology of Crohn's colitis distinguishing it from ulcerative colitis.

Following this report, many centres reviewed their inflammatory bowel disease patients, reclassifying many previously supposed 'ulcerative colitis' patients as having colonic Crohn's disease. Early reports of cancer in ulcerative colitis (prior to 1960) would therefore include some misclassified Crohn's disease cancers.

Small bowel cancer in Crohn's disease

Macroscopic Crohn's disease most commonly occurs in the terminal ileum, or terminal ileum and right colon (55–65% of all patients), although microscopic lesions may be present throughout the whole gastrointestinal tract.[3,4,16,19] If severe inflammatory change predisposes towards cancer, it might be expected that cancers develop mainly in the terminal ileum and right colon.

This is not seen in clinical practice, presumably because early surgical resection of this site results in dramatic relief of symptoms and improvement in health. Cancers have been reported in the small bowel in Crohn's disease, and also in the colon and rectum. The available evidence suggests (despite surgical resection of the most severely diseased bowel in most patients) that there is a considerably increased risk above the general population in developing cancer at both these sites (*Tables 7.21* and *7.22*).

The small bowel seems remarkably resistant to developing cancer. Small bowel cancer in the general population is extremely rare with an incidence of 1 per 100 000 population per year.[1,30] If Crohn's disease of the small bowel did predispose patients to develop cancer, and even given a 100-fold increase in risk above the general population, the actual numbers of cancers observed in any large clinical series would be very small.

Greenstein *et al.*[26,28] reviewed the cancer risk in 579 Crohn's disease patients diagnosed at Mount Sinai Hospital between 1960 and 1976, when they observed four small bowel cancers. However, applying age- and sex-specific cancer rates for the general population to these patients over the review period, only 0.047 cancers would have been expected to occur, giving an *86-fold risk* of small bowel cancer above the general population. Therefore, although there is a very high 'relative risk' of cancer (observed cancers/expected cancers) the absolute number of cancers observed are small and do not pose a significant clinical problem.

Hawker *et al.* in 1982,[33] reviewing all small bowel cancers in Crohn's disease reported in the literature ($n = 61$) found that 41 (67%) of these reported cases occurred in the ileum, and 18 of these were in bypassed loops. In the general population small bowel cancers are more evenly distributed.[44] Most of these cancers occurred at the site of macroscopic disease.[2,15,22,28,43,48] The mean age at diagnosis of cancer was 47 years and there was a mean latent period of 18 years between diagnosis and the development of cancer. Small bowel cancers have been described in association with fistulas.[10,21,28,46]

Histopathology

Most of the small bowel cancers reported were adenocarcinomas, but other cell types such as carcinoid tumours, reticulum cell sarcomas and lymphomas occurred.

Survival

No 5-year survivors were reported. The mean survival time was less than 9 months.

CANCER OF THE COLON

The true cancer risk in patients with Crohn's colitis cannot be determined while surgical resection remains the most effective form of treatment. Patients with total Crohn's colitis usually have persistent or recurrent symptoms so that they tend to undergo surgery at a relatively early stage. If an effective medical therapy for Crohn's colitis became available, and patients were kept in good health for many years with the colon in situ, the cancer risk in these patients might be much greater than it appears today.

Even in a large hospital series under long-term review, the absolute number of colorectal cancers diagnosed is small (see *Tables 7.21* and *7.22*). However, cancers start to appear in any large series after a period from diagnosis of 15 years or more.

In a large series of Crohn's disease patients under review at the General Hospital, Birmingham ($n = 513$) between 1944 and 1976, nine patients developed colorectal cancer.[12,20,29] Some 12 years later (1988), when the series comprised 800 patients, 16 patients had developed colorectal cancer – a doubling of the number of cancers in the series over a 12-year review period (H.A. Andrews and R.N. Allan, personal communication). This demonstrates how, at a certain point in any series, the cancers become overt, and emphasizes the need for long-term review when studying the cancer risk.

In a recent population study from Uppsala Health Care Region in Sweden,[17] 1655 patients were diagnosed with Crohn's disease between the years 1965 and 1983. During this time 12 colorectal cancers were diagnosed. The mean follow-up for patients in this series was not stated, but from the data in the report (given that the yearly incidence rates were constant) nearly half the patients were followed for less than 10 years from diagnosis. Given a latent period from diagnosis of disease to cancer of around 20 years, one might therefore expect to diagnose many more cancers in this series in the next 10–20 years.

Characteristics: colorectal cancer in Crohn's disease

Hamilton *et al.*[31] reviewed the surgical pathology records at the Johns Hopkins Hospital, Baltimore, between 1949 and 1983 and found 11 patients with a diagnosis of colorectal cancer in Crohn's disease. They then searched the files between 1981 and 1982 for patients with non-colitic colorectal cancer, and used these 118 cases as a group for comparison.

RESULTS OF THE JOHNS HOPKINS STUDY

Age at cancer

Patients developing colorectal cancer in Crohn's disease develop cancer at an age some 10 years younger than patients without Crohn's disease (55 years vs 65 years). This young age at diagnosis was also found by Petras *et al.*[42] in their study from the Cleveland Clinic where the mean age at diagnosis of cancer was 47 years. This is similar to findings in patients with ulcerative colitis who also develop colorectal cancer at an age some 10 years younger than that found in the general population.

Multiple cancers

One patient had two colorectal cancers. As in ulcerative colitis, more multiple cancers are found than in the general population.[31,35,42,52]

Site of cancer

In Hamilton's study,[31] for the Johns Hopkins Hospital, Baltimore, the sites of the colorectal cancers were similar to those found in the general population, seven of the eleven cancers (65%) occurring in the sigmoid colon and rectum.

In the series from the General Hospital, Birmingham, 50% of the cancers occurred in the sigmoid colon and rectum.[29]

In the study from the Cleveland Clinic,[42] all seven colorectal cancers were in the sigmoid colon ($n = 2$) or rectum ($n = 5$). These are small numbers and it is not yet possible to draw any firm conclusions concerning the distribution of colorectal cancer in Crohn's disease.

Bypassed loops

Two of the eleven cancers occurred in bypassed loops, and many reports from other centres, particularly from the series reported from Mount Sinai[27] and the Cleveland Clinic,[28,42] show that bypassed loops are at particular risk of developing cancer. This has been confirmed in other reports.[9,38,44,46]

Site of macroscopic disease

Ten of the eleven colorectal cancers in Hamilton's series from the Johns Hopkins Hospital[31] occurred at the site of macroscopic disease. All seven patients in Petras's series from the Cleveland Clinic[42] had active macroscopic Crohn's disease. Other reports confirm this finding.[15,24,28,29,45,51]

Histopathology

Dysplasia was present in all 10 patients with colorectal cancer in the Johns Hopkins report.[31] In the report from the Cleveland Clinic[42] only six of the seven patients' sections were available for review of whom five had dysplasia adjacent to the cancer. Four of the six also showed dysplasia remote from the cancer and dysplasia.[11,13]

Both studies showed a high incidence of mucinous carcinoma of nearly 50% compared with 9% in noncolitic cancers.

CANCER IN CROHN'S DISEASE – REPORTS FROM HOSPITAL SERIES

Table 7.21 documents cancers in Crohn's disease reported in hospital series where no actuarial risk of cancer was calculated. *Table 7.22* summarises the hospital series where actuarial analyses of the cancer risk over time were made. *Table 7.23* documents the risk found in Scandinavian population studies.

The relative risk of developing colorectal cancer is significantly increased with a young age at disease. Weedon *et al.*,[51] in a series of 449 patients from the Mayo Clinic, all with onset of disease before 21 years of age, calculated a 27-fold risk above the general population for the development of colorectal cancer (see *Table 7.22*).

Ekbom,[17] in a population study for the Uppsala Region in Sweden, estimated a 21-fold increased risk of colorectal cancer in patients diagnosed with

Table 7.21 Cancer in Crohn's disease: reports of cancers observed in hospital series without actuarial analysis of risk

Authors	*Year*	*Ref. no.*	*Centre*	*Review period*	*No. of patients in series*	*Total number of cancers observed*	*Colorectal*	*Small bowel*
Van Patter *et al.*	1954	49	Mayo Clinic	1912–1949	600	1	1	0
Atwell *et al.*	1965	5	Leeds	1934–1962	212	3	3	0
Farmer *et al.*	1975	18	Cleveland Clinic, Ohio }	1955–1971	466	3	1	2
Petras *et al.*	1987	42	Cleveland Clinic, Ohio }	1975–1984	3500	11	7	4
Darke *et al.*	1973	15	The London Hospital	1948–1973	167	3	2	1
Perret *et al.*	1968	41	Ratcliffe Infirmary, Oxford	1938–1970	303	4	4	0
Truelove and Pena	1976	47						
Hamilton	1985	31	Johns Hopkins, Baltimore	1949–1983	NK	11	10	NS
Cooke *et al.*	1980	12	General Hospital, Birmingham	1944–1976 (patients followed for 20 years or more)	176	4	3	1
Harper *et al.*	1987	32	Cleveland Clinic, Ohio	Diagnosis before 1965 (patients followed for 15 years or more)	139	4	3	1

NK = not known.
NS = not stated.

Table 7.22 Cancers in Crohn's disease: actuarial analysis in hospital series of patients

Authors	*Year*	*Ref.*	*Centre*	*Diagnostic period*	*No. of patients in series*	*Total*	*Colorectal*	*Small bowel*	*Relative risk (O/E)**
Weedon *et al.*	1973	51	Mayo Clinic	1919–1965	449 (onset of disease before age 21 years)	9	8	1	Colon O/E = $\frac{8}{0.3}$ = 26.6
Gyde *et al.*	1980	29	General Hospital, Birmingham	1944–1976	513	18	9	1	Colon O/E = $\frac{9}{2.26}$ = 4.0
Greenstein *et al.*	1980	28	Mount Sinai Hospital, New York	1960–1976	597	17	7	4	Colon O/E = $\frac{7}{1.01}$ = 6.9; Small bowel O/E = $\frac{4}{0.046}$ = 85.8
Kvist *et al.*	1986	37	Rigshospitalet, Copenhagen	1964–1983	473	5	3	2	O/E = $\frac{5}{2.3}$ = 2.2

*Relative risk is the risk of developing cancer in the group under review relative to risk of developing cancer in the general population. This is calculated by dividing the cancers observed in the group under review by the cancers which might have been expected to occur in a similar group in the general population.
Relative risk = $\frac{\text{Observed cancers}}{\text{Expected cancers}}$ = O/E.

Table 7.23 Cancer in Crohn's disease – Scandinavian population studies

Authors	*Year*	*Ref. no.*	*Geographical area*	*Review period*	*Population*	*No. of cases*	*No. of cancers observed*
Brame *et al.*	1975	8	City of Malmo/	1958–1973	217 330	191	0
Binder *et al.*	1985	7	Copenhagen County	1960–1978	500 000	185	1 (small bowel)
Ekbom *et al.*	1990	17	Uppsala/Sweden	1965–1983	1.2 million	1469	12 (colorectal)
Gollop *et al.*	1988	25	Olmsted County/ Minnesota	1943–1983		103	1 (rectum) 1 (ileum) (leiomyosarcoma)*

*Leiomyosarcoma (Gollop *et al.*) followed radiation for Crohn's disease 1940s to 1950s.

Crohn's disease before the age of 30 years. Two-thirds (66%) of the patients in the Birmingham Hospital series were diagnosed before the age of 30 years but in this study the increase in risk in the group as a whole was only fourfold.

RELATIVE RISK OF DEVELOPING CANCER RELATED TO SITE OF MACROSCOPIC CROHN'S DISEASE

The Ekbom study from Uppsala Health Region,[17] Sweden, was of great interest in that calculations were made for the relative risk of developing cancer by site of macroscopic disease. The relative risk by site of disease at diagnosis reported were as shown in *Table 7.24*.

Although the numbers of cancers were small, there seems to be a differential cancer risk related to the site of macroscopic disease at onset of disease. The prospective Scandinavian population studies[7,8] will, in time, together with the continuing follow-up of patients from the retrospectively defined cohort of incident cases in the Uppsala study, provide the most reliable data on the cancer risk in Crohn's disease. The studies for Malmo and Copenhagen[7,8] have relatively small numbers of patients and relatively short follow-up so far, but even so they do show a very small risk of cancer compared with either hospital studies or the retrospectively defined cohort from Uppsala.[17]

Table 7.24 Relative risk of developing cancer by site of disease at diagnosis

Site	*Number*
Terminal ileum	1
Terminal ileum and parts of colon	3.2
Colon alone	5.6
Colon only (diagnosis before age of 30 years)	20.9
Colon only (diagnosis after the age of 30 years)	2.2

SCREENING FOR CANCER IN CROHN'S DISEASE

There do not seem to be any grounds at present for initiating a randomized trial to test the effectiveness of screening for cancer in Crohn's disease.

The numbers of cancers observed in large series of patients under long-term review have been so small that such an approach could not be justified as either of potential benefit to the patient or a good use of limited resources.

Clinicians should be aware that cancer is a rare late complication of this disease and more common in patients at a young age (before the age of 30 years).

All bypassed loops of bowel should be suspect and, if surgery is required for other reasons, the bypassed loop should be examined for cancer, if possible without undue risk to the patient.

CANCER OF THE BILIARY TRACT AND GALLBLADDER

Cancer of the gallbladder and biliary tract has been reported in association with Crohn's disease, but no increased relative risk of cancer at these sites has been reported, as distinct from ulcerative colitis where an increased risk has been shown.[6,34]

REFERENCES

1. Ackerman, L.V. and Del Regato, J.A. (1962) *Cancer Diagnosis, Treatment and Prognosis*, 3rd Ed., p. 626. St Louis: Mosby.
2. Adler, S.N., Lyon, D.T. and Sullivan, P.D. (1982) Adeno-carcinoma of the small bowel. *American Journal of Gastroenterology*, **7**, 326–330.
3. Allan, R.N., Steinberg, D.N., Dixon, K. and Cooke, W.T. (1975) Changes in bidirectional sodium flux across the intestinal mucosa in Crohn's disease. *Gut*, **15**, 201–204.
4. Andrews, H.A. and Allan, R.N. (1990) Crohn's

disease of the small intestine. *Inflammatory Bowel Diseases*, 2nd Ed., p. 329. Edinburgh: Churchill Livingstone.
5. Atwell, J.D., Duthie, H.L. and Goligher, J.C. (1965) The outcome of Crohn's disease. *British Journal of Surgery*, **52**, 966–972.
6. Berman, M.D., Falchuk, K.R. and Trey, C. (1980) Carcinoma of the biliary tree complicating Crohn's disease. *Digestive Diseases and Sciences*, **25**, 795–797.
7. Binder, V., Hendriksen, C. and Kreiner, S. (1985) Prognosis in Crohn's disease based on results from a regional patient group from the County of Copenhagen. *Gut*, **26**, 146–150.
8. Brahme, F., Lindstrom, C. and Wenckert, A. (1975) Crohn's disease in a defined population. An epidemiological study of incidence, prevalence, mortality and secular trends in the City of Malmo, Sweden. *Gastroenterology*, **69**, 342–351.
9. Buchmann, P., Allan, R.N., Thompson, H. and Alexander-Williams, J. (1980) Carcinoma in a rectovaginal fistula in a patient with Crohn's disease. *American Journal of Surgery*, **140**, 462–463.
10. Burbige, E.J., Bedine, M.S. and Handelsman, J.C. (1977) Adenocarcinoma of the small intestine in Crohn's disease involving the small bowel. *Western Journal of Medicine*, **127**, 43–45.
11. Butt, J.H. and Morson, B. (1981) Dysplasia and cancer in inflammatory bowel disease. *Gastroenterology*, **80**, 865–867.
12. Cooke, W.T., Mallas, E., Prior, P. and Allan, R.N. (1980) Crohn's disease: course, treatment and long term prognosis. *Quarterly Journal of Medicine*, **195**, 363–384.
13. Craft, C.F., Mendelsohn, G., Cooper, H.S. and Yardley, J.H. (1981) Colonic 'precancer' in Crohn's disease. *Gastroenterology*, **80**, 578–584.
14. Crohn, B.B., Ginsberg, L. and Oppenheimer, D.G. (1932) Regional enteritis: a pathological and clinical entity. *Journal of the American Medical Association*, **99**, 1323–1328.
15. Darke, S.G., Parks, A.G., Grogono, J.L. and Pollock, D.J. (1973) Adenocarcinoma and Crohn's disease: a report of two cases and analysis of the literature. *British Journal of Surgery*, **60**, 169–175.
16. Dunne, W.T., Allan, R. and Cooke, W.T. (1976) Enzymatic and quantitative histological evidence for Crohn's disease as a diffuse lesion of the gastrointestinal tract (Abstract). *Gut*, **17**, 399.
17. Ekbom, A., Helmick, C., Zack, M. and Adami, H.O. (1990) Increased risk of large bowel cancer in Crohn's disease with colonic involvement. *The Lancet*, **336**, 357–359.
18. Farmer, R.G., Hawk, W.A. and Turnbull, R.B. (1975) Clinical patterns in Crohn's disease. A statistical study. *Gastroenterology*, **68**, 627–635.
19. Ferguson, R., Allan, R.N. and Cooke, W.T. (1975) A study of the cellular infiltrate of the proximal jejunal mucosa in ulcerative colitis and Crohn's disease. *Gut*, **16**, 205–208.
20. Fielding, J.F., Prior, P., Waterhouse, J.A. and Cooke, W.T. (1972) Malignancy in Crohn's disease. *Scandinavian Journal of Gastroenterology*, **7**, 3–7.
21. Fleming, K.A. and Pollock, A.C. (1975) A case of Crohn's carcinoma. *Gut*, **16**, 533–537.
22. Frank, J.D. and Shorey, B.A. (1973) Adenocarcinoma of the small bowel as a complication of Crohn's disease. *Gut*, **14**, 120–124.
23. Ginzburg, L., Schneider, K.M., Dreisin, D.H. and Levinson, C. (1956) Carcinoma of the jejunum occurring in a case of regional enteritis. *Surgery*, **39**, 347–351.
24. Glotzer, D.J. (1985) The risk of cancer in Crohn's disease. *Gastroenterology*, **89**, 438–441.
25. Gollop, J.H., Phillips, S.F., Melton, L.J. III and Zinsmeister, A.R. (1988) Epidemiologic aspects of Crohn's disease: a population-based study in Olmstead County, Minnesota, 1943–1982. *Gut*, **29**, 49–56.
26. Greenstein, A.J. and Sachar, D.B. (1983) Cancer in Crohn's disease. In *Inflammatory Bowel Diseases* (Ed.) Allan, R.N., Keighley, M.R.B., Alexander-Williams, J. and Hawkins, C.F. pp. 332–337. Edinburgh: Churchill Livingstone.
27. Greenstein, A.J., Sachar, D., Pucillo, A. *et al.* (1978) Cancer in Crohn's disease after diversionary surgery. A report of seven carcinomas occurring in excluded bowel. *American Journal of Surgery*, **135**, 86–90.
28. Greenstein, A.J., Sachar, D.B., Smith, H. *et al.* (1980) Patterns of neoplasia in Crohn's disease and ulcerative colitis. *Cancer*, **46**, 403–407.
29. Gyde, S.N., Prior, P., Macartney, J.C. *et al.* (1980) Malignancy in Crohn's disease. *Gut*, **21**, 1024–1029.
30. Haffner, J.F.W. and Semb, L.S. (1969) Malignant tumours of the small intestine. *Acta Chirurgica Scandinavica*, **135**, 543–548.
31. Hamilton, S.R. (1985) Colorectal carcinoma in patients with Crohn's disease. *Gastroenterology*, **89**, 398–407.
32. Harper, P.H., Fazio, V.W., Lavery, I.C. *et al.* (1987) The long term outcome of Crohn's disease. *Diseases of the Colon and Rectum*, **30**, 174–179.
33. Hawker, P.C., Gyde, S.N. and Allan, R.N. (1982) Adenocarcinoma of the small intestine complicating Crohn's disease. *Gut*, **23**, 188–193.
34. Joffe, N. and Antonioli, D.A. (1981) Primary carcinoma of the gall bladder associated with chronic inflammatory bowel disease. *Clinical Radiology*, **32**, 319–324.
35. Keighley, M.R.B., Thompson, H. and Alexander-Williams, J. (1975) Multifocal colonic carcinoma and Crohn's disease. *Surgery*, **78**, 534–537.
36. Korelitz, B.I. (1981) Epidemiological evidence for a hereditary component in Crohn's Disease. In *Recent Advances in Crohn's Disease* (Ed.) Pena, A.S., Weterman, I.T., Booth, C.C. and Strober, W. pp. 208–212. The Hague: Martinus Nijhoff.
37. Kvist, N., Jacobsen, O., Norgaard, P. *et al.* (1986) Malignancy in Crohn's disease. *Scandinavian Journal of Gastroenterology*, **21**, 82–86.

38. Lightdale, C.J., Sternberg, S.S., Posner, G. and Sherlock, P. (1975) Carcinoma complicating Crohn's disease. Report of seven cases and review of the literature. *American Journal of Medicine*, **59**, 262–268.
39. Lockhart-Mummery, H.E. and Morson, B.C. (1960) Crohn's disease (regional enteritis) of the large intestine and its distinction from ulcerative colitis. *Gut*, **1**, 87–105.
40. McConnell, R.B. (1980). Inflammatory bowel disease: newer views of genetic influences. In *Developments in Digestive Disease*, Vol. 3 (Ed.) Berk, J.E. pp. 271–278. Philadelphia: Lea and Febiger.
41. Perrett, A.D., Truelove, S.C. and Massarella, G.R. (1968) Crohn's disease and carcinoma of the colon. *British Medical Journal*, **2**, 466–468.
42. Petras, R.E., Mir-Madjlessi, S.D. and Farmer, R.G. (1987) Crohn's disease and intestinal carcinoma. *Gastroenterology*, **93**, 1307–1314.
43. Rochlin, D.B. and Longmire, W.P. Jr (1961) Primary tumours of the small intestine. *Surgery*, **50**, 586–592.
44. Simpson, S., Traube, J. and Riddell, R.H. (1981) The histological appearance of dysplasia (precarcinomatous change) in Crohn's disease of the small and large intestine. *Gastroenterology*, **81**, 492–501.
45. Smiddy, F.G. and Goligher, J.C. (1957) Results of surgery in treatment of cancer of the large intestine. *British Medical Journal*, **1**, 793–796.
46. Traube, J., Simpson, S., Riddell, R.H. *et al.* (1980) Crohn's disease and adenocarcinoma of the bowel. *Digestive Diseases and Sciences*, **25**, 939–944.
47. Truelove, S.C. and Pena, A.S. (1976) Course and prognosis of Crohn's disease. *Gut*, **17**, 192–201.
48. Valdes-Dapena, A., Rudolph, I., Hidayat, A. *et al.* (1976) Adenocarcinoma of the small bowel in association with regional enteritis. Four new cases. *Cancer*, **37**, 2936–2947.
49. Van Patter, W.N., Bargen, J.A. and Dockerty, M.B. (1954) Regional enteritis. *Gastroenterology*, **26**, 347–450.
50. Warren, S. and Sommers, S.C. (1948) Cicatrizing enteritis (regional enteritis) as a pathologic entity. *American Journal of Pathology*, **24**, 475–501.
51. Weedon, D.D., Shorter, R.G., Ilstrup, D.M. *et al.* (1973) Crohn's disease and cancer. *New England Journal of Medicine*, **289**, 1099–1103.
52. Zinkin, L.D. and Brandwein, C. (1980) Adenocarcinoma in Crohn's colitis. *Diseases of the Colon and Rectum*, **23**, 115–117.

PERIANAL CROHN'S DISEASE

(V.W. Fazio, N. Hyman and J.A. Procaccino)

When Crohn *et al.* first described the entity of regional ileitis no mention was made of perianal involvement.[9] Two years later, in 1934, Bissel[4] described the association recognized several years later by Crohn as well.[44] In 1959 Morson and Lockhart-Mummery described anal lesions in almost half of the Crohn's disease patients presenting to St Mark's Hospital and emphasized the importance of distinguishing the granulomatous changes of tuberculosis from those of Crohn's disease.[40] Interestingly, Gabriel had described the finding of multinucleated giant cells in non-tuberculous anal fistulas in 1921.[18] The St Mark's group went on further to describe and refine the clinical and pathological features of lesions occurring around the anus in patients with Crohn's disease.[36,41]

Perianal complications are now a well-recognized component of Crohn's disease. They may be the major cause of disability in some patients, a secondary cause of substantial morbidity in others, or they may be entirely asymptomatic. Reports of various treatments for the perianal complications are often confusing and ambiguous. The dilemma has occurred because of the uncertain nature of Crohn's disease and the generic 'lumping' of the various perianal complications leading to the paradoxical reports of success and failure with definitive therapy – especially that directed towards perianal fistulas. Thus, aggressive surgery for patients with the combination of active rectal disease and anal fistulas is to be deplored as much as an attitude of therapeutic nihilism for those with severe symptoms and surgically treatable lesions.

INCIDENCE

There is a wide variation in the reported incidence of perianal pathology in patients with Crohn's disease, depending on the inclusion criteria used. When all perianal abnormalities are included, even ordinary looking tags or haemorrhoids, the reported incidence is quite high. Skin tags and haemorrhoids are quite common in the general public and may or may not be related to the presence of Crohn's disease. However, in a study of 26 patients with Crohn's disease of the large and/or small bowel, in whom perianal skin tags were removed, 9 had granulomata present.[56] Findings such as perianal irritation or even fissures may simply be related to the diarrhoea experienced by patients with upstream intestinal disease. Using broad criteria, Fielding described perianal disease occurring in 80% of 167 patients.[14] Of these 24% had an abscess, sinus or fistula, 51% had anal fissure and 50% (contrasting with 36% in a control group) had skin tags.

When only anal fissures, fistulas or abscesses are included the reported incidence tends to be much lower. In the National Co-operative Crohn's Disease Study (NCCDS),[47] 36% of patients with Crohn's disease had a history of perianal disease. Williams *et al.* reported a 22% incidence in patients seen at the Lahey Clinic with the diagnosis of Crohn's disease.[60] In a paediatric series 49% of children and adolescents with Crohn's disease were found to have perianal lesions.[37]

Patients with large bowel involvement have a higher incidence of perianal disease than those with small bowel disease. In the NCCDS experience, 46.7% of patients with colonic disease had perianal manifestations versus 25.5% in the small bowel disease only group. Combined small and large bowel involvement had an intermediate incidence. In the Lahey Clinic report, 52% of patients with Crohn's colitis had an anal lesion, whereas only 14% with small bowel disease had such lesions.

In attempts to assess the incidence of perianal pathology in Crohn's disease patients, the length of follow-up must be considered. Patients may have many years of intestinal inflammatory activity before developing perianal symptomatology. So, if patients are only followed for short periods of time, the true incidence of perianal disease will be underestimated. In addition, lesions may heal with treatments primarily intended for the intestinal disease, or may resolve spontaneously. The importance of long-term follow-up is demonstrated by the Cleveland Clinic report in which 24% of patients with Crohn's disease developed perianal disease more than 15 years after diagnosis.[20] Not surprisingly, the reported incidence of perianal disease was 56% in this series, higher than reports using similar inclusion criteria but with shorter follow-up. Perianal lesions may occur before, concomitant with or many years after the onset of intestinal symptomatology. It may also be difficult to assess whether the perianal lesions are related directly to active anal Crohn's disease, the presence of a chronic diarrhoeal illness or an incidental finding.

Possible aetiological factors include the preponderance of lymphoid aggregates in the intersphincteric plane that elsewhere in the gastrointestinal tract are targeted by the Crohn's disease process.[43]

Hughes and Taylor[26] have speculated that this narrow part of the intestinal tract is perhaps vulnerable, as other sites of relative narrowing (e.g. the ileum proximal to the ileocaecal valve and the intestine proximal to anastomosis) are also prone to inflammatory activity.

CLINICAL PRESENTATION

Perianal manifestations may either complicate the management of Crohn's disease patients many years after the onset of intestinal disease or be a presenting sign of Crohn's disease. Williams reported that 64% of patients had intestinal symptomatology preceding perianal disease, whereas 36% had a perianal fistula, abscess or fissure at the initial presentation;[60] 26% of patients followed with intestinal involvement and developed anal complications more than 10 years after the onset of disease. However, 96% of those presenting initially with an anal complication had intestinal manifestations within 5 years, over half of which developed within the first year. Although intestinal symptoms frequently precede perianal disease by many years, patients with apparently isolated perianal lesions are likely rapidly to develop intestinal disease as well.

The perianal lesions include fissures, fistulas (including rectovaginal fistulas), abscesses, oedematous skin tags, ulcerations and bluish discoloration of the perianal skin.[35] Perianal fissures, fistulas, abscesses or combinations thereof are seen with almost equal frequency. Teenagers or young adults with unusual fissures, fistulas or abscesses should be suspected of having Crohn's disease.[63] In the paediatric population, haemorrhoids are rarely seen, so oedematous tags should raise suspicion in this age group (*Figure 7.44*).[37]

The diagnosis in patients with known intestinal involvement should be straightforward. An appropriate level of suspicion is required for previously undiagnosed patients with atypical perianal lesions. Venereal diseases, leukaemia, tuberculosis and anal carcinoma should be considered in this setting.[8] All suspicious perianal lesions should be biopsied. Histologically, non-caseating granulomata may be seen. Other causes of granulomatous reaction include fungal or bacterial infections, such as tuberculosis, foreign body reactions, sarcoidosis, chronic granulomatous disease (in children), and necrobiotic granulomata.[29]

The evidence of perianal involvement is usually obvious on simple inspection, digital examination, anoscopy and proctoscopy in patients with Crohn's disease. Early disease may be diagnosed by double-contrast enema before it manifests clinically.[11] Yousem[64] found abnormalities in 82% of 200 consecutive Crohn's disease patients undergoing a CT scan directed at the perirectal/perianal area, utilizing oral and rectal contrast; 73% had inflammation of the fat planes, 30% had bowel thickening, 22% had fistulas or sinus tracts identified, and 24% had abscesses. Because 37% of patients had computed tomography (CT) manifestations of Crohn's disease below the symphysis pubis, the authors argued for extending scanning sequences to the perineum. Likewise, there have been proponents of magnetic resonance imaging (MRI) for patients with anal fistulas and Crohn's disease.[32] MRI demonstrated the fistulas in

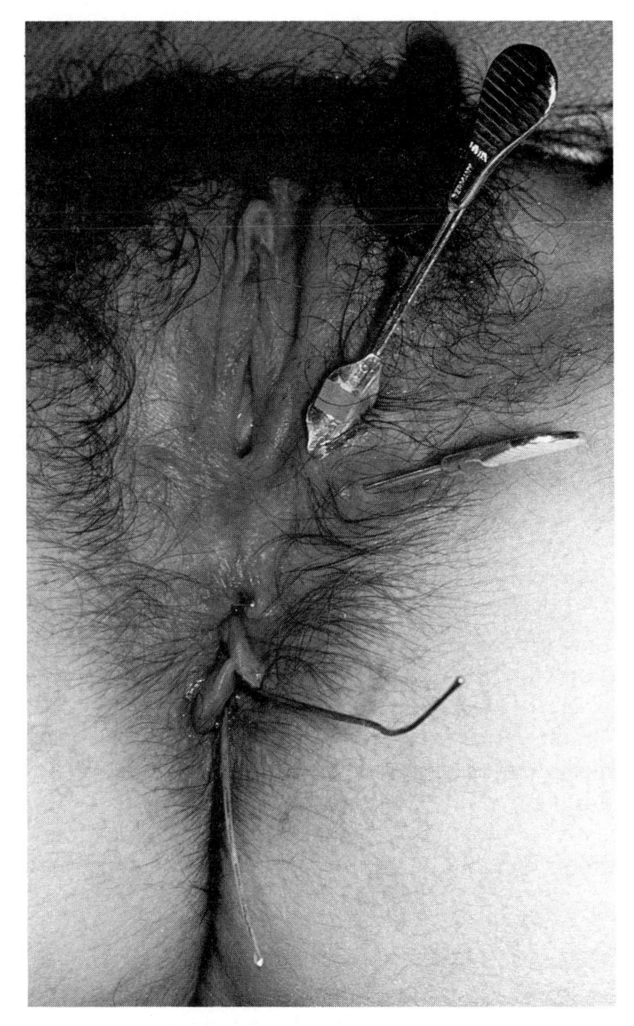

Figure 7.44 Indurated perianal skin tags with associated perianal fistulas.

14 of 17 cases and was accurate in showing fluid collections within fistulas and extraintestinal tissue. The particular value of MRI, according to the authors, was the uniformly successful demonstration of the fistula/sinus tract relative to the levator ani. Despite the apparent value of these imaging techniques, the authors cannot recommend their routine use and find that they add little to a well-conducted examination under anaesthesia.

PATHOPHYSIOLOGY

As the causative factor(s) responsible for Crohn's disease still need to be defined, the cause of the associated perianal lesions is also uncertain. As the anus is part of the gastrointestinal tract, a perianal fissure may simply represent another site of primary bowel activity in the anal mucosa. Patients with perianal disease, small bowel disease and no intervening colonic or rectal disease could be said to have a 'skip' lesion. Abscesses and fistulas may result from deep penetrating ulcers of the anal canal, thereby providing access for stool to the inter- or extrasphincteric planes. However, Hobbiss and Schofield assessed 26 fistulas and concluded that only 4 were likely to have arisen by this process.[24]

Hughes and Taylor[26] have argued that classification and, therefore, a better understanding of perianal lesions and their manifestations are facilitated by considering these lesions as primary and secondary. Thus a primary lesion such as anal fissure leads to secondary skin tags, an ulcerated oedematous pile leads to anal/rectal stricture, and a cavitating ulcer leads to perianal abscess/fistula or fistula into the vagina. This may occur in many, or most, patients, but fails to explain those fistulas without associated ulcer which resemble non-Crohn's disease fistulas of cryptoglandular origin. Likewise, the response of certain anorectal strictures to drainage (treatment of infection) indicates a complication relating to a deep ulcer or fistula.

Some of these lesions may represent extraintestinal cutaneous manifestations of Crohn's disease. In the NCCDS study there was a positive association between perianal disease and extraintestinal manifestations, which suggests that perianal disease can be an extraintestinal manifestation or so-called metastatic lesion of Crohn's disease. Patients with Crohn's disease can develop 'metastatic' cutaneous lesions (containing granulomata) in a wide array of locations including the vulva,[12] inguinal region, submammary area, axilla, oral cavity[38] and the penis.[50] Patients may even have involvement of the mouth and anus without any intervening gastrointestinal lesion.[58]

The role of a chronic diarrhoeal illness must also be considered in perianal disease. Chronic diarrhoea may promote the occurrence of perianal disease through the usual mechanisms of cryptoglandular obstruction and disease. Any or all of these mechanisms may be important and their recognition may lead to a more rational approach to management for an individual patient based on the mechanism of injury inducing each lesion.

PRINCIPLES OF MANAGEMENT

Appropriate treatment must be considered for each patient with perianal Crohn's disease based on certain management principles. The patient and the physician must have a clear understanding of the goals of any treatment. Decisions are made in the context of the extent and severity of gastrointestinal tract disease and symptomatology elsewhere.[30] Central to management is an accurate diagnosis of the nature and extent of the local disease as well as the proximal intestinal disease. This will usually require examination of the anorectum with anaesthesia, if local assessment is in any way inadequate.

The goals of treatment depend on the particular situation, the particular patient, the response to therapy and the passage of time. An ideal goal is total healing and, therefore, permanent symptomatic relief. But this is unrealistic in the patient with extensive scrotal or perineal fistulas accompanied by significant rectal disease. There is therefore a need for the clinician to provide realistic goals for the patient, explaining the reasons carefully. Common goals are relief of pain and reducing the frequency of or preventing abscess formation, avoiding procedures liable to produce incontinence and deferring–delaying or obviating the need for either rectal excision or faecal diversion. Thus treatment may range from simple (sometimes repeated) abscess drainage to fistulotomy which allows for healing of a simple fistula, to proctocolectomy for the incontinent patient whose sphincter has been destroyed by the disease. Therefore, the goal is usually palliation of symptoms through the simplest approach that will make the patient comfortable. Lesions that look painful to the examiner may be totally asymptomatic to the patient and need no treatment. Lesions may also remit spontaneously. In the European Co-operative Crohn's Disease Study (ECCDS), spontaneous remission rates of up to 60% were noted within 5 months of the patients' treatment with placebo.[54]

Conservative approaches as initial therapy of patients with perianal disease are generally advised. The principle of 'first, do no harm' is an imperative that applies to all medical and surgical treatment but is particularly pertinent to the treatment of perianal Crohn's disease. Excessively enthusiastic surgery frequently results in an outcome worse than the disease itself.

The effect of resecting upstream intestinal disease on the healing of anal lesions is controversial. Some have claimed that perianal manifestations are closely related to the inflammatory process in the bowel as are many of the extraintestinal manifestations, and that perianal lesions heal if the foci of intestinal activity are removed. Heuman and colleagues found that 80% of existing perianal lesions healed spontaneously after bowel resection in patients without recurrent intestinal disease, whereas they remained active among those who suffered from recurrence after resection.[23] Wolff *et al.* also noted the persistence or recurrence of perianal disease, if active proximal involvement remained or recurred after resection.[62]

However, in children Orkin and Telander found improvement in perianal disease in only 5 out of 17 patients after resection of intestinal disease and primary anastomosis.[42] Buchman *et al.* asserted that persistence or healing of perianal lesions was unrelated to intestinal activity. Based on available data, resection of intestinal Crohn's disease for the sole purpose of achieving perianal healing cannot be recommended.[6]

Similarly, faecal diversion does not alter the long-term course of perianal Crohn's disease. In one series, only 2 of 11 improved with a defunctioning procedure and none had intestinal continuity restored.[42] In another series only two of nine patients treated by defunctioning ileostomy for fistulous perianal disease subsequently had intestinal continuity restored.[57] Cohen treated 12 patients with perianal fistulas and an ileostomy, none of whom had a successful closure.[8]

At the Cleveland Clinic, the authors have been disappointed with the long-term effects of ileostomy for perianal disease. Of 22 patients undergoing faecal diversion only 6 had resolution of symptomatic anorectal disease after 3–5 years.[65] In Harper's report of the effect of 32 split ileostomies on 29 patients with symptomatic perianal Crohn's disease, improvement occurred in 23 (72%).[21] However, only six patients subsequently underwent ileostomy closure, eight underwent proctocolectomy and fifteen remained diverted.

A defunctioning stoma does not alter the natural history or dramatically improve the complications of perianal Crohn's disease. Despite the fact that an ileostomy is not a definitive procedure, it may allow for improvement of perianal sepsis in some patients before proctectomy and allow a patient the chance to adapt to an ileostomy. The authors rarely use ileostomy alone in this context.

SPECIFIC ENTITIES

Abscesses

The diagnosis of an abscess is usually straightforward as patients present with a tender fluctuant mass. Abscesses should be suspected when patients with chronic fistulas or fissures present with increased pain. An abscess may not be obvious in such a setting. If a thorough examination is not possible because of pain, patients should be examined under anaesthesia.

When an abscess is identified, an incision (made as close to the anus as possible) and drainage should be performed and a mushroom catheter left in place. These are generally well tolerated and can be left for long periods of time. There is little place for primary fistulotomy in this setting.

An apparent superficial but chronic abscess that undermines the perianal skin for several centimetres

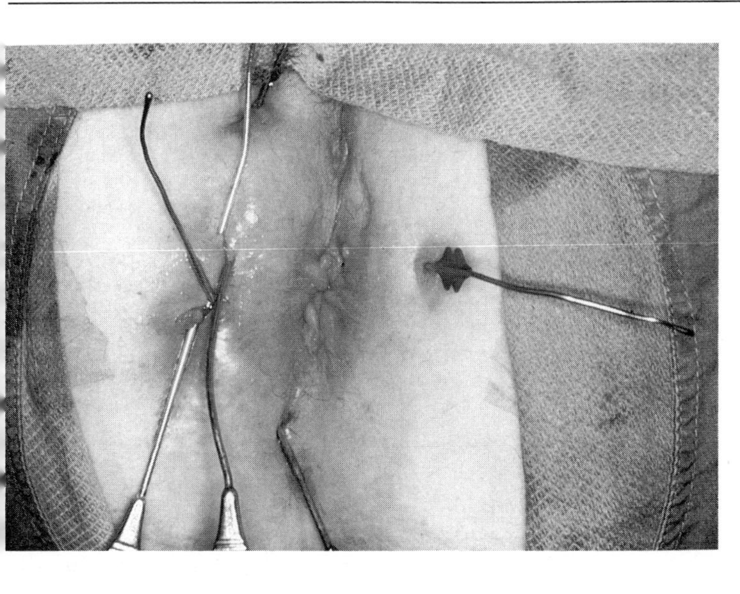

Figure 7.45 Abscess–fistula complex in perianal Crohn's disease. Note the brawny erythema around the opening near the three probes. This 'superficial' abscess is treated by excision of the rather thin, almost necrotic, skin that is undermined, and then by catheter drainage of the fistula.

(*Figure 7.45*) can be treated by placing a seton through the medial end of the cavity and into the internal opening. The outer component is then excised with the overlying skin. Antibiotics may be indicated to treat surrounding cellulitis.

Fistulas

The treatment of anal fistulas can be the most challenging of all of the perianal complications of Crohn's disease (*Figure 7.46*). A variety of timely medical and surgical treatments may be necessary and few patients will ultimately come to proctectomy. Conservative palliative approaches are usually recommended but certain subgroups are being successfully treated in a definitive manner.

VanDongen and Lubbers reviewed 55 Crohn's disease patients with perianal fistulas;[57] 13 patients required no treatment; 28 patients were managed with fistulotomy with a 79% success rate and no incontinence; 9 patients were treated with a defunctioning stoma of which 4 fistulas healed eventually; 5 patients underwent a primary proctectomy. It is important to note that a quarter of the patients required no treatment and that spontaneous healing does occur.

Recently, there has been a trend towards more aggressive treatment of some fistulas. Fuhrman and Larach treated 19 out of 26 fistulas in their series with fistulotomy, 18 of which ultimately healed.[17] Three patients healed spontaneously. All patients were treated postoperatively with metronidazole and the average time to healing was 48 days. They advocate early fistulotomy before the fistula becomes a more complex management problem. Similarly, Sohn *et al.* treated 20 patients for fistulas and recurrent abscesses by fistulotomy or internal anal sphincterectomy with good results.[52] They emphasized the utility of sulphasalazine in promoting wound healing. The drug was started 2 weeks postoperatively and continued until the wounds were healed.

In the Ochsner Clinic's report,[39] of 35 patients with anorectal fistulae and Crohn's disease, 29 had low intermuscular fistulas and 6 had high intermuscular (supralevator) fistulas. Fistulotomy alone was performed in 19 and 8 patients had partial fistulotomy and seton insertion. Five had fistulotomy following faecal diversion. Of the 32 patients having fistulotomy, 30 had complete healing, although 7 required more than one operation. The success was attributed to the absence of rectal disease and quiescent disease elsewhere in the intestine.

At the Ferguson Clinic,[33] 37 of 47 patients with Crohn's disease and anorectal fistulas achieved complete healing or minimal disability. In 29 patients the fistulotomy site healed primarily. The outcome was especially good in the group with no rectal involvement; 18 of 21 such patients achieved an excellent result.

Selective fistulotomy is not always satisfactory.[31] Of patients referred to the unit only 1 of 12 fistulotomy patients healed and 6 had been rendered incontinent. Where fistulotomy is successful, the healing time is similar to that for non-Crohn's anal fistulas.[24] However, a delayed or non-healing indolent wound is the price paid by some patients undergoing fistulotomy, especially for high fistulas associated with rectal Crohn's disease (*Figure 7.47*).

In the author's view, the evidence would favour fistulotomy for patients with low or intersphincteric fistulas, where the rectum appears normal and where incontinence is an unlikely sequel. Thus, the

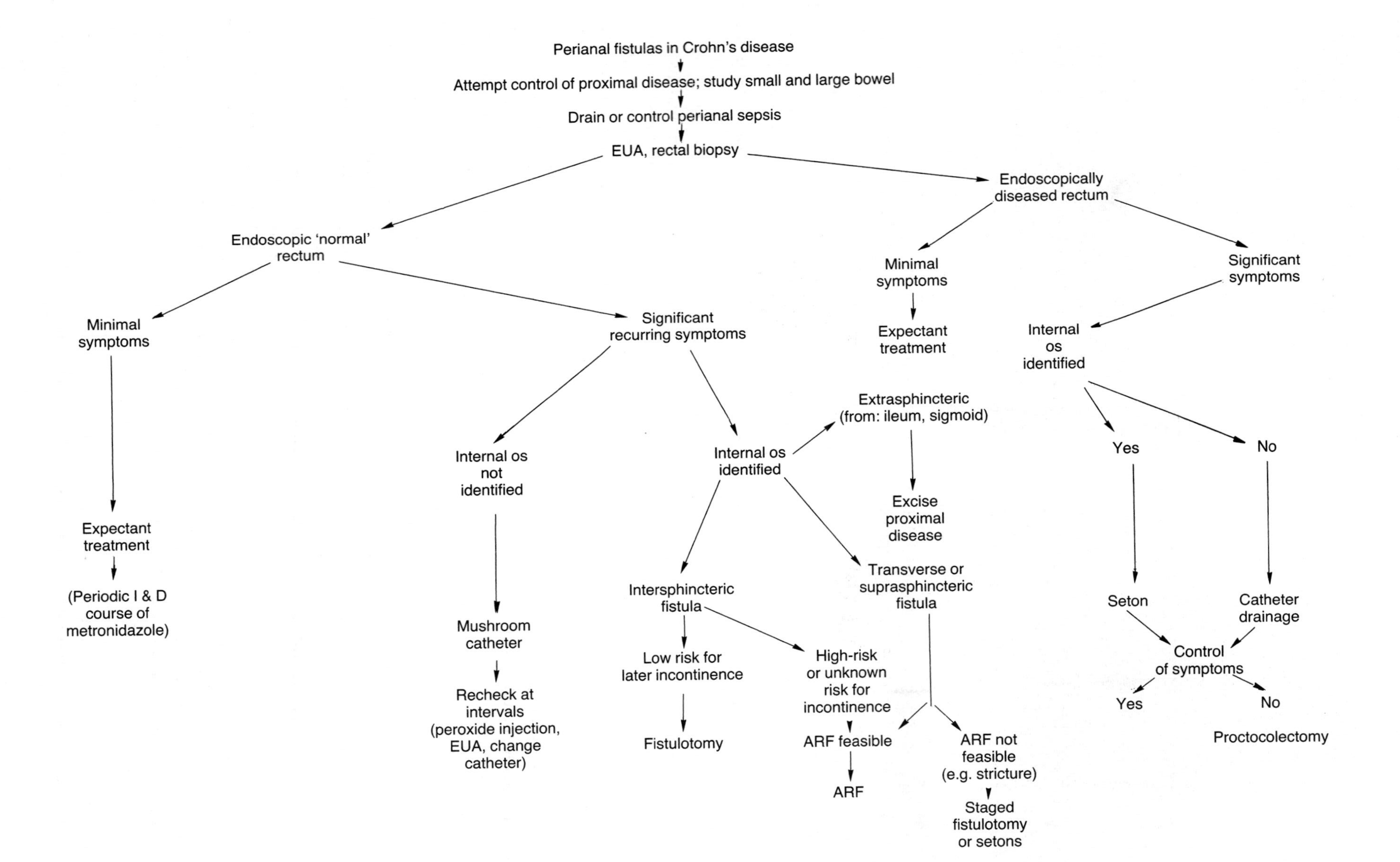

Figure 7.46 Treatment of perianal fistulas in Crohn's disease. EUA = examination under anaesthesia; ARF = advancement rectal flap.

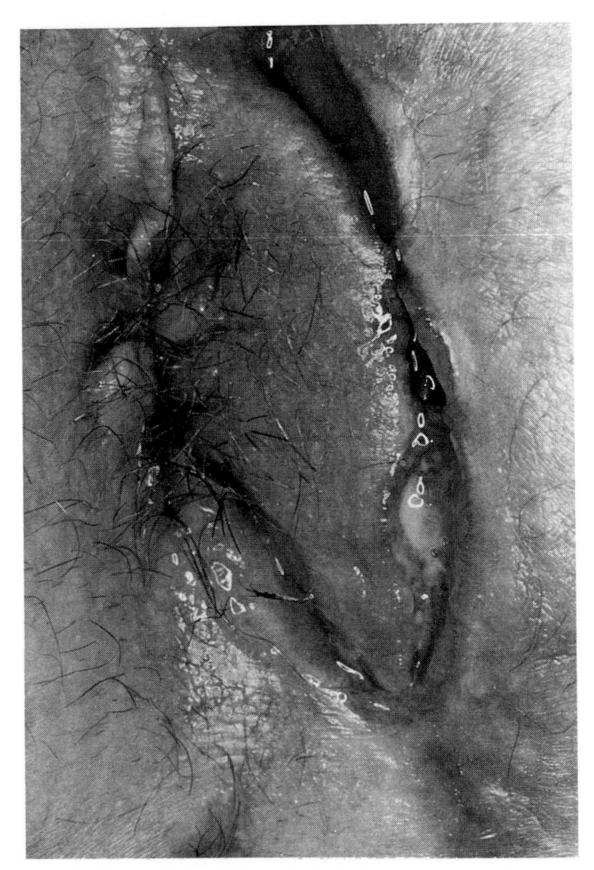

Figure 7.47 Indolent non-healing fistulotomy wound in a patient with Crohn's disease.

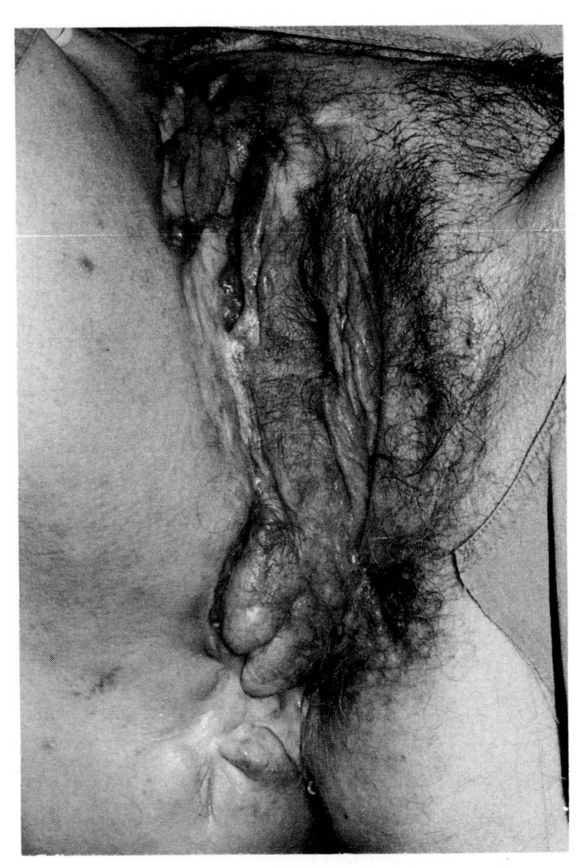

Figure 7.48 Severe inguinovulval destruction by fistula tract extension.

impact of coexistent diarrhoea, previous fistula surgery or obstetric injury must be considered and perhaps sphincter manometric studies added when choosing fistulotomy as definitive treatment. If adverse factors are present, advancement rectal flap operation (where the rectum appears normal) or use of seton would be preferable. The rare patient with inguinal, scrotal or vulval extensions is treated by catheter or seton drainage of the primary fistula and unroofing curettage of the extension (*Figure 7.48*).

The use of multiple techniques to deal with fistulas is demonstrated by the experience of Fry *et al.* who reported 73 patients undergoing 156 anorectal operations for anal or perineal sepsis.[16] The most common procedure was incision and drainage of abscess; 13 anal fistulotomies were carried out for simple intersphincteric fistulas and all healed within 4 months; 6 patients were treated with seton drainage and 6 patients were treated with endorectal advancement flaps; 5 of 12 patients treated by diversion had intestinal continuity restored.

The importance of preserving the sphincter mechanism must be emphasized. As such, fistulotomy seems to be an acceptable approach for low fistulas. However, it is the management of high fistulas that requires considerably more care and procedures that do not compromise the sphincters. In this situation seton drainage or endorectal advancement flaps are valuable.

With respect to use of setons (*Figure 7.49*), the surgeon must recall the goals of therapy. For the most part the value of long-term setons is in providing drainage of fistulous tracts, the prevention of recurrent abscess and relief of pain while avoiding sphincter division. Setons are used especially when there is rectal disease and/or a significant risk of incontinence with fistulotomy. Patients may be rendered comfortable, but there are occasions when setons can be an irritant – even when loosely applied Silastic bands are used. Small mushroom catheters placed in the tract may be better tolerated (*Figure 7.50*). In one report of ten cases of complex fistulas, excellent palliation was obtained after follow-up of 4 months to 7 years using setons.[59] Despite severe proctitis in six patients, none had required proctocolectomy. Small Silastic vessel loops function very well as setons. They can be left in situ for long periods and are generally well tolerated by the patient. When an overly aggressive fistulotomy has been performed or the patient otherwise becomes

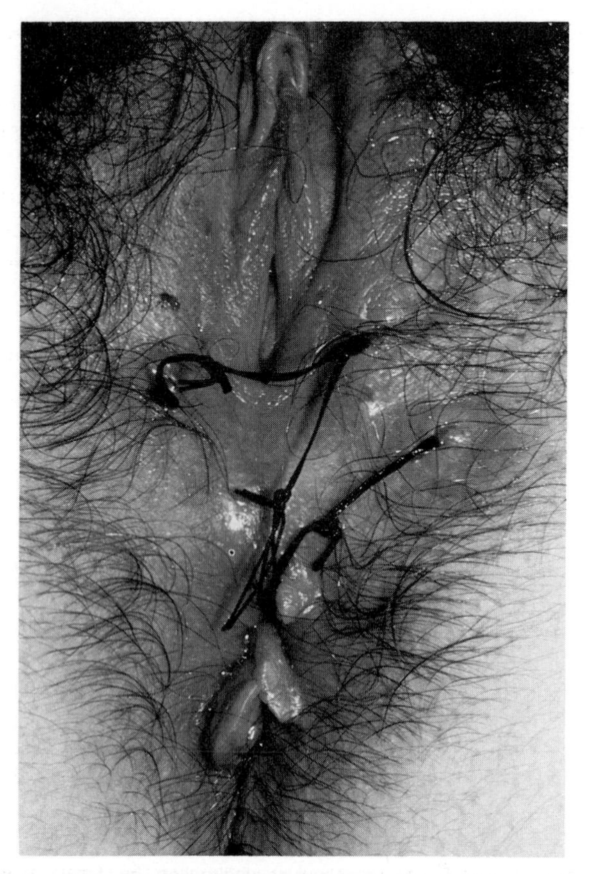

Figure 7.49 Perianal Crohn's disease with multiple fistulas, indurated tags and rectal disease. Loosely placed silk (here) or Silastic setons help reduce the occurrence of painful recurrent abscesses.

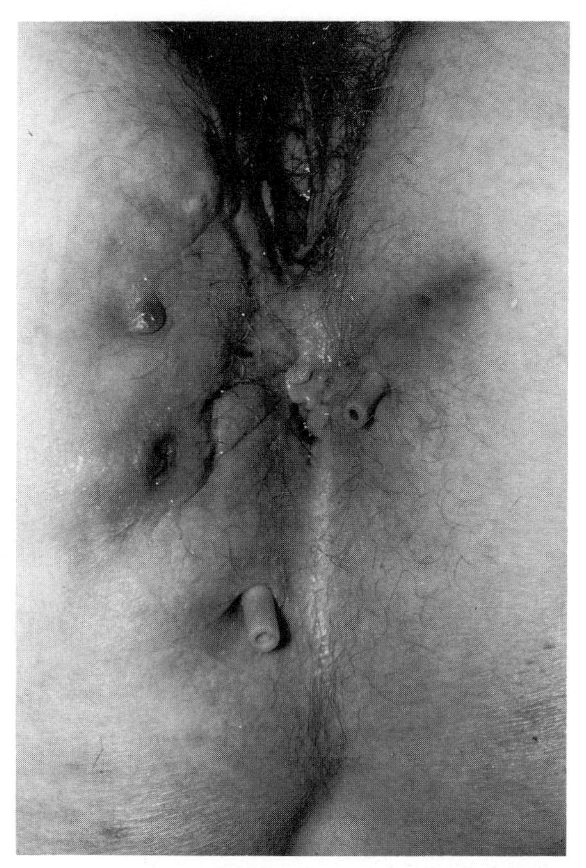

Figure 7.50 Perianal fistulas in Crohn's disease treated by mushroom catheter drainage. One of these fistulas was extrasphincteric. The patient had been free of recurrent abscesses and pain for 11 years before ultimately undergoing proctocolectomy.

incontinent, good results have been reported in selected patients with overlapping sphincter repair and temporary proximal diversion.[49]

The medical management of anal fistulas has included steroids, azathioprine, sulphasalazine and metronidazole. The NCCDS study suggested that sulphasalazine may be effective and there are proponents of these medications.[47] The use of metronidazole has been the subject of the most intense interest. Bernstein *et al.* noted 'dramatic improvement' in all 21 consecutive patients with chronic unremitting perianal disease, 10 of whom healed.[3] Jakobovits and Schuster treated eight patients with metronidazole 1000–1500 mg/day and noted a twentyfold decrease in the number of draining fistulas and a 50% decrease in the number of non-draining fistulous openings.[27] However, treatment must be continued for 4–6 months and up to half the patients experience paraesthesiae. Unfortunately, in a follow-up study the drug was only withdrawn in 28% of patients because the disease recurred when the medication was stopped.[5] When the potential mutagenic effects of metronidazole are considered the need for long-term therapy is of concern. Streptococcal liver abscess has been reported in a patient with streptococcal perianal abscess while on metronidazole.[22]

Treatment with an elemental diet has been described in a small number of patients with some improvement.[7] However, all patients were on other medications and of course spontaneous remissions may occur. As even a diverting intestinal stoma is of limited value, it would be surprising if elemental diets were of major value.

Rectovaginal fistulas (*Figure 7.51*)

This particularly distressing complication usually occurs because of deep penetration of an ulcer through the rectal wall or anal canal into the vagina. Patients commonly have severe rectal disease which requires proctectomy. Recently, however, the use of endoanal rectal advancement flaps has been advocated to deal with rectovaginal fistulas and complicated anoperineal fistulas in selected patients. This method is especially appealing be-

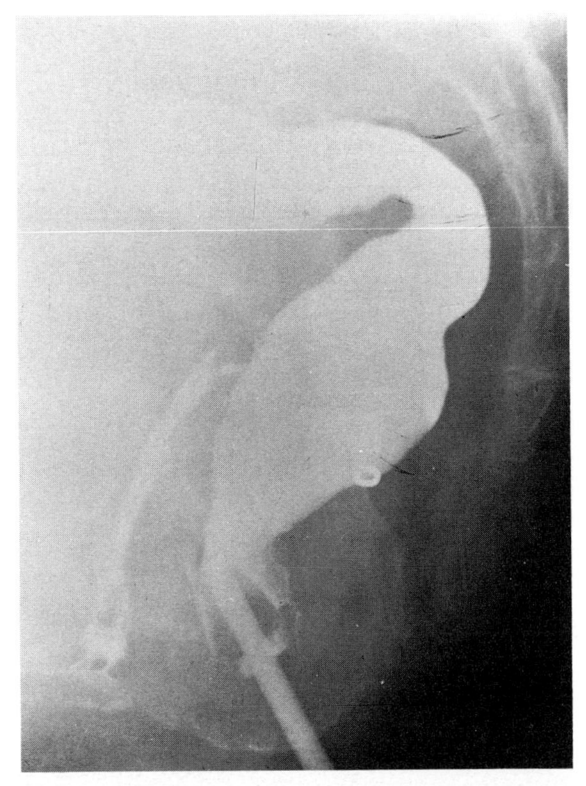

Figure 7.51 Contrast radiograph of rectum demonstrating a rather rigid diseased rectum and high rectovaginal fistula. This is *not* suitable for direct repair.

cause no sphincter division is required and even a failed advancement flap does not adversely affect the situation. Anovaginal or rectovaginal fistulas are sometimes associated with perianal fistulas as well where there is a common internal anorectal opening. This situation lends itself to the advancement flap technique when the rectum appears normal and there is no stricture present.

Crim from the Cleveland Clinic reported 28 transanal rectal advancement flaps performed in 23 patients with rectovaginal or complex anoperineal fistulas (unpublished data). Patients with florid proctitis were excluded. Ten of 14 rectovaginal fistulas ultimately healed after a mean follow-up of 15 months. There was no postoperative incontinence noted or change in anorectal manometric parameters.

Francois *et al.*[15] reported direct lay open excision and repair of nine patients with rectovaginal fistula. All healed, but three were incontinent for liquid stool or flatus. In the St Mark's Hospital series,[46] 90 of 886 women with Crohn's disease had anovaginal or rectovaginal fistulas; 12 patients (13%) had non-surgical management; another 12 patients underwent repair of whom 8 were cured. The remainder underwent a variety of procedures, mostly faecal diversion with abdominal colectomy or proctectomy.

Rectovaginal fistulas frequently occur in the context of severe disease which ultimately requires rectal excision. However, for those in whom the rectovaginal fistula is the major source of morbidity, and who do not have severe gross rectal disease or anal canal with a cavitating ulcer, advancement flap is a good option.

Although rare, rectourethral fistulas occur in patients with Crohn's disease. The authors reported on 3 such cases successfully treated by the advancement rectal flap technique.[13]

Fissures

Fissures are frequently pain-free and require no treatment. In contrast to the more common fissures found in the general population, those associated with Crohn's disease are frequently quite deep and wide with undermined edges. They may not be in the midline. In contrast to the high anal pressures seen in non-Crohn's disease fissures, the basal anal sphincter pressure in Crohn's disease-associated fissures is similar to that of normal control subjects.[55] These fissures may represent true activity of Crohn's disease in the anal canal, but no disease activity elsewhere.

Conservative approaches are best. In a 10-year follow-up, Buchman *et al.* reported that only 10 of 53 fissures were still present.[6] If associated pain is a feature then an abscess should be considered and examination under anaesthesia performed. There is some suggestion from the NCCDS study that fissures respond to prednisone or azathioprine.[47] Hughes treated seven patients suffering severe perianal symptomatology refractory to standard medical therapy with local depot injections of methylprednisolone, five of whom had dramatic relief.[25]

As noted by others,[26] the fissures/ulcers are of several varieties. By far the most important is the painful wide penetrating ulcer of the anal canal which may extend from the anal verge to the anorectal ring (*Figure 7.52*), and may even be circumferential. This latter entity is not suitable for local surgery. Most ultimately require faecal diversion although, like Hughes, the authors have used intralesional prednisolone (and azathioprine by mouth) with significant relief of pain.

For the non-cavitating, anal verge, 'simple' fissures that respond poorly to topical agents and bowel management programmes, the authors have used conservative dilatation (two fingers) and even partial sphincterotomy, if resting tone is high.

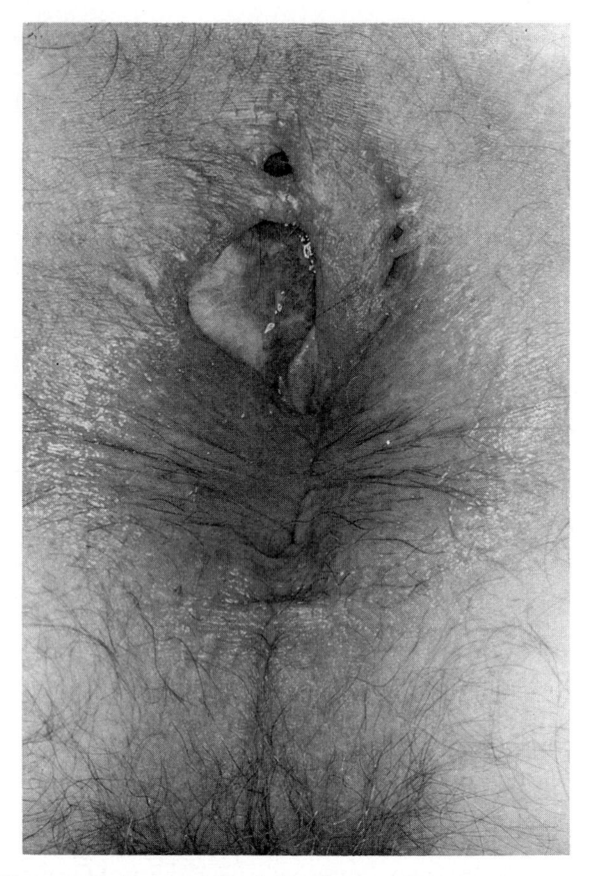

Figure 7.52 Large perianal ulcer/fissure with secondary fistula formation.

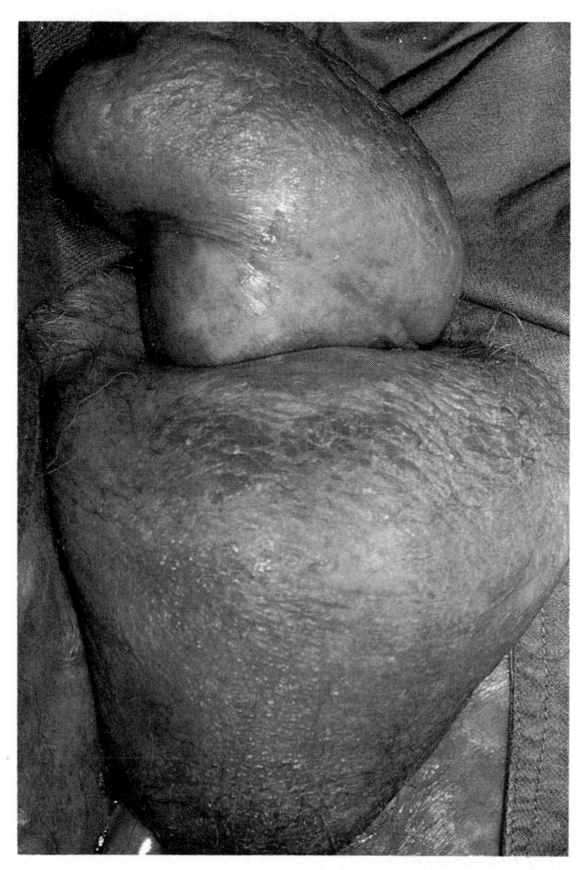

Figure 7.53 Gross scrotal and penile oedema following excision of inguinoscrotal fistula extension in a man with Crohn's disease.

Strictures

Most strictures result from the healing of fissures or fibrosis from chronic sepsis. As many patients have loose stools, anorectal strictures are frequently asymptomatic. Linares *et al.* reported on the management of 48 strictures in 44 patients.[34] Five required no treatment, 6 were treated with proctectomy (generally for associated proctitis) and 33 were dilated. Most dilatations were performed digitally, although on five occasions a coaxial balloon was used and two patients were treated with Hegar dilators. Fifteen required a single dilatation, eight required two dilatations, and ten required three or more. They noted that the strictures rarely give rise to symptoms unless complicated by perianal sepsis or fistulas. Associated perianal disease and proctitis are commonly seen. Greenstein *et al.* found a 7.5% incidence of strictures in most cases associated with complex fistulas.[19] The dilatations in these patients should be gentle to avoid damaging the sphincters. Strictures of skin following wide excision of groin, scrotal or vulval fistula extensions can lead to alarming deformity and lymphoedema (*Figure 7.53*).

Haemorrhoids/tags

True internal haemorrhoids are rarely seen in patients with Crohn's disease. Lesions labelled as haemorrhoids are usually large external tags. Haemorrhoids should be treated conservatively with control of bowel dysfunction and local soothing measures.[38] Jeffery *et al.* reported complications in 11 out of 26 Crohn's disease patients treated for haemorrhoids, 6 of whom required proctectomy.[28] The same non-surgical conservative approach should apply to skin tags.

Occasionally, otherwise asymptomatic patients without a previous diagnosis of Crohn's disease are seen where the haemorrhoidectomy wounds have not only failed to heal but the ulcer defects have coalesced. This represents a 'red flag' for the presence of occult Crohn's disease and requires complete endoscopic and radiological evaluation of the intestinal tract. On three such occasions the authors have found aphthous ulcers in the proximal colon and healing occurred with oral corticosteroids.

Proctectomy

Despite the frequent occurrence of perianal lesions in Crohn's disease patients, only a small number come to proctectomy for treatment of perianal complications. Williams and Hughes reviewed nine patients in whom the indication for proctectomy was perianal disease.[61] All nine had undergone multiple previous procedures. During the same period 55 other patients with perianal involvement were managed with local procedures and 17 underwent proctocolectomy for colorectal disease.

The proctectomy rate required to manage perianal complications is approximately 5%. At least that many patients with incidental perianal Crohn's disease will undergo proctectomy for colorectal disease. Keighley has described high anal fistulas, deep ulcerations, rectovaginal fistulas and supralevator abscesses as those lesions most likely to necessitate proctectomy.[32] When proctectomy is required, the main problem becomes management of the perineal wound. In Williams' experience, only one of nine wounds heals within 3 months and six patients required further surgery to achieve perineal healing. Three wounds remained unhealed.

In this setting, it is useful to perform an intersphincteric dissection, although the procedure can be difficult because of previous scarring. The levators are sutured to reconstitute the pelvic floor. Septic foci are unroofed or excised at the time of proctectomy. The septic perineal wound should be left open and treated with careful dressing changes. When the infection is controlled, split-thickness skin grafting can expedite closure, if a significant defect remains. The cardinal rule is to avoid the development of a presacral sinus. This 'high' sinus occurs when the levators are not closed or the closure breaks down. A further cause is that of incomplete excision of rectal mucosa – especially prone to occur when proctectomy is undertaken for severe chronic supralevator sepsis. Presacral sinuses which remain significantly symptomatic may require abdominoperineal excision (author's preference) or muscle graft.

Cancer (*Figure 7.54*)

Patients with Crohn's disease have a somewhat higher risk of developing gastrointestinal malignancies. A variety of perianal carcinomas has been reported in patients with Crohn's disease of the perianal region, perhaps related to chronic inflammation or irritation. This rare complication should be kept in mind and any suspicious lesion should be biopsied.

Several reports of squamous cell carcinomas of the anus exist,[45,51] including squamous cell carcinoma in a skin tag.[53] Adenocarcinomas arising in fistulas or located in the anus have been described.[1,48] There have also been reports of in situ[2,10] and invasive cloacogenic carcinomas.[51]

SUMMARY

Perianal complications are a frequent finding in patients with Crohn's disease. They are more frequently seen in patients with colorectal involvement. A minority of patients will have a perianal lesion as their presenting sign of Crohn's disease with intestinal disease developing within 5 years.

Many lesions are asymptomatic and require no treatment. The onset of pain associated with a chronic lesion usually mandates examination under anaesthesia to rule out an abscess. Although a conservative approach is advocated, certain lesions, such as low anal fistulas, may be definitively treated with good results. High fistulas can be treated with seton drainage or an endorectal advancement flap. A few patients will ultimately require proctectomy when emphasis must be placed on methods for obtaining perineal wound healing.

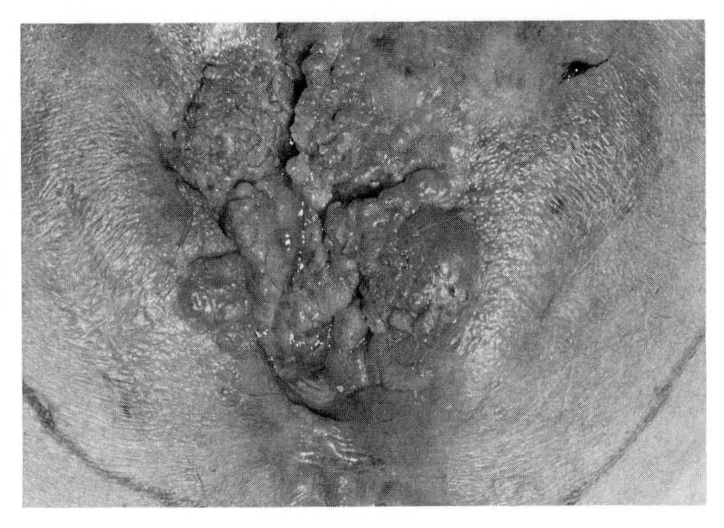

Figure 7.54 Squamous cell carcinoma of the anus complicating long-standing perianal Crohn's disease.

REFERENCES

1. Ball, C.S., Wujanto, R., Haboubi, N.Y. and Schofield, P.F. (1981) Carcinoma in anal Crohn's disease: Discussion paper. *Journal of the Royal Society of Medicine*, **81**, 217–219.
2. Beck, D.E., Harford, F.J. and Roettger, R.H. (1980) Perianal Bowen's disease associated with Crohn's colitis. Report of a case. *Diseases of the Colon and Rectum*, **32**, 252–255.
3. Bernstein, L.H., Frank, M.S. and Brandt, L.J. (1980) Healing of perianal Crohn's disease with metronidazole. *Gastroenterology*, **79**, 357–365.
4. Bissell, A.D. (1934) Localized chronic ulcerative ileitis. *Annals of Surgery*, **99**, 957–966.
5. Brandt, L.J., Bernstein, L.H. and Boley, S.J. (1982) Metronidazole therapy for perineal Crohn's disease: A follow-up study. *Gastroenterology*, **83**, 383–387.
6. Buchmann, P., Keighley, M.R., Allan, R.N., Thompson, H. and Alexander-Williams, J. (1980) Natural history of perianal Crohn's disease. Ten year follow-up: A plea for conservatism. *American Journal of Surgery*, **140**, 642–644.
7. Calam, J., Crooks, P.E. and Walker, R.J. (1980) Elemental diets in the management of Crohn's perianal fistulae. *Journal of Parenteral and Enteral Nutrition*, **4**, 4–8.
8. Cohen, Z. and McLeod, R.S. (1987) Perianal Crohn's disease. *Gastroenterology Clinics of North America*, **16**, 175–189.
9. Crohn, B.B., Ginzburg, L. and Oppenheimer, G.D. (1932) Regional enteritis: A pathologic and clinical entity. *Journal of the American Medical Association*, **99**, 1323–1329.
10. Daly, J.J. and Madrazo, A. (1980) Anal Crohn's disease with carcinoma in situ. *Digestive Diseases and Science*, **25**, 464–466.
11. DuBrow, R.A. and Frank, P.H. (1983) Barium evaluation of anal canal in patients with inflammatory bowel disease. *American Journal of Roentgenology*, **140**, 1141–1157.
12. Duhra, P. and Paul, C.J. (1988) Metastatic Crohn's disease responding to metronidazole. *British Journal of Dermatology*, **119**, 87–91.
13. Fazio, V.W., Jones, I.T., Jagelman, D.G. and Weakley, F.L. (1987) Rectourethral fistulas in Crohn's disease. *Surgery, Gynecology and Obstetrics*, **164**, 148–150.
14. Fielding, J.F. (1972) Perianal lesions in Crohn's disease. *Journal of the Royal College of Surgeons (Edinburgh)*, **17**, 32–37.
15. Francois, Y., Descos, L. and Vignal, J. (1990) Conservative treatment of low rectovaginal fistula in Crohn's disease. *International Journal of Colorectal Disease*, **5**, 12–14.
16. Fry, R.D., Shemesh, E.I. and Timmcke, A. (1989) Techniques and results in the management of anal and perianal Crohn's disease. *Surgery, Gynecology and Obstetrics*, **168**, 42–48.
17. Fuhrman, G.M. and Larach, S.W. (1989) Experience with perirectal fistulas in patients with Crohn's disease. *Diseases of the Colon and Rectum*, **32**, 847–848.
18. Gabriel, W.B. (1921) Results of an experimental and histologic investigation into 75 cases of rectal fistulae. *Proceedings of the Royal Society of Medicine*, **14**, 156–161.
19. Greenstein, A.J., Sachar, D.B. and Kark, A.E. (1975) Stricture of the anorectum in Crohn's disease involving the colon. *Annals of Surgery*, **181**, 207–212.
20. Harper, P.H., Fazio, B.W., Lavery, I.C. *et al.* (1987) The long-term outcome in Crohn's disease. *Diseases of the Colon and Rectum*, **30**, 174–179.
21. Harper, P., Kettlewell, M. and Lee, E. (1982) The effect of split ileostomy on perianal Crohn's disease. *British Journal of Surgery*, **69**, 608–610.
22. Hatoff, D.E. (1983) Perineal Crohn's disease complicated by pyogenic liver abscess during metronidazole therapy. *Gastroenterology*, **85**, 194–195.
23. Heuman, R., Bolin, T., Sjödahl, R. and Tagesson, C. (1981) The incidence and course of perianal complications and arthralgia after intestinal resection with restoration of continuity for Crohn's disease. *British Journal of Surgery*, **68**, 528–530.
24. Hobbiss, J.H. and Schofield, P.F. (1982) Management of perianal Crohn's disease. *Journal of the Royal Society of Medicine*, **75**, 414–417.
25. Hughes, L.E., Donaldson, D.R., Williams, J.G., Taylor, B.A. and Young, H.L. (1988) Local depot methylprednisolone injection for painful anal Crohn's disease. *Gastroenterology*, **94**, 709–711.
26. Hughes, L.E. and Taylor, B.A. (1990) Perianal lesions in Crohn's disease. In *Inflammatory Bowel Disease* (Ed.) Allan, R.N., Keighley, M.R., Alexander-Williams, J. and Hawkins, C.F. pp. 351–361. New York: Churchill-Livingstone.
27. Jakobovits, J. and Schuster, M.M. (1984) Metronidazole therapy for Crohn's disease associated fistulae. *American Journal of Gastroenterology*, **79**, 533–540.
28. Jeffery, P.J., Ritchie, J.K. and Parks, A.G. (1977) Treatment of haemorrhoids in patients with inflammatory bowel disease. *The Lancet*, **2**, 1084–1085.
29. Kauffman, C.L., Peterman, A.R. and Barnett, N.K. (1986) Perianal skin plaque in a child. *Archives of Dermatology*, **122**, 1065–1066.
30. Keddie, N. (1980) Anorectal manifestations of inflammatory bowel disease. *British Journal of Hospital Medicine*, **284**, 296–297.
31. Keighley, M.R. and Allan, R.N. (1986) Current status and influence of operation on perianal Crohn's disease. *International Journal of Colorectal Disease*, **1**, 104–107.
32. Koebel, G., Schmeidl, U., Majer, M. *et al.* (1989) Diagnosis of fistulae and sinus tracts in patients with Crohn's disease: Value of M.R. imaging. *American Journal of Roentgenology*, **152**, 999–1003.
33. Levien, D., Surrell, J. and Mazier, W. (1989)

Surgical treatment of anorectal fistula in patients with Crohn's disease. *Surgery, Gynecology and Obstetrics*, **169**, 133–136.
34. Linares, L., Moreira, L.F., Andrews, J.H., Allan, R.N., Alexander-Williams, J. and Keighley, M.R. (1988) Natural history and treatment of anorectal strictures complicating Crohn's disease. *British Journal of Surgery*, **75**, 653–655.
35. Lockhart-Mummery, H.E. (1985) Anal lesions in Crohn's disease. *British Journal of Surgery*, **72** (suppl.), 595–596.
36. Lockhart-Mummery, H.E. and Morson, B.C. (1960) Crohn's disease (regional enteritis) of the large intestine and its distinction from ulcerative colitis. *Gut*, **1**, 87–105.
37. Markowitz, J., Daum, F., Aiges, H., Kahn, E., Silverberg, M. and Fisher, S.E. (1984) Perianal disease in children and adolescents with Crohn's disease. *Gastroenterology*, **86**, 829–833.
38. Marks, C.G. (1990) Anal lesions in Crohn's disease. *Annals of the Royal College of Surgeons of England*, **72**, 158–159.
39. Morrison, J.G., Gathright, J.B., Ray, J.E., Ferrari, B.T., Hicks, T.C. and Timmcke, A. (1989) Surgical management of anorectal fistulas in Crohn's disease. *Diseases of the Colon and Rectum*, **32**, 492–496.
40. Morson, B.C. and Lockhart-Mummery, H.E. (1959) Anal lesions in Crohn's disease. *The Lancet*, **2**, 1122–1123.
41. Morson, B.C. (1990) Pathology of Crohn's disease. *Annals of the Royal College of Surgeons of England*, **72**, 150–151.
42. Orkin, B.A. and Telander, R.L. (1985) The effect of intra-abdominal resection or fecal diversion on perianal disease in pediatric Crohn's disease. *Journal of Pediatric Surgery*, **20**, 343–347.
43. Parks, A.G. and Morson, B.C. (1962) The pathogenesis of fistula-in-ano. *Proceedings of the Royal Society of Medicine*, **55**, 751–754.
44. Penner, A. and Crohn, B.B. (1938) Perianal fistulae as a complication of regional ileitis. *Annals of Surgery*, **108**, 867–869.
45. Preston, D.M., Fowler, E.G., Lennard-Jones, J.E. and Hawley, P.R. (1983) Carcinoma of the anus in Crohn's disease. *British Journal of Surgery*, **70**, 346–347.
46. Radcliffe, A.G., Ritchie, J.K., Hawley, P.R., Lennard-Jones, J. and Northover, J.M. (1988) Anovaginal and rectovaginal fistulas in Crohn's disease. *Diseases of the Colon and Rectum*, **31**, 94–99.
47. Rankin, G.B., Watts, H.P. and Melnyk, C.S. (1979) National Co-operative Crohn's disease study: Extraintestinal manifestations and perianal complications. *Gastroenterology*, **77**, 914–920.
48. Roe, A.M. and Mortensen, N.J. (1989) Perineal reconstruction with rectus abdominis flaps after resection of anal carcinoma in Crohn's disease. *Journal of the Royal Society of Medicine*, **82**, 369–370.
49. Scott, A., Hawley, P.R. and Phillips, R.K. (1989) Results of external sphincter repair in Crohn's disease. *British Journal of Surgery*, **76**, 959–960.
50. Slaney, G., Muller, S., Clay, J., Sumathipala, A.H., Hillenbrand, P. and Thompson, H. (1986) Crohn's disease involving the penis. *Gut*, **27**, 329–333.
51. Slater, G., Greenstein, A. and Aufses, A.J. Jr. (1984) Anal carcinoma in patients with Crohn's disease. *Annals of Surgery*, **199**, 348–350.
52. Sohn, N., Korelitz, B.I. and Weinstein, M.A. (1980) Anorectal Crohn's disease: Definitive surgery for fistulas and recurrent abscesses. *American Journal of Surgery*, **139**, 394–397.
53. Somerville, K.W., Langman, M.J., DaCruz, D.J., Balfour, T.W. and Sully, L. (1984) Malignant transformation of anal skin tags in Crohn's disease. *Gut*, **25**, 1124–1125.
54. Steinhardt, H.J., Loeschke, K., Kasper, H., Holtermüller, K.H. and Schafer, H. (1985) *Digestion*, **31**, 97–108.
55. Sweeney, J.L., Ritchie, J.K. and Nicholls, R.J. (1988) Anal fissure in Crohn's disease. *British Journal of Surgery*, **75**, 56–57.
56. Taylor, B.A., Williams, G.T., Hughes, L.E. and Rhodes, I. (1989) The histology of 'anal' skin tags in Crohn's disease: An aid to the confirmation of the diagnosis. *International Journal of Colorectal Disease*, **4**, 197–199.
57. VanDongen, L.M. and Lubbers, E.J. (1986) Perianal fistulas in patients with Crohn's disease. *Archives of Surgery*, **121**, 1187–1190.
58. Ward, C.S., Dunphy, E.P., Jagoe, W.S. and Sheahan, D.G. (1985) Crohn's disease limited to the mouth and anus. *Journal of Clinical Gastroenterology*, **7**, 516–521.
59. White, R.A., Eisenstat, T.E., Rubin, R.J. and Salvati, E.P. (1990) Seton management of complex anorectal fistulas in patients with Crohn's disease. *Disease of the Colon and Rectum*, **33**, 587–589.
60. Williams, D.R., Coller, J.A., Corman, M.L., Nugent, F.W. and Veidenheimer, M.C. (1981) *Diseases of the Colon and Rectum*, **24**, 22–24.
61. Williams, J.G. and Hughes, L.E. (1990) Abdomino-perineal resection for severe perianal Crohn's disease. *Disease of the Colon and Rectum*, **33**, 402–407.
62. Wolff, B.G., Culp, C.E., Beart, R.W. Jr., Ilstrup, D.M. and Ready, R.L. (1985) Anorectal Crohn's disease. A long-term perspective. *Diseases of the Colon and Rectum*, **28**, 709–711.
63. Wolff, B.G. (1986) Crohn's disease: The role of surgical treatment. *Mayo Clinic Proceedings*, **61**, 292–295.
64. Yousem, D.M., Fishman, E.K. and Jones, B. (1988) Crohn's disease: Perirectal and perianal findings at CT. *Radiology*, **167**, 331–334.
65. Zelas, P. and Jagelman, D. (1980) Loop ileostomy in the management of Crohn's colitis in the delibitated patient. *Annals of Surgery*, **191**, 164–168.

EXTRAINTESTINAL MANIFESTATIONS OF INFLAMMATORY BOWEL DISEASE

C. O'Morain

Extraintestinal manifestations are frequent and common to both forms of inflammatory bowel disease, pointing perhaps to a common pathogenesis for both diseases. The complications often influence therapeutic and management decisions. In a minority of patients they are the presenting feature and precede symptoms referable to the gastrointestinal tract. The extraintestinal symptoms may improve with effective medical treatment or surgical resection but this is not always true.

The complications are many and varied. Some may result from drug therapy and electrolyte or nutritional imbalance. The reported incidence rates differ. This may be due to variations in length of follow-up, the criteria for defining complications or different attitudes to screening for asymptomatic extraintestinal manifestations. Extraintestinal manifestations are more common in Crohn's colitis than in ileocaecal or small bowel disease.

The extraintestinal manifestations which may occur in inflammatory bowel disease can be classified into two major groups: activity related or autoimmune.[64]

THE LIVER

Liver disease is one of the most important extracolonic manifestations in terms of morbidity and mortality. The spectrum of liver disease extends from minor abnormalities of the biochemical profile to established cirrhosis, and includes fatty change, pericholangitis, chronic active hepatitis, cirrhosis, granulomata, amyloidosis, hepatic abscess, gallstones and carcinoma of the biliary tree.

A recent observation using a monoclonal antibody showed that there is a shared and unique epitope in human colon, skin and biliary tract epithelium. The shared epitope is related to a molecular weight of 40 000 which acts as an autoantigen in patients with ulcerative colitis.[23] This could explain the biliary and skin complications of inflammatory bowel disease.

INCIDENCE

In careful microscopic studies of liver biopsies obtained from patients undergoing colectomy for either ulcerative colitis or Crohn's disease, histological abnormalities were found in nearly 90%.[28,30] In a survey from Birmingham of 1200 patients with inflammatory bowel disease, abnormal liver function tests were present at some time in approximately 8% of patients, but in many cases they developed transiently after surgery, associated with abdominal sepsis. One-fifth of patients with abnormal liver function tests had pericholangitis.[25]

FATTY CHANGE

The most common lesion is fatty infiltration but sepsis and undernutrition may contribute to this finding. In one study, marked liver function abnormalities correlated with extent and severity, but not duration of the disease, and persisted despite therapy, whereas mildly abnormal liver function tests did not correlate with extent, activity or duration of ulcerative colitis and were usually self-limiting processes.[58]

PERICHOLANGITIS

Pericholangitis, also called triaditis, is recognized histologically by cellular infiltration of the portal tracts, portal fibrosis and concentric fibrosis around the intrahepatic and extrahepatic ducts (*Figure 7.55*).

The aetiology of pericholangitis is unknown but possible causes include immunological, toxic and infective mechanisms. It is not related to blood transfusion, drug treatment or other systemic manifestations.[28] An infective theory has been proposed as pathogens have been cultured from the portal vein.[29] Experimentally induced chronic portal bacteraemia in calves led to portal inflammation similar, but not identical, to pericholangitis.[90] Portal vein bacteraemia could be a consequence of invasion of the bowel flora through a damaged ulcerated bowel wall. Intestinal bacteria are involved in a variety of potential hepatotoxic events including deconjugation of bile salts, endogenous alcohol production, inactivation of hepatic lipotrophs such as choline, release of endotoxin and peptidoglycan–polysaccharide polymers. In an experimental rat model of small bowel, bacterial overgrowth caused significant hepatic inflammation.[57]

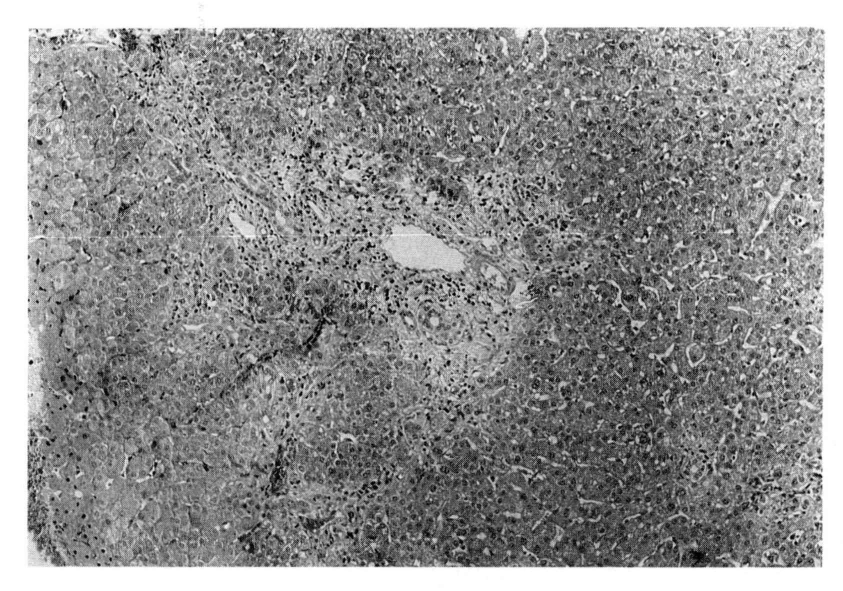

Figure 7.55 Sclerosing pericholangitis (also called triaditis), showing cellular infiltration of the portal tracts and fibrosis of the portal intra- and extrahepatic ducts.

PRIMARY SCLEROSING CHOLANGITIS

Primary sclerosing cholangitis occurs more frequently in association with ulcerative colitis than any other condition, commonly in patients with severe and extensive disease. The extent of the sclerosing cholangitis can be readily identified by endoscopic retrograde cholangiography. Light and electron microscopic studies of biopsies show that the main feature is mesenchymal proliferation involving phagocytic, fibroblastic and immunocytic cells, suggestive of an immunological type of liver injury which may attack bile duct epithelial cells.[63]

Beneficial results of aggressive treatment aimed at promoting biliary drainage and eradication of the biliary infection to prevent progression of the disease have been reported.[94] This was achieved by stenting and appropriate antibiotic therapy (cephalosporin or gentamicin plus metronidazole). The stent was left in place for 12–18 months but its care was managed on an outpatient basis.

CIRRHOSIS OF THE LIVER

Cirrhosis of the liver was found in 3 out of 517 patients with Crohn's disease and 11 out of 720 patients with ulcerative colitis.[25] Hepatoma occasionally complicates cirrhosis of the liver associated with ulcerative colitis.

OTHER CONDITIONS

Biliary tract carcinoma is a well-recognized complication of ulcerative colitis which, in the early stages, is often difficult to distinguish from sclerosing cholangitis.

Chronic active hepatitis, amyloidosis, granulomata and hepatic abscess are rare. An incidence of 1–2% of patients has been reported in several large studies.

TIME SEQUENCE

Liver abnormalities may precede symptomatic inflammatory bowel disease so that this possibility must be considered in the differential diagnosis of liver disease. Drug therapy for inflammatory bowel disease, particularly sulphasalazine, and total parenteral nutrition can cause liver function abnormalities.

THE SKIN

Erythema nodosum and pyoderma gangrenosum are important cutaneous manifestations and may be of diagnostic value. The incidence of cutaneous manifestations varies from 2% to 34%. The latter reports include drug hypersensitivity reactions, perianal and oral lesions. Erythema multiforme has been documented in association with Crohn's disease but may be a chance occurrence.[11] Patients with inflammatory bowel disease also have a higher incidence of atopic skin disease than controls.

PYODERMA GANGRENOSUM

Pyoderma gangrenosum can be recognized as a painful necrotic ulcer with an advancing rolled or determined border and a pustular centre. Preceding local trauma can be identified in 40% of cases.[6] The lesion most commonly occurs on the pre-tibial surface of the lower limbs but may occur elsewhere.

In one large series, 50% of patients with pyoderma gangrenosum had underlying ulcerative colitis.[72] It may also complicate Crohn's disease. The differential diagnosis of pyoderma gangrenosum includes rheumatoid arthritis, pulmonary infection, diverticulosis, leukaemia, Hodgkin's disease, polycythaemia rubra vera, myeloma, myelofibrosis, Behçet's disease and chronic active hepatitis. Pyoderma gangrenosum can occur spontaneously without underlying systemic disease, particularly in the elderly.[87]

Decreased neutrophil chemotaxis in vitro has been described in pyoderma gangrenosum due to either an intrinsic neutrophil leukocyte defect or inhibitory serum factors.[45,82] Neutrophil abnormalities have also been described in Crohn's disease and ulcerative colitis where the number of neutrophils accumulating in response to inflammation is reduced.[68,92] Defective complement function has also been reported in pyoderma gangrenosum.[21] Autoantibodies to skin and intestinal antigens have been demonstrated in patients with inflammatory bowel disease and pyoderma gangrenosum.

ERYTHEMA NODOSUM

The reported incidence of erythema nodosum in inflammatory bowel disease varies from 0.5% to 9%. Erythema nodosum is a form of panniculitis characterized by red nodules up to several centimetres in diameter, which are painless but tender to touch, on the anterior aspect of the lower limbs. Other sites include the thighs, arms and hands. Women are more commonly affected than men. Unlike pyoderma gangrenosum, the appearance of the nodules usually coincides with an active phase of the disease. Erythema nodosum may precede or coincide with the bowel symptoms. In other patients it only occurs many years after the onset of gastrointestinal disease.[6] Arthralgia or arthropathy commonly coexist. Significant skin involvement may be accompanied by fever and malaise. The lesions may occasionally ulcerate, but usually fade to a bronze discoloration when the underlying bowel disease goes into remission.

Erythema nodosum is probably due to a delayed hypersensitivity reaction whilst that of pyoderma gangrenosum is considered to be an impaired immune response to some antigens.[22] Skin lesion has been described, in two patients with Crohn's disease, which resembles erythema nodosum but runs a different clinical course independent of the activity of Crohn's disease. Steroid therapy proved effective.[26] The histological features were also different in that necrobiotic collagen (necrobiosis) was prominent. This variant may have been overlooked because skin biopsy is rarely performed in erythema nodosum. Cutaneous polyarteritis nodosum, which has also been described in Crohn's disease, may be mistaken for erythema nodosum.[48]

CUTANEOUS POLYARTERITIS NODOSUM

Cutaneous polyarteritis nodosum is characterized by a panarteritis of the subcutis and adjacent dermis which occasionally involves vessels of the peripheral nerves and skeletal muscle. Clinically, there may be red subcutaneous nodules of the lower extremities which have a tendency to ulcerate. Peripheral neuropathy, myalgia or arthritis may also be present. In most patients there is a complete spontaneous resolution of the arteritis, whereas in the remainder cutaneous nodules persist despite resolution of the associated myositis and polyneuritis. Corticosteroids and sulphasalazine may be beneficial. This complication is unrelated to the activity of the underlying intestinal disease. Histological examination of biopsies from the lesions shows granulomata with epithelioid cell formation in the vessel wall similar to that observed in Crohn's disease.

PSORIASIS

Psoriasis, although not related to disease activity, occurred in one series in 7% of patients with Crohn's disease. It must be considered as an associated condition in both forms of inflammatory bowel disease.[35,64]

APHTHOUS STOMATITIS

Aphthous stomatitis is seen in 4% of patients with inflammatory bowel disease.[37] The clinical picture is of ulcers on the floor of the mouth, gums, lower and upper lip, palate and uvula.[7] Their presence usually indicates active disease. Aphthous stomatitis is associated with Behçet's disease, which can involve the gastrointestinal tract. Many cases labelled as Behçet's disease could be Crohn's disease. Aphthous ulceration of the gastrointestinal tract is one of the earliest lesions of Crohn's disease.

ARTHRITIS

Inflammatory bowel disease is often complicated by two types of arthritis: an enteropathic arthritis and sacroiliitis or ankylosing spondylitis.[38,60,96] The reported incidence varies between 4% and 45% (average 37%) but this may be explained in part by the selected use of special radiographs of the sacro-iliac joints to exclude sacroiliitis.[97] Enteropathic arthritis is an inflammatory synovitis limited to a few large joints. The serum from these patients is negative for IgM and rheumatoid factor. Any joint may be affected but most commonly the joints of the lower limbs are involved. An acute, sometimes relapsing asymmetrical arthritis is characteristic and can precede, coincide with or develop in established bowel disease. The radiological findings of joints involved by enteropathic arthritis are minimal, such as minor joint narrowing, juxta-articular periostitis and, rarely, erosions. Significant permanent joint disease is rare but may occur and is exacerbated by injury to the inflamed joint. Enteropathic arthritis is more common in Crohn's disease patients with localized colonic disease, but an incidence of 14% has been recorded in patients with small bowel involvement.[38]

Arthritis is also observed after intestinal bypass operations for morbid obesity.[93] Cryoprotein complexes may be identified in the serum from these patients including IgG, IgM, IgA, complement components C3, C4, and C5, and IgG antibody against *Escherichia coli* and *Bacillus fragilis*. Circulating cryoprotein complexes can activate both the classic and the alternative complement pathways which may be important in the pathogenesis of the arthritis. Improvement follows treatment with metronidazole or taking down of the bypass in patients treated for morbid obesity, which suggests that bacterial byproducts originating in the excluded bowel may be important in the aetiology. Endotoxaemia has been found in patients with active inflammatory bowel disease, which may play a role in the development of extraintestinal manifestations.[18] There are similarities with the active arthritis associated with *Yersinia*, *Campylobacter* and *Chlamydia* spp., and other enteric infections. Both types are transient, asymmetrical in distribution of a non-deforming synovitis and have a predeliction for involvement of large joints.

Enteropathic arthritis improves following treatment of the inflammatory bowel disease. Colectomy in a case of fulminant ulcerative colitis led to rapid remission of the concomitant arthritis.[59] Surgical resection of Crohn's disease does not always result in a remission of the associated arthritis.[28] The enteropathic arthritis is usually self-limiting but symptomatic treatment with non-steroidal anti-inflammatory drugs may be necessary. Sulphasalazine is also effective treatment.[62] Recent data suggest that the 5-aminosalicylic acid moiety of sulphasalazine is the active component in the bowel, whereas sulphapyridine is active in synovial inflammation.[50]

SACROILIITIS AND ANKYLOSING SPONDYLITIS

Sacroiliitis is an early manifestation of ankylosing spondylitis. It is frequently asymptomatic, the diagnosis being made on radiological grounds. Ankylosing spondylitis predominantly affects males (male : female ratio is 4 : 1), but the sex ratio of those with spondylitis complicating inflammatory bowel disease is almost equal. The association between ankylosing spondylitis and the histocomptability antigen HLA-B27 was first noted by Brewerton *et al.*[14] Ninety per cent of patients with sporadic ankylosing spondylitis are HLA-B27 positive, whereas in spondylitis associated with inflammatory bowel disease only 35% are positive for HLA-B27.[31] HLA-B27 does not predispose to the development of Crohn's disease or ulcerative colitis. The prevalence of inflammatory bowel disease and B27-negative spondylitis in family studies suggests that a non-HLA-linked genetic predisposition to inflammatory bowel disease exists, which also confers susceptibility to spondylitis, even in the absence of expression of bowel disease.

Spondylitis does not correlate with disease activity and is slowly progressive. Effective medical treatment of the inflammatory bowel disease and even colectomy does not alter the clinical course.[34] Treatment regimens include pain relief with analgesic anti-inflammatory drugs such as indomethacin and propionic acid derivatives. Exercise is encouraged and the physiotherapist should recommend back exercises as well as correct posture during working and leisure. Radiotherapy has been used in difficult cases.

CLUBBING OF THE FINGERS

The association between finger clubbing and inflammatory bowel disease is well recognized. The reported prevalence of finger clubbing in Crohn's disease varies between 31.5% and 58% and 4% and 13% in ulcerative colitis.[51,75] Hypertrophic osteoarthropathy occurs occasionally. Active disease is significantly associated with finger clubbing in both Crohn's disease and ulcerative colitis. Disease activity, although important in the pathogenesis of the disease, is not the only factor, because finger clubbing may be found in inactive disease. The vagus nerve and possibly other autonomic nerves may act as the afferent pathway of a reflex inducing finger clubbing. The focal stimuli are mucosal inflammatory changes and fibrosis. The efferent pathway of the finger-clubbing reflex has not been established. The focal changes include increased blood flow and amount of fibrous connective tissue. Finger clubbing in patients with Crohn's disease tends to regress after resection of macroscopic disease.[51]

OCULAR LESIONS

The reported frequency of eye changes varies widely but was 4% in patients with ulcerative colitis and 13% in patients with granulomatous colitis in a series of 700 cases of inflammatory bowel disease.[37] The most common eye condition is uveitis, the next most common being episcleritis. Retrospective studies report a lower incidence, but in these studies the eyes were not checked routinely. Conjunctivitis is uncommon but three patients have been described with inflammatory bowel disease and papillary hypertrophy with fibrovascular membrane formation, pyoblepharoconjunctivitis and eosinophilic microabscess formation.[95] Unilateral corneal lesions have also been described in inactive inflammatory bowel disease.[80] These lesions are small, peripheral, subepithelial infiltrates of white blood cells associated with mild irritative symptoms. No signs of staphylococcal infection are present. The corneal lesions clear rapidly with topical corticosteroids or systemic indomethacin. They may be due to a leukocyte infiltrate which migrates to a site of antigen–antibody reaction.[17]

Uveitis has been reported as a complication in 4% of patients with inflammatory bowel disease, but a higher incidence is suspected in Crohn's disease localized to the large bowel.[24,37] There have been associations of uveitis with other systemic disorders. In a review of 100 patients with uveitis, 33 had other systemic disease. More than half the patients with uveitis were positive for HLA-B27 antigen.[13] The patient may be asymptomatic or may complain of blurred vision, eye pain, photophobia and headache. Examination of the eye may show ciliary congestion, extreme turbidity of the aqueous and adhesions in the irides.

Uveitis can precede the onset of gastrointestinal symptoms and has been reported after colectomy and in inactive inflammatory bowel disease. Uveitis responds to systemic and local steroid therapy.

HAEMATOLOGICAL DISEASE

A wide range of haematological abnormalities has been described in association with inflammatory bowel disease, ranging from nutritional anaemias to acute myeloid leukaemia. The association of inflammatory bowel disease and malignancy is well described (see pages 1116, 1181). In a series of 400 patients with ulcerative colitis recently reported, 5 patients developed acute myelogenous leukaemia.[33]

AUTOIMMUNE HAEMOLYTIC ANAEMIA

Autoimmune haemolytic anaemia is a rare complication of inflammatory bowel disease, with less than 20 cases recorded in the literature.[3] The diagnosis is based on anaemia, reticulocytosis and a positive Coombs' test. Sulphasalazine can induce these changes and must therefore be excluded. Gastrointestinal haemorrhage and poor nutrition may contribute to the anaemia. Patients with autoimmune haemolytic anaemia associated with ulcerative colitis should be treated in a similar way to idiopathic autoimmune haemolytic anaemia. Half the patients will respond to corticosteroid therapy. The addition of immunosuppressive therapy to the non-responding corticosteroid-treated patients may induce a remission. Splenectomy produces a remission in the majority of patients.[81] Autoimmune haemolytic anaemia is not an indication for colectomy, because severe haemolysis has been reported many years after the colectomy.[2]

THROMBOSIS

Arterial and venous thromboses have been described in association with inflammatory bowel disease. The incidence is about 4% with overt clinical signs, but the incidence in postmortem studies is as high as 31%.[5] Extensive thrombosis is a grave complication of both forms of inflammatory bowel disease. There have been four reports of Budd–Chiari syndrome complicating ulcerative colitis with only one patient surviving.[12] Various sites of venous thrombus formation have been recorded, including the cerebral, thoracoepigastric, ileofemoral, portal and pulmonary veins. Arterial thrombosis is a more serious and poorly understood complication. It has occurred in the carotid, retinal, glans penis, femoral, subclavian, trachial, radial and ulnar arteries. Local vascular factors probably determine the site and whether arterial or venous thrombosis occurs.[10]

Symptomatic evaluation has revealed a hypercoaguable state in most patients with inflammatory bowel disease.[65] Increased platelet count, accelerated platelet aggregation and platelet retention rate, and increased fibrinogen content, factor VIII and factor IX activity were found. The high platelet count could be due to the associated anaemia.

In another study, antithrombin III, an important inhibitor of coagulation, was decreased in patients with inflammatory bowel disease compared with hospitalized controls.[55] Decreased levels could predispose to a hypercoaguable state. The levels of clotting factors correlated with the activity of the disease because they are acute phase reactants and decrease with successful medical treatment of the underlying inflammatory bowel disease. However, there is no direct evidence that elevated factors predispose to thrombotic formation.[43] Steroids were originally thought to play a role but this theory has now been discredited.[87] Other possible factors include stasis from bed rest, toxaemia, dehydration and immunological mechanisms inducing changes in the vessel wall leading to a vasculitis.

Conversely, thrombocytopenia and purpura have also been reported in ulcerative colitis.[54] Sulphasalazine may be responsible, so platelet counts should be checked at intervals. Malnutrition causing combined iron and vitamin B_{12} deficiency may contribute to thrombocytopenia. In a study examining baseline coagulation factors in patients with mild or inactive colitis, routine coagulation studies were normal but there was a high incidence of abnormalities of fibrinolysis and circulating immune complexes.[20]

The Hemansky–Pudlak syndrome consists of tyrosine-positive albinism, a defect in the second phase of platelet aggregation and an accumulation of ceroid-like pigment in tissue. This syndrome has been described in patients with inflammatory bowel disease and suggests that patients with inflammatory bowel disease might have a genetic predisposition to acquiring this condition.[78,79]

VASCULITIS

Isolated cases of vasculitis complicating inflammatory bowel disease have been described. Dermal vasculitis with necrotic skin lesions and pulmonary vasculitis are complications of many systemic diseases, but have also been described in ulcerative colitis.[4,19] Circulating immune complexes may play a role in initiating the vasculitis. Vasculitis has been postulated as the cause of Crohn's disease affecting maximally the gastrointestinal tract.[89] A pathogenic sequence of events in Crohn's disease has been postulated – vascular injury, focal arteritis, fibrin deposition, arterial occlusion mainly at the level of the muscularis propria, followed by tissue infarction or neovascularization. These features were confined to segments of intestine affected by Crohn's disease and did not occur in normal bowel. The findings suggest that Crohn's disease is mediated by multifocal gastrointestinal infarction.[91]

Takayasu's disease is a rare condition complicating both Crohn's disease and ulcerative colitis probably with an autoimmune basis.[8,16] Less than ten cases of this association have been published; all the affected patients were females of child-bearing age and the disease was characterized by a generalized arteritis. Patients with Takayasu's disease without bowel involvement have other manifestations including peripheral arthritis, skin lesions, erythema nodosum, pyoderma gangrenosum and uveitis. The arteritis usually responds to high-dose corticosteroid therapy. Some of the histological findings in Crohn's disease, such as granuloma formation, are seen in Takayasu's disease.

BRONCHOPULMONARY DISEASE

Pulmonary function tests performed on fit patients with underlying inflammatory bowel disease showed a significant decrease in the carbon monoxide transfer factor (*T*LCO).[15] The observed reduction in *T*LCO was similar whether or not patients were taking sulphasalazine. The reduction was still observed when *T*LCO was corrected for the haemoglobin levels.[47] A report described seven patients with lung disease. In three, rapidly progressive bronchiectasis developed within 1 year of proctocolectomy. In two it developed in association with an exacerbation of colitis, and in the other two a milder limited colitis postdated the start of the lung disease. All seven patients had an arthropathy or skin rash, and a high incidence of personal or family history of autoimmune diseases. Antinuclear antibodies were detected in six of the patients and smooth muscle antibodies in five. There was no evidence of hepatic dysfunction. These findings and the clinical reponse to corticosteroid therapy were highly suggestive of an autoimmune aetiology.

Some patients with inflammatory bowel disease were non-smokers and yet had a productive cough and exertional dyspnoea. Bronchial epithelial biopsies from these patients revealed basal cell hyperplasia, basement membrane thickening and submucosal inflammatory change.[39] There are some morphological and developmental similarities between colonic and bronchial epithelium. Both are derived from the primitive gut, and both have columnar epithelial and goblet cells, and submucous glands. The non-specific inflammatory changes beneath the bronchial epithelium are similar to those seen in colonic epithelium in colitis. It is possible that a systemic factor is responsible for the common response at both epithelial sites in patients with colitis. Alternatively, it may be due to contact hypersensitivity to inhaled allergens in the case of bronchial epithelium or ingested allergens in the gut epithelium. Drugs used in the treatment of inflammatory bowel disease may cause lung disease, e.g. sulphasalazine can cause fibrosing alveolitis.

CARDIOVASCULAR DISEASE

Only 16 examples of pericarditis complicating inflammatory bowel disease have been described in the literature,[56,87] and it can result in life-threatening cardiac tamponade. It is usually associated with active disease but may predate the onset of bowel symptoms and can occur after colectomy. Pericarditis responds to high-dose corticosteroid therapy but may relapse when the dose is reduced. Pleural effusions have also been noted in these patients.

RENAL DISEASE

The incidence of urolithiasis in inflammatory bowel disease is 15%.[53] The pathogenesis of stone formation includes dehydration, corticosteroid treatment, urinary tract infection, and hydronephrosis secondary to ureteric obstruction of the right ureter. The tendency to stone formation is increased following small bowel resection. Bile salt absorption is reduced after ileal resection and their presence in the colon enhances oxalate absorption. However, there is also a high incidence of urolithiasis among ileostomy patients, so that other mechanisms must be involved. Steatorrhoea precipitates calcium which normally binds oxalate in the intestine and therefore enhances oxalate absorption. Curiously, a recent study found a similar incidence of urolithiasis in groups of patients with inflammatory bowel disease with hyperoxaluria and normal urinary oxalate excretion.[41]

Dehydration leading to low urinary volume and pH increases uric acid precipitation. The percentage of uric acid stones rises following colectomy, half of the stones containing uric acid compared to an incidence of 10% in the normal population.[61]

Pyelonephritis occurs in 2–4% of patients with ulcerative colitis. The incidence is higher in Crohn's disease due to ureteric obstruction and enterovesical fistulas.[84]

AMYLOIDOSIS

Less than 30 cases of amyloidosis complicating Crohn's disease have been reported in the literature. Only a few patients had the diagnosis made during life. The association between amyloid and ulcerative colitis is even rarer. The patients often present in renal failure and may require renal transplantation. It was once thought to occur only with ileal involvement, but a report of seven patients, all of whom had had previous resection, makes this untenable.[32] Regression of amyloidosis has followed surgical resection and some think that it is an indication for surgical resection of the underlying inflammatory bowel disease.

ENDOCRINE DISEASE

There are several reports of coexisting inflammatory bowel disease and hyperthyroidism.[42] Eight per cent had a palpable goitre and 4% had thyrotoxicosis in one large series of patients with ulcerative colitis.[46] Exacerbations of the thyroid disease and ulcerative colitis occurred together and made patient management difficult. Janerot has reported abnormalities of iodine metabolism in patients with inflammatory bowel disease. He noted a decreased 24-hour urine iodine excretion and increased 24-hour ^{131}I uptake, suggesting iodine deficiency.[45] As thyroxine (T_4) is protein bound, and patients with inflammatory bowel disease often have low serum albumin, they also tend to have low levels of thyroxine binding prealbumin and albumin, and a higher thyroglobulin compared to controls. These data may erroneously suggest hyperthyroidism so that radio-immunoassay of thyroid hormones should be used in patients with weight loss and diarrhoea if thyroid disease is suspected.

PATHOGENESIS

The exact mechanism by which the systemic manifestations occur is not known. An immune mechanism has been implicated although this fails to explain all of the manifestations, nor why only a minority of patients develop them. No linkage with common genetic markers such as blood group or secretor status has been found, and there is no strong association with any of the histocompatibility locus antigens (HLA) apart from those who have ankylosing spondylitis, uveitis and primary sclerosing cholangitis. The strength of the association between HLA-B27 and inflammatory bowel disease is less strong than in idiopathic spondylitis; this suggests a non-HLA genetic predisposition to inflammatory bowel disease which also confers susceptibility to spondylitis, even in the absence of expression of bowel disease.

There is a high frequency of HLA-D8 and HLA-DR3 antigens among patients with primary sclerosing cholangitis. This association is also found in other diseases such as insulin-dependent diabetes, dermatitis herpetiformis, Graves' disease, Sjögren's syndrome or disease, myasthenia gravis and coeliac disease. A recent study showed that the association of HLA-DRw52a with primary sclerosing cholangitis was total and the HLA might be helpful in differentiating this condition from primary biliary cirrhosis. They also found that primary sclerosing cholangitis, in combination with ulcerative cholitis, is found primarily in patients with the extended haplotype AI, B8, Cw7, DRw17, DQw2 and DRw52a, suggesting that at least one form of ulcerative colitis is a manifestation of the autoimmune haplotype.[74]

Using a monoclonal antibody an intriguing observation has been made that a shared and unique epitope exists in human colon, skin and biliary tract, the extraintestinal organs being commonly involved in ulcerative colitis. The shared epitope is related to a colonic protein of molecular weight 40 000 which acts as an autoantigen in patients with ulcerative colitis.[23] The monoclonal antibody did not react with other epithelial organs including small intestinal tissue. Further work is being carried out on the possible role for this protein/shared epitope in the pathogenesis of ulcerative colitis and the extraintestinal manifestations of inflammatory bowel disease.

In experimental serum sickness, the arthritis, uveitis, glomerulonephritis and skin lesions which occur may be due to circulating immune complexes. As similar lesions can occur as extraintestinal manifestations in inflammatory bowel disease, circulating immune complexes formed within the inflamed mucosa may play a role in their initiation. The presence of immune complexes within the intestinal mucosa of patients with inflammatory bowel disease has been inferred from immunofluorescence studies. Increased circulating immune complexes have been described in Crohn's disease using different assay techniques.[40] Some methods of measuring immune complexes may simply be measuring aggregated IgG. When an essay is performed so as to exclude measurement of aggregated IgG, no circulating immune complexes are found in patients with inflammatory bowel disease even among those with extraintestinal manifestations.[83] In a more recent study no association of concentrations of circulating immune complexes with disease activity or presence of extraintestinal manifestations was found.[52]

Perpetuation of inflammatory changes in inflammatory bowel disease may be due to complement activation. Immune complexes can activate complement through both the classic and alternative pathways. Evidence for complement activation has come from studies showing the presence of complement breakdown products,[86] antibodies to fixed complement,[71] and increased synthesis and catabolism of C3 and C1q.[73] Complement may be activated by immune complexes and deposited at extravascular sites such as the gastrointestinal tract skin and joints. Most tests for the presence of immune complexes and antigen–antibody complexes are indirect. They depend upon the biochemistry of complement. This is especially so when the antigen is unknown. The antigen in inflammatory bowel disease could be an infective agent, a dietary component or altered tissue reaction. Patients who have jejunoileal bypass operations for morbid obesity may also develop hepatic and arthritic manifestations. This is probably due to bacteria or bacterial toxins which proliferate in the isolated bowel, enter the circulation and are deposited as antigen–antibody complexes which activate complement and lead to tissue damage. Their symptoms respond to treatment with antibiotics and remit after taking down the bypass.

PHAGOCYTIC FUNCTION

The process of localization and elimination of foreign material can be termed an 'immune effector function' and is largely mediated by an immunologically initiated inflammatory response. The local accumulation of immune effector cells such as lymphocytes, macrophages or polymorphonuclear (PMN) leukocytes is instrumental in the localization and destruction of antigens. A defective effector mechanism may explain some of the extraintestinal manifestations of inflammatory bowel disease (*Figure 7.56*). A neutrophil defect has been described in Crohn's disease, in that they fail to migrate to a site of inflammation.[68] Neutrophil selective enzyme activities are lower and 5′-nucleotidase synthesized by activated macrophages is high in non-involved Crohn's disease tissue.[70] This

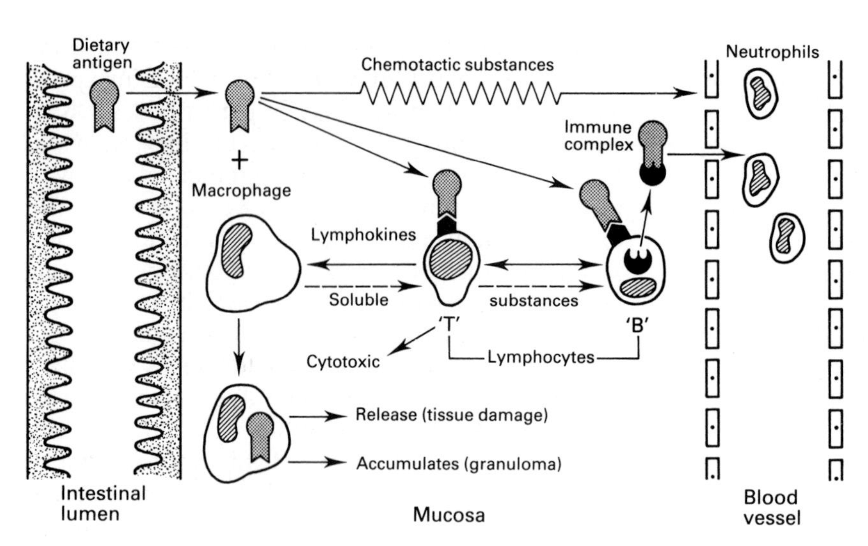

Figure 7.56 Hypothesis of the pathogenesis of Crohn's disease. A dietary antigen penetrates the mucosa. Chemotactic factors are not released in sufficient amounts to attract neutrophils. The dietary antigen persists and interacts with macrophages and lymphocytes. This results in accumulation of macrophages leading to granulomatous formation and lymphocyte activation and tissue damage.

indicates that, in the absence of neutrophils, the macrophage has an important role in the pathogenesis of the disease.

The gastrointestinal tract is exposed to multiple antigens in a normal diet. Many of these antigens penetrate the epithelial surface of the gut; most are eliminated by body defence mechanisms. However, patients with Crohn's disease are unable to accumulate sufficient neutrophils to phagocytose foreign material. This may be due to mucosal cells not liberating sufficient amounts of chemotatic factor to attract neutrophils, because the neutrophils have normal migration and phagocytic ability in vitro. This host immune mechanism could be genetically determined, which could account for the increased familial and racial incidence of the disease. It is probable that only some food components, by virtue of their size, configuration or physical state, have this effect and may be food additives. This could account for the increased incidence of the disease in developed Western countries. The dietary component would act as an antigen and cause B cells to secrete antibody, which would escape into the circulation and initiate the extraintestinal manifestation.

An elemental diet is effective treatment in removing the offending dietary antigen, for not only do the patients respond clinically but their extraintestinal manifestations also resolve.[67] Patients with Crohn's disease have an increased intestinal mucosal permeability as assessed by different probes including chromium-labelled ethylenediamine tetraacetic acid (EDTA) and polyethylene glycol (PEG).[9,66,76,77] Relatives of patients with Crohn's disease have increased permeability to PEG but not to chromium-labelled EDTA, suggesting a primary abnormality.[1,49] Patients treated with an elemental diet who have high urinary excretion of chromium-labelled EDTA before institution of the diet therapy have normal urinary excretion levels following treatment.[85] This suggests than an elemental diet has a direct beneficial effect on the mucosa.

In patients with ulcerative colitis leukocytes are mobilized in normal numbers immediately after eliciting the inflammatory reaction, indicating a normal inflammatory response, but mobilization of neutrophils into skin window chambers is subsequently reduced.[93] This could be due to an intrinsic neutrophil defect or exhaustion of locally produced chemotactic substance. Lysosomal enzyme markers are decreased in rectal biopsies from patients with ulcerative colitis indicating that their release may be important in the pathogenesis of the disease and the extraintestinal manifestations.[36,69,70] The failure of neutrophils to continue to accumulate would allow antigens which are normally cleared by innate body defences to persist and set up a secondary immunological reaction.

SUMMARY

The wide variety and similarity of extraintestinal manifestations in both forms of inflammatory bowel disease suggest that a common pathogenesis is involved, most probably immunological. It is possible that ulcerative colitis and Crohn's disease are generalized diseases in which the major manifestations are in the gastrointestinal tract.

REFERENCES

1. Ainswood, M., Eriysen, J., Waevr-Rasmussen, T. *et al.* (1989) 51Cr-labelled ethylenediamine tetraacetic acid in patients with Crohn's disease and

their healthy relatives. *Scandinavian Journal of Gastroenterology*, **24**, 993–998.
2. Altman, A.R., Maltz, C. and Janowitz, H.D. (1979) Autoimmune haemolytic anaemia in ulcerative colitis. *Digestive Diseases and Sciences*, **24**, 282–285.
3. Balford, J. and Shiner, M. (1974) Evidence of cytoxicity in ulcerative colitis from immunofluorescent staining of rectal mucosa. *The Lancet*, **1**, 1014–1017.
4. Ball, G.V. and Goldman, L.N. (1970) Chronic ulcerative colitis, skin necrosis and cryofibrinogenemia. *Annals of Internal Medicine*, **85**, 464–466.
5. Bargen, I.A. and Barker, N.W. (1936) Extensive arterial and venous thrombosis complicating chronic ulcerative colitis. *Archives of Internal Medicine*, **58**, 17–31.
6. Basler, R.S.W. (1980) Ulcerative colitis and the skin. *Medical Clinics of North America*, **64**, 941–954.
7. Basu, M.K. and Asquith, P. (1980) Oral manifestations of inflammatory bowel disease. *Clinics in Gastroenterology*, **9**, 307–322.
8. Beau, B., Colasse, W., Bihan, G. and Bourreillo, J. (1980) Association d'une maladie de Takayasu et d'une colite inflammatoire. *Semaine de Hospitaux Paris*, **56**, 1841–1845.
9. Bjarnasson, I., O'Morain, C., Levi, A.J. and Peters, T.J. (1983) Absorption of 51 chromium labelled EDTA in inflammatory bowel disease. *Gastroenterology*, **85**, 318–322.
10. Braverman, D. and Bogoch, A. (1978) Arterial thrombosis in ulcerative colitis. *Digestive Diseases*, **23**, 1148–1150.
11. Brenner, S.M. and Delany, H.M. (1972) Erythema multiforme and Crohn's disease of the large intestine. *Gastroenterology*, **62**, 479–482.
12. Brinson, R.R., Curtis, W.D., Schuman, B.M. and Mills, I.R. (1989) Recovery from hepatic vein thrombosis (Budd–Chiari syndrome) complicating ulcerative colitis. *Digestive Diseases and Sciences*, **33**, 1615–1620.
13. Brewerton, D.A., Caffrey, M., Nicholls, A. and Walters, D. (1973) Acute anterior uveitis and HL-AW227. *The Lancet*, **2**, 994–996.
14. Brewerton, D.A., Hart, F.D., Nicholls, A. *et al.* (1973) Anklyosing spondylitis and HLA-B27. *The Lancet*, **1**, 1904.
15. Butland, R.J.A., Cole, P., Citron, K.M. and Turner-Warwick, M. (1981) Chronic bronchial suppuration and inflammatory bowel disease. *Quarterly Journal of Medicine*, **50**, 63–75.
16. Chapman, R., Dawe, C., Whorwell, P.J. and Wright, R. (1978) Ulcerative colitis in association with Takayasu's Disease. *Digestive Disease*, **23**, 660–662.
17. Chignall, A.H., Easty, D.L., Chesterton, J.R. and Tomsitt, J. Marginal ulceration of the cornea. *British Journal of Ophthalmology*, **54**, 443–444.
18. Colin, R., Grancher, T., Lemeland, J.F. *et al.* (1979) Recherche d'une endotoxinemie dans les entero-colites inflammatoire cryptogenetiques. *Gastroenterologie Clinic et Biologique*, **3**, 15–19.
19. Collins, W.J., Bendig, B.W. and Taylor, W.F. (1979) Pulmonary valculitis complicating childhood ulcerative colitis. *Gastroenterology*, **77**, 1091–1093.
20. Conlon, M.G., Haire, W.D. and Burnett, D.A. (1989) Prothrombotic abnormalities in inflammatory bowel disease. *Digestive Diseases and Sciences*, **34**, 1084–1093.
21. D'Amelio, R., Rossi, P., Le Moles, S. *et al.* (1981) In vitro studies in cellular and humoral chemotasis in Crohn's disease using the under agarose gel technique. *Gut*, **22**, 566–570.
22. Danzi, T.J. (1988) Extraintestinal manifestations of idiopathic inflammatory bowel disease. *Archives of Internal Medicine*, **148**, 247–321.
23. Das, K.M., Vecchi, M. and Sukamuki, S. (1990) A shared and unique epitope(s) on human colon, skin and biliary epithelium detected by a monoclonal antibody. *Gastroenterology*, **98**, 464–469.
24. Daum, F., Gould, H.B., Gold, D. *et al.* (1979) Asymptomatic transient uveitis in children with inflammatory bowel disease. *American Journal of Diseases of Children*, **133**, 170–171.
25. Dew, M.J., Thompson, H. and Allan, R.N. (1979) The spectrum of hepatic dysfunction in inflammatory bowel disease. *Quarterly Journal of Medicine*, **48**, 113–135.
26. Du Boulay, C. and Whorwell, P.J. (1982) Nodular necrobiosis; a new cutaneous manifestation of Crohn's disease. *Gut*, **23**, 712–715.
27. Eade, O.E., Smith, C.L., Alexander, J.R. and Whorwell, P.J. (1980) Pulmonary function in patients with inflammatory bowel disease. *American Journal of Gastroenterology*, **73**, 154–156.
28. Eade, M. (1970) Liver disease of ulcerative colitis. *Annals of Internal Medicine*, **72**, 475–487.
29. Eade, M.N. and Brooke, B.N. (1969) Portal bacteremia in cases of ulcerative colitis submitted to colectomy. *The Lancet*, **1**, 1008–1009.
30. Eade, M.N., Cooke, W.T., Brooke, B.N. and Thompson, H. (1971) Liver disease in Crohn's colitis. A study of 21 consecutive patients having colectomy. *Annals of Internal Medicine*, **74**, 518.
31. Enlow, R.W., Bias, W.B. and Arnett, F.C. (1980) The spondylitis of inflammatory bowel disease. *Arthritis and Rheumatism*, **23**, 1359–1365.
32. Fausa, O., Nygaard, K. & Elgio, K. (1977) Amyloidosis and Crohn's disease. *Scandinavian Journal of Gastroenterology*, **12**, 657–662.
33. Fabry, T.L., Sachar, D.B. and Janowitz, H.D. (1980) Acute myelogenous leukemia in patients with ulcerative colitis. *Journal of Clinical Gastroenterology*, **2**, 225–227.
34. Ferguson, R.H. (1981) Arthritis associated with inflammatory bowel disease. *Minnesota Medicine*, **64**, 165–166.
35. Gebbers, J. and Otto, H.F. (1978) Immunohisto- and ultracytochemical observations on the early lesion in ulcerative colitis. *Gut*, **19**, 989.

36. Fielding, J.F. (1986) Clinical features of Crohn's disease in Ireland. *American Journal of Gastroenterology*, **81**, 524–528.
37. Greenstein, A.J., Janowitz, H.D. and Sinclair, D.B. (1976) The extra-intestinal complications of Crohn's disease and ulcerative colitis. *Medicine*, **55**, 401–412.
38. Haslock, I. (1973) Arthritis and Crohn's disease – a family study. *Annals of the Rheumatic Diseases*, **32**, 479.
39. Higenbottam, T., Cochrane, G.M., Clarke, T.J.H. *et al.* (1980) Bronchial disease in ulcerative colitis. *Thorax*, **35**, 581–585.
40. Hodgson, H.J.F., Potter, B.J. and Sewell, D.P. (1979) Immune complexes in ulcerative colitis and Crohn's disease. *Clinical and Experimental Immunology*, **29**, 187–196.
41. Hylander, E., Jarnum, S. and Frandsen, I. (1979) Urolithiasis and hyper-oxaluria in chronic inflammatory bowel disease. *Scandinavian Journal of Gastroenterology*, **14**, 475–479.
42. Iyer, S.K. and Karlstadt, R.G. (1980) Hyperthyroidism and ulcerative colitis report of two cases and a review of the literature. *Journal of the National Medical Association*, **72**, 127–131.
43. Iyer, S.K., Handler, L.J. and Jounston, J.S. (1981) Thrombophlebitis migrans in association with ulcerative colitis. *Journal of the National Medical Association*, **73**, 987–989.
44. Jacobs, J.C. and Goezl, E.J. (1975) Streaking leucocyte factor, arthritis and pyoderma gangrenosum. *Pediatrics*, **56**, 570–578.
45. Janerot, G. (1975) The thyroid in ulcerative colitis and Crohn's disease. Part 1. Thyroid radioiodide uptake and urinary codine excretion. *Acta Medica Scandinavica*, **197**, 83–87.
46. Janerot, G., Khan, A. and Spendlove, S. (1925) The thyroid in ulcerative colitis. Part 2: Thyroid enlargement and hyperthyroidism in ulcerative colitis. *Acta Medica Scandinavia*, **197**, 83–87.
47. Johnson, N., McImee, A.S., Jewell, D.P. and Clarke, S.W. (1978) Pulmonary function in inflammatory bowel disease. *Digestion*, **18**, 416–418.
48. Kahn, E., Daum, F., Aiges, H.W. and Silverberg, M. (1980) Cutaneous polyarteritis nodosa associated with Crohn's disease. *Diseases of the Colon and Rectum*, **23**, 258–262.
49. Katz, K.O., Hollander, D., Vadheim, C.M. *et al.* (1989) Intestinal permeability in patients with Crohn's disease and their healthy relatives. *Gastroenterology*, **97**, 927–931.
50. Kirsner, J.B. and Shorter, R.G. (1982) Recent developments in non-specific inflammatory bowel disease. *New England Journal of Medicine*, **306**, 775–785.
51. Kitis, G., Thompson, H. and Allan, R.N. (1979) Finger clubbing in inflammatory bowel disease: its prevalence and pathogenesis. *British Medical Journal*, **2**, 825–828.
52. Knoflach, P., Vladutu, A.O., Swierczynsku, Z., Weiser, M.M. and Albini, B. (1986) Lack of circulating immune complexes in inflammatory bowel disease. *International Archives of Applied Immunology*, **80**, 9–16.
53. Knudsen, L., Marcussen, H., Fleckenstein, P. *et al.* (1978) Urolithiasis in chronic inflammatory bowel disease. *Scandinavian Journal of Gastroenterology*, **13**, 433–436.
54. Kocoshis, S.A., Gartner, J.C., Gaffney, P.C. and Gryboski, J.D. (1979) Thrombocytopenia in ulcerative colitis. *Journal of Pediatrics*, **95**, 83–84.
55. Lam, A. and Borda, I.T. (1975) Coagulation studies in ulcerative colitis and Crohn's disease. *Gastroenterology*, **68**, 245–251.
56. Levin, E.N., Hirschfeld, D.S. and Herch, R.A. (1979) Pericarditis in association with ulcerative colitis. *Western Journal of Medicine*, **130**, 369–370.
57. Lichtman, S.N., Surton, R.B., Keku, J. and Schwab, J.H. (1990) Hepatic inflammation in rats with experimental small intestinal bacterial overgrowth. *Gastroenterology*, **98**, 418–423.
58. Lupmetti, M., Mehigan, D. and Cameron, J.L. (1980) Hepatobiliary complications of ulcerative colitis. *American Journal of Surgery*, **139**, 113–118.
59. McCullock, D.K., Fraser, D.M. and Turner, A.L. (1980) Arthritis preceding fulminant ulcerative colitis and responding to colectomy. *British Medical Journal*, **1**, 839.
60. Macrae, I.F. and Wright, V. (1973) A family of ulcerative colitis with particular reference to ankylosing spondylitis and sacro-ileitis. *Annals of the Rheumatic Diseases*, **32**, 10.
61. Maratka, Z. and Nedba, J. (1964) Urolithiasis as a complication of the surgical treatment of ulcerative colitis. *Gut*, **5**, 414–417.
62. Miclants, H. and Veys, E.M. (1985) HLA-B27 related arthritis and bowel inflammation. Sulfasalazine in HLA-B27 related reactive arthritis. *Journal of Rheumatology*, **12**, 287–293.
63. Mihas, A.A., Murad., T.M. and Hirschowitz, B.I. (1978) Sclerosing cholangitis associated with ulcerative colitis; light and electron microscopy studies. *American Journal of Gastroenterology*, **70**, 614–619.
64. Monsen, U., Sorstad, J., Hellers, G. and Johansson, C. (1990) Extracolonic diagnosis in ulcerative colitis. An epidemiological study. *American Journal of Gastroenterology*, **85**, 711–716.
65. Mori, K., Watanabe, H., Hiwatashi, N. *et al.* (1980) Studies on blood coagulation in ulcerative colitis and Crohn's disease. *Tohoku Journal of Experimental Medicine*, **132**, 93–101.
66. O'Morain, C., Abelow, A.C., Chervil, L.R., Fleischner, G.M. and Das, K. (1986) Chromium 51-ethylenediamine tetraacetate test: A useful test in the assessment of inflammatory bowel disease. *Journal of Laboratory and Clinical Medicine*, **108**, 430–435.
67. O'Morain, C., Segal, A.W. and Levi, A.J. (1980) Elemental diets in the treatment of acute Crohn's disease. *British Medical Journal*, **1**, 1173–1175.

68. O'Morain, C., Segal, A.W., Walker, D. and Levi, A.J. (1981) Abnormalities of neutrophils function to not cause the migration defect in Crohn's disease. *Gut*, **22**, 817–822.
69. O'Morain, C., Smethurst, P., Levi, A.J. and Peters, T.J. (1984) Organelle pathology in ulcerative colitis with special reference to the lysosomal alterations. *Gut*, **25**, 455–459.
70. O'Morain, C., Smethurst, P., Levi, A.J. and Peters, T.J. (1983) Biochemical analysis of enzymic markers of inflammation in rectal biopsies from patients with ulcerative colitis and Crohn's disease. *Journal of Clinical Pathology*, **36**, 1312–1316.
71. Pepys, M.B., Druguet, M., Klass, H.J. *et al.* (1977) Immunological studies in inflammatory bowel disease. In *Immunology of the Gut: Ciba Foundation Symposium*, pp. 283–297. Amsterdam: Elsevier.
72. Perry, H.O. (1969) Pyoderma gangrenosum. *Southern Medical Journal*, **62**, 899–908.
73. Potter, B.J., Mee, A.S., Hodgson, H.J.F. and Jewell, D.P. (1978) C1q metabolism in patients with inflammatory bowel disease. *Gut*, **19**, A443.
74. Prochazka, E.J., Terasaki, P.I., Min Sik Park, D.V.M., Goldstein, L.I. and Busuttil, R.W. (1990) Association of primary sclerosis cholangitis with HLA-DRw52a. *New England Journal of Medicines*, **332**, 1842–1848.
75. Rankin, G. (1990) Extraintestinal and systemic manifestations of inflammatory bowel disease. *Medical Clinics of North America*, **74**, 39–49.
76. Sanderson, I.R., Boulton, P. Menzies, B.I. and Walker Smith, J.A. (1987) Improvement of abnormal lactulose/rhamnose permeability in active Crohn's disease of the small bowel by an elemental diet. *Gut*, **28**, 1073–1076.
77. Schafflitzky De Muckaell, O.B., Ainsworth, M., Eriksen, J. and Waever-Rasmussen, J. (1989) 51Cr labelled ethylenediaminotetraacetic acid in patients with Crohn's disease and their healthy relatives. *Scandinavian Journal of Gastroenterology*, **24**, 933–998.
78. Schmella, R., Greco, A., Corbert, B., Denmark, L. and Cox, R. (1980) Hemansky–Pudlak syndrome with granulomatous colitis. *Annals of Internal Medicine*, **92**, 20–23.
79. Shanahan, F., Randolph, L., King, R. *et al.* (1988) The Hemansky–Pudlak syndrome. An immunological assessment of 15 cases. *American Journal of Medicine*, **85**, 823–828.
80. Schulman, M.F. and Sugar, A. (1981) Peripheral corneal infiltrates in inflammatory bowel disease. *Annals of Ophthalmology (New York)*, **13**, 109–111.
81. Shashaty, G.G., Rath, C.F. and Britt, E.J. (1977) Autoimmune hemolytic anemia associated with ulcerative colitis. *American Journal of Hematology*, **3**, 199–208.
82. Shore, R.N. (1976) Pyoderma gangrenosum, defective neutrophilchemotoxin and leukemia. *Archives of Dermatology*, **112**, 1792–1793.
83. Soltis, R.D. (1981) Circulating immune complexes in Crohn's disease. In *Recent Advances in Crohn's Disease* (Ed.) Pena, A.S., Waterman, I.T., Booth, C.C. and Strober, W. pp. 328–377. The Hague: Martinus Nijhoff.
84. Smith, J.N. and Winship, D.H. (1980) Complications and extraintestinal problems in inflammatory bowel disease. *Medical Clinics of North America*, **64**, 1161–1171.
85. Teahon, K., Bjarnasson, I. and Levi, A.J. (1991) The effect of elemental diet on intestinal permeability and inflammation in Crohn's disease. *Gastroenterology*, **101**, 84–89.
86. Teisberg, P. and Gjone, E. (1975) Humoral immune system activity in inflammatory bowel disease. *Scandinavian Journal of Gastroenterology*, **10**, 545–550.
87. Thompson, D.G., Lennard Jones, J.E., Swarbrick, E.T. and Bown, R. (1979) Pericarditis and inflammatory bowel disease. *Quarterly Journal of Medicine*, **67**, 93–97.
88. Thornton, J.R., Teague, R.H., Low-Beer, T.S. *et al.* (1980) Pyoderma gangrenosum and ulcerative colitis. *Gut*, **21**, 247–248.
89. Truelove, S.C. and Witts, L.J. (1955) Cortisone in ulcerative colitis. Final report on a therapeutic trial. *British Medical Journal*, **2**, 1041–1048.
90. Vinnick, I.E., Kern, F., Struthers, J.E. *et al.* (1964) Experimental chronic portal vein bacteremia. *Proceedings of the Society of Experimental Biology and Medicine*, **115**, 311–314.
91. Wakefield, A.J., Sawyerr, A.M., Dhillon, A.P. *et al.* (1989) Pathogenesis of Crohn's disease: multifocal gastrointestinal infection. *The Lancet*, **2**, 1057–1062.
92. Wandall, J.H. and Binder, V. (1982) Leucocyte function in ulcerative colitis, quantitative leucocyte mobilisation to skin windows and in vitro function of blood leucocytes. *Gut*, **23**, 758–765.
93. Wands, J.R., La Mont, J.T., Mann, E. and Isselbacher, K.J. (1976) Arthritis associated with intestinal bypass procedure for morbid obesity, complement activation and characterization of circulating cryoproteins. *New England Journal of Medicine*, **294**, 121–124.
94. Wood, A.R.B. and Cuschieri, A. (1980) Is sclerosing cholangitis complicating ulcerative colitis a reversible condition. *The Lancet*, **2**, 716–718.
95. Wright, P. (1980) Conjunctival changes associated with inflammatory disease of the bowel. *Transactions of the Ophthalmic Society*, **100**, 96–97.
96. Wright, V. and Watkinson, G. (1965) The arthritis of ulcerative colitis. *British Medical Journal*, **2**, 670.
97. Wright, R., Lumsden, K., Luntz, M.H. *et al.* (1965) Abnormalities of the sacro-iliac joints and uveitis in ulcerative colitis. *Quarterly Journal of Medicine*, **34**, 229.

INFLAMMATORY BOWEL DISEASE IN CHILDHOOD

B.S. Kirschner

Inflammatory bowel disease often becomes evident during childhood and adolescence. Of 844 patients with ulcerative colitis and 489 patients with Crohn's disease diagnosed at the University of Chicago, 40% in each group developed symptoms before 20 years of age and 20% were under 15 years old.[51] The peak ages of onset for both conditions in this retrospective study were 16–20 years. Most children are currently diagnosed between 10 and 18 years of age. Presentation under 10 years has been observed in 12.8% of children with ulcerative colitis and 5.6% with Crohn's disease.[43] Chong *et al.* reported two cases of ulcerative colitis and two cases of Crohn's disease in children less than 3 years of age, out of a total population of 106 children with chronic inflammatory bowel disease.[9] The relative prevalence of these two disorders varies in different countries. At the author's institution, Crohn's disease is now more common than ulcerative colitis and accounts for approximately two-thirds of the children with inflammatory bowel disease. However, 10–15% of paediatric cases are initially categorized as indeterminate colitis.[8] Ulcerative colitis and Crohn's disease have become important causes of chronic gastrointestinal disease in children.

EPIDEMIOLOGY

Epidemiological factors related to the aetiology of inflammatory bowel disease in children were investigated in an international multicentre study which included 499 children with inflammatory bowel disease and 998 age-matched controls.[19] A family history of inflammatory bowel disease occurred significantly more often in patients than in controls. No significant differences were noted between groups with regard to the prevalence of breast feeding, type of formula feeding or formula intolerance, gastroenteritis requiring hospitalization or major stressful life events (parental divorce or death or major financial difficulties).

Barton *et al.* observed that, despite an 18% fall in the population aged less than 16 years, the incidence of Crohn's disease in the paediatric population in Scotland increased threefold between 1968 and 1983.[3] In contrast, the frequency of newly diagnosed cases of chronic ulcerative colitis showed a marginal fall.

CLINICAL FEATURES

The signs and symptoms of childhood inflammatory bowel disease show great individual variation; the subtle features of Crohn's disease may delay the correct diagnosis for many months or years.[7] Ulcerative colitis is usually diagnosed more rapidly because of the history of rectal bleeding. Prominent clinical findings are summarized in *Table 7.25.*

ABDOMINAL PAIN

Abdominal pain is the most common symptom of inflammatory bowel disease in children. In Crohn's disease, pain is often postprandial. The terminal ileum is affected in at least 80% of children with Crohn's disease, either as ileocolitis or isolated small bowel disease.[22] When disease involves the colon, pain characteristically occurs immediately before defaecation. Perianal disease is present in 49% of children and adolescents with Crohn's disease.[40] In most of these patients (70%), the findings consist of skin tags or fissures, but 14% have fistulas and 16% abscesses.

Table 7.25 The presenting signs and symptoms of children with inflammatory bowel disease

	Crohn's disease (%) (n = *52)*	*Ulcerative colitis (%)* (n = *22)*
Abdominal pain	88	95
Altered stool pattern	81	91
Rectal bleeding	54	100
Weight loss	87 (x = 5.7 kg)	68 (x = 4.1 kg)
Fever	44	41
Fall in height percentile	36	14

STOOL PATTERNS

A change in stool pattern is the second most common symptom (*Table 7.25*). Diarrhoea is not observed in 20% of children with Crohn's disease, particularly when disease is limited to the terminal ileum. Rectal bleeding occurred in all patients with ulcerative colitis but in only half of those with Crohn's disease.

SYSTEMIC SIGNS OF INFLAMMATORY BOWEL DISEASE

Recurrent fever (oral temperature more than 38°C) was infrequent in the author's young patients at the time of diagnosis.[32] However, low-grade temperature elevations may go unrecognized.

JOINT INVOLVEMENT

Arthralgias and arthritis are frequently reported,[36,48] Passo *et al.* reporting that joint pain occurred in 40% of 102 children with inflammatory bowel disease, with most having arthralgias.[48] Arthritis occurred in 13 out of 44 (9%) children with ulcerative colitis and 9 out of 58 (10%) with Crohn's disease.[36] Most instances involved a few peripheral joints (especially ankles, knees, elbows and hips) and tended to follow the onset of intestinal symptoms. The episodes were usually short-lived (lasting an average of 30 days in most patients). No child developed chronic persistent arthropathy. In most children the intestinal disease was active concurrently with the joint symptoms. Lindsley and Schaller[36] observed spondylitis in 4% of their patients which did not necessarily occur when the intestinal symptoms were active. This form of arthritis was progressive, resulting in permanent joint damage.

SKIN INVOLVEMENT

Cutaneous and mucocutaneous lesions have been described, including aphthous ulcers of the oral mucous membranes, erythema nodosum and pyoderma gangrenosum. These complications may be more frequent in ulcerative colitis than in Crohn's disease.[2] Resolution usually coincides with satisfactory response of the bowel disease to medical management. Clubbing of the fingers occurs in up to 25% of children with Crohn's disease.[22] The prevalence is greatest (66%) in children with extensive small bowel disease. It may improve or disappear following remission of disease in activity in the intestine.

VASCULAR COMPLICATIONS

Vascular complications, such as arteritis or thromboembolic disease, occur in approximately 3% of children with chronic inflammatory bowel disease.[38] Paediatric patients appear to have a higher frequency of cerebrovascular involvement than deep-vein thrombosis.[38,41] In a recent review of seven reported cases, six of the children had ulcerative colitis.[38] Most of these children recovered, although residual deficits were observed occasionally.

HEPATOBILIARY MANIFESTATIONS

Hepatobiliary disease is seen in 3% of children with inflammatory bowel disease.[37] Of 160 paediatric patients reviewed by Lloyd-Still and Cahan, 5 children (all with ulcerative colitis) had 'clinically significant' liver disease. The types of disorders noted were sclerosing cholangitis (3), chronic active hepatitis (1) and fatty liver (1). Several case reports have documented the presence of hepatobiliary disease (especially sclerosing cholangitis) either before or coincident with the diagnosis of inflammatory bowel disease, which in most instances was ulcerative colitis.[10,12,25,37]

OPTHALMOLOGICAL COMPLICATIONS

Eye findings including conjunctivitis, iritis and episcleritis are uncommon. These are seen in only 4% of patients with ulcerative colitis but in up to 13% in the subgroup of children with Crohn's colitis.[14]

GROWTH FAILURE

Children attempt to decrease gastrointestinal symptoms by diminishing their dietary intake.[1,27–29] Weight loss occurs in 68% of children with ulcerative colitis and the average loss is 9.1 kg. This finding is more frequent in Crohn's disease (87% of patients) and is more marked (12.5 kg).[32]

Growth failure is a serious complication of childhood inflammatory bowel disease. This finding (based on a fall in height percentile for age >1 standard deviation) was observed at the time of diagnosis in 14% of the children with ulcerative colitis and in 36% of those with Crohn's disease. The prevalence varies in reports from different centres, occurring in 2.5–21% of children with ulcerative colitis and 13–58% with Crohn's disease.[28] However, when prepubertal children with Crohn's disease are analysed for growth velocity, impairment in linear growth is observed in 60–88% of these patients.[26,34] The reasons for these discrepancies include differing definitions of growth failure and utilization of past growth records, referral patterns and the inclusion of steroid-treated patients.

GENETIC SHORT STATURE

By definition 3% of the normal population will be at the third height percentile for age. These children have genetic short stature and are not growth impaired. They have normal growth velocity although their height remains at the lower end of normal. Skeletal age is similar to chronological age and there is usually a family history of short stature.

ASSESSMENT OF IMPAIRED GROWTH

The child shows an abnormal growth velocity, defined as a subnormal increase in linear growth. Most normal children and teenagers (prior to sexual maturation) increase their height by at least 4.0 cm/year.[58] If abnormal growth velocity persists for an extended period, a fall in height percentile will follow. Children whose height percentile is normal for age at the time of diagnosis may still have growth impairment if the height percentile has fallen from previous levels. Skeletal age, assessed radiologically, in these children is usually 18–24 months behind the chronological age. There is unequivocal evidence that inflammatory bowel disease itself causes growth impairment prior to starting any corticosteroid therapy.[7,22,26–29,42]

CAUSES OF GROWTH FAILURE

Several explanations for the growth failure have been proposed. These include malabsorption,[4] secondary hypopituitarism with impaired growth hormone secretion,[42] zinc depletion,[55] and increased protein and energy requirements.[35] Studies from several centres have shown important areas of agreement. First, most children with growth failure do not have malabsorption based on measurements of D-xylose absorption, Schilling tests or faecal fat excretion.[27,29,35] Plasma zinc levels are not consistently low in children with growth failure[22,27,29] and appear to reflect serum albumin concentration.[55]

Provocative tests for growth hormone secretion in growth-retarded children, studied prior to receiving corticosteroids, have shown consistently normal or even elevated levels of growth hormone.[20,29,60] However, more sensitive tests of nocturnal growth hormone secretion, using continuous venous sampling during sleep, have shown a normal pulsatile pattern but reduced amplitude in some growth-impaired patients with Crohn's disease.[15] The peripheral effects of growth hormone may be blunted in these children. The author's group has recently shown that somatomedin C (insulin-like growth factor I) levels are lower in growth-impaired children with inflammatory bowel disease than in normally growing patients.[31] Furthermore, levels rise after treatment and precede improved growth velocity.

There is no evidence to suggest that protein or energy requirements are increased above those needed in healthy children. The basal metabolic rate and nitrogen flux, including protein synthesis and catabolism and nitrogen retention, are similar to those of normal control children.[27,46]

Nutritional intervention has resulted in improved growth velocity and allowed some children to reach their pre-illness height percentiles. Early studies utilized 4–6 weeks' total parenteral nutritional support.[35] Similar results have been obtained using oral liquid supplements,[29] continuous nasogastric infusions with elemental formulas,[5,45,47,53] and home parenteral nutritional support.[57] Growth velocity data in two studies, one using parenteral nutrition and the other using oral supplements, were similar.[27,29] Growth velocity increased from 1.8–1.9 cm/year before treatment to 6.2–6.4 cm/year in both centres. Although growth velocity may improve, a return to the pre-illness height percentile may not occur. Three to four years of improved growth velocity may be necessary before the original height percentile is reached.[29] During this interval, disease activity must be controlled, particularly if adequate energy and protein intake are to be achieved by oral means. Recently, two nutritional approaches which use either supplemental nasogastric infusion of formulas on a nightly basis[1] or exclusively elemental diet for one month out of every four[5] have resulted in enhanced growth velocity in comparison with pretreatment periods.

INVESTIGATIONS

Radiological evaluation of patients suspected of having inflammatory bowel disease is considered elsewhere (see page 1141). A discussion of the findings in children with Crohn's disease was reported by MacFarlane *et al.*[39]

Table 7.26 illustrates the frequency of abnormal results in selected blood tests which are useful in

Table 7.26 Abnormal laboratory tests at diagnosis in children with inflammatory bowel disease

	Crohn's disease (%) (n = 52)	*Ulcerative colitis (%) (n = 22)*
ESR > 20 mm/h	90 (x = 40 mm/h)	67 (x = 30 mm/h)
PCV < 33%	38	50
< 36%	64	64
Iron < 50 μg/dl	68	55
Albumin < 3.3 g/dl	46	45
Folate < 3.6 ng/dl	34	44

ESR = erythrocyte sedimentation rate.
PCV = packed cell volume.

following children with inflammatory bowel disease. The erythrocyte sedimentation rate is a more reliable indicator of disease activity in children than in adults, and correlates more closely with symptoms in Crohn's disease than in ulcerative colitis. Additional studies which may be informative include platelet count (thrombocytosis) and the percentage unsegmented polymorphonuclear cells. Measures of intestinal absorptive capacity (D-xylose absorption, Schilling test and quantitative faecal fat) or nutritional status (folate, vitamin B_{12}, vitamin A, vitamin D, zinc) are obtained as indicated. Enteric protein losses are increased in virtually all patients with active disease, and there is evidence that protein losses diminish as inflammation decreases.[57]

Lactose intolerance should be considered in order to exclude the possibility that intestinal symptoms are produced by milk products. Dairy products are important sources of energy, protein and calcium, and may improve nutrient intake. Children with extensive small bowel disease are most likely to have lactose intolerance. In the others, genetic factors are important regardless of whether disease is localized to the small bowel or colon.[30] Patients belonging to population groups with a high prevalence of lactose deficiency should be tested for lactose intolerance.

TREATMENT

MEDICAL

The medical management of children with inflammatory bowel disease is in many ways similar to adults (*Table 7.27*).

Sulphasalazine

This is used as primary therapy and to minimize the corticosteroid dose. Hypersensitivity reactions are not unusual in children, with 15% developing dermatological lesions and 2.5% manifesting signs of haemolytic anaemia.[22] In these situations, metronidazole[61] may be indicated for active Crohn's disease. The risk of complications resulting from long-term continuous metronidazole administration in children is unknown. Some of the newer salicylate derivatives may be useful in ulcerative colitis and Crohn's disease. A recent multicentre double-blind study of olsalazine and sulphasalazine in children with mild ulcerative colitis demonstrated a greater need for prednisone in the olsalazine group.[16] Addi-

Table 7.27 Medical therapy of active ulcerative colitis (UC) and Crohn's disease (CD) in children

Drug	*Dose*	*Indications*
Sulphasalazine	50–75 mg/kg per day	Mild/moderate UC Ileocolonic/colonic CD
Prednisone/methylprednisolone	1.0–2.0 mg/kg per day	Moderate/severe UC or CD
Topical corticosteroid	1–2 times daily	Anal/left colon UC or CD
Topical 4′- or 5′-aminosalicylic acid	bedtime	Rectal/left colon UC or CD
Metronidazole	15–20 mg/kg per day	Perianal CD/sulphasalazine intolerance
Azathioprine	2.0 mg/kg per day	Steroid dependent or
6-Mercaptopurine	1.5 mg/kg per day	unresponsive CD or UC
Cyclosporin A	2 mg/kg i.v. every 12 h 5–8 mg/kg p.o. every 12 h	Severe chronic CD Selected cases/severe UC

tional studies are required to determine the relative effectiveness of these medications.

Corticosteroids

Corticosteroids are the most effective drugs for children with moderately active disease. Once symptoms are controlled with daily administration, the gradual change to an alternate-day regimen has definite advantages. Sadeghi-Nejad and Senior[52] reported that growth in children with ulcerative colitis 'approached normal' using an alternate-day regimen. Others have described similar findings for children with Crohn's disease.[65] The duration of daily administration varies according to the severity of symptoms. The initial dose of prednisone or methylprednisolone is usually 1.0–2.0 mg/k body weight daily for approximately 4–6 weeks and then tapered by 2.5–5.0 mg every 1–2 weeks on the alternate day.[32] Occasionally the daily regimen continues for a longer period. The maintenance dose of prednisone given on the alternate day is usually 20 mg or less.

Azathioprine and 6-mercaptopurine

Azathioprine (or 6-mercaptopurine) has been used in adults with Crohn's disease with varying degrees of success.[49] The author's group has given these drugs in selected children to improve symptoms or to reduce the corticosteroid dose. Verhave *et al.* reported their results with azathioprine in 21 children with either progressive disease while taking corticosteroid medications or steroid toxicity.[62] Partial or complete remission rates were observed in 9 of 12 children (75%) with Crohn's disease and 7 of 9 patients (77%) with chronic ulcerative colitis. The dose administered was 2.0 mg/kg per day for 3–36 months. Side effects included a decrease in leukocyte count in two patients and increased aminotransferase levels in five; however, therapy was continued. The problem of long-term safety remains unanswered in children. Therefore, there is a tendency to restrict its use to children with extensive small bowel disease, particularly if they have had a previous intestinal resection, or to other patients with dependency on or complications of corticosteroids.

Cyclosporin

Cyclosporin is being evaluated as a potential therapeutic modality in children with intractable inflammatory bowel disease, who are unresponsive to other medications. Two reports which used cyclosporin in a total of seven children with severe ulcerative colitis showed divergent results.[24,33] Remission and avoidance of colectomy in two patients were reported in one study,[24] whilst colectomy (either during the hospitalization or subsequently following a relapse) was necessary in four of five patients studied in the second report.[33]

NUTRITIONAL INTERVENTION

Collection of baseline anthropometric measurements

Serial height and weight measurements are plotted on standard growth charts. The parents' heights should also be recorded. If there is any question of growth impairment, a bone age determination should be performed to document the delay in skeleton maturation and to estimate growth potential.

Assessment of nutrient intake and goals

When weight gain is unsatisfactory, energy and protein intake should be evaluated from food diaries. The energy intake should approach that recommended for normal children of similar age and sex.[1,29] This is usually 30–45% above the mean daily energy intake reported for untreated symptomatic children.[27,29,45–47] Some authors recommend energy intakes based upon body weight and suggest 310–335 kJ/kg (75–80 kcal/kg).[35,46,47] Concomitant protein intakes of 1.6–3.0 g/kg daily are associated with improved growth. Initially, liquid formula supplements may provide an additional source of nutrients. In addition to energy and protein intake, other nutrients must be provided if tests indicate specific deficiencies. These include iron, folate, vitamin B_{12}, vitamins A and D, and zinc. Because of the wide range of deficiencies reported in these patients, the author's group advises a multivitamin preparation once daily for all children with Crohn's disease. Folate supplementation is given to patients receiving sulphasalazine.

Monitoring patient response

The response to treatment is determined by clinical signs and symptoms including weight and height gains and selected laboratory tests (see Table 7.26). If clinical improvement does not occur, additional therapeutic manoeuvres may be necessary. A period of bowel rest and parenteral nutritional (TPN) support or prolonged nasogastric infusion of an elemental diet may initiate a remission, particularly in Crohn's disease.[5,27,35,45,47,53,57] The results of total parenteral support in severe ulcerative colitis are usually disappointing.[13] Response may occur within 2 weeks, but is more likely during the first attack (83%) than subsequent severe episodes (31%).[54,63] Unfortunately, it is impossible to predict which children will respond to this form of intervention.[54,63] The availability of home total parenteral nutrition allows children with extensive Crohn's disease the opportunity to resume normal growth and to participate in normal social activities without prolonged hospitalization.[57]

SURGICAL

Ulcerative colitis

Most indications for surgery in children with ulcerative colitis are similar to those for adults: haemorrhage, suspected perforation or abscess, toxic megacolon and medical intractability. The latter may be caused by proximal extension of the disease process, which occurs more frequently in children than in adults.[44] In children, impaired growth which persists despite medical management is another reason for considering surgery. A fall in the surgical rate for children from 49.2% to 26.6% for the decades 1955–1964 and 1965–1974 was observed by Michener *et al.*[43] This was attributed to earlier recognition of the disease and better supportive medical care.

There has been renewed interest in mucosal resection and ileoanal anastomosis in children.[6,18,59] Complications of the ileoanal anastomosis are nocturnal incontinence and inflammation of the pouch in some patients. Even in centres with considerable experience in paediatric inflammatory bowel disease, approximately 10% of children who are thought to have ulcerative colitis at the time of colectomy (based on endoscopic, histological and radiological criteria) are subsequently shown to have Crohn's disease.[6] Despite these reservations, these procedures are a promising alternative to the permanent standard or continent ileostomy.

Crohn's disease

The high risk of recurrence following surgery is higher in children than in adults with Crohn's disease. The indications for surgery in children need careful consideration. The frequency of recurrence depends upon the site of involvement and the length of follow-up after surgery.[11,17,21,56,64] Fonkalsrud *et al.* studied recurrence in 50 children with Crohn's disease, an average of 4–5 years following surgery.[17] Disease recurred in 7 out of 20 children (25%) with ileocaecal disease after resection of the terminal ileum and ascending colon and reanastomosis. The results were worse in children with colorectal diseases, 64% having recurrence after proctocolectomy. Only two patients had primary small bowel (terminal ileal) resections and one of these had a recurrence. These authors reported that the severity and extent of recurrent disease was greater with colorectal disease than with ileocolitis. These observations differ from those reported in adults and may reflect the greater risk for recurrence in younger patients.[11,21,56] High recurrence rates (57%) were also observed in 30 children with Crohn's disease after a follow-up period averaging 6.3 years.[64] Studies in adult patients have suggested a clinical recurrence rate of 94% and a reoperation rate of 89% for the fifteenth year after surgery.[21] For these reasons, medical management, including total parenteral nutritional support, is suggested when absolute indications for surgery (e.g. suspected abscess or bowel obstruction) are not present.

When there is growth impairment that does not respond to medical therapy, surgical intervention must be considered. This is particularly true when there is evidence of localized disease amenable to resection. The effect of surgery upon growth is controversial. This is caused by different definitions of growth and 'catch-up growth' and the substitution of weight gain for linear growth. The degree of skeletal maturation and the period of time available for growth before sexual maturation are of critical importance. If puberty advances rapidly, bone maturation may be accelerated and sufficient time may not be available to permit a return to the pre-illness height percentile. Improved linear growth and growth velocity usually occur but the achievement of pre-illness height percentile is variable. Homer and Grand reported that only 2 of 14 prepubertal children with growth retardation reached their pre-illness height percentile following surgery.[23] Wesson showed that two-thirds of children will manifest improved growth velocity, but height percentiles were not reported.[63] Children who are prepubertal or in early stages of sexual development demonstrate greater linear growth than do adolescents who are in the later stages of sexual maturation.

SUMMARY

Ulcerative colitis and Crohn's disease in children may present with subtle clinical signs and symptoms which may themselves be overshadowed by extra-intestinal complications. Despite the high risk of surgical resection, the long-term prognosis for many paediatric patients with Crohn's disease is good. Puntis *et al.* reviewed the outcome of 67 children followed for an average of 15 years.[50] They showed that 38 patients were asymptomatic with no evidence of recurrent disease, whereas 14 others were well although having radiological evidence of residual disease. The management of inflammatory bowel disease during childhood requires an assessment of the extent and severity of the intestinal disease as well as any extraintestinal manifestations. An integrated, individualized approach which includes medication, nutritional intervention and emotional support for the child and family, is necessary to help paediatric patients respond, as well as possible, to therapy for these disorders.

REFERENCES

1. Aiges, H., Markowitz, J., Rosa, J. and Daum, F. (1989) Home nocturnal supplement nasogastric feedings in growth-retarded adolescents with Crohn's disease. *Gastroenterology*, **97**, 905–910.
2. Ament, M.E. (1975) Inflammatory disease of the colon: Ulcerative colitis and Crohn's disease. *Journal of Pediatrics*, **86**, 322–334.
3. Barton, J.R., Gillion, S. and Ferguson, A. (1989) Incidence of inflammatory bowel disease in Scottish children between 1968 and 1983; marginal fall in ulcerative colitis, three-fold rise in Crohn's disease. *Gut*, **30**, 618–622.
4. Beeken, W. (1973) Absorptive defects in young people with regional enteritis. *Pediatrics*, **52**, 69–74.
5. Belli, D.C., Seidman, E., Bouthillier, L., Weber, A.M., Roy, C.C., Pletincx, M., Beaulieu, M. and Morin, C.L. (1988) Chronic intermittent elemental diet improves growth failure in children with Crohn's disease. *Gastroenterology*, **94**, 603–610.
6. Berry, R., Perrault, J. and Telander, R.L. (1987) Postoperative development of Crohn's disease (CD) in young patients undergoing endorectal pull-through procedure for ulcerative colitis (CUC) (Abstract). *Gastroenterology*, **92**, 1315.
7. Burbige, E.J., Huang Shi-Shung and Bayless, T.M. (1975) Clinical manifestations of Crohn's disease in children and adolescents. *Pediatrics*, **55**, 866–871.
8. Chong, S.K.F., Blackshaw, A.J., Boyle, S., Williams, C.B. and Walker-Smith, J. (1985) Histological diagnosis of chronic inflammatory bowel disease in childhood. *Gut*, **26**, 55–59.
9. Chong, S.K.F., Blackshaw, A.J., Boyle, S., Williams, C.B. and Walker-Smith, J. (1986) Prospective study of colitis in infancy and early childhood. *Journal of Pediatric Gastroenterology and Nutrition*, **5**, 352–358.
10. Classen, M., Gotze, H., Richter, H.-J. and Bender, S. (1987) Primary sclerosing cholangitis in children. *Journal of Pediatric Gastroenterology and Nutrition*, **6**, 197–202.
11. de Dombal, F.T., Burton, I. and Goligher, J.C. (1971) The early and late results of surgical treatment for Crohn's disease. *British Journal of Surgery*, **58**, 805–816.
12. El-Shabrawi, M., Wilkinson, M.L., Portmann, B. *et al.* (1987) Primary sclerosing sholangitis in childhood. *Gastroenterology*, **92**, 1226–1235.
13. Elson, C.O., Layden, T.J., Nemchausky, B.A. *et al.* (1980) An evaluation of total parenteral nutrition in the management of inflammatory bowel disease. *Digestive Diseases and Sciences*, **25**, 42–48.
14. Farmer, R.G. and Michener, W.M. (1979) Prognosis of Crohn's disease with onset in childhood or adolescence. *Digestive Diseases and Sciences*, **24**, 752–759.
15. Farthing, M.J.G., Campbell, C.A., Walker-Smith, J., Edwards, C.R.W., Rees, L.H. and Dawson, A.M. (1981) Nocturnal growth hormone and gonadotrophin secretion in growth-retarded children with Crohn's disease. *Gut*, **22**, 933–938.
16. Ferry, G., Grand, R., Kirschner, B.S. *et al.* (1990) Results of the Pediatric Gastroenterology Collaborative Research Group (CPGGRG) – clinical trial comparing olsalazine (Dipentum®, Pharmarcia, Inc.) with sulfasalazine in mild to moderate childhood ulcerative colitis (Abstract). *Gastroenterology*, **98**, A169.
17. Fonkalsrud, E.W., Ament, M.E., Fleisher, D. and Bryne, W. (1979) Surgical management of Crohn's disease in children. *American Journal of Surgery*, **138**, 15–20.
18. Fonkalsrud, E.W., Ament, M.E. and Byrne, W.J. (1979) Clinical experience with total colectomy and endorectal mucosal resection for inflammatory bowel disease. *Gastroenterology*, **77**, 156–160.
19. Gilat, T., Hacohen, D., Lilos, P. and Langman, M.J.S. for the International IBD Study Group (1987) Childhood factors in ulcerative colitis and Crohn's disease: an international cooperative study. *Scandinavian Journal of Gastroenterology*, **22**, 1009–1024.
20. Gotlin, R.W. and Dubois, R.S. (1973) Nyctohemeral growth hormone levels in children with growth retardation and inflammatory bowel disease. *Gut*, **14**, 191–195.
21. Greenstein, A.J., Sachar, D.B., Paternack, B.S. and Janowitz, H.D. (1975) Reoperation and recurrence in Crohn's colitis and ileocolitis. *New England Journal of Medicine*, **293**, 685–690.
22. Gryboski, J.D. and Spiro, H.M. (1978) Prognosis in children with Crohn's disease. *Gastroenterology*, **74**, 807–817.
23. Homer, D.R., Grand, R.J. and Colodny, A.H. (1977) Growth course and prognosis after surgery after Crohn's disease. *Pediatrics*, **59**, 717–725.
24. Hyams, J.S. and Treem, W.R. (1989) Cyclosporin treatment of fulminant colitis. *Journal of Pediatric Gastroenterology and Nutrition*, **9**, 383–387.
25. Kane, W., Miller, K. and Sharp, H.L. (1980) Inflammatory bowel disease presenting as liver disease during childhood. *Journal of Pediatrics*, **97**, 775–778.

26. Kanof, M.E., Lake, A.M. and Bayless, T.M. (1988) Decreased height velocity in children and adolescents before the diagnosis of Crohn's disease. *Gastroenterology*, **95**, 1523–1527.
27. Kelts, D.G., Grand, R.J., Shen, G. *et al.* (1979) Nutritional basis of growth failure in children and adolescents with Crohn's disease. *Gastroenterology*, **76**, 720–727.
28. Kirschner, B.S., Voinchet, O. and Rosenberg, I.H. (1978) Growth retardation in children with inflammatory bowel disease. *Gastroenterology*, **75**, 504–511.
29. Kirschner, B.S., Klich, J.R., Kalman, S.S. *et al.* (1981) Reversal of growth retardation in Crohn's disease with therapy, emphasizing oral nutritional restitution. *Gastroenterology*, **80**, 10–15.
30. Kirschner, B.S., deFavaro, M.V. and Jensen, W. (1981) Lactose malabsorption in children and adolescents with inflammatory bowel disease. *Gastroenterology*, **81**, 829–832.
31. Kirschner, B.S. and Sutton, M.M. (1986) Somatomedin-C levels in growth-impaired children and adolescents with chronic inflammatory bowel disease. *Gastroenterology*, **91**, 830–836.
32. Kirschner, B.S. (1988) Inflammatory bowel disease in children. *Pediatric Clinics of North America*, **35** 189–208.
33. Kirschner, B.S., Whitington, P.F. and Malfeo-Klein, R. (1989) Experience with cyclosporin A (CyA) in severe non-specific ulcerative colitis (UC) (Abstract). *Pediatric Research*, **25**, 117A.
34. Kirschner, B.S. (1990) Special aspects of inflammatory bowel disease in children. In *Inflammatory Bowel Disease and Coeliac Disease in Children* (Ed.) Hadziselimovic, F., Herzog, B. and Burgin-Wolff, A. Lancaster: Kluwer.
35. Layden, T., Rosenberg, T., Nemchawsky, B., Elson, C. and Rosenberg, I.H. (1976) Reversal of growth arrest in adolescents with Crohn's disease after parenteral alimentation. *Gastroenterology*, **70**, 1017–1026.
36. Lindsley, C.B. and Schaller, J.G. (1974) Arthritis associated with inflammatory bowel disease in children. *Journal of Pediatrics*, **84**, 16–20.
37. Lloyd-Still, J.D. and Cahan, J. (1987) Liver disease associated with childhood inflammatory bowel disease (IBD) (Abstract). *Hepatology*, **7**, 1088.
38. Lloyd-Still, J.D. and Tomasi, L. (1989) Neurovascular and thromboembolic complications of inflammatory bowel disease in childhood. *Journal of Pediatric Gastroenterology and Nutrition*, **9**, 461–466.
39. MacFarlane, R.I., Miller, V. and Ratcliffe, J.F. (1986) Clinical and radiological diagnosis of Crohn's disease in children. *Journal of Pediatric Gastroenterology and Nutrition*, **5**, 87–92.
40. Markowitz, J., Daum, F., Aiges, H., Kahn, E., Silverberg, M. and Fisher, S.E. (1984) Perianal disease in children and adolescents with Crohn's disease. *Gastroenterology*, **86**, 829–833.
41. Markowitz, R.L., Ment, L.R. and Gryboski, J.D. (1989) Cerebral thromboembolic disease in pediatric and adult inflammatory bowel disease: case report and review of the literature. *Journal of Pediatric Gastroenterology and Nutrition*, **8**, 413–420.
42. McCaffery, T.D., Nasr, K., Lawrence, A.M. and Kirsner, J.B. (1970) Severe growth retardation in children with inflammatory bowel disease. *Journal of Pediatrics*, **45**, 386–393.
43. Michener, W.H., Whelan, G., Greenstreet, R.L. and Farmer, R.G. (1982) Comparison of the clinical features of Crohn's disease and ulcerative colitis with onset in childhood or adolescence. *Cleveland Clinic Quarterly*, **49**, 13–16.
44. Mir-Madjlessi, S.H., Michener, W.H. and Farmer, R.G. (1986) Course and prognosis of idiopathic ulcerative proctosigmoiditis in young patients. *Journal of Pediatric Gastroenterology and Nutrition*, **5**, 570–575.
45. Morin, C.L., Roulet, M., Roy, C.C. and Weber, A. (1980) Continuous elemental enteral alimentation in children with Crohn's disease and growth failure. *Gastroenterology*, **79**, 1205–1210.
46. Motil, K.J., Grand, R.J., Maletskos, C.J. and Young, V.R. (1982) The effect of disease, drug and diet on whole body protein metabolism in adolescents with Crohn's disease and growth failure. *Journal of Pediatrics*, **101**, 343–351.
47. Navarro, J., Vargas, J., Cezard, J.P. *et al.* (1982) Prolonged constant rate elemental enteral nutrition in Crohn's disease. *Journal of Pediatric Gastroenterology and Nutrition*, **1**, 541–546.
48. Passo, M.H., Fitzgerald, J.F. and Brandt, K.D. (1986) Arthritis associated with inflammatory bowel disease in children. *Disease Sciences*, **31**, 491–497.
49. Present, D.H., Korelitz, B.I., Wisch, N. *et al.* (1980) Treatment of Crohn's disease with 6-mercaptopurine. *New England Journal of Medicine*, **302**, 981–987.
50. Puntis, J., McNeish, A.S. and Allan, R.N. (1984) The long term prognosis of Crohn's disease with onset in childhood and adolescence. *Gut*, **25**, 329–336.
51. Rogers, B.H.G., Clark, L.M. and Kirsner, J.B. (1971) The epidemiologic and demographic characteristics of inflammatory bowel disease: an analysis of a computerized file of 1400 patients. *Journal of Chronic Diseases*, **24**, 743–773.
52. Sadeghi-Nejad, A. and Senior, B. (1968) The treatment of ulcerative colitis in children with alternate-day corticosteroids. *Pediatrics*, **43**, 840–845.
53. Sanderson, I.R., Udeen, S., Davies, P.S.W., Savage, M.O. and Walkersmith, J.A. (1987) Remission induced by elemental diet in small bowel Crohn's disease. *Archives of Diseases in Childhood*, **61**, 123–127.
54. Seashore, J.H., Hillemeier, A.C. and Gryboski, J.D. (1982) Total parenteral nutrition in the management of inflammatory bowel disease in children: a limited role. *American Journal of Surgery*, **143** 504–507.
55. Solomons, N.W. Rosenberg, I.H., Sandstead, H.H.

and Vo-Khactu, K.P. (1977) Zinc deficiency in Crohn's disease. *Digestion*, **16**, 87–95.
56. Steinberg, D.M., Allan, R.N., Thompson, H. *et al.* (1974) Exicisional surgery with ileostomy for Crohn's colitis with particular reference to factors affecting recurrence. *Gut*, **15**, 845–851.
57. Strobel, C.T., Byrne, W.J. and Ament, M.E. (1979) Home parenternal nutrition in children with Crohn's disease: an effective management alternative. *Gastroenterology*, **77**, 272–279.
58. Tanner, J.M., Whitehouse, R.H. and Takaishi, M. (1966) Standards from birth to maturity for height, weight, height velocity, and weight velocity. British children, 1965, Part II. *Archives of Diseases of Childhood*, **41**, 613–635.
59. Telander, R.L. and Perrault, J. (1980) Total colectomy with rectal mucosectomy and ileoanal anastomosis for chronic ulcerative colitis in children and young adults. *Mayo Clinic Proceedings*, **55**, 420–424.
60. Tenore, A., Berman, W.F., Parks, J.S. and Bongiovannie, A.M. (1977) Basal and stimulated serum growth hormone concentrations in inflammatory bowel disease. *Journal of Clinical Endocrinology and Metabolism*, **44**, 622–628.
61. Ursing, B., Alm, T., Barany, F. *et al.* (1982) A comparative study of metronidazole and sulfasalazine for active Crohn's disease: the cooperative Crohn's disease study in Sweden. *Gastroenterology*, **83**, 550–562.
62. Verhave, M., Winter, H.S. and Grand R.J. (1990) Azathioprine in the treatment of children with inflammatory bowel disease. *Journal of Pediatrics*, **117**, 809–814.
63. Werlin, S.L. and Grand, R.J. (1977) Severe colitis in children and adolescents: diagnosis course and treatment. *Gastroenterology*, **73**, 828–832.
64. Wesson, D.E. and Shandling, B. (1981) Results of bowel resection for Crohn's disease in the young. *Journal of Pediatric Surgery*, **16**, 449–452.
65. Whitington, P.F., Barns, H.V. and Bayless, T.M. (1977) Medical management of Crohn's disease in adolescence. *Gastroenterology*, **72**, 1338–1344.

INFLAMMATORY BOWEL DISEASE AND PREGNANCY

C.P. Willoughby

In the past patients with inflammatory bowel disease were often advised to avoid pregnancy if at all possible, because conception was likely to result in a marked deterioration in the mother's health, with potential risks for both her life and that of the fetus.[1] Fortunately, more recent experience suggests that childbearing in both ulcerative colitis and Crohn's disease is not particularly hazardous and a favourable outcome to pregnancy is highly probable. This section will summarize current knowledge of the effects of inflammatory bowel disease on pregnancy, and vice versa, and suggest guidelines on management.

FERTILITY AND INFLAMMATORY BOWEL DISEASE

FERTILITY IN WOMEN

Ulcerative colitis

Nearly all studies in women patients with ulcerative colitis show that fertility is normal. For example, a survey from Oxford showed that the involuntary infertility rate among 147 married women with the disease was only 6.8%, which is no higher than the infertility rate in the general population.[20] Reduced fertility may be more common in patients with chronic continuous colitis, but the routine use of medical maintenance therapy or early recourse to surgery if drugs prove ineffective makes this an uncommon situation nowadays.

Crohn's disease

Most reports imply that fertility is impaired to some extent in women with Crohn's disease.[10] Subfertility may be particularly common in patients with colonic involvement, but not all authors agree on this point.[13] Several factors may contribute to reduced fertility, including tubal involvement by the inflammatory reaction, dyspareunia, general ill-health interfering with the normal ovulatory cycle, and possibly vitamin B_{12} deficiency.

If a remission of the Crohn's disease can be induced by medical treatment fertility may improve, but sometimes resection of diseased bowel seems to give a better chance of subsequent conception.

FERTILITY IN MEN

There is no evidence that ulcerative colitis in itself affects male fertility. However, in men with Crohn's

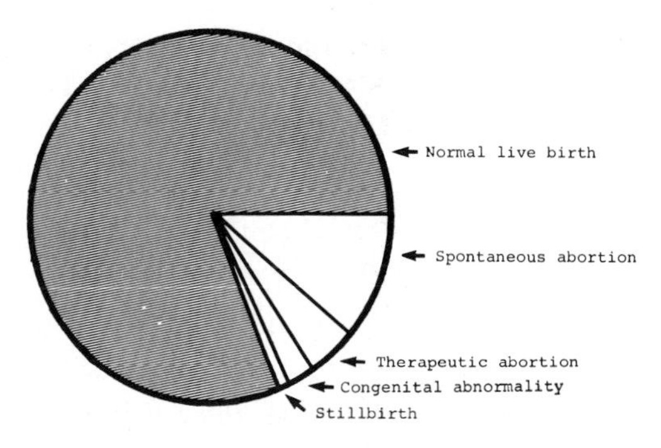

Figure 7.57 Outcome of 456 pregnancies in women with Crohn's disease.

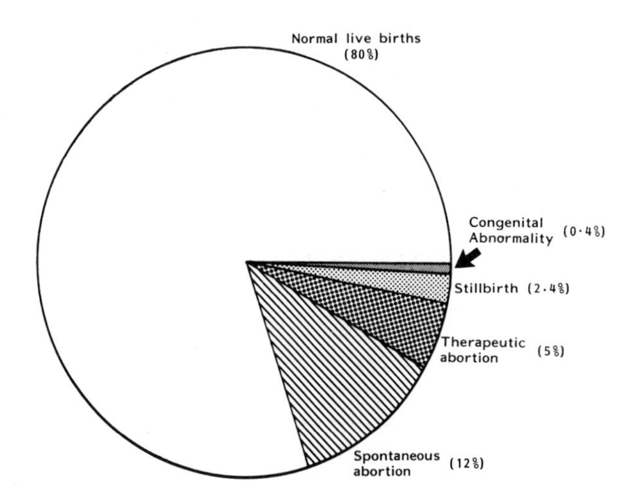

Figure 7.58 Outcome of 209 completed pregnancies in women with ulcerative colitis.

disease, general ill-health and poor nutrition can lead to oligospermia.[7] Two particular circumstances may reduce fertility in men with inflammatory bowel disease.

First, it is now well recognised that maintenance treatment with sulphasalazine interferes with spermatogenesis in a significant proportion of men. Sperm counts and motility are reduced, and there is an increased frequency of abnormal spermatozoal forms.[18] This subfertility is reversible; if sulphasalazine can be withdrawn, all semen qualities are usually restored after about 8 weeks and normal pregnancies have then commonly followed. The toxic element in the drug is probably its sulphapyridine moiety, as the substitution of 5-aminosalicylic acid preparations by mouth or as enemas for sulphasalazine treatment can also reverse the seminal abnormalities.[2,3]

Secondly, impaired fertility may occur in men with inflammatory bowel disease treated by proctocolectomy. Wide operative excisions of the rectum may damage the nerves controlling erection and ejaculation, and lead to permanent impotence. However, this problem can almost invariably be avoided if modern surgical techniques involving close dissection of the rectum are used (*Figure 7.57*).

THE IMPACT OF INFLAMMATORY BOWEL DISEASE ON PREGNANCY

ULCERATIVE COLITIS

Most published studies agree that ulcerative colitis does not reduce the chance of a women producing a normal health baby. The data from the Oxford survey[20] are summarized in *Figure 7.58*. The outcome of the 209 completed pregnancies was almost identical to that expected for the general population of the UK. Other studies in North America, Germany and Scandinavia, as well as in the UK, have given very similar results.[19] Vaginal delivery is the general rule in pregnancies which proceed to term, and the incidence of instrumental or operative deliveries is not increased.

The prognosis for a normal live birth is particularly favourable if the mother's colitis is in established remission when conception occurs. Active disease at the start of pregnancy has, in some studies, been associated with a marginally higher chance of abortion, prematurity or stillbirth. Even if a first attack of ulcerative colitis develops during pregnancy, control of symptoms can almost invariably be achieved with current medical treatment and a normal infant is the usual outcome.

CROHN'S DISEASE

Figure 7.58 summarises the results of six studies into the outcome of pregnancy in women with Crohn's disease.[19] The chance of a normal live birth seems good, and in most series has been 75–85%.[9,10] A survey on pregnancies in married women with Crohn's disease attending the Oxford inflammatory bowel disease clinic showed a rather lower success rate (70%), but the results were biased by one patient prone to recurrent spontaneous abortions.[12] The incidence of congenital abnormality and stillbirth was not increased.

The state of the Crohn's disease seems to influence the pregnancy outcome, in that active disease at conception may raise the risk of spontaneous abortion[12] whilst first attacks of Crohn's disease during pregnancy have often been accompanied by a poor prognosis for a normal live birth.[10]

THE EFFECT OF PREGNANCY ON INFLAMMATORY BOWEL DISEASE

ULCERATIVE COLITIS

Women who conceive when their ulcerative colitis is in stable remission have no excess risk of a flare-up of their disease during pregnancy or the puerperium. Approximately one-third of the patients will develop an exacerbation of their colitis during this period, but this is no higher than the expected recurrence rate for a comparable group of non-pregnant women. Any relapses of ulcerative colitis which do occur are particularly likely during the first trimester of pregnancy, but can easily be controlled by conventional medical treatment in most instances, and nowadays there should be no risk to the mother's life. Exacerbations of colitis were considered likely in the puerperium, but recent studies suggest that this is no longer the case.

The outlook is rather less favourable when the disease is active at the time of conception. Over two-thirds of the patients remain symptomatic or become worse during pregnancy and the puerperium, whilst the remainder may improve or go into remission. Worsening symptoms are most common early in pregnancy, but severe attacks can usually be prevented by standard medical therapy. At one time, therapeutic abortion was held to be a reliable method of halting relapses of colitis,[1,4] but there is little clear evidence to support this view and termination of pregnancy cannot be justified purely for this reason.

Sometimes ulcerative colitis starts during pregnancy, and this is especially common during the first trimester. Early studies suggested that this was a grave situation, with a high probability of severe disease and a substantial maternal mortality. More recent studies provide a more optimistic view, in that the colitis usually responds to energetic medical treatment, and maternal deaths have not been observed.

A similar improvement in outlook applies to first attacks of ulcerative colitis in the puerperium. Although these also used to carry a poor prognosis and an appreciable material risk, nowadays the attacks tend to be mild and readily controlled.

CROHN'S DISEASE

Pregnancy seems to have little effect on the course of Crohn's disease.[16] In general the patients do well, particularly if the disease is quiescent at conception. Such women have a 60–70% chance overall of remaining symptom-free, and the proportion is probably even higher if the Crohn's disease has been treated surgically before pregnancy.[5,6] If relapse does occur, the most common time for recurrence of symptoms seems to be after delivery.

Active disease at conception behaves in a very similar way to active ulcerative colitis in pregnancy, with the majority of patients continuing to have symptoms but a small proportion showing improvement, particularly as the pregnancy progresses.[8]

First attacks of Crohn's disease may coincide with pregnancy, but very few such cases have been reported; the available data imply that the condition often follows a severe course under such circumstances. The same may be true for the onset of Crohn's disease in the puerperium, but again the available information is very limited.

DRUG TREATMENT DURING PREGNANCY

Corticosteroids and sulphasalazine are the most important agents for the treatment of inflammatory bowel disease. Both drugs carry a theoretical risk of teratogenicity (on the basis of animal experiments), but no evidence at all has emerged of any increased incidence of congenital abnormality in the babies of mothers treated for inflammatory bowel disease with conventional dosages.[12,15,20]

It has been suggested that corticosteroid treatment might lead to impaired placental function and an increased chance of stillbirth or delivery preterm, but again no evidence to support this view has been provided by clinical surveys.

Sulphasalazine and sulphapyridine cross the placenta and could possibly increase the risk of bilirubin displacement from albumin in the neonate, with consequent kernicterus. Neonatal jaundice is not more common in babies of mothers treated with sulphasalazine, and no cases of kernicterus have been reported. Sulphasalazine and its metabolites are secreted into breast milk, and a similar argument might suggest a theoretical risk of kernicterus in breast-fed babies whose mothers took the drug. However, the binding sites for sulphasalazine, sulphapyridine and bilirubin on albumin are different, and the bilirubin-displacing effects of the parent drug and its derivatives are insignificant.[11] There seems no reason, therefore, to advise women who take sulphasalazine to discontinue the drug near to parturition or while they are breastfeeding.

Other drugs such as azathioprine and metronidazole are occasionally used in the treatment of inflammatory bowel disease. Pregnancy is inadvisable in women taking azathioprine because of its potential teratogenic effects. No adverse effects of metronidazole on the fetus have been reported, but as usual it seems sensible to avoid the use of any drug in pregnancy unless there are strong positive reasons for its employment.

A few uneventful pregnancies have been reported in women taking the new 5-aminosalicylic acid preparations such as mesalazine and olsalazine, but no formal studies into the safety of these compounds in pregnancy have yet been undertaken.

SURGICAL TREATMENT DURING PREGNANCY

Surgical intervention during pregnancy is rarely necessary, as even severe attacks can now usually be controlled by medical treatment. Emergency colectomy in cases of severe ulcerative colitis carries a substantial risk to mother and child, but sometimes has to be undertaken because of life-threatening disease. Case reports in recent years imply a more favourable prognosis than was once the case.

PREGNANCY AFTER SURGICAL TREATMENT FOR INFLAMMATORY BOWEL DISEASE

The outlook for a normal pregnancy is very good for women who have a permanent ileostomy. Vaginal delivery is usually possible, although perineal scarring may increase the chance of caesarean section, particularly in women with Crohn's disease. Minor degrees of ileostomy prolapse are not uncommon as the abdomen enlarges late in pregnancy, but the only other problem which has been reported with any frequency is acute or subacute intestinal obstruction.

Uneventful pregnancies have also been reported in women previously treated by colectomy and ileoanal pouch anastomosis.[14,17]

CONCLUSIONS

Fertility is normal in women with ulcerative colitis, but may be impaired in some women with Crohn's disease. The most common cause of subfertility in men with inflammatory bowel disease is probably sulphasalazine treatment.

In general, a normal outcome to pregnancy can be expected in women with ulcerative colitis or Crohn's disease. Neither disorder should prevent a woman from embarking on a pregnancy if she so wishes, but ideally she should be symptom-free at the time of conception. If the inflammatory bowel disease is quiescent at the start of pregnancy, there is little or no excess chance of relapse. Any exacerbations which do occur can usually be controlled by medical means, and the commonly used drugs seem to be quite safe. Therapeutic abortion does not help in inducing remission of active disease during pregnancy. Surgical intervention during pregnancy may be hazardous but necessary. Pregnancy in women after surgical treatment usually presents no major problems.

REFERENCES

1. Abramson, D., Jankelson, I.R. and Milner, L.R. (1951) Pregnancy in idiopathic ulcerative colitis. *Americal Journal of Obstetrics and Gynecology*, **61**, 121–129.
2. Cann, P.A. and Holdsworth, C.D. (1984) Reversal of male infertility on changing treatment from sulphasalazine to 5-aminosalicylic acid. *The Lancet*, **1**, 1119.
3. Chatzinoff, M., Guarino, J.M., Corson, S.L., Batzer, F.R. and Friedman, L.S. (1988) Sulphasalazine-induced abnormal sperm penetration assay reversed on changing to 5-aminosalicylic acid enemas. *Digestive Diseases and Sciences*, **33**, 108–110.
4. Crohn, B.B., Yarnis, H., Crohn, E.B., Walter, R.I. and Gabrilove, L.J. (1956) Ulcerative colitis and pregnancy. *Gastroenterology*, **30**, 391–403.
5. Crohn, B.B., Yarnis, H. and Korelitz, B.I. (1956) Regional enteritis complicating pregnancy. *Gastroenterology*, **31**, 615–628.
6. de Dombal, F.T., Watts, J.M., Watkinson, G. and Goligher, J.C. (1965) Ulcerative colitis and pregnancy. *The Lancet*, **2**, 599–602.
7. Farthing, M.J.G. and Dawson, A.M. (1983) Impaired semen quality in Crohn's disease – drugs, ill health or undernutrition? *Scandinavian Journal of Gastroenterology*, **18**, 57–60.
8. Fielding, J.F. and Cooke, W.T. (1970) Pregnancy and Crohn's disease. *British Medical Journal*, **2**, 76–77.
9. Ganchrow, M.I. and Benjamin, H. (1975) Inflammatory colorectal disease and pregnancy. *Diseases of Colon and Rectum*, **18**, 706–709.
10. Jarnerot, G. (1982) Fertility, sterility and pregnancy in chronic inflammatory bowel disease. *Scandinavian Journal of Gastroenterology*, **17**, 1–4.
11. Jarnerot, G., Anderson, S., Esbjorner, E., Sandstrom, B. and Brodersen, R. (1981) Albumin

reserve for binding of bilirubin in maternal and cord serum under treatment with sulphasalazine. *Scandinavian Journal of Gastroenterology*, **16**, 1049–1055.
12. Khosla, R., Willoughby, C.P. and Jewell, D.P. (1984) Crohn's disease and pregnancy. *Gut*, **25**, 52–56.
13. Mayberry, J.F. and Weterman, I.T. (1986) European survey of fertility and pregnancy in women with Crohn's disease: a case-control study by European collaborative group. *Gut*, **27**, 821–825.
14. Metcalf, A., Dozois, R.R., Beart, R.W. and Wolff, B.G. (1985) Pregnancy following ileal pouch–anal anastomosis. *Diseases of Colon and Rectum*, **28**, 859–861.
15. Mogadam, M., Dobbins, W.O., Korelitz, B.I. and Ahmed, S.W. (1981) Pregnancy in inflammatory bowel disease: effect of sulphasalazine and corticosteroids on fetal outcome. *Gastroenterology*, **80**, 72–76.
16. Nielsen, O.H., Andreasson, B., Bondesen, S., Jacobsen, O. and Jarnum, S. (1984) Pregnancy in Crohn's disease. *Scandinavian Journal of Gastroenterology*, **19**, 724–732.
17. Pezim, M.E. (1984) Successful childbirth after restorative proctocolectomy with pelvic ileal reservoir. *British Journal of Surgery*, **71**, 292.
18. Toovey, S., Hudson, E., Hendry, W.F. and Levi, A.J. (1981) Sulphasalazine and male infertility: reversibility and possible mechanism. *Gut*, **22**, 445–451.
19. Willoughby, C.P. (1990) Fertility, pregnancy and inflammatory bowel disease. In *Inflammatory Bowel Diseases*, 2nd Ed. (Ed.) Allan, R.N., Keighley, M.R.B., Hawkins, C.F. and Alexander-Williams, J., pp. 547–558. Edinburgh: Churchill Livingstone.
20. Willoughby, C.P. and Truelove, S.C. (1980) Ulcerative colitis and pregnancy. *Gut*, **21**, 469–474.

COLLAGENOUS COLITIS

I. Hamilton

Collagenous colitis, once considered rare, is now increasingly being recognized with the growing use of colonoscopy and mucosal biopsy in the investigation of patients with diarrhoea. The relationship of collagenous colitis to other forms of inflammatory bowel disease, particularly to the clinically indistinguishable entity of microscopic colitis, is now being clarified.[13,20,23]

The characteristic feature of collagenous colitis is the deposition of a collagenous band beneath the subepithelial basement membrane of the colon. Collagen deposition at this site, however, is not specific for collagenous colitis because it occurs in association with other colonic lesions, such as adenoma, colonic carcinoma and Crohn's disease or ulcerative colitis.[9,25] The diagnosis of collagenous colitis is, therefore, a clinicopathological one, demanding the coexistence of appropriate clinical features as well as the morphological lesion.

CLINICAL FEATURES

Lindstrom in 1976 described a case of watery diarrhoea in which colonic biopsy revealed the presence of linear eosinophilic thickening of the subepithelial basement membrane – he termed this 'collagenous colitis', analogous to collagenous sprue.[16] Subsequently, numerous case reports, and a small number of larger series, have defined the clinical features of collagenous colitis. It is a chronic, relapsing condition, usually in middle-aged women. About 20% of cases occur in men. Childhood cases and familial clustering have been described.[4,24] The principal symptom is diarrhoea, typically watery and intermittent, recurring over several years before the diagnosis is established. Diarrhoea may be of large volume with up to 20 stools daily with a stool volume of 2–4 l/24 h. Isolated cases presenting with bloody diarrhoea also have other pathology, e.g. colonic adenoma, where there is secondary collagen deposition. Abdominal pain, distension, anorexia, flatulence, weight loss, nausea and, occasionally, vomiting may also be present. General health is usually unaffected and physical examination is normal.

Stool microscopy and culture are normal. Measurement of osmolality suggests a secretory diarrhoea. Faecal fat excretion, D-xylose absorption, the Schilling test and the [^{14}C]glycocholate breath test are usually normal, and pancreatic function is also normal.[20] Radiology of both the large and the small bowel are normal, as are sigmoidoscopy and colonoscopy. Indeed the diagnosis cannot be entertained in the presence of macroscopic evidence of abnormal colonic epithelium.

Rarely collagenous colitis coexists with small intestinal villous atrophy, which usually, but not invariably, responds to a gluten-free diet.[23]

Collagenous colitis has been reported in patients maintained on a gluten-free diet without recurrence of small intestinal disease,[10] suggesting an association between collagenous colitis and coeliac disease. Collagenous colitis is also associated with thyroid disease[20] and polyarthritis, particularly rheumatoid arthritis.[19] It may coexist with diabetes mellitus, pernicious anaemia or with positive antinuclear antibodies, suggesting an autoimmune pathogenesis.[20] Occasional cases have been associated with hypertension or pulmonary fibrosis.[23] There is no consistent relationship with HLA phenotype.[23]

Microscopic colitis is a clinically similar entity, in which middle-aged or elderly women present with long-standing watery diarrhoea. An association with coeliac disease has also been described. Whilst anaemia, hypoalbuminaemia and iron deficiency have characterized some series,[14] laboratory investigations are usually normal.[3] Because the colonic mucosa may appear macroscopically normal in other forms of idiopathic inflammatory bowel disease (e.g. Crohn's disease) and yet have clear histological evidence of inflammation, the term 'lymphocytic colitis' is to be preferred to 'microscopic colitis',[15] but has not yet gained wide acceptance.

In view of the close similarity between the histological features of collagenous colitis and microscopic colitis, with chronic inflammation as the unifying feature, and the demonstration of high faecal levels of an inflammatory mediator in a patient with collagenous colitis, it seems probably that both are chronic idiopathic inflammatory diseases of the colon in which diarrhoea follows ionic secretion by the colonic mucosa secondary to inflammation. Furthermore, the observed differences between the two conditions may represent differences in interpretation rather than in pathology, and they may represent different stages in the evolution of a single disease process.[12] The subsequent development of collagen deposition in patients initially diagnosed as having microscopic colitis, the spontaneous regression of subepithelial collagen and the patchy distribution of collagen within the colon all support this concept. Observed differences in the pattern of ion transport by the colonic mucosa, however, are difficult to reconcile with this view.

PATHOLOGY AND PATHOPHYSIOLOGY

Although the colonic mucosa appears macroscopically normal in collagenous colitis, light and electron microscopic examinations reveal the pathognomonic abnormality of collagen deposition beneath the subepithelial basement membrane. The collagen band is confined to the intercryptal area and is patchily distributed throughout the bowel, but particularly in the proximal colon.[13] The thickness of the collagen band should exceed 10 μm, to establish the diagnosis because there is considerable variation in the structure of the normal subepithelial collagen.[9]

Ultrastructurally, there is mature collagen with irregularly arranged fibrils of diameter 30–34 nm and a periodicity of 64 nm, intimately fused to the basement membrane.[1,26] Occasional spindle-shaped cells within the collagen band have been identified immunohistochemically as myoid cells,[26] as have the pericryptal cells from which the collagen band seems to originate and which is abnormally separated from the epithelium. The cause of this separation of the epithelial-mesenchymal junction has not been elucidated, but, in contrast to mere thickening of the subepithelial collagen plate, it is unique to collagenous colitis.[11]

The nature of the collagen laid down beneath the basement membrane is unclear. It has been classified by ultrastructural studies as type III collagen consistent with an origin from the pericryptal cells,[2,7] but organ culture of affected colonic biopsies has synthesized predominantly type VI collagen, a relatively low-molecular-weight form not normally found in the colon.[17]

Histological evidence of epithelial cell damage and a chronic inflammatory cell infiltrate in the lamina propria are invariable features of collagenous colitis and not seen when collagen deposition is secondary to other pathology.[25] The epithelial cell injury is characterized by focal degeneration and detachment of cells, and a patchy infiltrate consisting principally of lymphocytic and plasma cells with occasional eosinophils.[20,25] Occasional cases are reported as demonstrating large numbers of mucosal mast cells,[18] but there is no consistent increase in the mast cell population.[26] Normal crypt architecture is preserved but there is chronic inflammatory infiltration of the crypts also, although without crypt abscess formation. These changes are typical of microscopic colitis.[15] In some cases, histological abnormality in the rectum may be confined to chronic inflammation with typical collagen deposition prominent in the more proximal colon, and patients with microscopic colitis may subsequently develop collagenous colitis in the same part of the bowel.[22]

The pathogenesis of the diarrhoea in collagenous colitis has been established in vivo by colonic perfusion studies which have found active secretion of chloride ion into the colonic lumen with subsequent sodium secretion down an electrochemical gradient, and an increased lumen-negative transmucosal potential difference. Net lumen-to-plasma sodium flux was reduced, with an increased plasma-to-lumen sodium flux. Levels of prostaglandin E_2 in faecal dialysate were increased.[21] In vitro studies on colonic biopsies in culture have confirmed active sodium secretion.[17]

Similar perfusion studies in microscopic colitis have demonstrated abnormal ionic transport, with reduction in lumen-to-plasma fluxes of chloride, sodium and water, but plasma-to-lumen ion flux was unaffected with maintenance of a net absorption of water and ions, although at a reduced level. Transmucosal potential difference was normal.[3]

TREATMENT

The variable and unpredictable course of collagenous colitis makes assessment of treatment difficult. Symptoms may subside spontaneously, and the mucosal inflammation, and even the collagen deposition, may remit.[5] However, response to sulphasalazine has now been described sufficiently frequently for this to be recommended as primary treatment. Anecdotal evidence suggests that 5-aminosalicylic acid may also be effective. Corticosteroids have induced remission after failure of sulphasalazine (Salazopyrine). Mepacrine is only occasionally useful. Antidiarrhoeals will relieve symptoms in some, but not all, cases.

REFERENCES

1. Balazs, M., Egerszegi, P., Vadasz, G. and Kovacs, A. (1988) Collagenous colitis: an electron microscopic study including comparison with the chronic fibrotic stage of ulcerative colitis. *Histopathology*, **13**, 319–328.
2. Bogomoletz, W.V., Adnet, J.J., Birembaut, P., Feydy, P. and Dupont, P. (1980) Collagenous colitis: an unrecognised entity. *Gut*, **21**, 164–168.
3. Bo-Linn, G.W., Vendrell, D.D., Lee, E. and Fordtran, J.S. (1985) An evaluation of the significance of microscopic colitis in patients with chronic diarrhoea. *Journal of Clinical Investigation*, **75**, 1559–1569.
4. Busuttil, A. (1989) Collagenous colitis in a child. *American Journal Diseases of Childhood*, **143**, 998–1000.
5. Debongnie, J.C., De Galocsy, C., Caholessur, M.O. and Haot, J. (1984) Collagenous colitis: a transient condition? *Diseases of The Colon and Rectum*, **27**, 672–676.
6. Fausa, O., Foerster, A. and Hovig, T. (1985) Collagenous colitis: A clinical, histological, and ultrastructural study. *Scandinavian Journal of Gastroenterology*, **20** (suppl. 107), 8–23.
7. Flejou, J.F., Grimaud, J.A., Molas, G., Baviesa, E. and Potet, F. (1984) Collagenous colitis: Ultrastructural study and collagen immunotyping of 4 cases. *Archives of Pathology and Laboratory Medicine*, **108**, 977–982.
8. Giardiello, F.M., Bayless, T.M., Jessurun, J., Hamilton, S.R. and Yardley, J.H. (1987) Collagenous colitis: physiologic and histopathologic studies in seven patients. *Annals of Internal Medicine*, **106**, 46–49.
9. Gledhill, A. and Cole, F.M. (1984) Significance of basement membrane thickening in the human colon. *Gut*, **25**, 1085–1088.
10. Hamilton, I., Sanders, S., Hopwood, D. and Bouchier, I.A.D. (1986) Collagenous colitis associated with small intestinal villous atrophy. *Gut*, **27**, 1394–1398.
11. Hwang, W.S., Kelly, J.K., Shaffer, E.A. and Hershfield, N.B. (1986) Collagenous colitis: a disease of pericryptal fibroblast sheath? *Journal of Pathology*, **149**, 33–40.
12. Jessurun, J., Yardley, J.H., Lee, E.L., Vendrell, D.D., Schiller, L.R. and Fordtran, J.S. (1986) Microscopic and collagenous colitis: different names for the same condition? *Gastroenterology*, **91**, 1583–1584.
13. Jessurun, J., Yardley, J.H., Giardiello, F.M., Hamilton, S.R. and Bayless, T.M. (1987) Chronic colitis with thickening of the subepithelial collagen layer (collagenous colitis): histopathologic findings in 15 patients. *Human Pathology*, **18**, 839–848.
14. Kingham, J.G.C., Levison, D.A., Ball, J.A. and Dawson, A.M. (1982) Microscopic colitis – a cause of chronic watery diarrhoea. *British Medical Journal*, **285**, 1601–1604.
15. Lazenby, A.J., Yardley, J.H., Giardiello, F.M., Jessurun, J. and Bayless, T.M. (1989) Lymphocytic ('microscopic') colitis: a comparative histopathologic study with particular reference to collagenous colitis. *Human Pathology*, **20**, 18–28.
16. Lindstrom, C.G. (1976) 'Collagenous colitis' with watery diarrhoea – A new entity? *Pathology, Europe*, **11**, 87–89.
17. Loo, F.D., Wood, C.M., Soergel, K.H. *et al.* (1985) Abnormal collagen deposition and ion transport in collagenous colitis (abstract). *Gastroenterology*, **88**, 1481.
18. Molas, G.J.-M., Flejou, J.F. and Potet, F. (1990) Microscopic colitis, collagenous colitis and mast cells. *Digestive Diseases and Sciences*, **35**, 920.
19. Palmer, K.R., Berry, H., Wheeler, P.J. *et al.* (1986) Collagenous colitis – a relapsing and remitting disease. *Gut*, **27**, 578–580.
20. Rams, H., Rogers, A.I. and Ghandur-Mnaymneh, L. (1987) Collagenous colitis. *Annals of Internal Medicine*, **106**, 108–113.
21. Rask-Madsen, J., Grove, O., Hansen, M.G.J., Bukhave, K. and Henrik-Nielsen, R. (1983) Colonic transport of water and electrolytes in a

patient with secretory diarrhoea due to collagenous colitis. *Digestive Diseases and Sciences*, **28**, 1141–1145.

22. Teglbjaerg, P.S., Thaysen, E.H. and Jensen, H.H. (1984) Development of collagenous colitis in sequential biopsy specimens. *Gastroenterology*, **87**, 703–709.
23. Sylwestrowicz, T., Kelly, J.K., Hwang, W.S. and Shaffer, E.A. (1989) Collagenous colitis and microscopic colitis: the watery diarrhoea-colitis syndrome. *American Journal of Gastroenterology*, **84**, 763–768.
24. Van Tilburg, A.J.P., Lam, H.G.T., Selden Rijk, C.A. and Stel, H.V. (1990) Familial occurrence of collagenous colitis. A report of two families. *Journal of Clinical Gastroenterology*, **12**, 279–285.
25. Wang, H.H., Owings, D.V., Antonioli, D.A. and Goldman, H. (1988) Increased subepithelial collagen deposition is not specific for collagenous colitis. *Modern Pathology*, **1**, 329–335.
26. Widgren, S., Jlidi, R. and Cox, J.N. (1988) Collagenous colitis: histologic, morphometric, immunohistochemical and ultrastructural studies. Report of 21 cases. *Virchows Archiv A, Pathological Anatomy and Histopathology*, **413**, 287–296.

CHAPTER 8

SYSTEMIC DISEASES AND SKIN DISORDERS

VASCULITIC AND CONNECTIVE TISSUE DISORDERS

A.R. Myers and D. DeMarco

Involvement of the gastrointestinal tract may accompany the connective tissue disorders and explain a vast array of symptoms that suggest abnormal gastrointestinal function. On occasion, significant gastrointestinal symptoms may precede the clinical diagnosis of a specific connective tissue disorder. More commonly, gastrointestinal symptoms present late in the course of the disease. The literature is replete with information describing the different patterns of gastrointestinal involvement in progressive systemic sclerosis (scleroderma), systemic lupus erythematosus, polymyositis/dermatomyositis, polyarteritis nodosa and rheumatoid arthritis. Although all of these disorders involve connective tissue and vascular channels, each is probably distinct aetiologically and pathogenically.

The gastrointestinal involvement of this group of diseases includes not only the entire visceral gastrointestinal tract extending from the mouth to the anus, but also some of the parenchymal organs such as the liver, biliary tract and pancreas. Scleroderma and polymyositis are prototypal diseases in which predominantly smooth and striated muscles, respectively, are involved. In contrast, the majority of the gastrointestinal manifestations due to polyarteritis nodosa are associated with inflammation and occlusion of vascular channels.

This review will consider the organ distribution, associated symptoms, and treatment of the gastrointestinal manifestations of the major connective tissue disorders. Those at the more vasculitic end of the spectrum – polyarteritis nodosa and Henoch–Schönlein purpura – are also described. Although it would be convenient if each of these disorders were well defined in its gastrointestinal involvement, readers will note that there are significant overlapping features which may lead to confusion.

PROGRESSIVE SYSTEMIC SCLEROSIS (SCLERODERMA) *(A.R. Myers and D. DeMarco)*

The gastrointestinal tract is preceded only by the skin and joints in the frequency of organ system involvement in progressive systemic sclerosis (or scleroderma). Serious gastrointestinal involvement is present in approximately 50% of patients.[7] Oesophageal involvement in systemic sclerosis was initially described in 1903[11] with subsequent radiological demonstration in 1916. Thereafter, changes in the small bowel were described by Rake[26] and colonic involvement by Hale and Schatzki.[13] Although the earlier descriptions of gastrointestinal involvement by systemic sclerosis used radiological techniques, manometric methods for studying intraluminal pressures within gastrointestinal organs were first employed to study this disorder in 1954.[10] Subsequent physiological approaches have included the measurement of myoelectrical activity and scintigraphic quantitation of aboral movement of an ingested bolus.[38]

In general, clinical gastrointestinal manifestations of progressive systemic sclerosis occur late in its course.[9] This delay in presentation is probably related to the pathogenesis of the disease which presumably involves an initial vascular abnormality followed by physiological alterations progressing ultimately to tissue changes. Therefore, gastrointestinal studies in asymptomatic individuals with systemic sclerosis will frequently yield evidence of altered physiology and provide a basis for preventive therapy (e.g. gastro-oesophageal reflux) leading to reduction in complications (e.g. stricture). Occasionally, however, systemic sclerosis occurs in the absence of obvious skin manifestations and in these instances the gastrointestinal findings may predominate.[12,29]

Commonly, the skin around the mouth may become sclerotic, producing a characteristic appearance and restricting the introduction of food into the mouth. Hypertrophy of periodontal ligaments may cause characteristic changes around dental roots. The gums may become indurated, friable or even atrophic. In advanced cases, the buccal mucosa and tongue may appear atrophic. On occasion, aphthous ulcerations due to candidiasis may complicate the clinical picture. All of these disorders may contribute to feeding problems.

OESOPHAGUS

In systemic sclerosis, the oesophagus is the most commonly involved gastrointestinal organ, occurring in approximately 80% of patients.[30,41] Raynaud's phenomenon occurs in 90–95% of these cases.[12,40] Abnormal oesophageal motility may be one of the earliest manifestations of scleroderma. This occurs secondary to involvement of the smooth muscle of the lower oesophageal sphincter and the distal two-thirds to four-fifths of the oesophageal body.[32] The abnormalities in motility are demonstrated best by manometric examination[36,39] and include decreased resting lower oesophageal sphincter pressure and feeble non-progressive contractions in the smooth muscle portion of the oesophagus, but normal contractions in the proximal (striated muscle) portion of the oesophagus and the oropharynx (*Figure 8.1*). The radiologist may

Figure 8.1 Oesophageal manometric tracings from different segments of the oesophagus in a patient with progressive systemic sclerosis. Pressure recordings from proximal, middle and distal leads spaced at 5-cm intervals are shown in the top three tracings, respectively. Recordings of swallows and respiration are also shown. Dark squares represent 1 cm withdrawal of the tube assembly. (a) The tube assembly is withdrawn across the lower oesophageal sphincter (arrows). A mean pressure of approximately 6 mmHg (normal 12–26 mmHg) is demonstrated. (b) Pressure recordings from the distal 10 cm of the oesophagus. Note that all oesophageal contractions are feeble and non-progressive. (c) Pressure recordings from the upper oesophageal sphincter, the proximal 5 cm of the oesophagus, and the mid-oesophagus 5 cm distally, respectively. A normal upper oesophageal sphincter with a normal resting pressure and complete post-deglutition relaxations is shown in the proximal pressure lead. In the middle lead, normal oesophageal contractions (arrows) from the proximal oesophagus are demonstrated. More distally, feeble oesophageal contractions are observed. In (c), the paper speed is faster than in (a) and (b).

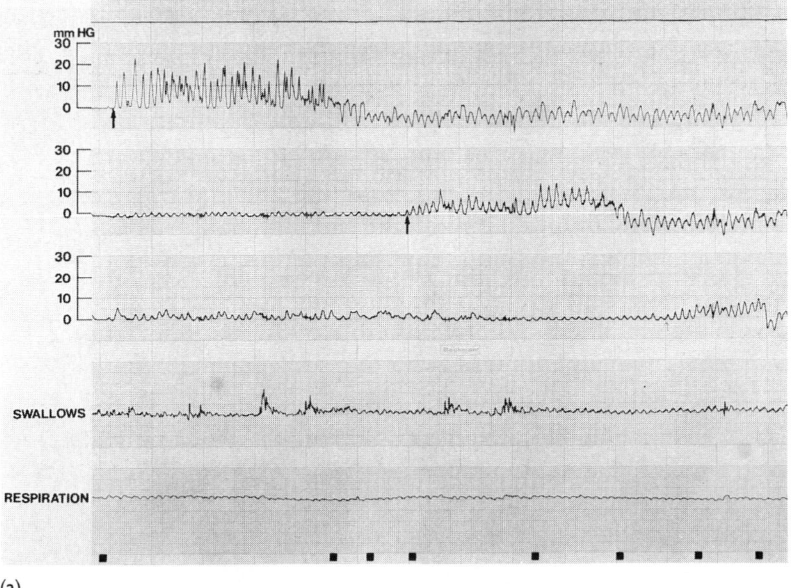
mm HG
30
20
10
0
30
20
10
0
30
20
10
0
SWALLOWS
RESPIRATION

(a)

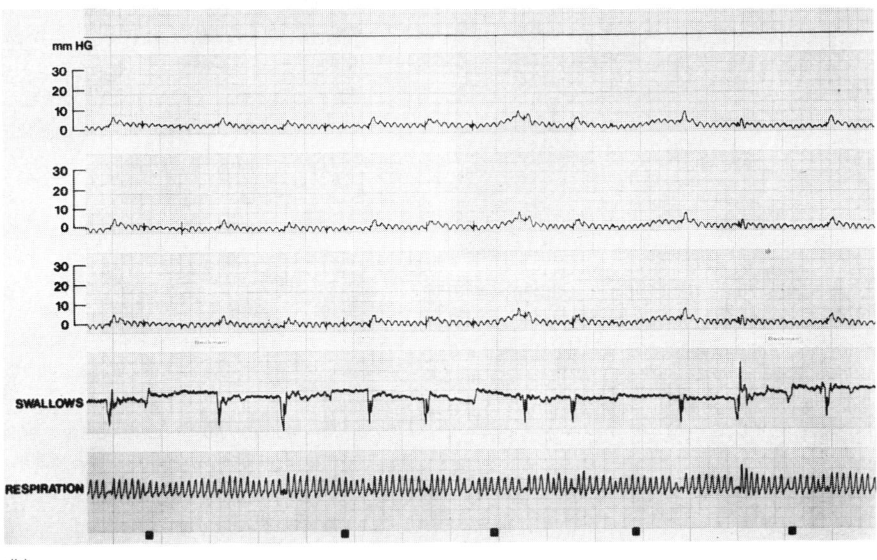
mm HG
30
20
10
0
30
20
10
0
30
20
10
0
SWALLOWS
RESPIRATION

(b)

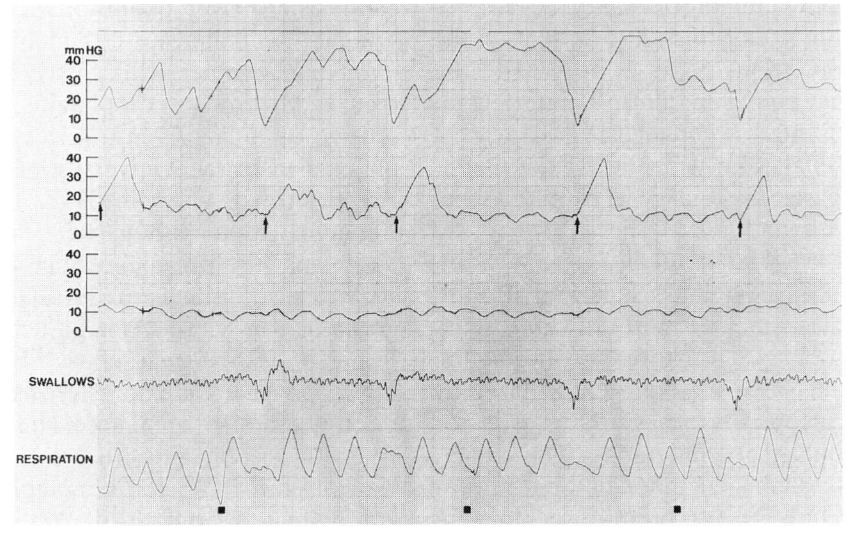
mm HG
40
30
20
10
0
40
30
20
10
0
40
30
20
10
0
SWALLOWS
RESPIRATION

(c)

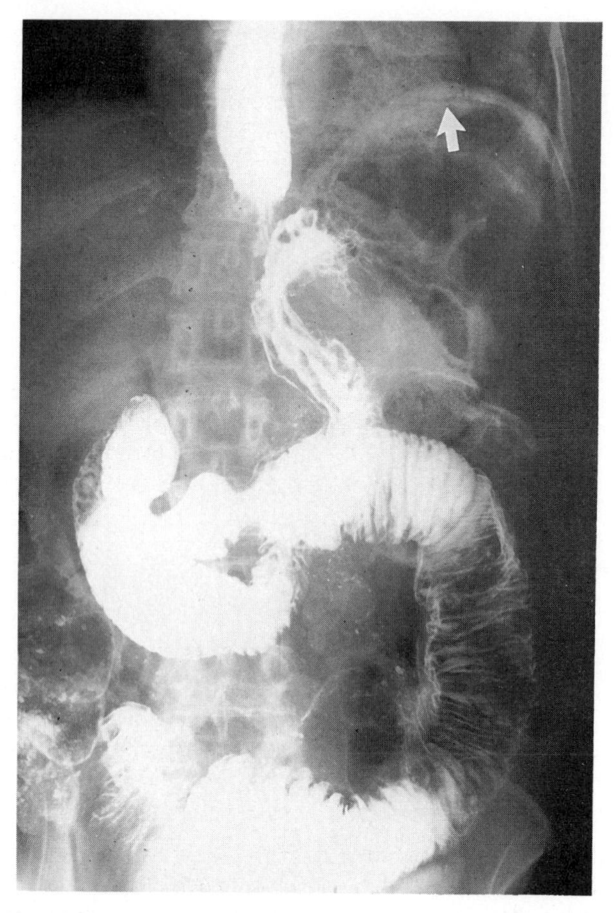

Figure 8.2 Upper gastrointestinal tract in a patient with scleroderma. Note the focal dilatation of the distal oesophagus with a stricture at the gastro-oesophageal junction, the dilatation in the second and third portions of the duodenum and the dilatation and prominent valvulae conniventes resembling a coiled spring in the jejunum. The apparent free air under the left diaphragm (arrow) represents pneumatosis coli.

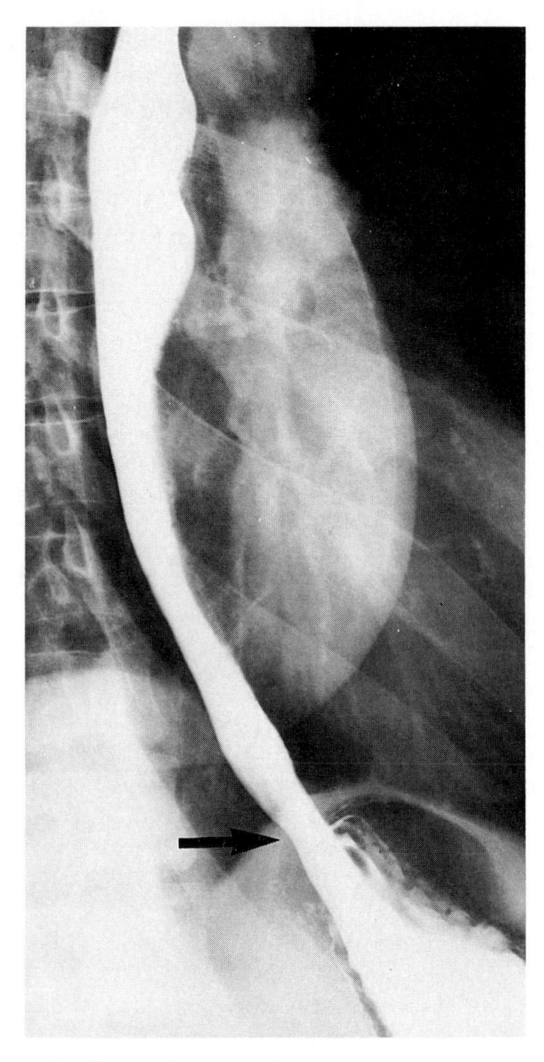

Figure 8.3 Non-motile, non-dilated oesophagus of early scleroderma. The oesophagogastric junction (arrow) is patulous.

report feeble contractions in the distal oesophagus associated with poor emptying of swallowed barium. Care must be taken to examine these patients in the prone or supine positions because, otherwise, the force of gravity may empty the contrast material into the stomach. Other oesophageal radiological findings include dilatation, widening of the diaphragmatic hiatus, gastro-oesophageal reflux and strictures (*Figures 8.2* and *8.3*). The body of the oesophagus may be dilated slightly or distension may be so marked as to simulate achalasia. Differentiation from achalasia may be most difficult when a benign distal oesophageal stricture complicates the picture. Significant gastro-oesophageal reflux may be detected fluoroscopically by acid reflux testing or using gastro-oesophageal scintigraphy. The combination of gastro-oesophageal reflux and poor oesophageal contractility may predispose to the formation of benign oesophageal strictures. Poor oesophageal emptying has been demonstrated recently using newer, quantitative, oesophageal scintigraphic techniques.[38] Inadequate oesophageal emptying together with gastro-oesophageal reflux may lead to erosive oesophagitis. The prevalence of erosive oesophagitis in a series of 53 scleroderma patients from the University of California at Los Angeles (UCLA) was 60%. In those patients with frequent symptoms of gastro-oesophageal reflux or dysphagia, the prevalence increased to more than 70%. These findings are in marked contrast to a group of non-scleroderma patients with symptomatic gastro-oesophageal reflux.[42] Endoscopic findings in oesophageal systemic sclerosis range from a normal mucosa to severe mucosal inflammation consistent with oesophagitis. In a retrospective study by Katzka *et al.*[19] Barrett's metaplasia was found in approximately one-third of systemic sclerosis patients undergoing endoscopy. These patients could not be differentiated on the basis of age, sex, presence of proximal skin involvement, digital ulceration and pulmonary involvement. Patients with Barrett's metaplasia had a longer duration of heartburn and dysphagia, an increased incidence of the CREST variant of systemic sclerosis and they tended to have greater impairment of lower oesophageal sphincter pressure (CREST syndrome = calcinosis, Raynaud's phenomenon, oesophageal dysmotility, sclerodactyly, and telangiectasia). Clinical, manometric, laboratory and radiological features were found to be poor predictors for Barrett's metaplasia. The presence of Barrett's metaplasia in this study was associated with the presence of both benign and malignant complications. Four of the nine patients with Barrett's metaplasia had benign oesophageal strictures; two patients who had no other risk factors developed adenocarcinoma.

The typical histological findings associated with oesophageal systemic sclerosis are muscle atrophy within the oesophageal mucosa with ultimate replacement by fibrous tissue.[7] However, early in the course of disease, no fibrotic or atrophic histological abnormalities may be seen despite marked oesophageal motor dysfunction.[39] In such early cases of oesophageal systemic sclerosis, the lower oesophageal sphincter pressure has been reported to increase in response to direct cholinergic stimulation but not in response to indirect cholinergic stimulation.[6] These findings suggest that a neural defect may be the earliest manifestation of gastrointestinal systemic sclerosis. However, as time progresses, this physiological dysfunction is supplanted by muscle atrophy and fibrosis in the distal oesophagus, leading to dilatation and the other changes.

Clinical features

Characteristic complaints attributable to oesophageal systemic sclerosis are: heartburn due to gastro-oesophageal reflux of the gastric contents; dysphagia, usually for both solids and liquids; chest fullness, especially after meals; and episodes of nocturnal coughing associated with aspiration of refluxed gastric contents while the patient is in the supine or prone position during sleep.[21]

Treatment

A vigorous antireflux regimen is the focus of treatment for oesophageal systemic sclerosis.[25,27] This includes sleeping with the trunk of the body elevated in order to use the force of gravity to minimize reflux episodes, acid neutralization with common antacids or an alginic acid–antacid combination; antisecretory treatment with H_2-receptor blocking agents; and specific antireflux treatment with cholinomimetic agents, such as bethanechol and metoclopramide, or the alginic acid–antacid combination that mechanically impedes gastro-oesophageal reflux. In very severe cases, antireflux surgery may be considered.[16] In view of the oesophageal motility dysfunction associated with systemic sclerosis, surgery should be performed only as a last resort. In the case of systemic sclerosis complicated by benign oesophageal stricture, treatment by an antireflux regimen and serial oesophageal bougienage (dilatation) is usually effective. On occasion, surgical correction of the stricture may be coupled with an antireflux procedure.

STOMACH

Of the visceral gastrointestinal tract, systemic sclerosis seems to involve the stomach least frequently (5%). Stomach involvement usually manifests itself as gastroparesis, i.e. delayed gastric emptying in the absence of a mechanical gastric outlet obstruction.[13] Delayed gastric emptying and gastric atony may be responsible for symptoms such as early satiety, postprandial nausea and vomiting, and epigastric pain. Gastroparesis may be demonstrated radiologically by a dilated stomach with retained barium for many hours. Recently, scintigraphic techniques have become the standard techniques for measuring gastric emptying of solids and liquids simultaneously[14] and perhaps, if applied widely, sclerodermatous gastropathy will be found to be more frequent than has been recognized previously.

SMALL INTESTINE

Small intestinal involvement has been identified in 40% of unselected patients with systemic sclerosis by barium examination.[7] Histopathologically, muscle atrophy with little fibrosis is characteristic, but occasionally extensive collagen deposition has been observed. Nerve cells generally appear normal.

Physiological abnormalities have been recognized which may explain the clinical disorder of small bowel function noted in systemic sclerosis. DiMarino *et al.*[9] evaluated duodenal myoelectrical activity and observed small intestinal motor dysfunction analogous to that seen in the oesophagus. Rees *et al.*[28] found abnormal interdigestive motor activity in scleroderma patients with clinical evidence of small bowel involvement. Certainly, stasis of small bowel contents and its resultant complications could result from these defects.

Clinical features

Evidence of malabsorption has been found in 10–25% of patients and intestinal pseudo-obstruction is the next most frequent complication.[35] Whilst small intestinal involvement may be asymptomatic, the most striking symptoms associated with small intestinal systemic sclerosis are diarrhoea, steatorrhoea, abdominal pain, abdominal distension and weight loss. These symptoms are due to a combination of vascular obstruction, altered motility, impairment of the intestinal lymphatics and bacterial overgrowth. Of these, bacterial overgrowth is probably most important. Overgrowth may be associated with dehydroxylation and deconjugation of bile salts, coupled with direct damage to the small intestinal mucosa. These alterations may lead to fat malabsorption, decreased absorption of fat-soluble vitamins, vitamin B_{12} deficiency, diarrhoea and weight loss. Less commonly, systemic sclerosis involving the small intestine may present with more acute findings associated with true intestinal infarction, perforation, haemorrhage or ulcerations. There have been a number of reports of pneumatosis cystoides intestinalis in systemic sclerosis. This otherwise uncommon disorder occurs frequently in systemic sclerosis secondary to bowel hypomotility leading to bacterial overgrowth and bowel distension. Intraluminal pressure becomes elevated and forces gas into the intestinal wall forming subserosal or submucosal cysts. The stasis and small vessel involvement in progressive systemic sclerosis may affect the mucosal lining as well. Oral or intravenous hyperalimentation solutions, often used in the management of systemic sclerosis with bowel involvement, could encourage bacterial overgrowth in a hypomotile bowel because of their high carbohydrate content. This may also precipitate pneumatosis cystoides intestinalis by the same mechanism discussed above.[33]

Investigations

Radiological abnormalities involving the entire length of the small intestine have been well described. Dilatation and stasis are noted most prominently in the second and third portions of the duodenum and in the proximal jejunum.[3] In addition to dilatation, loops of the jejunum may appear thickened with an approximation of the valvulae conniventes resulting in a typical wire-spring configuration (*Figures 8.2, 8.4 and 8.5*).[18] Delayed

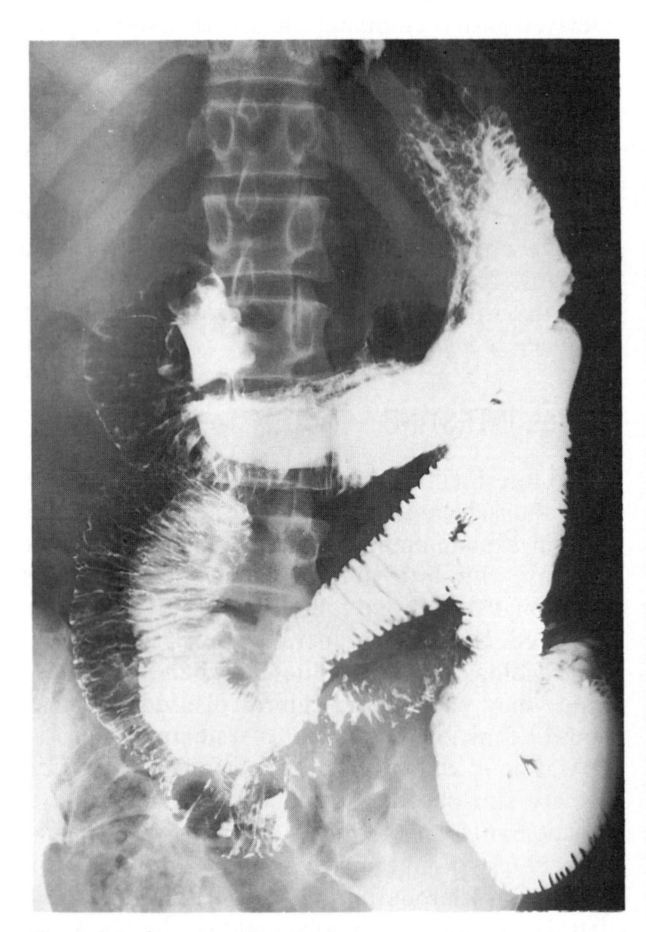

Figure 8.4 Characteristic duodenal and jejunal pattern of scleroderma. Note the focal dilatation of the second and third portions of the duodenum. The jejunum is also dilated with a prominence of the valvulae conniventes resembling a coiled spring.

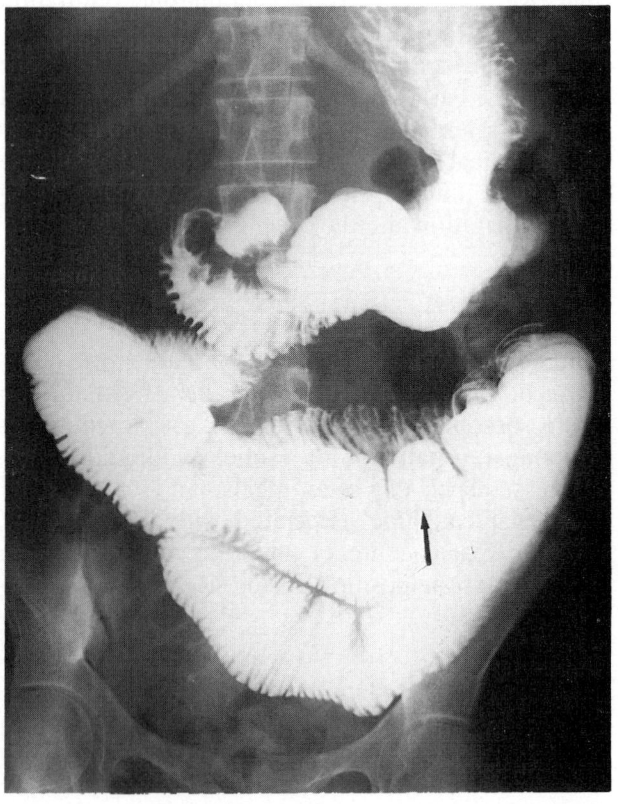

Figure 8.5 Small bowel changes in scleroderma. Note dilated second and third portions of the duodenum and the sacculations of the jejunum (arrow) which closely resemble colonic haustrations.

small intestinal transit of contrast material and associated segmentation and flocculation of barium may be seen. At times the extensive dilatation of the sclerodermatous small bowel may simulate a mechanical obstruction (pseudo-obstruction).

Treatment

The treatment of the small intestinal disorder of systemic sclerosis requires awareness of the various complications. Bacterial overgrowth must be treated aggressively with antibiotics (tetracycline 250 mg four times daily for 10–14 days initially) in order to correct maldigestion and malabsorption of fats and vitamins. The recognition of pseudo-obstruction is imperative in order to avoid unnecessary and ineffective surgical intervention. Conservative measures, including suction, bowel rest and hydration, are usually effective. Intravenous hyperalimentation has been used successfully in scleroderma patients with malnutrition, malabsorption and intestinal pseudo-obstruction. Ng *et al.* evaluated 15 patients with severe scleroderma bowel disease who received home central venous hyperalimentation. They found an improved quality of life in 11 of the 15 patients and also a low incidence of complications from the treatment.[24]

COLON

Although colonic involvement in patients with progressive systemic sclerosis is common (one-third of patients), symptoms referable to the large bowel are not prominent. However, severe complications may occur. Usually, the colonic changes in systemic sclerosis accompany other gastrointestinal involvement. Radiological features of colonic systemic sclerosis may be striking and include the virtually pathognomonic, wide-mouthed diverticula seen especially on the antimesenteric border of the transverse and descending colon (*Figure 8.6*). Wide-mouthed diverticula also may be found in the jejunum and ileum of scleroderma patients (see *Figure 8.5*).[15,23] Generalized dilatation may be present as well as hypomotility and loss of haustrations. The symptoms of colonic scleroderma may include abdominal bloating, a change in the calibre of the stools, diarrhoea, constipation and obstipation. Pathologically, atrophy and fibrosis of the colonic musculature may be found with colonic systemic sclerosis. These changes are similar to those found in the oesophagus and small intestine. Complications of colonic systemic sclerosis include pseudo-obstruction, perforation, infarction, megacolon and volvulus.[4] On occasion, mechanical obstruction may supervene due to a faecal impaction. Colonic telangiectasias have also been reported in patients with systemic sclerosis and can be the source of significant gastrointestinal blood loss.[1] Treatment of colonic involvement in systemic sclerosis is non-specific, ranging from a high-fibre diet and the use of various laxatives, to colonic resection in severe cases.

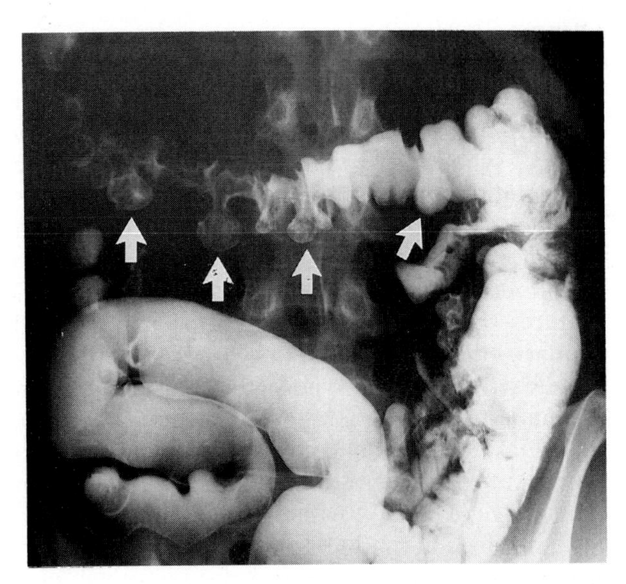

Figure 8.6 Large bowel in a patient with scleroderma. Note the characteristic large mouth diverticula (arrows) primarily located in the transverse colon.

Studies of colonic motility in patients with systemic sclerosis revealed findings similar to those found in other parts of the gastrointestinal tract. The majority of patients with systemic sclerosis do not exhibit the normal postprandial gastrocolonic response which is a cholinergic reflex. There is a normal response to the direct smooth muscle stimulants neostigmine and metoclopramide in those patients with mild disease but no response as disease progresses. These findings suggest a latent neurogenic defect early in the disease with a myopathic process evolving due to atrophy and fibrosis, resulting in symptomatic hypomotility.[35]

ANAL SPHINCTER

In addition to constipation and diarrhoea, faecal incontinence may be encountered in patients with systemic sclerosis. Impaired internal anal sphincter function has been observed[5,17] and may account for significant constipation or faecal incontinence. Rectal prolapse has also been reported and may be a complication of chronic constipation.[8] Treatment of anal sphincter dysfunction is very difficult but behavioural techniques and electrical stimulation may be helpful.

LIVER

The association between primary biliary cirrhosis and progressive systemic sclerosis, particularly the CREST syndrome, is well recognized.[31] The clinical presentation of these patients includes pruritus, jaundice, hepatomegaly, marked elevation of alkaline phosphatase and high titres of serum antimitochondrial antibodies in addition to the CREST features. In studying a group of 100 patients with primary biliary cirrhosis, three patients were noted to have the CREST syndrome.[34] In comparison, evaluation of 29 patients with CREST syndrome yielded 11 with evidence of primary biliary cirrhosis.[20] Anticentromere antibodies, found in a high percentage of patients with the CREST syndrome,[37] have also been found in up to one-third of patients with primary biliary cirrhosis.[20,22]

References

1. Baron, M. and Srolovitz, H. (1986) Colonic telangiectasias in a patient with PSS. *Arthritis and Rheumatism*, **29**, 282–285.
2. Battle, W.M., Snape, W.J., Jr, Wright, S. *et al.* (1981) Abnormal colonic motility in progressive systemic sclerosis. *Annals of Internal Medicine*, **94**, 749–752.
3. Bluestone, R., MacMahon, M. and Dawson, J.M. (1969) Systemic sclerosis and small bowel involvement. *Gut*, **10**, 185–195.
4. Brandwein, M. and Schwartz, I.S. (1988) Megacolon and volvulus complicating progressive systemic sclerosis. *Mount Sinai Journal of Medicine*, **55**, 343–345.
5. Cerulli, M., Nikoomanesh, P. and Schuster, M.M. (1976) Effect of progressive systemic sclerosis on electrical and motor activity of the internal anal sphincter. *Clinical Research*, **24**, 282.
6. Cohen, S., Fisher, R., Lipshutz, W. *et al.* (1972) The pathogenesis of esophageal dysfunction in scleroderma and Raynaud's disease. *Journal of Clinical Investigation*, **51**, 2663–2668.
7. Cohen, S., Laufer, I., Snape, W.J., Shiau, Y.F., Levine, G.M. and Jimenez, S.J. (1980) The gastrointestinal manifestations of scleroderma: Pathogenesis and management. *Gastroenterology*, **70**, 155–166.
8. D'Angelo, G., Stern, H.S. and Myers, E. (1985) Rectal prolapse in scleroderma: Case report and review of the colonic complications of scleroderma. *Canadian Journal of Surgery*, **28**, 62–63.
9. DiMarino, A.J., Carlson, G., Myers, A. *et al.* (1973) Duodenal myoelectric activity in scleroderma. *New England Journal of Medicine*, **289**, 1220–1223.
10. Dornhurst, A.C., Pierce, J.W. and Whimster, I.W. (1954) The oesophageal lesion in scleroderma. *The Lancet*, **1**, 698–699.
11. Ehrmann, S. (1903) Uber die Bezichung des sklerodermie zu den autotoxischen erythemen. *Wiener Medizinische Wochenschrift*, **53**, 1097–1102.
12. Goldbraber, M.B. and Kirshner, J.B. (1957) Scleroderma of the gastrointestinal tract. *Archives of Pathology*, **64**, 255–265.
13. Hale, C.H. and Schatzki, R. (1944) The roentegenographic appearance of the gastrointestinal tract in scleroderma. *American Journal of Roentgenology and Radium Therapy*, **51**, 407–414.
14. Heading, R.C., Tothill, P. and McGloughlin, G.P. (1976) Gastric emptying rate measurement in man: a dual isotope scanning technique for simultaneous study of liquid and solid components of a meal. *Gastroenterology*, **71**, 45–50.
15. Heinz, E.R., Steinberg, A.J. and Sackner, M.A. (1963) Roentgenographic and pathologic aspects of intestinal scleroderma. *Annals of Internal Medicine*, **59**, 822–831.
16. Henderson, R.D. and Pearson, F.G. (1973) Surgical management of esophageal scleroderma. *Journal of Thoracic and Cardiovascular Surgery*, **66**, 686–692.
17. Hogan, W.J., Kahn, M.A., Nelson, J.W. and Winship, D.H. (1971) Impairment of anal sphincter function in progressive systemic sclerosis. *Clinical Research*, **19**, 394.
18. Horowitz, A.L. and Meyers, M.E. (1973) The 'hidebound' small bowel of scleroderma: characteristic mucosal fold pattern. *American Journal of Roentgenology, Radium Therapy and Nuclear Medicine*, **119**, 332–334.
19. Katzka, D.A., Reynolds, J.F., Saul, S.H. *et al.* (1987) Barrett's metaplasia and adenocarcinoma of the esophagus in scleroderma. *American Journal of Medicine*, **82**, 46–51.
20. Klatskin, G. and Kantor, F.S. (1972) Mitochondrial antibody in primary biliary cirrhosis and other diseases. *Annals of Internal Medicine*, **77**, 533–541.
21. Lorber, S.H. and Zarafonetis, C.J.D. (1963) Esophageal transport studies in scleroderma. *American Journal of Medical Science*, **245**, 654–667.
22. Makinen, D., Fritzler, M., Davis, P. and Sherlock, S. (1983) Anticentromere antibodies in primary biliary cirrhosis. *Arthritis and Rheumatism*, **26**, 914–917.
23. Meszaros, W.T. (1959) The colon in systemic sclerosis (scleroderma). *American Journal of Roentgenology, Radium Therapy and Nuclear Medicine*, **82**, 1000–1011.
24. Ng, S.C., Clements, P.J., Berquist, W.E., Furst, D.E. and Paulus, H.E. (1989) Home central venous hyperalimentation in fifteen patients with severe scleroderma bowel disease. *Arthritis and Rheumatism*, **32**, 212–216.
25. Petrokubi, R.J. and Jeffries, G.H. (1978) Cimetidine versus antacid in scleroderma with reflux esophagitis. A randomized double blind controlled study. *Gastroenterology*, **74**, 1077–1080.
26. Rake, S.G. (1931) On the pathology and

pathogenesis of scleroderma. *Johns Hopkins Hospital Bulletin*, **48**, 212–227.
27. Ramirez-Mata, M., Ibanex, G. and Alarcon-Segovia, D. (1977) Stimulatory effects of metoclopramide on the esophagus and lower esophageal sphincter of patients with progressive systemic sclerosis. *Arthritis and Rheumatism*, **20**, 30–34.
28. Rees, W.D.W., Leigh, R.J., Christofides, N.D. *et al.* (1982) Interdigestive motor activity in patients with systemic sclerosis. *Gastroenterology*, **83**, 575–580.
29. Rodnan, G.P. and Fennell, R.H., Jr (1962) Progressive systemic sclerosis sine scleroderma. *Journal of the American Medical Association*, **180**, 665–670.
30. Saladin, T.A., French, A.B., Zarafonetis, C.J.D. and Volland, H. (1966) Esophageal motor abnormalities in scleroderma and related diseases. *American Journal of Digestive Diseases*, **11**, 522–535.
31. Schaffner, F. (1979) Primary biliary cirrhosis as a collagen disease. *Postgraduate Medical Journal*, **65**, 97–102.
32. Schneider, H.A., Yonder, R.A., Longley, S., Katz, P., Mathias, J. and Panush, R.S. (1984) Scleroderma esophagus: A nonspecific entity. *Annals of Internal Medicine*, **100**, 848–850.
33. Sequeira, W. (1990) Pneumatosis cystoides intestinalis in systemic sclerosis and other diseases. *Seminars in Arthritis and Rheumatism*, **19**, 269–277.
34. Sherlock, S. and Scheurer, P.J. (1973) The presentation and diagnosis of 100 patients with primary biliary cirrhosis. *New England Journal of Medicine*, **289**, 674–678.
35. Stafford-Brady, F.J., Kahn, H.J., Ross, T.M. and Russell, M.L. (1988) Advanced scleroderma bowel: Complications and management. *Journal of Rheumatology*, **15**, 869–874.
36. Stevens, M.B., Hookman, P., Seigel, C.I. *et al.* (1964) Aperistalsis of the esophagus in patients with connective tissue disorders and Raynaud's phenomenon. *New England Journal of Medicine*, **270**, 1218–1222.
37. Tan, E.M., Rodnan, G.P., Garcia, I., Moroi, Y., Fritzler, M.J. and Peebles, C. (1980) Diversity of antinuclear antibodies in PSS: anticentromere antibody and its relationship to CREST syndrome. *Arthritis and Rheumatism*, **23**, 617–625.
38. Tolin, R., Malmud, L.S., Reilly, J. and Fisher, R.S. (1979) Esophageal scintigraphy to quantitate esophageal transit. *Gastroenterology*, **76**, 1402–1408.
39. Treacy, W.L., Baggenstoss, A.H., Slocumb, C.H. and Code, F.H. (1963) Scleroderma of the esophagus: correlation of histologic and physiologic findings. *Annals of Internal Medicine*, **59**, 351–356.
40. Tuffanelli, D.L. and Winklemann, R.K. (1961) Systemic scleroderma: a clinical study of 727 cases. *Archives of Dermatology*, **84**, 359–371.
41. Turner, R., Lipshutz, W.H., Miller, W. *et al.* (1973) Esophageal dysfunction in Collagen disease. *American Journal of Medical Sciences*, **265**, 191–199.
42. Zamost, B.J., Hirschberg, J., Ippoliti, A.F., Furst, D.E., Clements, P.J. and Weinstein, W.M. (1987) Esophagitis in scleroderma. *Gastroenterology*, **92**, 421–428.

SYSTEMIC LUPUS ERYTHEMATOSUS

(A.R. Myers and D. DeMarco)

Gastrointestinal symptoms in patients with systemic lupus erythematosus are common and include anorexia, dysphagia, nausea, vomiting, abdominal pain and diarrhoea.[7] Often these symptoms are of limited significance and difficult to ascribe to specific organ involvement. Occasionally, however, gastrointestinal complications in systemic lupus erythematosus present as an acute surgical abdomen[10,23] which may be secondary to a variety of problems including ulceration, haemorrhage, perforation, obstruction, ischaemic colitis or sterile peritonitis.[5]

Delay in diagnosis is common; Zizic *et al.*[23] noted that abdominal pain was present in two-thirds of patients with systemic lupus erythematosus for an average of 34 days before the acute abdominal crisis. Abdominal pain may be the presenting manifestation of lupus, making accurate diagnosis extremely difficult. Patients with known systemic lupus erythematosus are often taking high doses of corticosteroids or immunosuppressive agents which may mask abdominal symptomatology. Also symptoms initially may be attributed to medication such as non-steroidal anti-inflammatory agents, corticosteroids or hydroxychloroquine, all of which can cause gastrointestinal upset.

OESOPHAGUS

Clinical, radiological[21] and manometric[15,20] data indicate that oesophageal function may be altered in 25–35% of patients with systemic lupus erythematosus. Radiological findings in the oesophagus include diffuse or focal dilatation and decreased aboral movement of contrast material. Oesophageal manometric studies have shown that the amplitude of oesophageal contractions may be decreased and contractions may be non-progressive (i.e. aperistaltic). These abnormalities may be diffuse or they may be confined to specific segments of the oesophageal body. In some patients, the resting lower oesophageal sphincter pressure may be diminished. The relationship of the oesophageal dysfunction to

Raynaud's phenomenon has been emphasized by Stevens *et al.*[20]

Oesophageal symptoms such as dysphagia are less common. The oesophageal findings in systemic lupus erythematosus may be similar to, but less severe than, those found in scleroderma. On occasion, the proximal or striated muscle portions of the oesophagus may be involved alone or in combination with the distal oesophagus. Pharmacological studies of the type performed in scleroderma have not been done; thus, the presence of a neural defect has not been suggested. Extensive pathological studies of the oesophagus are not available. Superimposed inflammatory or candidal oesophagitis may complicate systemic lupus erythematosus.

STOMACH AND INTESTINE

The predominant lesion in the stomach and intestine appears to be a small vessel vasculitis. This may progress to ischaemic enteritis and eventually to bowel infarction with peritonitis. Early on, plain abdominal radiographs may show only an ileus or pseudo-obstruction pattern which may be due to ischaemia, sepsis or uraemia. Other radiological abnormalities include a distended atonic stomach or frank ulceration in the stomach and duodenum. If progression of ischaemia occurs, bowel wall oedema becomes manifest with oedematous haustra and valvulae conniventes. True perforation of the small intestine can also occur.[4,19] Rarely, pneumatosis cystoides intestinalis may occur. It may be benign, as in other diseases such as progressive systemic sclerosis, or it may be associated with a necrotizing enterocolitis.[11,14]

Other aetiologies for abdominal pain in systemic lupus erythematosus may also occur. Colon involvement is well recognized and may present as perforation secondary to arteritis.[24] The coexistence of systemic lupus erythematosus with Crohn's disease has been reported and although rare, patients with systemic lupus erythematosus showing gastrointestinal manifestations might require evaluation for that disease.[9] Malabsorption and protein losing enteropathy have been seen in systemic lupus erythematosus with evidence of immune deposits in intestinal vessels and basement membranes.[2,22]

LIVER AND SPLEEN

Involvement of the liver, spleen and pancreas may also occur in systemic lupus erythematosus. Spontaneous rupture of the liver and spleen has been reported.[6,8] Functional asplenia has also been reported but the mechanism of this disorder is unclear. No evidence of vasculitis has thus far been found. Hepatic involvement secondary to systemic lupus erythematosus has been recognized relatively recently.[3,17] Previously, liver disease found in systemic lupus erythematosus patients was most often ascribed to intercurrent illnesses or to pharmacological agents. While many drugs may produce hepatotoxicity, aspirin appears to the most common toxicant in patients with systemic lupus erythematosus.[18] However, the liver toxicity is entirely reversible. Excluding drug-induced hepatotoxicity and other obvious causes, histological abnormalities such as fatty infiltration, chronic active hepatitis and even cirrhosis have been demonstrated in systemic lupus erythematosus.[3,17] Both progression of systemic lupus erythematosus-related liver disease and death due to liver failure have been reported.[17] Subclinical and overt liver disease may be a more common concomitant of systemic lupus erythematosus than previously recognized.

PANCREAS

Hyperamylasaemia is common in systemic lupus erythematosus[16] and has been most frequently attributed to corticosteroid therapy despite occasional recognition of arteritis as an aetiology.[1] Careful evaluation for pancreatitis as a cause of abdominal pain in lupus erythematosus revealed that it was not a rare occurrence and that frequently it may be due to the inflammatory disease itself rather than any associated therapy such as corticosteroids.[16]

References

1. Baron, M. and Brisson, M. (1982) Pancreatitis in systemic lupus erythematosus. *Arthritis and Rheumatism*, **25**, 1006–1009.
2. Casteneda, S., Moldenhauer, F., Herrero-Beaumont, G. and Yanez, R. (1985) Protein losing enteropathy as the initial manifestation of SLE. *Journal of Rheumatology*, **12**, 1210–1212.
3. Gibson, T. and Myers, A.R. (1981) Subclinical liver disease in systemic lupus erythematosus. *Journal of Rheumatology*, **8**, 752–759.
4. Gore R.M., Calenoff, L. and Rogers, L.F. (1979) Roentgenographic manifestations of ischemic colitis. *Journal of American Medical Association*, **241**, 1171–1173.
5. Gore, R.M., Marn, C.S., Ujiki, G.T., Craig, R.M. and Marquardt, J. (1983) Ischemic colitis associated with SLE. *Diseases of Colon and Rectum*, **26**, 449–451.
6. Haslock, I. (1973) Spontaneous rupture of the liver in SLE. *Annals of Rheumatic Diseases*, **33**, 482–484.

7. Hoffman, B.I. and Katz, W.A. (1980) The gastrointestinal manifestations of systemic lupus erythematosus: a review of the literature. *Seminars in Arthritis and Rheumatism*, **9**, 237–247.
8. Huttonen, R., Seppala, A. and Mokka, R. (1975) Spontaneous rupture of the liver and spleen: report of a successfully treated case with immunopathologic reaction. *Surgery*, **77**, 722–725.
9. Johnson, D.A., Diehl, A.M., Finkelman, F.D. and Cattau, E.L. (1985) Crohn's disease and SLE. *American Journal of Gastroenterology*, **80**, 869–870.
10. Jovaisas, A. and Kraag, G. (1987) Acute gastrointestinal manifestations of systemic lupus erythematosus. *Canadian Journal of Surgery*, **30**, 185–188.
11. Laing, T.J. (1988) Gastrointestinal vasculitis and pneumatosis intestinalis due to SLE: Successful treatment with pulse intravenous cyclophosphamide. *American Journal of Medicine*, **85**, 555–558.
12. Miller, M.H., Urowitz, M.B., Gladman, D.D. and Blendis, L.M. (1984) The liver in SLE. *Quarterly Journal of Medicine*, **53**, 401–409.
13. Nagata, M., Ogawa, Y., Hisano, S. and Ueda, K. (1989) Crohn disease in SLE: A case report. *European Journal of Pediatrics*, **148**, 525–526.
14. Pruitt, R.E., Tumminello, V.V. and Reveille, J.D. (1988) Pneumatosis cystoides intestinalis and benign pneumoperitoneum in a patient with ANA negative SLE. *Journal of Rheumatology*, **15**, 1575–1577.
15. Ramirez-Mata, M., Reyes, P.A., Alarcon-Segovia, D. and Garza, R. (1974) Esophageal motility in systemic lupus erythematosus. *American Journal of Digestive Diseases*, **19**, 132–136.
16. Reynolds, J.F., Inman, R.D., Kimberly, R.P. *et al.* (1982) Acute pancreatitis in systemic lupus erythematosus: report of twenty cases and a review of the literature. *Medicine*, **61**, 25–32.
17. Runyon, B.A., LaBrecque, D.R. and Anuras, S. (1980) the spectrum of liver disease in systemic lupus erythematosus: Report of 33 histologically proved cases and review of the literature. *American Journal of Medicine*, **69**, 187–194.
18. Seaman, W.E., Ishak, K.G. and Plotz, P.H. (1974) Aspirin-induced hepatotoxicity in patients with systemic lupus erythematosus. *Annals of Internal Medicine*, **80**, 1–8.
19. Shapeero, L.G., Myers, A., Oberkircher, P.E. and Miller, W.T. (1974) Acute reversible lupus vasculitis of the gastrointestinal tract. *Radiology*, **112**, 569–574.
20. Stevens, M.B., Hookman, P., Siegel, C.I. *et al.* (1964) Aperistalsis of the esophagus in patients with connective tissue disorders and Raynaud's phenomenon. *New England Journal of Medicine*, **270**, 1218–1222.
21. Tatelman, M. and Keech, M.R. (1966) Esophageal motility in systemic lupus erythematosus, rheumatoid arthritis and scleroderma. *Radiology*, **86**, 1041–1045.
22. Weiser, M.M., Andres, G.A., Brentjens, J.R. *et al.* (1981) Systemic lupus erythematosus and intestinal venulitis. *Gastroenterology*, **81**, 570–579.
23. Zizic, T.M., Classen, J.N. and Stevens, M.B. (1982) Acute abdominal complications of systemic lupus erythematosus and polyarteritis nodosa. *American Journal of Medicine*, **73**, 525–531.
24. Zizic, T.M., Shulman, L.E. and Stevens, M.B. (1975) Colonic perforations in systemic lupus erythematosus. *Medicine*, **54**, 411–426.

POLYMYOSITIS/DERMATOMYOSITIS

(A.R. Myers and D. DeMarco)

Polymyositis/dermatomyositis is a chronic disease characterized by degenerative and inflammatory changes in skeletal (striated) muscles. Associated characteristic dermal involvement occurs in 40% of cases. Polymyositis/dermatomyositis is frequently associated with extramuscular disorders and gastrointestinal tract involvement is common. Pathological examination of the oesophagus in polymyositis/dermatomyositis reveals infrequent evidence of smooth muscle atrophy or fibrosis as seen in scleroderma but mucosal ulceration is common.[3] Complicating oesophageal candidiasis may supervene.

CLINICAL FEATURES

Dysphagia for solid and liquid foods is the most common digestive symptom in polymyositis/dermatomyositis and occurs in about 60% of cases.[7] One group reported that the highest frequency of dysphagia is found among patients with associated malignancy.[4] Most commonly dysphagia is due to involvement of the oropharynx; however, the proximal oesophagus is also frequently involved. Dysphagia may be associated with a nasal quality in the voice, regurgitation, and tracheal aspiration, related to weakness of pharyngeal and cricopharyngeal muscles.[1] Although polymyositis/dermatomyositis is regarded as a disease of the striated muscles, there are now several reports documenting abnormal distal oesophageal motility and functionally decreased amplitude of lower oesophageal contractions as well.[3,5] The relationship to Raynaud's phenomenon requires further study.

Radiological studies may reveal pooling of contrast material in the vallecula, tracheal aspiration and/or decreased peristalsis. Studies in which oesophageal manometric examinations have been performed have yielded conflicting results. Some have demonstrated decreased amplitudes of pharyngeal and oesophageal contractions confined to striated muscles, but more recent studies have shown manometric abnormalities of both smooth and striated muscles.[5] No studies utilizing pharmacological manipulation attempting to identify the lesion have been reported.

A disturbing but still controversial aspect of polymyositis/dermatomyositis is the association with malignancy, especially in the lung and gastrointestinal tract.[4] The frequency of malignancy among adult patients with polymyositis/dermatomyositis varies from 7% to 24%. Patients with polymyositis/dermatomyositis and an associated malignancy tend to be older than those without malignancy. It does not appear that malignancy is more common in men than in women, but it appears that malignancy is more common with dermatomyositis than with polymyositis. There is not, however, universal agreement about this association in the literature. There have been several studies comparing patients with myositis to various age- and sex-matched control populations which did not show an increase in the incidence of malignancy and many of the studies that do show an association have been criticized for their small numbers and poor statistical analysis.[6,8]

Coexistent gastrointestinal cancers occur most commonly in the stomach, but have also been found in the gallbladder, colon, rectum, oesophagus and pancreas. Signs and symptoms of dermatomyositis may precede the discovery of the tumour by up to 1 year, and resection of the tumour may result in resolution of the myositic process. It has been suggested that patients with polymyositis/dermatomyositis as part of an overlap syndrome are unlikely to have malignancies but there are now several reports to the contrary.[2,9]

TREATMENT

Treatment of the gastrointestinal manifestations of polymyositis/dermatomyositis relate mainly to the control of the myopathy for which corticosteroids are generally employed. Cricopharyngeal and proximal oesophageal involvement may lead to aspiration which must be protected against until control of the generalized disorder is achieved. Oesophageal ulceration may be inhibited by an antacid and antireflux programme.

References

1. Bohan, A. and Peter, J.B. (1975) Polymyositis and dermatomyositis. *New England Journal of Medicine*, **292**, 344–347.
2. Callen, J.P. (1984) Dermatomyositis and malignancy. *Clinical Rheumatic Diseases*, **10**, 117–130.
3. DeMerieux, P., Verity, M.A., Clements, P.J. and Paulus, H.E. (1983) Esophageal abnormalities and dysphagia in polymositis and dermatomyositis. Clinical radiologic and pathologic features. *Arthritis and Rheumatism*, **26**, 961–968.
4. Hochberg, M.G., Feldman, D. and Stevens, M.B. (1986) Adult onset PM/DM: An analysis of clinical and laboratory features and survival in 76 patients with a review of the literature. *Seminars in Arthritis and Rheumatism*, **15**, 168–178.
5. Jacob, H., Berkowitz, D., McDonald, E., Bernstein, L.H. and Beneventano, T. (1983) The esophageal motility disorder of polymyositis. *Archives of Internal Medicine*, **143**, 2262–2264.
6. Manchul, L. A., Jin, A., Pritchard, K.I. *et al.* (1985) The frequency of malignant neoplasms in patients with PM/DM. *Archives of Internal Medicine*, **145**, 1835–1839.
7. Pearson, C.M. (1985) Polymyositis and dermatomyositis. In *Arthritis and Allied Conditions* 10th edn (Ed.) McCarty, D., pp. 971–993. Washington: Lea and Febiger.
8. Plotz, P.H., Dalakas, M., Leff, R.L., Love, L.A., Miller, F.W. and Cronin, M.E. (1989) Current concepts in the idiopathic inflammatory myopathies: PM, DM and related disorders. *Annals of Internal Medicine*, **111**, 143–157.
9. Sakon, M., Monden, M., Fujimoto, Y. *et al.* (1989) Gastric carcinoma associated with dermatomyositis. *Acta Chirurgica Scandinavia*, **155**, 365–366.

VASCULITIS (*A.R. Myers and D. DeMarco*)

POLYARTERITIS NODOSA

The vasculitic syndromes may be separated on the basis of vessel size and histopathological features.[8] Although gastrointestinal manifestations have been reported with most systemic vasculidites, they occur most commonly in polyarteritis nodosa. Polyarteritis nodosa is characterized by inflammation involving medium-sized arteries often with aneurysmal dilatation. It is a necrotizing panarteritis which occurs most commonly in men in their mid-forties but can effect males or females of any age. There may be involvement of multiple organs and a lethal outcome is the rule without treatment. Pathogenesis is not completely understood but immune complexes appear to play a role. Hepatitis B surface antigen is associated with polyarteritis nodosa in 30% of cases[5] and hypersensitivity to drugs and infectious agents has also been shown.

Clinical features

Although the disease can involve any organ, the gastrointestinal tract is involved in 50% of autopsy cases. Systemic symptoms of weight loss, fever and malaise are found along with more specific gastrointestinal manifestations including abdominal pain or bleeding. Abdominal pain, often in the right upper quadrant or periumbilical area, along with diarrhoea and minor gastrointestinal bleeding occur in 30–50% of cases.[2] These complaints are frequently the presenting symptoms of polyarteritis nodosa.[6] The pain may be non-specific or may herald an abdominal catastrophe such as necrotizing enterocolitis, bowel infarction with perforation, peritonitis or shock[9,12] often with a fatal outcome. Patients may also present with cholecystitis or necrotizing pancreatitis.

Arteries of the liver are involved in 60% of cases at autopsy but clinically apparent liver disease such as cirrhosis, hepatic infarction, and intrahepatic or perihepatic bleeding, is infrequently encountered.[1]

Investigations

In the majority of patients with polyarteritis nodosa, laboratory abnormalities occur but are non-specific. They include: polymorphonuclear leukocytosis, anaemia (usually normocytic/normochromic) and an elevated erythrocyte sedimentation rate.[6] These are seen along with other indicators of acute inflammation such as thrombocytosis, elevated serum complement and hypergammaglobulinaemia. Hepatitis B surface antigen is found in 30% of patients.[5] Anti-neutrophil cytoplasmic antibody may also be detected.[4]

Definitive diagnostic procedures should be pursued in patients with suspected polyarteritis nodosa because of the high incidence of fatal outcome in untreated disease as well as the potential morbidity of the treatment itself. If there is evidence of clinical involvement, diagnosis of polyarteritis nodosa may be pursued by muscle biopsy or sural nerve biopsy.[4,14] Yield is high in carefully selected patients and there is minimal morbidity. Angiography is the diagnostic test of choice when easily accessible tissues are not clinically involved or when the main findings point towards intra-abdominal involvement. The morbidity of this test is low despite its invasive nature and in 70–80% of patients with polyarteritis nodosa, abdominal angiography which includes renal, coeliac and mesenteric arteries, will be diagnostic.[13] The most characteristic lesions are multiple aneurysms at the bifurcations of medium-sized arteries.

Pathological examination of involved arteries shows pan-mural necrotizing inflammation, often at areas of vessel bifurcation. The inflammatory infiltrate is composed predominantly of polymorphonuclear leukocytes. Aneurysmal dilatation is common.

Treatment

Treatment must be individualized depending upon the extent of disease and the organs involved. Steroids are the mainstay of therapy but, despite their use, 5-year survival has remained at about 60% since the 1960s. The usual starting dose is 60 mg prednisone or its equivalent per day in divided doses.[3] If there is life-threatening or rapidly progressive disease despite high doses of oral steroids, then pulse intravenous methylprednisolone should be used.[11] If disease control is not attained with glucocorticoids, or if disease recurs with steroid taper, addition of a cytotoxic agent should be considered. There is evidence that either cyclophosphamide or azathioprine may be efficacious in severe disease.[7,10]

References

1. Alleman, M.J.A., Janssens, A.R., Spoelstra, P. and Kroon, H.M.J.A. (1986) Spontaneous intrahepatic hemorrhages in PAN. *Annals of Internal Medicine*, **105**, 712–713.
2. Camilleri, M., Pusey, C.D., Chadwick, V.S. and Rees, A.J. (1983) Gastrointestinal manifestations of systemic vasculitis. *Quarterly Journal of Medicine*, **52**, 141–149.
3. Conn, D.L. (1990) Polyarteritis. *Rheumatic Diseases Clinics of North America*, **16**, 341–362.
4. Dahlberg, P.J., Lockhart, J.M. and Overholt, E.L. (1989) Diagnostic studies of systemic necrotizing vasculitis. *Archives of Internal Medicine*, **149**, 161–165.
5. Duffy, J., Lidsky, M.D., Sharp, J.T. *et al.* (1976) Polyarteritis nodosa and hepatitis B. *Medicine*, **56**, 255–286.
6. Fan, P.T., Davis, J.A., Somer, T., Kaplan, L. and Bluestone, R. (1980) A clinical approach to systemic vasculitis. *Seminars in Arthritis and Rheumatology*, **9**, 248–304.
7. Fauci, A.S., Katz, P., Haynes, B.F. and Wolff, S.M. (1979) Cyclophosphamide therapy of severe systemic necrotizing vasculitis. *New England Journal of Medicine*, **301**, 235–238.
8. Gilliam, J.N. and Smiley, J.D. (1976) Cutaneous necrotizing vasculitis and related disorders. *Annals of Allergy*, **37**, 328–329.
9. Karp, D.R., Kantor, O.S., Halverson, J.D. and Atkinson, J.P. (1988) Successful management of gastrointestinal involvement in PAN. *Arthritis and Rheumatism*, **31**, 683–687.
10. Leib, E.S., Restivo, C. and Paulus, H.E. (1979) Immunosuppression and corticosteroid therapy of PAN. *American Journal of Medicine*, **67**, 941–947.

11. Neild, G.H. and Lee, H.A. (1977) Methylprednisolone pulse therapy in the treatment of PAN. *Postgraduate Medical Journal*, **53**, 328–387.
12. Roikjaer, O. (1987) Perforation and necrosis of the colon complicating PAN. *Acta Chirurigica Scandinavia*, **153**, 385–386.
13. Travers, R.L., Allison, D.J., Brettle, R.P. and Hughes, G.R.V. (1979) PAN: A clinical and angiographic analysis of 17 cases. *Seminars in Arthritis and Rheumatism*, **8**, 184–199.
14. Wees, S.J., Sunwoo, I.N. and Oh, S.J. (1981) Sural nerve biopsy in systemic necrotizing vasculitis. *American Journal of Medicine*, **71**, 525–532.

CRYOGLOBULINAEMIA

Cryoglobulins are serum immunoglobulins that precipitate a low temperature. Three major types have been identified[3] on the basis of their immunoglobulin content. Type I cryoglobulins are monoclonal proteins, usually IgG or IgM. They are usually associated with lymphoproliferative diseases and account for about 25% of cryoglobulins.[3] Type II cryoglobulins are composed of a monoclonal immunoglobulin (usually IgM) that has rheumatoid factor activity, and a polyclonal immunoglobulin. They account for 15–25% of all cryoglobulins. Finally, type III cryoglobulins, which account for 50% of all cases, are composed entirely of polyclonal immunoglobulins. The IgM component has rheumatoid factor activity. Types II and III cryoglobulins are called mixed cryoglobulins and are associated with a variety of diseases including infections, inflammatory diseases (especially bacterial endocarditis) and connective tissue diseases, such as systemic lupus erythematosus, Sjögren's syndrome, rheumatoid vasculitis and polyarteritis nodosa. Essential mixed cryoglobulinaemia, in which no other major disease can be identified, is found in about 30% of patients.[4]

Clinical features

Clinical features of essential mixed cryoglobulinaemia (referred to as cryoglobulinaemia throughout) are varied but usually include recurrent palpable purpura or petechiae and arthralgia. Renal disease, often presenting as oedema and hypertension, is found in 50% of cases of cryoglobulinaemia. Most patients have liver disease[6] which in many cases is associated with hepatitis B infection. Liver involvement may be asymptomatic and pathology has ranged from minimal triaditis to chronic active hepatitis or cirrhosis.[7] Hepatomegaly and splenomegaly are seen in 50–70% of patients. The most frequent liver function test abnormality is elevated alkaline phosphatase.[4]

Gastrointestinal involvement other than liver disease is found in about 20% of patients with cryoglobulinaemia. It is usually manifested by abdominal pain which may be severe enough to require hospitalization. The mechanism of pain is not known but may be secondary to intestinal vasculitis in some patients.

Treatment

Treatment of cryoglobulinaemia should be directed at the underlying inflammatory or malignant disease if present. Treatment for patients with cryoglobulinaemia is based on the severity of disease but no controlled studies are available. Corticosteroids, cytotoxic agents and plasmapheresis have all been used with variable degrees of success.

Cryoglobulinaemia has been reported during the acute phase of hepatitis A infection with resolution as the liver disease improves.[8] Although extrahepatic features of hepatitis A are rare, there are reports of patients with arthritis and cryoglobulinaemia occurring during relapsing hepatitis A.[5] The aetiological role of cryoglobulins in hepatitis A remains unknown.

References

1. Baxter, R., Nino-Murcia, M., Bloom, R.J. and Kosek, J. (1988) Gastrointestinal manifestations of essential mixed cryoglobulinemia. *Gastrointestinal Radiology*, **13**, 180–182.
2. Case records of Massachussetts General Hospital (1984) *New England Journal of Medicine*, **311**, 904–911.
3. Brouet, J.C., Clauvel, J.P., Danon, F., Klein, M. and Seligman, M. (1974) Biologic and clinical significance of cryoglobulins: A report of 86 cases. *American Journal of Medicine*, **57**, 775–788.
4. Gorevic, P.D., Kassab, H.J., Levo, Y. *et al.* (1980) Mixed cryoglobulinemia: Clinical aspects and long term follow up of 40 patients. *American Journal of Medicine*, **69**, 287–303.
5. Inman, R.D., Hodge, M., Johnston, M.E.A., Wright, J. and Heathcote, J. (1986) Arthritis, vasculitis and cryoglobulinemia associated with relapsing hepatitis A virus infection. *Annals of Internal Medicine*, **105**, 700–703.
6. Levo, Y., Gorevic, P.D., Kassab, H.J., Tobias, H. and Franklin, E.C. (1977) Liver involvement in the syndrome of mixed cryoglobulinemia. *Annals of Internal Medicine*, **87**, 287–292.
7. Scully, R.E., Mark, E.J., McNeely, W.F. and McNeely, B.U. (Ed.) (1989) Weekly clinicopathological exercises: Mixed cryoglobulins: *New England Journal of Medicine*, **320**, 718–728.

8. Shalit, M., Wollner, S. and Levo, Y. (1982) Cryoglobulinemia in acute type A hepatitis. *Clinical Experimental Immunology*, **47**, 613–616.

RHEUMATOID ARTHRITIS

The issue of abnormal gastrointestinal mucosa in rheumatoid arthritis patients remains controversial. There is an apparent increase in gastric ulceration in patients with rheumatoid arthritis but it is not clear if this is due to the disease itself or secondary to disease therapy.

Malone *et al.*[4] evaluated hospitalized rheumatoid arthritis and osteoarthritis patients by questionnaire for peptic ulcer disease history. They questioned patients about treatment with non-steroidal anti-inflammatory drugs, aspirin, steroids, alcohol and cigarette use and defined definite peptic ulcer disease if confirmed surgically, radiologically or endoscopically. They found similar rates of peptic ulcer disease in both patient groups and concluded that the reported increase in its incidence is secondary to drug therapy.

Farah *et al.*[3] however, found an increased incidence of peptic ulcer disease in rheumatoid arthritis patients compared to non-rheumatoid arthritis controls, despite similar use of non-steroidal anti-inflammatory drugs. They compared the gastrointestinal symptoms, smoking history, use of non-steroidal anti-inflammatory drugs and endoscopic findings. The increase in peptic ulcer disease could not be accounted for by age or quantity of non-steroidal anti-inflammatory drugs used, although smoking was strongly associated with peptic ulcer disease in the rheumatoid arthritis patients. An interesting finding of this study is that peptic ulcer disease is most often asymptomatic in these patients.

Histological change of the gastric mucosa is a common finding in rheumatoid arthritis patients but is non-specific.[2] Superficial and atrophic gastritis are common findings and similar non-specific inflammatory changes are seen in the colon and rectum. These changes may also be age related. It remains unclear at this point if the changes in gut mucosa in rheumatoid arthritis cause increased susceptibility to effects of anti-inflammatory drugs.

Intestinal involvement secondary to medium vessel vasculitis may also occur in rheumatoid arthritis.[5] Visceral lesions may present with intermittent abdominal pain, bleeding or an acute abdomen secondary to perforation. Vasculitis usually occurs only in those patients with severe, erosive rheumatoid arthritis.

Juvenile chronic arthritis may be associated with splenomegaly in about 25% of cases. Although the degree of splenomegaly may be extreme it is not usually associated with Felty's syndrome (rheumatoid arthritis, neutropenia and splenomegaly). Hepatomegaly is less common but children with juvenile chronic arthritis appear to have an increased susceptibility to salicylate-induced hepatotoxicity.[1]

References

1. Athreya, B.H., Moser, G., Cecil, H.S. *et al.* (1975) Aspirin induced hepatotoxicity in juvenile rheumatoid arthritis. A prospective study. *Arthritis and Rheumatism*, **18**, 347–352.
2. Doube, A. and Collins, A.J. (1988) Editorial: Is the gut intrinsically abnormal in RA? *Annals of Rheumatic Diseases*, **47**, 617–619.
3. Farah, D., Sturrock, R.D. and Russell, R.I. (1988) Peptic ulcer in RA. *Annals of Rheumatic Diseases*, **47**, 478–480.
4. Malone, D.E., McCormick, P.A., Daly, L. *et al.* (1986) PUD in RA patients – Intrinsic or related to drug therapy? *British Journal of Rheumatology*, **25**, 342–344.
5. Schneider, H.A., Yonger, R.A., Katz, P., Longley, S. and Panush, R.S. (1985) Rheumatoid vasculitis: Experience with 13 patients and review of the literature. *Seminars in Arthritis and Rheumatism*, **14**, 280–286.

SJÖGREN'S SYNDROME

Sjögren's syndrome is a multisystem disease defined by the presence of at least two of the following criteria: keratoconjunctivitis sicca, xerostomia and a connective tissue disease, usually rheumatoid arthritis.[1] Primary Sjögren's syndrome refers to the presence of the occular and oral manifestations alone while secondary Sjögren's syndrome refers to the sicca complex associated with a connective tissue disease such as rheumatoid arthritis, systemic lupus erythematosus, polymyositis, chronic active hepatitis, primary biliary cirrhosis or progressive systemic sclerosis.

The lacrimal and salivary glands are the major target organs of primary Sjögren's syndrome but involvement of other organs such as the oesophagus, pancreas or stomach may lead to clinical symptoms.[9] The frequency of gastrointestinal manifestations of primary Sjögren's syndrome is difficult to estimate but dysphagia is thought to occur in about 30% of patients and is usually secondary to xerostomia.[4] Less commonly, the dysphagia may be secondary to abnormal motility of the oesophagus with aperistalsis or decreased amplitude of contractions in the upper oesophagus.[8]

Atrophic gastritis occurs in about 80% of patients with Sjögren's syndrome;[6] this is in marked contrast to an age-matched control population in which it occurs in 41% of subjects[10] and an age-matched rheumatoid arthritis population in which atrophic gastritis was found in 35%.[6] Gastric studies have revealed abnormal acid secretion,[2] hypopepsinogenaemia,[5] autoantibodies to parietal cells[2] and inflammatory cell infiltration in gastric mucosa.[2,3] Although serological and immunogenetic differences exist between primary and secondary Sjögren's syndrome,[7] the gastric findings are indistinguishable.[6] The severity of gastritis appears to correlate with some serological parameters such as elevated sedimentation rate, high IgA level and high SS-B antibody titre.[6] No obvious relationship has been observed between medication and histological findings in Sjögren's syndrome.

Other gastrointestinal findings in Sjögren's syndrome include hepatomegaly, chronic active hepatitis, biliary cirrhosis, acute pancreatitis and decreased pancreatic endocrine secretion. The incidence of lymphoma is increased 44-fold in Sjögren's syndrome[12] but location in the gastrointestinal tract has been rarely reported.[11]

References

1. Bloch, K.J., Buchanan, W.W., Wohl, M.J. and Bunim, J.J. (1965) Sjögren's syndrome. A clinical, pathological and serological study of sixty-two cases. *Medicine*, **44**, 187–231.
2. Buchanan, W.W., Cox, A.G., Harden, R.M., Glen, A.I.M., Andersen, J.R. and Grey, K.G. (1966) Gastric studies in Sjögren's syndrome. *Gut*, **7**, 351–354.
3. Kilpi, A., Bergroth, V., Konttinen, Y.T., Maury, C.P.J., Reitamo, S. and Wegelius, O. (1983) Lymphocyte infiltrations of the gastric mucosa in Sjögren's syndrome: An immunoperoxidase study using monoclonal antibodies in the avidin–biotin–peroxidase method. *Arthritis and Rheumatism*, **26**, 1196–1200.
4. Mason, A.M., Gumpel, J.M. and Golding, P.L. (1973) Sjögren's syndrome. A clinical review. *Seminars in Arthritis and Rheumatism*, **2**, 301–331.
5. Maury, C.P.J., Rasanen, V., Teppo, A.M., Helve, T. and Wegelius, O. (1982) Serum pepsinogen I in rheumatic disease: Reduced levels in Sjögren's syndrome. *Arthritis and Rheumatism*, **25**, 1059–1063.
6. Maury, C.P.J., Tornroth, T. and Teppo, A.M. (1985) Atrophic gastritis in Sjögren's syndrome. *Arthritis and Rheumatism*, **28**, 388–394.
7. Moutsopoulos, H.M., Chused, T.M., Mann, D.L. *et al.* (1980) Sjögren's syndrome (sicca syndrome): Current issues. *Annals of Internal Medicine*, **92**, 212–226.
8. Ramirez-Mata, M., Pena-Ancira, F.F. and Alarcon-Segovia, D. (1976) Abnormal esophageal motility in primary Sjögren's syndrome. *Journal of Rheumatology*, **3**, 63–69.
9. Shearn, M.A. (1977) Sjögren's syndrome. *Medical Clinics of North America*, **61**, 271–282.
10. Siurala, M., Isokoski, M., Varis, K. and Kekki, M. (1968) Prevalence of gastritis in a rural population: Biopsy study of subjects selected at random. *Scandinavian Journal of Gastroenterology*, **3**, 211–223.
11. Takasugi, M., Hayakawa, A., Hirakata, H., Hiyama, T., Tominaga, K. and Ibayashi, H. (1979) Gastric involvement in Sjögren's syndrome simulating early gastric carcinoma. *Endoscopy*, **11**, 263–266.
12. Talal, N., Sokoloff, L. and Barth, W.F. (1967) Extrasalivary lymphoid abnormalities in Sjögren's syndrome (reticulum cell sarcoma, 'pseudo-lymphoma', macroglobulinemia). *American Journal of Medicine*, **43**, 50–65.

HENOCH–SCHÖNLEIN PURPURA

(*H.J.F. Hodgson*)

The classic case of Henoch–Schönlein purpura is unmistakable, with a full symptom complex of palpable purpura, colicky abdominal pain, arthralgias and acute nephritis in a child or adolescent. To the gastroenterologist, diagnostic problems arise when the syndrome is incomplete, particularly if the gastrointestinal symptoms are the first manifestations. The management of the abdominal complications may also be clinically taxing.

AETIOLOGY AND PATHOGENESIS

Henoch–Schönlein purpura is the best characterized of the multisystem vasculitic disorders. From the histological appearances of the skin it is classified as a leukocytoclastic vasculitis because of the characteristic perivascular accumulation of leukocytes (polymorphonuclear leukocytes and monocytes) and nuclear fragments, around small blood vessels, particularly postcapillary venules, in the corium.[1] The histological appearances of the gut also show a vasculitis, with secondary areas of haemorrhage and oedema. The kidneys usually show a focal glomerulonephritis, with proliferation of mesangial cells within the glomerulus often being a striking feature, and occasionally a prominent necrotizing arteritis is seen affecting interlobular arteries and arterioles.

IgA has been implicated in the pathogenesis of these changes, which are commonly viewed as an inflammatory response to the deposition of IgA immune complexes in the tissues. IgA deposits can be detected by immunfluorescence in skin, gut and renal biopsies. IgA deposits can be found in both clinically affected and unaffected areas, in vessel walls in skin and intestine, and generally throughout the mesangium in the kidney. IgA levels in the blood are often increased and 70% of patients have detectable circulating IgA–immune complexes. However, as the immune complexes may contain IgA rheumatoid factors (antiglobulins) combined with IgG, and IgG deposition can also occur in vasculitic areas, IgA and IgG probably have an interrelated role.[10] Studies of the IgA subtype have attempted to determine whether the IgA immune response is likely to have arisen within the local mucosal immune system (where IgA is largely dimeric and equally divided between subclasses IgA1 and IgA2) or in the systemic immune system (where IgA is monomeric and largely of the IgA1 subclass), but consensus has not been reached.

The initiating events for the episode of Henoch–Schönlein purpura are unclear. A variety of antecedents – upper respiratory tract infection, drugs, food allergy and insect biles – has been reported, with infections reported in 80–90% of most series in children. Serological or culture evidence of streptococcal infection does not, however, have a higher incidence than in a general hospital paediatric population, although a classic pattern of recurrent attacks following streptococcal throat infections, preventable by penicillin prophylaxis, is reported in children.

CLINICAL FEATURES

The peak incidence is in children, up to the age of 15, and the onset is rare in adults. The rash – effectively by definition – is present in all patients, arthritis in 60–75% in large series, gastrointestinal involvement in 50–90%, and renal involvement in 30–50%.

The rash commences in erythematous macular lesions on extensor surfaces of the arms and legs, buttocks and over the back. They may become raised and haemorrhagic, and persist for up to 2 weeks before fading. They appear in crops and may recur over a period of weeks.

The joint involvement is a transient non-migrating polyarthritis mainly affecting ankles, knees, wrists and elbows, which resolves completely. It normally occurs at the same time as the skin rash.

The nephritis may present only with transient proteinuria or haematuria (occasionally macroscopic). Very rarely nephritis leads to rapidly progressive renal failure. Sometimes, hypertension is the only manifestation of renal involvement. Long-term minor urinary abnormalities (haematuria and proteinuria) may frequently persist for a long time, although only a small minority of patients develop chronic renal failure. This appears to be more common when the age of onset is 12 years.

Other rare manifestations of the acute episode include neurological complications such as fits, cerebral haemorrhage or cranial nerve palsy (in the absence of hypertension), pulmonary haemorrhage and carditis.

GASTROINTESTINAL MANIFESTATIONS

Clinical gut involvement occurs in one-quarter to two-thirds of affected individuals; the higher incidence is in children and young adults.[2,4] The cardinal clinical feature is colicky abdominal pain, reflecting subacute obstruction from areas of submucosal oedema and haemorrhage in the small intestine. Nausea, vomiting and diarrhoea occur in the majority of patients. Bleeding into the gastrointestinal tract can be detected by faccal testing in over three-quarters of patients, but significant haemorrhage is less common. In some series, however, between 10% and 20% of individuals experience haematemesis, melaena or rectal bleeding.[14] Areas of submucosal haemorrhage or oedema may on occasion initiate intussusception – in 6% of one series of children.[3] Perforation and infarction of the intestine can occur but rarely.[12] Vasculitic infarction on the gallbladder and pancreas may occur, adults being at greater risk.[8]

In approximately 15% of individuals, gastrointestinal disease may be the initial manifestation, without the diagnostically helpful rash or other features. The presentation as an acute abdomen at this stage understandably has frequently lead to surgical exploration.

INVESTIGATIONS

Clinical investigations may confirm the areas of vasculitis and oedema in the gastrointestinal tract. Gastritis and duodenitis are visible at endoscopy, with haemorrhage and necrosis, and either diffuse or perivascular inflammation on biopsy. Jejunal biopsies have shown diffuse villous atrophy, but are usually not clinically indicated. Barium follow-through examination may show easily recognizable 'thumb printing' areas of the oedema and haemorrhage (*Figure 8.7*) with areas of spasm, ulceration or pseudotumour, but the appearances may also be non-specific, highly reminiscent of Crohn's disease or unremarkable.[5] CT appearances of small bowel wall thickening and luminal narrowing have been reported.[11] Visceral angiography demonstrates nor-

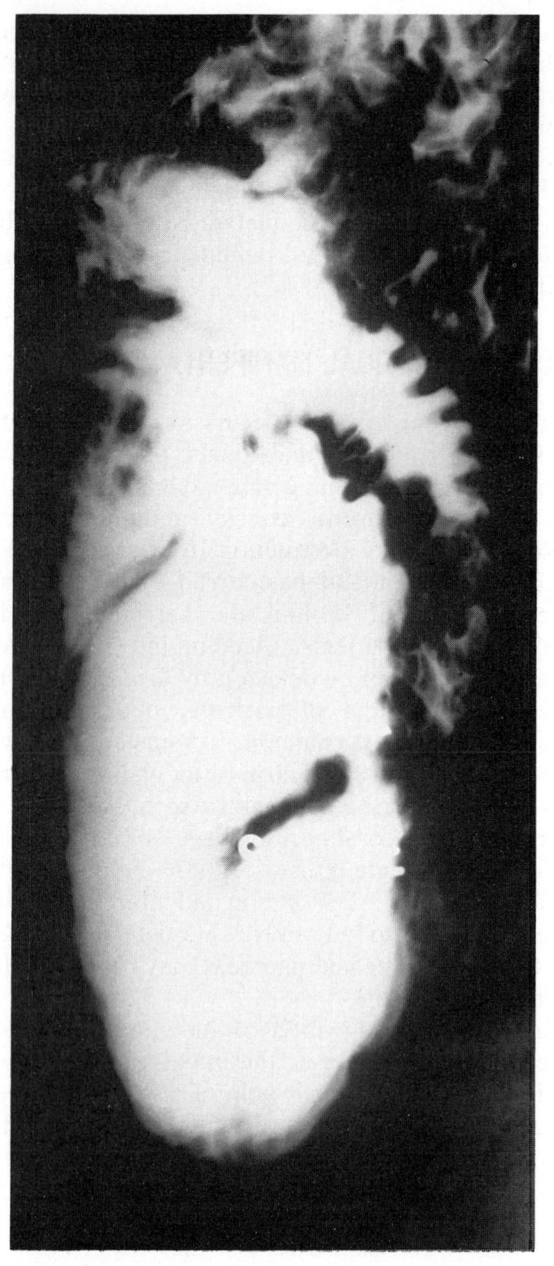

Figure 8.7 Barium follow-through examination showing terminal ileum and caecum in a case of Henoch–Schönlein purpura, with oedema and 'thumb-printing' of ileal mucosa.

mal mesenteric vessels. Hypoproteinaemia may occur reflecting a combination of both urinary protein loss and protein-losing enteropathy.

Diagnosis can usually be made on clinical grounds. The leukocyte count tends to show moderate elevation, with a normal platelet count, and a normal or elevated erythrocyte sedimentation rate. Autoantibodies and abnormalities of complement levels are usually absent. In a patient with a multisystem disease, where doubt still exists, skin biopsy showing IgA deposition may be of help and if there is renal involvement the finding of mesangial IgA deposits restricts the diagnostic possibilities to Henoch–Schönlein purpura, subacute bacterial endocarditis or systemic lupus erythematosus.

TREATMENT

No specific form of therapy has gained acceptance in Henoch–Schönlein purpura. Anecdotally, high doses of steroids appear to be of benefit in patients with severe vasculitis. However, when the main manifestations are visceral, and local abdominal signs point to severe local inflammation which is potentially a site of bowel perforation the decision to use corticosteroids is clinically taxing. A retrospective survey of the use of corticosteroids in children with Henoch–Schönlein purpura and abdominal pain suggested that these drugs, when introduced usually within 4 days of the onset of abdominal pain, resulted in relief of symptoms within 24–48 hours. Symptom relief occurred slightly later in patients not receiving steroids, but by 72 hours pain had been relieved in 75% of all patients whether or not they had received these drugs.[9] With conservative management the whole episode usually resolves within a couple of weeks to a month, although relapses are common. A prime management responsibility of the gastroenterologist is to bear in mind the possibility of perforation, intussusception or infarction as these of course would indicate surgical intervention.[7,13]

PROGNOSIS

Unlike many other vasculitic conditions Henoch–Schönlein purpura is usually a benign and self-limited disease, although there is a tendency to relapse. Importantly, the gastrointestinal involvement is reversible as healing usually occurs without fibrosis. Very rarely subsequent chronic subacute obstruction due to ileal stricture has been reported.[6,14] The major factor accounting for the morbidity and mortality of Henoch–Schönlein purpura is nephritis, but even in this group over 90% of patients survive more than 15 years.

References

1. Agha, F.P., Nostrant, T.T. and Keren, D.F. (1986) Leucocytoclastic vasculitis (hypersensitivity angiitis) of the small bowel presenting with severe gastrointestinal haemorrhage. *American Journal of Gastroenterology*, **81**, 195–198.
2. Balf, C.L. (1951) The alimentary lesions in Henoch–Schönlein purpura. *Archives of Disease in Childhood*, **26**, 20–27.
3. Brust, N.M. (1982) Ileo-ileal intussusception

associated with Henoch–Schönlein purpura. *Archives of Paediatrics*, **69**, 212–218.
4. Feldt, R.H. and Stickler, G.B. (1962) The gastrointestinal manifestations of anaphylactoid purpura in children. *Staff Meeting of Mayo Clinics*, **37**, 465–473.
5. Handle, J. and Swartz, G. (1957) Gastrointestinal manifestations of Henoch–Schönlein purpura. *American Journal of Roentgenology*, **78**, 645–652.
6. Lombard, K.A., Shah, P.C., Thrasher, T.V. and Grill, B.B. (1986) Ileal stricture as a late complication of Henoch–Schönlein purpura. *Pediatrics*, **77**, 396–398.
7. Martinez-Frontanilla, L.A., Haase, G.M. *et al.* (1984) Surgical complications in Henoch–Schönlein purpura. *Journal of Pediatric Surgery*, **19**, 434–436.
8. Puppala, A.R., Cheng, J.F. and Steinheber, F.U. (1979) Pancreatitis: a rare complication of Schönlein–Henoch purpura. *American Journal of Gastroenterology*, **69**, 101–104.
9. Rosenblum, N.D. and Winter, H.S. (1987) Steroid effects on the course of abdominal pain in children with Henoch–Schönlein purpura. *Pediatrics*, **79**, 1018–1021.
10. Saulsbury, F.T. (1987) The role of IgA_1 rheumatoid factor in the formation of IgA-containing immune complexes in Henoch–Schönlein purpura. *Journal of Clinical and Laboratory Immunology*, **23**, 123–127.
11. Siskind, B.N. Burrell, M.I., Pun, H., Russo, R. Jr and Levin, W. (1985) CT demonstration of gastrointestinal involvement in Schönlein–Henoch syndrome. *Gastrointestinal Radiology*, **10**, 352–354.
12. Smith, H.J. and Krupski, W.C. (1980) Spontaneous intestinal perforation in Henoch–Schönlein purpura. *Southern Medical Journal*, **73**, 603–610.
13. Weber, T.R., Grosfeld, J.L., Bergstein, J. *et al.* (1983) Massive gastric haemorrhage: an unusual complication of Henoch–Schönlein purpura. *Journal of Pediatric Surgery*, **18**, 576–578.
14. Young, D.G. (1964) Chronic intestinal obstruction following Henoch–Schönlein disease. *Clinical Pediatrics*, **3**, 737–740.

BEHÇET'S SYNDROME (*M. Ninkovic*)

Behçet's syndrome is a chronic, relapsing, inflammatory disorder which affects multiple organs and which may persist over many years. Its multifocal nature may require the participation of several medical specialists in its management. Although gastroenterological manifestations are well documented it is unusual for patients to present initially to this specialty. Pathological findings are nonspecific in Behçet's syndrome. Although a predominantly small vessel, non-granulomatous vasculitis is often a prominent feature; large vessel arteritis or venous thrombosis also occur.

According to Hippocrates, the characteristic clinical triad of this syndrome – oral and genital ulceration in association with a chronic inflammation of the eye – was endemic in Ancient Greece.[14] Behçet identified the condition in 1937. Current knowledge suggests that an as yet unidentified virus may be the trigger for the development of this clinical syndrome in genetically susceptible individuals, although its aetiology and subsequent pathogenesis are still obscure.

EPIDEMIOLOGY AND GENETICS

There is a striking geographical variation in the incidence of Behçet's syndrome.[29] It is most common in Japan with a prevalence of 1 in 10 000; The Middle East, Greece, Turkey, Italy and Israel also have a relatively common prevalence. The syndrome is rare in the United Kingdom (prevalence 1 in 170 000)[8] and even rarer in the USA (prevalence 1 in 800 000).[33]

Behçet's syndrome may develop at any age but the most common onset is in the third decade. There is a male predominance which varies from 2:1 in Japan to 9:1 in the Middle East. An increased familial prevalence of the syndrome is well documented although rare, and this does not comply with any obvious inheritance pattern. There is also an increased incidence of simple oral ulceration in consanguineous relatives of patients with the syndrome.[25]

Behçet's syndrome is associated with the histocompatibility locus antigen HLA-B5 (particularly the HLA-BW51 subset)[7] for Japanese, Turkish, Israeli and French patients but not for British or Americans.[25] The association is strongest in Turkey with 84% of Behçet's syndrome patients being HLA-B5 positive, as compared to only 27% of controls. Conversely, if a Turkish individual is HLA-B5 positive they have a twentyfold increased relative risk of developing the syndrome. In Japan there is a sevenfold increased risk.

Among British patients there was no significantly increased frequency of HLA-B5 overall compared to controls. In contrast, HLA-B27 and B12 were more frequent.[26] Analysis of clinical subsets showed a significant relationship between HLS-B5 and the 'ocular type' of Behçet's syndrome, whilst HLA-B27 was most common in the 'arthritis type', and HLA-B12 in the 'mucocutaneous type'. The spectrum of organs involved in Behçet's syndrome may therefore be determined by factors residing in the HLA locus of individual patients, and HLA markers may be useful in aiding diagnosis.

AETIOLOGY

Since the time of Behçet himself, infection has been considered as an aetiological factor in provoking the syndrome. However, no infectious agent has been isolated and attempts to pass it to experimental animals have been unsuccessful. The HLA associations may indicate that an abnormal immunological response to a commonly encountered infective agent may be important.

As orogenital ulceration is the most usual manifestation of Behçet's syndrome the potential role of herpes simplex viruses has been considered. The virus has not been demonstrated in lesions and there are no raised antibody titres in serum. However, in some patients part of the herpes simplex viral genome is transcribed in peripheral blood mononuclear cells,[13] and lymphocytes from patients do not permit replication of the virus in a cultured system which may imply viral infection in these cells.[10] This effect is not, however, specific to Behçet's syndrome.

Further infective possibilities considered have included bacteria, in particular streptococci, which are implicated because of the high incidence in Behçet's syndrome in those suffering childhood tonsillitis and tonsillectomy.[9] In a proportion of patients it is possible to induce a clinical relapse following a streptococcal antigen skin-prick test.[29] However, the evidence for streptococcal involvement in the aetiology of Behçet's syndrome is inconclusive.

PATHOLOGY

The pathological hallmark of the disease is small vessel vasculitis, although this is not always convincing in mucocutaneous lesions. These show lymphocytic invasion of the prickle cell layer of the epidermis and often invasion of dermal vessels. Occasionally necrotizing vasculitis is seen. Frank vasculitis is more commonly seen in genital ulcers and in subcutaneous small vessels.

CLINICAL FEATURES

In addition to Behçet's original triad of oral ulceration, genital ulceration and uveitis, many other additional features of the syndrome are now recognized. These include synovitis, skin lesions, meningoencephalitis, phlebitis and arteritis.[24,34] Patients may present to the gastroenterologist with discrete ulceration of the gastrointestinal tract or with Budd–Chiari syndrome. Diagnosis is often delayed as key clinical features appear asynchronously and can present many years after the first clinical sign which is usually oral ulceration. The most serious complications are uveitis, meningoencephalitis and large vessel disease. There are no pathognomonic, pathological or serological tests and the diagnosis therefore remains entirely clinical (*Table 8.1*).

Table 8.1 Frequency of major end organ lesions in Behçet's syndrome[34]

Lesion or involvement	*Percentage*
Aphthous stomatitis	100
Genital ulcerations	75
Uveitis	60–80
Synovitis	50
Cutaneous lesions	56
Central nervous system	10–30
Major vessel occlusions or aneurysms	10–37

In 1969, Mason and Barnes[27] first suggested a series of diagnostic criteria which should be satisfied before a diagnosis of Behçet's syndrome could be made:

1. *Major criteria*
   Buccal ulceration
   Genital ulceration
   Eye lesions
   Skin lesions
2. *Minor criteria*
   Gastrointestinal lesions
   Thrombophlebitis
   Cardiovascular lesions
   Arthritis
   Central nervous system lesions
   Family history

Three major or two major and two minor criteria are required for diagnosis.

However, since then different groups of clinicians have devised further lists of criteria.[3,32] This has hampered international comparisons of the syndrome and has hindered the interpretation of therapeutic trials. The International Study Group for Behçet's Disease has devised a rational set of criteria[18] which appear to have diagnostic specificity and are to be universally used (*Table 8.2*).

Oral ulceration

Recurrent oral aphthous ulceration forms the cornerstone in the diagnosis of Behçet's syndrome and is commonly the earliest manifestation.[23] Ulceration occurs on the buccal mucosa, lips, tongue and pharynx, but can be found anywhere in the intestinal tract. Ulcers are usually multiple, painful and occur

Table 8.2 International Study Group (ISG) for Behçet's Disease:[18] Criteria for diagnosis (findings applicable only in absence of other clinical explanations)

Recurrent oral ulceration	Minor aphthous, major aphthous, or herpetiform ulceration observed by physician or patient which recurred at least three times in one 12-month period
Plus any two of:	
Recurrent genital ulceration	Aphthous ulceration or scarring observed by physician or patient
Eye lesions	Anterior uveitis, posterior uveitis or cells in vitreous on slit-lamp examination; or retinal vasculitis observed by ophthalmologist
Skin lesions	Erythema observed by physician or patient, pseudofolliculitis or papulopustular lesions or acneiform nodules observed by physician in post-adolescent patients not on corticosteroid treatment
Positive pathergy test	Read by physician at 24–48 hours

in crops with healing occurring over 3–30 days. The ulcers heal without scarring.

Genital ulceration

Recurrent multiple ulcers occur in the vagina, cervix and vulva of female patients and on the scrotum or penis in male patients. These resemble oral ulcers and are usually painful but may be asymptomatic and, therefore, missed.

Ocular disease

Ocular involvement in Behçet's syndrome is a serious problem in Japan and Turkey where it is one of the most common causes of blindness. It is a much less common cause of blindness in the UK (0.3% of new patients with uveitis).[11] Relapsing anterior uveitis with hypopyon and retinal vascular lesions occurs with both eyes eventually involved in 90% of cases, and useful vision lost in half of these over 4 years.[11] Uveitis is seldom the presenting feature and may occur years after the first manifestation. Fluorescein angiography may be used to detect early vascular retinal lesions. If left untreated, or treated solely with corticosteroids, retinal infarcts progress to blindness, with other late features including cataracts, secondary glaucoma and optic atrophy.

Skin involvement

Skin lesions in Behçet's syndrome are varied and include acneiform pustules, nodules or pseudofolliculitis on the trunk and arms. Erythema nodosum and superficial thrombophlebitis are also found and are all considered to be non-specific manifestations of cutaneous vasculitis. Skin sensitivity to simple trauma, such as a needle-stick injury, occurs in Behçet's syndrome (Behçetin reaction, or pathergy test).[49] It forms part of the International Study Group's criteria for diagnosis. A positive test produces a 3–10 mm nodule or pustule when read 24–48 h after the oblique insertion of a gauge 20 or smaller needle under sterile conditions. The test has a 60% sensitivity but 90% specificity for the syndrome.[18] It is present in up to 75% of Japanese and Turkish patients but is less common in North Americans and north European patients.[51]

Synovitis

Subacute or chronic synovitis is experienced in 50–60% of patients. There is characteristically a non-erosive, seronegative mono- or oligoarthritis which commonly affects the knees and ankles.[34] Sacro-iliitis is rare and thus contrasts Behçet's syndrome with the enteropathic arthritis, which is normally erosive and axial. Patients with features of Behçet's syndrome in combination with relapsing polychondritis have been described.[15]

Neurological involvement

Neurological complications occur in 10–30% of patients and the mean interval of onset of Behçet's syndrome to CNS involvement is 1.3 years. Patients may develop meningoencephalitis, the neurological deficits including brain-stem, cerebellar or cortico-spinal tract signs.[44] Intracranial venous sinus thromboses can occur. Cerebrospinal fluid typically shows a lymphocytosis in association with a mild elevation of protein but no oligoclonal bands. Although early reports of CNS involvement indicated a grave prognosis, it is now possible to arrest and prevent recurrence with immunosuppressants.[36]

Venous and arterial involvement

Venous abnormalities include superficial thrombophlebitis, deep vein thrombosis, superior and inferior vena caval obstruction, which may not be prevented by anticoagulation.[35] This is not surprising when considering that histological examination often reveals vasculitis. Venous occlusion can produce the Budd–Chiari syndrome (see below).

Large vessel arteritis may rarely produce acute myocardial infarction, fatal limb ischaemia, stroke and renovascular disease. Behçet's syndrome stands apart from other vasculitides by being associated with multiple pulmonary artery aneurysms which may present with massive haemoptysis.[40] Pulmonary angiography is needed to differentiate this cause of haemoptysis from pulmonary embolism, as anticoagulation is contradicted if pulmonary aneurysms exist.

Other organs

Renal involvement is rare but may be manifest as glomerulonephritis or amyloidosis.[50] Other abnormalities attributed to Behçet's syndrome have been described in many organs but are extremely rare.

Gastroenterological manifestations

The incidence of gastrointestinal morbidity in Behçet's syndrome is variable. It is much more common in Japan than in the West.[5] The usual pattern is of colonic or ileal ulcers which develop after several years of recurrent oral ulceration. They may manifest themselves acutely as intestinal perforation or massive haemorrhage or in a more protracted course with bloody diarrhoea and malaise.

Several general points can be made. Gastrointestinal manifestations can occur in any patient with Behçet's syndrome irrespective of clinical severity or disease spectrum. Gastrointestinal problems, even if not the predominant manifestation of this condition, can be a significant cause of mortality, particularly in patients with intestinal perforation or massive haemorrhage secondary to small bowel ulceration. It may be difficult to differentiate gastrointestinal Behçet's syndrome from inflammatory bowel disease which clearly may be complicated by uveitis, arthralgia, oral ulceration and skin rashes.

Although gastrointestinal manifestations of Behçet's syndrome may be difficult to separate from inflammatory bowel disease, several discriminating features do exist (*Table 8.3*).

In an epidemiological survey in Japan nearly 10% of 3000 patients with Behçet's syndrome had evidence of gastrointestinal lesions,[2] mostly discrete ulceration of the ileocaecal region, although ulceration of any part from the oesophagus to the rectum may occur.[30] Up to 75% of patients in one Japanese study reported abdominal symptoms of pain, diarrhoea, vomiting or flatulence.[47] By contrast Israeli patients rarely develop gastrointestinal problems.[6]

Mason and Barnes[27] reviewed patients in the UK and found that of a total of 33 patients three had duodenal ulceration and one had 'classic ulcerative colitis', no patients having ileocaecal ulceration. Sladen and Lehner[48] found only 1 patient from a total of 70 with small intestinal ulceration, 2 patients with rectal ulceration and two with anal ulcers or

Table 8.3 Comparison of gastrointestinal involvement in Behçet's syndrome and Crohn's disease

	Behçet's disease	*Crohn's disease*
Site of involvement		
Predominant site	Variable, often right-sided or discontinuous	Variable, often right-sided or discontinuous
Total colon involvement	Occasional	Uncommon
Rectal involvement	About 50% in Western World Rare in Japan	About 50% in Western World
Anal involvement	Occasional	Common
Terminal ileal involvement	Sometimes	Common
Histology		
Granulomata	Uncommon	Common
Vasculitis	Occasional lymphocytic venulitis	Rare granulomatous vasculitis
Transmural lymphoid aggregates	Uncommon	Usual
Extraintestinal features		
Oral ulcers	Usual	Occasional
Genital ulcers	Usual	Rare

Adapted from Lee.[22]

fistulation. They also reported a single patient with associated coeliac disease. Other reports in the Western literature document universal or left-sided colitis with features often indistinguishable from ulcerative colitis, or clinical and histological findings resembling a granulomatous colitis.[31] Western patients with Behçet's syndrome may indeed have a different spectrum of gastrointestinal manifestations to Japanese patients, but it may be that in the West such patients are more like to be classified as having inflammatory bowel disease with extra-intestinal manifestations resembling Behçet's syndrome.

Kasahara *et al.*[20] reviewed over 100 cases of gastrointestinal ulceration in surgical patients with Behçet's syndrome. Overall, less than 1% of all patients with Behçet's syndrome require intestinal surgery, and the interval between diagnosis and laparotomy was extremely variable ranging from a month to up to 30 years. Features that led to laparotomy included pain mimicking appendicitis, intestinal perforation, fistulation or haemorrhage. They described two patterns of ulceration: a localized pattern and a diffuse pattern. In the localized group ulcers were found to involve the terminal ileum, ileocaecal region or caecum in 76% of cases, with less frequent ulceration being found in other areas including the stomach, duodenum and colon. As compared to Crohn's disease, there is less inflammation surrounding localized ulcers and they penetrate deeply to the serosa. Less than 20% of cases showed diffuse involvement with ulceration affecting almost the entire colon in a proportion. Over three-quarters of cases had multiple ulceration. Fistulation, usually rectovaginal, and perianal ulcers are occasionally seen.

Histological examination of gastrointestinal ulceration shows no specific diagnostic features.[2,22] Macroscopically, ulceration can be variable ranging from shallow superficial ulcers to deep ulcers that perforate the serosa. Shallow ulcers may extend laterally into the submucosa, forming a 'collar-button' profile.[22] Ulcers are frequently multiple and there may be swelling around ulcer margins. Inflammation is transmural and may extend to the serosal surface, although there are no transmural lymphoid aggregates. The surrounding intestinal mucosa is usually normal and there are usually no granulomata. A vasculitis with perivascular mononuclear infiltration, often a venulitis with thrombosis of vessels around the ulcer, may be seen, but is not a consistent finding, and whether vasculitis is primary or secondary is subject to debate. Fibrinoid necrosis consistent with vasculitis may be seen.[2]

Marked lymphangiectasia has been reported in jejunal biopsies of 4 of 15 Japanese patients with Behçet's syndrome who otherwise had no associated protein-losing enteropathy or malabsorption.[1]

Radiological investigation of gastrointestinal Behçet's syndrome illustrates the variable spectrum of disease with evidence of punched-out colonic and ileal ulcers, mucosal irregularity and ileal narrowing with fistula formation. Ulcers tend to be deeper than in Crohn's disease. Barium enema may show skip lesions with haustral preservation in a pattern that may resemble Crohn's disease. In addition, radiology of the small bowel may show dilated loops with flocculation of barium and strictures.[38] Radioactively labelled white cell scans may be useful in defining intestinal activity.[21]

Colonoscopic examination again generally demonstrates discrete ulceration with normal surrounding mucosa which may resemble peptic ulceration in appearance;[22,41] occasionally an ulcerative colitis type of picture may be seen.

Management has been, in the main, surgical with the suggestion that at least 1 metre of intestine be resected at the time of surgery in order to attempt the prevention of recurrent ulceration and subsequent complications.[20] However, prognosis is not always favourable with 10% of deaths associated with resection. Recurrence rates of up to 65% over a 6-month period are reported with ulceration or fistulation occurring at the site of the anastomosis. No comparative trials of medical therapy in Behçet's syndrome enteritis exists. Systemic steroids are useful but may predispose to silent perforation. Sulphasalazine has been used on an empirical basis to some effect.[42]

Hepatic disease

Although major blood vessel occlusion occurs in up to one-third of Behçet's syndrome patients (see *Table 8.1*), hepatic vein thrombosis or Budd–Chiari syndrome is an uncommon but well-documented manifestation.[4] Hepatic vein thrombosis in Behçet's syndrome is said to have several distinctive features when compared to that occurring in the context of, for example, primary myeloproliferative disorders. It predominantly affects male patients (male:female 19:1) and is more often fatal due to early hepatic failure (25%). Furthermore, in 90% of cases it was found to be associated with inferior vena caval thrombosis which may be the site of initial thrombosis that then extends to the hepatic veins.

INVESTIGATIONS

Serum levels of the acute phase reactants, C-reactive protein and α_1-antitrypsin increase during disease activity, along with the erythrocyte sedimentation rate. Circulating immune complexes are found in 40–60% of patients and IgA levels are often elevated.[24] Serum complement levels are usually normal or elevated, although they have been reported to fall preceding an attack of uveitis, suggesting complement consumption.[46] In addition, histochemistry has shown immunoglobulin and complement deposition in blood vessel walls. Autoantibodies are generally not detected although anticardiolipin antibodies are found in 15–35% of patients.[12] There is evidence of abnormal cell-mediated immunity with cytophilic IgA bound to CD4 and CD8 T cells which may affect their function.[16]

In view of the thrombotic tendency seen in Behçet's syndrome, many studies have focused on the possibility of abnormal fibrinolysis. Protein C and antithrombin III levels are normal but, in the acute phase, there may be reduced plasma fibrinolysis, or a defective release of tissue plasminogen activator.[19]

TREATMENT

Multidisciplinary approaches are needed in the management of patients with Behçet's syndrome with perhaps ophthalmological, rheumatological and neurological participation. A variety of topical and systemic drugs have been used (*Table 8.4*). Large multicentre trials comparing various therapies have in general not been performed and treatment advice stems largely from extrapolation of results of smaller studies. In most patients the disease runs a chronic indolent course with high morbidity but low mortality. In Japanese patients there is a 3–4% associated mortality, with death precipitated by vascular, neurological or intestinal complications.[47]

Table 8.4 Drug treatments in Behçet's syndrome

Corticosteroids	Tropical and systemic
Cytotoxic drugs	Azathioprine
	Chlorambucil
	Cyclophosphamide
Cyclosporin	
Colchicine	
Anticoagulation	Heparin/warfarin
	aspirin
Others	Dapsone
	Thalidomide
	5-Aminosalicylic acid
	Sulphasalazine
	Plasma exchange
	Interferon-γ

Traditionally, mucocutaneous lesions have been treated with topical steroids. Oral colchicine (0.6 mg three times daily) is also useful. Further treatments have included topical 5-aminosalicylic acid,[39] oral dapsone[45] or thalidomide.[17] High-dose corticosteroid therapy (up to 60 mg oral prednisolone daily) is effective in suppressing mucosal, skin and joint inflammation but has only a palliative effect on uveitis or neurological manifestations. It is clear that steroids alone do not, therefore, prevent blindness from uveitis or recurrence of meningoencephalitis. Patients with more severe disease have been treated with oral prednisolone in various combinations with immunosuppressants, such as azathioprine,[52] cyclosporin,[28] cyclophosphamide or chlorambucil.[37]

Although cytotoxic drugs are indicated for the treatment of the serious complications of ophthalmic or neuro-Behçet's syndrome, they are rarely indicated for the other complications of the syndrome, apart from large vessel arteritis. Currently there is little consensus as to the treatment of major venous or arterial disease, although large vessel arteritis necessitates immunosuppression with steroids and cytotoxic agents. Anticoagulants and aspirin are also given but should be avoided when pulmonary arteritis is present because of the risk of catastrophic haemorrhage from pulmonary artery aneurysmal rupture.[35]

References

1. Asakura, H., Morita, A., Morishita, T. *et al.* (1973) Histopathological and electron microscopic studies of lymphangiectasia of the small intestine in Behçet's disease. *Gut*, **14**, 196–203.
2. Baba, S., Maruta, M., Ando, K. *et al.* (1976) Intestinal Behçet's disease: report of five cases. *Disease of the Colon and Rectum*, **19**, 428–440.
3. Behçet's Disease Research Committee of Japan. (1974) Behçet's disease: guide to diagnosis of Behçet's disease. *Japanese Journal of Ophthalmology*, **18**, 291–294.
4. Bismuth, E., Hadengue, A., Hammel, P. *et al.* (1990) Hepatic vein thrombosis in Behçet's disease. *Hepatology*, **11**, 969–974.
5. Boe, J., Dalgaard, J.D. and Scott, D. (1958) Mucocutaneous – ocular syndrome with intestinal involvement. *American Journal of Medicine*, **25**, 857–867.
6. Chajek, T. and Fainaru, M. (1975) Behçet's disease. Report of 41 cases and a review of the literature. *Medicine*, **54**, 179–196.

7. Chajek, T. (1987) HLA-B51 may serve as an immunogenetic marker for a subgroup of patients with Behçet's syndrome. *American Journal of Medicine*, **83**, 666–671.
8. Chamberlain, M.A. (1977) Behçet's syndrome in 32 patients in Yorkshire. *Annals of the Rheumatic Diseases*, **36**, 491–499.
9. Cooper, C., Pipperard, E.C., Sharp, H., Wickham, C., Chamberlain, M.A. and Barker, D.J.P. (1989) Individual risk factors for Behçet's disease. *Annals of Rheumatic Disease*, **48**, 421–423.
10. Denman, A.M., Fialkow, P.J. and Pelton, B.K. (1980) Lymphocyte abnormalities in Behçet's syndrome. *Clinical Experimental Immunology*, **42**, 175–185.
11. Dinning, W. (1979) Behçet's disease and the eye: epidemiological considerations. In *Behçet's syndrome: Clinical and Immunological Features*, pp. 179–189. (Ed.) Lehner, T. and Barnes, C.G. New York, London: Academic Press.
12. Efthimiou, J. (1985) Negative anticardiolipin antibodies and vascular complications in Behçet's syndrome. *Annals of Rheumatology*, **44**, 425–726.
13. Eglin, R.P., Lehner, T. and Subak-Sharpe, J.H. (1982) Detection of RNA complementary to Herpes-Simplex virus in mononuclear cells from patients with Behçet's syndrome and recurrent oral ulcers. *The Lancet*, **2**, 1356–1361.
14. Feigenbaum, A. (1956) Description of Behçet's syndrome in the Hippocratic third book of endemic diseases. *British Journal of Ophthalmology*, **40**, 355–357.
15. Firestein, G.S., Gruber, H.E., Weisman, M.H., Zvaifler, N.J., Barber, J. and O'Duffy, J.D. (1985) Mouth and genital ulcers with inflamed cartilage: MAGIC syndrome. Five patients with features of relapsing polychondritis and Behçet's disease. *American Journal of Medicine*, **79**, 65.
16. Fortune, F., Walker, J. and Lehner, T. (1990) The expression of gamma delta T cell receptor and the prevalence of primed, activated and IgA-bound T cells in Behçet's syndrome. *Clinical and Experimental Immunology*, **82**, 326–332.
17. Hamza, M. (1990) Behçet's disease, palmoplantar pustulosis and HLA-B27 treatment with thalidomide. *Clinical Experimental Rheumatology*, **8**, 427.
18. International Study Group for Behçet's disease (1990) Criteria for diagnosis of Behçet's disease. *The Lancet*, **335**, 1078–1080.
19. Jordan, J.M., Allen, N.B. and Pizzo, S.V. (1987) Defective release of tissue plasminogen activator in systemic and cutaneous vasculitis. *American Journal of Medicine*, **82**, 397–400.
20. Kasahara, Y., Tanaka, S., Nishino, M. *et al.* (1981) Intestinal involvement in Behçet's disease: review of 136 surgical cases in the Japanese literature. *Diseases of the Colon and Rectum*, **24**, 103–106.
21. Keshavarzian, A., Saverymuttu, S.H., Chadwick, V.S. *et al.* (1984) Noninvasive investigation of the gastrointestinal tract in collagen-vascular disease. *American Journal of Gastroenterology*, **79**, 873–877.
22. Lee, R.G. (1986) The colitis of Behçet's syndrome. *The American Journal of Surgical Pathology*, **10**, 888–893.
23. Lehner, T. (1977) Oral ulceration and Behçet's syndrome. *Gut*, **18**, 491–511.
24. Lehner, T. (1986) Behçet's syndrome. In *The Oxford Textbook of Medicine*, pp. 24.13–24.15. (Ed.) Weatherall, D.J., Ledingham, J.G.G. and Warrell, D.A. Oxford: Oxford Medical Publications.
25. Lehner, T. and Barnes, C.G. (1979) Criteria for diagnosis and classification of Behçet's syndrome. In *Behçet's syndrome: Clinical and Immunological Features*, pp. 1–9. (Ed.) Lehner, T. and Barnes, C.G. New York, London: Academic Press.
26. Lehner, T. and Batchelor, J.R. (1979) Classification and an immunogenetic basis of Behçet's syndrome. In *Behçet's syndrome: Clinical and Immunological Features*, pp. 13–32. (Ed.) Lehner, T. and Barnes, C.G. New York, London: Academic Press.
27. Mason, R.M. and Barnes, C.G. (1969) Behçet's syndrome with arthritis. *Annals of the Rheumatic Diseases*, **28**, 95–103.
28. Masuda, K., Nakajima, A., Urayama, A. *et al.* (1989) Double-masked trial of cyclosporin versus colchicine and long-term open study of cyclosporin in Behçet's disease. *The Lancet*, **2**, 1093–1096.
29. Mizushima, Y. (1989) Skin hypersensitivity to streptococcal antigens and the induction of systemic symptoms by the antigens in Behçet's disease – A multicenter study. *Journal of Rheumatology*, **16**, 506.
30. Mori, S., Yoshihira, A., Kawamura, H. *et al.* (1983) Esophageal involvement in Behçet's disease. *American Journal of Gastroenterology*, **78**, 548–553.
31. Nilsen, K.H., Jones, S.M. and Shorey, B.A. (1977) Behçet's syndrome with perforation of the colon. *Postgraduate Medical Journal*, **53**, 108–110.
32. O'Duffy, J.D. (1974) Suggested criteria for diagnosis of Behçet's disease. *Journal of Rheumatology*, **1** (suppl. 1), 18.
33. O'Duffy, J.D. (1978) Summary of international symposium on Behçet's disease. *Journal of Rheumatology*, **5**, 229–233.
34. O'Duffy, J.D. (1989) Behçet's disease. In *Textbook of Rheumatology*, pp. 1209–1214. (Ed.) Kelley, W.N., Harris, E.D., Ruddy, S. and Sledge, C.B. Philadelphia: W.B. Saunders.
35. O'Duffy, J.D. (1990) Vasculitis in Behçet's disease. *Rheumatic Diseases Clinics of North America*, **16**, 423–430.
36. O'Duffy, J.D. and Goldstein, N.P. (1976) Neurological involvement in seven patients with Behçet's disease. *American Journal of Medicine*, **61**, 170–178.
37. O'Duffy, J.D., Robertson, D.M. and Goldstein, N.P. (1984) Chlorambucil in the treatment of

uveitis and meningoencephalitis of Behçet's disease. *American Journal of Medicine*, **77**, 75–84.
38. Oshima, Y., Shimizu, T., Yokohari, R. *et al.* (1963) Clinical studies on Behçet's syndrome. *Annals of Rheumatological Disease*, **22**, 36–45.
39. Ranzi, T., Campanini, M. and Bianchi, P.A. (1989) Successful treatment of genital and oral ulcers in Behçet's disease, with topical 5-aminosalicylic acid (5-ASA). *British Journal of Dermatology*, **120**, 471–472.
40. Raz, I., Okon, E. and Chajek-Shaul, T. (1989) Pulmonary manifestations in Behçet's syndrome. *Chest*, **95**, 585–589.
41. Reuben, A., Russell Jones, R. and Lovell, D. (1980) Behçet's syndrome with colonic involvement and arterial thrombosis. *Journal of the Royal Society of Medicine*, **73**, 520–524.
42. Sawyer, A., Walker, T.M. and Teery, S.I. (1978) Behçet's syndrome with ileal involvement – the beneficial effect of sulphasalazine. *West Indian Medical Journal*, **28**, 218–221.
43. Sayek, I., Aran, O., Uzunalimoglu, B. *et al.* (1991) Intestinal Behçet's Disease: Surgical experience in seven cases. *Hepato-gastroenterology*, **38**, 81–83.
44. Shakir, R.A., Sulamain, K., Kahn, R.A. and Rudwan, M. (1990) Neurological presentation of neuro-Behçet's syndrome: clinical categories. *European Neurology*, **30**, 249–253.
45. Sharquie, K.E. (1984) Suppression of Behçet's disease with dapsone. *British Journal of Dermatology*, **110**, 493–494.
46. Shimada, K., Kogura, M., Kawashima, T. and Nishioka, K. (1974) Reduction of complement in Behçet's disease and drug allergy. *Medical Biology*, **52**, 234–239.
47. Shimuzu, T., Ehrlich, G.E., Inaba, K. and Hayashi, K. (1979) Behçet's disease (Behçet's syndrome). *Seminars in Arthritis and Rheumatism*, **8**, 223–260.
48. Sladen, G.E. and Lehner, T. (1979) Gastro-intestinal disorders in Behçet's syndrome and a comparison with recurrent oral ulcers. In *Behçet's Syndrome: Clinical and Immunological Features*, pp. 151–158. (Ed.) Lehner, T. and Barnes, C.G. New York, London: Academic Press.
49. Sobel, J.D., Haim, S., Shafrir, A. and Gellei, B. (1973) Cutaneous hyperreactivity in Behçet's disease. *Dermatologica*, **146**, 350–356.
50. Tasdemir, I., Sivri, B., Turgan, C., Emri, S., Yasavul, U. and Caglar, S. (1989) The expanding spectrum of a disease: Behçet's disease associated with amyloidisis. *Nephron*, **52**, 154–157.
51. Yazici, H., Chamberlain, M.A., Tuzan, Y. and Muftuolu, A. (1984) A comparative study of the pathergy reaction among Turkish and British patients with Behçet's disease. *Annals of Rheumatic Disease*, **43**, 74–75.
52. Yazici, H., Pazarli, H., Barnes, C.G. *et al.* (1990) A controlled trial of azathioprine in Behçet's syndrome. *The Lancet*, **322**, 281–285.

MISCELLANEOUS VASCULITIC AND OTHER CONDITIONS *(H.J.F. Hodgson)*

GIANT CELL (TEMPORAL) ARTERITIS

This is a systemic vasculitis best known for its ability to cause blindness following involvement of the ophthalmic arteries with a granulomatous vasculitis, usually but not invariably associated with an elevated erythrocyte sedimentation rate. On rare occasions this can clinically affect intra-abdominal vessels.[10] Chronic abdominal pain due to ischaemia may result, although this is difficult to substantiate. More definitively, the presentation of gut involvement may be as an abdominal emergency due to gut infarction.[17,21] The prognosis in giant cell arteritis adequately treated with corticosteroids is good.[2]

VASCULITIS SECONDARY TO GASTROINTESTINAL DISEASE

Coeliac disease,[1,4,19] ulcerative colitis[22] and Crohn's disease[5] have all been reported as associated with a systemic vasculitis, associated in some cases with cryoglobulinaemia.

COARCTATION OF THE AORTA

After surgical relief of coarctation of the aorta, older series reported the not infrequent development of abdominal symptoms within a few days. The clinical picture varied from mild, with some abdominal pain and distension, to a full-blown intestinal infarction.[20] This was attributed to the response of the visceral vessels to the sudden increase in perfusion pressure, resulting in dilatation, perivascular inflammation and arteriolar thrombosis. This is now infrequent, and current thought suggests that these are delayed manifestations of gut ischaemia incurred during cross-clamping of the aorta, and avoided by temporary bypass. Should it occur, and surgery not be required, medical management includes resting the gut and control of hypertension.

MALIGNANT ATROPHIC PAPULOSIS (KÖHLMEIER–DEGOS DISEASE)[6]

This is a rare but recognizable condition in which a small vessel vasculitis involves the skin and gut. Most patients are young men, only a quarter being female. One pair of affected relatives (mother–son) suggests a genetic basis, but the aetiology is unknown. The characteristic presentation is with scattered skin lesions, initially pink papules but evolving a characteristic 'porcelain-like' area of grey–white atrophy centrally. Lesions are from a few millimetres to 15 cm in diameter. The gut vasculitis is predominantly submucosal, and ischaemia and fibrosis lead to episodes of abdominal cramp and diarrhoea.[24] Involvement of the retroperitoneum may lead to chylous ascites from lymphatic obstruction and leakage. Half the reported cases have died within 3 years of presentation, usually after perforation through a subserosal fibrotic plaque; both more rapid and more indolent evolution of the disease may occur. Vessels elsewhere, notably in the brain, may also be involved.

TAKAYUSU'S ARTERITIS

This chronic aortitis is best recognized in the Orient, particularly in young women, but occurs sporadically world wide.[9,15] 'Pulseless disease' epitomizes one major sign, reflecting both obliteration and ectasia of the aorta and its main branches.[12] Although the disease may be confined to the aortic arch (type 1), the descending aorta may be involved instead (type 2) or in addition (type 3). Although the involvement of retinal and renal vessels, and the aortic root, often dominates symptomatology, gastrointestinal symptoms may occur reflecting involvement of the coeliac or mesenteric vessels (*Figures 8.8* and *8.9*).[13] Abdominal as well as other bruits are common. The slow progression of the inflammation usually means that collateral supply is developed, and gastrointestinal symptoms are more likely to be intermittent pain rather than the acute emergency of intestinal infarction.

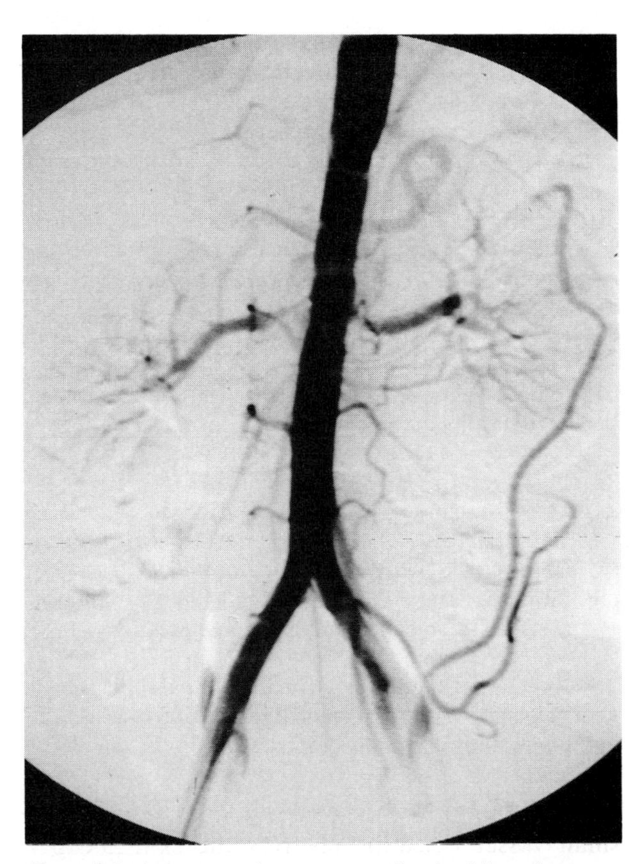

Figure 8.8 Anteroposterior aortogram showing bilateral stenoses of renal arteries, with delayed filling of the superior mesenteric artery and collateral filling from the inferior mesenteric artery.

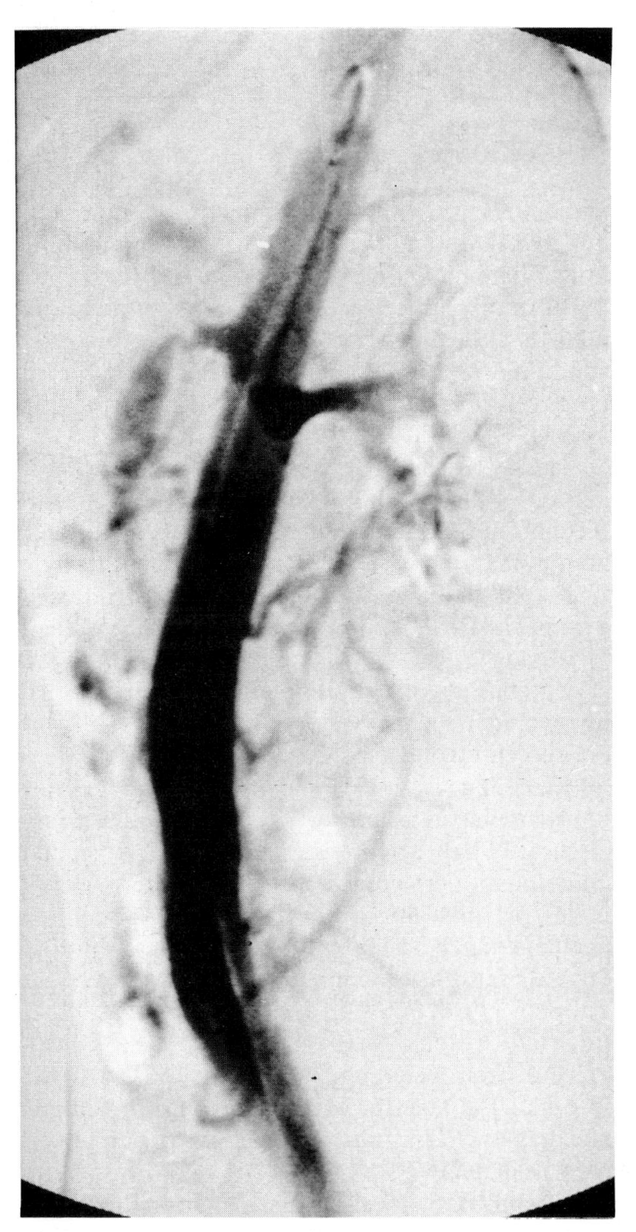

Figure 8.9 Lateral aortogram showing stenosis with poststenotic dilatation of the superior mesenteric artery.

Medical therapy involves the control of the inflammatory process by corticosteroids, possibly with other immunosuppressants, but fibrotic obliteration of vessels may necessitate surgery. Angioplasty of mesenteric vessels or the descending aorta has been used. An association of the condition with Crohn's disease has been noted.[9]

OTHER CAUSES OF VASCULITIS

Systemic vasculitis clinically affecting the gut may be associated with complement deficiencies, chronic bacteraemias, Kawasaki's disease, and occurs as part of a rare familial syndrome associated with renal and retinal vessel disease, intracerebral calcification and premature hair greying.[17]

SARCOIDOSIS

Sarcoidosis is a chronic inflammatory condition of unknown aetiology, characterized by granulomatous inflammation most commonly in lung, lymph nodes and spleen, with a variety of skin and other manifestations associated. Compared with other conditions in this section, sarcoid is relatively common, yet clinical involvement of the gut in sarcoid is rare.[14]

Gastric sarcoidosis may be symptomatic, reflecting antral ulceration or thickening. A 1985 survey recognized only 20 cases in the literature, although granulomata may be reported asymptomatically in that area in patients with systemic sarcoidosis.[3] Symptoms are those of pain or less frequently bleeding, and the most common gastric radiological appearance is akin to linitis plastica. Small intestinal involvement seems even less frequent. A 1984 report accepted only eight cases from the literature as fully meeting histological and other criteria for intestinal sarcoidosis as part of a systemic picture of the disease.[23] Less rigorous reports cover isolated granulomatous involvement of mesenteric lymph nodes or small intestine. Weight loss, abdominal pain and diarrhoea are prominent in the few reports of small intestinal sarcoid, with a few cases of villous atrophy. Protein-losing enteropathy has been reported. Colonic sarcoidosis is also rare, clinical presentations including bloody diarrhoea, with diffuse mucosal abnormality, or polypoid or tumour-like masses.[7,11] In contrast, hepatic granulomata are present in about 60% of cases of sarcoidosis.

Systemic sarcoidosis when symptomatic merits corticosteroid therapy, and gastrointestinal involvement usually responds to such therapy, whereas hepatic involvement usually does not.

References

1. Alegre, V.A., Winkelmann, R.K., Diez-Martin, J.L. and Banks, P.M. (1988) Adult coeliac disease, small and medium vessel cutaneous necrotizing vasculitis, and T-cell lymphoma. *Journal of the American Academy of Dermatology*, **19**, 973–978.
2. Andersson, R. (1988) Giant cell arteritis. *Acta Medica Scandinavia*, **224**, 193–194.
3. Chinitz, M.A., Brandt, L.J., Frank, M.S., Frager, D. and Sablay, L. (1985) Symptomatic sarcoidosis of the stomach. *Digestive Diseases and Sciences*, **30**, 682–688.
4. Doe, W.F., Evans, D., Hobbs, J.R. and Booth, C.C. (1972) Coeliac disease, vasculitis and cryoglobulinaemia. *Gut*, **13**, 112–123.
5. Duker, J.S. (1987) Retinal vasculitis in Crohn's disease. *American Journal of Ophthalmology*, **103**, 604–608.
6. Evans, G.H. and Ribeiro, B.F. (1987) Degos' disease. A rare cause of multiple intestinal perforations. *Journal of the Royal College of Surgeons of Edinburgh*, **32**, 371–372.
7. Ell, S.R. and Frank, P.H. (1981) Spectrum of lymphoid hyperplasia: colonic manifestations of sarcoidosis, infectious mononucleosis, and Crohn's disease. *Gastrointestinal Radiology*, **6**, 329.
8. Gorevic, P.D., Kassab, H.J., Levo, Y. *et al.* (1980) Mixed cryoglobulinaemia: clinical aspects and long term follow up of 40 patients. *American Journal of Medicine*, **69**, 287–303.
9. Hall, S., Barr, W., Lie, J.T. *et al.* (1985) Takayusu's arteritis. A study of 32 North American patients. *Medicine*, **64**, 89–99.
10. Klein, R.G., Hunder, G.G., Stevenson, A.W. and Sheps, S.G. (1975) Large artery involvement in giant cell activity. *Annals of International Medicine*, **83**, 806–812.
11. Kohn, N.N. (1980) Sarcoidosis of the colon. *Journal of the Medical Society of New Jersey*, **77**, 517–519.
12. Lande, A. and Rossi, P. (1975) The value of total aortography in the diagnosis of Takayasu's arteritis. *Radiology*, **114**, 287–297.
13. Lupi-Herrera, E., Sanchez-Torres, G., Marcushamer, J., Mispireta, J., Horwitz, S. and Vela J.E. (1977) Takayasu's arteritis: clinical study of 107 cases. *American Heart Journal*, **93**, 94–103.
14. Mora, R.G. and Gullung, W.H. (1980) Sarcoidosis: a case with unusual manifestations. *Southern Medical Journal*, **73**, 1064–1066.
15. Nakao, K., Ikeda, M., Kimata, S. *et al.* (1967) Takayasu's arteritis: clinical report of 84 cases and immunological studies of 7 cases. *Circulation*, **35**, 1141–1155.
16. Patsner, B., Pitzele, S., Mann, W.J. and Chalas, E. (1989) Temporal arteritis and intestinal perforation. *New York State Journal of Medicine*, **89**, 476–477.
17. Rambaud, J.C., Galian, A., Touchard, G. *et al.* (1986) Digestive tract and renal small vessel hyalinosis, idiopathic nonarteriosclerotic intra-

cerebral calcification, retinal ischemic syndrome and phenotypic abnormalities. A new familial syndrome. *Gastroenterology*, **90**, 930–938.
18. Reza, M.J., Roth, B.E., Pops, M.A., Goldberg, L.S. (1974) Intestinal vasculitis in essential mixed cryoglobulinaemia. *Annals of Internal Medicine*, **81**, 632–634.
19. Rush, P.J. (1986) Isolated vasculitis of the central nervous system in a patient with coeliac disease. *American Journal of Medicine*, **81**, 1092–1094.
20. Sealey, W.G., Harris, J.A., Young, W.H. and Callaway, H.A. (1957) Paradoxical hypertension following resection of coarctation of aorta. *Surgery*, **42**, 135–147.
21. Smith, J.A., O'Sullivan, M., Gough, J. and Williams, B.D. (1988) Small intestinal performation secondary to localised giant-cell arteritis of the mesenteric vessels. *British Journal of Rheumatology*, **27**, 236.
22. Speiser, J.C., Moore, T.L. and Zuckner, J. (1985) Ulcerative colitis with arthritis and vasculatitis. *Clinical Rheumatology*, **4**, 343.
23. Sprague, R., Harper, P, McClari, S. *et al.* (1984) Disseminated gastrointestinal sarcoidosis. Case report and review of the literature. *Gastroenterology*, **87**, 421–425.
24. Strole, W.E., Clark, W.H. and Isselbacher, K.J. (1967) Progressive arterial occlusive disease (Kohlmeier-Degos). *New England Journal of Medicine*, **276**, 195.

MANIFESTATIONS OF CHRONIC RENAL FAILURE

Geoffrey I. Sandle

The development of varied and often non-specific symptoms in patients with chronic uraemia usually heralds severe renal dysfunction (i.e. glomerular filtration rate less than 20 ml/min). Cardiovascular, neurological and musculoskeletal complications of chronic uraemia are well recognized and tend to improve with the introduction of dialysis and specific pharmacological modalities. However, the gastrointestinal manifestations of chronic uraemia often persist or develop when the other multisystem manifestations of the uraemic syndrome have been largely corrected. In addition to gastrointestinal symptoms of uraemia, renal failure and gastroenterology interact via gastrointestinal complications of dialysis, and the effects of renal failure on the pharmacokinetics of gastrointestinal drugs and gastrointestinal function.

GASTROINTESTINAL SYMPTOMS SECONDARY TO CHRONIC URAEMIA

NAUSEA AND VOMITING

Nausea and vomiting occur frequently in patients with advanced renal failure. When persistent these symptoms may reduce protein and calorie intake, resulting in progressive weight loss and malnutrition. Although the underlying causes of nausea and vomiting in chronic uraemia are unclear, several gastrointestinal factors may be involved. Impaired gastric motor function may play a role, although the evidence for this is conflicting. In one study, gastric emptying of a semi-solid meal was markedly delayed in each of the ten severely uraemic adults who were not undergoing haemodialysis.[19] In contrast, emptying patterns were normal in three out of four haemodialysis patients, suggesting that gastric stasis may be confined to non-dialysed patients.[19] Normal gastric emptying of liquids and solids has in fact been demonstrated in haemodialysis patients, irrespective of the presence of nausea and vomiting,[37] and in nine out of ten continuous ambulatory peritoneal dialysis (CAPD) patients when the abdomen was drained of dialysate.[4] However, normal liquid and solid gastric emptying times have also been reported in nine non-dialysed patients with severe uraemia.[10] The lack of uniformity among these studies suggests that other factors may play a role in the development of nausea and vomiting in chronic uraemia. In this regard, it should be noted that in diabetic patients with end-stage renal failure, autonomic dysfunction leading to gastroparesis and diarrhoea occurs in about 10% of cases undergoing peritoneal dialysis.[25] In addition, endoscopic evaluation of 60 patients on haemodialysis revealed nodular gastritis in 60% which correlated significantly with the presence of nausea and vomiting.[18] Although end-stage uraemia can be complicated by generalized mucositis, in current practice the gastric and duodenal ulcers formerly reported to be common in patients with end-stage renal failure are less frequently seen. In one series with a 60% incidence of gastritis, only two out of six patients had peptic ulceration.[32]

Plasma concentrations of gastrointestinal polypeptide hormones are often raised in uraemic patients, and may also contribute to the development of symptoms. Both fasting and postcibal increases in plasma gastrin concentration have been shown to be four times greater in uraemic patients than in control subjects.[20] Although exogenous gastrin stimulates gastric antral contractility,[7] it has the paradoxical effect of slowing gastric emptying of liquids[7] and solids.[17] Any relationship between raised postcibal plasma gastrin concentrations and delayed gastric emptying in uraemic patients is difficult to predict, because eating invokes other neurohumoral factors which may modify the effect of gastrin on gastric motility. Similarly, fasting and postcibal increases in plasma gastric inhibitory polypeptide concentration were substantially higher in uraemic patients undergoing haemodialysis than in control subjects.[22] The association between these changes and the production of nausea and vomiting is unclear, but exogenous gastric inhibitory polypeptide inhibits gastric secretion and motility,[3] and inhibits the resting and pentagastrin-stimulated lower oesophageal sphincter pressure.[31] Increased circulating concentrations of secretin[6] and glucagon[30] have also been reported in patients with chronic renal failure. Again, the importance of these changes to the pathogenesis of nausea and vomiting is tenuous, but in normal subjects exogenous secretin inhibits both gastric emptying[34] and upper small bowel motility,[11] and exogenous glucagon inhibits both the resting and pentagastrin-stimulated lower oesophageal sphincter pressure[14] and small intestinal motility.[25] In the light of these findings, it is perhaps not surprising that there appear to be no clear-cut links between nausea and vomiting, and disorders of oesophago-gastroduodenal motility in uraemia.

HICCOUGHS

Hiccoughs are a common manifestation of uraemia, and persistent bouts in a dialysis patient suggest inadequate dialysis.

DIARRHOEA

Diarrhoea occurs occasionally as part of the uraemic syndrome, and its pathogenesis is often unclear. However, in diabetic patients undergoing peritoneal dialysis, diarrhoea may be a manifestation of autonomic neuropathy in 10% of cases.[25]

GASTROINTESTINAL COMPLICATIONS OF DIALYSIS

CONSTIPATION

Constipation occurs commonly in dialysis patients owing to dietary restrictions and oral iron therapy. Agents that increase stool bulk (e.g. ispaghula) or produce softening of the stool (e.g. lactulose) are preferred and are generally effective in preventing constipation despite the continuation of iron therapy. Aluminium hydroxide (which also produces constipation) is now used less frequently to retard intestinal phosphate absorption owing to the risk of aluminium toxicity.

OCCULT BLOOD LOSS

Occult bleeding from otherwise asymptomatic oesophageal, gastric or duodenal mucosal lesions often occurs in dialysis patients, and may be promoted by anticoagulation during haemodialysis. Chromium-labelled red blood cell studies indicate blood losses of approximately 6 ml/day in dialysis patients (compared with 3 ml/day in undialysed uraemic patients, and less than 1 ml/day in normal subjects).[24] Drugs that impair the mucus–bicarbonate 'mucosal protective barrier' (e.g. corticosteroids, non-steroidal anti-inflammatory drugs, aspirin, alcohol), possibly combined with uraemia-associated defects in platelet function,[5] may predispose to gastrointestinal blood loss.

OVERT BLOOD LOSS

Overt bleeding from the gastrointestinal tract is relatively common in dialysis patients and may be caused by or associated with a variety of mucosal abnormalities. Radiological and endoscopic evidence for reflux oesophagitis has been found in 8–13% of dialysis patients.[18] Prolonged vomiting may produce Mallory–Weiss tears of the distal oesophagus. Radiology often reveals hypertrophic mucosal folds in the stomach (12% of dialysis patients) and duodenum (42% of patients), whilst gastritis and duodenitis may occur in up to 60% of cases.[18] Gastric and duodenal ulcers are probably no more prevalent in uraemic patients than in the general population. It is unclear why dialysis patients are prone to upper gastrointestinal bleeding, but the use of ulcerogenic drugs, platelet abnormalities and intermittent anticoagulation during haemodialysis may be contributory factors. Bleeding from colonic ischaemia is also being recognized more frequently as more elderly uraemic patients are maintained on long-term dialysis.

DIVERTICULAR DISEASE OF THE COLON

Colonic diverticulosis has been reported in 83% of patients with polycystic disease of the kidneys, compared with much lower incidence in other dialysis patients (32%) and age- and sex-matched normal controls (38%). Patients with polycystic disease of the kidneys may have an increased risk of developing diverticulitis, gross colonic perforation and faecal peritonitis.[28]

ASCITES

Although it occurs only rarely, persistent ascites in patients undergoing long-term haemodialysis appears to be unrelated to cardiac or hepatic dysfunction, or infection of the peritoneal cavity. The underlying cause of refractory ascites is unclear, but a history of previous peritoneal dialysis in many cases suggests a change in peritoneal membrane permeability. The protein content of the ascitic fluid is usually high, and patients may be hypoalbuminaemic. Treatment with fluid restriction, intensive dialysis, albumin infusion and high protein diets is generally unsuccessful, although some success may be achieved by renal transplantation, ascitic fluid reinfusion via a La Veen shunt, or the intraperitoneal application of non-absorbable steroid after ascitic fluid drainage.[1,9]

PERITONEAL INFECTION

Peritonitis is a constant hazard of chronic ambulatory peritoneal dialysis and accounts for up to 50% of treatment failures and 25% of deaths in patients undergoing this type of dialysis. Contamination of the peritoneal cavity may arise from exit site infections, contamination during fluid exchange (although newer techniques such as the disconnect systems have reduced this likelihood), and bacterial migration from the gut. Patients maintained on intermittent peritoneal dialysis are less prone to peritonitis as the peritoneal cavity is empty between dialyses, and normal peritoneal defences come into play. Peritonitis may be frequent and recurrent, or more severe and sporadic and related to fungal infection or faecal contamination. Patients often complain of abdominal pain and altered bowel frequency (in which case Gram-negative infection should be suspected), but these symptoms may be absent in the early stages. The dialysate is cloudy, contains more than 100 leukocytes/ml (of which more than 50% are polymorphs), and positive cultures are obtained in 95% of cases. Gram-positive organisms (usually species of staphylococci and streptococci) are present in approximately 70% of cases, whereas Gram-negative organisms (e.g. *Escherichia coli*, *Klebsiella*, *Proteus*, and *Pseudomonas* spp.) are responsible for 25–30% of cases. Fungal and mycobacterial species are isolated only rarely, and then usually in patients who have received antibiotics for the treatment of bacterial peritonitis or other infections. Faecal peritonitis, with its high rate of morbidity and mortality, is suggested by the presence of both aerobic and anaerobic organisms, and often occurs against a background of colonic diverticular disease. Although the management of peritonitis varies between dialysis units, intraperitoneal (and occasionally systemic) antibiotics provide the main therapeutic options, the choice of antibiotic(s) depending on the results of the Gram stain and culture of the peritoneal fluid.[29]

SCLEROSING ENCAPSULATING PERITONITIS

Sclerosing encapsulating peritonitis is a distinct syndrome which occurs in some patients receiving peritoneal dialysis. Patients develop nausea, vomiting, anorexia, malnutrition, intermittent bowel obstruction (often without typical radiological appearances), and impaired peritoneal transport of water and solutes.[2] The small intestine, which may itself appear normal, is encapsulated by a thick fibrous layer. The overall prognosis in these patients is poor, with a mortality of 50% rising to almost 80% in those requiring laparotomy for bowel obstruction. Many diverse causes have been implicated in the development of sclerosing encapsulating peritonitis, but the use of acetate (rather than lactate)-containing dialysis solutions may be the most important predisposing factor.[2]

HERNIAS

Hernias may occur in peritoneal dialysis patients, especially those on chronic ambulatory peritoneal dialysis.[8] The chronic increase in intra-abdominal pressure may cause tight herniation at sites of weakness in the abdominal wall (e.g. inguinal canal, previous surgical incision), resulting in intestinal obstruction. Herniation at catheter insertion sites now occurs less commonly since the introduction of new inserting techniques (e.g. paramedian via the rectus muscle rather than midline). Multiparous women are particularly liable to develop hernias during chronic ambulatory peritoneal dialysis.

Ideally, any obvious weakness of the abdominal wall should be repaired before the patient commences peritoneal dialysis, and over distension of the abdomen should be avoided in high-risk patients.

USE OF GASTROINTESTINAL DRUGS IN CHRONIC URAEMIA

Most of the drugs that act on the gastrointestinal tract require modification of their dose and frequency of administration in the presence of severe renal impairment (i.e. glomerular filtration rate less than 20 ml/min).[23] In general there is little information available regarding the effect of chronic uraemia on intestinal drug absorption, but the bioavailabilities of most drugs that have been evaluated are unchanged or increased. The following drugs should be avoided or used with extreme caution: codeine (increased and prolonged effect which may cause severe narcosis in uraemic patients); tripotassium dicitratobismuthate (De-Nol and De-Noltab); ispaghula husk (as Fybogel each sachet contains 7 mmol potassium): sodium alginate–sodium bicarbonate–calcium carbonate preparations (Gaviscon); magnesium salts; mercaptopurine; mesalazine (metabolite excreted via kidneys); metoclopramide (increased risk of extrapyramidal side effects); neomycin (ototoxic and nephrotoxic); potassium salts; and potassium-sparing diuretics. Drugs that may be used at reduced dose and frequency of administration include: azathioprine; cimetidine, ranitidine and famotidine (increase risk of confusion); cisapride; domperidone; metronidazole (increased risk of neurotoxicity); and sulphasalazine (increased risk of rashes, blood dyscrasias and crystalluria).

EFFECTS OF CHRONIC URAEMIA ON GASTROINTESTINAL PHYSIOLOGY

POLYPEPTIDE HORMONES

In normal individuals, large amounts of low- and medium-molecular-weight polypeptide hormones are extracted by the kidneys and catabolized in the renal parenchyma. The plasma concentrations of a variety of polypeptide hormones are therefore raised in many patients with end-stage renal failure. It is by no means clear whether these changes are linked to abnormalities of gastrointestinal function, because the immunoreactive components of many hormones may have minimal biological activity.[15] Nevertheless, changes in the plasma concentrations of secretin,[6] gastrin[20] and gastric inhibitory polypeptide[22] are worthy of mention.

Plasma secretin concentrations in the fasting state are higher in patients with uraemia than in normal subjects.[6] Secretin administered intravenously disappears more rapidly from the plasma of normal subjects than of patients with chronic renal failure, and the mean half-life of secretin has been reported to be 6 minutes in uraemic patients compared with 2.4 minutes in healthy controls. These observations suggest that decreased catabolism of secretin by the diseased kidneys may contribute to high fasting plasma secretin concentrations in patients with chronic renal failure. However, the relatively fast clearance of intravenously administered secretin seen in uraemic patients suggests that secretin is also catabolized at extrarenal sites.[33]

Fasting and meal-stimulated plasma gastrin concentrations have been reported to be substantially higher in young adult patients with chronic renal failure than in age-matched controls.[20] The rates of both basal and maximal gastric acid secretion were also significantly lower in the uraemic patients than in the control subjects, and within the uraemic group the highest plasma gastrin concentrations were seen in those patients with hypochlorhydria. These findings suggest that hypergastrinaemia in uraemia may reflect decreased gastrin catabolism (particularly of the G34 fragment) by the kidneys, and an impairment of the negative feedback mechanism between gastric acid production and gastrin secretion,[21] as seen in pernicious anaemia. In addition, there is experimental evidence that nephrectomy reduces the clearance of gastrin at extrarenal sites.[16]

Fasting and meal-stimulated plasma gastric inhibitory polypeptide concentrations have also been shown to be eight times higher in uraemic patients undergoing haemodialysis than in control subjects.[22] Plasma gastric inhibitory polypeptide concentrations remained elevated in uraemic patients 3 hours after the meal when the polypeptide concentrations in control subjects had returned to fasting levels. These observations and the results of other physiological studies[22] suggest that the kidneys play an important role in the inactivation or clearance of gastric inhibitory polypeptide from the circulation. Although exogenous gastric inhibitory polypeptide inhibits gastric acid secretion and gastric motility in normal subjects,[3] it remains to be seen whether raised plasma polypeptide concentrations contribute significantly to the hypochlorhydria and delayed gastric emptying which occurs in some patients with chronic renal failure.

Table 8.5 Potassium excretory pathways in normal subjects and patients undergoing continuous ambulatory peritoneal dialysis

	Normal subjects	*CAPD* patients*
Dietary potassium intake (mmol/day)	80–100	70–80
Urinary potassium excretion (mmol/day)	70–90	Negligible
Estimated peritoneal potassium loss (mmol/day)	Nil	30
Faecal potassium excretion (mmol/day)	10	40–50

CAPD = Chronic ambulatory peritoneal dialysis.
*Ten normokalaemic (mean plasma potassium concentration 4.1 mmol/l) CAPD patients undergoing peritoneal dialysis with 2 litres dialysate containing 0.7 mmol/l potassium (dwell-time 6–8 hours).

COLONIC POTASSIUM ADAPTATION

Potassium adaptation is an important property of colonic epithelia, and colonic potassium transport processes respond readily to changes in dietary potassium intake and other disturbances of potassium homoeostasis (e.g. chronic renal failure).[13] In healthy individuals most of the normal dietary potassium intake (80–100 mmol/day) is excreted by the kidneys, and faecal potassium excretion amounts to only 10 mmol/day. Although hyperkalaemia eventually develops in all patients with end-stage renal failure despite dietary potassium restriction, hyperkalaemia is a relatively late complication of uraemia as surviving nephrons increase their capacity for potassium secretion and, in addition, the colon becomes a significant potassium excretory pathway. In the 1960s, metabolic balance studies performed in normal subjects and patients with varying degrees of renal impairment showed that faecal potassium excretion increased appreciably to maintain potassium balance at a point (creatinine clearance less than 5 ml/min) when compensatory increases in potassium secretion by surviving nephrons became maximal.[12] Total faecal potassium excretion in uraemic patients was directly related to wet stool weight and dietary potassium intake, but returned to normal after renal transplantation.[12] More recently, transport studies have demonstrated increased net potassium secretion in the proximal rectum in three groups of patients with chronic renal failure: (1) normokalaemic patients with normal dietary potassium intakes (80–100 mmol/day);[26] (2) normokalaemic patients on chronic ambulatory peritoneal dialysis with potassium intakes of 70–80 mmol/day and normal total body potassium contents (TBK);[27] and (3) chronic haemodialysis patients with moderately restricted potassium intakes (60–70 mmol/day) and normal TBK.[27] Increased potassium secretion in all three groups was not associated with increases in sodium absorption, transmucosal electrical potential difference (a simple indicator of electrogenic sodium transport) or plasma potassium concentration and, contrary to previous studies,[36] there was no evidence that enhanced potassium secretion was linked to secondary hyperaldosteronism.[27] As the ability to augment their capacity for potassium secretion (e.g. in response to dietary potassium loading and during chronic uraemia) is an inherent feature of all segments of the mammalian colon, it seems likely that increased potassium secretion in uraemic patients occurs throughout the large intestine and is not limited to the rectum. It would therefore appear that in end-stage renal failure, the colon is transformed into an important alternative potassium excretory pathway. Increased faecal potassium excretion may in fact be the main determinant of potassium homoeostasis in many uraemic patients, because in the absence of undue dietary potassium restriction, potassium losses achieved by chronic ambulatory peritoneal dialysis represent less than 50% of the daily potassium intake (*Table 8.5*).[27]

REFERENCES

1. Arismendi, G.S., Izard, M.W., Hampton, W.R. and Maher, J.F. (1976) The clinical spectrum of ascites associated with maintenance dialysis. *American Journal of Medicine*, **60**, 46–51.
2. Bargman, J.M. and Oreopoulos, D.G. (1989) Complications other than peritonitis or those related to the catheter and the fate of uremic organ dysfunction in patients receiving peritoneal dialysis. In *Peritoneal Dialysis* pp. 289–318 (Ed.) Nolph, K.D. Dordrecht: Kluwer Academic Publishers.
3. Brown, J., Dryburgh, J., Ross, S. and Dupre, J. (1975) Identification and actions of gastric inhibitory polypeptide. *Recent Progress in Hormone Research*, **31**, 487–532.

4. Brown-Cartwright, D., Smith, H.J. and Feldman, M. (1988) Gastric emptying of an indigestible solid in patients with end-stage renal disease on continuous ambulatory peritoneal dialysis. *Gastroenterology*, **95**, 49–51.
5. Castaldi, P.A., Rozenberg, M.C. and Stewart, J.H. (1966) The bleeding disorder of uraemia. A qualitative platelet defect. *The Lancet*, **2**, 66–69.
6. Chey, W.Y., Chang, T.M., Lee, K.Y. and Rominger, J. (1979) Secretin in normal and abnormal states. In *Gut Peptides. Secretion, Function and Clinical Aspects*, pp. 367–375. (Ed.) Miyoshi, A. Tokyo: Kodansha Ltd; Amsterdam: Elsevier North-Holland Biomedical Press.
7. Cooke, A.R., Chvasta, T.E. and Weisbrodt, N.W. (1972) Effect of pentagastrin on emptying and electrical and motor activity of the dog stomach. *American Journal of Physiology*, **223**, 934–938.
8. Digenis, G.E., Khanna, R., Mathews, R. and Oreopoulos, D.G. (1982) Abdominal hernias in patients undergoing continuous ambulatory peritoneal dialysis. *Peritoneal Dialysis Bulletin*, **2**, 115–117.
9. Epstein, M. (1982) Peritoneovenous shunt in the management of ascites and the hepatorenal syndrome. *Gastroenterology*, **82**, 790–799.
10. Freeman, J.G., Cobden, I., Heaton, A. and Keir, M. (1985) Gastric emptying in chronic renal failure. *British Medical Journal*, **291**, 1048.
11. Gutierrez, J., Chey, W. and Dinoso, V. (1974) Actions of cholecystokinin and secretin on the motor activity of the small intestine in man. *Gastroenterology*, **67**, 35–41.
12. Hayes, C.P., McLeod, M.E. and Robinson, R.R. (1967) An extrarenal mechanism for the maintenance of potassium balance in severe chronic renal failure. *Transactions of the Association of American Physicians*, **80**, 207–216.
13. Hayslett, J.P. and Binder, H.J. (1982) Mechanisms of potassium adaptation. *American Journal of Physiology*, **243**, F103–F112.
14. Jaffer, S., Makhlouf, G., Schorr, G. and Zfass, A. (1974) Nature and kinetics of inhibition of lower oesophageal sphincter pressure by glucagon. *Gastroenterology*, **67**, 42–46.
15. Katz, A.I. and Emmanouel, D.S. (1978) Metabolism of polypeptide hormones by the normal kidney and in uremia. *Nephron*, **22**, 69–80.
16. Loly, J., Depressen, J., Brassinne, A. and Nizet, A. (1982) Renal control of the peripheral uptake of exogenous gastrin in the dog. *European Journal of Physiology*, **395**, 171–174.
17. MacGregor, I.L., Wiley, Z.D. and Martin, P.M. (1978) Effect of pentagastrin infusion on gastric emptying rate of solid food in man. *American Journal of Digestive Diseases*, **23**, 72–75.
18. Margolis, D.M., Saylor, J.L., Geisse, G., DeSchryver-Kecskemeti, K., Harter, H.R. and Zuckerman, G.R. (1978) Upper gastrointestinal disease in chronic renal failure. A prospective evaluation. *Archives of Internal Medicine*, **138**, 1214–1217.
19. McNamee, P.T., Moore, G.W., McGeown, M.G., Doherty, C.C. and Collins, B.J. (1985) Gastric emptying in chronic renal failure. *British Medical Journal*, **291**, 310–311.
20. Muto, S., Asano, Y., Hosoda, S. and Miyata, M. (1988) Hypochlorhydria and hypergastrinaemia and their association with gastrointestinal bleeding in young patients with chronic renal failure. *Nephron*, **50**, 5–9.
21. Muto, S., Murayama, N., Asano, Y., Hosoda, S. and Miyata, M. (1985) Hypergastrinaemia and achlorhydria in chronic renal failure. *Nephron*, **40**, 143–148.
22. O'Dorisio, T.M., Sirinek, K.R., Mazzaferri, E.L. and Cataland, S. (1977) Renal effects of serum gastric inhibitory polypeptide (GIP). *Metabolism*, **26**, 651–656.
23. Prescribing in renal impairment (1984) In *British National Formulary*, pp. 10–11. London: British Medical Association and The Pharmaceutical Press.
24. Rosenblatt, S.G., Drake, S., Fadem, S., Welch, R. and Lifschitz, M.D. (1982) Gastrointestinal blood loss in patients with chronic renal failure. *American Journal of Kidney Diseases*, **1**, 232–236.
25. Rottembourg, J. (1989) Peritoneal dialysis in diabetics. In *Peritoneal Dialysis*, pp. 365–379. (Ed.) Nolph, K.D. Dordrecht: Kluwer Academic Publishers.
26. Sandle, G.I., Gaiger, E., Tapster, S. and Goodship, T.H.J. (1986) Enhanced rectal potassium secretion in chronic renal insufficiency: evidence for large intestinal potassium adaptation in man. *Clinical Science*, **71**, 393–401.
27. Sandle, G.I., Gaiger, E., Tapster, S. and Goodship, T.H.J. (1987) Evidence for large intestinal control of potassium homoeostasis in uraemic patients undergoing long-term dialysis. *Clinical Science*, **73**, 247–252.
28. Scheff, R.T., Zuckerman, G., Harter, H.R., Delmez, J. and Koehler, R. (1980) Diverticular disease in patients with chronic renal failure due to polycystic kidney disease. *Annals of Internal Medicine*, **92**, 202–204.
29. Schoenfeld, P. (1985) Care of the patient on peritoneal dialysis. In *Introduction to Dialysis*, pp. 172–178. (Ed.) Cogan, M.G. and Garovoy, M.R. New York: Churchill Livingstone.
30. Sherwin, R.S. Bastl, C., Finkelstein, F.O., Black, H., Hindler, R. and Felig, P. (1976) Influence of uremia and haemodialysis on the turnover and metabolic effects of glucagon. *Journal of Clinical Investigation*, **57**, 722–731.
31. Sinar, D., O'Dorisio, T., Mazzaferri, E., Mekhjan, H., Caldwell, J. and Thomas, F. (1978) Effect of gastric inhibitory polypeptide on lower esophageal sphincter pressure in cats. *Gastroenterology*, **75**, 263–267.
32. Tami, N., Harasawa, S. and Suzuki, S. (1980) Lesions of upper gastrointestinal tract in patients

with chronic renal failure. *Gastroenterology Japan*, **15**, 148–152.
33. Thompson, J.C., Llanos, O.L., Schafmayer, A., Teichmann, R.K. and Rayford, P.L. (1978) Mechanisms of release and catabolism of secretin. In *Gut Hormones*, pp. 176–181. (Ed.) Bloom, S.R. Edinburgh, London and New York: Churchill Livingstone.
34. Vagne, M. and Andre, C. (1971) The effect of secretin on gastric emptying in man. *Gastroenterology*, **60**, 421–424.
35. Whalen, G. (1974) Glucagon and the small gut. *Gastroenterology*, **67**, 1284–1286.
36. Wilson, D.R., Ing, T.S., Metcalfe-Gibson, A. and Wrong, O.M. (1968) The chemical composition of faeces in uraemia, as revealed by in-vivo faecal dialysis. *Clinical Science*, **35**, 197–209.
37. Wright, R.A. Clemente, R. and Wathen, R. (1984) Gastric emptying in patients with chronic renal failure receiving haemodialysis. *Archives of Internal Medicine*, **144**, 495–496.

CARDIAC DISEASE: THE INTERFACE BETWEEN CARDIOLOGY AND GASTROENTEROLOGY

John G.F. Cleland

It has often been said that the way to a man's heart is through his stomach! This has become a reality with the use of the gastroepiploic artery to revascularize the myocardium. Equally, several cardiac conditions have important effects on the gastrointestinal tract and its appendages. However, no bodily system exists in isolation and many other conditions affect both equally. This chapter is devoted to those areas of practice where knowledge of both cardiology and gastroenterology is required.

PRIMARY GASTROINTESTINAL CONDITIONS THAT LEAD TO CARDIOLOGICAL PROBLEMS

ULCERATIVE COLITIS

Ulcerative colitis may be associated with a recurrent myopericarditis, which may present with classic pericarditic symptoms or merely as non-specific ST segment changes on the ECG.[10] More rarely a clinical picture consistent with a dilated cardiomyopathy may be seen. Endomyocardial biopsy may reveal an increase in inflammatory cells, but a true myocarditis picture with myocyte necrosis is rarely seen. There is anecdotal evidence that steroids and immunosuppressive agents may be useful.

In patients with associated polyarthritis, a small proportion develop aortic regurgitation. Anatomically the aortic ring appears to dilate; histologically inflammatory changes are followed by fibrosis and scarring. It is not clear what proportion of these patients have the HLA-B27 histocompatibility antigen, which is of course associated with ankylosing spondylitis. HLA-B27 is also associated with an increased incidence of atrioventricular conduction defects.

WHIPPLE'S DISEASE

Patients may develop mitral or aortic regurgitation due to valve fibrosis, and rarely heart failure due to additional myocardial dysfunction.[9] Large macrophages with PAS-positive granules may be found in cardiac tissues (PAS = periodic acid–Schiff). Pericardial, myocardial and valvular fibrosis may develop. Cardiac lesions appear unrelated to the duration or severity of the disease.

LIVER CIRRHOSIS

Liver cirrhosis leading to hypoalbuminaemia, oedema and ascites may occasionally be mistaken for heart failure, and can complicate the clinical picture and treatment when both diagnoses exist. Heart failure does not lead to true liver cirrhosis. Liver cirrhosis is associated with a reduction in systemic and pulmonary vascular resistance and an increase in cardiac output, which may obscure milder degrees of cardiac dysfunction. Occasionally liver cirrhosis may result in a sufficient degree of pulmonary arteriovenous shunting to result in a central cyanosis. Patients may also present in high output heart failure due to a systemic arteriovenous shunt. This is often attributed to thiamine deficiency, but is probably multifactorial.

Alcohol has been widely implicated in the induction of both heart and liver disease. However, the existence of a true syndrome of alcohol heart muscle disease has not been established. Patients with dilated cardiomyopathy do appear to drink more than matched controls and heavy alcohol consumption may predispose to the development of coronary artery disease, but many life-long drinkers have excellent ventricular function. Alcoholic 'cardiomyopathy', if it does exist, like alcoholic liver cirrhosis must be idiosyncratic. Some observers suggest that cirrhosis and severe ventricular dysfunction rarely coexist in patients who drink heavily.[1]

Liver cirrhosis may increase the risk of infective endocarditis.[14] This relationship may be more association than cause and effect, but the diseased liver may be less effective in clearing bacteria from the blood stream, whilst many alcoholic patients are also immunocompromised.

CARCINOID SYNDROME

Exposure of the heart to 5-hydroxytryptamine (serotonin) is necessary for the production of cardiac lesions in carcinoid syndrome.[6] The heart is not usually affected until there are extensive liver metastases, because a large tumour mass is needed to secrete enough serotonin, and the liver (and lung) can efficiently remove serotonin from the circulation.

Carcinoid tumours that do not secrete serotonin (e.g. rectal) or do not metastasize to the liver (e.g. appendiceal) do not produce the carcinoid syndrome. A combination of serotonin excess, hepatic impairment and tryptophan deficiency appears necessary to produce cardiac lesions in animal models.

Histology reveals subendothelial fibrosis. This resists myocardial deformation during systole, preventing normal contraction of the involved ventricle. Affected valves become thickened and rigid.

Liver metastases lead to involvement of the right ventricle, and to a lesser extent right atrium, and tricuspid and pulmonary valves. The tricuspid valve leaflets and associated chordae tendineae become rigid, shortened and immobile. The valve becomes relatively fixed in a half-open position. Regurgitation usually predominates. The pulmonary valve also becomes fixed and rigid, but with predominant stenosis. Right ventricular involvement may be extensive and result effectively in a restrictive myopathy. Occasionally high cardiac output due to continuous release of vasodilator substances or high flow rates in the tumour itself may exacerbate the cardiac problems.

Clinically the classic signs of tricuspid regurgitation may be observed, including large V waves in the jugular venous pulse, a pansystolic murmur over the lower sternum, accentuated by manoeuvres that increase venous return, such as leg raising or inspiratory effort (especially if against a closed glottis). Tricuspid stenosis may be revealed by an early to mid diastolic rumble. Right ventricular involvement may be manifest by a rapid early diastolic collapse of the venous pressure and an early diastolic sound, indicating the abrupt cessation of right ventricular filling. Pulmonary stenosis is denoted by an ejection systolic murmur loudest in the pulmonary area. Lesions on the mitral and aortic valves may occur if there is extensive right-sided involvement, if an interatrial shunt exists or if the tumour originates in the bronchus. Echocardiography is the initial investigation of choice. Invasive studies, especially angiography, can precipitate a carcinoid crisis but, if deemed necessary, should be appropriately covered by steroids and somatostatin analogue (and H_1- and H_2-receptor antagonists if the tumour is also thought to secrete histamine).

Valvuloplasty may be helpful if pulmonary stenosis is severe, but as the tricuspid valve is usually stuck in the half-way position tricuspid valvuloplasty is of limited benefit. If right ventricular involvement is extensive then neither procedures for correction of the valve problems – or surgery to the ventricle itself has much to offer.

In one study the mean survival from the time of identification of cardiac involvement was 1.9 years, and surgery seemed to have little influence.[6] Hepatic failure, heart failure and bowel obstruction appear to be the common forms of death. Reduction of the tumour mass by resection or embolization may slow progress of the disease, but is unlikely to be of benefit in patients with advanced cardiac disease.

MALNUTRITION AND MALABSORPTION

Malabsorption in itself rarely leads to cardiac problems, but may contribute in cases of heart failure to the overall debility of the patient. Dietary thiamine deficiency is commonly associated with alcoholism in Western countries and is occasionally seen in patients on chronic parenteral nutrition, when vitamin supplements have been omitted. Patients may present with breathlessness and signs of fluid overload with a hyperdynamic circulation or in circulatory shock, often accompanied by a metabolic acidosis.

If high-output heart failure due to thiamine deficiency is suspected, administration of thiamine may reduce the systemic vasodilatation rapidly causing the failing ventricle further problems due to the increased afterload. Treatment of the heart failure with diuretics and digoxin is recommended immediately prior to giving thiamine.

CARDIOVASCULAR PROBLEMS THAT LEAD TO GASTROINTESTINAL PROBLEMS

The most common form of heart disease in developed countries is ischaemic heart disease. Atheroma is rarely confined to the coronary vasculature and associated disease of the mesenteric circulation is common.

CHEST PAIN OF UNCERTAIN ORIGIN

Pain of gastrointestinal origin may be indistinguishable from pain due to myocardial ischaemia or pericarditis.

Pain may arise both from irritation of the oesophageal mucosa or abnormal oesophageal motility.[12] Heartburn, a hot burning sensation usually felt diffusely over the precordium, is regularly relieved by antacids and is often easy to distinguish from angina. However, oesophageal disorders can give rise to pain that is oppressive, substernal, severe and that may radiate to the neck, jaw or arms. The character and radiation of the pain may be indistinguishable from that due to angina or myocardial infarction. The relative importance of acid reflux and disordered oesophageal motility in the production of this pain is disputed. In about half the cases, there will also be complaints of heartburn. Antacids are much less effective in relieving this oppressive oesophageal discomfort. Exercise can precipitate gastro-oesophageal reflux and oesophageal spasm, whereas nitrates may relieve pain of oesophageal origin, further mimicking the picture of angina pectoris. Often there is a history that relates the pain to the ingestion of food or medication (which may lodge in the oesophagus and cause ulceration), but a history of dysphagia may be revealed only after close questioning. Angina is not infrequently precipitated by food, and exacerbation of exertional angina after meals is the rule rather than the exception. Induction of pain by cold liquids is said to suggest an oesophageal origin, but such manoeuvres may also cause coronary vasoconstriction. A prolonged dull ache after the main episode of pain is over is also thought to suggest an oesophageal origin. The past medical history and the presence of risk factors for coronary disease can sometimes be helpful.

The pathophysiology of pain arising from the oesophagus appears to be complex. Pain may arise directly from the oesophagus either as a result of stimulation of tension receptors or due to muscle ischaemia from prolonged contraction. As the pain fibres enter the spinal cord at the same level as those from the heart, pain from both organs appear to be similar. However, others have suggested that disorders of oesophageal motility may be associated with abnormalities of the coronary microcirculation.

Pain from peptic ulceration is less frequently confused with cardiac pain as the site and radiation tend to be different. Pain from peptic ulceration is usually relieved by antacids and food. Pain originating from the gallbladder can also be difficult to distinguish from cardiac pain on occasion. Other regions of the gastrointestinal tract, such as the colon, are less frequently recognized as causing chest pain.

Patients may present with a first episode of prolonged chest pain to the accident and emergency department, in which case a distinction between pain of cardiac or gastrointestinal origin has to be made. The electrocardiogram (ECG) is rarely normal in patients with myocardial infarction, but is not uncommonly so in patients with unstable angina once the pain has settled. If the patient is still in pain and the ECG normal, this provides strong presumptive evidence that the pain is not cardiac in origin. A trial of antacids is indicated. If this fails to settle the pain then admission for further evaluation is indicated. Serial ECGs and cardiac enzymes will help exclude myocardial infarction. Viral titres are not going to be helpful for many weeks and elevated titres are found at a later date in only the minority of cases of pericarditis presumed to be viral in origin. Further ECGs during pain, including leads placed on the right side of the chest (V4r) or the back (V8, V9), are probably the most valuable determinant of the presence of myocardial ischaemia. A low-grade fever and/or a pericardial rub may indicate pericarditis or a transmural myocardial infarction. A therapeutic trial of sublingual or intravenous nitrates versus antacids may also be valuable, though the former may not be entirely specific.

If the pain does not recur frequently enough to make a diagnosis in this way, then exercise testing is indicated. This is also the strategy to be adopted in patients with recurrent chest pain who present in the out-patient department. This may precipitate pain accompanied by classic horizontal or down-sloping ST segment depression of more than 1.5 mm (or occasionally elevation) persisting beyond the first minute of the recovery period, in which case myocardial ischaemia is likely. If the patient exercises well without symptoms or ST segment depression and achieves more than 80% of his or her predicted heart rate (approximated by the formula 200 – age in years) then coronary disease is unlikely. Any other response must be deemed equivocal, including ST segment *depression* in the absence of typical pain. Typical pain in the absence of ST segment changes and with a good exercise tolerance indicates a good prognosis, but does not exclude the possibility of coronary disease. ST segment change is a poorly understood epiphenomenon of myocardial ischaemia. The diagnostic accuracy of exercise testing in different series varies between 70% and 100%. Accepting a grey area where the exercise test is equivocal, and keeping to the above criteria, the accuracy of the test approaches the latter figure.

In equivocal cases alternative techniques may be employed. Thallium scintigraphy has been employed to image defects in myocardial perfusion, which may be fixed (suggesting myocardial infarction) or reversible with rest (suggesting angina). The diagnostic accuracy of this technique has recently been called into question and outside a few specialized centres the results appear to be unreliable. Radionuclide ventriculography (blood pool scanning) at rest and during the induction of pain, usually by exercise, may reveal regional wall motion abnormalities and a failure of ejection fraction to rise if the patient has angina. However, in patients with ventricular dysfunction for reasons other than coronary disease, and in women, the diagnostic criteria worked out for 'ideal' male subjects do not hold true. Stress echocardiography is still in its infancy. Results in 'ideal' subjects look promising but results from more general application are awaited. Thus specialized, non-invasive, cardiac imaging techniques are helpful in some cases when correctly applied, but are of limited use in many patients.

In the absence of a prognostically adverse exercise test (i.e. good exercise tolerance, no major or persistent ST segment changes), and when doubt persists, then pursuit of a gastrointestinal cause for pain may be helpful. Identification of gastro-oesophageal reflux, hiatus hernia or peptic ulceration will lead to appropriate therapy. If the patient's symptoms abate this is diagnostically useful. If the patient's symptoms are not relieved then additional cardiac pathology should be considered. If gallstones are identified, it may be appropriate to remove them pharmacologically or with minimally invasive techniques. However, if there is any possibility of a cardiac origin for the pain this should be excluded prior to major operative intervention, which could precipitate myocardial infarction, attended by a high mortality in the perioperative period.

In patients where no gastrointestinal disease is obvious, tests of oesophageal motility and provocation of pain by instillation of dilute hydrochloric acid may help. Saline (with the chill taken off) should be instilled prior to dilute acid to exclude a (positive) placebo response. Only production of the pain in question should be regarded as positive. Induction of heartburn rather than oppressive retrosternal pain should be regarded as negative. Large studies are few, but 30% or more of patients presenting with retrosternal chest pain without evidence of cardiac disease may have an oesophageal origin for their pain. Twenty-four-hour monitoring of oesophageal pH and pressures has also been used to identify coincidence of pain and an oesophageal abnormality, but this is cumbersome and requires more sophisticated technology. Edrophonium may provoke oesophageal spasm in up to 30% of patients with otherwise unexplained chest pain, without producing a high incidence of side effects due to its short duration of action.

In the absence of evidence of serious cardiac or gastrointestinal pathology, a therapeutic trial may help in making a diagnosis. Although oesophageal pain may be relieved by glyceryl trinitrate, striking therapeutic benefit is more suggestive of angina. Antacids are effective in about half of cases with oesophageal pain. H_2-receptor antagonists are also successful in just over half of cases with a pain considered to be of oesophageal origin. Proton pump inhibitors may offer more benefit, but this still has to be properly substantiated. Calcium antagonists have been used to relieve oesophageal spasm with mixed results. Antidepressants have been used by those who believe that psychological problems may be at the root of the problem. These appear to improve overall well-being, but do not reduce the frequency or severity of episodes.

Ultimately cardiac catheterization may be required to define the presence and extent of coronary disease. However, the mere demonstration of an obstacle to coronary flow does not indicate that the patient has angina or even myocardial ischaemia. The mortality or major morbidity from coronary angiography is in excess of 0.1%, and from angioplasty or coronary surgery under optimal conditions tenfold that of angiography. Reasonable evidence that coronary obstruction is the cause of the patient's symptoms is necessary to justify these risks. Careful consideration of the possible results of the test and the consequences for the patient, and his or her therapy, should be given before angiography is performed. Angiography is *not* indicated if the tests have shown clear evidence of angina and the patient has responded to medical therapy, unless the exercise test is strongly positive at a low workload. Angiography is *not* indicated if the patient has a prognostically good exercise test in the absence of persisting symptoms. Angiography is indicated in the presence of continuing symptoms without a clear diagnosis or if the exercise test indicates a poor prognosis. Demonstration of normal coronary arteries has often been found not to allay the patient's fears, in contrast to a positive diagnosis of oesophageal disease.

HEART FAILURE

As the gastrointestinal tract is richly supplied with blood it is no surprise that heart failure may result in a variety of gastrointestinal problems, some of which may even obscure the diagnosis of the cardiac condition.

Elevation of right atrial pressure due to either tricuspid valve disease or right ventricular failure (which is usually secondary to left heart failure) usually results in hepatomegaly, which may pulsate in the presence of tricuspid regurgitation. Marked increases in hepatic venous pressure can result in jaundice and, especially if attended by hypotension, pulmonary oedema and hypoxaemia, can cause hepatic enzymes to increase markedly. Although the spleen is often enlarged, causes other than heart failure should be sought if it is palpable (e.g. endocarditis). Marked elevations in venous pressure, especially if due to tricuspid valve disease or constrictive pericarditis, may lead to ascites.

Hypoalbuminaemia, weight loss and cachexia may mimic the signs of chronic liver disease or malignancy. Although lean body mass is lost, fat mass is reduced even more.[4] The patient becomes subjectively and objectively weak, and cell-mediated immunity may be disturbed. Reduced appetite is a major factor in cachexia, and is probably due to hepatic or gastric congestion, and mental depression. Venous congestion of the gut may contribute to malabsorption. Although D-xylose absorption tests have been reported as normal, malabsorption of fats and amino acids has been found in patients with cardiac cachexia.[2,7] Elevations in venous or lymphatic pressure within the bowel wall may lead to a protein-losing enteropathy. Hepatic albumin synthesis rates appear to be increased to try and compensate for increased losses. Patients with heart failure have an elevated basal metabolic rate which may further exacerbate weight loss. Digoxin may contribute to anorexia and impair sugar and amino acid transport across the gut wall.

Cardiac cachexia is an ominous sign. The underlying cardiac problem should be sought and corrected if possible, although surgical mortality is increased in these patients. It is not clear if digoxin or diuretics make any difference to the course of the cachexia, although initial studies indicate that angiotensin-converting enzyme inhibitors may do so.

INFECTIVE ENDOCARDITIS

This commonly presents with general malaise and weight loss, whilst anaemia and hepatosplenomegaly may suggest an underlying gastrointestinal problem. Fever, cardiac murmurs and 'embolic' phenomena may not be prominent at presentation.

ARRHYTHMIAS

Mesenteric ischaemia is common in patients with cardiac disease. Acute obstruction of the mesenteric artery may follow aortic dissection, a period of hypotension or, more rarely, systemic embolization. The acute onset of an arrhythmia may result in a period of hypotension and bowel infarction in the presence of mesenteric atheroma. Patients with heart failure, especially if already hypotensive, may be particularly prone to such complications. Arrhythmias may also result in systemic emboli to the mesenteric circulation.

AORTIC STENOSIS: ANGIOMATOUS DYSPLASIA

Angiodysplasia is a common problem in the elderly patient, and so is aortic stenosis. It is likely that the two conditions are associated with the ageing process. However, patients with aortic stenosis, possibly related to relative hypotension and hypoperfusion, are more likely to bleed from these colonic arteriovenous malformations. Most appear to be located in the right side of the colon. If significant bleeding occurs then surgery is indicated when possible.

DISEASES THAT AFFECT BOTH THE CARDIOVASCULAR AND GASTROINTESTINAL SYSTEMS

HAEMOCHROMATOSIS AND HAEMOSIDEROSIS (*see also* page 1281)

Iron overload causes similar abnormalities of cardiac function regardless of the aetiology. Iron is deposited within the myocytes and conduction tissue, but only causes dysfunction when present in large amounts. The rate of accumulation rather than the absolute amount may be more important. Cardiac involvement parallels that in other organs only roughly, is clinically apparent in half of all cases at diagnosis and is thought to be more common in younger subjects. The exact mechanism by which iron overload causes cardiac dysfunction is unknown, but defects in myocyte contraction as well as interstitial fibrosis occur. Arrhythmias (usually atrial), conduction disturbances and heart failure may all occur. In a Swedish population, 3 of 232 men requiring a pacemaker for atrioventricular block had evidence of iron overload on liver biopsy, considerably higher than in the general population.[13] Cardiac failure remains a common cause of death in these syndromes and usually occurs within a few years of the appearance of significant cardiac dysfunction, although effective treatment may modify the course of the disease.

The ECG shows diminished voltages and non-specific T-wave changes. Echocardiography in the earlier stages of the disease shows a non-dilated, hypertrophied ventricle with a reduced filling rate; in the late stages of the disease the ventricle is usually dilated and indistinguishable from dilated cardiomyopathy, more rarely the restrictive picture (resembling constrictive pericarditis) may persist.

The presence of diabetes mellitus or of haematological conditions requiring frequent blood transfusions, in the presence of heart failure, should alert to the possibility of iron overload. Hepatomegaly is almost universal, but skin pigmentation may be absent. Serum ferritin levels are usually grossly elevated. Endomyocardial biopsy can establish the diagnosis.

Venesection and iron chelation can reverse iron accumulation over a period of years.[3] Regression of the symptoms and signs of heart disease has been reported with such treatment. During iron depletion therapy, tissue stores may still be high when serum ferritin levels have fallen. Serial endomyocardial biopsy (the routine use of this technique to monitor patients frequently after cardiac transplantation for signs of early rejection has demonstrated its safety) may be employed to monitor regression of iron stores.[11] Endomyocardial biopsy may be useful in identifying cardiac infiltration at an early stage in those at risk of iron overload.

AMYLOIDOSIS

Clinical cardiac involvement is extremely rare with amyloidosis associated with chronic inflammatory disease or familial mediterranean fever (AA-amyloid), but is common (40% or more) in AL-amyloid, the type associated with deposition of immunoglobulin light chains and monoclonal proliferation of plasma cell lines. It is also found in amyloid due to deposition of pre-albumin (familial amyloidosis and senile amyloidosis).[5]

Amyloidosis may affect the gastrointestinal tract directly (AA- or AL-amyloid), or indirectly through the involvement of the autonomic nerves (usually AL-amyloid). It is mainly the latter that causes gastrointestinal symptoms. Rarely an atrial myxoma may cause AA-amyloid affecting the gut.

Cardiac infiltration with amyloid may result in heart failure. The ECG is usually of low voltage and Q waves may be present. Arrhythmias and conduction abnormalities are frequent. Echocardiography usually reveals a non-dilated, thick-walled ventricle with reduced systolic function and impaired filling, the predominant haemodynamic defect.[8] The myocardium characteristically has a 'sparkling' appearance. The low ECG voltages contrast with the echocardiographic appearance of hypertrophy. Apart from the echocardiographic features described above, amyloid may also affect the coronary vasculature. Non-invasive diagnostic procedures using radioactively-labelled serum amyloid component P can image amyloid deposits in other organs, but usually fails to image cardiac deposits. This may be because the heart is relatively deep and therefore more difficult to image, or because amyloid deposits that are sufficiently gross to appear on a scan are incompatible with life.

Endomyocardial biopsy is diagnostic but not all cases demonstrate typical apple-green birefringence when stained with Congo red. Electron microscopy reveals characteristic amyloid fibrils. Small amounts of amyloid are common in the hearts of elderly patients and may play a role in the decline of cardiac function with age, but senile amyloidosis appears to run an indolent course. Medical treatment is of limited efficacy and the prognosis grave, with most patients dying within a year of the onset of heart failure. If appropriate, cardiac transplantation is advisable sooner rather than later. Although histological evidence of amyloid may occur within months, overt cardiac dysfunction may not occur for much longer, and cardiac transplantation is not a ticket to immortality even in those without amyloid. Recently liver transplantation has been suggested as a treatment for arresting the progress of amyloidosis. Combined heart and liver transplants have been successful in conditions such as familial hypercholesterolaemia, and may be suitable for the treatment of amyloidosis when the prognosis is not limited by the presence of malignant disease. Diuretics or agents to reduce the preload on the failing heart will reduce pulmonary and venous congestion but will lead to a fall in cardiac output which may lead to hypotension and uraemia, especially if there is associated autonomic neuropathy or renal involvement.

BEHÇET'S SYNDROME

Cardiovascular involvement includes myopericarditis, thrombophlebitis and aneurysm formation in large systemic and/or pulmonary arteries. Myocarditis may lead to heart failure, conduction disturbances and valvular regurgitation. Thrombophlebitis may lead to myocardial infarction and rupture of pulmonary or systemic aneurysms to severe haemorrhage.

CARDIOVASCULAR DRUGS ASSOCIATED WITH GASTROINTESTINAL SIDE EFFECTS

ANTICOAGULANTS

These may cause exacerbation of gastrointestinal blood loss.

DRUGS USED FOR ARRHYTHMIAS

Nausea and vomiting are common with most antiarrhythmic agents, and are sometimes the first indication of excessive dosing. Most of these agents can cause hepatitis and/or cholestatic jaundice.

Amiodarone

Hepatitis is rare, and elevation in liver enzymes is more usually due to problems associated with the underlying heart disease. A reduction in amiodarone dose is recommended if patients present with abnormal liver function, or if transient elevations in liver enzymes occur. Amiodarone should be withdrawn as appropriate if liver enzymes are persistently elevated. The liver histology is variable, and has included cirrhosis, although it is difficult to attribute this directly to the drug. Very rarely hepatitis may progress despite withdrawal of the drug, which may be related to the long elimination half-life of amiodarone deposited in adipose tissues.

Disopyramide

Anticholinergic side effects such as a dry mouth are common; cholestatic jaundice is rare. The half-life of disopyramide is increased in patients with liver disease.

Digoxin

Nausea and vomiting may be valuable signs of drug toxicity. Constipation is a less well-recognized side effect.

DRUGS USED FOR HYPERTENSION

Methyldopa

Methyldopa may cause a Coombs' positive, haemolytic anaemia in 10–20% of cases, but this rarely manifests as jaundice. Methyldopa may rarely cause hepatitis and hepatic necrosis.

DRUGS USED FOR ANGINA

Verapamil

Constipation is common if enquired after, but is rarely severe and often improves with continued therapy, perhaps secondary to alterations in the diet.

B-Blockers

This class of agents has been associated with the production of retroperitoneal fibrosis. Practolol, one of the B-blockers most commonly associated with this side effect, has now been withdrawn. Other B-blockers have very rarely been associated with this side effect.

DRUGS USED FOR HEART FAILURE

Angiotensin converting enzyme (ACE) inhibitors

The renin–angiotensin system is important in blood pressure control especially during periods of salt and water depletion. Vomiting and diarrhoea may result in hypotension, prerenal renal failure and occasionally shock in such patients.

DIURETICS

Constipation may occur associated with relative dehydration.

PHOSPHODIESTERASE INHIBITORS

The inotropic and vasodilator agents such as amrinone, milrinone and enoximone have been licensed for intravenous use at present only in several countries. Nausea, vomiting and diarrhoea are common with these agents, and may respond to a reduction in dosage.

REFERENCES

1. Ahmed, S.S., Howard, M., ten Hove, W., Leevy, C.M. and Regan, T. (1984) Cardiac function in alcoholics with cirrhosis: absence of overt cardiomyopathy – myth or fact? *Journal of American College of Cardiologists*, **3**, 696–702.
2. Buchanan, N., Keen, R.D. and Kingsley, R. (1977) Gastrointestinal absorption studies in cardiac cachexia. *Intensive Care Medicine*, **3**, 89–91.
3. Candell-Riera, J., Lu, L., Seres, L. *et al.* (1983) Cardiac haemochromatosis: beneficial effects of iron removal therapy. *American Journal of Cardiology*, **52**, 824–829.
4. Cleland, J.G.F., Dargie, H.J., Robertson, I., Robertson, J.I.S. and East, B.W. (1987) Total body electrolyte composition in patients with heart failure: a comparison with normal subjects and patients with heart failure. *British Heart Journal*, **58**, 230–238.
5. Gertz, M.A. and Kyle, R.A. (1989) Primary systemic amyloidosis – a diagnostic primer. *Mayo Clinic Proceedings*, **64**, 1505–1519.
6. Himelman, R.B. and Schiller, N.B. (1989) Clinical echocardiographic comparison of patients with the carcinoid syndrome with and without carcinoid heart disease. *American Journal of Cardiology*, **63**, 347–352.
7. Jones, R.V. (1961) Fat malabsorption in congestive heart failure. *British Medical Journal*, **1**, 1276–1278.
8. Kinoshita, O., Hongo, M., Yamada, H. *et al.* (1989) Impaired left ventricular diastolic filling in patients with familial amyloid polyneuropathy: a pulsed doppler echocardiographic study. *British Heart Journal*, **61**, 198–203.
9. McAllister, H.A. and Fenoglio, J.J. (1975) Cardiac involvement in Whipple's Disease. *Circulation*, **52**, 152–159.
10. Mowat, N.A.G., Bennet, P.N., Finlayson, J.K., Brunt, P.W. and Lancaster, W.M. (1974) Myopericarditis complicating ulcerative colitis. *British Heart Journal*, **36**, 724–729.
11. Olson, L.J., Edwards, W.D., Holmes, D.R., Miller, F.A., Nordstrom, L.A. and Baldus, W.P. (1989) Endomyocardial biopsy in haemochromatosis: clinicopathological correlates in six cases. *Journal of the American College of Cardiologists*, **13**, 116–120.
12. Pope, C.E. (1989) Chest pain and the oesophagus. In *Topics in Gastroenterology*, pp. 13–26. (Ed.) Jewell, J.P. and Lowes, J.R. Oxford: Blackwell Scientific.
13. Rosenqvist, M. and Hultcrantz, R. (1989) Prevalence of haemochromatosis among men with clinically significant bradyarrhythmias. *European Heart Journal*, **10**, 473–478.
14. Snyder, N., Atterbury, C.E., Correia, J.P. and Conn, H.F. (1977) Increased occurrence of cirrhosis in bacterial endocarditis. *Gastroenterology*, **73**, 1107–1113.

PULMONARY ASSOCIATIONS OF GASTROINTESTINAL DISEASE

N.J. Douglas

The lung and the foregut have a common embryological origin and remain both connected and in close proximity throughout life. This results in many diseases of the gastrointestinal tract affecting the lung.

CONGENITAL

Tracheo-oesophageal fistulas probably develop around 5 weeks after conception. In 90% of cases, there is a proximal blind-ending oesophagus and usually a connection between the distal oesophagus and the trachea. In the remaining 10% of cases, an 'H'-type fistula occurs which may remain undetected until investigation of the resulting bronchiectasis in adulthood. Respiratory complications following surgical correction of tracheo-oesophageal fistulas are rare. Foregut duplication cysts are often asymptomatic; those that are not usually present in childhood with dyspnoea, dysphagia or infections.

HEREDITARY DISORDERS

Lung and gastrointestinal disease coexist in several such conditions, including cystic fibrosis, α_1-antitrypsin deficiency and hereditary haemorrhagic telangiectasia. The latter may produce gastrointestinal bleeding in a third of patients and pulmonary arteriovenous malformations in a fifth.[21] The pulmonary arteriovenous malformations (*Figure 8.10*) may give rise to hypoxaemia, bleeding and the intracerebral complications of emboli and abscess

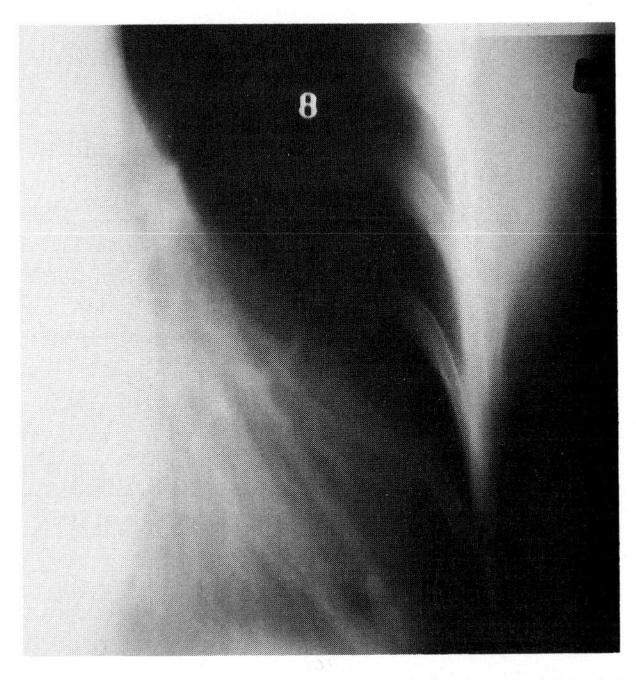

Figure 8.10 Arteriovenous malformation on tomography of the left lung base in a patient with hereditary haemorrhagic telangiectasia.

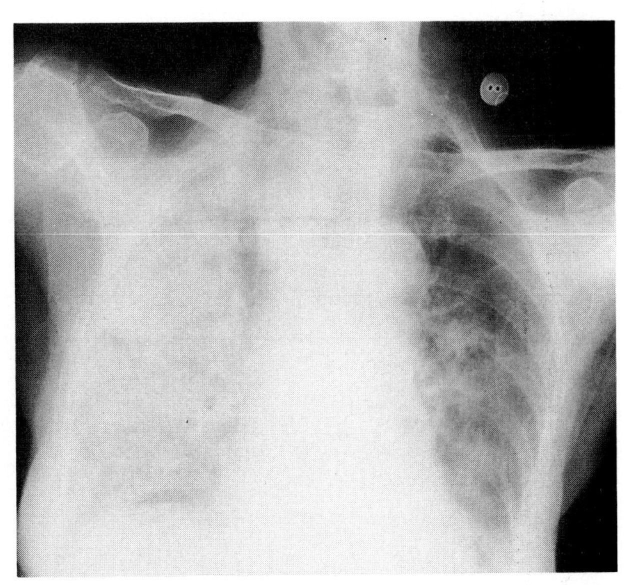

Figure 8.11 Aspiration pneumonia as a result of spill-over from an oesophageal pouch. The fluid level in the pouch can be seen at the level of the first thoracic vertebra.

formation. Percutaneous transcatheter embolization is now the treatment of choice[4] although resection of isolated lesions is still carried out in some centres.

OESOPHAGEAL DISEASE

A wide variety of oesophageal and pharyngeal disorders has been associated with lung disease, including hiatus hernia, achalasia, oesophageal atresia and pharyngeal pouch[2] (*Figure 8.11*). Patients with these conditions may not have any direct oesophageal symptoms and may present with cough, wheeze, dyspnoea or recurrent production of purulent sputum. These oesophageal conditions may cause pneumonia, bronchiectasis, lung abscess and airway obstruction. Gastro-oesophageal reflux was believed to cause pulmonary effects by two mechanisms: first, oesophageal contents may reflux into the airways causing pulmonary infections; secondly, the presence of acid in the oesophagus may cause vagally mediated bronchoconstriction but the clinical importance of this mechanism is debatable.[20] It is usually difficult – indeed impossible – to make an absolute diagnosis of reflux-associated lung disease. Barium swallow, oesophageal motility and oesophageal endoscopy studies will all show evidence of reflux in over 40% of adults with respiratory disease, and oesophageal pH monitoring may show reflux in almost all such patients. Ultimately the diagnosis will rest on clinical suspicion, supportive – but not diagnostic – investigation and a successful response to treatment.

Oesophagoscopy can also result in respiratory problems when perforation occurs (*Figure 8.12*). This may produce communication with either the pleural space or the lung initiating an inflammatory reaction (*Figure 8.13*).

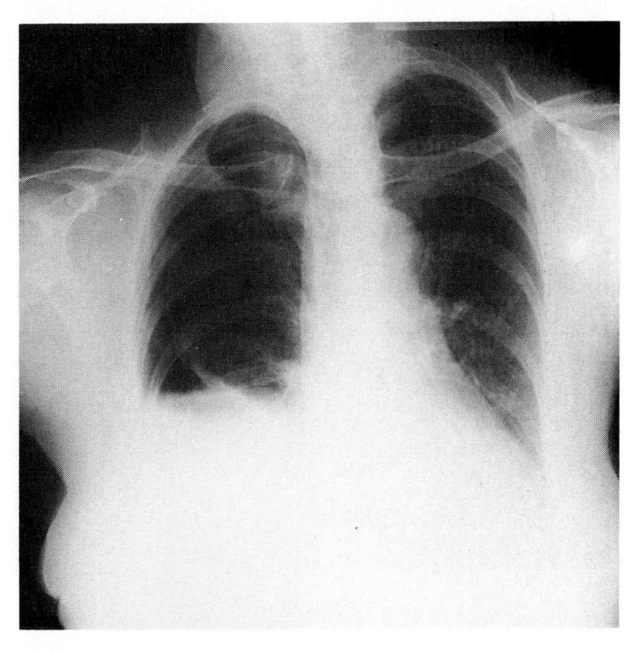

Figure 8.12 Right hydropneumothorax resulting from oesophageal perforation at oesophagoscopy.

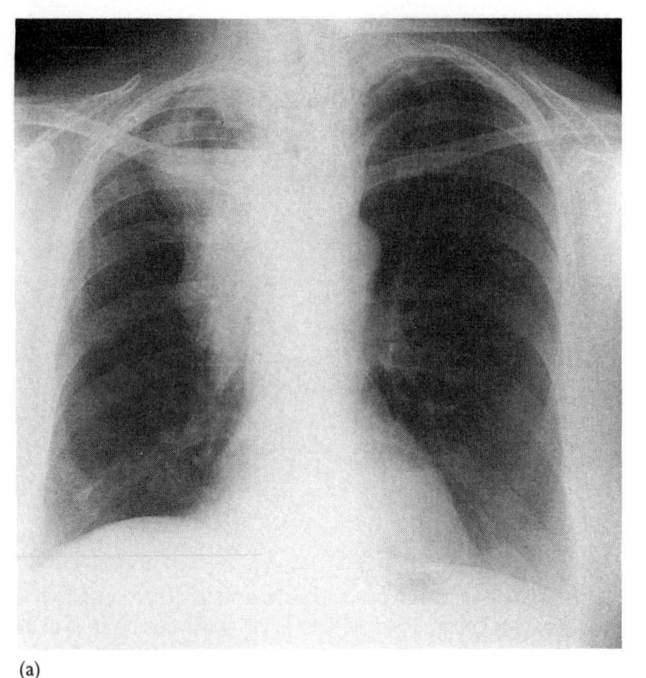

(a)

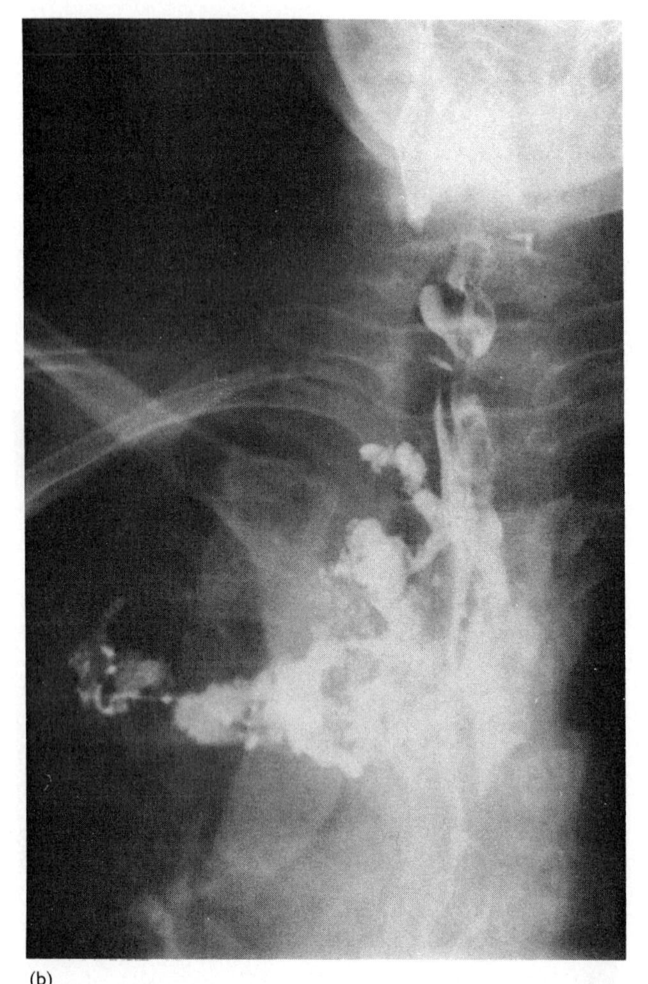

(b)

Figure 8.13 Right pulmonary abscess and mediastinal widening following oesophageal perforation at oesophagoscopy. The contrast study shows the fistula created.

Pulmonary complications of endoscopic sclerotherapy

Aspiration pneumonia, pleural effusion and pulmonary infiltrates can all occur following sclerotherapy of oesophageal varices. Usually these complications follow the use of sodium morrhuate as the sclerosing agent. Reactions to this agent may include bronchospasm and transient pulmonary hypertension, and the latter may be blunted by indomethacin in animals.

ASPIRATION OF STOMACH CONTENTS

Aspiration of gastric contents following vomiting produces Mendelson's syndrome characterized by dyspnoea, cyanosis and crepitations (crackles). The clinical and radiological features progress rapidly in the hours after aspiration and may quickly result in full-blown adult respiratory distress syndrome. The severity of the illness relates to both the acidity and the volume of fluid aspirated. Treatment is by oxygen and ventilatory support, as required. Neither prophylactic antibiotics nor steroids are helpful.

Aspiration of fluids of neutral pH usually only causes transient respiratory distress. However, the aspiration of large volumes of hypertonic fluid such as enteral feeds may cause extensive pulmonary epithelial damage and sustained hypoxaemia. Aspiration of small food particles may result in aspiration pneumonia. Large food particles may obstruct the airways, the largest ones causing laryngeal obstruction and then requiring the Heimlich manoeuvre to clear the airway.

INTESTINAL DISEASE

Inflammatory bowel disease is associated with pulmonary disease. Early retrospective studies showed this to be an infrequent connection[10] with only 3 of 1400 patients with inflammatory disease being found to have concurrent, unexplained, lung disease.[10,17] However, prospective studies have shown relatively high rates of abnormality of pulmonary function tests.[3,6] In addition to direct effects of the disease on the lungs, inflammatory bowel disease may reduce oxygen carriage by reducing haemoglobin, and impaired nutrition may adversely affect respiratory muscle function.[5]

ULCERATIVE COLITIS

Ulcerative colitis is occasionally causally associated with lung disease, in addition to the development of alveolitis caused by sulphasalazine (see below). The main lung problem seems to be an inflammatory reaction affecting the airways resulting in persistent cough and, in about one-third of those affected, bronchiectasis. Bronchial biopsies have been performed in two patients with bronchitis and in two with bronchiectasis, and in all four there was epithelial and basement membrane thickening and submucosal inflammatory infiltration.[9] These changes are similar to those found in the colonic mucosa and it has been suggested that there is a common immune reaction affecting both the bowel and the bronchi in these patients.[3,9] Although, pulmonary function tests are not consistently abnormal in patients with ulcerative colitis, compared to normals matched for age, sex, smoking and haemoglobin, recent evidence suggests that, in some patients, functional residual capacity may be raised and gas transfer impaired during exacerbations, both abnormalities settling as the bowel disease becomes inactive.[6] In addition, respiratory symptoms may improve with therapy for the bowel disease, steroids improving cough and dyspnoea, and reducing sputum volume in 7 out of 10 patients.[3]

Pulmonary fibrosis has been occasionally reported in patients with ulcerative colitis, but it is not clear whether this is merely a chance association. Ankylosing spondylitis can be associated with apical fibrosis, but only one patient with ulcerative colitis, ankylosing spondylitis and pulmonary fibrosis has been reported.

CROHN'S DISEASE

Pulmonary manifestations in Crohn's disease seem to be less common than in ulcerative colitis but alveolitis, bronchiectasis and pleural effusion have all been reported. Cough and chest infections from recurrent aspiration may occur in patients with Crohn's disease of the oesophagus which has resulted in oesophageal stricture. Lung function testing has shown functional residual capacity to be raised and gas transfer to be impaired during exacerbations of the bowel disease.[6]

Bronchoalveolar lavage has shown increases in lymphocytes in two-thirds of Crohn's disease patients[22] with other studies showing that this increase particularly affects CD4 lymphocytes.[18] These studies suggest that most patients with Crohn's disease have some pulmonary involvement. There are also biopsy reports of granuloma formation in the airways and in the alveoli of patients with Crohn's disease. The respiratory symptoms and the respiratory function abnormalities in patients with Crohn's disease have been reported to improve with steroid therapy.[6]

Lung complications of sulphasalazine

Cough, fever and dyspnoea with eosinophilia and diffuse pulmonary shadowing on chest radiograph can result from sulphasalazine therapy.[1] Pathological changes include vasculitis, alveolitis, pulmonary infiltration and fibrosis. Challenge testing indicates that the hypersensitivity reaction is due to the sulphapyridine moiety. The idiosyncratic alveolitis seems to arise only in those treated for more than 2 months with doses greater than 2 g/day. Withdrawal of treatment may result in improvement in both symptoms and radiological features.

WHIPPLE'S DISEASE

Cough, dyspnoea, pleuritic pain and pleural effusion can all be major features of this rare disorder. Although the predominant intestinal and joint manifestations are attributed to intestinal infection, the pulmonary manifestations may be the result of an inflammatory reaction to locally deposited immune complexes containing bacterial antigens.[19] The pulmonary manifestations may mimic pulmonary sarcoidosis.

COELIAC DISEASE

Pulmonary fibrosis has been thought to be associated with coeliac disease[12] but no causal connection has been proven. Routine pulmonary function testing is no different in patients with coeliac disease than in matched normals,[14] but there is recent evidence of increased pulmonary epithelial permeability in coeliac disease.[16]

PANCREATITIS

Pulmonary effects of acute pancreatitis are both common and clinically important. They are major factors in around a quarter of deaths in this condition, and contribute significantly to a further third.[15] The development of respiratory symptoms indicates a poor prognosis, with around 60% of deaths in the first week being associated with respiratory failure.[15] The most common chest radiograph manifestation of pancreatitis is diaphragmatic elev-

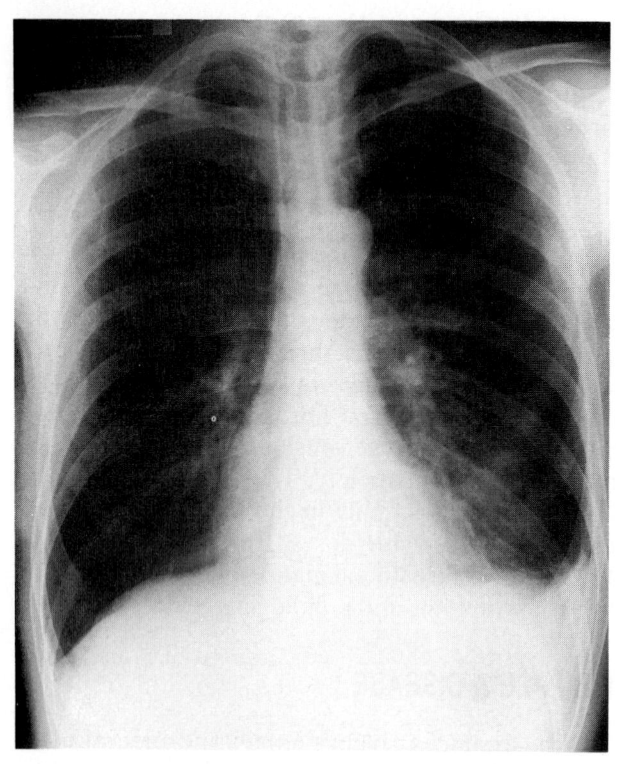

Figure 8.14 Left pleural effusion, left basal atelectasis and minor pulmonary infiltration in a patient with acute pancreatitis.

ation found in about a third of patients. Basal atelectasis is almost as frequent, with pneumonitis and pleural effusion less common (*Figure 8.14*). Around 15% of patients with acute pancreatitis develop the adult respiratory distress syndrome which is particularly common in those with haemorrhagic pancreatitis.[15] Breathlessness and tachypnoea develop within a week of onset, and are associated with diffuse abnormalities on the chest radiograph and arterial hypoxemia.

The hypoxemia may be difficult to detect clinically because the haemoglobin dissociation curve may be shifted to the left. Pulmonary histology in adult respiratory distress syndrome is indistinguishable from other causes with interstitial and alveolar oedema, hyaline membrane formation and alveolar type 2 cell proliferation. This is then followed by organization and interstitial fibrosis. The cause of adult respiratory distress syndrome in acute pancreatitis is not known, although many explanations have been proposed. It is possible that neutrophil activation results from the pancreatitis and these primed neutrophils aggregate in the lung causing damage by release of reactive oxygen species.[8] Treatment of the adult respiratory distress syndrome is by oxygen and ventilatory support, if indicated. There is no role for prophylactic steroids. Antibiotics should only be used once a pathogen has been identified.

Pleural effusions can occur in patients with acute or chronic pancreatitis and in association with pancreatic abscesses and pseudocysts. At least 5% of patients with acute pancreatitis will have radiological evidence of pleural effusions and an incidence of up to 40% has been reported. Three-quarters of such effusions occur on the left side, presumably reflecting proximity to the pancreas. Lymphatic connections may be involved in the transdiaphragmatic spread, although direct communication has also been invoked. Pleural amylase is high in 90% of cases, a useful aetiological pointer in the clinical context. However, pleural effusion amylase may also be raised in effusions caused by lung carcinoma or oesophageal rupture. Pleural effusions normally subside as acute pancreatitis resolves and persistence of the effusion after 2 weeks should suggest the possibility of pancreatic abscess or pseudocyst. Pleural effusions are much less common in chronic pancreatitis. In this situation, the fluid is an exudate usually with a very high polymorph count and a very high amylase level. Such effusions are often large and symptomatic, and thus require intermittent or continuous drainage. Pancreatopleural fistulas may occur and may require surgical closure.[13] Rarely, decortication may be required to control recurrent effusions or resultant gross pleural thickening.[13]

LIVER DISEASE

Both acute and chronic liver disease are associated with hypoxaemia due at least in part to intrapulmonary vascular dilatation.[7] The respiratory manifestations of liver disease are outside the scope of this book but have been recently reviewed.[11]

REFERENCES

1. Averbuch, M., Halpern, Z., Hallak, A. *et al.* (1985) Sulphasalazine pneumonitis. *American Journal of Gastroenterology*, **80**, 343–345.
2. Belsey, R. (1960) The pulmonary complications of oesophageal disease. *British Journal of Diseases of the Chest*, **54**, 342–348.
3. Butland, R.J.A., Cole, P., Citron, K.M. *et al.* (1981) Chronic bronchial suppuration and inflammatory bowel disease. *Quarterly Journal of Medicine*, **197**, 63–75.
4. Chilvers, E.R., Whyte, M.K.B., Jackson, J.E., Allison, D.J. and Hughes, M.B. (1990) Effects of percutaneous trans-catheter embolization on pulmonary function, right to left shunt and arterial oxygenation in patients with pulmonary arteriovenous malformations. *American Review of Respiratory Disease*, **142**, 420–425.

5. Christie, P.M. and Hill, G.L. (1990) Effect of intravenous nutrition on nutrition and function in acute attacks of inflammatory bowel disease. *Gastroenterology*, **99**, 730–736.
6. Douglas, J.G., McDonald, C.F., Leslie, M.J., Gillon, J., Crompton, G.K. and McHardy, G.J. (1989) Respiratory impairment in inflammatory bowel disease: Does it vary with disease activity? *Respiratory Medicine*, **83**, 389–394.
7. Edell, E.S., Cortese, D.A., Krowka, M.J. and Rehder, K. (1989) Severe hypoxemia in liver disease. *American Review of Respiratory Disease*, **140**, 1631–1635.
8. Guice, K.S., Oldham, K.T., Wolfe, R.R. *et al.* (1987) Lung injury in acute pancreatitis: primary inhibition of phospholipid synthesis. *American Journal of Surgery*, **153**, 54–60.
9. Higenbottom, T., Cochrane, G.M., Clark, T.J.H. *et al.* (1980) Bronchial disease in ulcerative colitis. *Thorax*, **35**, 581–585.
10. Kraft, S.C., Earle, R.H., Rosler, M. *et al.* (1973) Unexplained bronchopulmonary disease with inflammatory bowel disease. *Archives of Internal Medicine*, **136**, 454–459.
11. Krowka, M.J. and Cortese, D.A. (1989) Pulmonary aspects of liver disease and liver transplantation. *Clinics in Chest Medicine*, **10**, 593–616.
12. Lancaster Smith, M.J., Benson, M.K. and Strickland, I.D. (1971) Coeliac disease and diffuse interstitial lung disease. *The Lancet*, **1**, 473–475.
13. Light, R.W. (1985) Exudative pleural effusions secondary to gastrointestinal disease. *Clinics in Chest Medicine*, **6**, 103–111.
14. Neilly, J.B., Main, A.N.H., McSharry, C., Murray, J., Russell, R.I. and Moran, F. (1989) Pulmonary abnormalities in Crohn's disease. *Respiratory Medicine*, **83**, 487–491.
15. Renner, I.G., Savage, W.T., Pantoja, J.L. *et al.* (1985) Death due to acute pancreatitis: A retrospective analysis of 405 autopsy cases. *Digestive Diseases and Sciences*, **30**, 1005–1008.
16. Robertson, D.A., Taylor, N., Sidhu, H., Briten, A., Smith, C.L. and Holdstock, G. (1989) Pulmonary permeability in coeliac disease in inflammatory bowel disease. *Digestion*, **42**, 98–103.
17. Rogers, B.H.G., Clark, L. and Kirsher, J.P. (1971) The epidemiologic and demographic characteristics of inflammatory bowel disease: An analysis of a computerized file of 1400 patients. *Journal of Chronic Diseases*, **24**, 743–773.
18. Smlejan, J.M., Cosnes, J., Chollet-Martin, S. *et al.* (1986) Sarcoid-like lymphocytosis of the lower respiratory tract in patients with active Crohn's disease. *Annals of Internal Medicine*, **104**, 17–21.
19. Symmons, D.P.M., Shepard, A.N., Boardman, P.L. *et al.* (1985) Pulmonary manifestations of Whipple's disease. *Quarterly Journal of Medicine*, **56**, 497–504.
20. Tan, W.C., Martin, R.J., Pandey, R. and Ballard, R.D. (1990) Effects of spontaneous and simulated gastroesophageal reflux on sleeping asthmatics. *American Review of Respiratory Disease*, **141**, 1394–1399.
21. Vase, P., Holm, M. and Arendrup, H. (1985) Pulmonary arteriovenous fistulas in hereditary haemorrhagic telangiectasia. *Acta Medica Scandinavica*, **218**, 105–109.
22. Wallaert, B., Colombel, J.F., Tonnel, A.B. *et al.* (1985) Evidence of lymphocytic alveolitis in Crohn's disease. *Chest*, **87**, 363–367.

LIPID ABNORMALITIES

G.R. Thompson

LIPOPROTEIN PHYSIOLOGY

The gastrointestinal tract plays an important role in the metabolism of plasma lipoproteins.[17] Dietary fat, mainly triglyceride, is first emulsified in the stomach and then undergoes hydrolysis by pancreatic lipase and solubilization by bile salts. The resultant fatty acids and monoglycerides, together with some free cholesterol and lysophosphatidylcholine (lysoPC), become incorporated into mixed micelles and are then taken up by the jejunal mucosa, whereas bile salts get reabsorbed later in the ileum. Subsequent resynthesis of triglyceride, and partial re-esterification of cholesterol and reacylation of lysophosphatidylcholine leads to the formation of chylomicrons, which comprise a core of triglyceride and cholesterol esters enclosed in a surface coat of free cholesterol, phosphatidylcholine and various apoproteins (apo). The latter include apoB48, apoA-I, apoA-II, apoA-IV and the apoC group. All are synthesized in the small intestine and are constituents both of chylomicrons and of the similar but smaller particles in lymph known as intestinal very-low-density lipoprotein (VLDL). In addition apoA-I is a major constituent of high-density lipoprotein (HDL) of intestinal origin, in contrast to HDL of hepatic origin which is rich in apoE.

After traversing the thoracic duct lymph chylomicrons enter the plasma and acquire apoE and additional apoC peptides from HDL, including apoC-II, the activator of lipoprotein lipase. This enzyme is situated mainly in capillaries serving adipose tissue and muscle and effects the hydrolysis of chylomicron and VLDL triglyceride. During this process, chylomicrons decrease in size and lose much of their apoA-I, apoA-IV and apoC together with some of the polar lipids in their surface coat. The resultant chylomicron remnants are taken up by the liver, probably via receptors that bind apoE, where they serve to regulate the activity of hydroxymethylglutaryl coenzyme A (HMG-CoA) reductase and thus control endogenous cholesterol synthesis. All the apoB48 gets removed from plasma but some free cholesterol and phosphatidylcholine transfer from chylomicrons to HDL_3, promoting its conversion to HDL_2 by providing substrate for lecithin:cholesterol acyltransferase (LCAT). This enzyme functions in plasma to esterify free cholesterol with an unsaturated fatty acid derived from the position 2 of phosphatidylcholine. HDL_3 is the major substrate for this reaction, which is activated by apoA-I.

Some of the free fatty acid released during peripheral lipolysis of chylomicrons is bound to albumin and transported to the liver, where it is converted into triglyceride and secreted back into plasma as VLDL of hepatic origin. The latter contains apoB100 and is hydrolysed in the periphery in a similar manner to chylomicrons, resulting in the formation of VLDL remnants which eventually get converted to low-density lipoproteins (LDL) via the action of hepatic lipase. VLDL remnants and LDL contain apoB100 but not apoB48 and interact with a receptor that recognizes both apoE and apoB100, the co-called LDL receptor. A simplified scheme of the various events which occur during lipoprotein metabolism is shown in *Figure 8.15*.

LIPOPROTEIN DISORDERS

The relationship between abnormalities of lipoprotein metabolism and the gastrointestinal tract is complex. Primary, genetically determined defects of lipoprotein metabolism can lead to hypocholesterolaemia and malabsorption, as in abetalipoproteinaemia, or to severe hypertriglyceridaemia and acute pancreatitis, as in familial type I hyperlipoproteinaemia. More commonly, however, changes in serum lipids are secondary manifestations either of malabsorption caused by disease or surgical intervention, or of excessive alcohol intake. The changes in serum lipids which accompany diabetes will not be considered in this section. For the sake of clarity both primary and secondary abnormalities of lipoprotein metabolism have been sub-divided according to whether they are primarily associated with malabsorption or with pancreatitis.

MALABSORPTION

Primary Hypolipoproteinaemia

Abetalipoproteinaemia

This rare, recessively inherited disease is characterized by the onset during infancy of malabsorption and anaemia accompanied by the development in later childhood of progressively severe ataxia and of retinitis pigmentosa. Examination of the blood shows the presence of acanthocytosis and the absence from plasma of chylomicrons, VLDL and LDL. Serum cholesterol and triglyceride levels are both very low, usually in the range 0.5–2 mmol/l, and apoB is undetectable.[16] Nearly all the cholesterol in plasma is present as HDL, mainly as HDL_2.

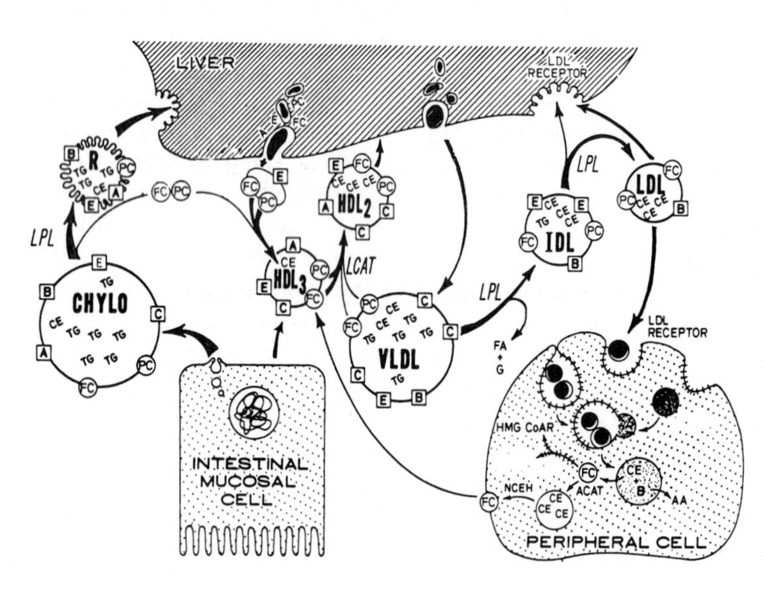

Figure 8.15 A schematic diagram of lipoprotein metabolism. CHYLO = chlyomicron; IDL = intermediate-density lipoprotein; R = remnant; LPL = lipoprotein lipase; FC = free cholesterol; CE = cholesterol ester; TG = triglyceride; FA = fatty acid; G = glycerol; HDL = high-density lipoprotein; LDL = low-density lipoprotein; VLDL = very-low-density lipoprotein. A, B, C, E refer to respective apo proteins. (Reproduced with permission from Davignon *et al.*[8])

Serum phospholipids are also markedly decreased, as is the phosphatidylcholine: sphingomyelin ratio. Postheparin lipolytic activity (which reflects mobilization of lipoprotein lipase and hepatic lipase) and LCAT activity are both reduced.

The clinical and biochemical features of this disorder have been reviewed by Herbert *et al.*[18] The majority of patients described seem to be males and at least half of them were the result of consanguineous unions. Obligate heterozygotes, however, show no signs of disease and have normal serum lipids. Homozygotes usually present with failure to grow and steatorrhoea in early childhood, with a differential diagnosis of either coeliac disease or cystic fibrosis of the pancreas. Jejunal biopsy shows the characteristic lipid-filled but otherwise normal looking villi.[20] Immunofluorescent studies have failed to demonstrate the presence of any apoB in the intestinal mucosa[13] or in the liver, which also contains excess fat. It had been assumed that the underlying defect was an inherited inability to synthesize both apoB48 and apoB100, and thus a failure to form either intestinal chylomicrons or hepatic VLDL. Linkage studies suggest, however, that the genetic abnormality responsible does not involve the apoB gene but another gene, possibly one involved in synthesis or secretion of apoB-containing lipoproteins.[35]

Malabsorption of triglyceride, although less marked than that of fat-soluble vitamins, leads to decreases in the linoleate and arachidonate content of plasma lipids. Osteomalacia has been reported[21] but deficiency of vitamin D is less common than of vitamins A, E and K.[18] The fluidity and filterability of red cells is decreased and this has been attributed to an increase in the sphingomyelin: phosphatidylcholine ratio of the red cell membrane.

Abetalipoproteinaemia represents the most severe vitamin E deficiency state known in humans. There is good evidence that vitamin E supplementation prevents the development of neurological symptoms if given in early childhood, and improves neurological function or prevents further deterioration if disability is present prior to starting treatment.[23]

Untreated neurological symptoms, of which the first tends to be ataxia, occur during the first decade of life in one-third of patients and by the age of 20 in the rest. The reflexes are often hypoactive before symptoms develop. The complete neurological picture consists of dysarthria, cerebellar ataxia of the limbs and of gait, areflexia, distal loss of vibration and joint position sense, pes cavus and scoliosis. Generalized muscle weakness is quite common. The plantar responses may be flexor or extensor. Ptosis and external ophthalmoplegia have been described. The disorder is progressive and relatively few patients are still ambulant after the age of 30.

Nocturnal amblyopia occasionally develops prior to ataxia but visual symptoms are very variable and many never arise. Pigmentary retinal degeneration has been seen in children aged 10 years or less and is usually evident during the second decade of life. The peripheral part of the retina contains hyperpigmented and depigmented areas with 'bone spicules'. These changes later spread to affect the macula with resulting loss of visual activity. The visual fields become progressively restricted.

Therapy for this disorder consists of a diet low in long-chain triglyceride, but containing 5–10 g linoleic acid daily, and supplements of vitamins A, E and K. Medium-chain triglyceride supplements are absorbed normally but have side effects which limit their usefulness. Perhaps the most encouraging feature of therapy is the probability that large doses of oral vitamin E (100 mg/kg per day) given from an early age may prevent or modify the neurological and retinal complications of abetalipoproteinaemia.[23]

Familial hypobetalipoproteinaemia

In the homozygous form this disorder presents in a manner either identical to or as a milder version of abetalipoproteinaemia. It differs in that heterozygotes have hypocholesterolaemia and LDL levels which are about 25% of normal. Thus the disorder appears to be inherited in an autosomal dominant manner.[6] It has been suggested that heterozygotes are protected from coronary heart disease by their low LDL levels and that this leads to enhanced longevity.[15] Reduced synthesis of apoB has been demonstrated in such individuals.[33]

Recently, it has been shown that hypobetalipoproteinaemia can result from mutation of the apoB gene, the severity of clinical manifestations correlating inversely with the length and amount of apoB synthesized, as reviewed by Innerarity.[19] At least 10 different mutations have been described so far, resulting in truncated forms of apoB which represent 25–89% of normal apoB100.

Normotriglyceridaemic abetalipoproteinaemia

Malloy *et al.*[22] described a young girl with ataxia in whom VLDL and LDL were absent but who was able to absorb triglyceride normally and produce chylomicrons in response to dietary fat. Jejunal biopsy was normal. It was subsequently shown that this patient was homozygous for an apoB50 mutation, which enabled her to produce apoB48 but not apoB100.[19]

Secondary hypolipoproteinaemia

Hypocholesterolaemia secondary to malabsorption ('sprue syndrome') was first described in adults by Adlersberg *et al.*[1] and similar findings were subsequently reported in children with coeliac disease.[27] Decreases in both LDL and HDL concentration in the face of normal or increased levels of VLDL were observed in a varied group of malabsorbers by Thompson and Miller[36] who noted that LDL levels were inversely correlated with the extent of steatorrhoea. These authors also observed changes in LDL composition, with a decreased proportion of cholesterol ester and a reciprocal increase in triglyceride. Such patients were subsequently shown to have reduced amounts of linoleic acid in lipoprotein lipids,[32] and in three instances overt essential fatty acid deficiency was documented following massive intestinal resection.[26] Decreased concentrations of LDL, HDL and linoleate have also been documented in children with pancreatic steatorrhoea due to cystic fibrosis.[37]

Hypocholesterolaemia can be induced surgically by ileal resection or by creating a partial ileal bypass.[3] The latter procedure results in a mean reduction in serum cholesterol of 40% and appears to be especially useful in the treatment of patients with heterozygous familial hypercholesterolaemia in whom it lowers LDL levels by stimulating receptor-mediated LDL catabolism,[34] thus helping to counteract the underlying metabolic defect. Its superiority over anion exchange resins seems to be due to the more marked increase in bile acid excretion, and presumably bile acid synthesis, which results from the surgical procedure. Partial ileal bypass necessitates the administration of parenteral vitamin B_{12} on a life-long basis and may also decrease the absorption of calcium but promote that of oxalate.[10] The POSCH (Programme on the Surgical Control of Hyperlipidaemia) trial recently demonstrated the beneficial effect of this procedure on hypercholesterolaemic coronary heart disease.[4]

PANCREATITIS

Although acute pancreatitis was originally thought to be the cause of the hyperlipaemia (i.e. gross hypertriglyceridaemia) which commonly accompanies it, evidence of this explanation is somewhat slender.[38] Studies by Cameron *et al.*[5] involving careful follow-up of patients with acute pancreatitis and hyperlipaemia revealed defects in lipid metabolism which persisted long after their attack of pancreatitis had subsided, which suggested that hyperlipaemia was the cause rather than the consequence of acute pancreatitis. Most of their patients exhibited a type V lipoprotein phenotype (excess chylomicrons and VLDL) during the acute episode but subsequently this phenotype often changed, either to a type IV phenotype (excess VLDL) or, less commonly, to a type I (excess chylomicrons) or type III (excess chylomicron and VLDL remnants) phenotype.

The mechanism whereby extreme hypertriglyceridaemia induces acute pancreatitis is uncertain. One possibility is that some of the triglyceride undergoes hydrolysis by pancreatic lipase, with release of free fatty acids and consequent damage to the gland.[28] Alternatively it is possible that pancreatic ischaemia is caused by the hyperviscosity which results from the presence of high concentrations of chylomicrons and VLDL in plasma.[31]

Primary hyperlipoproteinaemia

Familial lipoprotein lipase deficiency

This rare inherited disorder, also known as familial type I hyperlipoproteinaemia, is characterized by the onset in childhood of recurrent attacks of abdominal pain, acute pancreatitis and by eruptive xanthomas and hepatosplenomegaly. The condition is due to deficiency of lipoprotein lipase and a consequent inability to catabolize chylomicrons, which leads to marked hypertriglyceridaemia. Fasting chylomicronaemia is accompanied by normal or decreased levels of VLDL and by marked decreases in both LDL and HDL. The diagnosis depends upon establishing the presence in post-heparin plasma of levels of lipoprotein lipase less than 10% of normal. Discrimination between lipoprotein lipase and the other lipases released into plasma by heparin, notably hepatic lipase, is essential and is best achieved by an immunochemical method or by affinity chromatography.

The condition is usually considered to be due to an autosomal recessive gene, although measurements of postheparin lipoprotein lipase levels in the siblings of affected patients shows bimodality.[24] The risk of acute pancreatitis is minimal as long as plasma triglyceride levels are kept below 15–20 mmol/1; this is best achieved by a fat diet of less than 50 g. Establishing the diagnosis of acute pancreatitis during an episode of acute abdominal pain is made difficult through the interference by triglyceride with the assay for serum amylase.

Familial apoprotein C-II deficiency

This rare, recessively inherited disorder usually presents in adult life and is due to deficiency of apoC-II, the activator of lipoprotein lipase. Nineteen patients with this disorder have been described so far[24] among whom recurrent attacks of acute pancreatitis have been a common feature, in one instance progressing to chronic pancreatic insufficiency. The lipoprotein phenotype is type V and the diagnosis can sometimes be made by demonstrating absence or anomalies of apoC-II on isoelectric focusing of delipidated VLDL.

The first report of apoC-II deficiency[2] described a man with a type V phenotype whose hypertriglyceridaemia improved dramatically after a blood transfusion. Further investigations revealed detectable amounts of lipoprotein lipase in postheparin plasma, which became evident only after addition of apoC-II in vitro. Infusions of normal plasma containing apoC-II dramatically reduce plasma triglyceride levels in affected subjects, albeit temporarily. At least four functionally inactive forms of apoC-II have now been described.

Hepatic lipase deficiency

This rare disorder is characterized by both hypercholesterolaemia and hypertriglyceridaemia, due to accumulation of VLDL remnants. The HDL fraction contains triglyceride-rich HDL_2 but HDL_3 is absent.

Familial type V hyperlipoproteinaemia

This disorder is characterized by the onset in adult life of attacks of abdominal pain, eruptive xanthomas and peripheral neuropathy. The abdominal pain can be due to pancreatitis, which occurs in 40–60% of patients,[24] or to hepatic or splenic enlargement. Hypertriglyceridaemia is due to a combination of chylomicronaemia and increased levels of VLDL, and is exacerbated by factors which promote triglyceride synthesis, notably oestrogens, alcohol and being male.

The disorder is probably inherited in an autosomal dominant manner. There is an increased prevalence of type IV phenotypes among first-degree relatives. The exact nature of the biochemical defect is uncertain; postheparin lipoprotein lipase levels are usually normal but the activity of this enzyme is often subnormal in adipose tissue and muscle, which is compatible with a defect of triglyceride clearance. However, turnover studies suggest that VLDL synthesis is increased which makes it difficult to know whether the accompanying decrease in fractional catabolic rate is a primary or secondary phenomenon. Glucose intolerance, often leading to frank diabetes, and hyperuricaemia are common accompaniments of type V hyperlipoproteinaemia.

Treatment of this disorder is difficult, necessitating reductions in both total calories and fat intake. Possibly the most useful drugs are nicotinic acid or large doses of W-3 fatty acid-rich fish oil.[25] There have been several instances of patients with this condition in whom repeated attacks of acute pancreatitis eventually led to chronic pancreatic insufficiency.[11] It is debatable whether patients with type V hyperlipoproteinaemia have an increased prevalence of coronary heart disease, as has been claimed.

Secondary hyperlipoproteinaemia

Acquired type I hyperlipoproteinaemia has been described in systemic lupus erythematosus, due to the presence in plasma of an IgG antibody which blocked the release into plasma of lipoprotein lipase.[24] Oestrogens, given as replacement therapy[14] or as oral contraceptives,[7] can induce severe hypertriglyceridaemia and acute pancreatitis in patients with previously undiagnosed type IV or V hyperlipoproteinaemia. In one instance a similar effect has been attributed to β-blockers, which were shown to markedly impair triglyceride clearance.[9] But by far the most common cause of secondary type V hyperlipoproteinaemia is alcohol, which was the precipitating factor in more than 50% of the patients with hyperlipaemia and acute pancreatitis reported by Cameron *et al.*[5] Alcohol is preferentially oxidized by the liver which results in increased amounts of free fatty acid becoming available for triglyceride synthesis, thus increasing VLDL synthesis. Whether the magnitude of the hypertriglyceridaemic response to alcohol is genetically determined remains to be seen. The recent discovery of apoE polymorphism and the apparent increase in the apoE4 allele in type V patients[12] compared with normolipidaemic or type IV subjects, in whom the apoE3 allele predominates, offers a potentially fruitful line of enquiry, especially in view of the well-established relationship between inheritance of the apoE2 allele and type III hyperlipoproteinaemia.

REFERENCES

1. Adlersberg, D., Wang, C.I. and Bossak, E.T. (1957) Disturbances in protein and lipid metabolism in malabsorption syndrome. *Journal of the Mount Sinai Hospital*, **24**, 206.
2. Breckenridge, W.C., Little, A., Steiner, G. *et al.* (1978) Hypertriglyceridaemia associated with deficiency of apo-lipoprotein C-II. *New England Journal of Medicine*, **298**, 1265–1273.
3. Buchwald, H. (1964) Lowering of cholesterol resorption and blood levels by ileal exclusion. *Circulation*, **XXIX**, 713–720.
4. Buchwald, H., Varco, R.L., Matts, J.P. *et al.* (1990) Effect of partial ileal bypass surgery on mortality and morbidity from coronary heart disease in patients with hypercholesterolaemia. *New England Journal of Medicine*, **323**, 946–955.
5. Cameron, J.L., Capuzzi, D.M., Zuidema, G.D.

and Margolis, S. (1974) Acute pancreatitis with hyperlipemia. Evidence for a persistent defect in lipid metabolism. *American Journal of Medicine*, **56**, 482–487.
6. Cottrill, C., Glueck, C.J., Leuba, V. *et al.* (1974) Familial homozygous hypobetalipoproteinemia. *Metabolism*, **23**, 779–791.
7. Davidoff, F., Tishler, S. and Rosoff, C. (1973) Marked hyperlipidemia and pancreatitis associated with oral contraceptive therapy. *New England Journal of Medicine*, **289**, 552–555.
8. Davignon, J., Dufour, R. and Cantin, M. (1983) Atherosclerosis and hypertension. In *Hypertension, Physiopathology and Treatment* (Ed.) Genest, G., Kuchel, O., Hamet, P. and Cantin, M. New York: McGraw-Hill.
9. Durrington, P.N. and Cairns, S.A. (1982) Acute pancreatitis: a complication of beta-blockade. *British Medical Journal*, **284**, 1016.
10. Faegerman, O., Meinertz, H., Hylander, E. *et al.* (1982) Effects and side-effects of partial ileal by-pass surgery for familial hypercholesterolaemia. *Gut*, **23**, 558–563.
11. Fallat, R.W. and Glueck, C.J. (1976) Familial and acquired type V hyperlipoproteinemia. *Atherosclerosis*, **23**, 41–62.
12. Ghiselli, G., Schaefer, E.J., Zech, L.A. *et al.* (1982) Increased prevalence of apolipoprotein E_4 in type V hyperlipoproteinemia. *Journal of Clinical Investigation*, **70**, 474–477.
13. Glickman, R.M., Green, P.H.R., Lees, R.S. *et al.* (1979) Immunofluorescence studies of apolipoprotein B in intestinal mucosa. Absence in abetalipoproteinemia. *Gastroenterology*, **76**, 288–292.
14. Glueck, C.J., Scheel, D., Fishback, J. and Steiner, P. (1972) Estrogen-induced pancreatitis in patients with previously covert familial type V hyperlipoproteinemia. *Metabolism*, **21**, 657–666.
15. Glueck, C.J., Gartside, P., Fallat, R.W. *et al.* (1976) Longevity syndromes: familial hypobeta and familial hyperalpha lipoproteinemia. *Journal of Laboratory and Clinical Medicine*, **88**, 941–957.
16. Gotto, A.M., Levy, R.I., John, K. and Fredrickson, D.S. (1971) On the protein defect in abetalipoproteinemia. *New England Journal of Medicine*, **284**, 813.
17. Green, P.H.R. and Glickman, R.M. (1981) Intestinal lipoprotein metabolism. *Journal of Lipid Research*, **22**, 1153–1173.
18. Herbert, P.N., Assman, G., Gotto, A.M. and Fredrickson, D.S. (1983) Familial lipoprotein deficiency abetalipoproteinemia, hypobetalipoproteinemia, and Tangier disease. In *The Metabolic Basis of Inherited Disease* (Ed.) Stanbury, J.B., Wyngaarden, J.B., Fredrickson, D.S. *et al.*, 5th edn, pp. 589–621. New York: McGraw-Hill.
19. Innerraity, T.L. (1990) Familial hypobetalipoproteinaemia and familial defective apolipoprotein B100: genetic disorders associated with apolipoprotein B. *Current Opinion in Lipidology*, **1**, 104–109.
20. Isselbacher, K.J., Scheig, R., Plotkin, G.R. and Caulfield, J.B. (1964) Congenital β-lipoprotein deficiency: an hereditary disorder involving a defect in the absorption and transport of lipids. *Medicine (Baltimore)*, **43**, 347.
21. Lamy, M., Frezal, J., Polonovski, J. *et al.* (1963) Congenital absence of beta-lipoproteins. *Pediatrics*, **31**, 277–289.
22. Malloy, M.J., Kane, J.P., Hardman, D. *et al.* (1981) Normotriglyceridemic abetalipoproteinemia. Absence of the B-100 apolipoprotein. *Journal of Clinical Investigation*, **67**, 1441–1450.
23. Muller, D.P.R., Lloyd, J.K. and Bird, A.C. (1977) Long-term management of abetalipoproteinaemia. *Archives of Diseases in Childhood*, **52**, 209–214.
24. Nikkila, E.A. (1983) Familial lipoprotein lipase deficiency and related disorders of chylomicron metabolism. In *Metabolic Basis of Inherited Disease* (Ed.) Stanbury, J.B., Wyngaarden, J.B., Fredrickson, D.S. *et al.* 5th edn, pp. 622–642. New York: McGraw-Hill.
25. Phillipson, B.E., Rothrock, D.W., Connor, W.E., Harris, W.S. and Illingworth, D.R. (1985) Reduction of plasma lipids, lipoproteins and apoproteins by dietary fish oils in patients with hypertriglyceridemia. *New England Journal of Medicine*, **312**, 1210–1216.
26. Press, M., Kikuchi, H., Shimoyama, T. and Thompson, G.R. (1974) Diagnosis and treatment of essential fatty acid deficiency in man. *British Medical Journal*, **2**, 247–250.
27. Rey, J. (1965) Modifications des lipides plasmatiques dans les troubles de l'absorption intestinale. *Revue Européene d'Etudes Cliniques et Biologiques*, **10**, 488.
28. Saharia, P., Margolis, S., Zuidema, G.D. and Cameron J.L. (1977) Acute pancreatitis with hyperlipemia: studies with an isolated perfused canine pancreas. *Surgery*, **82**, 60–67.
29. Scott, B.B., Miller, J.P. and Losowsky, M.S. (1979) Hypobetalipoproteinaemia – a variant of the Bassen–Kornzweig syndrome. *Gut*, **20**, 163–168.
30. Scott, H.W., Dean, R.H., Younger, R.K. and Butts, W.H. (1974) Changes in hyperlipidemia and hyperlipoproteinemia in morbidly obese patients treated by jejunoileal bypass. *Surgery, Gynecology and Obstetrics*, **138**, 353–358.
31. Seplowitz, A.H., Chien, S. and Smith, F.R. (1981) Effects of lipoproteins on plasma viscosity. *Atherosclerosis*, **38**, 89–95.
32. Shimoyama, T., Kikuchi, H., Press, M. and Thompson, G.R. (1973) Fatty acid composition of plasma lipoproteins in control subjects and in patients with malabsorption. *Gut*, **14**, 716–722.
33. Sigurdsson, G., Nicoll, A. and Lewis, B. (1977) Turnover of apolipoprotein-B in two subjects with familial hypobetalipoproteinemia. *Metabolism*, **26**, 25–31.

34. Spengel, F.A., Jadhav, A., Duffield, R.G.M. *et al.* (1981) Superiority of partial ileal bypass over cholestyramine in reducing cholesterol in familial hypercholesterolaemia. *The Lancet*, **2**, 768–770.
35. Talmud, P.J., Lloyd, J.K., Muller, D.P.R., Collins, D.R., Scott, J. and Humphries, S. (1988) Genetic evidence from two families that the apolipoprotein B gene is not involved in abetalipoproteinemia. *Journal of Clinical Investigation*, **82**, 1803–1806.
36. Thompson, G.R. and Miller, J.P. (1973) Plasma lipid and lipoprotein abnormalities in patients with malabsorption. *Clinical Science and Molecular Medicine*, **45**, 583–592.
37. Vaughan, W.J., Lindgren, F.T., Whalen, J.B. and Abraham, S. (1978) Serum lipoprotein concentrations in cystic fibrosis. *Science*, **199**, 783–786.
38. Zieve, L. (1968) Relationship between acute pancreatitis and hyperlipemia. *Medical Clinics of North America*, **52**, 1493–1501.

HAEMOCHROMATOSIS

P.C. Hayes

Iron is present in a normal adult in quantities of 3–4 g; of this approximately 65% is present as haemoglobin, 30% as non-haem iron storage compounds, such as haemosiderin and ferritin, and approximately 3% as myoglobin.

Transferrin, the principal iron carriage protein, is synthesized in the liver and has a molecular weight of 80 000. It is present in the plasma at a concentration of 45–72 μmol/l and carries 3–4 mg iron with a serum concentration of 10–32 μmol/l. Transferrin binds two atoms of iron which can be transported into cells from transferrin after it is bound to membrane transferrin receptors. Ferritin was thought principally to be an intracellular, iron-binding protein. However, it is present in the serum at concentrations of 8–350 μg/l, and in situations of iron deficiency the serum ferritin level falls whereas in iron overload, it may rise considerably. Ferritin is capable of carrying over 4000 atoms of iron. Two other iron-binding proteins are present in blood – haptoglobin which binds haem iron and haemopexin which binds haem.

Pathological accumulation of iron in tissues may occur in certain circumstances resulting in haemosiderosis, but when such overload is severe enough to cause parenchymal injury haemochromatosis results. Iron overload results from a failure to maintain normal iron homoeostasis due to either (1) iron absorption in excess of body requirements, i.e. genetic, idiopathic or primary haemochromatosis, or (2) excessive iron administration or hyperabsorption secondary to blood disorders, acquired or secondary haemochromatosis. Irrespective of the mechanism involved, iron overload results in widespread tissue damage, especially of the liver, heart and pancreas.

PRIMARY HAEMOCHROMATOSIS

AETIOLOGY, PREVALENCE AND PATHOPHYSIOLOGY

This is an autosomal recessive disorder,[9,18] the gene of which is associated with the histocompatibility locus on the short arm of chromosome 6.[18] A disproportionately high frequency of the haplotypes of the histocompatibility locus antigen (HLA) – HLA-A3, HLA-B7 and HLA-B14 – occurs in homozygotes. Although the association is not close enough to be useful diagnostically, it may be useful in family studies. The frequency of homozygosity for haemochromatosis is 0.0045 with a gene frequency in the population of 0.067 – nearly 7% of the population. Not all subjects homozygous for the gene have clinical features of haemochromatosis. The proportion is lower in women, presumably due to iron loss with pregnancy and menstruation. A small proportion of heterozygotes develop features of iron overload.[10]

The genetic defect in primary haemochromatosis, in which iron absorption and tissue deposition continues unchecked despite an increase in total body iron, is incompletely understood. Two sites of iron uptake – the small intestine and the hepatocyte – have been intensively studied. A recent immunohistochemical study has demonstrated that, in untreated primary haemochromatosis, epithelial cells expressed transferrin receptors in the basolateral subnuclear region in similar concentrations to normal subjects. In patients with secondary iron overload, such receptors were absent in this region although present in duodenal crypt cells. These findings were attributed to a failure of down-regulation of the villous enterocyte transferrin receptor, resulting in an inability to control iron absorption in primary haemochromatosis.[14] On the hepatocytes, however, absorption of transferrin-bound iron by means of high-affinity transferrin receptor binding has been shown to be saturatable and down-regulation of these receptors has been demonstrated in primary haemochromatosis.[13,20] A second, non-saturatable, low-affinity internalization of transferrin-bound iron is known to exist.[20]

As well as transferrin, ferritin which has a high capacity for iron carriage may be involved in iron overload. A recent animal study has demonstrated that rapid uptake of ferritin by the liver takes place despite iron overload and, because serum ferritin is very high in primary haemochromatosis, this may be an important mechanism mediating hepatic iron overload.[1] These two factors – the increased intestinal absorption with lack of down-regulation under situations of iron excess and the inability of hepatocytes to reduce ferritin-transported iron – may be important in the pathogenesis of primary haemochromatosis. However, other abnormalities have been implicated, such as reticuloendothelial dysfunction. An inability to remove excess iron from the body, an impaired uptake of iron into reticuloendothelial cells and a reduced ability of cells in this system to synthesize ferritin have all been identified[4,21] (*Figure 8.16*).

The exact mechanism by which iron produces cellular injury is incompletely understood, although its electrochemical reactivity is probably important. The catalytically active form exists in the hepatic cytosolic pool as low-molecular-weight iron. Changes in the oxidation state of iron atoms are believed to be accompanied by formation of oxygen radicals, which results in lipid peroxidation of cellular membranes and intracellular organelles. The accumulation of intracellular ferritin and haemosiderin also probably damages lysosomes resulting in intracellular enzyme leakage.[17] This process affects hepatocytes, pancreatic acinar and islet cells, and myocardial cells, as well as those in salivary, sweat and Brunner's glands, the anterior pituitary, parathyroids, thyroid testes and adrenal zona glomerulosa.

It has been known for some time that a disproportionate number of subjects suspected or known to abuse alcohol are identified as having significant iron overload. Sometimes the iron content of the alcoholic beverage can explain this, but many such subjects are heterozygotes for the haemochromatosis gene. A recent animal study has demonstrated

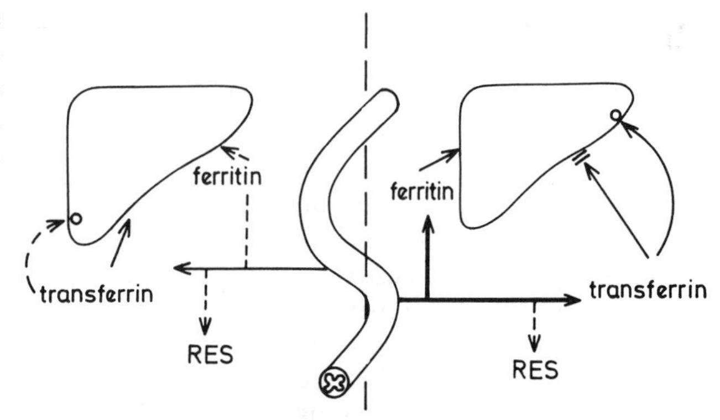

Figure 8.16 An idealized scheme of the mechanism of iron overload in primary haemochromatosis (on the right) compared with normal (on the left) under situations of adequate iron intake. Excessive iron absorption occurs as a result of impaired down-regulation of intestinal transferrin receptors and inappropriate hepatic uptake due to non-saturatable, low-affinity, transferrin internalization (despite down-regulation of high-affinity transferrin receptors) and increased ferritin uptake.

that iron overload in itself increases susceptibility to alcohol, resulting in such patients presenting earlier with liver damage. Similarly, alcohol may enhance iron absorption as well as affecting erythropoiesis by associated folate deficiency and abnormal pyridoxine metabolism. It may also be that, by raising serum ferritin concentrations, alcohol abuse increases non-transferrin iron uptake in the liver.

SECONDARY HAEMOCHROMATOSIS

This occurs when excess iron is ingested orally as in beers prepared in metal pots (for example, by the Bantu) and in some red wines, or more often when received parenterally in the form of blood transfusions. As each unit of blood contains 250 mg iron which takes approximately 8 months to excrete, transfusional iron overload readily occurs, unless, and sometimes even in spite of, concurrent treatment with desferrioxamine. In blood disorders with ineffective erythropoiesis, e.g. sideroblastic anaemia and thalassaemia, profound iron overload may result as a consequence of inappropriate hyperabsorption of dietary iron.[15]

In secondary haemochromatosis serum ferritin measurements correlate with the degree of iron overload, but do not differentiate it from haemosiderosis (i.e. iron overload without parenchymal damage). This differentiation requires histology and/or measurement of hepatic iron content. In secondary haemochromatosis, reticuloendothelial overload (e.g. by Kupffer cells) is characteristic.

CLINICAL FEATURES

Secondary iron overload affects men and women similarly, dependent upon the underlying disease. Primary haemochromatosis, although genotypically carried equally in men and women, is principally expressed in men, because of the protective effect of iron loss through menstruation and pregnancy. Although the prevalence increases with age, most patients are recognized between the ages of 40 and 60 years.[11] Presentation is usually with lethargy, abdominal pain, arthralgia and reduced libido, accompanied by such signs as hepatomegaly, skin pigmentation, reduced body hair, splenomegaly and less often jaundice, gynaecomastia, testicular atrophy and ascites.

GASTROINTESTINAL MANIFESTATIONS

Hepatic

Involvement of the liver in haemochromatosis is universal and hepatomegaly is present in most. Hepatic fibrosis and cirrhosis develop with increasing iron overload and are accompanied by portal hypertension, although this is seldom marked. Oesophageal varices occur in approximately 15% of those with cirrhosis. Treatment by venesection results in the disappearance of iron overload, the reduction in the inflammatory cell infiltrate and hepatocellular death, and occasionally in regression of fibrosis. Primary hepatocellular carcinoma occurs 200 times more commonly in primary haemochromatosis, invariably in association with cirrhosis. Unfortunately, the risk of hepatocellular carcinoma probably does not reduce with venesection, in those with cirrhosis; indeed it has been reported in a patient with primary haemochromatosis in whom the cirrhosis had been reversed by venesection.[5]

Abdominal pain

This is common in primary haemochromatosis (58% of patients), particularly in those with cirrhosis (67%) and in many patients the cause cannot be found. Unlike alcoholic liver disease, pancreatitis and gallstone disease is uncommon and indeed it has been suggested that iron overload may have a protective effect on the development of gallstones.[12] The abdominal pain lessens in the majority during the initial treatment period.

Pancreatic dysfunction

Although endocrine pancreatic insufficiency is common (see below), the disturbance of exocrine function (hypersecretion of dilute pancreatic juice) is of little clinical significance.[2]

Gastrointestinal infection

Infection with *Yersinia enterocolitica* occurs with increased frequency in patients with iron overload.[6] Iron overload substantially increases the virulence of *Y. enterocolitica* which may produce disorders ranging from mild diarrhoea and vomiting to terminal ileitis, hepatic abscess or septicaemia.

EXTRA-GASTROINTESTINAL MANIFESTATIONS

Diabetes mellitus

In patients with primary haemochromatosis diabetes mellitus is found in 55% and impaired glucose tolerance in a further 10%.[16] Type I diabetes (insulin dependent) is more common than type II, particularly in those with cirrhosis. The relatively high frequency of diabetes in primary haemochromatosis is due to a genetic element, because diabetes is more common in relatives of patients with primary haemochromatosis and diabetes, than in those in whom glucose intolerance is absent; it is also due to pancreatic damage which occurs with iron overload and impaired glucose tolerance which accompanies cirrhosis. Unlike the diabetes which is commonly associated with other forms of cirrhosis, diabetic complications appear to be common.[7] Treatment of haemochromatosis may result in improved diabetic control.

Pigmentation

Bronzed or metallic grey skin pigmentation is apparent in most patients with haemochromatosis, particularly in areas exposed to sunlight. Pigmentation of the oral mucosa is present in the minority but is more specific. The colour is due to melanin, or melanin and iron deposition. The underlying mechanism for melanin deposition is unknown but it may regress with treatment of the iron overload. Pigmentation as a sign is, however, of limited value diagnostically, because many patients with alcoholic liver disease have a similar weathered appearance.

Arthropathy

Arthralgia is a symptom present at the time of diagnosis in primary haemochromatosis in approximately 40%. The second and third metacarpophalangeal joints are usually affected first with subsequent involvement of other hand joints, wrists, shoulders, knees and hips. Radiological changes include loss of cartilage and sclerosis of the metacarpal heads. Chondrocalcinosis (pseudo-gout) is well recognized and is due to deposition of calcium pyrophosphate crystals in the larger joints. The role of iron in the arthropathy is poorly understood and treatment of iron overload has little effect on the symptomatology.

Cardiomyopathy (*see also* page 1267)

This usually manifests itself as biventricular cardiac failure or cardiac arrhythmias in patients with untreated primary haemochromatosis. In less severe cases cardiac involvement may be apparent only on 24-hour ECG monitoring as minor arrhythmias. Both these and cardiac failure respond to venesection.[8] Occasionally constrictive pericarditis may be present.

INVESTIGATIONS AND SCREENING

The diagnosis of primary haemochromatosis in patients with liver disease is usually straightforward because individuals with haemochromatosis and hepatic fibrosis or cirrhosis have serum ferritin concentrations of more than 700 μg/l and transferrin saturation of more than 50%[3] (*Table 8.6*). The serum ferritin increases by approximately 65 μg/l per year in primary haemochromatosis homozygotes compared with heterozygotes and normal subjects.[3] Gross iron overload can be confirmed by measuring hepatic iron concentration where levels of more than 75 μmol/g dry weight (417 μg/100 mg) can be taken as clearly indicative of homozygosity for haemochromatosis.

The situation is, however, not so simple in younger subjects with no evidence of liver disease, usually undergoing screening because a first-degree relative has the disease. Because iron overload takes many years to develop, it is recommended that screening should not commence before the age of 10 years. HLA typing is also of value in identifying those with particular risk in a family, i.e. those with identical HLA haplotypes to the proband. In subjects in whom both serum ferritin and transferrin saturation are normal, it is unlikely even at a young age that iron overload exists. However, if either test is elevated the diagnosis can be confirmed by measuring the hepatic iron index (=hepatic iron concentration in μmol/g dry weight divided by age in years). An index of more than 1.9 identifies homozygous patients whilst heterozygotes or normals have an index of less than 1.5.[19] Although serum iron is often increased, this is not sensitive or specific. However, an increased urinary 24-hour iron excretion (i.e. >2 mg) following intramuscular desferrioxamine (10 mg/kg) indicates iron overload. Other tests which have been evaluated in patients with haemochromatosis include computer tomography and magnetic resonance imaging. Although they can be specific for iron overload their use is unlikely to be cost-effective.

TREATMENT

The average life expectancy of untreated primary haemochromatosis after it is clinically apparent is less than 5 years, the chief causes of death being cardiac failure, hepatic failure, upper gastrointestinal bleeding and hepatocellular carcinoma.

Table 8.6 Iron and iron-binding proteins in normal subjects and those with haemochromatosis

	Normal	*Haemochromatosis*
Total body iron (g)	3–4	10–40
Haemoglobin iron (g)	1.5–3	1.5–3
Serum iron (μmol/l)	10–32	35–70
Transferrin saturate (%)	10–60	40–100
Serum ferritin (μg/l)	8–350	>700*
Hepatic iron (μg/100 mg dry wt)	10–180	>400

*In patients with fibrosis or cirrhosis.

Removal of excess iron in primary haemochromatosis and prevention of continuing accumulation in secondary haemochromatosis improve the prognosis.

In primary haemochromatosis, except in patients in whom it is important to remove iron quickly, e.g. in those with cardiac failure, once- or twice-weekly venesection of 500 ml blood is usually appropriate. This regimen of venesection should be continued until either mild iron-deficiency anaemia develops, serum iron falls to normal, the serum ferritin falls below 12 μg/l or liver biopsy shows complete iron depletion. Thereafter, venesection every 3 months is usually sufficient to prevent reaccumulation of iron. Anaemia is rare in such patients, before iron stores are reduced towards normal, as a result of increased erythropoiesis. In a few patients, anaemia may develop early because of a poor erythroid response and this may respond to testosterone treatment. Patients treated in this way who have not developed cirrhosis have a normal life expectancy.[16] Patients successfully depleted of iron but who have progressed to cirrhosis continue to have a significant risk of death from hepatocellular carcinoma.

It is important in the adequate management of primary haemochromatosis that first-degree relatives are screened for the condition (see above).

In secondary haemochromatosis iron chelation therapy is generally indicated. The principal therapeutic agent is desferrioxamine which unfortunately requires parenteral administration. Co-administration of oral ascorbic acid 500 mg daily significantly increases the urinary excretion of iron during desferrioxamine treatment.

REFERENCES

1. Adams, P.C. and Chaw, L.A. (1990) Hepatic ferritin uptake and hepatic iron. *Hepatology*, **11**, 805–808.
2. Althausen, T.L., Doig, R.K., Weiden, S. *et al.* (1951) Hemochromatosis: an investigation of twenty-three cases with special reference to nutrition, to iron metabolism, and the studies of hepatic and pancreatic function. *Archives of Internal Medicine*, **88**, 553–570.
3. Basset, M.L., Halliday, J.W., Ferris, R.A. and Powell, L.W. (1984) Diagnosis of hemochromatosis in young subjects. Predictive accuracy of biochemical screening test. *Gastroenterology*, **87**, 628–633.
4. Blitzer, B.L., Weiss, G.B., Osbaldistone, G.E. *et al.* (1978) Early idiopathic hemochromatosis with absent stainable bone marrow iron stores. *Gastroenterology*, **75**, 886.
5. Bloomberg, R.F., Chopra, S., Ibrahim, R. *et al.* (1988) Primary hepato-cellular carcinoma in idiopathic hemochromatosis after reversal of cirrhosis. *Gastroenterology*, **95**, 1399–1402.
6. Cover, T.L. and Aber, R.C. (1989) *Yersinia enterolytica*. *New England Journal of Medicine*, **321**, 16–24.
7. Dymock, I.W., Casser, J., Pyke, D.A., Oakley, W.G. and Williams, R. (1972) Observations on the pathogenesis complications and treatment of diabetes in 115 cases of hemochromatosis. *American Journal of Medicine*, **50**, 203.
8. Easley, R.M. Jr, Schreiner, B.F. Jr, and Yu, P.N. (1972) Reversible cardiomyopathy associated with hemochromatosis. *New England Journal of Medicine*, **287**, 866.
9. Edwards, C.Q., Dadone, M.M., Skolnick, M.H. and Kushner, J.P. (1982) Hereditary haemochromatosis. *Clinical Haematology*, **11**, 411–435.
10. Edwards, C.Q., Griffin, L.M., Goldgar, D., Drummond, C., Skolnick, M.H. and Kushner, J.M. (1988) Prevalence of haemochromatosis among 11,065 presumably healthy blood donors. *New England Journal of Medicine*, **318**, 1355–1362.
11. Finch, S.C. and Finch C.A. (1955) Idiopathic hemochromatosis and iron storage disease. Iron metabolism in hemochromatosis. *Medicine*, **34**, 381.
12. Guyader, D., Robert, J-Y., Loreal, O. *et al.* (1990) Prevalence of gallbladder lithiasis in genetic haemochromatotic cirrhosis. *Hepatology*, **12**, 980, A570.
13. Lombard, M., Bomford, A., Hynes, M. *et al.* (1989) Regulation of the hepatic transferrin receptor in hereditary hemochromatosis. *Hepatology* **9**, 1–5.
14. Lombard, M., Bomford, A.B., Polson, R.J., Bellingham, A.J. and Williams, R. (1990) Differential expression of transferrin receptor in duodenal mucosa in iron overload. *Gastroenterology*, **98**, 976–984.
15. Peppard, M.J., Callander, S.T., Warner, G.T. and Wetherall, D.J. (1979) Iron absorption and loading in beta thalassaemia intermedia. *The Lancet*, **2**, 819–821.
16. Niederau, C., Fischer, R., Sonnenberg, A. *et al.* (1985) Survival and causes of death in cirrhosis and non-cirrhotic patients with primary hemochromatosis. *New England Journal of Medicine*, **313**, 1256–1262.
17. Seymour, C.A. and Peters, T.J. (1978) Organelle pathology in primary and secondary haemochromatosis with special reference to lysosomal changes. *British Journal of Haematology*, **40**, 239–253.
18. Simon, M., Bourel, M., Genetet, B. and Fauchet, R. (1977) Idiopathic hemochromatosis: demonstration of recessive transmission and early detection by family HLA typing. *New England Journal of Medicine*, **297**, 1017–1021.
19. Summers, K.M., Halliday, J.W. and Powell, L.W. (1990) Identification of homozygous

hemochromatosis subjects by measurement of hepatic iron index. *Hepatology*, **12**, 20–25.
20. Trinder, D., Morgan, E.H. and Baker, E. (1988) The effect of an antibody to the rat transferrin receptor and of rat serum albumin on the uptake of differic transferrin by rat hepatocytes. *Biochimica Biophysica Acta*, **9**, 440–446.
21. Valberg, L.S. (1978) Tissue iron distribution in idiopathic haemochromatosis. *Gastroenterology*, **75**, 915.

INTERNAL PARANEOPLASTIC SYNDROMES ASSOCIATED WITH CANCER

R.C.F. Leonard

In addition to the local symptoms of swelling, invasion and obstruction, malignant tumours can produce symptoms and signs at a distance from the primary tumour or from its metastases. These remote effects of cancer are described as paraneoplastic syndromes. Their importance should not be underestimated as they may significantly add to the disability caused by the cancer. Consequently their control, in the absence of cure of the basic disease process, will improve the quality of life of the patient.

Specific endocrine syndromes have been studied in greatest detail and have provided established mechanisms of causation of paraneoplastic syndromes. The secretion of polypeptide hormones by tumours has been recognized over many decades as a cause of paraneoplastic syndromes.[3] However, in the last 15 years a large number of previously undescribed polypeptide hormones have been discovered to be associated with central nervous system or gastrointestinal tract malignancies. These are mainly detected by specific antibodies using radioimmunoassays and specific examples of gastrointestinal tract APUDomas associated with paraneoplastic syndromes are described in Chapter 11 (APUD = amine precursor uptake and decarboxylation).

Although diagnosis of true ectopic endocrine syndromes depends strictly upon the recognition of elevated levels of hormone in the blood, in many cases detection of tumour products is an expensive and time-consuming effort. Very often it is sufficient to recognize the clinical features to make the diagnosis. The ectopic syndromes are often termed 'inappropriate' because the hormone secretion is not affected by the normal regulatory mechanism which operates physiologically. The reasons for the relative frequency of polypeptide hormone synthesis in association with particular cancers are unclear.[1]

The formal proof of ectopic hormone synthesis by a cancer depends upon one or more of the following observations:[5]

1. Detecting elevated blood levels of the hormone – not always easy or economical.
2. Disappearance of abnormal hormone with removal or control of the tumour.
3. Immunohistochemistry on the tumour biopsy to confirm the presence of hormone in the cells.
4. Demonstration of an arteriovenous gradient of hormone in the blood supply to and from the tumour.
5. Cultures of tumour cells in vitro producing detectable hormones in the supernatant.

This section concentrates on the internal paraneoplastic syndromes and does not include dermatological complications which are discussed later (see page 1336).

AETIOLOGY, PATHOGENESIS AND DIFFERENTIAL DIAGNOSIS OF PARANEOPLASTIC SYNDROMES

Paraneoplastic syndromes can arise in the following ways:

1. The production of biologically active proteins or polypeptides including the classic hormones.
2. Immune complex production, immunosuppression or autoimmune effects.
3. The synthesis of ectopic cellular receptors competing for normal circulating hormones.
4. Other mechanisms of uncertain nature.

This latter category would include the syndromes of central nervous syndrome (CNS) degeneration, myopathies, myasthenic syndromes, dermatological manifestations, some of the haematological syndromes, anorexia, weight loss and fever.

Table 8.7 Relative frequency of metabolic and paraneoplastic syndromes

Common clinical problems (5–50%)	
Cachexia/anorexia	Fever
Anaemia (various causes)	Leukocytosis
Hypercalcaemia (may be subclinical)	Hypomagnesaemia*
Various neurological syndromes (mainly metastatic)	Hyponatraemia
Uncommon clinical problems (1–5%)	
Lymphopenia/neutropenia	Thrombocytopenia
Lactic acidosis	Hypertrophic, pulmonary osteoarthropathy
Disseminated intravascular coagulation	
Rare complications (<1%)	
Polycythaemia	Hypoglycaemia
Amyloidosis	Endocarditis
Other endocrine products producing clinical features	

*Treatment-induced (*cis*-platinum).

It is important to make a differential diagnosis of the cause of a supposed paraneoplastic syndrome because other conditions such as metastatic disease or infection may be inappropriately labelled as paraneoplastic syndromes, perhaps leading to delays in appropriate therapy (*Table 8.7*). Other separate complications to be ascertained are obstruction due to the tumour or tumour products, vascular abnormalities, fluid and electrolyte disturbances, and the complications of therapy due to cytotoxic drugs, irradiation, antibiotics, and therapy with 'biological response modifiers', such as interferons, interleukins and growth factors. Side effects caused by the biological therapies are complex and diverse, often being immune mediated. They are important because these agents are being increasingly used in the management of a variety of cancers.

ANOREXIA, CACHEXIA AND FEVER

The gastrointestinal tract is a common site of primary malignancy and is secondarily affected in the small or large bowel or, more often, the liver by secondary tumours in the abdomen. Not surprisingly therefore the gastrointestinal tract is very frequently involved in complications due to malignancy. These complications may comprise local problems, such as bowel obstruction, perforation, and jaundice, but they also may involve much more generalized effects due to disturbances in nutritional balance.

Most of the common cancers, once disseminated, are not curable. The aim of treatment is often limited to temporary palliation, so that a complete and permanent reversal of gastrointestinal complications is not a realistic aim of treatment. Nevertheless, many of the agents used for treating cancer, whether cytotoxic drugs or irradiation, may temporarily exacerbate nutritional problems which can therefore appear to become intractable and worsened by treatment. This preamble suggests that the lay image of the cancer patient – gaunt, anorexic, lethargic and fatigued – truly represents the typical patient with widespread disease. However, anyone involved in the routine management of people with cancer knows that this is not the case. Not all cancers are associated with extreme nutritional problems and it is often possible effectively to reverse the problem of chronic weight loss and malnutrition. This is achieved in part by paying careful attention to supportive measures, but also by delivering effective, palliative therapy for the primary disease process.[10]

PATHOPHYSIOLOGY

Hospitalized cancer patients are commonly in negative nitrogen balance. This is true of 30–40% of patients with breast cancer or advanced sarcoma, 50–60% of the patient population with lung or colonic cancer and as many as 80–90% of patients with stomach and pancreatic cancer. In these more severe cases the features of weight loss, anorexia and lethargy are associated with severe muscle wasting, loss of fat, hypoproteinaemia and peripheral oedema. Across a variety of cancers the presence of the dominating problems of weight loss and general symptoms, such as pain and low energy, resulting in impaired functional capacity are associated with poor outcome, whether in terms of tumour response or overall survival. Indeed these 'non-specific' symptoms contributing to a scaled 'health performance status' (such as the Karnofsky scale) may be the dominant presenting prognostic feature for a variety of advanced cancers. Although not always dominant, cachexia, anorexia and weight loss are thus common features of malignant disease, especially in the metastatic state.

Despite the strong association with cachexia/anorexia in many cancers no single mechanism has been identified for this. Weight loss may be reversed when the tumour is controlled by adequate systemic therapy. In many instances it is possible to attribute weight loss to the toxic effects of treatment, metabolic disturbance such as hypercalcaemia or to clinical depression, which affects perhaps 20–30% of patients with cancer.

In humans, it is possible that the hypothalamus acts as the CNS control of appetite, but this possibility has not been thoroughly elucidated. Some of the peptides, e.g. vasoactive intestinal polypeptide (VIP), cholecystokinin and substance P, are detectable in the central nervous system and may act as neurotransmitters in addition to exerting their peripheral effects.[7] These peptides have profound effects on taste and appetite and cholecystokinin infused into rhesus monkeys produces anorexia. Other contributors to the cachectic state may include hypoalbuminaemia which could directly cause poor appetite, and reduced albumin synthesis, resulting in hypoalbuminaemia, could also occur in the absence of overt liver impairment. Occasionally, an increased metabolic state may be associated with the hyperthyroid effect of certain cancer-associated hormones. In particular human chorionic gonadotrophin (hCG) may mimic the effect of thyroid hormone by binding thyroid hormone receptors on cells and so acting as an inappropriate agonist. These observations suggest that a multiplicity of factors contribute to the problem of inadequate nutrition and weight loss.

TREATMENT

Anorexia or the feeling of easy and early satiety are common problems of cancer, occurring in approximately 40% of all patients; it is a feature of upper gastrointestinal tract cancers and tumours affecting the liver. It may also have specific causes which require specific remedies, including bowel obstruction, which is a common complication of ovarian cancer, as well as primary gastrointestinal malignancies. Anorexia may be a temporary side effect of chemotherapy and 'large field' irradiation or could be due to local problems such as ulceration in the mouth. This latter complication can have direct cytotoxic causation but frequently it can be caused by under-diagnosed causes such as fungal or herpetic infection. Both depression and anxiety can contribute to the problem of anorexia with a consequent improvement following adequate attention to psychological support. Physiological control of appetite is poorly understood. Among a variety of putative causes, the following have been postulated as important influences: the effects of blood glucose, the level of free fatty acids in the blood, the plasma amino acid concentration, the presence of gastrointestinal tract distension, and possibly the plasma levels of insulin, cholecystokinin and gastrin-releasing peptide (GRP). In cancer, the disturbance of some of these may be a partial explanation for anorexia. It is quite probable, however, that the effects of the levels of circulating lymphokines are even more important. This has been particularly well illustrated by clinical experience with the anticancer agent, tumour necrosis factor (TNF), which has been available as a cloned gene product for clinical trial in cancer medicine over the last few years. This substance, injected into experimental animals, produces profound cachexia and has been given the alternative name of cachexin. It is undoubtedly present in elevated levels in many patients who have cancer, and pharmacological doses produce profound disturbance of appetite and can result in marked weight loss following prolonged treatment.

Depressed appetite is thus a major problem and may be intractable despite strenuous efforts by the patient and his or her carers. It should be remembered that some of the weight loss is probably attributable to increasing energy expenditure, and about one-third of patients with cancer have been shown to be slightly hypermetabolic although one-third have a normal metabolic rate and about one-third are slightly hypometabolic.[5] However, because the intake level is frequently reduced, even a normal metabolic state may be too high for someone on an inadequate intake. Specific attention is therefore paid to the following aspects of management of weight loss.

Alteration of diet

Many cancer patients ask questions about the use of specific diets to control the cancer. Few seem to understand that calorie intake is itself a very important issue and in many cases patients actively have to be encouraged to pursue diets that they may have learned are inappropriate such as fatty and high carbohydrate foods. Undoubtedly the assistance of the dietician is very valuable in this respect.

Pain control

Pain suppresses appetite. Overdosage with opiates can also suppress appetite, induce nausea and produce profound constipation which again will adversely affect appetite. The issues therefore are careful control of pain and careful monitoring of the side effects of powerful analgesics.

Supportive measures for psychological problems

Increasingly units concerned with the care of cancer patients involve the expertise of a clinical psychologist or psychiatrist. Between 20% and 30% of patients present with depression or overt anxiety as complications of cancer, and these symptoms merit specific attention.

Oral infection

Infection of the mouth, and the trauma due to cytotoxic drugs or irradiation, can adversely affect food intake. Infection may be temporary or permanent. *Candida albicans* is often considered and is usually easily treatable with such agents as fluconazole or nystatin, although the problem of herpes infection is underestimated. Herpes simplex has been demonstrated almost as frequently as fungal infection,[12] and sometimes both infections are present simultaneously. There is a strong association between herpes simplex infection and a previous history of cold sores, so careful history taking is important. With patients who have had persistent oral ulceration, it is not necessary to obtain viral cultures but simply to treat with prophylactic oral antiviral agents, such as acyclovir.

Hormones

There have been many poorly controlled studies of anabolic steroids and glucocorticoids as appetite stimulants. Glucocorticoids can have a temporary beneficial effect on appetite, particularly in suppressing nausea – an undoubted benefit of drugs such as dexamethasone. However, such drugs cannot be used for more than a few weeks at standard doses (20 mg prednisolone or greater) and may only be useful as temporary adjuncts for patients on cytotoxic drugs or on radiotherapy, given for the duration of the pulsed treatments. Cannabinoids and anabolic steroids have also been recommended but they really are unproven as genuine appetite stimulants of long-term benefit. Alcohol likewise is often recommended on a pragmatic basis but its value is really unknown.

Nasogastric feeding

Some patients benefit from nasogastric feeding particularly when there are chronic obstructive or inflammatory problems in the upper gastrointestinal tract. However, generally nasogastric feeding is a second best alternative to oral feeding. Lactose-free whole protein preparations are available commercially which contain polysaccharides, fats, mineral, trace elements; these are usually delivered at a rate of about 75–100 calories/hour (1 cal/ml).[10] Simple elemental diets given as an oral liquid feed are sometimes recommended but many nauseous patients find the preparations unpalatable because of taste or smell.

Total parenteral nutrition

This is occasionally required as a temporary expedient. It is costly, and complicated by the risks of infection of an external line, particularly in patients who have treatment-induced myelosuppression in addition to immunosuppression due to nutritional state and disease. It is possible to deliver about 2–4.4 kcal/24 hours containing about 40 g nitrogen in 3 litres fluid.[10] With good nursing and medical care serious infections should be seen in less than 5% of cases. Occasionally patients can be maintained on total parental nutrition at home with the assistance of support from the GP and district nurse.

FUTURE

It is probable that future developments will depend upon a better understanding of the mechanisms of causation. The most interesting recent insight was the recognition of lymphokines in the host response as probable mediators of many gastrointestinal symptoms. Specific targeted remedies may therefore be developed in time.

FEVER

The aetiology of fever is also unclear, but it is a very common feature of many advanced malignancies, particularly Hodgkin's disease and aggressive non-Hodgkin's lymphomas. However, the multiplicity of mechanisms already mentioned suggest that although tumour necrosis factor, interleukin-1 and other lymphokines may be important, the isolation of one immunological response to cancer is unlikely to provide the whole explanation for the general problem of anorexia, weight loss and fever.

CALCIUM HOMEOSTASIS IN CANCER

MALIGNANT HYPERCALCAEMIA

Malignant hypercalcaemia was originally described as a pseudohyperparathyroidism and was assumed to be caused by ectopic synthesis of normal parathyroid hormone (PTH). Early radio-immunoassay techniques of low discriminatory capacity frequently detected elevated levels of immunoreactive parathyroid hormone in patients with malignant hypercalcaemia. With the advent of monoclonal antibodies, however, it is clear that endogenous parathyroid hormone is characteristically reduced in the serum of patients with malignant hypercalcaemia.

In 1980 Stewart *et al.*[16] reported that malignant hypercalcaemia was frequently associated with increased levels of urinary cyclic AMP (cAMP). This marker, characteristic of parathyroid hormone-like activity, is not, however, characteristically raised in the urine of hypercalcaemic breast cancer, myeloma or lymphoma patients. The generation of hypercalcaemia in most (though not all) cases of malignant hypercalcaemia has been illuminated by the detection of an immunoreactive serum polypeptide now designated parathyroid hormone-related polypeptide (PTHrP).[16,17] The action of PTHrP on bone is poorly understood and different from that of parathyroid hormone. The bone effects cannot be blocked by parathyroid hormone antagonists whereas the renal effects can. PTHrP is a polypeptide consisting of 141 amino acids and of approximate molecular weight 17 000, approximately twice the size of natural parathyroid hormone. Its amino-terminal end resembles the receptor-binding portion of parathyroid hormone. Parathyroid hormone and PTHrP behave similarly in vitro, stimulating cAMP production in either kidney plasma membrane or osteoclasts. There is some evidence, however, for supplementary targets for PTHrP, and possibly even specific receptors, although its main target appears to be the parathyroid hormone receptor on bone osteoclasts. A parathyroid hormone receptor antagonist is theoretically an active drug for preventing malignant hypercalcaemia in humans.

A specific assay is not currently available for the general monitoring of PTHrP levels in humans because radio-immunoassays are hampered by the variation in its molecular size of the PTHrP species of molecules. In around 75% of cases of malignant hypercalcaemia, elevated levels of PTHrP can be detected using available immunoassays, the levels broadly correlating with the level of serum calcium.

It is certain, however, that PTHrP is not the sole mediator of malignant hypercalcaemia. A number of metabolic features are quite unlike those induced by parathyroid hormone-like activity, including osteoclast-mediated bone resorption, absence of synthesis of new bone, inappropriately high urinary calcium excretion, low or normal calcitriol level, and finally a tendency to metabolic alkalosis. In brief, other major contenders as mediating factors include the following.

Transforming growth factor α (TGFα)

TGFα is one of several tumour-produced transforming growth factors which are capable of stimulating anchorage-independent growth of normal fibroblasts in vitro. TGFα is also an important mediator of bone resorption by stimulating osteoclasts and osteoclastic progenitors. It can also inhibit osteoblast formation and induce hypercalcaemia in mice. Its role in human malignant hypercalcaemia has not yet been demonstrated.

Transforming growth factor β (TGFβ)

This often appears to act as a growth inhibitor in tumour systems. Its effect on bone metabolism is complex but the sum of its effects may be a net increase in bone formation. Breast cancer cells may produce TGFβ and its synthesis is amplified by the antihormone agent tamoxifen.

Interleukin-1 (IL-1)

IL-1 stimulates osteoclastic progenitors and hence may be important in the generation of bone resorption.

Tumour necrosis factor α (TNFα)

TNFα is a potent osteoclast inhibitor and is also a stimulator of bone resorption. Although raised levels of TNFα are seen in a wide variety of malignant diseases, TNFα has specifically been seen at elevated levels in the serum of patients with malignant hypercalcaemia.

Osteoclast-activating factors (OAFs)

These may be more important in some diseases than in others. For instance, it seems that osteoclast-activating factors are important in myeloma whereas prostaglandins may be important in metastatic breast cancer.

Pathogenesis and clinical features

The control of serum calcium is partly a balancing act between absorption, bone turnover and renal excretion. The kidneys can add to the problem of hypercalcaemia by a reduced glomerular filtration rate and increased calcium reabsorption. Reduction of glomerular filtration rate is usually a problem of dehydration (i.e. prerenal cause) which will also tend to cause a compensatory increase in sodium and calcium tubular reabsorption. This tendency may be enhanced by the action of PTHrP but the importance of this is uncertain. From the evidence of the efficacy of modern agents in reducing hypercalcaemia (see below), the major contributor to hypercalcaemia appears to be increased bone resorption rather than reduced renal excretion. Nevertheless, there are some instances of malignant hypercalcaemia where the administration of a calciuretic compound can achieve the control which is not obtained by the standard bone resorption-blocking agents.

Metastatic bone involvement as a cause of malignant hypercalcaemia has not been thoroughly investigated. It seems probable that most of the bone destruction seen in metastatic bone disease is due to osteoclast activity. Osteoclast activating factors have been identified as tumour products in multiple myeloma and thus may be regarded as a paracrine hormonal effect. Finally, prostaglandins deserve mention as potential mediators of malignant hypercalcaemia, and their synthesis by metastatic breast cancer cells in bone may contribute to neoplastic osteolysis.[9]

Treatment

Generally hypercalcaemia is a treatable but potentially lethal complication of cancer. Regardless of its cause it may present as an acute medical emergency, but more characteristically it is insidious in onset, producing mental confusion, polyuria, polydypsia, nausea and vomiting, and culminating in variable degrees of clinical dehydration, contributing to prerenal uraemia. In many patients these symptoms may be attributed to the effects of metastases or the toxicity of cancer treatment, but the problem of hypercalcaemia should always be considered in a patient with malignant disease who becomes generally unwell, suffering from a multitude of seemingly unconnected symptoms. Patients with malignant hypercalcaemia may present to the gastroenterologist with nausea, vomiting, anorexia or constipation. Although a particular feature of breast cancer, hypercalcaemia is also seen in association with lung cancer, myeloma and less frequently in patients with lymphoma, renal cancer, cervical and ovarian cancers.[2] As many as 10% of patients with breast cancer may develop hypercalcaemia at some time in their illness. In recent years, an attitude of therapeutic nihilism has been replaced by a more activist philosophy with the recognition that treatment may produce a very satisfactory palliative result. Occasionally, however, the underlying condition may not justify strenuous efforts to reverse the effects of hypercalcaemia when this may be seen as an acceptable way for a patient to slip into unconsciousness with an untreatable malignancy.

For the purposes of active management, it is important to understand that malignant hypercalcaemia is only manifested when the kidneys are no longer able to clear the calcium load. As the load on the renal tubules increases, the maximum calcium output is exceeded and then the serum calcium rises. This reduces the ability of the tubule to secrete further calcium, and instead promotes sodium and water loss contributing to severe dehydration.

Although the potential areas for control of hypercalcaemia would appear to include restriction of intake, calcium diets have no useful effect on malignant hypercalcaemia. Indeed, there is a tendency to a rather low calcium absorption from the intestine. At the renal level it is possible to encourage excretion of calcium by loop diuretics such as frusemide. However, this is contraindicated in the typical patient due to dehydration, unless there is simultaneous vigorous rehydration with saline. The best tactic is to replace fluids lost through systemic dehydration immediately using physiological saline. A typical level of depletion is of the order of 2–4 litres of fluid which should be replaced over the first 24 hours. For many years the standard approach following this has been to use systemic corticosteroids. However, less than 50% of patients respond adequately to such treatment, and it often takes several days for steroids to exhibit their maximum and usually inadequate effects. Corticosteroids probably decrease osteoclastic activity, and chronic unwanted effects of high doses of steroids limit their ability to control the situation regardless of the immediate impact. Alternatively calcitonin, often given in the form of salmon calcitonin, promotes urinary excretion of calcium and is a partial inhibitor of osteoclasts. Despite its attractive pharmacological attributes, the clinical benefit conferred by calcitonin is very limited and generally it is unable to reduce the serum calcium by more than 0.5–0.6 mmol/l blood in the first 24 hours.

In recent years the management of hypercalcaemia has been transformed by the development of diphosphonates (bisphosphonates) which are potent inhibitors of osteoclastic bone resorption. The first in this class of compounds, disodium etidronate, has largely been replaced by compounds such as disodium clodronate, which is given over 5 days and disodium aminohydroxypropylidene (pamidronate). Either is given as a short 60-minute intravenous infusion, the latter at a dose of 30–60 mg. Unlike clodronate, pamidronate is usually active when given as just a single infusion and it produces normalization of the serum calcium in 90% of patients within the first 4 days. The effect may last for up to 4 weeks but usually repeat doses are required after 2–3 weeks.[6] Unfortunately the bioavailability of the oral preparation is extremely dubious and cannot be recommended for routine management. On occasions when the renal component is predominant, calcitonin can sometimes assist in the refractory patient with hypercalcaemia. Alternatively (increasing rarely), the cytotoxic agent, mithramycin, is a potent compound for controlling hypercalcaemia. Given either once daily as an infusion of 25 μg/kg (or at half this dose repeated daily for up to 4 days), the drug can produce profound nausea in addition to controlling hypercalcaemia. It has a further distinct disadvantage in that is produces dose-limiting myelosuppression, which in turn limits the use of cytotoxic drugs to control the underlying malignancy.

The overriding principle of management for the majority of patients is to treat hypercalcaemia in the patient with an established malignancy rather than investigating it. Once the calcium is at a 'safe' level, i.e. below 3 mmol/l, further investigations may be justified in order to plan definitive management. Rarely, a single area of lytic bone disease may partially explain the problem and justify local treatment with radiotherapy. However, it is important once again to stress that most cases are caused by a hormonal mechanism and that control of the generalized disease is the long-term aim of therapy.

Thus the recognition of hypercalcaemia in the hitherto well patient with chronic malignancy is an extremely important event. It is routinely amenable to treatment by agents which themselves are of relatively low toxicity and proven efficacy.

HYPOCALCAEMIA

Hypocalcaemia occurs more frequently in malignancy than hypercalcaemia – it occurs in more than 16% of all cancer cases. However, the condition leads only rarely to tetany or other symptoms from complications, although refined studies of neuromuscular function may indicate impairment due to hypocalcaemia in the absence of clinical problems. There is no direct evidence for ectopic calcitonin as the cause of hypocalcaemia and there is no indication for specific therapy other than control of the underlying condition.[5]

OTHER HORMONES

There is a particularly high frequency of certain ectopic syndromes in association with small cell lung cancer.[5,7,12] Neuroendocrine tumours arising in the gastrointestinal tract can also be associated with such syndromes. Recent molecular techniques may provide a more precise explanation of the causation of ectopic hormone synthesis at the genetic level.[9,20,24,25]

ECTOPIC ACTH

The major disease associated with ectopic ACTH is lung cancer, particularly small cell lung cancer (SCLC).[7,14,22,23] However, carcinoid tumours have also been associated with ectopic ACTH. The gene encoding these products is the pro-opiomelanocortin (POMC) gene on chromosome 11 producing the 'big ACTH' pro-hormone containing four repetitive sequences based on the ACTH–MSH core (MSH = melanocyte-stimulating hormone). Thus the targets are adrenocortical cells (to synthesize corticosteroids and androgens), melanocyte hyperpigmentation, and opiate-like activity due to the β-endorphin/metenkephalin product. Ectopic ACTH is not under feedback control and thus it blunts the normal diurnal cortisol rhythm. It is suppressed by exogenous dexamethasone, although the suppression may be incomplete. When ACTH is present in large excess, patients may develop overt Cushing's syndrome. More typically a hypokalaemic alkalosis is seen with hypotension, oedema and profound muscular weakness as the predominant features. Related peptides may be secreted such as β-lipotrophin, metenkephalin A and C and melanocyte-stimulating hormone. The clinical syndrome has been reported in up to 2% of lung cancer; contrasting with this, prospective studies of blood from patients with lung cancer show abnormal levels of ACTH in between 11% and 50%. In the overt syndrome, the plasma ACTH is in excess of 200 pg/l and direct measurement of the plasma cortisol routinely shows a level in excess of 40 μg/dl with loss of diurnal variation. In adrenal gland hyperplasia or primary adrenal carcinoma, the circulating ACTH level is low and in pituitary Cushing's syndrome, the ACTH level is usually suppressed by high-dose dexamethasone. The levels of ACTH in the cancer-related syndrome are, however, much higher than in classic Cushing's syndrome. Occasionally ectopic ACTH is suppressible by high-dose dexamethasone, although the reasons for this are not well understood. The overt ACTH syndrome frequently presents in association with extremely advanced malignancy and, in the author's experience, is an extremely adverse prognostic feature.

ECTOPIC ANTIDIURETIC HORMONE

Antidiuretic hormone (ADH) causes water retention by promoting reabsorption at the renal tubule. Inappropriate antidiuretic hormone production, being unregulated, results in inappropriately concentrated urine and a plasma of correspondingly low osmolality.

The syndrome of inappropriate antidiuretic hormone secretion (SIADH or the Schwartz–Bartter syndrome) was first described in 1957.[21] Arginine vasopressin (AVP) was first detected in association with cancer in 1963 – it was associated with a thoracic tumour – and it is a classic accompaniment of small cell lung cancer, its effects often being the presenting features of the disease. Water intoxication produces a variety of central nervous system effects: lethargy and/or confusion are common presentations. Severe hyponatraemia may cause such severe cerebral oedema that presenting features can vary from altered behaviour to psychotic syndromes and coma. It is important to differentiate this complication from cerebral metastases. Occult SIADH (as with occult ACTH syndromes) is probably a much more frequent occurrence than clinically apparent SIADH. Water-loading tests show an impaired response. Most cases of SIADH have a serum sodium level of 120–130 mmol/l at presentation. At levels above 130 mmol/l the hyponatraemia is often ignored.[12]

Treatment

Treatment depends upon controlling the underlying tumour. At levels above 130 mmol/l the serum sodium does not require specific treatment; below, symptomatic improvement may be temporarily achieved by either fluid restriction (around 500–1000 ml fluid/day or the concomitant use of tetracyclines (demeclocycline) which interfere with the action of antidiuretic hormone on the renal tubule.[8] In severe cases (serum sodium <110 mmol/l) it may be necessary to consider the administration of hypertonic saline. However, this can be hazardous, requiring close biochemical and cardiovascular monitoring. Ultimate control depends upon controlling the underlying disease.

Although SIADH is predominantly a feature of small cell lung cancer, hyponatraemia has other origins in patients with advanced cancer. Hepatic impairment, renal failure and even adrenal failure may complicate many cancers and can lead to hyponatraemia. This is further complicated by the occasional need for diuretics and the potential for some cytotoxic drugs, notably cyclophosphamide[11] and high doses of vincristine, to induce a degree of hyponatraemia. Hyponatraemia has been a striking feature of the (fortunately rare) instances of vincristine overdose.

TUMOUR HUMAN PLACENTAL LACTOGEN, GROWTH HORMONE, PROLACTIN AND THYROTROPHIC SUBSTANCE

Human placental lactogen (hPL) has been detected in 5–8% of patients with non-trophoblastic tumours; it may also be associated with elevated oestrogens and gynaecomastia. Growth hormone has been produced by gastric cancers as well as lung cancers, but it is uncommon. The natural history of the tumour is probably too short for the patients to develop acromegaly, but growth hormone is a speculative cause of hypertrophic pulmonary osteoarthropathy.[22]

Cancer patients frequently have an increased metabolic rate, rarely producing a state resembling hyperthyroidism. It appears that human chorionic gonadotrophin (hCG), which can be produced in spectacular quantities by some tumours, may have a thyroid-stimulating hormone-like activity.[5]

In addition to the classic production of βhCG by trophoblastic malignancies, a variety of other tumours also produce it. It has been detected in up to 20% of colorectal cancers, 50% of pancreatic cancers, 25% of gastric cancers, over 10% of small intestinal tumours and 20% of hepatomas. Again, as opposed to having an important end effect in itself, the tumour product may be regarded as a sensitive marker for disease presence or recurrence, but its real value as a tumour marker requires prospective study in diseases other than germ-cell neoplasia.

Calcitonin

Although not necessarily functionally important, calcitonin can be an extremely sensitive indicator of residual tumour in patients suffering from specific gastrointestinal-associated malignancies in addition to the multiple endocrine neoplasia type 2 syndrome (involving medullary carcinoma of the thyroid, phaeochromocytoma and parathyroid adenomas). Immunoreactive calcitonin has also been found in extracts of tissue from a wide variety of cancers.[5]

HYPOGLYCAEMIA

Various non-islet cell tumours can rarely cause clinical hypoglycaemia, including mesothelioma, some abdominal sarcomas, hepatomas, adrenal carcinomas and about 5% of gastrointestinal primary carcinomas. Although often associated with large tumours metastasizing to the liver, hypoglycaemia may be present before diagnosis of the cancer. Thus stupor, coma and occasional focal neurological signs associated with agitated behaviour may be the presenting features. A variety of mechanisms have been observed or postulated including the production of ectopic insulin, the production of a non-suppressible insulin-like activity (NSILA), utilization of sugar by the tumour and the stimulation of ectopic insulin release by some precursor material produced by the tumour. Finally, massive infiltration of the liver may of itself be an inhibitor of hepatic hexose synthesis. NSILA has been blamed for the vast majority of cases of cancer-associated hypoglycaemia and the substance appears to comprise four peptides and several larger proteins. Certainly, the inhibition of hepatic glycogenolysis would explain the development of hypoglycaemia in patients with hepatoma. It should be remembered that approximately half of the activity of 200 μU biologically active insulin and half of the insulin-like activity in normal human serum is related to NSILA/somatomedin activity. Occasionally insulin-like growth factors (IGF-I and IGF-II) have been identified as possible culprits. Initially, treatment of paraneoplastic hypoglycaemia may involve glucose infusion to control acute symptoms, but reducing tumour bulk by surgical resection should be carried out if possible. Alternatively, the following can be considered as treatments although their long-term effectiveness is uncertain:[5,15] glucagon (given intramuscularly), somatomedin/somatostatin (neutastatin), diazoxide or high doses of corticosteroids.

LACTIC ACIDOSIS

Metabolic acidosis with excessive blood lactate may be seen in malignant disease in the absence of infection and shock. In addition to lymphomas and leukemias, it is occasionally seen in colon cancer, breast and lung cancer.[4] The mechanisms are obscure but, as with other cases of metabolic acidosis, there is a strong compensatory respiratory drive so that tachypnoea may be prominent. The condition may be chronic and stable. An increased anion gap suggests the condition which is then confirmed by a blood lactate level above 2 mmol/l. Blood pH alone will not necessarily confirm the diagnosis, and the pH may even be normal or elevated due to respiratory over-compensation. In many cases liver impairment is present and undoubtedly contributes to the problem because the organ is responsible routinely for the catabolism of excess blood lactate. Although fluids and sodium bicarbonate can be used to correct the acidaemia in acute situations, the management of chronic lactic acidosis is less clear and essentially depends upon control of the underlying condition.

HYPERLIPIDAEMIA

This can be seen in patients with hepatoma and colon cancer as well as in those with myeloma. The mechanism of causation is obscure and its clinical effect seems unimportant.[5]

ELEVATION OF SERUM AMYLASE

This has been seen in some patients with gastrointestinal cancers and can misleadingly suggest acute pancreatitis. This uncertainty is further complicated by the observation of true acute pancreatitis as a non-metastatic complication – notably in some cancer patients, particularly those with small cell lung cancers.[5]

ADRENAL IMPAIRMENT

This is rare in advanced cancer, although the organs may be the sites of metastasis in a variety of conditions including breast, kidney, pancreas, stomach, melanoma and especially lung cancer. It appears that organ damage must be more than 90% before adrenal failure will be seen. Management of patients with known adrenal metastases usually involves control of the underlying condition and monitoring for features of hypoadrenalism, such as increasing nausea, potassium imbalance and a high index of suspicion in 'at risk' patients when other non-specific features present, e.g. weakness and lethargy.[5]

NEUROLOGICAL MANIFESTATIONS

Neurological problems are frequent complications of cancer. In one report 17% of patients with cancer had neurological symptoms and signs justifying neurological consultation. However, in patients with a range of cancers, true paraneoplastic syndromes account for only the minority of neurological problems, and paraneoplastic causes can be established only after other causes, particularly central nervous system metastases, have been excluded. Fluid and electrolyte abnormalities are also a frequent cause of neurological symptoms in cancer patients, and in this category hepatic encephalopathy and hypercalcaemia are important. In a study of 'stroke' in cancer patients, embolic infarction was detected in 27% of cases, thrombotic infarction in 19% (of which half were due to disseminated intravascular coagulation), and intraparenchymal haemorrhage in 32% that were seemingly tumour related in most instances. In most patients subdural haemorrhage, subarachnoid haemorrhage or superior sagittal sinus occlusion was noted. Thus, true paraneoplastic syndromes in the central nervous system are rather uncommon, although the incidences reported vary according to different studies. Peripheral neuromyopathies, detected in one survey in 7% of nearly 1500 cancer patients, were mostly associated with lung cancer. However, a patient who develops a neurological syndrome without overt cancer often merits evaluation for malignant causation; neurological syndromes include subacute cerebellar degeneration, subacute motor neuropathy, and dermatomyositis in addition to the Eaton–Lambert syndrome and a sensory dorsal root ganglion disorder. Most syndromes that have been established as associated with cancer run a course parallel to the tumour.[5]

SUBACUTE CEREBELLAR DEGENERATION

This has been seen mainly in association with lung cancer but has been reported with colorectal tumours as well as other abdominal neoplasms. Characteristically subacute, progressive, bilateral, cerebellar degeneration takes place causing ataxia, dysarthria and other characteristic cerebellar signs. There may be an element of dementia in addition. Pathologically there is evidence of cerebellar atrophy with loss of the Purkinje cells. Control of the underlying tumour can produce improvement in the syndrome.

DEMENTIA

This is a frequent abnormality but is often difficult to attribute directly to the development of malignancy. Characteristically limbic encephalitis is associated with progressive dementia and degenerative changes are seen on CT scan images. Pathologically degeneration is seen in the hippocampus, and there may be evidence of inflammation. The syndrome does not usually appear to improve with control of the primary tumour. Most commonly it has been associated with small cell lung cancer and Hodgkin's disease but cases have been seen where the probable primary tumour is of gastrointestinal origin.

PROGRESSIVE MULTIFOCAL LEUKOENCEPHALOPATHY

A viral aetiology has been well established for this and it is usually a rapidly progressive disorder of ataxia, dementia, paralysis, blindness and finally coma. Although the CSF is usually normal, progressive multifocal leukoencephalopathy is associated with impaired immunity disorders, particularly lymphomas. Pathologically there is demyelination of the white matter throughout the central nervous system and recent evidence suggests involvement of one of the papova viruses.

SPINAL CORD DISORDERS

Paraneoplastic syndromes account for only a small proportion of neurological syndromes but up to 10% of cases of the amyotrophic lateral sclerosis form of motor neuron disease had an underlying malignancy in one series reported by Norris and Engel. This again has a particularly strong association with lymphomas, with progressive lower motor neuron weakness in the absence of sensory changes.

PERIPHERAL NERVOUS EFFECTS

Paraneoplastic syndromes involving the peripheral nervous system are more frequent than central nervous system effects. Pure sensory neuropathy with dorsal route ganglion atrophy has a strong association with malignancy, particularly lung tumours and intestinal malignancy including carcinoma of the oesophagus. Subacute syndromes characterized by distal sensory loss, particularly proprioception, predominate. Muscle strength is often preserved. Neurological symptoms may precede the development of malignancy and unfortunately rarely improve despite control of the cancer. A variant of the Guillain–Barré syndrome has again been associated with lymphomas. Autonomic neuropathy is seen particularly with lung cancer and breast cancer and is usually associated with widespread disease. The most common symptom of this is orthostatic hypotension causing dizziness that may be sufficiently severe to render the patient bed-ridden. Neurogenic bladder, disordered peristalsis and pseudo-obstruction (Ogilvie syndrome) have also been reported with advanced malignancies.

NEUROMUSCULAR DISORDERS – DERMATOMYOSITIS AND POLYMYOSITIS

Between 7% and 35% of patients with dermatomyositis or polymyositis have been reported to have underlying malignancy. This is approximately five to seven times the incidence of malignancy in the general population. Clinically, the syndromes are characterized by progressive muscular weakness and may present for a period of up to a year or more before the tumour is revealed. Steroids can produce remissions of the syndrome before the tumour has been diagnosed, but even with adequate control of the tumour the dermatomyositis or polymyositis rarely remits completely.

MYASTHENIC SYNDROME (THE EATON–LAMBERT SYNDROME)

This has a particularly striking association with small-cell lung cancer and is characterized by weakness and fatigue particularly of the pelvic girdle. Severe forms may produce dysarthria, dysphagia, diplopia, paraesthesia and muscle pain. There is a poor response to edrophonium chloride (Tensilon) but the symptoms may be alleviated by exercise. Myasthenic syndromes usually improve if the cancer responds to treatment. This is particularly the case with small cell lung cancer, a chemosensitive tumour.

Other cancers which induce true myasthenia gravis include a variety of tumours of the pancreas and rectum in addition to thymoma.

HAEMATOLOGICAL MANIFESTATIONS

ANAEMIA

Gastrointestinal tumours routinely produce anaemia due to blood loss and iron deficiency. Poor nutrition and marrow involvement are two other contributing features in some cancers. However, a variety of other effects can occasionally contribute or may be the sole cause of anaemia. A chronic moderate anaemia with normocytic, normochromic or hypochromic features has no clear explanation in some malignancies, although in others the anaemia is clearly of the 'chronic disorders' type with impaired utilization of iron and a shortened red cell survival. The response of this type of anaemia to erythropoietin is poor. In some instances pure red cell aplasia has been reported in association with gastric cancer, as well as lung and breast malignancy. Occasionally a megaloblastic picture without folate or vitamin B_{12} deficiency can be seen in association with haematological malignancy, notably lymphomas and myeloma. Although hypersplenism is not a feature of gastrointestinal malignancy, autoimmune haemolytic anaemias can be found in association with malignant B-cell tumours of the bowel and, more rarely, in association with carcinomas of the stomach and colon.[12] In these cases the tumour-associated anaemia may be the presenting symptom with haemoglobin reduced to half the normal level. Control of the primary tumour may cause the anaemia to remit but sometimes splenectomy is indicated.

MICROANGIOPATHIC HAEMOLYTIC ANAEMIA

If primary haematological disease or renal failure has been excluded, internal malignancy has to be considered high on the list of causes of microangiopathic haemolytic anaemia (MAHA). It is a particular feature of mucinous adenocarcinomas. A high proportion of patients with MAHA develop evidence of disseminated intravascular coagulation. The haemolysis results from shearing of the erythrocytes in the microcirculation. MAHA may be severe with haemoglobin below 7 g/dl and evidence of increased marrow turnover including nucleated cells in the peripheral blood. The syndrome is associated with severe advanced malignancy and the prognosis is often very poor. Coombs' test is always negative and there is evidence of disseminated intravascular coagulation in up to 60% of cases. Some patients have a migratory thrombophlebitis. In one study, 55% of diagnosed cases were of proven gastric origin and 10% were uncertain. Lung cancer and breast cancer accounted for most of the others with isolated cases due to colon carcinoma, cholangiocarcinoma, hepatoma and one or two pelvic tumours. MAHA is easily diagnosed as a severe haemolytic anaemia associated with fragmentation of the red cells with a negative Coombs test. Of interest in the causation is the implication of sialomucin which is frequently a product of the associated carcinomas.[5]

POLYCYTHAEMIA

This may occur in patients with hepatoma and renal carcinoma, and it may antecede the development of neoplastic transformation in patients with existing cirrhosis. Erythropoietin production has been detected in such cases but prostaglandins produced by the tumour may enhance the effects of endogenous erythropoietin.

LEUKOCYTOSIS

The mechanisms of elevation of the peripheral white cell count have not been fully elucidated. However, 'leukaemoid reactions' due to neutrophil levels above 20×10^9/litre without overt infection or leukaemia may be seen in association with gastric and pancreatic tumours as well as lymphomas.[12] The main features distinguishing the paraneoplastic leukaemoid reaction from true chronic myelocytic leukaemia are the absence of splenomegaly, the presence of an elevated leukocyte alkaline phosphatase, and the absence of the Philadelphia chromosome. Also, characteristically, the white cell counts are in the range of $(20–40) \times 10^9$/litre and rarely above this level. In a study of serum and urine from 12 patients with cancer of several kinds, including hepatoma, there was a detectable haematological colony-stimulating factor in all patients. Thus, it is probable that many of the cases of granulocytosis are due to the production of specific colony-stimulating factors by tumours.

NEUTROPENIA AND LYMPHOPENIA

Usually a feature of treatment, a low white cell count may develop as a consequence of marrow involvement, although more frequently it is a feature of pancytopenia.[12]

PLATELET ABNORMALITIES

It is very characteristic for patients with cancer to have an increased platelet count at presentation. It is probable that there is megakaryocyte overproduction due to some tumour-associated product (colony-stimulating factors), but the level of platelet elevation is not usually thought to be important functionally.

A syndrome similar to idiopathic thrombocytopenic purpura is commonly seen in association with lymphoma. Although lymphomas predominate in reports of idiopathic thrombocytopenic purpura, carcinomas of the rectum and gallbladder have also been described as well as lung and breast cancers. In most cases the idiopathic thrombocytopenic purpura is clinically important, causing bleeding, petechiae and purpura. Some patients respond to steroids but in other cases splenectomy may be indicated after a trial of steroids and sometimes a trial of intravenous γ-globulin.

COAGULOPATHIES

An increased tendency to thrombosis occurs in a variety of cancers in association with abnormal blood clotting times, elevated clotting factors and/or fibrinogen degradation products. The most consistent finding is increased platelet and/or fibrinogen turnover. The clinical association between cancer and thrombophlebitis was first reported by Trousseau in association with a mucin-secreting adenocarcinoma of the gastrointestinal tract. The latter cancers remain the most common associated diseases, but patients with lung, breast, ovary or prostate cancer may also present with thrombophlebitis. The incidence of thrombophlebitis in pancreatic cancer is very high and probably exceeds 50%.[12] Chronic therapy with heparin or warfarin is often only partially successful.

DISSEMINATED INTRAVASCULAR COAGULATION

Abnormalities of blood coagulation may be seen in the majority of cancer patients but only rarely do the patients manifest the full syndrome of disseminated intravascular coagulation which is a characteristic of promyelocytic leukaemia and disseminated prostatic carcinoma. The mechanism for the enhanced thrombotic state include the following:

1. The activation of intrinsic pathway of coagulation possibly due to abnormal vascular endothelial lining or infection.
2. The activation of the extrinsic pathway by thromboplastin, possibly liberated by normal tissues destroyed by tumour.
3. The aggregation by tumours of platelets.
4. The production of pro-coagulant factors, such as mucous glycoprotein and trypsin which may activate an alternative cellular pathway other than the classic coagulation pathways.

Treatment of disseminated intravascular coagulation

Treating the underlying condition is of major importance but the detection of sepsis and other predisposing causes such as dehydration should be considered. The use of heparin remains controversial but only a minority of patients obtain control of the disseminated intravascular coagulation and the outlook is generally very poor.[13] The severity of disseminated intravascular coagulation in a chronic situation may vary with time and patients can be controlled temporarily with heparin while the condition waxes, and then be withdrawn from it as the tendency to thrombosis seems spontaneously to remit.

MARANTIC ENDOCARDITIS

Sterile subendocardial lesions may develop on the mitral and aortic valves in patients with cancer and may become a source of cerebral and other arterial emboli. Echocardiography may not detect the frequently small valve lesion. The control of the complication is determined by the success of control of the underlying condition.

RENAL MANIFESTATIONS OF MALIGNANCY

Apart from direct infiltration or compression of the urinary tract, damage to the kidneys can occur from hypercalcaemia or uric acid nephropathy. Similarly, severe dehydration and infection are common causes of renal complications as are the toxic side effects of drugs and radiotherapy. The characteristic paraneoplastic syndrome is, however, the nephrotic syndrome in association with cancer due to either renal vein thrombosis or amyloidosis. In one series of 101 patients with nephrotic syndrome, 11 were found to have cancer, the nephrotic syndrome often preceding the discovery of malignancy. Nephrotic syndrome due to systemic amyloid has been associated with carcinomas of the stomach, colon and gallbladder.

Membranous glomerulonephritis has been found in various cases of gastrointestinal malignancy including stomach and colon cancer, and sometimes attributed to deposition of tumour–antigen–antibody complexes. Rarely, disseminated intravascular coagulation due to cancer can cause glomerular microangiopathy producing a nephrotic syndrome.

Renal tubular dysfunction has been reported with pancreatic cancer and hypokalaemia-induced renal tubular damage in association with villous colonic tumours or via the ectopic production of ACTH due to carcinoid.

RHEUMATIC SYNDROMES

The best known associated malignancy with polyarthropathy is lymphoma with Sjögren's syndrome. Systemic lupus erythematosus has been associated with testicular and ovarian tumours. Cancers of the colon, liver and pancreas have been implicated as causing a carcinomatous arthritis with the joint symptoms becoming active on recurrence of disease.

HYPERTROPHIC PULMONARY OSTEOARTHROPATHY AND ACROMEGALY

Although hypertrophic pulmonary osteoarthropathy may be characteristic of any of the subtypes of lung cancer and carcinoids, it is seen occasionally in association with abdominal malignancies, especially tumours which metastasize to the lung. Typically the patient suffers pain and swelling of the ankle or wrist joints with radiological evidence of subperiosteal new bone at the distal ends of the tibia, fibula, radius or ulna. In some cases of hypertrophic, pulmonary osteoarthropathy, excessive levels of growth hormone have been detected in the blood. There are also documented instances of patients with cancer-associated acromegaly in whom skull radiographs show the presence of an enlarged pituitary fossa and acromegalic facies. Shalet *et al.*[22] has investigated this phenomenon and found that although the tumour does not necessarily produce growth hormone there may be a growth hormone-releasing hormone in the tumour cells. As in classic acromegaly, the growth hormone excess is unlikely to be suppressed by a glucose challenge.

HYPERTENSION AND HYPOTENSION

Malignant hypertension has been seen with some lung cancers and hypernephromas. Hypotension is seen usually as a feature of the autonomic neuropathy of advanced systemic malignancy.

AMYLOIDOSIS

About one patient in six with amyloidosis has underlying malignancy as the cause, most frequently myeloma or lymphoma but sometimes carcinoma. Epithelial tumours producing amyloid include bladder and kidney carcinomas, cervical cancer and biliary tract cancer. A characteristic pattern is the neuropathy, hypotension and impaired gastrointestinal motility syndrome. Occasionally a cardiomyopathy may develop. The diagnosis can be made by specific staining of skin or, preferably, rectal biopsy. The amyloid responds only poorly to supportive measures.

SUMMARY

Cancers produce a variety of metabolic complications via hormonal, putative humoral and other mechanisms. Many of these causes remain obscure and may be complicated by the toxic effects of the therapy. The overriding principle in the management of the paraneoplastic syndromes and other similar non-metastatic complications is the recognition that patients with cancers may have symptoms associated with the cancer that can be controlled by fairly simple measures. Non-toxic treatments may thus contribute in a meaningful way to the quality of life of patients whose underlying condition may not be curable.

REFERENCES

1. Abelhoff, M.D. (1987) Paraneoplastic syndromes: a window on the biology of cancer. *New England Journal of Medicine*, **317**, 1598–1600.
2. Allan, S.G., Lockhard, S.P., Leonard, R.C.F. and Smyth, J.F. (1984) Paraneoplastic hypercalcaemia in ovarian carcinoma. *British Medical Journal*, **288**, 1714–1715.
3. Blackman, M.R., Rosen, S.W. and Weintraub, B.D. (1978) Ectopic hormones. *Advances in Internal Medicine*, **23**, 85–113.
4. Block, J.B. (1974) Lactic acidosis in malignancy and observations on its possible pathogenesis. *Annals of the New York Academy of Sciences*, **230**, 94–102.
5. Bunn, P.A. and Minna, J.D. (1985) Paraneoplastics syndrome. In *Cancer Principles and Practices of Oncology*, 2nd edn, pp. 1797–1843. (Eds.) DeVita, V.T., Hellman, S. and Rosenberg, S.A. Philadelphia: Lippincott.
6. Coleman, R.E., Woll, P.J., Myles, M., Scrivner, W. and Rubens, R.D. (1988) Treatment of bone metastases from breast cancer with 3-amino, 1-hydroxypropylidene, 1-bisphosphonate (APD). *British Journal of Cancer*, **56**, 465–469.
7. Coombes, R.C. (1984) Paraneoplastic syndrome in lung cancer. In *Small Cell Lung Cancer*, pp. 150–171. (Ed.) Smyth, J. Oxford: Blackwell Scientific.
8. DeTroyer, A. (1977) Demeclocycline treatment for syndrome of inappropriate antidiuretic hormone secretion. *Journal of the American Medical Association*, **237**, 2823–2826.
9. Dickson, R.B. and Lippman, M.E. (1987) Estrogenic regulation of growth and polypeptide growth factor secretion in human breast carcinoma. *Endocrinology Review*, **8**, 29–43.
10. Fearon, K. (1988) Cachexia and weight loss in cancer patients. In *Medical Complications of Malignancy*, pp. 375–395. (Eds.) Kaye, S.B. and Rankin, E. London: Blackwell.
11. Harlow, P.J., DeClerk, Y.A., Shore, N.A., Ortega, J.A., Carranza, A. and Heuser, E. (1979) A fatal case of inappropriate ADH secretion induced by cyclophosphamide therapy. *Cancer*, **44**, 896–898.
12. Leonard, R.C.F. (1988) Metabolic complications of malignant disease. In *Medical Complications of Malignancy*, pp. 261–283. (Ed.) Kaye, S.B. and Rankin, E. London: Blackwell.
13. Leonard, R.C.F. (1991) Other medical complications of malignant disease. *Medicine*, series 5, in press.
14. Meador, C.K., Liddle, G.W., Island, B.P. *et al.* (1962) Cause of Cushing's syndrome in patients with tumour arising from non-endocrine tissue. *Journal of Clinical Endocrinology and Metabolism*, **22**, 693–698.
15. Moertel, C.J. (1987) Karnofsky Memorial Lecture. An Odyssey in the land of small tumours. *Journal of Clinical Oncology*, **5**, 1503–1522.
16. Mundy, G.R. (1990) Pathophysiology of cancer associated hypercalcemia. *Seminars in Oncology*, **17** (suppl. 5), 10–15.
17. Mundy, G.R. (1988) Hypercalcemia of malignancy revisited. *Journal of Clinical Investigations*, **82**, 1–6
18. ReMine, W.H., Chong, G.C. and Van Heerden, J.A. (1974) Current management of pheochromocytoma. *Annals of Surgery,* **179**, 740–746.
19. Ralston, S.H., Vogelman, I., Giardiner, M.D. and Boyle, I.T. (1984) Relative contribution of humoral and metastatic factors to the pathogenesis of hypercalcaemia in malignancy. *British Medical Journal*, **288**, 1404–1408.
20. Salomon, D.S. and Perroteau, I. (1986) Growth factors in cancer and their relationship to oncogenes. *Cancer Investigations*, **4**, 43–60.
21. Schwartz, W.D.F., Bennett, W., Curelop, S. and Bartter, F. (1957) A syndrome of renal sodium loss and hyponatremia probably resulting from inappropriate secretion of antidiuretic hormone. *American Journal of Medicine*, **23**, 529–542.
22. Shalet, S.M., Beardwell, C.J., Macfarlane, I.A. *et al.* (1979) Acromegaly due to production of a growth hormone releasing factor by a bronchial carcinoid tumour. *Clinical Endocrinology*, **10**, 61–64.
23. Skrabanek, P. and Powell, D. (1978) Unifying concept of non-pituitary ACTH secreting tumours: evidence of common origin of neural-crest tumours, carcinoids, and oat-cell carcinomas. *Cancer*, **42**, 1263–1269.
24. Sporn, M.B. and Roberts, A.B. (1985) Autocrine growth factors and cancer. *Nature*, **313**, 745–747.
25. Sporn, M.B. and Todaro, G.J. (1980) autocrine secretion and malignant transformation of cells. *New England Journal of Medicine*, **303**, 878–880.

26. Steward, A.F., Horst, R. and Deftos, L.J. (1980) Biochemical evaluation of cancer associate hypercalcemia evidence for humoral and non-humoral groups. *New England Journal of Medicine*, **303**, 1377–1383.

27. Vogelzang, N.J., Torkelson, J.L. and Kennedy, B.J. (1985) Hypomagnesemia, renal dysfunction and Raynaud's phenomenon in patients treated with cisplatin, vinblastine and bleomycin. *Cancer*, **56**, 2765–2700.

GRAFT-VERSUS-HOST DISEASE

Kerry Atkinson

Graft-versus-host disease (GVHD) occurs when the following circumstances obtain:

1. There is a genetically determined histocompatibility antigen difference between the transplant donor and the recipient.
2. There are immunocompetent cells present in the transplant that can recognize the foreign histocompatibility antigens present in the host and mount an immune attack on cells bearing those antigens.
3. There is an inability of the host to react against, and to reject, the donor transplant.

In clinical practice human graft-versus-host disease occurs almost exclusively after allogeneic bone marrow transplantation (usually for leukaemia), but has very rarely been reported after blood transfusion, and solid organ transplantation.

ACUTE GRAFT-VERSUS-HOST DISEASE

After marrow transplantation acute graft-versus-host disease is defined as that occurring in the first 100 days after the transplant. The three main clinically relevant target organs are the skin, the gastrointestinal tract and the liver, and a grading system for severity has been devised.[14] Skin involvement is most common, occurring in 90% of allogeneic transplant recipients. Gut and liver involvement is rarer occurring in approximately 10% of HLA-identical sibling marrow transplant recipients, but in approximately 60% of HLA-non-identical family member transplant recipients or in matched unrelated transplant recipients (HLA = human leucocyte antigen). Risk factors for acute graft-versus-host disease include increasing age of recipient, male recipients of female marrow and increasing parity of female donors. Studies of the pathogenesis have shown that the initiating event is the recognition by mature donor T cells in the marrow inoculum of foreign histocompatibility antigens in the recipient. The actual mediation of target cell damage is less clearly defined, but electron microscope studies have shown lymphocytes in close apposition to epithelial cells in the skin, bowel and bile duct. The incidence of acute graft-versus-host disease can be minimized by the prophylactic use of immunosuppressive therapy both before and after transplant; this is most commonly a combination of cyclosporin and methotrexate.[11] Elimination of mature T cells from the donor marrow prior to its infusion can also be effective. Both these measures, however, simultaneously decrease the therapeutically valuable graft-versus-leukaemia effect which contributes to the cure of the underlying haematological malignancy, with a subsequent increase in the risk of recurrent leukaemia after the transplant.[8]

ACUTE GRAFT-VERSUS-HOST DISEASE OF THE GASTROINTESTINAL TRACT

HISTOPATHOLOGY

Microscopically, individual crypt cell destruction giving the appearance of the 'exploding crypt cell' can lead on to crypt abscesses and finally a totally denuded mucosa. There is often little lymphocytic inflammatory infiltrate present.[9] Increased HLA-DR expression of gut epithelial cells has been demonstrated as has a decrease in the number of mucosal plasma cells bearing IgM or IgA. These biopsy findings are not useful until 3 weeks after the transplant, before which they may be mimicked by damage to the mucosa by the pre-transplant chemoradiotherapy regimen.

CLINICAL FEATURES[6,7]

The stomach, small bowel and large intestine are the main sites of involvement, with the ileocaecal region being the most severely affected. Clinical features include anorexia, nausea, vomiting, diarrhoea that is often marked and watery and sometimes haemorrhagic, and crampy abdominal pains.[7] Signs of peritonism are occasionally present; protein is lost in the diarrhoea. Endoscopic appearances can be normal or show a friable or frankly ulcerated and haemorrhagic mucosa. Recently, a predominantly upper gastrointestinal variant has been described with the cardinal features being anorexia, nausea and vomiting.[15] Severity is graded according to the volume of diarrhoea.[6,14] Occasionally, the mouth is involved, producing mucosal erythema.

INVESTIGATIONS

Diagnosis rests on the presence of the above clinical features, together with concomitant acute graft-versus-host disease of the skin or liver, and a negative stool culture for infectious agents particularly *Clostridium difficile* and *Campylobacter* spp., as well as exclusion of cytomegalovirus enteritis on gut biopsy. Radiological studies with barium show mucosal and submucosal oedema, especially over the distal small intestine, and transit time is rapid. None of the radiological, histopathological or clinical features are entirely specific for gut graft-versus-host disease.

TREATMENT

Severity of graft-versus-host disease is indicated best by volume of diarrhoea and the presence of macroscopic blood in the diarrhoea. The patient should be placed on a nil by mouth regimen and given intravenous total parenteral nutrition together with fluid and electrolyte replacement. Cyclosporin should be given intravenously because poor absorption of oral cyclosporin is present with diarrhoea of any cause.[1] Methylprednisolone ranging from 2 mg/kg per day to 1 g daily is usually used. If there is no response, a course of antithymocyte globulin should be given. Rapid treatment (or appropriate prophylaxis) should be instituted for any intercurrent infections, particularly with herpes simplex or cytomegalovirus, Gram-negative rods or fungi. Experimental treatment at the present time includes the use of monoclonal antibody to the interleukin-2 receptor and ultraviolet photopheresis. Moderate-to-severe acute graft-versus-host disease of the bowel (grade II–IV) has a mortality approaching 50%.

ACUTE GRAFT-VERSUS-HOST DISEASE OF THE LIVER

HISTOPATHOLOGY

Abnormalities consist of bile duct atypia, lymphocytic endothelialitis of the hepatic portal vein and hepatocyte damage. However, liver biopsy is seldom carried out for diagnostic reasons due to the risk of bleeding associated with thrombocytopenia early after the transplant. Liver biopsy (or bowel biopsy) should not be attempted with a platelet count of less than 50×10^9/l.

CLINICAL FEATURES

Hepatic graft-versus-host disease is characterized by a cholestatic jaundice and mild hepatomegaly. Ascites is rare as is subsequent liver failure. Liver function tests show an increase in (predominantly) conjugated bilirubin, a marked rise in serum alkaline phosphatase and a lesser rise in transaminase levels.

DIFFERENTIAL DIAGNOSIS

The diagnosis is based on the above clinical features together with the presence of concomitant skin or gut acute graft-versus-host disease. Differential diagnosis includes hepatic veno-occlusive disease which has an identical liver function test profile, but is characterized by the presence of ascites and weight gain and usually occurs within the first 3 weeks after the transplant. The most common cause of jaundice after marrow transplantation is cyclosporin hepatoxicity characterized by a raised conjugated bilirubin, but with minimal elevation of alkaline phosphatase or transaminase values.[2] Viral hepatitis is usually easy to differentiate from hepatic graft-versus-host disease due to the characteristically marked elevation of transaminase levels. Other causes of jaundice after marrow transplantation include haemolysis associated with ABO incompatible transplants, septicaemia and treatments such as co-trimoxazole and parenteral nutrition.

TREATMENT

Management is similar to that described for gastrointestinal acute graft-versus-host disease. The slower rate of metabolism of drugs such as cyclosporin, methotrexate and opiates in patients with hyperbilirubinaemia should be remembered.

CHRONIC GRAFT-VERSUS-HOST DISEASE

Chronic graft-versus-host disease is defined as that occurring 100 days or later after the transplant.[10,12] It occurs at a median of 3–4 months after the transplant with a range from 70 days to 15 months. It has a wider spectrum of organ involvement than the acute form and resembles a systemic, multiorgan, connective tissue disorder. Organs involved include skin, mouth, liver, eye, oesophagus, sinus, and less commonly small and large intestine, lung, vagina and serosal surfaces. Wasting may be present, as well as cytopenias. It may develop after a quiescent period free of acute graft-versus-host disease, or the acute form of graft-versus-host disease may progressively merge into the chronic form, or chronic graft-versus-host disease can occur without prior acute symptoms. The chronic form also occurs as a 'flare' following the tapering of prophylactic immunosuppression, particularly with cyclosporin. The disease is marked by a considerable susceptibility to infections, especially Gram-positive coccal infections.[4] This reflects the marked immune deficiency of many parameters of T- and B-cell function present in these patients, but not in their healthy long-term counterparts without chronic graft-versus-host disease.[6] It occurs in approximately 50% of recipients of HLA-identical sibling transplants surviving 6 months or more after the transplant. Risk factors include preceding acute graft-versus-host disease, as well as increasing recipient age, and female marrow donors for male recipients. Besides allogeneic T cells the pathogenesis includes a role for autoreactive T cells, abnormal self-regulatory T cells and a variety of cytokines, some of which mediate the fibrosis characteristic of chronic graft-versus-host disease.[6] Again there is an important graft-versus-leukaemia effect associated with the chronic form which contributes to cure of the underlying haematological malignancy.[8]

CHRONIC GRAFT-VERSUS-HOST DISEASE OF THE GASTROINTESTINAL TRACT

HISTOPATHOLOGY

The three distinct abnormalities detected are epithelial cell damage, a mononuclear cell inflammatory infiltrate predominantly of the CD8-positive cells and epithelial and subepithelial fibrosis. In the mouth both the mucosa and the ducts of the minor salivary glands are involved with glandular loss.

CLINICAL FEATURES[6,10,12]

Mouth

A sicca syndrome often develops with dry mouth; lichen planus-like striae are common and mucosal ulceration can sometimes become severe and painful. These changes eventually lead to atrophy of the tongue and gums.

Oesophagus

This is now uncommon, but occasionally a desquamative oesophagitis occurs with difficulty in swallowing produced by an upper oesophageal web, and retrosternal pain produced by acid influx. Abnormal motility has been demonstrated.

Small intestine and large intestine

Involvement of these organs is much less common than with acute graft-versus-host disease. However, the clinical features are the same. Initially observed, but rarely seen now due to better immunosuppression and earlier interventionist treatment, are malabsorption secondary to extensive fibrosis in the submucosal and subserosal regions, and a bacterial stasis syndrome resulting in diarrhoea and malabsorption.

The diagnosis is based on the clinical findings and histopathological biopsy features. In the clinical setting of allogeneic marrow transplantation it is usually straightforward.

TREATMENT

This depends on the extent of involvement and organs involved and can range from no treatment with asymptomatic disease restricted to the liver, reinstitution of cyclosporin if development of chronic graft-versus-host disease has occurred with the patient on a tapering dose of cyclosporin or, for more severe disease, prednisone which has been shown to be better than a combination of prednisone and azathioprine.[13] The most commonly used regimen currently is a combination of cyclosporin and prednisone. The dose of prednisone is usually 1 mg/kg on alternate days. An important component of treatment is the institution of prophylactic therapy against both Gram-positive coccal infections and *Pneumocystis carinii* pneumonia. This can be achieved by the use of co-trimoxazole. Second-line immunosuppressive treatment includes thalidomide and psoralen ultraviolet A phototherapy which is especially effective for dry mouth.[5]

CHRONIC GRAFT-VERSUS-HOST DISEASE OF THE LIVER

This occurs in 80% of patients with chronic graft-versus-host disease. The clinical features are similar to those of the acute form of the liver. The serum alkaline phosphatase may be increased up to twenty-fold. Involvement may be prolonged without general patient deterioration. Histopathological features again show small bile duct atypia and damage leading to necrosis and drop-out. This is a reasonably sensitive, but not a specific, indicator of the disease. It is difficult to distinguish histologically from chronic hepatitides. Treatment can range from no active management other than the use of prophylactic co-trimoxazole to orthotopic liver transplantation for end-stage liver damage.

REFERENCES

1. Atkinson, K., Biggs, J.C., Britton, K., Farrell, C., Concannon, A. and Dodds, A.J. (1984) Oral administration of cyclosporin A for recipients of allogeneic bone marrow transplants: implications of clinical gut dysfunction. *British Journal of Haematology*, **56**, 223–231.
2. Atkinson, K., Biggs, J.C., Dodds, A.J. and Concannon, A.J. (1983) Cyclosporin A associated hepatotoxicity after allogeneic bone marrow transplantation: differentiation from other causes of post transplant liver disease. *Transplantation Proceedings*, **15**, 2761–2767.
3. Atkinson, K., Horowitz, M.M., Gale, R.P. *et al.* (1990) Risk factors for chronic graft-versus-host disease after HLA-identical sibling bone marrow transplantation. *Blood*, **75**, 2459–2464.
4. Atkinson, K., Storb, R., Prentice, R.L. *et al.* (1979) Analysis of late infections in 89 long term survivors of bone marrow transplantation. *Blood*, **53**, 720–731.
5. Atkinson, K., Weller, P., Ryman, W. and Biggs, J.C. (1986) PUVA therapy for drug-resistant graft-versus-host disease. *Bone Marrow Transplantation*, **1**, 227–236.
6. Burakoff, S.J., Deeg, H.J., Ferrara, J. and Atkinson, K. (Eds.) (1990) *Graft-versus-host disease*. New York: Marcel Dekker.
7. Glucksberg, H., Storb, R., Fefer, A. *et al.* (1974) Clinical manifestations of graft-versus-host disease in human recipients of marrow from HLA-matched sibling donors. *Transplantation*, **18**, 295–304.
8. Horowitz, M.M., Gale, R.P., Sondel, P.M. *et al.* (1990) Graft-versus-leukaemia reactions after bone marrow transplantation. *Blood*, **75**, 555–562.
9. Lerner, K.G., Kao, G.F., Storb, R., Buckner, C., Clift, R. and Thomas, E. (1974) Histopathology of graft-versus-host reaction (GVHR) in human recipients from HLA-matched sibling donors. *Transplantation Proceedings*, **6**, 367–371.
10. Shulman, H.M., Sullivan, K.M., Weiden, P.L. *et al.* (1980) Chronic graft-versus-host syndrome in man. A long term clinicopathological study of 20 Seattle patients. *American Journal of Medicine*, **69**, 204–217.
11. Storb, R., Deeg, H.J., Whitehead, J. *et al.* (1986) Marrow transplantation for leukemia. Methotrexate and cyclosporine compared with cyclosporine alone for prophylaxis of acute graft-versus-host disease after marrow transplantation for leukemia. *New England Journal of Medicine*, **314**, 729–735.
12. Sullivan, K.M., Shulman, H.M., Storb, R. *et al.* (1981) Chronic graft-versus-host disease in 52 patients: adverse natural course and successful treatment with combination immunosuppression. *Blood*, **57**, 267–276.
13. Sullivan, K.M., Witherspoon, R.P., Storb, R. *et al.* (1988) Prednisone and azathioprine compared with prednisone and placebo for treatment of chronic graft-versus-host disease: prognostic influence of prolonged thrombocytopenia after allogeneic marrow transplantation. *Blood*, **72**, 546–554.
14. Thomas, E.D., Storb, R., Clift, R. *et al.* (1975) Bone marrow transplantation. *New England Journal of Medicine*, **292**, 895–902.
15. Weisdorf, D.J., Snover, D.C., Haake, R. *et al.* (1990) Acute upper gastrointestinal graft-versus-host disease: clinical significance and response to immunosuppressive therapy. *Blood*, **76**, 624–629.

SYSTEMIC ENDOCRINE DISORDERS

R.G. Long

PARATHYROID DISEASES

The four parathyroid glands secrete the 84 amino acid polypeptide hormone, parathyroid hormone. In the presence of a normal plasma magnesium, parathyroid hormone maintains the plasma calcium in the normal range of 2.05–2.55 mmol/l. When the plasma calcium is low, parathyroid hormone mobilizes calcium from bone, increases absorption of dietary calcium by stimulation of the activity of 25-hydroxy-vitamin D 1-hydroxylase, and causes decreased urinary calcium and increased urinary phosphate secretion.

Fluctuations in plasma calcium affect gut function. Experimentally raising the plasma calcium causes gastrin release and raises basal gastric acid secretion, a phenomenon unaffected by atropine; a fall in plasma calcium results in a fall in gastrin level and gastric acid secretion. A rise in plasma calcium to the supranormal range also has an inhibitory effect on gut motility. These effects appear to be mediated directly through plasma calcium because parathyroid hormone infusions alone have no effect.

HYPERPARATHYROIDISM

Primary hyperparathyroidism

The clinical spectrum of primary hyperparathyroidism is changing as many patients are now identified with minimal or no symptoms when hypercalcaemia and hypophosphataemia are discovered on a multichannel biochemical analyser. Patients are therefore usually diagnosed much earlier than in the past and advanced cases with long-standing complications are rarely seen.

The main gastrointestinal complications of primary hyperparathyroidism are thought to be peptic ulcers, acute and chronic pancreatitis and constipation. All are probably primarily related to the hypercalcaemia, although as patients are now being diagnosed by biochemical screening, the association between these clinical features and hyperparathyroidism is becoming less strong. The constipation may be very severe, and reduced gastric emptying and small intestinal mobility along with colonic atony are reported. Other gastrointestinal symptoms include anorexia, nausea, vomiting, weight loss and diarrhoea. Obscure abdominal pain not due to peptic ulcer disease, pancreatitis or renal stones may also be a feature.[7]

Peptic ulcer disease

The incidence of peptic ulcers in primary hyperparathyroidism has been estimated at 8–30% compared with about 2.5–3.2% in the normal population.[4] The increase is solely in duodenal ulcers, with no change in the incidence of gastric ulcer. The high incidence of duodenal ulcer is associated with raised plasma gastrin levels, and increased gastric acid and pepsin secretion; these all fall after successful parathyroidectomy.

It has been suggested that the raised plasma gastrin levels are associated with increased antral G-cell numbers. The presence of an associated chronic pancreatitis with reduced pancreatic bicarbonate output might also contribute to the pathogenesis of duodenal ulcer. Linos *et al.*[12] suggested in a series of 46 patients that there is no association between ulcers and hyperparathyroidism, but as this was a retrospective study with small numbers, and in view of the previous evidence, a prospective study is now needed to clarify the situation. Meanwhile, patients with persistent or recurrent peptic ulceration should have their plasma calcium and phosphate levels measured to search for hypercalcaemia due to primary hyperparathyroidism, with or without an associated gastrinoma.[17]

Duodenal ulcers associated with primary hyperparathyroidism should respond to H_2 receptor antagonists. It has been shown that cimetidine may also reduce plasma parathyroid hormone levels so a double effect may be expected.[20] Despite this some patients may not respond to cimetidine but make a good response to excision of the parathyroid adenoma.[14]

A specific problem with duodenal ulcers and primary hyperparathyroidism is the possible presence of a coexistent gastrinoma as part of a multiple endocrine neoplasia (MEN) syndrome (see also later). The release of gastrin from gastrinomas is highly sensitive to the serum calcium level and, after parathyroidectomy, plasma gastrin may return to normal despite a persisting gastrinoma. Under these circumstances a paradoxical rise in plasma gastrin with intravenous calcium or secretin suggests a gastrinoma. It is generally accepted that, in the context of MEN, it is best to perform a parathyroidectomy as the first procedure. If gastric acid output and plasma gastrin levels (including with secretin or calcium provocation) are normal after parathyroidectomy it should be possible to reduce or stop H_2-receptor antagonists or proton pump inhibitor drugs; if symptoms of peptic ulceration return, a further gastroscopy should be performed and the patient reinvestigated fully if ulceration is present.[18] If the tests remain abnormal, attempts to localize a gastrinoma by gastroduodenoscopy, retrograde pancreatography, selective pancreatic, and duodenal arteriography and portal venous sampling should be considered.[10,15]

Pancreatic disease

Both acute and chronic pancreatitis are thought to be associated with primary hyperparathyroidism. However, in the presence of an acute attack of pancreatitis the plasma calcium levels may become normal or even subnormal, so it is important to carry out an estimation of the plasma calcium after the patient has fully recovered. Possible aetiological links between hyperparathyroidism and pancreatitis include calcium stones in the pancreatic duct, increased trypsin activation due to increased pancreatic calcium secretion (trypsinogen conversion to trypsin is calcium dependent), and vasculitis; this last hypothesis is based on the observation that experimental animals treated with parathyroid hormone have developed a thromboendarteritis. In some patients, pancreatic calcification seen on plain abdominal radiographs may be particularly marked.

The consequences of pancreatitis – steatorrhoea, diabetes mellitus, pain and other complications – should be treated in the standard manner.

The association between primary hyperparathyroidism and pancreatitis is standard teaching but has been challenged. Bess *et al.*[1] retrospectively studied 1153 Mayo Clinic patients and found only 17 who had evidence of pancreatitis, 11 of whom had evidence of a gallstone and/or alcoholic aetiology. As this is similar to the incidence of pancreatitis in a control hospital population, they suggest that the association may not exist.

Cases of acute pancreatitis continued to be reported, especially when hypercalcaemia is moderate or severe, but there are sometimes other risk factors such as previous gastric surgery, alcohol abuse or treatment with azathioprine and corticosteroids after renal transplantation. The association of pregnancy, primary hyperparathyroidism and acute pancreatitis is described in a few cases.[8] Parathyroidectomy should be performed if indicated and may improve the prognosis for recurrent pancreatitis.[21]

An association between hyperparathyroidism and gallstones has also been claimed, but in a prospective study of Stockholm council workers 82 were found to have primary hyperparathyroidism and the frequency of cholelithiasis on oral cholecystography was the same in the patients as in 82 age- and sex-matched controls.[3] Clearly, a large prospective series is needed of hyperparathyroid patients without evidence of pancreatic endocrine tumours in whom full gastric, biliary and pancreatic assessment has been performed.

Secondary hyperparathyroidism

When there is chronic steatorrhoea, calcium and vitamin D malabsorption often ensue. This causes a reduction in the plasma calcium, and parathyroid hormone is consequently secreted in large amounts from hyperplastic glands. Patients may then develop osteomalacia with the biochemical and bone changes of secondary hyperparathyroidism. Conditions associated with this problem include coeliac disease, Crohn's disease, postgastrectomy, the short bowel syndrome, jejunoileal bypass for morbid obesity and chronic cholestatic liver disease.[5,16]

Clinically, patients with severe disease may develop bone pains and pseudofractures. These along with radiological bone thinning indicate osteomalacia; subperiosteal resorption, particularly on the hand phalanges, suggest secondary hyperparathyroidism. Biochemical changes include a low or low/normal fasting plasma calcium and phosphate, a low serum 25-hydroxy-vitamin D and a raised plasma bony-type alkaline phosphatase isoenzyme level. Biochemical changes more specifically suggesting secondary hyperparathyroidism are raised plasma immunoreactive parathyroid hormone levels, raised plasma and 24-hour urinary hydroxyproline levels and evidence of increased phosphate excretion in the presence of hypophosphataemia (by demonstrating a reduced maximum tubular reabsorption of phosphate related to glomerular filtration rate). However, the most definite way of making a diagnosis is by bone biopsy including the examination of calcification fronts using in vivo tetracycline labelling. The changes of osteomalacia are increased osteoid tissue and reduced calcification fronts; those of secondary hyperparathyroidism are increased osteoclastic resorption and increased fibrous tissue (osteitis fibrosa). Severe untreated cases may result in radiographs showing multiple, well-marginated, mixed lytic and sclerotic lesions of bone which histologically can be shown to be brown tumours of bone.[6]

Treatment involves correction of the malabsorption, if feasible. In patients with coeliac disease, a careful gluten-free diet alone may lead to full resolution. In other patients oral vitamin D supplements will allow resolution; increased exposure to ultraviolet light (from the sun or an ultraviolet lamp), vitamin D_2 or D_3 supplements and 1α-hydroxy-vitamin D_3 may all be effective. When there is biochemical evidence of magnesium or severe calcium deficiency, supplements of these ions may be helpful. Basic treatment monitoring can be done by estimating the plasma calcium and phosphate levels, but the only accurate way is by bone biopsy, perhaps every 6–12 months, because many patients have normal biochemical and radiological markers but grossly abnormal bone histology.

Pseudohyperparathyroidism and tertiary hyperparathyroidism

Hypercalcaemia may result from the 138 amino acid parathyroid hormone-related protein which is produced by carcinomas, most commonly of the bronchus or breast; this condition is usually termed 'pseudohyperparathyroidism'.[2] In patients with secondary hyperparathyroidism an autonomous parathyroid-hormone-secreting adenoma may develop in the hyperplastic parathyroid glands and cause hypercalcaemia (tertiary hyperparathyroidism). The most common gastrointestinal complication of these problems is severe constipation. Treatment of the hypercalcaemia with tumour excision or by medical means (saline diuresis with frusemide, corticosteroids, calcitonin, diphosphonates or mithramycin) usually relieves the symptoms.

Hypoparathyroidism

The usual presenting symptoms of hypoparathyroidism are cramps, tetany and steatorrhoea. A familial association with Addison's disease, diabetes mellitus and hypothyroidism is described.[13] Some of these patients will have an immunodeficiency syndrome, which may initiate multiple causes of gastrointestinal disease. Biochemical changes include hypocalcaemia, hyperphosphataemia and immeasurable immunoreactive parathyroid hormone levels. When the plasma calcium is less than 1.75 mmol/l, achlorhydria is usually present. Gastric acid secretion becomes normal as the plasma calcium is corrected.

The steatorrhoea is usually modest but may be very high, e.g. more than 352 mmol (100 g) daily. Reduced absorption of xylose, glucose and fat-soluble vitamins is documented. The cause of the steatorrhoea which is corrected by successful treatment is controversial. Most small bowel biopsies have been reported as normal, but villous atrophy responding to treatment of the hypocalcaemia has been described.[19] Other suggested factors in the pathogenesis of the steatorrhoea are intestinal candidiasis and bacterial overgrowth due to associated immunodeficiency and reduced bile acid secretion due to associated liver disease. Barium follow-through studies show delayed gastric emptying, and small intestinal transit associated with dilated intestinal loops and flocculation of the barium; these changes resolve with successful vitamin D and calcium treatment. Pancreatic enzymes are unhelpful but medium-chain triglyceride supplements have been shown to improve calcium balance.

Pseudohypoparathyroidism is a rare, probably X-linked, dominant condition with similar symptoms and signs to hypoparathyroidism. However, plasma parathyroid hormone levels are high but may be suppressed by calcium infusions; there is a reduced response to exogenous parathyroid hormone indicating an increased peripheral resistance. The patients have short stature, with shortened tubular bones, and may develop cataracts, mental handicap, tetany and ectopic calcification. The previously memorable condition 'pseudo-pseudohypoparathyroidism' now appears not to be distinguishable.[9] Similar gastrointestinal problems might be expected to those seen with hypoparathyroidism but to date they are poorly documented.

References

1. Bess, M.A., Edis, A.J. and Van Heerden, A. (1980) Hyperparathyroidism and pancreatitis – chance or a causal association. *Journal of the American Medical Association*, **343**, 246–247.
2. Burtis, W.J., Brady, T.G., Orloff, J.J. *et al.* (1990) Immunochemical characterization of circulating parathyroid hormone-related protein in patients with humoral hypercalcemia of cancer. *New England Journal of Medicine*, **322**, 1106–1112.
3. Christensson, T. and Einarsson, K. (1977) Cholelithiasis in subjects with hypercalcaemia and primary hyperparathyroidism detected in the health screening. *Gut*, **18**, 543–546.
4. Christianssen, J. (1974) Primary hyperparathyroidism and peptic ulcer disease. *Scandinavian Journal of Gastroenterology*, **9**, 111–114.
5. Compston, J.E., Horton, L.W.L., Laker, M.F. *et al.* (1978) Bone disease after jejuno-ileal bypass for obesity. *The Lancet*, **2**, 1–4.
6. Ehrlich, G.W., Gennant, H.K. and Kolb, F.O. (1983) Secondary hyperparathyroidism and brown tumours in the patient with gluten enteropathy. *American Journal of Roentgenology*, **141**, 381–383.
7. Eversman, J.J., Farmer, R.G. and Brown, C.H. (1967) Gastrointestinal manifestations of hyperparathyroidism. *Archives of Internal Medicine*, **119**, 605–609.
8. Fabrin, B. and Eldon, K. (1986) Pregnancy complicated by concurrent hyperparathyroidism and pancreatitis. *Acta Obstetrica et Gynecologica Scandinavica*, **65**, 651–652.
9. Fitch, N. (1982) Albright's hereditary osteodystrophy – a review. *American Journal of Medical Genetics*, **11**, 11–29.
10. Glowniak, J.V., Shapiro, B., Vinik, A.I. *et al.* (1982) Percutaneous transhepatic venous sampling of gastrin: value in sporadic and familial islet-cell tumours and G-cell hyperfunction. *New England Journal of Medicine*, **307**, 293–297.
11. Gogel, H.K., Buckman, M.T., Cadieux, D. and McCarthy, D.M. (1985) Gastric secretion and hormonal interactions in multiple endocrine neoplasia type I. *Archives of Internal Medicine*, **145**, 855–859.
12. Linos, D.A., Van Heerden, J.A., Abboud, C.F. and Edis, A.J. (1978) Primary hyperparathyroidism and peptic ulcer disease. *Archives of Surgery*, **113**, 384–386.
13. Lorenz, R. and Burr, I.M. (1974) Idiopathic hypoparathyroidism and steatorrhea: a new aid in management. *Journal of Pediatrics*, **85**, 522–525.
14. McCarthy, D.M., Peikin, S.R., Lopatin, R.N. *et al.* (1979) Hyperparathyroidism – a reversible cause of cimetidine resistant gastric hypersecretion. *British Medical Journal*, **1**, 1765–1766.
15. McGuigan, J.E., Colwell, J.A. and Franklin, J. (1974) Effect of parathyroidectomy and hypercalcaemic hypersecretory peptic ulcer disease. *Gastroenterology*, **66**, 269–272.

16. Melvin, K.E.W., Hepner, G.W., Bordier, P. *et al.* (1970) Calcium metabolism and bone pathology in adult coeliac disease. *Quarterly Journal of Medicine*, **39**, 83–113.
17. Mowat, E., Gunn, A. and Paterson, C.R. (1981) Hyperparathyroidism in peptic ulcer patients. *British Journal of Surgery*, **68**, 455–458.
18. Norton, J.A., Cornelius, M.J., Doppman, J.L., Maton, P.N., Gardner, J.D. and Jensen, R.T. (1987) Effect of parathyroidectomy in patients with hyperparathyroidism, Zollinger–Ellison syndrome and multiple endocrine neoplasia type I: a prospective study. *Surgery*, **102**, 958–966.
19. Russell, R.I. (1967) Hypoparathyroidism and malabsorption. *British Medical Journal*, **3**, 781–782.
20. Sherwood, J.K., Ackroyd, F.W. and Garcia, M. (1980) Effect of cimetidine on circulating parathyroid hormone in primary hyperparathyroidism. *The Lancet*, **2**, 616–620.
21. Sitges-Serra, A., Alonso, M., de Lecea, C., Gores, P.F. and Sutherland, D.E.R. (1988) Pancreatitis and hyperparathyroidism. *British Journal of Surgery*, **75**, 158–160.

THYROID DISEASES *(R.G. Long)*

Thyroxine and triiodothyronine are secreted by the thyroid gland and are normally under the control of thyroid-stimulating hormone (TSH) from the anterior pituitary. The thyroid hormones have a major effect on gut motility, as well as other lesser effects, and consequently hyperthyroidism and hypothyroidism are associated with numerous gastrointestinal features.[14] However, it should be stressed that it is very rare for gastrointestinal symptoms to be present without some of the other usual systemic symptoms and signs of thyroid disease.

An association between ulcerative colitis and a history of thyrotoxicosis, hypothyroidism and simple goitre has been demonstrated. A relationship between thyrotoxicosis and coeliac disease is also claimed. Under normal circumstances, the thyroid hormones are bound in plasma to thyroxine-binding globulin (TBG) (75%), thyroxine-binding prealbumin (15%) and albumin (10%). In protein-losing enteropathy states, levels of these proteins fall. In ulcerative colitis and Crohn's disease, there is evidence for iodine deficiency and reduced plasma albumin and prealbumin concentrations. Plasma thyroxine-binding globulin levels are raised in mild and moderate inflammatory bowel disease but fall with severe corticosteroid-treated disease. In general, active ulcerative colitis is often associated with a small goitre but neither active ulcerative colitis nor Crohn's disease is associated with hyperthyroidism or hypothyroidism. However, thyroid uptake tests should be interpreted with care in both conditions because iodine deficiency is common and results in increased uptake which suggests a misleading diagnosis of thyrotoxicosis.[12]

HYPERTHYROIDISM

The most common gastrointestinal symptom of hyperthyroidism is diarrhoea, which occurs in about 25% of thyrotoxic patients. The symptom is usually modest and the patient notices only a slight increase in the frequency of bowel movements, along with some softening of the faeces. Profuse watery diarrhoea is unusual. On occasions patients may notice steatorrhoea. Conversely, if marked hypercalcaemia occurs, which is rare in thyrotoxicosis, constipation may occur. A large appetite with hyperphagia usually occurs, but some patients have severe anorexia which contributes to rapid weight loss. Nausea and vomiting may be prominent in the absence of hypercalcaemia and it has been suggested that this is a central effect.[17] Other rare symptoms are hyperbilirubinaemia (possibly reflecting hepatic fatty change or the unmasking of Gilbert's disease), abdominal pain and oedema which can be associated with either normal or low serum protein concentrations.

The gastrointestinal aspects of hyperthyroidism are usually modest. The final diagnosis rests on the usual thyroid function tests including serum thyroxine, triiodothyronine, thyroid uptake of radioactive iodine and a flat response of TSH to intravenous thyrotrophin-releasing hormone (TRH). Investigation in the majority of patients shows a slight increase above the upper limit of normal of the faecal fats (18 mmol/24 h) but this is rarely above 90 mmol/24 h. There are numerous studies of the effect of hyperthyroidism on various parts of the gut and these are outlined below.

Proximal skeletal myopathy is well recognized and this effect is thought to occur sometimes in the oesophagus. There is a decrease in oesophageal propulsion and closure. Recurrent aspiration pneumonia due to oesophageal incoordination with tracheal overspill is reported; when the thyrotoxicosis was recognized and treated with carbimazole there was no recurrence of the pneumonia.[13]

Gastric acid secretion varies greatly but mean acid outputs in thyrotoxic patients are reduced and gastric histology shows a marked gastritis. Initially, despite the hypochlorhydria, it was suggested that patients had an increased incidence of duodenal ulcers but subsequently this has been disproved. Wiersinga and Touber[21] have shown that high plasma gastrin levels occur in both Graves' disease and toxic nodular goitre, and that they are associated with reduced acid secretion. In patients with hypochlorhydria the acid secretion and gastrin levels are corrected with treatment but, in five patients with achlorhydria, only one recovered although the other four all had parietal cell antibodies; this suggests the presence of established atrophic gastritis.

The gastric emptying rate has been shown to be increased using barium sulphate and it has long been assumed that some of the malabsorption was exacerbated by rapid emptying of meals into the small intestine. Wiley *et al.*[22] used technetium-99m sulphur colloid-labelled chicken's liver in a mixed meal in four patients and suggested that physiological gastric emptying was similar in controls and hyperthyroidism. Further studies using a mixed nutrient meal have shown no change in gastric secretion, gastric emptying and pancreatic secretion in a group of thyrotoxic patients. It seems probable that the main causes of the diarrhoea and steatorrhoea reside distal to the duodenum.[15]

Barium studies of small intestinal transit in thyrotoxicosis have suggested that transit times are greatly reduced due to increased peristaltic activity. In a rat experimental model of hyperthyroidism, it has been shown that small intestinal weight, villus height, total mucosal thickness, mucosal protein content and brush border enzymes are increased.[14] If this effect occurs in human hyperthyroidism it would explain the minimal malabsorption seen in a situation where there is probably gross intestinal hurry. Thomas *et al.*[19] found steatorrhoea in 60% of patients studied and related it to an increased fat intake (mean 873 mmol (248 g) 24 h) and increased intestinal hypermotility associated with a mild degree of malabsorption. Propranolol was shown to reduce faecal fat excretion by 50%. In contrast, glucose absorption is increased from isolated rat intestinal sacs by thyroxine administration and rapid absorption has been shown in thyrotoxic humans. In thyrotoxicosis, the urinary D-xylose excretion is increased but this is a renal effect and is seen whether the xylose is given orally or intravenously, and overall intestinal absorption appears normal. Other parameters of absorption and jejunal histology are normal.

Two cases of secretory diarrhoea associated with thyrotoxicosis have been reported. Stool volumes were up to 5 litres/day and were unaffected by fasting. Treatment with antithyroid drugs and radioactive iodine returned the patients to a normal bowel habit. These observations fit with previous physiological studies of the Thiery–Vella fistula model in dogs where thyroxine induced jejunal secretion. It is known that triiodothyronine increases plasma cyclic AMP and binds to erythrocyte membranes producing a rise in intracellular cyclic AMP; it is possible that thyroid hormones can also bind to small intestinal enterocytes and cause activation of the adenylate cyclase system in a similar way to vasoactive intestinal polypeptide and the toxin of *Vibrio cholerae*.[2,6]

Calcium malabsorption commonly occurs and there is a negative calcium balance associated with increased urinary and faecal loss. Some patients are also in negative phosphate balance. Calcium malabsorption occurs at low and high intestinal luminal concentrations but there is a particular reduction in active calcium absorption. The plasma concentrations of the active metabolite of vitamin D – 1,25-dihydroxy-vitamin D_3, – are low. Bone histology shows osteoporosis with thin trabecula and this is related to calcium loss from bone; there is no evidence of osteomalacia or hyperparathyroidism. When the patients are treated with either drugs or radioactive iodine, calcium balance and absorption, and 1,25-dihydroxy-vitamin D_3 levels, become normal.[4,9,16]

Biliary and pancreatic function may also change in thyrotoxicosis. Total bile acids are normal but there is an increase in the dihydroxy fraction, particularly taurochenodeoxycholic acid. The response of pancreatic bicarbonate to intravenous secretin is normal but trypsin output to a standard meal has been reported as reduced. This finding may be related to increased sympathetic activity because intravenous isoprenaline infusion has a similar effect and thyrotoxic steatorrhoea improves with administration of propranolol.[22] Another study reported normal pancreatic secretion including trypsin and a reduction in bile acid output. At present it seems reasonable to conclude that there may be changes in biliary and pancreatic secretion but their clinical effects are likely to be relatively minor.[15]

HYPOTHYROIDISM

Major gastrointestinal symptoms of hypothyroidism include reduced appetite without weight loss and a mild-to-severe constipation. Some of the other non-gastrointestinal symptoms are nearly always present. Other symptoms include rectal prolapse, spurious diarrhoea due to faecal impaction and ascites. The ascites is a clear, straw-coloured exudate with a protein electrophoretic strip pattern similar to that of plasma, and it occurs in the absence of cardiac, hepatic, renal or peritoneal disease; on occasions there may be concurrent pleural and pericardial effusions.

In the oesophagus, the peristaltic wave pressure and velocity are reduced and the peristaltic wave duration is prolonged in the distal three-quarters, but normal in the proximal one-quarter. This shows that non-striated muscle is more affected than striated muscle. In some patients this can result in dysphagia and can be demonstrated by most voluntary wet swallows producing non-propagated, simultaneous repetitive contractions. These abnormalities disappear with treatment.[3]

Gastric acid secretion is variable but in general is normal, as are plasma gastrin levels. However, as a result of the association with pernicious anaemia, some patients have achlorhydria, hypergastrinaemia and positive parietal cell antibodies. Gastric histology usually shows gastritis and oedema of the mucosal muscles. Gastric emptying is markedly delayed.

The duodenum is the most affected part of the small intestine and in severe hypothyroidism may become dilated and atonic; rarely this may spread to the rest of the small bowel. On occasions frank intestinal obstruction with fluid levels may be seen. Histologically a diffuse mucoid infiltration, especially of the submucosa, is seen in duodenal, jejunal and colonic specimens. Jejunal biopsies may show subtotal villous atrophy and there may be associated mild steatorrhoea. Small bowel motility is reduced. Peroral radiotelemetry capsules in the jejunum have shown greatly reduced rhythm, wave amplitude and other indices of motility. A flat glucose tolerance curve is common and partially reflects slow gastric emptying. D-xylose excretion is reduced when it is given intravenously and consequently it is impossible to assess D-xylose intestinal absorption.

The colon is another major site of severe mucoid infiltration; atony, dilatation and sometimes a gross megacolon may occur. Histological examination of Auerbach's and Meissner's plexus is normal. Motility probes have been introduced into the colon and low motility indices found. It there is some response to parasympathetic stimulation with the muscarinic drug urecholine the prognosis for recovery with thyroxine is good but otherwise it is poor. Surgical decompression has been advocated.[18] However, if fluid levels are seen and laparotomy undertaken in an undiagnosed case of myxoedema, death may be precipitated.

MEDULLARY CARCINOMA OF THE THYROID

These tumours are derived from thyroid parafollicular C cells which synthesize calcitonin and somatostatin. The most common initial presentation of a sporadic case is as a solid thyroid mass which may be bilateral. Mascroscopically the tumours are grey and firm, usually lack a capsule and may diffusely infiltrate the local tissues. Histologically there are sheets of tumour cells with connective tissue septa forming nests; the number of mitoses varies and amyloid is often present. Metastases are initially to cervical lymph nodes and the mediastinum, but later in the disease process may involve the lungs, liver, adrenals and bone. The tumours may occur sporadically or in families; the presence of familial cases in an area may increase the incidence of these tumours to about 10% of thyroid malignancies, but usually it is less than this. The familial cases may have raised plasma biochemical markers of a tumour (in particular, calcitonin) for many years before the tumour becomes palpable or symptomatic. The prognosis is very variable but total thyroidectomy and the general surgical excision of tumour mass may be very helpful; some patients survive for many years whereas others die within a year of diagnosis.

Numerous active substances have been found in the plasma and/or tumour extracts of patients with medullary carcinoma of the thyroid and these include the following:

- Calcitonin
- Prostaglandin E_2
- Prostaglandin F_2
- Carcinoembryonic antigen
- Histaminase
- 5-Hydroxytryptamine
- Adrenocorticotrophic hormone
- Kallikrein
- Somatostatin
- Neurotensin
- β-Endorphin
- Substance P

Calcitonin is a 32 amino acid polypeptide which lowers plasma calcium and phosphate levels and may play a role in preserving the skeleton and preventing osteoporosis; pharmacological infusions decrease gastrin levels and gastric acid secretion, and increase ileal secretion of sodium, chloride, potassium and water.[10] Calcitonin is always secreted by medullary carcinomas, and plasma levels usually, but not always, correlate with the tumour mass.[20] Plasma calcitonin radio-immunoassay is widely used in patient diagnosis and follow-up, and is particularly helpful in the management of presymptomatic familial cases. In doubtful situations, calcitonin provocation tests with whisky, pentagastrin or calcium may be useful. Regular prospective screening of patients with multiple endocrine neoplasia type 2 for medullary carcinoma of the thyroid and early surgery are thought to improve the prognosis.[8] In some patients tumour mass may also be monitored by plasma prostaglandin, carcinoembryonic antigen or histaminase values, or 24-hour urinary 5-

hydroxyindole acetic acid levels. Rarely adrenocorticotrophic hormone secretion may result in the clinical and biochemical manifestation of Cushing's syndrome. The other listed substances do not have any definite clinical roles, or yet play a part in diagnosis or follow-up.

The main gastrointestinal symptoms of medullary carcinoma of the thyroid are dysphagia due to local cervical infiltration and diarrhoea which occurs at some stage in 30% of patients and may precede the presence of a palpable thyroid mass. Other occasional symptoms are weight loss, borborygmi and colicky abdominal pain. The diarrhoea may be modest or profuse and watery with more than 1 litre of stool daily, resulting in hypokalaemia. Steatorrhoea is usually minimal and rarely more than 50 mmol fatty acid per day. Triple lumen tube studies in the jejunum have shown normal transport of electrolytes, and normal mucosal permeability and transit time, but in the ileum there is a failure to absorb sodium and chloride against a concentration gradient, an abnormal mucosal permeability and a rapid transit time.[11] The variability of the diarrhoea observed is probably dependent on the colonic ability to cope with the increased ileocaecal flow.

There is evidence that both calcitonin and prostaglandins play a role in the pathogenesis of the diarrhoea because infusions of both into healthy volunteers can cause intestinal secretion. When pharmacological doses of calcitonin are given to patients with Paget's disease, some 12% develop diarrhoea. Cox *et al.*[5] studied a patient with diarrhoea, increased distal ileal flow and very high plasma calcitonin concentrations. Large amounts of plasma were obtained by plasmapheresis and infused into dogs in whom an inhibition of small intestinal absorption was seen. These workers also showed that the diarrhoea is not associated with activation of the adenylate cyclase/cyclic AMP system because the mucosal cyclic AMP levels are normal and there is no response to anti-cyclic AMP drugs such as nicotinic acid and colchicine.

The evidence for prostaglandins mediating the diarrhoea is incomplete because many patients fail to respond to antiprostaglandin drugs. Exogenous prostaglandin $F_{2\alpha}$ ($PGF_{2\alpha}$) infusion into normal volunteers can cause ileal secretion of sodium, chloride and water. It was initially shown that some patients with diarrhoea have raised plasma and/or tumour prostaglandin levels.[23] The diarrhoea of some patients responds to nutmeg (e.g. one teaspoonful nine times a day); this charmingly medieval substance, from *Myristica fragrans*, contains volatile oils, fats, myristin, elemicin and safrol, and has anticholinergic, sympathomimetic and occasionally hallucinogenic, as well as antiprostaglandin, effects.[1] The more specific antiprostaglandin drug, indomethacin 25–50 mg three times a day, is effective in controlling diarrhoea in some patients but ineffective in most. It must be concluded that the precise pathogenesis of the diarrhoea in these patients is unknown.

References

1. Barrowman, J.A., Bennett, A., Hillenbrand, P. *et al.* (1975) Diarrhoea in thyroid medullary carcinoma: role of prostaglandins and therapeutic effect of nutmeg. *British Medical Journal*, **3**, 11–12.
2. Charney, D.I. and Mercedo, D.L. (1987) Secretory diarrhoea and thyrotoxicosis. *Annals of Internal Medicine* **106**, 332.
3. Christensen, J. (1967) Esophageal manometry in myxedema (Abstract). *Gastroenterology*, **52**, 1130.
4. Cook, P.B., Nassim, J.R. and Collins, J. (1959) The effects of thyrotoxicosis upon the metabolism of calcium, phosphorus, and nitrogen. *Quarterly Journal of Medicine*, **28**, 505–529.
5. Cox, T.M., Fagan, E.A., Hillyard, C.J. *et al.* (1979) Role of calcitonin in diarrhoea associated with medullary carcinoma of the thyroid. *Gut*, **20**, 629–633.
6. Culp, K.S. and Piziak, V.K. (1986) Thyrotoxicosis presenting with secretory diarrhoea. *Annals of Internal Medicine*, **105**, 216–217.
7. Duret, R.L. and Bastenie, P.A. (1971) Intestinal disorders in hypothyroidism. Clinical and manometric study. *American Journal of Digestive Diseases*, **16**, 723–727.
8. Gagel, R.F., Tashjian, A.H., Cummings, T. *et al.* (1988) The clinical outcome of prospective screening for multiple endocrine neoplasia type 2a. *New England Journal of Medicine*, **318**, 476–484.
9. Haldimann, B., Kaptein, E.M., Singer, F.R., Nicoloff, J.T. and Massry, S.G. (1980) Intestinal calcium absorption in patients with hyperthyroidism. *Journal of Clinical Endocrinology and Metabolism*, **51**, 995–997.
10. Hunter, L.A. and Heath, H. III (1981) Calcitonin: physiology and pathophysiology. *New England Journal of Medicine*, **304**, 269–278.
11. Isaacs, P., Whitaker, S.M. and Turnberg, L.A. (1974) Diarrhoea associated with medullary carcinoma of the thyroid: studies of intestinal function in a patient. *Gastroenterology*, **67**, 521–526.
12. Jarnerot, G., Kagedal, B., von Schenck, H. and Truelove, S.C. (1976) The thyroid in ulcerative colitis and Crohn's disease V. Triiodothyronine. Effects of corticosteroids and influence of severe disease. *Acta Medica Scandinavica*, **199**, 229–232.
13. Marks, P., Anderson, J. and Vincent, R. (1980) Thyrotoxic myopathy presenting as dysphagia. *Postgraduate Medical Journal*, **56**, 669–670.
14. Middleton, W.R. (1971) Thyroid hormones in the gut. *Gut*, **12**, 172–177.

15. Miller, L.J., Owyang, C., Malagelada, J.R., Gorman, C.A. and Go, V.L.W. (1980) Gastric, pancreatic and biliary responses to meals in hyperthyroidism. *Gut*, **21**, 695–700.
16. Peerenboom, H., Keck, E., Kruskemper, H.L. and Strohmeyer, G. (1984) The defect of intestinal calcium transport in hyperthyroidism and its response to therapy. *Journal of Clinical Endocrinology and Metabolism*, **59**, 936–940.
17. Rosenthal, F.D., Jones, C. and Lewis, S.I. (1976) Thyrotoxic vomiting. *British Medical Journal*, **2**, 209–211.
18. Solano, F.X., Starling, R.C. and Levey, G.S. (1985) Myxedema megacolon. *Archives of Internal Medicine*, **145**, 231.
19. Thomas, F.B., Caldwell, J.H. and Greenberger, N.J. (1973) Diarrhoea in thyrotoxicosis. *Annals of Internal Medicine*, **78**, 669–675.
20. Trump, L., Mendelsohn, G. and Baylin, S.B. (1979) Discordance between plasma calcitonin and tumor-cell mass in medullary thyroid carcinoma. *New England Journal of Medicine*, **301**, 253–255.
21. Wiersinga, W.M. and Touber, J.L. (1980) The relation between gastrin, gastric acid and thyroid function disorders. *Acta endocrinologica (Copenhagen)*, **95**, 341–349.
22. Wiley, Z.D., Lavigne, M.E., Liu, K.M. and MacGregor, I.L. (1978) The effect of hyperthyroidism on gastric emptying rates and pancreatic exocrine and biliary secretion in man. *American Journal of Digestive Diseases*, **23**, 1003–1008.
23. Williams, E.C., Karim, S.M.M. and Sandler, M. (1968) Prostaglandin secretion by medullary carcinoma of the thyroid: a possible cause of the associated diarrhoea. *The Lancet*, **1**, 22–23.

PITUITARY DISEASE *(R.G. Long)*

The pituitary is divided into anterior and posterior parts and has been nicknamed the leader of the endocrine orchestra because its hormones control most adrenocortical, thyroid and gonadal hormone secretions as well as many other endocrine and metabolic functions. The pituitary hormones include:

Anterior pituitary:
- adrenocorticotrophic hormone (ACTH)
- thyrotrophin-stimulating hormone (TSH)
- growth hormone (GH)
- follicle-stimulating hormone (FSH)
- luteinizing hormone (LH)
- prolactin

Posterior pituitary:
- arginine vasopressin

However, the term 'leader' is something of a misnomer because secretion of the anterior pituitary hormones is itself controlled by stimulatory hypothalamic peptides (e.g. corticotrophin-releasing hormone, thyrotrophin-releasing hormone and gonadotrophin-releasing hormone) and in the case of growth hormone by both stimulatory and inhibitory hormones (growth hormone-releasing hormone and somatostatin).

The pituitary hormones have major effects on the gut. Adrenocorticotrophic hormone (ACTH) stimulates cortisol secretion and enhances brush border enzyme activity and thyrotrophin-stimulating hormone (TSH) causes thyroxine secretion with major effects on gut motility. Growth hormone causes intestinal villous growth and enhances absorption. There is no good evidence for the gonadotrophins having a physiological effect on the gut. In pregnancy and during lactation many animals develop intestinal mucosal growth and an increased absorptive capacity, but evidence for prolactin, the obvious candidate, mediating this adaptive response has not been confirmed in experimental models of hyperprolactinaemia.[2]

PITUITARY TUMOURS

Pituitary tumours secrete ACTH (Cushing's disease), growth hormone (acromegaly) and prolactin (prolactinomas) whilst some appear to be non-secretory. They have two major types of effect: those due to excessive hormone being secreted and those of secondary failure to excrete other hormones, resulting from expansion of the tumour and loss of neighbouring normal cells. In general, the effects of hypersecretion appear to spare the gut. In acromegaly, increased intestinal mucosal growth occur and negative calcium balance is thought to be a factor in the pathogenesis of acromegalic osteoporosis, along with hypogonadism, muscle weakness and inactivity.

A colonoscopic or double-contrast barium enema study in 17 acromegalics[1] found adenomatous polyps in five patients, hyperplastic polyps in three patients and unclassified polyps in one patient. The adenomatous polyps were small and varied in number from one to five; as no control group was included, this study needs expansion and confirmation before a clinically important association between acromegaly and adenomatous colonic polyps is accepted.

HYPOPITUITARISM

This may occur as a result of an expanding primary or secondary tumour, a vascular accident, infection (e.g. tuberculosis) or a granulomatous process (e.g.

sarcoidosis or the Hand–Schüller–Christian syndrome). The gonadotrophins are usually the hormones to be lost first, and ACTH, TSH, prolactin and growth hormone follow; as a result, sexual dysfunction (amenorrhoea or impotence) is usually an early symptom. Subsequent common symptoms of hypopituitarism include lethargy, anorexia and weight loss; these symptoms are similar to those seen in some patients with anorexia nervosa and primary gastrointestinal problems such as inflammatory bowel disease and coeliac disease. Diarrhoea may be a major feature in hypopituitary patients and, if treatment is not rapidly initiated, death may ensue associated with Addisonian crisis. Most of the symptoms can be reversed by standard physiological cortisone and thyroxine replacement therapy. In children growth failure is also present and growth hormone supplements are required.

References

1. Klein, I., Parveen, G., Gavaler, J.S. and Thiel, D.H. (1982) Colonic polyps in patients with acromegaly. *Annals of Internal Medicine*, **97**, 27–30.
2. Muller, E. and Dowling, R.H. (1981) Prolactin and the small intestine: effect of hyperprolactinaemia on mucosal structure in the rat. *Gut*, 558–565.

ADRENAL DISORDERS

The adrenal cortex secretes glucocorticosteroids and mineralocorticosteroids, and the adrenal medulla secretes primarily the catecholamines, noradrenaline and adrenaline. Glucocorticosteroids bind to specific cytoplasmic receptors on the enterocyte and the activated receptor–steroid complex is then translocated to the nucleus and causes new messenger RNA synthesis. They increase the absorptive capacity of the small intestine without increasing the number of cells in the normal individual. Studies of the ileum after jejunal resection in the rat have shown that the addition of pharmacological doses of prednisolone results in increased levels of ileal epithelial cell DNA, RNA and brush-border enzymes (i.e. α-glucosidase, leucyl-2-naphthylamidase and α-glutamyl transferase), but there is no increase in cell numbers or in lysosomal and mitochondrial enzymes. Glucocorticosteroids, occasionally used to improve diarrhoea in patients with the short bowel syndrome, appear to act in that context by enhancing brush-border membrane digestive capacity.[6] In coeliac disease, where absorptive capacity is also increased, there is an improvement in villous architecture.

CUSHING'S SYNDROME

Cushing's syndrome may be due to Cushing's disease (an ACTH-secreting tumour in the pituitary), ectopic ACTH syndrome (a tumour elsewhere, commonly the bronchi or pancreas, secreting ACTH), or to benign or malignant cortisol-secreting tumours of the adrenal cortex. Cushing's disease may be associated with multiple endocrine adenomatosis type 1, and reported associations include gastrinoma, parathyroid adenoma, phaeochromocytoma and medullary carcinoma of the thyroid (see below).

The role of corticosteroid therapy in the pathogenesis of peptic ulcer disease remains controversial[2,5] and there is currently no objective evidence for Cushing's syndrome being associated with an increased incidence of peptic ulcers. Theoretically absorption would be expected to be improved in Cushing's syndrome as a result of cortisol inducing the brush-border membrane enzymes, but diarrhoea has been reported. In general the intestine appears to be hardly affected by Cushing's syndrome.

ADRENOCORTICAL INSUFFICIENCY

Primary adrenocortical failure (Addison's disease) is usually either associated with autoimmunity or due to tuberculosis. Weight loss, anorexia, dehydration, pigmentation, hypotension and hyponatraemia are features that are shared with severe coeliac disease, and there is evidence that the two diseases may sometimes be associated. Other associations with Addison's disease include hypothyroidism, pernicious anaemia, hypoparathyroidism, diabetes mellitus, vitiligo and primary ovarian failure.

Adrenocortical insufficiency is associated with steatorrhoea, hypoglycaemia and normal jejunal histology. Faecal fats of up to 114 mmol (32.5 g)/day are reported but the values return to normal with glucocorticosteroid and mineralocorticosteroid replacement.[4] This response is compatible with the known effects of glucocorticosteroids on the small intestine.

PHAEOCHROMOCYTOMA

Phaeochromocytomas are catecholamine-secreting tumours of the adrenal glands and sympathetic chain. Reported gastrointestinal manifestations include nausea, vomiting, abdominal pain, diarrhoea and constipation, paralytic ileus and ischaemic colitis due to vasoconstriction. Phaeochromocytomas vary greatly in size and on occasion may be palpable as a large abdominal mass, for example, mimicking a primary liver cell carcinoma. Catecholamines inhibit gut smooth muscle contraction and infusions do not cause diarrhoea. Phaeochromocytomas have been reported sometimes to secrete calcitonin[8] and enkephalin[7] and it is possible that hypersecretion of these two peptides may respectively contribute to the development of diarrhoea and constipation in some patients. The diagnostic exercise for a suspected phaeochromocytoma before surgery is complex and in most patients with high urinary 4-hydroxy-3-methoxymandelic acid or vanillylmandelic acid (VMA) excretion should include plasma adrenaline and noradrenaline assays before and after pentolinium administration and abdominal computed tomography. In extra-adrenal cases, arteriography and venous sampling may also be needed.[1]

GANGLIONEUROBLASTOMAS

Ganglioneuromas and ganglioneuroblastomas arise from similar anatomical sites to phaeochromocytomas but differ histologically. They most commonly present in childhood with an intra-abdominal mass and are found to have raised 24-hour urinary vanillylmandelic acid concentrations. Profuse secretory diarrhoea has been recognized in some patients for more than 30 years but there is no correlation with catecholamine secretion. In 1973 it was shown that the diarrhoea was associated with high plasma and tumour vasoactive intestinal polypeptide levels, and subsequently it has been shown that vasoactive intestinal polypeptide causes secretory diarrhoea and most of the other features of this syndrome, including weight loss, abdominal colic, spontaneous cutaneous flushing, dehydration, hypokalaemic acidosis and reduced gastric acid secretion (see Chapter 11). In contrast to the usual bad prognosis of ganglioneuroblastomas, seven out of ten of the author's series of VIP-secreting tumours were successfully operated on and apparently cured[3] and consequently it must be concluded that this is an important diagnosis for gastroenterologists to make.

References

1. Allison, D.J., Brown, M.J., Jones, D.H. and Timmis, J.B. (1983) Role of venous sampling in locating a phaeochromocytoma. *British Medical Journal*, **286**, 1122–1124.
2. Conn, H.O. and Blitzer, B.L. (1976) Nonassociation of adrenocorticosteroid therapy and peptic ulcer. *New England Journal of Medicine*, **294**, 473–479.
3. Long, R.G., Bryant, M.G., Mitchell, S.J. *et al.* (1981) Clinicopathological study of pancreatic and ganglioneuroblastoma tumours secreting vasoactive intestinal polypeptide (vipomas). *British Medical Journal*, **282**, 1767–1771.
4. McBrien, D.J., Jones, R.V. and Creamer, B. (1963) Steatorrhea in Addison's disease. *The Lancet*, **i**, 25–26.
5. Messer, J., Reitman, D., Sacks, H.S., Smith, H. and Chalmers, T.C. (1983) Association of adrenocorticosteroid therapy and peptic ulcer disease. *New England Journal of Medicine*, **309**, 21–24.
6. Scott, J., Batt, R.M. and Peters, T.J. (1979) Enhancement of ileal adaptation by prednisolone after proximal small bowel resection in the rat. *Gut*, **20**, 858–864.
7. Sullivan, S.N., Bloom, S.R. and Polak, J.M. (1978) Enkephalin in peripheral neuroendocrine tumours. *The Lancet*, **1**, 986–987.
8. Weinstein, R.S. (1980) Immunoreactive calcitonin in pheochromocytomas. *Proceedings of the Society for Experimental Biology and Medicine*, **165**, 215–217.

MULTIPLE ENDOCRINE NEOPLASIA

(R.G. Long)

Multiple endocrine neoplasia (MEN) or adenomatosis (MEA) is divided into two main types: type 1 (MEN1) or Wermer's syndrome and type 2 (MEN2) or Sipple's syndrome:

MEN1 (Wermer's syndrome)
- pancreatic endocrine tumour
- pituitary tumour
- parathyroid tumour

MEN2 (Sipple's syndrome)
- medullary carcinoma of the thyroid
- phaeochromocytoma
- parathyroid tumour

However, occasionally the features of the two syndromes may overlap, resulting in loss of this distinction. Both are inherited as an autosomal dominant trait with variable penetrance but sporadic cases are sometimes seen. Other features can include benign and malignant carcinoid tumours, multiple lipomas, schwannomas and thymomas.

Recently, there has been a great deal of study into the genetics of the MEN syndromes. The gene associated with MEN1 is located on chromosome 11 (11q13); tumours may develop after a phase of polyclonal hyperplasia. There is a single inherited locus on chromosome 11 causing the syndrome, and the monoclonal development of parathyroid and pancreatic tumours involves similar allelic deletions on chromosome 11.[4,10] A plasma protein with parathyroid mitogenic activity has been found in patients with MEN1 and it has been postulated that this may be the humoral cause of primary hyperparathyroidism in these patients.[2] MEN2A is the usual form of Sipple's syndrome and has been localized to chromosome 10. MEN2B involves additional phenotypical abnormalities and a more aggressively behaving medullary thyroid carcinoma; there is a third subdivision of 'medullary thyroid carcinoma only' tumours where the onset is late and the tumours are hardly ever fatal. These last two types probably also arise from chromosome 10.[12]

Wermer's syndrome is more common than Sipple's syndrome. The pancreatic endocrine tumours may excrete one or more of the following: insulin, pancreatic glucagon, gastrin, vasoactive intestinal polypeptides, somatostatin, pancreatic polypeptide, adrenocorticotrophic hormone and parathyroid hormone. The usual clinical presentation is as described in Chapter 11. The pituitary tumours may secrete growth hormone, prolactin or adrenocorticotrophic hormone, or they may be apparently nonsecretory. The parathyroid adenomas secrete parathyroid hormone and present with hypercalcaemia. The most common presentation of MEN1 is with primary hyperparathyroidism; subsequently other tumours manifest themselves.[1] It has been suggested that primary hyperparathyroidism in MEN1 may have a more benign course than hyperparathyroidism alone but, in fact, MEN1 patients appear to be younger, to have multiple glands involved more often and to have more recurrences after surgery.[3]

The diagnosis of pancreatic endocrine tumours can usually be made through a clinical diagnosis and then measurement of the appropriate regulatory peptide by radio-immunoassay. Pancreatic polypeptide-secreting tumours are not associated with a specific metabolic syndrome but are usually co-secreted with other peptides that produce symptoms. Gastrinomas may be diagnosed by fasting hypergastrinaemia, high gastric acid output and inappropriate gastrin increases to intravenous calcium and secretin.[5] In patients at risk for MEN1, if one tumour develops it is usual for tumours to develop in the other characteristic sites later.[8] In the presence of any pancreatic endocrine tumour, it is always advisable to screen the pituitary radiologically, to check the fasting plasma calcium and phosphate levels and, if there is any doubt, to measure the hormone levels.

The treatment of MEN1 must be considered individually in each case. In general the tumour producing the most symptoms should be treated first; the exception to this is a gastrinoma in the presence of primary hyperparathyroidism when the problems of the gastrinoma such as duodenal ulcers and diarrhoea usually settle with removal of the parathyroid adenoma.[7]

Sipple's syndrome (MEN2) can present with any of the three tumour types; as a result of the familial basis, early presymptomatic cases are often monitored biochemically and a gradual rise in the tumour marker seen. Some of the patients also have a Marfanoid appearance with long limbs, poor muscular development, a high arched palate and pes cavus. Both the medullary carcinomas of the thyroid and the phaeochromocytomas may present with diarrhoea, but occasionally a third cause of diarrhoea, constipation or intestinal obstruction is seen; this may be related to intestinal ganglioneuromas that can occur in all layers of the gut wall in some patients. Other problems of MEN2B include tongue nodules, dilatation of the colon and adenomatous polyps in the colon, duodenum and stomach.[3,11]

Medullary carcinoma of the thyroid should be monitored by plasma calcitonin levels (with whisky, pentagastrin or calcium stimulation), phaeochromocytomas by 24-hour urinary vanillylmandelic acid excretion, and plasma adrenaline and noradrenaline levels before and after pentolinium administration, and parathyroid adenomas by plasma calcium, phosphate and parathyroid hormone values. If one tumour is present, it is important to screen for the other two types. Phaeochromocytomas in MEN2 tend to secrete a very high proportion of adrenaline compared to noradrenaline and also to be bilateral in about 70% of cases.

If a phaeochromocytoma is present it is important to treat this first to avoid a hypertensive crisis. The patient is treated by α- and β-adrenergic blockade and, after precise preoperative tumour localization, the tumour(s) is removed. The medullary carcinomas of the thyroid should be treated by total thyroidectomy and regional lymph node dissection when clinically indicated (some of the tumours are very slow growing) and the parathyroid adenomas should be localized by venous sampling, radioactive isotopic scanning or other methods[13] and excised.

Once a diagnosis of a case of multiple endocrine neoplasia has been made, it is imperative to screen at-risk relatives for this autosomal dominant condition. This requires a combination of pedigree analysis and, now that the chromosomal location of the genetic abnormality has been recognized, DNA-linkage analysis and hormone screening tests. The last of these may involve routine plasma and urine sampling and, particularly when the family history involves medullary carcinoma of the thyroid, provocation tests.[9]

References

1. Betts, J.B., O'Malley, B.P. and Rosenthal, F.D. (1980) Hyperparathyroidism: a prerequisite for

Zollinger–Ellison syndrome in multiple endocrine adrenomatosis Type I – report of a further family and a review of the literature. *Quarterly Journal of Medicine*, **73**, 69–76.
2. Brandi, M.L., Aurbach, G.D., Fitzpatrick, L.A. *et al.* (1986) Parathyroid mutogenic activity in plasma from patients with familial multiple endocrine neoplasia type 1. *New England Journal of Medicine*, **314**, 1287–1293.
3. Demos, T.C., Blonder, J., Schey, W.L., Braithwaite, S.S. and Goldstein, P.L. (1983) Multiple endocrine neoplasia syndrome Type IIb: gastrointestinal manifestations. *American Journal of Roentgenology*, **140**, 73–78.
4. Friedman, E., Sakaguchi, K., Bale, A.E. *et al.* (1989) Clonality of parathyroid tumors in familial multiple endocrine neoplasia type I. *New England Journal of Medicine*, **321**, 213–218.
5. Lamers, C.B., Bois, J.T. and van Tongeren, J. (1977) Secretin-stimulated serum gastrin levels in hyperparathyroid patients from families with multiple endocrine adenomatosis Type I. *Annals of Internal Medicine*, **86**, 719–724.
6. Lamers, C.B. and Froeling, P.G. (1978) Clinical significance of hyperparathyroidism in familial multiple endocrine adenomatosis type I (MEA I). *American Journal of Medicine*, **66**, 422–424.
7. McCarthy, D.M., Peikin, S.R., Lopatin, R.N. *et al.* (1979) Hyperparathyroidism – a reversible cause of cimetidine-resistant gastric hypersecretion. *British Medical Journal*, **1**, 1765–1766.
8. Majewski, J.T. and Wilson, S.D. (1979) The MEA I syndrome: an all or none phenomenon. *Surgery*, **86**, 475–484.
9. Mathew, C.G.P., Easton, D.F., Nakamura, Y. and Ponder, B.A.J. and the MEN2a International Collaborative Group (1991) Presymptomatic screening of multiple endocrine neoplasia type 2a with linked DNA markers. *The Lancet*, **337**, 7–11.
10. Thakker, R.V., Bouloux, P., Wooding, C. *et al.* (1989) Association of parathyroid tumours in multiple endocrine neoplasia type I with loss of alleles on chromosome 11. *New England Journal of Medicine*, **321**, 218–224.
11. Perkins, J.T., Blackstone, M.O. and Riddell, R.H. (1985) Adenomatous polyposis coli and multiple endocrine neoplasia type IIb. *Cancer*, **55**, 375–381.
12. Ponder, B. (1990) Multiple endocrine neoplasia type 2 – the search for the gene continues. *British Medical Journal*, **300**, 484–485.
13. Young, A.E., Gaunt, J.I., Croft, D.N. *et al.* (1983) Location of parathyroid adenomas by thallium-201 and technetium-99m subtraction scanning. *British Medical Journal*, **286**, 1384–1386.

DIABETES MELLITUS *(B.T. Cooper)*

Patients with long-standing diabetes mellitus may have considerable derangement of gastrointestinal function which can lead to severe and intractable symptoms. Such problems are usually, but not exclusively, seen in insulin-dependent diabetics. The mechanisms leading to these abnormalities are uncertain but suggested causes include autonomic neuropathy, microangiopathy, hyperglycaemia, electrolyte abnormalities, and abnormalities in blood levels or release of insulin, glucagon, or other hormones, e.g. gastric inhibitory peptide, motilin.

ABDOMINAL PROBLEMS OF DIABETIC KETOACIDOSIS

Acute diabetic ketoacidosis can also be associated with largely unexplained gastrointestinal problems. Anorexia, nausea and vomiting occur in up to 75% of patients with ketoacidosis. Nasogastric aspiration is often recommended on the grounds that these symptoms reflect gastric stasis, but gastric emptying has never been properly studied during ketoacidosis. Acute gastric dilatation may occur but its frequency is unknown. During nasogastric aspiration, small amounts of blood are commonly seen, although frank haematemesis is rare. Bleeding usually results from acute erosions or acute haemorrhagic gastritis; endoscopy is not routinely necessary unless bleeding is severe or persists after correction of the metabolic derangements. The aetiology of the gastritis is unknown, but retention of acid or urea has been blamed.[18]

Severe abdominal pain, caused by ketoacidosis, occurs in about 8% of patients and is more common in diabetic children than in adults. It seems to be related to acidosis and settles with its correction. It may be severe enough to suggest an acute abdomen and diagnosis may be difficult, especially as ketoacidosis is often associated with neutrophilia and hyperamylasaemia. Thus acute pancreatitis may either be missed, or incorrectly assumed to be present. A diabetic with ketoacidosis and abdominal pain should have the metabolic disorder treated and his or her abdomen closely observed, provided no obvious intra-abdominal catastrophe, such as perforation, has occurred. Early exploratory laparotomy without definite indications should be steadfastly avoided. Identification of isoamylases in diabetic ketoacidosis shows that in fact the elevated amylase is usually of the salivary type, rather than the pancreatic type associated with pancreatitis.[57]

OESOPHAGUS IN DIABETES

Minor gastro-oesophageal reflux symptoms are reported by one-third of diabetics but are just as common than in non-diabetics. However, significant abnormalities of oesophageal motility are found in diabetics often in the absence of symptoms.[22,24,34,51] Manometric abnormalities reported include reduced amplitude of pharyngeal contractions and oesophageal peristalsis, increased frequency of spontaneous (tertiary) contractions, delayed oesophageal emptying and delayed relaxation of the lower oesophageal sphincter. Most studies show a decrease in resting lower oesophageal sphincter pressure.[22,24,34,51] Rarely, the appearances of the oesophagus may resemble diffuse oesophageal spasm.[22]

The prevalence of these abnormalities is unknown but they have been found in randomly selected insulin-dependent diabetics and up to 40% of insulin-dependent diabetics may have delayed oesophageal emptying of a solid bolus.[24]

There is no correlation between oesophageal dysfunction and symptoms, age or length of diabetic history. Most diabetics with oesophageal motor abnormalities are asymptomatic, but gastro-oesophageal reflux symptoms and dysphagia may occur and, if they do, other oesophageal disorders must be excluded (see Chapter 1).

The aetiology of these motility abnormalities is uncertain but there is a strong association with the presence of neuropathy,[22,51] and vagal damage with demyelination occur in diabetics with neuropathy.[50] Patients with symptoms may benefit from standard antireflux measures or by treatment with bethanecol or pro-kinetic drugs (metoclopramide, domperidone, cisapride) which may improve some of the motility disturbances.[25,51]

Oesophageal candidiasis is seen in poorly controlled diabetics or in diabetics with chronic renal failure who may present with dysphagia or odynophagia; it is readily diagnosed by barium swallow and endoscopy (see Chapter 1).

GASTRIC SECRETION, GASTRITIS AND PERNICIOUS ANAEMIA

In most diabetics, basal, food-stimulated and maximal acid outputs are normal, even in those with neuropathy.[15,26] Acid secretion is impaired in response to hypoglycaemia in patients with long-standing, insulin-dependent diabetes, most of whom will have evidence of neuropathy.[26] This suggests vagal dysfunction which is supported by impaired acid secretion to sham feeding.[15] However, reduced or absent acid output has been found in as many as 10% of diabetics studied.[26] As in non-diabetic patients, achlorhydria is associated with the development of chronic atrophic gastritis[1] which may develop at a younger age than in normal individuals.[31] The cause may be related to the development of gastric antibodies or diabetic microangiopathy.[1] There is an increased prevalence of gastric parietal cell and intrinsic factor antibodies in diabetics; the increase in parietal cell antibodies is most marked in young insulin-dependent diabetics, whereas the increase in intrinsic factor antibodies is seen particularly in insulin-dependent females more than 40 years of age (4% of such patients).[27] Thus a significant association between diabetes and pernicious anaemia seems to exist; the estimated prevalence of pernicious anaemia among diabetics is 0.98% and of diabetes in pernicious anaemia is 2.1%.[27] Latent cases of pernicious anaemia are often found, e.g. six cases among nine diabetics with intrinsic factor antibodies and atrophic gastritis.[27] There is no relationship between neuropathy and the presence of antibodies, atrophic gastritis or achlorhydria. In spite of the known malignant potential of atrophic gastritis, diabetics do not appear to be at increased risk of gastric carcinoma.

PEPTIC ULCER AND DIABETES

The prevalence of duodenal ulcer is said to be reduced among diabetics.[13,59] The data on which this view is based were collected before diagnosis by fibreoptic endoscopy and are suspect. However, the thesis may be correct because atrophic gastritis and achlorhydria can occur in diabetics. In contrast, the prevalence of gastric ulcer is said to be normal,[13] although this is also unproven as is the view that duodenal ulcer complications are more frequent and severe than in non-diabetics.[59]

DIABETIC GASTROPARESIS

Diabetic gastroparesis is seen in severe long-standing insulin-dependent diabetes, usually with evidence of neuropathy.[60] Patients may be asymptomatic and therefore the estimated prevalence of 1 in 1000 diabetics[60] may be an under-estimate. Symptoms are unexplained weight loss, vague epigastric or generalized abdominal pain or discomfort, nausea, epigastric bloating or fullness and, occasionally, halitosis. Severe or intractable vomiting occurs in severe cases. Vomit can contain food eaten more than 24 hours previously and bezoars can form. The clinical picture may mimic pyloric obstruction but a succussion splash is rare.[60] Usually, diabetic control has been poor and good control is often difficult to achieve; indeed, this may be the presenting complaint. A few cases may be complicated by gastric bacterial overgrowth and candidiasis.

Barium studies show an atonic stomach with

delayed gastric emptying and few peristaltic waves.[30] Structural pyloric obstruction is excluded by the patulous appearance of the pylorus and manual expression of barium into the duodenum. Retained gastric contents may resemble filling defects and duodenal dilatation can be seen. Radioactive isotopic studies confirm delayed gastric emptying for both solids and liquids.[5,24,25] Manometric studies show a marked decrease in sporadic motor activity, an abnormal antral component of the interdigestive motor complex, continuous low-amplitude antral activity and high-amplitude pyloric contractions.[16,35,41,50] Abnormalities of intestinal motility are also seen.[4] The motility disturbances are strongly related to the presence of autonomic neuropathy and are similar to those in the vagotomized stomach. However, there is evidence that delayed gastric emptying can be related to hyperglycaemia although the mechanisms are unknown.[5,24]

Diagnosis of gastroparesis is suggested at barium meal, with the stomach being normal endoscopically.[35] However, the diagnosis is confirmed by radioactive isotopic gastric emptying studies. Treatment is unsatisfactory. Some patients improve symptomatically with good diabetic control, and small regular and frequent meals. Pro-kinetic drugs improve gastric emptying acutely[5,23,25,35] but after 4–6 weeks' therapy, emptying (especially of solids) seems to return to the pre-treatment state.[23,47] Erythromycin, which may be a motilin agonist, also improves gastric emptying acutely but continues to show benefit after 4 weeks' therapy.[28] Most clinical reports are anecdotal but cholinergics (e.g. bethanecol, neostigmine) and pro-kinetic drugs have incurred improvement in symptoms. Surgical procedures such as pyloroplasty have not been helpful. Prognosis is poor; in one series,[60] a third died within 3 years of the diagnosis of gastroparesis. However, the deaths were due to vascular and renal complications of diabetes, indicating that symptomatic gastroparesis occurs when diabetic complications are quite advanced.

Less severe delays in gastric emptying have been reported in 20–50% of diabetics[5,24,45] but these figures may be overestimates.

CONSTIPATION IN DIABETICS

Constipation among diabetics is common, being reported in 16% of diabetics compared to 5% of non-diabetics.[39] It has been reported in 42% of diabetics with neuropathy and 51% of such patients required regular enemas to prevent impaction.[43] Thus, constipation can be severe, disabling, lead to symptoms mimicking large bowel obstruction and cause stercoral ulceration. Radiological studies may show an atonic and often greatly dilated colon with massive faecal retention and impaction. Motility studies show impaired or absent colonic motor responses to feeding.[3] Microangiopathy can be seen in rectal biopsies from severe diabetics, but there is no definite evidence to link this with colonic motor abnormalities. Constipation is probably another manifestation of autonomic neuropathy.[16,39] Neostigmine and pro-kinetic drugs can improve colonic motility and may ease constipation in some patients.[3]

DIABETIC DIARRHOEA

Diarrhoea is a relatively common complaint among diabetics; 7% of diabetics complained of it compared to 2% of non-diabetic controls.[39] True 'diabetic diarrhoea' is much less common. This is the severe and occasionally disabling diarrhoea that is seen in severe diabetics and for which no cause is apparent apart from the diabetes itself. Diabetic diarrhoea occurs in adults at any age but is most common in middle age and among men. It is typically seen in insulin-dependent diabetics of long standing. Poor control before the onset of diarrhoea is common. Rare cases of acute-onset diabetes with diarrhoea have been recorded. At presentation, about 75% of patients have evidence of neuropathy, especially autonomic neuropathy, and 33% have retinopathy.[36] Diarrhoea is described in up to 20% diabetics with neuropathy.[43]

Diarrhoea may be persistent or intermittent and may alternate with episodes of constipation. The stool is often watery, large in volume, and may contain undigested food. The diarrhoea may be explosive and incontinence may occur. Nocturnal diarrhoea is characteristic and in one series 50% of patients only had diarrhoea at night.[36] Attacks of diarrhoea may be preceded by abdominal distension, discomfort and rumbling but pain is rare. There is usually no obvious precipitating factor and attacks can last from several hours to months or even years. Diarrhoea persists in a few patients but in most cases, there is a tendency to spontaneous improvement over the years. Apart from the diarrhoea, patients are usually reasonably well.

Gastroparesis is seen in up to 30% of patients. With a small bowel meal, intestinal transit may be normal, rapid or delayed and the mucosal pattern is usually normal. Most patients have no evidence of malabsorption with normal faecal fat excretion, pancreatic function, and absorption of vitamin B_{12}, folic acid, iron and xylose. However, up to a third of patients have steatorrhoea[58] and they may have the non-specific malabsorption pattern on small bowel meal. Other causes of steatorrhoea must be excluded, especially coeliac disease and chronic pancreatitis. All patients with diabetic diarrhoea have normal small bowel biopsy appearances.[10,11,37]

Aetiology of diabetic diarrhoea

It is widely thought that diabetic diarrhoea and steatorrhoea result from motility disturbances caused by autonomic neuropathy because of frequent association between diarrhoea and neuropathy, although it has been suggested that glucagon may play a role.[18] Jejunal distension in diabetics with diarrhoea does not induce pain, suggesting afferent nerve damage.[58] The small intestine responds normally to methacholine, suggesting intact parasympathetic and efferent sympathetic pathways.[40,58] Autopsy studies show giant sympathetic neurons and dendritic swelling of postganglionic neurons in the pre- and paravertebral ganglia.[21] Diabetic rats with diarrhoea have impaired adrenergic regulation of mucosal ion transport leading to a postsynaptic denervation hypersensitivity and fluid secretion, both of which can be reversed by α_2-adrenergic agonists.[8] Human diabetic diarrhoea may respond to clonidine.[14] Manometric studies show markedly abnormal small intestinal motility,[4] although orocaecal transit times may be normal, increased or decreased.[10,11] Colonic motility may also be abnormal.

Other factors causing diarrhoea are bacterial overgrowth in the small intestine and bile salt malabsorption. Indirect evidence for the former is the relief of symptoms by antimicrobials in up to 70% of patients,[36] although the actual prevalence is unknown. Objective evidence for bacterial overgrowth is provided by jejunal juice colony count,[17] [^{14}C]glycocholate breath test,[46] and glucose hydrogen breath test.[10,11] In some patients, diabetic diarrhoea is relieved by cholestyramine suggesting that bile acid malabsorption is present; faecal bile acid loss and a reduced bile salt pool have been reported.[42]

There is no evidence that diabetic diarrhoea is caused by pancreatic insufficiency because pancreatic function tests are normal even if the patient has steatorrhoea[58] and there is no response to pancreatic supplements. Intestinal permeability studies suggest reduction in small intestinal absorptive area,[10,11] although jejunal sodium and water absorption is normal.[58]

Diagnosis and treatment of diabetic diarrhoea

Diagnosis is by exclusion and investigation should include serum folate, iron and vitamin B_{12}, faecal fat measurement, plain abdominal radiology, small bowel meal and biopsy, and pancreatic function tests.

Treatment is empirical and assessment of response to treatment is complicated by the tendency of the diarrhoea to occur in self-limiting attacks and to improve with time. Strict diabetic control is necessary in every case and may help symptoms. Diets containing more or less fibre or carbohydrate have not been helpful. However, a low-fat diet will help to alleviate symptoms in patients with steatorrhoea. Opiates, e.g. codeine phosphate, and cholinergics may be helpful. Clonidine is of great potential benefit and short-term clinical trials have been encouraging.[14]

Cholestyramine is worth a trial, especially if bile acid malabsorption has been demonstrated, but it can precipitate or aggravate steatorrhoea. Steroids are of no value. Antimicrobials, e.g. tetracycline or metronidazole, are indicated in the presence of bacterial overgrowth of the small intestine and are worth a therapeutic trial in other cases. Treatment may need to be continued, often intermittently, for many months or years.

COELIAC DISEASE AND DIABETES

In diabetics with diarrhoea and steatorrhoea, coeliac disease must be considered as a diagnosis because the two disorders often coexist.[56] Both are associated with HLA-B8. Precise prevalence figures are not known. Clinical clues to coexisting coeliac disease are a family history of coeliac disease, frequent swings from hypo- to hyperglycaemia on small doses of insulin, a childhood history of diarrhoea, anaemia and failure to thrive, unexplained diarrhoea and anaemia before the onset of diabetes, and features of malabsorption on physical examination.[56] Infertility may be a problem in female diabetic coeliacs. Folate deficiency and hypoalbuminaemia are not features of diabetic diarrhoea and should suggest coeliac disease.[10,11,56] All diabetics with diarrhoea must have a small bowel biopsy. Treatment with a strict gluten-free diet will usually relieve symptoms and improve diabetic control, although daily insulin requirements usually increase.[56]

INCONTINENCE IN DIABETICS

Diabetics, especially those with autonomic neuropathy, may suffer from incontinence which can be present in those passing solid stool as well as those with diarrhoea. There is significant impairment of all aspects of anal function.[49,55] Drug therapy is usually unhelpful but biofeedback therapy may re-establish continence.[55]

OTHER GASTROINTESTINAL MANIFESTATIONS OF DIABETIC NEUROPATHY

Diabetic radiculopathy (diabetic plexus neuropathy), which is secondary to neuropathy involving the thoracic roots, is unique to diabetes.[33] It causes chronic severe abdominal pain which is often associated with weight loss and anorexia. The picture simulates malignancy, especially pancreatic carcinoma, so unnecessary diagnostic laparotomies are often performed. The patients are usually insulin dependent and have peripheral neuropathy. It is diagnosed by electromyography, the treatment is symptomatic and the symptoms often gradually subside over 6–20 months.

Diabetics with neuropathy have been described who get attacks of severe sharp epigastric pain with vomiting lasting a few hours to several days.[43] These are similar clinically to the gastric crises of tabes dorsalis. Postprandial facial sweating is said to be a specific manifestation of diabetic autonomic neuropathy, although this is disputed. It is most profuse after spicy food and may be treated by anticholinergics if troublesome.

EFFECTS OF DIABETES AND INSULIN ON JEJUNAL FUNCTION

Perfusion studies in diabetics have shown that glucose absorption is either increased[54] or normal.[12] Sodium and water absorption[12] and brush border disaccharidase, peptidase and alkaline phosphatase activities[6] are normal. Blood insulin levels do not influence glucose, sodium or water absorption in diabetics or normal subjects.[12,54]

ORAL HYPOGLYCAEMIC DRUGS AND THE GUT

Biguanides

These drugs inhibit glucose absorption from the small intestine. There are conflicting data on whether this inhibition is selective or not. Reports of inhibition of xylose absorption by metformin and sodium absorption by phenformin have not been confirmed by other studies. Metformin and (to a lesser extent) phenformin inhibit vitamin B_{12} absorption. Up to 30% of patients taking metformin for two or more years show vitamin B_{12} malabsorption,[53] although this rarely leads to megaloblastic anaemia. Vitamin B_{12} malabsorption may be a consequence of bacterial overgrowth secondary to poor intestinal motility caused by biguanides, because vitamin B_{12} absorption improves after antibiotic therapy and patients taking biguanides have evidence of bile salt deconjugation in the small intestine.[7]

Biguanides commonly cause anorexia, nausea, vomiting, abdominal pain and diarrhoea. As many as 25% of patients on phenformin complain of gastrointestinal disturbances. Phenformin has been blamed for causing acute pancreatitis, impaired pancreatic exocrine function and delayed gastric emptying.

Sulphonylureas

These drugs do not affect glucose absorption but do cause minor nausea, epigastric pain and occasional vomiting.

DIABETES MELLITUS AND THE PANCREAS

(see Chapter 11)

Pancreatic exocrine function

Abnormalities of pancreatic exocrine function have been found in 20–70% of all diabetics[9] although many of these patients may have had diabetes secondary to pancreatic disease. Reduced total volume, reduced amylase and bicarbonate concentrations have been found individually and together. Suggested causes include autonomic neuropathy, the wasting of uncontrolled diabetes, the inhibitory action of glucagon and the lack of stimulation by insulin. These abnormalities of pancreatic secretion are rarely severe and are not usually associated with steatorrhoea.

Acute pancreatitis

Hyperglycaemia occurs in 10–80% of patients with acute pancreatitis, but it is usually transient, lasting at most a few months and rarely requires specific treatment. Lasting diabetes mellitus is uncommon after an episode of acute pancreatitis, occurring in about 1% of cases. Confusion arises because diabetes with ketoacidosis may have transient hyperamylasaemia or even frank acute pancreatitis. Acute pancreatitis seems to be more common in diabetics than in non-diabetics and has a higher mortality.

Chronic pancreatitis

There is no evidence that chronic pancreatitis is more common among diabetics than normals. However chronic pancreatitis, particularly when associated with calcification, can lead to secondary diabetes mellitus when more than 90% of the gland is destroyed. In one series, 30% of patients with chronic pancreatitis had overt diabetes and a further 20% had impaired glucose tolerance.[2] If calcification was present, 70% of patients had diabetes and 20% had impaired glucose tolerance.

Pancreatic carcinoma

Diabetes occurs in 25–40% of patients with carcinoma of the pancreas. The development of diabetes at the onset of symptoms related to carcinoma is a common occurrence or it can predate the onset of symptoms of carcinoma by a year or more. Some patients with carcinoma of the pancreas develop diabetes after the onset of symptoms related to the carcinoma.[19] Diabetes is most commonly manifested by abnormal glucose tolerance rather than glycosuria or hyperglycaemia. The diabetes may be unstable and the mechanism by which the carcinoma causes diabetes is unknown.[29] Pancreatic carcinoma should be considered in all new diabetics over 40 years of age, especially if they have no family history of diabetes, in deteriorating or unstable older diabetics or in older diabetics with abdominal symptoms.

This association has complicated the answer to the question of whether diabetes mellitus pre-disposes to pancreatic carcinoma. Among 21 447 diabetics, the standard mortality ratio for pancreatic carcinoma was increased significantly for females at 2.13 and for males at 1.47.[32] However, if cases where carcinoma developed within a year of the diagnosis of diabetes were excluded, the ratio was only significant for females.

Pancreatic islet cell tumours (see Chapter 11)

Glucagonomas and somatostatinomas cause hyperglycaemia which is usually mild but can occasionally require insulin. The syndrome of watery diarrhoea with hypokalaemia (Verner–Morrison syndrome) is associated with VIP producing islet cell tumours and 15% of patients have hyperglycaemia which may require insulin. The mechanism of diabetes is unknown.

DIABETES MELLITUS AND THE BILIARY TRACT

In diabetics, especially those with autonomic neuropathy, the gallbladder on cholecystography tends to be large with poor filling and poor contraction after a fat meal[19] and gallbladder emptying in response to cholecystokinin-octapeptide is impaired on radionuclide scanning.[52] These findings have no clinical relevance provided that no gallstones are present.

The prevalence of gallstones among diabetics is about twice that of non-diabetics, the increase being entirely due to cholesterol stones. Maturity-onset, but not juvenile-onset, diabetics tend to have supersaturated bile but this is related to obesity rather than to diabetes.[20]

In diabetics, acute cholecystitis is severe, tends to suppuration and has a mortality of 10–20%.[48] Moreover, 20% of patients with emphysematous cholecystitis are diabetics. Early surgery is advised but postoperative complications are still common. A case has been made for elective cholecystectomy in diabetics with asymptomatic gallstones because operative mortality is not increased,[48] although postoperative complications seem to be more common than in non-diabetics.[44]

REFERENCES

1. Angervall, L., Dotevall, G. and Lehmann, K.E. (1961) The gastric mucosa in diabetes mellitus. A functional and histopathological study. *Acta Medica Scandinavica*, **169**, 339–349.
2. Bank, S., Marks, I.N. and Vinik, A.I. (1975) Clinical and hormonal aspects of pancreatic diabetes. *American Journal of Gastroenterology*, **64**, 13–22.
3. Battle, W.M., Snape, W.J., Alavi, A. *et al.* (1980) Colonic dysfunction in diabetes mellitus. *Gastroenterology*, **79**, 1217–1211.
4. Camilleri, M. and Malagelada, J.R. (1984) Abnormal intestinal motility in diabetics with gastroparesis syndrome. *European Journal of Clinical Investigation*, **14**, 420–427.
5. Campbell, I.W., Heading, R.C., Tothill, P. *et al.* (1977) Gastric emptying in diabetic autonomic neuropathy. *Gut*, **18**, 462–467.
6. Caspary, W.F., Winckler, K. and Creutzfeldt, W. (1974) Intestinal brush border enzyme activity in juvenile and maturity onset diabetes mellitus. *Diabetologia*, **10**, 353–355.
7. Caspary, W.F., Zavada, I., Reimold, W. *et al.* (1977) Alterations of bile acid metabolism and vitamin B_{12} absorption in diabetics on biguanides. *Diabetologia,* **13**, 187–193.
8. Chang, E.B. (1986) Experimental diabetic diarrhea in rats. Intestinal mucosal denervation hypersensitivity and treatment with clonidine. *Gastroenterology*, **91**, 564–569.
9. Chey, W.Y., Shay, H. and Shuman, C.R. (1963) External pancreatic secretion in diabetes mellitus. *Annals of Internal Medicine*, **59**, 812–821.
10. Cooper, B.T., O'Brien, I.A.D., Ukabam, S.O. *et al.* (1983) Abnormal small intestinal permeability in patients with diabetic diarrhoea. *Clinical Science*, **64**, 16P.
11. Cooper, B.T., Ukabam, S.O., O'Brien, I.A.D.,

O'Hare, J.P. and Corrall, R.J.M. (1987) Intestinal permeability in diabetic diarrhoea. *Diabetic Medicine*, **4**, 49–52.
12. Costrini, N.V., Ganneshappa, K.P., Wu, W. *et al.* (1977) Effect of insulin, glucose and controlled diabetes mellitus on human jejunal function. *American Journal of Physiology*, **233**, E181–E187.
13. Dotevall, G. (1959) Incidence of peptic ulcer in diabetes mellitus. *Acta Medica Scandinavica*, **164**, 463–477.
14. Fedorak, R.N., Field, M. and Chang, E.B. (1985) Treatment of diabetic diarrhea with clonidine. *Annals of Internal Medicine*, **102**, 197–199.
15. Feldman, M., Corbett, D.B., Ramsey, E.J. *et al.* (1977) Abnormal gastric function in long standing insulin dependent diabetic patients. *Gastroenterology*, **77**, 12–17.
16. Fox, S. and Behar, J. (1980) Pathogenesis of diabetic gastroparesis; a pharmacologic study. *Gastroenterology*, **78**, 757–763.
17. Goldstein, F., Wirts, C.W. and Knowlessar, O.D. (1970) Diabetic diarrhoea and steatorrhoea. Microbiologic and clinical observations. *Annals of Internal Medicine*, **72**, 215–218.
18. Goyal, R.K. and Spiro, H.M. (1971) Gastrointestinal manifestations of diabetes mellitus. *Medical Clinics of North America*, **55**, 1031–1044.
19. Grodski, M., Mazurkiewicz-Rozinska, E. and Czyzyka, A. (1968) Diabetic cholecystopathy. *Diabetologia*, **4**, 345–348.
20. Haber, G.B. and Heaton, K.W. (1979) Lipid composition of bile in diabetics and obesity matched controls. *Gut*, **20**, 518–522.
21. Hensley, G.T. and Soergel, K.H. (1968) Neuropathologic findings in diabetic diarrhoea. *Archives of Pathology*, **85**, 587–597.
22. Hollis, J.B., Castell, D.O. and Braddon, R.L. (1977) Esophageal function in diabetes mellitus and its relation to peripheral neuropathy. *Gastroenterology*, **73**, 1098–1102.
23. Horowitz, M., Harding, P.E., Chatterton, B.E., Collins, P.J. and Shearman, D.J.C. (1985) Acute and chronic effects of domperidone on gastric emptying in diabetic autonomic neuropathy. *Digestive Diseases and Science*, **30** 1–9.
24. Horowitz, M., Harding, P.E., Maddox, A. *et al.* (1986) Gastric and oesophageal emptying in insulin dependent diabetes mellitus. *Journal of Gastroenterology and Hepatology*, **1**, 97–113.
25. Horowitz, M., Maddox, A. and Harding, P.E. (1987) Effect of cisapride on gastric and esophageal emptying in insulin-dependent diabetes mellitus. *Gastroenterology*, **92**, 1899–1907.
26. Hosking, D.J., Moody, F., Stewart, I.M. and Atkinson, M. (1975) Vagal impairment of gastric secretion in diabetic autonomic neuropathy. *British Medical Journal*, **2**, 588–590.
27. Irvine, W.J., Clarke, B.F., Scarth, L. *et al.* (1970) Thyroid and gastric auto antibodies in patients with diabetes mellitus. *The Lancet*, **2**, 163–168.
28. Janssens, J., Peeters, T.V. and Vantrappen, G. (1990) Improvement of gastric emptying in diabetic gastroparesis. *New England Journal of Medicine*, **322**, 1029–1031.
29. Karmody, A.J. and Kyle, J. (1969) The association between carcinoma of the pancreas and diabetes mellitus. *British Journal of Surgery*, **56**, 362–364.
30. Kassander, P. (1958) Asymptomatic gastric retention in diabetics (gastroparesis diabeticorum). *Annals of Internal Medicine*, **48**, 797–812.
31. Katz, L.A. and Spiro, H.M. (1966) Gastrointestinal manifestations of diabetes. *New England Journal of Medicine*, **275**, 1350–1361.
32. Kessler, I.I. (1970) Cancer mortality among diabetics. *Journal of the National Cancer Institute*, **44**, 673–686.
33. Longstreth, G.F. and Newcomer, A.D. (1977) Abdominal pain caused by diabetic radiculopathy. *Annals of Internal Medicine*, **86**, 166–168.
34. Loo, F.D., Dodds, W.J., Soergel, K.H., Armdorfer, R.C., Helm, J.F. and Hogan, W.J. (1985) Multipeaked esophageal peristaltic pressure waves in patients with diabetic neuropathy. *Gastroenterology*, **88**, 485–491.
35. Malagelada, J.R., Rees, W.D.W., Mazzotta, L.J. and Go, V.L.W. (1980) Gastric motor abnormalities in diabetic and post vagotomy gastroparesis: effect of metoclopramide and bethanechol. *Gastroenterology*, **78**, 286–293.
36. Malins, J.M. and French, J.M. (1957) Diabetic diarrhoea. *Quarterly Journal of Medicine*, **26**, 467–480.
37. Malins, J.M. and Mayne, N. (1969) Diabetic diarrhoea. A study of 13 patients with jejunal biopsy. *Diabetes*, **18**, 858–866.
38. Mandelstam, P. and Lieber, A. (1967) Esophageal dysfunction in diabetic neuropathy-gastropathy. *Journal of the American Medical Association*, **201**, 582–586.
39. Mayne, N. (1965) Neuropathy in the diabetic and non-diabetic populations. *The Lancet*, **2**, 1313–1316.
40. McNally, E.F., Reinhard, A.E. and Schwartz, P.E. (1969) Small bowel motility in diabetics. *American Journal of Digestive Diseases*, **14**, 163–169.
41. Mearin, F., Camilleri, M. and Malagelada, J.R. (1986) Pyloric dysfunction in diabetics with recurrent nausea and vomiting. *Gastroenterology*, **90**, 1919–1925.
42. Molloy, A.M. and Tomkin, G.H. (1978) Altered bile in diabetic diarrhoea. *British Medical Journal* **ii**, 1462–1463.
43. Rundles, R.W. (1945) Diabetic neuropathy. General review with report of 125 cases. *Medicine (Baltimore)*, **24**, 111–160.
44. Sandler, R.S., Maule, W.F. and Baltin, M.E. (1986) Factors associated with post-operative complications in diabetics after biliary tract surgery. *Gastroenterology*, **91**, 157–162.
45. Scarpello, J.H.B., Barber, D.C., Hague, R.V. *et al.* (1976) Gastric emptying of solid meals in diabetics. *British Medical Journal*, **ii**, 671–673.

46. Scarpello, J.H.B., Hague, R.V., Cullen, D.R. and Sladen, G.E. (1976) The ^{14}C-glycocholate test in diabetic diarrhoea. *British Medical Journal*, **ii**, 673–675.
47. Schade, R.R., Dugas, M.C., Lhotsky, D.M., Gavalier, J.S. and Van Thiel, D.H. (1985) Effect of metoclopramide on gastric liquid emptying in patients with diabetic gastroparesis. *Digestive Diseases and Sciences*, **30**, 10–15.
48. Schein, C.J. (1969) Acute cholecystitis in the diabetic. *American Journal of Gastroenterology*, **51**, 511–515.
49. Schiller, L.R., Santa Ana, C.A., Schmulen, C., Hendler, R.S., Harford, W.V. and Fordtran, J.A. (1982) Pathogenesis of fecal incontinence in diabetes mellitus. Evidence for internal anal sphincter dysfunction. *New England Journal of Medicine*, **307**, 1666–1671.
50. Smith, B. (1974) Neuropathy of the oesophagus in diabetes mellitus. *Neurology, Neurosurgery and Psychiatry*, **37**, 1151–1154.
51. Stewart, I.M., Hosking, D.J., Preston, B.J. and Atkinson, M. (1976) Oesophageal motor changes in diabetes mellitus. *Thorax*, **31**, 278–283.
52. Stone, B.G. (1988) Impairment of gallbladder emptying in diabetes mellitus. *Gastroenterology*, **95**, 170–176.
53. Tomkin, G.H., Hadden, D.R., Weaver, J.A. and Montgomery, D.A.D. (1971) Vitamin B_{12} status of patients on long term metformin therapy. *British Medical Journal*, **ii**, 685–687.
54. Vinnik, I.E., Kern, F.J. and Sussman, K.E. (1965) The effect of diabetes mellitus and insulin on glucose absorption by the small intestine in man. *Journal of Laboratory and Clinical Medicine*, **66**, 131–136.
55. Wald, A. and Tunuguntla, A.K. (1984) Ano-rectal sensorimotor dysfunction in fecal incontinence and diabetes mellitus. *New England Journal of Medicine*, **310**, 1282–1287.
56. Walsh, C.H., Cooper, B.T., Wright, A.D. *et al.* (1978) Diabetes mellitus and coeliac disease: a clinical study. *Quarterly Journal of Medicine*, **47**, 89–100.
57. Warshaw, A.L., Feller, E.R. and Lee, K.H. (1977) On the cause of raised serum amylase in diabetic keto-acidosis. *The Lancet*, **1**, 929–930.
58. Whalen, G.E. Soergel, K.H. and Greenen, J.E. (1969) Diabetic diarrhoea. A clinical and pathophysiological study. *Gastroenterology*, **56**, 1021–1032.
59. Wood, M.N. (1947) Chronic peptic ulcer in 94 diabetics. *American Journal of Digestive Diseases*, **14**, 1–11.
60. Zitomer, B.R., Gramm, H.F. and Kozak, G.P. (1968) Gastric neuropathy in diabetes mellitus: clinical and radiologic observations. *Metabolism*, **17**, 199–211.

THE ACUTE PORPHYRIAS

K.E.L. McColl, S. Dover and M.R. Moore

There are six classic forms of porphyria, each being due to a single enzyme defect in the pathway of haem biosynthesis. The acute porphyrias (acute intermittent porphyria, hereditary coproporphyria and variegate porphyria) present with intermittent attacks of neurovisceral dysfunction which may be precipitated by various drugs and other exogenous factors. Patients with variegate porphyria or hereditary coproporphyria may in addition develop photosensitive skin lesions. The non-acute porphyrias (cutaneous hepatic porphyria, erythropoietic protoporphyria and congenital porphyria) present solely with cutaneous manifestations and will therefore not be dealt with further in this text.

ACUTE INTERMITTENT PORPHYRIA

This is the most common and most severe form of the acute porphyrias. Although the genetic trait is inherited in an autosomal dominant fashion, manifest disease is more common in females, with a female:male ratio of around 5:1 – this is probably due to hormonal fluctuations precipitating clinical attacks. The highest incidence of onset of symptoms is between puberty and 30 years of age, and attacks are most common in the third decade. In one-third of reported cases there is no family history, the condition probably having remained latent or unidentified for several generations.

The frequency and severity of attacks vary considerably from patient to patient. In a proportion, the disease remains latent throughout life, even in the presence of precipitating factors. Other patients experience frequent and sometimes life-endangering attacks even in the absence of extrinsic precipitating factors.

UNDERLYING BIOCHEMICAL DISORDER

The basic defect in acute intermittent porphyria is partial deficiency of the enzyme porphobilinogen deaminase.[9] As a result, there is excess formation and urinary excretion of the porphyrin precursors δ-aminolaevulinic acid and porphobilinogen which are formed prior to the enzyme defect. There is also increased excretion of uroporphyrin in the urine. Excretion of these haem precursors is always increased during clinical attacks but may be normal or remain increased during clinical remission.

CLINICAL FEATURES

Gastrointestinal manifestations

Abdominal pain is the most frequent complaint, occurring in 95% of attacks of acute porphyria; it can often be so severe that parenteral opiate analgesics are required. The pain is usually felt diffusely over the abdomen and often radiates round the back. Abdominal examination may be normal or reveal mild generalized tenderness, sometimes associated with a degree of muscle guarding. Bowel sounds are normal. Anorexia usually occurs and there is often associated nausea and vomiting. Some patients develop marked delayed gastric emptying and a succussion splash may be elicited. Constipation is usually present. Abdominal radiographs are usually normal though in some patients dilatation of the colon may be seen.

Patients presenting with their first attack may be misdiagnosed as suffering from an acute abdomen. Unnecessary anaesthetic and laparotomy may result in a fatal outcome.

Neuropathy

Neuropathy may be the presenting feature and complicates more than 50% of porphyric attacks. Motor involvement is most common but paraesthesiae may also occur. The paralysis usually starts peripherally and then spreads proximally; however, in some patients shoulder girdle involvement may be the first manifestation. The neuropathy may progress rapidly, resulting in respiratory embarrassment.

Psychiatric manifestations

Psychiatric manifestations are also a common feature of the porphyric attack and may result in a patient being misdiagnosed as suffering from a primary psychiatric disorder. Agitation, mania, depression, hallucinations and schizophrenic-like behaviour may occur.

Autonomic dysfunction

Tachycardia and hypertension disproportionate to the pain are usually present. Other manifestations of autonomic dysfunction such as profuse sweating, pallor and pyrexia may occur. Severe hyponatraemia due to inappropriate secretion of antidiuretic hormone complicates a proportion of attacks, and sometimes presents with convulsions or deterioration in conscious level following commencement of intravenous fluids.

INVESTIGATIONS

The most important factor in determining a satisfactory outcome for a patient presenting in acute porphyric crisis is early diagnosis. The disorder should be considered in any patient presenting with unexplained abdominal pain. A helpful clue to the diagnosis is the passage of dark urine due to the excessive excretion of haem precursors. If the urine is left standing in the light, the discoloration becomes more pronounced. The diagnosis is confirmed by demonstrating excess porphobilinogen in the urine. A useful side-room test for excess porphobilinogen is to add an equal volume of Ehrlich's aldehyde reagent to the patient's urine. This causes a red discoloration which remains in the upper aqueous layer following the further addition of chloroform.

RELATIONSHIP BETWEEN BIOCHEMICAL DISORDER AND CLINICAL FEATURES OF THE PORPHYRIC ATTACK

All the clinical features of the attack of acute porphyria can be explained by neurological dysfunction affecting the central, peripheral and autonomic nervous system. The abdominal pain, vomiting and constipation are all thought to be the result of dysfunction of the autonomic control of the gastrointestinal tract. The mechanism by which the abnormal haem biosynthesis results in the functional alterations of the nervous system remains to be elucidated.[13]

FACTORS THAT MAY PRECIPITATE ACUTE PORPHYRIA

Various factors may precipitate attacks of acute porphyria in subjects with the genetic trait and great care must be taken to prevent exposure to them. Drugs are the most common precipitating agents.[10] A list of drugs (listed alphabetically) believed to be unsafe in patients with acute porphyria is given in *Table 8.8*. A list of drugs believed to be safe (also alphabetically listed) is given in *Table 8.9*.

Other factors that may trigger attacks include alcohol ingestion, reduced caloric intake due to

Table 8.8 Drugs *unsafe* for use in acute porphyria

Aminoglutethimide
Aminophylline
Amiodarone
(Amitriptyline)
(Amphetamines)
*__Amylobarbitone__
Antipyrine
Aurothiomalate
Azapropazone

Baclofen
*__Barbiturates__
*__Bemegride__
Bendrofluazide
Benoxaprofen
Bromocriptine
Busulphan

Captopril
*__Carbamazepine__
*__Chloramphenicol__
*__Chlordiazepoxide__
Chloroform
*__Chlorpropamide__
Cinnarizine
Clonidine hydrochloride
Cyclophosphamide
Cycloserine
Cyclosporin

Danazol
Dapsone
Dextropropoxyphene
*__Dichloralphenazone__
Diclofenac sodium
Dihydralazine
*__Dihydroergotamine__
Diltiazem
*__Dimenhydrinate__
Diphenhydramine
Doxycycline

Enalapril
Enflurane
*__Ergot compounds__
*__Erythromycin__
*__Ethanol__
Ethosuximide
Etidocaine
Etomidate

Fenfluramine
*__Flufenamic acid__
Flupenthixol
Flurazepam

*__Glutethimide__
Gramicidin
*__Griseofulvin__

*__Halothane__
*__Hydantoins__
Hydralazine
Hydroxyzine
Hyoscine

*__Imipramine__
Iproniazid

Ketoconazole

Lignocaine
Lofepramine

Mebeverine hydrochloride
Megestrol acetate
Mepivacaine
*__Meprobamate__
Mercaptopurine
Mestranol
Methotrexate
Methoxyflurane
*__Methyldopa__
*__Methyl sulphanol__
*__Methyprylone__
Methysergide
Metyrapone
Mianserin hydrochloride
Miconazole
Minoxidil

Nalidixic acid
*__Nifedipine__
*__Nikethamide__
Nitrazepam
(Nitrofurantoin)
Novobiocin

*__Oral contraceptives__
*__Orophenadrine__
Oxytetracycline

*__Pentazocine__
Perhexiline
Phenacetin
Phenelzine
*__Phenobarbitone__
Phenoxybenzamine
Phensuximide
Phenylhydrazine
*__Phenytoin__
Piroxicam
*__Pivampicillin__
Prenylamine
*__Primidone__
(Probenecid)
*__Progesterone__
Promethazine
*__Pyrazinamide__

Quinalbarbitone

Rifampcin

Spironolactone
Stanozolol
Succinimides
Sulphonamides
*__Sulphasalazine__
Sulphonylureas

Tamoxifen
Terfenadine
Tetrazepam
*__Theophylline__
*__Thiopentone__
Tolbutamide
Tranylcypromine
Trazodone hydrochloride
Trimethoprim
Troxidone

Valpromide
Verapamil
Viloxazine hydrochloride

Zuclopenthixol

These drugs have been classified as 'unsafe' because all have been shown to be porphyrinogenic in animals or in vitro systems.
*Those marked in **bold** with an asterisk have been associated with acute attacks of porphyria in humans.

fasting or dieting, and infection; in addition, hormones are important.[8] Attacks are more common in females and rarely occur before puberty or after the menopause. Pregnancy and oral contraceptives may also precipitate attacks and some women experience regular attacks commencing in the week prior to the onset of menstruation.

TREATMENT

An attack of acute porphyria still carries significant mortality. A successful outcome largely depends on early diagnosis, removal of precipitating factors and provision of intensive supportive therapy.

Steps should be taken to ensure that the patient

Table 8.9 Drugs thought to be safe for use in acute porphyria

Acetazolamide	Desferrioxamine	Ketoprofen	Quinidine
Actinomycin *D*	Dexamethasone		Quinine
Acyclovir	Diamorphine	Labetalol	
Alclofenac	Diazoxide	Lithium salts	Reserpine
Allopurinol	Dicyclomine	Loperamide	
Amiloride	hydrochloride		Salbutamol
Aminoglycosides	Digoxin	Metformin	Sodum fusidate
Amoxycillin	Dihydrocodeine	Methadone	Sorbitol
Amphotericin	Dimercaprol	Methyluracil	Streptomycin
Ampicillin	Diphenoxylate	Metoprolol	Sulindac
Ascorbic acid	hydrochloride	Mianserin	Sulfadoxine
Aspirin	Dipyridamole	Morphine	Suxamethonium
Atenolol	Domperidone		
Atropine	Doxorubicin	Neostigmine	Temazepam
Azathioprine	hydrochloride	Nitrous oxide	Thiouracil
	Droperidol		Triamterene
Beclomethasone		OxytocinParacetamol	Triazolam
Benzhexol hydrochloride	Ethacrynic acid	Paraldehyde	Trifluoperazine
Beta-carotene	Ethambutol	Penicillamine	Tubocurarine
Biguanides		Penicillin	
Bumetanide	Famotidine	Pentolinium	Vancomycin
Bupivacaine	Fenbrufen	Pethidine	
Buprenorphine	Fenoprofen	Phenformin	Warfarin sodium
Buserelin	Fentanyl	Phenoperidine	
	Flucytosine	Phentolamine	
Canthaxanthin	Flumazenil	Pirenzepine	
Carbimazole	Flurbiprofen	Pizotifen	
Chloral hydrate	Folic acid	Primaquine	
Chlorpheniramine	Fusidic acid	Procainamide	
Chlorpromazine		Procaine	
Cisplatin	Gentamicin	Prochlorperazine	
Clofibrate	Glipizide	Proguanil	
Cloxacillin	Glucagon	Promazine	
Codeine phosphate	Glyceryl trinitrate	Propantheline	
Colchicine	Guanethidine	Propofol	
Coumarins		Propanolol	
Cyclizine	Heparin	Propylthiouracil	
Cyclopenthiazide		Pseudoephedrine	
Cyclopropane	Ibuprofen	hydrochloride	
	Indomethacin	Pyridoxine	
	Insulin		
	Iron		

has an adequate carbohydrate intake. In mild attacks, this may be done by ensuring an adequate intake of glucose polymer drinks, such as Caloreen or Hycal. In more severe cases, 2 litres 20% dextrose should be infused every 24 hours into a large peripheral vein or via a central line.

Control of pain

For severe pain, pethidine, morphine or diamorphine may be required. There is a danger of addiction in patients experiencing frequent attacks and those requiring large amounts of opiate analgesics; every attempt should be made to withdraw all opiates between attacks.

In a few unfortunate patients the pain is refractory to even very large doses of intravenous opiate analgesics, and signs of respiratory and cardiovascular system depression appear before pain relief is obtained. Some of our patients report that the only time the pain goes away is when they are asleep. This observation may be used to advantage by encouraging sleep for several hours through combination of chlorpromazine or promazine with the analgesics and leaving the patients relatively undisturbed in a darkened room.

Some patients continue to complain of chronic abdominal pain unaccompanied by any other symptom between attacks. This can be very difficult to manage and the risk of opiate addiction in these patients is high. Although, in some cases, a psychological element may be a factor, in others the pain is clearly genuine and presumably a manifestation of residual neurological damage.

Tachycardia and hypertension

These are features of most attacks, and they are thought to be the result of sympathetic over-activity and should be controlled with propranolol. The dose should be titrated against its effect on the cardiovascular system; frequently a very large dose is required. Pulse and blood pressure should be closely monitored because they tend to be labile and a marked postural effect is commonly seen.

Convulsions

These are not infrequent at the peak of an attack. Their onset may be a sign of hyponatraemia due to inappropriate antidiuretic hormone secretion, and plasma osmolality and electrolyte values should be checked. If hyponatraemia is the underlying cause it should be corrected by fluid restriction. Convulsions occurring during the attack usually settle as the attack resolves and therefore therapy should be aimed at treating the underlying disease process. However, some patients continue to suffer convulsions outside the acute attack. As all the commonly employed anticonvulsants are porphyrinogenic, management of chronic epilepsy in porphyric patients is extremely difficult.

Neuropathy

All patients should be examined regularly for evidence of developing peripheral neuropathy. This may progress rapidly leading to quadriplegia, and bulbar and ventilatory paralysis. When signs of peripheral neuropathy are present, the expiratory peak flow rate should be monitored regularly. If there is any reduction in this, blood gases should be checked and the patient nursed in an intensive care unit with facilities for assisted ventilation. Even in patients in whom there is widespread paralysis requiring assisted ventilation for many months, good functional recovery can still be expected. The usual attention should be given to splinting of the joints and appropriate physiotherapy in the paralysed patient.

Haematin therapy

It is possible to improve the underlying biochemical disturbance by the administration of the end-product of the haem biosynthetic pathway.[12] Haem preparations administered in this way bind to haemopexin and albumin in the plasma, and are taken up by the liver. They supplement the depleted intracellular free haem pool, thus suppressing activity of the initial and rate-controlling enzyme of the pathway δ-aminolaevulinic acid synthetase, thereby reducing the over-production of porphyrins and the precursors formed prior to the enzyme block. The administration of haem preparations results in a marked and consistent reduction in porphyrin precursor excretion.[5,6] The most suitable haem preparation for the treatment of acute porphyria is haem arginate (Normosang) because it is stable when stored in solution.

The clinical response to haem therapy is more difficult to assess. There has only been one placebo-controlled trial of haem arginate therapy and it did not show a statistically significant benefit for the active therapy, although there was a trend in favour of it.[3] The lack of significant effect may, however, be due to the small numbers studied and the variability of severity of attacks. The overall impression is that the marked improvement of biochemistry is accompanied by a significant, though less dramatic, clinical response.

Haem arginate is administered in a dose of 3 mg/kg per day for 3 or 4 days. It is given intravenously over 15 minutes into a slow-running intravenous infusion. In some patients the treatment results in phlebitis around the injection site.

PREVENTION OF ATTACKS

Patients who have experienced a clinical attack of porphyria should be carefully counselled concerning the avoidance of precipitating factors. They should be given a booklet indicating which drugs are safe and which are unsafe to take. It is also important to ensure that their family doctor is fully informed about the disease and given advice about prescribing drugs. In addition, they should wear a bracelet or necklace indicating that they have porphyria.

Some women experience regular attacks in the week prior to the onset of menstruation. The use of the contraceptive pill to suppress ovulation and prevent these attacks cannot be recommended because all forms of contraceptive pill may, themselves, trigger attacks. The authors, and others, have found some benefit from treating these patients with the long-acting analogue of luteinizing hormone-releasing hormone, buserelin, which can be administered nasally.[1,4]

Pregnancy may precipitate attacks of acute porphyria with attacks being most common in early pregnancy and during the puerperium. When attacks occur during pregnancy they should be treated in the usual manner. No information is available concerning the effects of haem arginate on the fetus. The vast majority of patients with acute porphyria tolerate pregnancy well with a successful outcome for mother and child.[2]

Surgery and anaesthetics

Provided that appropriate precautions are taken, most patients with acute porphyria can tolerate surgery and general anaesthesia. Patients with acute porphyria have undergone such major surgery as coronary artery bypass grafts, hip replacement and cholecystectomy without any complications. Care must be taken in selecting safe anaesthetic agents.[11] Atropine or morphine may be used as a premedication. Intravenous ketamine has been found to be a safe alternative to thiopentone as an anaesthesia-inducing agent. Cyclopropane and ether are safe inhalational agents in respect of the porphyria but they suffer the disadvantage of being potentially explosive and inducing postoperative vomiting. Nitrous oxide used in conjunction with intravenous opiates may be a more acceptable alternative. Suxamethonium and d-tubocurarine can be used as muscle relaxants and diamorphine, morphine, pethidine or fentanyl are suitable opiates for controlling postoperative pain. In some situations, epidural anaesthesia may be preferable to general anaesthesia in which case bupivacaine is the local anaesthetic of choice. To prevent an attack being induced by fasting, an intravenous infusion of dextrose should be commenced prior to surgery and continued until the patient is able to take an adequate diet.

Screening of relatives

Blood relatives should also be screened for latent disease. Urinalysis will only pick up 50% of latent cases of porphyria and, therefore, analysis of the activity of the relevant deficient enzyme in the peripheral blood cells must be performed.[7]

HEREDITARY COPROPORPHYRIA AND VARIEGATE PORPHYRIA

These may present clinically with attacks identical to those seen in acute intermittent porphyria. They are provoked by the same precipitating factors and patients should be managed in exactly the same way as those with acute intermittent porphyria.

Because of the over-production of formed porphyrins, patients with hereditary coproporphyria and variegate porphyria may, in addition, develop cutaneous photosensitivity. These forms of porphyria are also inherited in an autosomal dominant fashion and relatives should be screened for the condition and given advice about prevention of attacks.

REFERENCES

1. Anderson, K.E., Spitu, I.M., Bardin, C.W. and Kappas, A. (1990) A gonadotrophin releasing hormone analogue prevents cyclical attacks of porphyria. *Archives of Internal Medicine*, **150**, 1469–1474.
2. Brodie, M.J., Moore, M.R., Thompson, G.G., Goldberg, A. and Low, R.A.L. (1977) Pregnancy and the acute porphyrias. *British Journal of Obstetrics and Gynaecology*, **84**, 726–731.
3. Herrick, A.L., McColl, K.E.L., Moore, M.R., Cook, A. and Goldberg, A. (1989) Controlled trial of haem arginate in acute hepatic porphyria. *The Lancet*, **i**, 1295–1297.
4. Herrick, A.L., McColl, K.E.L., Wallace, A.M., Moore, M.R. and Goldberg, A. (1990) LHRH Analogue treatment for the prevention of premenstrual attacks of acute porphyria. *Quarterly Journal of Medicine, New Series 75*, **276**, 355–363.
5. Lamon, J.L., Frykholm, B.C., Hess, R.A. and Tschudy, D.P. (1979) Haematin therapy for acute porphyria. *Medicine*, **58**, 252–269.
6. McColl, K.E.L., Moore, M.R., Thompson, G.G. and Goldberg, A. (1981) Treatment with haematin in acute hepatic porphyria. *Quarterly Journal of Medicine, New Series L*, **198**, 161–174.
7. McColl, K.E.L., Moore, M.R., Thompson, G.G. and Goldberg, A. (1982) Screening for latent acute intermittent porphyria: The value of measuring both leucocyte δ-aminolaevulinic acid synthase and erythrocyte uroporphyrinogen-L-synthase activities. *Journal of Medical Genetics*, **19**, 271–276.
8. McColl, K.E.L., Wallace, A.M., Moore, M.R., Thompson, G.G. and Goldberg, A. (1982) Alterations in haem biosynthesis during the female menstrual cycle: Studies in normal subjects and patients with acute intermittent porphyria. *Clinical Science*, **62**, 183–191.
9. Meyer, U.A., Strand, L.J., Doss, M., Rees, A.C. and Marver, H.S. (1972) Intermittent acute porphyrika – demonstration of a genetic defect in porphobilinogen metabolism. *New England Journal of Medicine*, **286**, 1277–1286.
10. Moore, M.R. and McColl, K.E.L. (1987) Drugs and the acute porphyrias. *Bulletino Dell'instituto Dermatologico S. Gallicano*, **13**, 151–158.

11. Parikh, R.K. and Moore, M.R. (1978) The effects of certain anaesthetic agents on the activity of rat hepatic delta aminolaevulinate synthase. *British Journal of Anaesthesia*, **50**, 1099–1103.
12. Watson, C.J., Dhar, G.J., Bossemaier, I., Cardinal, R. and Petryko, Z.J. (1973) Effect of haematin in acute porphyric relapse. *Annals of Internal Medicine*, **79**, 80–92.
13. Yeung Laiwah, A.C., Moore, M.R. and Goldberg, A. (1987) Pathogenesis of acute porphyria. *Quarterly Journal of Medicine*, **63**, 377–392.

SKIN DISEASE IN GASTROENTEROLOGY

W.G. Phillips and J.R. Marsden

It is important to recognize the cutaneous signs found in association with many gastrointestinal disorders as these can greatly facilitate diagnosis and management. The dermatological manifestations described in this section are also cross-referenced to other sections of this book.

INHERITED DISORDERS

POLYPOSES

Familial adenomatous polyposis (*see also* Chapter 4)

Probands of familial adenomatous polyposis (FAP) usually present with either extraintestinal manifestations in childhood or intestinal lesions as young adults. Multiple epidermoid cysts (commonly misnamed sebaceous cysts) appear as smooth dome-shaped swellings within the skin, sometimes with a central punctum. Their diameter ranges from a few millimetres to several centimetres. Osteomas of the skull and jaw and dental abnormalities should be sought through appropriate radiographs. Osteomas are present in the majority of patients but rarely cause problems. Fundi should be examined for hypertrophy of the retinal pigment epithelium which is present in at least 90% of affected individuals. DNA marker linkage analysis should be used in addition to clinical screening in order to quantify the probability of the familial adenomatous polyposis gene being present in each family member.[14]

Peutz–Jeghers syndrome (*see also* Chapter 3)

Peutz–Jeghers syndrome is an autosomal dominant disorder characterized by mucocutaneous melanin pigmentation and polyposis of the gastrointestinal tract. The skin lesions are pigmented macules (lentigines) on the buccal mucosa, lips (*Figure 8.17*), around the mouth and sometimes on the dorsum of fingers and toes. Lesions are usually several millimetres in diameter; they may be present at birth or develop in early childhood. The lentigines fade with age and may disappear, whilst those on the buccal mucosa persist.

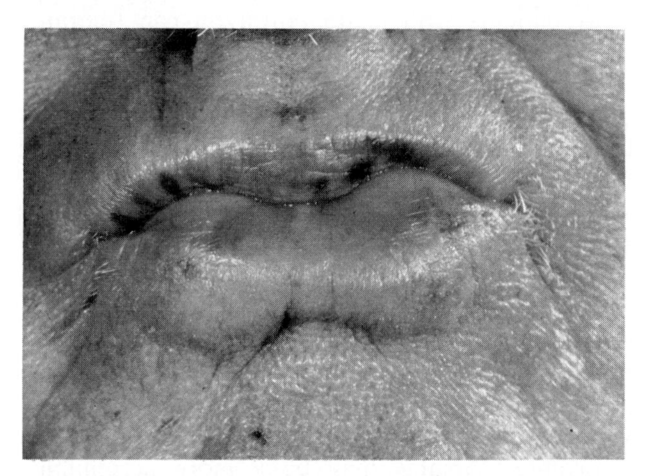

Figure 8.17 Pigmented macules on the lips of a patient with Peutz–Jeghers syndrome.

Recent reports suggest an increased incidence of gastrointestinal and other malignancies in patients with Peutz–Jeghers syndrome.[21] Therefore, once Peutz–Jeghers syndrome has been identified in a proband, other family members should be screened for cutaneous signs of the disorder and, if found to be affected, should receive genetic counselling. In addition to gastroenterological follow-up, female patients require careful gynaecological surveillance for the early detection of ovarian and cervical neoplasms.[8,13]

VASCULAR MALFORMATIONS

Hereditary haemorrhagic telangiectasia (Osler–Weber–Rendu syndrome (see also Chapter 5)

This autosomal dominant disorder is characterized by telangiectasia of the skin, mucous membranes,

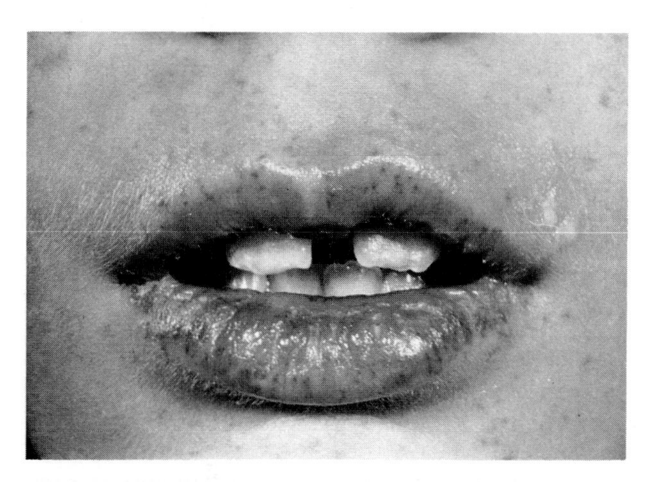

Figure 8.18 Hereditary haemorrhagic telangiectasia showing perioral telangiectasia.

gastrointestinal tract and other viscera. Skin lesions are usually macular telangiectasia a few millimetres in diameter which appear after puberty and increase in number with age. They are found on the lips, face, fingers, oral and nasal mucous membranes, and are prone to ulceration and haemorrhage (*Figure 8.18*). Spider naevi and linear telangiectasis may also be found, as may pulmonary arteriovenous fistulas, ectatic hepatic vessels and vascular malformations of the central nervous system.

Patients present with epistaxis, haematemesis, haemoptysis, melaena, haematuria or iron-deficiency anaemia. Less common presentations occur as a result of pulmonary arteriovenous fistulas in childhood (dyspnoea on exertion, cyanosis, clubbing) or with septic emboli complicating such a lesion. Subarachnoid haemorrhage from berry aneurysms, and other consequences of vascular malformations of the central nervous system also occur. The diagnosis is usually made on the basis of a family history, cutaneous lesions and haemorrhage.

Patients should be investigated to exclude an associated coagulopathy which may be von Willebrand's disease.[2] Therapy is primarily supportive although oestrogens may be of benefit in some patients.[16]

Blue rubber bleb naevus syndrome

This rare disorder presents in infancy or childhood with cyanotic, rubbery, lobulated swellings (*Figure 8.19*) up to several centimetres in diameter protruding from the skin of the trunk and proximal part of the limbs. Familial cases have been reported.[38] The lesions may be tender and empty on gentle compression. Similar lesions occur in the gastrointestinal tract and can cause recurrent gastrointestinal bleeding.

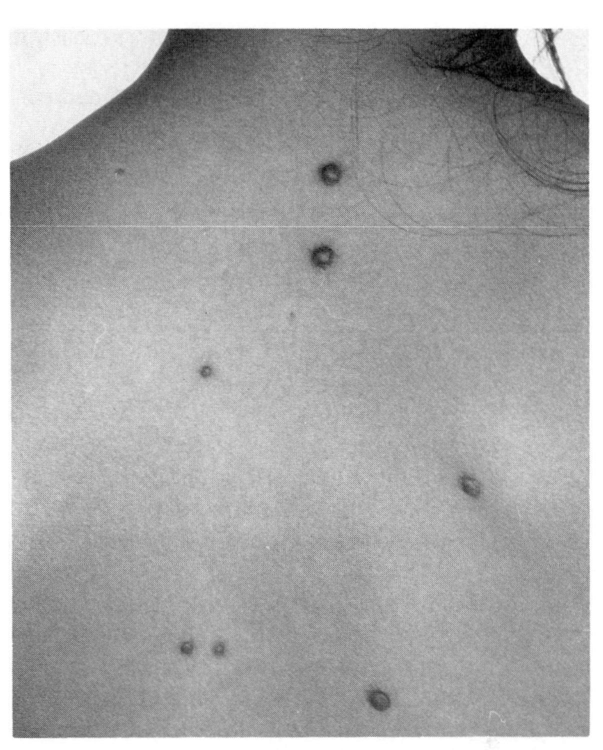

Figure 8.19 Rubbery cyanotic swellings which empty with gentle pressure on the back of a patient with blue rubber bleb naevus syndrome.

CONNECTIVE TISSUE DISORDERS

Ehlers–Danlos syndrome

Ehlers–Danlos syndrome is a term covering a group of diseases characterized by hyperextensibility of skin and joints, and poor wound healing. Umbilical, inguinal and hiatus herniation are common. Easy bruising, very fragile skin, gastrointestinal bleeding, intestinal perforation and arterial rupture are particular features of the very rare Ehlers–Danlos syndrome type IV, which has autosomal dominant and autosomal recessive forms that are both due to a defect in the synthesis of type III collagen.[32] Arteriography should be avoided where possible for the investigation of gastrointestinal bleeding because of an increased risk of arterial dissection and arterial rupture.

Pseudoxanthoma elasticum

This rare group of genetic disorders is characterized by progressive calcification and degeneration of elastin fibres in skin, retina, medium-size and small arteries. It is present in 0.6 per 100 000 population. Clinical signs develop in the second or third decades and may be found in patients presenting with gastrointestinal bleeding – a well recognized but in-

Table 8.10 The characteristics of the four types of pseudoxanthoma

Type	*Mode of inheritance*	*Gastrointestinal bleeding (%)*	*Skin*	*Vascular*	*Eyes*
1	Autosomal dominant	8	Peau d'orange flexural	Severe	Severe
2	Autosomal dominant	3.8	Yellow maccules	Infrequent	Mild
3	Recessive	15.8	Peau d'orange flexural	Moderate	Moderate
4	Recessive	–	–	?	Nil

frequent complication. Pope subclassified pseudoxanthoma elasticum into four types on the basis of the mode of inheritance and the clinical features (*Table 8.10*).[32]

The neck, axillary folds, umbilicus, groin, penis and facial folds are affected by infiltrative yellowish dermal papules or plaques resembling xanthomas. In several affected patients the skin becomes loose and inelastic (*Figure 8.20*). Histological examination shows fragmentation and calcification of elastic fibres in the deep and mid-dermis. Angioid streaks result from breaks in Bruch's membrane and are present in most affected subjects. These grey streaks are larger in diameter than the retinal vessels and radiate from the optic disc. Retinal ischaemia with consequent neovascularization, haemorrhage and fibrosis may lead to blindness. This disorder can be treated with laser photocoagulation in its early stages and routine ophthalmological review is required. Fragmentation of the elastin in the media of arteries with surrounding oedema may result in renovascular hypertension, absent or reduced peripheral pulses, and ischaemic heart disease. Patients should be reviewed regularly to detect and treat hypertension, and to optimize other cardiovascular risk factors.

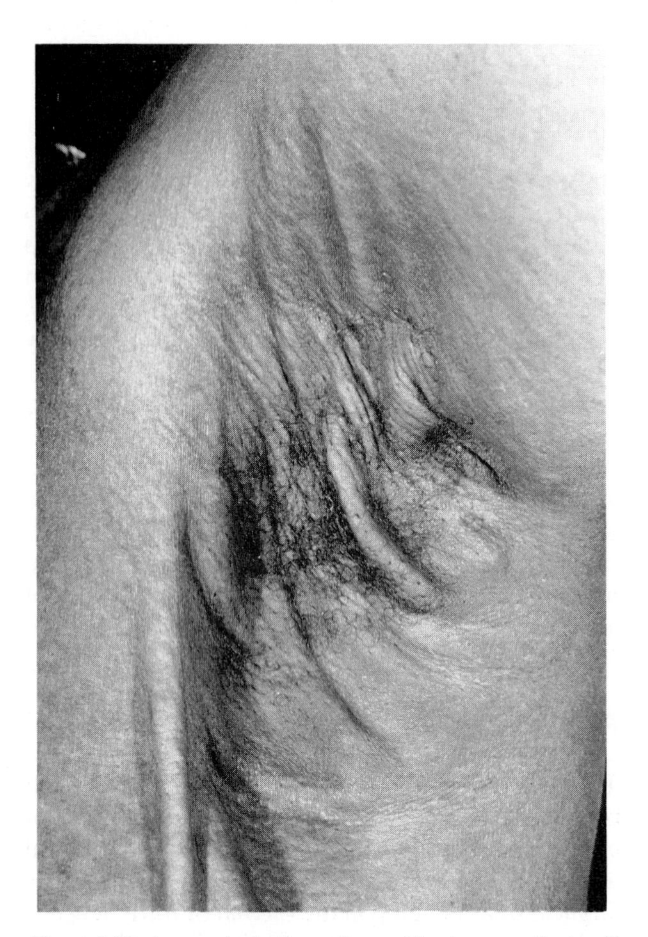

Figure 8.20 Loose inelastic axillary skin in a patient with pseudoxanthoma elasticum.

Gastrointestinal bleeding may occur either as a result of other pathologies, such as hiatus hernia or peptic ulcer disease, or as the result of spontaneous rupture of diseased submucosal vessels in otherwise normal mucosa.[5] Haematemesis is more common in affected females than in males and is especially common in pregnancy. Patients should be managed with particular care in view of the high incidence of ischaemic heart disease and thus their poor tolerance of hypovolaemia.

METABOLIC

Haemochromatosis (*see also* page 1281)

Generalized hyperpigmentation occurs in over 90% of patients. The skin colour may be bronze or blue–grey due to the relative increase of melanin and haemosiderin in the skin. Hyperpigmentation is accentuated on sun-exposed areas and on the genitalia, nipples, flexures and scars. Mucous membrane involvement is seen in a minority of patients and may resemble those changes seen in Addison's disease. The hyperpigmentation may appear before cirrhosis and diabetes develop, when diagnosis and treatment reduce morbidity and mortality. Later cutaneous changes include those seen in cirrhosis.

MALABSORPTION

Acrodermatitis enteropathica

This rare autosomal recessive disorder is the result of zinc malabsorption.

Clinical features

The clinical presentation varies with age but there is a basic triad of signs: dermatitis, diarrhoea and alopecia. Symptoms occur within a few weeks of birth in bottle-fed infants and shortly after weaning in breast-fed infants. The dermatitis is a progressively severe eczematous eruption particularly around the mouth, anus, scalp, perineum, hands and feet, often complicated by secondary infection. Paronychia is prominent as is involvement of the creases on palms and soles. Other symptoms include anorexia, diarrhoea, irritability, failure to thrive, anaemia and recurrent infections.[40] Rare features include photophobia, hypo-osmia, hypogonadism and impaired wound healing.

The natural history of this disorder was 20% mortality in childhood, the remainder improving at puberty. Fertility was low in those who survived to adulthood and congenital malformations, especially affecting the central nervous system, were common in their offspring.[24]

Investigations

Zinc levels are usually low in serum, urine and hair but some patients with acrodermatitis enteropathica have normal serum zinc levels.[29] Radioactively-labelled zinc absorption tests are available which have greater specificity for acrodermatitis enteropathica. A therapeutic trial of zinc is useful if there is doubt as to the diagnosis.

Treatment

Treatment is with oral zinc sulphate elixir 100 mg daily, increasing to 400 mg daily.[30]

Hereditary angioneurotic oedema

This rare autosomal dominant disorder is caused by C1 esterase inhibitor deficiency and characterized by recurrent episodes of painful tender oedema affecting subcutaneous tissue, skin, oropharynx, larynx and gut. Acute laryngeal oedema can cause sudden death by asphyxia. The reduction in C1 esterase inhibitor activity allows excessive activation of the classic pathway of complement as evidenced by reduced levels of complement C4. Episodic subcutaneous oedema may occur spontaneously or after minor trauma via activation of factor XII.[20] It is distinguishable from idiopathic urticaria in which lesions develop within minutes; they are itchy, primarily involve the dermis and usually last less than 24 hours. Most patients have symptoms in childhood which deteriorate during adolescence and continue into adult life.

Intestinal oedema causes abdominal pain, diarrhoea and vomiting. Plain abdominal radiographs show marked separation of loops of small bowel due to mural oedema which may be sufficiently intense to produce intestinal obstruction. It is important to make this diagnosis to spare the patient an unnecessary laparotomy and the risks of acute laryngeal oedema caused by endotracheal intubation.

Patients usually have low levels of C1 esterase inhibitor as well as of complement C4 and a low value for the assay of the total haemolytic titre of complement (CH50); some have normal levels of C1 esterase inhibitor but its function is impaired. C4 and CH50 are still reduced in these patients.

C1 esterase inhibitor concentrate is the treatment of choice for laryngeal oedema.[1] It has yet to gain a product licence and is only available on a named patient basis in the United Kingdom. Fresh frozen plasma is an alternative although it also supplies substrate to sustain the complement cascade. Adrenaline, corticosteroids and antihistamines are ineffective. Long-term prophylaxis is important in view of the risk of laryngeal obstruction. The two groups of drugs used are inhibitors of plasminogen activation and androgen analogues. Tranexamic acid, one of the former, is well tolerated but less effective than stanozolol or danazol which increase the concentration of C1 esterase inhibitor.

Acquired C1 inhibitor deficiency occurs very rarely in association with an underlying malignancy, particularly lymphoma.

NEUROFIBROMATOSIS 1

This autosomal dominant disorder is occasionally associated with gastrointestinal manifestations including neurofibromas, duodenal carcinoids and rhabdomyosarcomas.[25] It is distinguished from neurofibromatosis 2, the dominant feature of which is the development of acoustic neuromas. Cutaneous signs of neurofibromatosis 1 (NF1) include the presence of six or more café-au-lait patches larger than 5 mm before puberty or 15 mm after puberty, axillary or inguinal freckling, and cutaneous neurofibromas.[17]

DERMATOLOGICAL ASSOCIATIONS OF INFLAMMATORY BOWEL DISEASE

ERYTHEMA NODOSUM

Clinical features

This clinical syndrome consists of acute tender erythematous nodules involving skin and subcutaneous tissue often associated with fever, malaise and arthropathy. Lesions usually range from 2 to 5 cm in diameter, although they may be much larger (*Figure 8.21*). They are typically found on the anterior and lateral aspects of the lower limbs, although they may occur elsewhere on the skin including the arms, neck and face. The colour of the nodules evolves from erythema in the first week through a violaceous blue in the second week to a yellow bruise before they disappear without scarring by 6 weeks.

Investigations

There may be no abnormality on routine laboratory testing although erythrocyte sedimentation rate is often elevated. A skin biopsy is only indicated if it is not possible to reach a confident diagnosis on clinical grounds. An ellipse of skin should be taken through the edge of a lesion less than 5 days old and include associated subcutaneous fat. Histology will show varying involvement of small veins, interlobular septae and lobular fat with either an acute or chronic inflammatory infiltrate.

Investigation is then directed towards identifying any of the known precipitating factors which include the following:

Gastrointestinal
- ulcerative colitis
- Crohn's disease
- Behçet's syndrome
- *Yersinia enterocolitica* infection
- leptospirosis
- tuberculosis

Other
- streptococcal infections
- sarcoidosis
- leprosy
- infectious mononucleosis
- sulphonamides
- radiotherapy
- psittacosis
- cat-scratch disease
- lymphogranuloma venereum
- histoplasmosis
- coccidioidomycosis
- blastomycosis
- lymphoma
- leukaemia

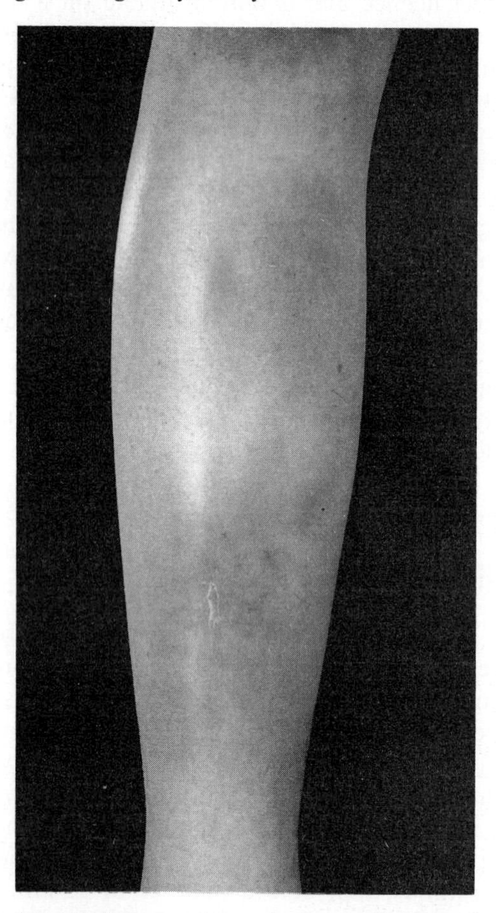

Figure 8.21 Erythema nodosum: tender erythematous nodules and plaques on the shins.

In the United Kingdom, routine investigation includes a full blood count and film, biochemical indices of renal and hepatic function, throat swab for bacterial culture, antistreptolysin O titre, and chest radiograph. A weak correlation exists between the presence of erythema nodosum and the activity of associated inflammatory bowel disease.

Non-steroidal anti-inflammatory drugs relieve fever, pain from cutaneous lesions and arthralgia. Oral corticosteroids are very effective in shortening the course of the illness, but should only be used in circumstances where they will not obscure the diagnosis of or exacerbate any underlying disease.

PYODERMA GANGRENOSUM

Clinical features

This uncommon skin disease presents with one or more painful erythematous nodules or pustules in the skin, which break down to form rapidly enlarg-

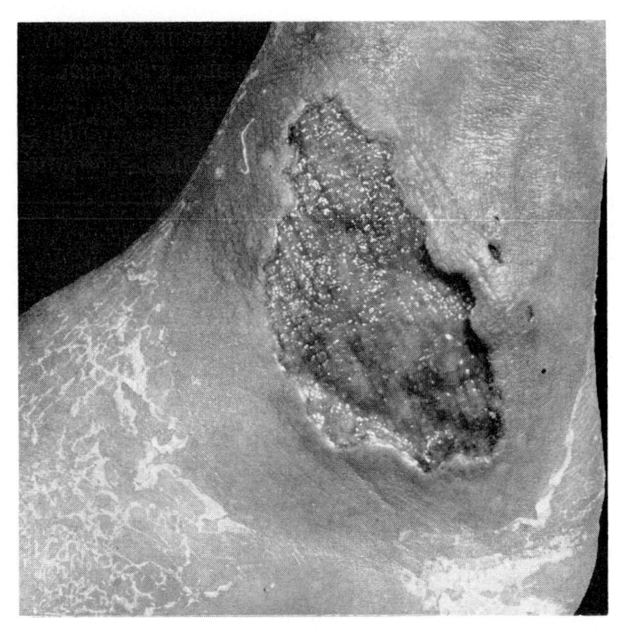

Figure 8.22 Rapidly enlarging ulcers with irregular purple borders undermined by a necrotic base in a patient with pyoderma gangrenosum.

ing ulcers with elevated borders or irregular purplish tissue undermined by a necrotic base (*Figure 8.22*). There is a marked erythema around the advancing edge and pus may be expressed from this. Fever and malaise are common. Lesions are most frequently seen on the lower limbs, buttocks, trunk and face but they may occur anywhere on the skin, including stoma sites as well as sites of trauma (pathergy). The incidence of pyoderma gangrenosum in patients with inflammatory bowel disease is between 1% and 5%, usually being found in patients with active gastrointestinal disease. The relative frequencies of disorders associated with pyoderma gangrenosum reported in published data vary considerably and can be divided into common and uncommon associations, as follows:

Disorders commonly associated with pyoderma gangrenosum:
- ulcerative colitis
- Crohn's disease
- rheumatoid arthritis
- seronegative rheumatoid-like arthritis
- IgA monoclonal gammopathy

Disorders occasionally associated with pyoderma gangrenosum:
- myeloma
- leukaemia
- myelofibrosis
- Behçet's syndrome
- chronic active hepatitis
- primary biliary cirrhosis

Investigations

The following tests should be performed: full blood count and film (which often shows an elevated white cell count), indices of renal and hepatic function, rheumatoid factor, plasma protein electrophoresis, urinary Bence-Jones protein and hepatitis serology. Investigation of the bowel for inflammatory disease should be performed if there are suggestive symptoms and if no other predisposing cause is evident. Skin biopsy from the margin of the spreading lesion shows dense infiltration of the dermis by neutrophils, abscess formation and necrosis. There is associated dermal oedema, haemorrhage and thrombosis of small and medium-size vessels.

Treatment

Intralesional corticosteroids are sometimes effective but are very painful to administer. Oral prednisolone 50–100 mg/day is usually effective in relieving pain and stopping progression of the lesions, often within a few days when the dose can be reduced and the drug stopped on healing. Patients who have not responded to oral prednisolone should either be treated with pulsed methyl prednisolone 1G intravenously for 5 days,[27] or by the addition of dapsone or azathioprine. Sulphasalazine, sulphapyridine and minocycline have also been used; the efficacy of these agents is not yet clear. Topical treatment is directed at keeping the ulcers clean and free from secondary infection.

In patients with pyoderma gangrenosum secondary to inflammatory bowel disease the effect of resection of diseased bowel is unpredictable, and it should not be performed unless there are other specific indications.[37] The clinical course of pyoderma gangrenosum is variable as is the steroid requirement.

CUTANEOUS VASCULITIS

Cutaneous vasculitis can occur in association with active inflammatory bowel disease. This usually presents as palpable purpura on the lower limbs. Histological examination of the skin shows a necrotizing vasculitis. This is not usually associated with vasculitis in other organs and having excluded other causes of necrotizing cutaneous vasculitis (see list below), management should be directed towards controlling the activity of the inflammatory bowel disease. Causes of necrotizing cutaneous vasculitis include the following:

Drug reactions

Infection, e.g. hepatitis B, herpes simplex virus, cytomegalovirus
Henoch–Schönlein purpura
Rheumatoid arthritis
Systemic lupus erythematosus
Sjögren's syndrome
Wegener's granulomatosis
Polyarteritis nodosum
Mixed cryoglobulinaemia
Tumour-associated
Idiopathic

SWEET'S SYNDROME (acute febrile neutrophilic dermatosis)

This rare disorder is characterized by the sudden onset of painful red oedematous papules which coalesce into plaques associated with fever, arthralgia, marked malaise and a polymorph leukocytosis. Histological examination reveals a neutrophilic infiltrate of the lower dermis with perivascular leukocytoclasis. The most important association of Sweet's syndrome is with acute myeloid leukaemia, although there are reports of its association with inflammatory bowel disease.[3]

CUTANEOUS CROHN'S DISEASE (see Chapter 7)

Perianal, oral and enterocutaneous Crohn's disease are discussed in other chapters. Cutaneous Crohn's disease is a rare condition characterized by erythematous nodules, plaques or ulcers with granulomatous histology. These occur on skin distant from the gastrointestinal tract in patients with gastrointestinal Crohn's disease. Cutaneous disease usually coincides with active Crohn's disease elsewhere. Treatment is with potent topical steroids or systemic steroids;[35] metronidazole has also been used successfully.

OTHER INFLAMMATORY DISORDERS

DERMATITIS HERPETIFORMIS (see page 540)

This is a chronic pruritic papulovesicular disease associated with gluten intolerance in most, if not all, patients. It presents most frequently in the second to fourth decades of life although it may occur in children or the elderly. Itch is intense and may occur some hours before any lesion is visible on the skin. The primary lesions are vesicles or papules often grouped together in a manner reminiscent of herpes simplex. Lesions are distributed over the elbows, knees, lower back and shoulders. Secondary changes including excoriation and lichenification may dominate the clinical appearance.

Histological examination of early lesions shows neutrophil microabscesses in the dermal papillae which progress to subepidermal blisters. Immunofluorescence of unaffected skin (usually taken from the buttock) shows granular deposits of IgA in the dermal papillae; fibrin, IgG, IgM and C3 may also be found.

Dermatitis herpetiformis is strongly associated with coeliac disease. In a recent review of 86 patients taking a normal diet, 25% of patients had subtotal villous atrophy, 50% of patients had partial villous atrophy and 25% of patients had normal jejunal biopsies.[19] Two patients were identified with clinical and biochemical evidence of malabsorption.

Dapsone at an initial adult dose of 100–200 mg once daily relieves itch within 24 hours. It prevents new lesions from developing but has no effect on the presence of IgA in the dermal papillae. The dose can then be reduced to the minimum necessary to prevent symptoms, sometimes as little as 25 mg weekly, although this is very variable. Symptoms recur rapidly after discontinuing treatment. For those patients who are unable to take dapsone, sulphapyridine 1–1.5 g daily is an alternative.

Strict adherence to a gluten-free diet will produce clinical remission in 6 months to 1 year.[33] Intestinal lesions will respond to gluten withdrawal in the same way as coeliac disease. Following such a diet requires motivation and some patients decide to take dapsone and continue with a normal diet.

There is an increase in the incidence of small bowel lymphoma. It is probable, but unproven, that a gluten-free diet may reduce this risk in dermatitis herpetiformis as has been found in coeliac disease.

CRONKHITE–CANADA SYNDROME

In 1955 Cronkhite and Canada described a syndrome of generalized gastrointestinal polyposis, hyperpigmentation, hair loss and nail atrophy.[10] This is a sporadic disorder of unknown aetiology. Patients are usually over the age of 50 years when they present with symptoms, secondary to polyposis or protein-losing enteropathy such as diarrhoea, weight loss and recurrent abdominal pain. Pigmentary abnormalities develop several months later and most commonly consist of lentigines on the face, palms and soles, although other areas of skin may be involved. Patchy alopecia, thinning and splitting of the nail plate and onycholysis may occur before the development of overt gastrointestinal disease. The prognosis is poor; approximately 40% of published cases have died from cachexia, postoperative complications and complications of debility such as bronchopneumonia and thromboembolic disease. Nutritional support is helpful. Corticosteroids, anabolic steroids and antibiotics have all been associated with remission in limited numbers of cases. Surgery is performed for complications such as gastroduodenal ulceration and polyps causing obstruction or other symptoms.[11]

SYSTEMIC SCLEROSIS (*see also* page 1230)

Cutaneous signs include oedema, tightening of the skin which loses its elasticity initially over the fingers (sclerodactyly), hands and face, telangiectasia, subcutaneous calcification and dilated nail-fold capillaries. The dermatological signs are usually marked by the time the patients develop dysphagia or other gastroenterological disorders.

POLYARTERITIS NODOSA (*see also* page 1240)

This is a multisystem disorder that can involve both the skin and gut. Livedo reticularis (a mottled cyanosis affecting the skin of the trunk and limbs), palpable purpura and vasculitic ulcers on the lower limbs are common. Skin histology shows leukocytoclastic vasculitis of dermal vessels, with more characteristic necrotizing vasculitis of muscular arteries in the deep dermis or subcutaneous fat.

HENOCH–SCHÖNLEIN PURPURA

For this condition, see page 1244)

BOWEL BYPASS SYNDROME (*see also* Chapter 3, page 666, 'Jejunoileal bypass')

This is characterized by recurrent fever, polyarthritis, tenosynovitis and skin lesions in patients who have had jejunoileal bypass surgery for morbid obesity. Erythematous papules up to 1 cm in diameter evolve through vesicles to pustules. Acral distribution of the lesions is common although they may be generalized. Histological examination of the skin reveals a dense neutrophil infiltrate in the dermis. Erythema nodosum and cryoglobulinaemia can also occur. The disorder is thought to be a response to bacterial peptidoglycans and responds to treatment with tetracycline, metronidazole or low-dose steroids.[15]

AMYLOIDOSIS (*see also* Chapter 3, page 591, 'Amyloidosis')

Cutaneous amyloid deposition may be found in association with systemic light chain amyloidosis. Such amyloidosis occurs in association with multiple myeloma and as a primary disorder. Involvement of the heart, kidneys, tongue, bowel and skin are seen. Common skin signs include purpura and waxy papules and plaques, often around the eyes and misdiagnosed as xanthalasmas. Alopecia and bullous lesions are rare. The tongue is enlarged and stiffened by amyloid infiltration. When suspected, the diagnosis should be histologically proven and the patient investigated for multiple myeloma. Other forms of systemic amyloidosis may involve the skin histologically but clinical manifestations are rare; cutaneous amyloidosis can occur without systemic involvement.

ACUTE PANCREATITIS

Acute pancreatitis is associated with bruising in the flanks (Grey Turner's sign) and around the umbilicus (Cullen's sign). Lobular panniculitis without vasculitis presents with tender subcutaneous nodules similar to erythema nodosum; it can occur as a complication of acute pancreatitis although there are numerous other causes.

PATTERSON–KELLY–PLUMMER–VINSON SYNDROME (*see also* Chapter 1, page 11 'Mouth')

Cutaneous signs consist of angular stomatitis, pale atrophic facial skin and koilonychia, whilst the buccal mucosa is also pale and atrophic. The tongue may show glossitis, papillary atrophy and white patches (leukoplakia).

TYLOSIS

Palmoplantar keratosis is a manifestation of several genodermatoses. The well-known association of palmoplantar keratosis with oesophageal carcinoma is based on reports of only two kindreds. Patients without a family history of associated oesophageal cancer are not at increased risk.

MASTOCYTOSIS

This disorder is due to a pathological proliferation of mast cells. Cutaneous lesions consist of brown–yellow macules or patches which become erythematous and urticariate within a few minutes of gentle scratching (Darier's sign). Clinical involvement is confined to the skin in over 90% of children and resolves spontaneously before adolescence.[39] Mastocytosis is not self-limiting in adults who are more likely to have diffuse cutaneous lesions and develop symptomatic systemic involvement. Systemic symptoms consist of paroxysmal headache, flushing, hypotension, vomiting, diarrhoea and wheezing due to the release of histamine, heparin and prostaglandin D_2. Organ infiltration by mast cells can cause weight loss, malabsorption, hepatomegaly, portal hypertension, lytic bone lesions and pancytopenia. Mast cell leukaemia develops in a small minority of patients.

KAPOSI'S SARCOMA (*see also* Chapter 9, page 1484)

This malignant neoplasm arises from endothelial cells. It is strongly associated with human immunodeficiency virus (HIV) infection. Skin lesions are typically dermal papules and plaques which are purple–red in Caucasians and purple–blue in dark-skinned races (*Figure 8.23*). Similar lesions may be seen in the mouth. Kaposi's sarcoma may involve other organs including the bowel, where it is a cause of gastrointestinal bleeding.

PRIMARY MALIGNANT MELANOMA

Although the primary neoplasm usually arises in the skin, it can occur in the anal canal (1% of all malignant melanomas). Metastatic disease frequently involves the liver and small bowel although it may involve any part of the gastrointestinal tract. Unfortunately, when visceral spread has occurred the prognosis is very poor and treatment is palliative.

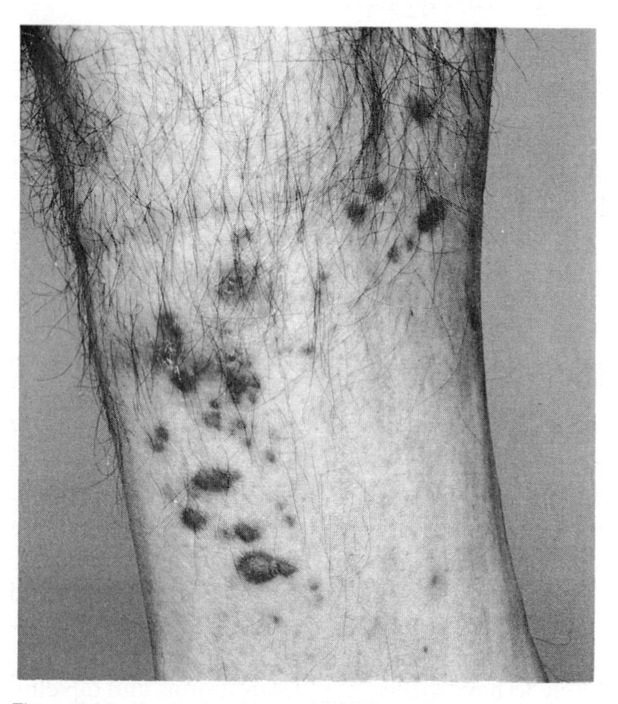

Figure 8.23 Purple dermal papules of Kaposi's sarcoma.

NON-METASTATIC EFFECTS

DERMATOMYOSITIS

Dermatomyositis is a rare inflammatory disorder involving skin and proximal muscles. The systemic manifestations are discussed earlier under 'polymyositis/dermatomyositis'. Oedema and heliotrope erythema of periorbital and forehead skin is the characteristic skin sign. This is usually combined with an erythematous maculopapular eruption over the forehead, neck and extensor aspects of the extremities. Gottron's sign consists of localization of this rash over the extensor aspect of the knuckles, often associated with similar lesions over the elbows and knees. The proximal nail folds show erythema, telangiectasia and haemorrhage whilst splinter haemorrhages may be present in the nail bed.

ACANTHOSIS NIGRICANS

This disorder is characterized by the presence of symmetrical, velvety, grey–brown plaques often with pedunculated skin tags in the axillae, groins, nape of the neck and mucous membranes. When associated with malignancy, occult or otherwise, the onset tends to be rapid involving large areas of skin and mucous membranes. Other causes are associated with insidious onset and localized disease, causes including the following:

- Idiopathic
- Obesity
- Endocrine
  - insulin-resistant diabetes mellitus
  - polycystic ovary syndrome
  - Addison's disease
  - pituitary tumours
  - pinealoma
- Drugs
  - Nicotinic acid
  - glucocorticoids
  - diethylstilboestrol
- Adenocarcinoma
  - 80% intra-abdominal
  - 60% stomach
- Lymphoma

Unfortunately, the majority of patients with tumour-associated acanthosis nigricans have advanced disease at the time of presentation.[34]

Thrombophlebitis migrans is associated with carcinoma of the stomach (Trousseau's sign), pancreas, prostate, colon, lung, liver, gallbladder and ovary, as well as haematological malignancies.

NECROLYTIC MIGRATORY ERYTHEMA

This rare dermatosis consists of superficial annular or arcuate erythematous lesions with peripheral blistering, epidermal necrosis and scaling. Lesions occur around body orifices, in the flexures, on the trunk and limbs. There is usually an associated stomatitis. Skin histology shows epidermal necrosis with dyskeratotic cells in the superficial epidermis. Although this eruption is classically found in patients with glucagonomas, similar lesions have been described in patients with cirrhosis, chronic pancreatitis,[22] zinc deficiency and essential fatty acid deficiency.

Investigation and treatment should be directed towards the underlying glucagonoma as outlined in detail in Chapter 11, Tumours of the Endocrine Pancreas. Zinc and essential fatty acids should be measured to exclude their deficiency disorders.

HYPERTRICHOSIS LANUGINOSA

Increased growth of lanugo hair initially on the face and ears, but spreading to the rest of the skin, is a very rare complication of malignancy which can occur in association with gastrointestinal cancer.

SISTER JOSEPH'S NODULE

Sister Joseph's nodule occurs when an intra-abdominal adenocarcinoma metastasizes to the umbilicus. The primary lesion is usually found in the large bowel and is believed to have metastasized via the falciform ligament.

CUTANEOUS METASTASES

These occur from many gastrointestinal tumours. They are usually seen in patients with advanced disease but can be a presenting feature. They are skin-coloured, subcutaneous or pink dermal papules or nodules.

ACQUIRED ICTHYOSIS

This disorder occurs in association with lymphomas. It is occasionally a presenting feature although it more commonly occurs when disease is advanced. Other rare causes include carcinomas of the lung, cervix and breast, Kaposi's sarcoma and leiomyosarcoma.

INFECTIONS

HERPES ZOSTER

Before the characteristic segmental erythematous macules, papules and vesicles appear, herpes zoster presents with an unusual burning or stinging pain exacerbated by light touch of the affected dermatome. It is important to be aware of the possibility of an underlying neoplasm or immunosuppressive disorder in patients with widespread lesions.

ORAL DISEASE AND THE SKIN (see Chapter 1)

ORAL ULCERATION

Behçet's syndrome is covered in detail on page 1235. Painful orogenital and anal ulceration is a common feature. Ulcers affect any part of the oral mucosa. Genital ulceration, erythema nodosum, pyoderma gangrenosum and thrombophlebitis may all be seen, as may erythematous papules and pustules. Pathergy may be demonstrable with skin lesions appearing at the sites where the skin has been damaged, such as by cannula insertion; the ability to demonstrate pathergy depends on needle size and requires at least a gauge 20 needle.

LUPUS ERYTHEMATOSUS

The butterfly rash of lupus erythematosus may be isolated or associated with systemic disease including gastrointestinal involvement (see page 1237).

LICHEN PLANUS (see page 1236)

This common disorder of adults presents with 2–10 mm diameter, flat-topped polygonal papules whose violaceous surface is crossed by fine interlacing white lines known as Whickam's striae. Papules are found on the flexor aspect of the wrists, the lower limbs, the trunk, the penis and scalp where they may cause scarring alopecia. They may occur at sites of minor skin trauma (Koebner's phenomenon). Nail changes range from longitudinal ridging to complete destruction of the nail.

Approximately two-thirds of patients presenting with cutaneous lesions also have disease affecting the oral mucous membrane, whilst only 30% of patients presenting with oral disease will have skin signs at presentation. The oral lesions are divided into four groups: (1) asymptomatic hyperkeratotic papules and lace-like lesions of the buccal mucosa; (2) vesicobullous lesions; (3) atrophic lesions that are often asymptomatic and usually found on the tongue and gums; and (4) erosive lesions that are painful, usually extensive and respond poorly to treatment. Similar lesions can occur on perianal skin.

Treatment with topical intralesional or systemic steroids is effective in relieving itch and may hasten healing.

PEMPHIGUS VULGARIS (see page 1247)

This is a chronic autoimmune disorder causing blistering and erosion of skin and mucous membranes by impairing keratinocyte–keratinocyte adhesion.

Clinical features

It is most often seen in patients in their forties and fifties although it may affect any age group. Patients frequently present with flaccid blisters containing clear fluid on the mucosal surfaces which rupture easily to form painful erosions, often covered by a yellow–grey sloughy membrane. The patient may be unaware of the blistering phase and present complaining of mouth ulcers. Uninvolved mucosa looks normal but may show Nikolsky's sign (formation of bullae on pressure). Similar flaccid bullae and erosions occur on the skin, pharynx, larynx, conjunctiva and perineum. Early diagnosis is important because delay in starting treatment may be associated with the development of much more extensive disease.

Investigations

A skin biopsy should be taken including a blister less than 24 hours old and perilesional skin. Histology shows suprabasal acantholysis (keratinocytes in the mid-epidermis failing to stick to each other) and bulla formation with a layer of intact basal cells on the basement membrane. Direct immunofluorescence of perilesional mucous membrane or skin reveals intercellular immunoglobulin, usually IgG, in the prickle cell region of the epidermis. Indirect immunofluorescence commonly shows a circulating antibody to the intercellular cement of normal squamous epithelium.

Treatment

Corticosteroids have revolutionized the prognosis in this disease which was usually fatal before their introduction. Oral prednisolone may be started at an initial dose of 60 mg daily; there is no convincing evidence that the very large doses sometimes prescribed are any more effective. Meticulous nursing care is important for those with extensive lesions whether in the mouth, skin or conjunctiva. Once established lesions are healing and no new lesions are emerging, the dose of prednisolone should be tapered to a maintenance dose. Immunomodulatory and immunosuppressive agents, such as sodium aurothiomalate and azathioprine respectively, may be used alone or as steroid-sparing agents. Relapse is common necessitating long maintenance therapy.

BULLOUS PEMPHIGOID

Bullous pemphigoid is characterized by 1–5 cm, tense, fluid-filled subepidermal bullae which may also be blood-filled. There is linear staining of the basement membrane on direct immunofluorescence for immunoglobulin and complement C3. Unlike pemphigus vulgaris, this disorder does not present with oral ulceration, although bullous lesions of the oral mucosa develop in up to 30% of patients at some time. Cutaneous manifestations dominate the clinical course and management.

PERIANAL SKIN DISEASES

Many skin diseases affect the perianal skin. Here are briefly considered some of the more common and important conditions, many of which may also be found at stoma sites.

Irritant and allergic contact dermatitis are important causes of pruritis ani. It is important to take a detailed history of what applications the patient is using on the perianal skin. Patients may not volunteer such information and may not realize that both over-the-counter remedies, especially antiseptic and local anaesthetic creams, as well as prescribed medications, can cause contact dermatitis. Contact allergic dermatitis requires patch-testing for accurate diagnosis.

Lichen sclerosus et atrophicus has a predilection for the vulva, penis and perianal skin. Early lesions are sharply demarcated, ivory-coloured, flat or atrophic macules with fine cigarette paper surface. In males this may progress to the thickened fibrotic foreskin of balanitis xerotica obliterans. Histological examination reveals an atrophic epidermis with a loss of the normal rete ridges and a hyalinized oedematous dermis. Potent topical steroid therapy may both relieve itch and improve the appearance but should only be used with dermatological supervision. There is an increased risk of cutaneous squamous carcinoma at involved sites.

Psoriasis should be suspected when a clearly defined shiny erythematous plaque is found on the perianal skin. Evidence of psoriasis should be sought on skin elsewhere, particularly other flexures, umbilicus, scalp, trunk, limbs and nails. Mild or moderately potent topical steroids improve symptoms but usually do not improve the disease.

Intertrigo is a non-specific inflammatory disorder found in areas where skin lies against skin and secondary infection occurs, particularly with *Candida* spp. Treatment should include simple hygienic measures combined with effective anticandidal treatment and mild topical steroids.

Lichen simplex chronicus is skin thickening due to persistent rubbing or scratching. This is a common finding in pruritus ani. The lesions are poorly defined lichenified plaques sometimes with excorations. An explanation that there is no serious skin disease present is important. A short course of potent topical steroids may be helpful. Long-term prevention of itching and scratching is rarely possible.

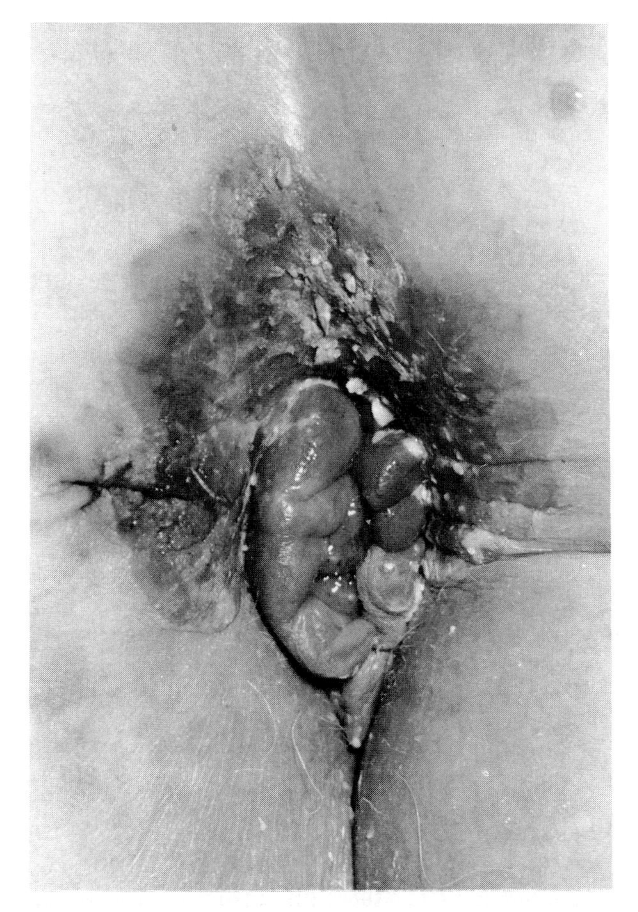

Figure 8.24 A clearly demarcated fixed scaly erythematous patch of perianal Paget's disease.

EXTRAMAMMARY PAGET'S DISEASE

This is a rare disorder of patients over 50 presenting with a slow-growing, clearly demarcated, itchy, scaly, erythematous patch, usually on the perineum. Histology shows intraepidermal infiltration of large, pale or eosinophilic tumour cells. Lesions which may extend on to the vaginal or anal mucosa are due to contiguous spread of a carcinoma that has arisen in a sweat gland, cervix, prostate, anus or rectum (*Figure 8.24*). Investigation should be directed to finding the underlying tumour. Surgical excision is the preferred treatment.

REFERENCES

1. Agostone, A. (1989) Inherited C1 inhibitor deficiency. *Complement and Inflammation*, **6**, 112–118.
2. Ahr, D.J., Rickles, F.R., Hoyer, L.W., O'Leary, D.S. and Conrad, M.E. (1977) Von Willebrand's disease and hemorrhagic telangiectasia: association of two complex disorders of haemostasis resulting in life threatening haemorrhage. *American Journal of Medicine*, **62**, 452–458.
3. Allegue, F., Soria, C., Munoz, Z.E., Gil, G.L., Freire, M.P. and Ledo, A. (1989) Neutrophilic dermatosis in inflammatory intestinal disease. *Revista Clinica Espanola (Madrid)*, **185**, 250–252.
4. Altman, A.R., Tschen, J.A. and Rice, L. (1989) Treatment of malignant carcinoid syndrome with a long-acting somatostatin analogue. *Archives of Dermatology*, **125**, 394–396.
5. Belli, A. and Cawthorne, S. (1988) Visceral angiographic findings in pseudoxanthoma elasticum. *British Journal of Radiology*, **61**, 368–371.
6. Bickers, D.R. and Pathak, M.A. (1987) The porphyrias. In: *Dermatology in General Medicine*, 3rd edn, pp. 1666–1715. (Ed.) Fitzpatrick, T.B., Eisen, A.Z., Wolff, K., Freedberg, I.M. and Austen, K.F. New York: McGraw-Hill.
7. Burg, G., Vieluf, D. and Stolz, W. (1989) Malignant atrophic papulosis. *Hautarzt*, **40**, 480–485.
8. Chen, K.T.K. (1986) Female genital tract tumors in Peutz–Jeghers syndrome. *Human Pathology*, **17**, 858–861.
9. Cox, N.H., Lawrence, C.L., Langtry, J.A.A. and Ive, A. (1990) Dermatomyositis. Disease associations and an evaluation of screening investigations for malignancy. *Archives of Dermatology*, **126**, 61–65.
10. Cronkhite, L.W. Jr and Canada, W.J. (1955) Generalised gastrointestinal polyposis. *New England Journal of Medicine*, **252**, 1011–1015.
11. Daniel, E.S., Shelly, L.L., Lewin, K.J., Ruprecht, R.M., Rajacich, G.M. and Schwabe, A.D. (1982) The Cronkhite–Canada syndrome. An analysis of

clinical and pathologic features and therapy in 55 patients. *Medicine (Baltimore)*, **61**, 293–309.
12. Dienstag, J.L., Rhodes, A.R., Bhan, A.K., Dvorak, A.M., Mihm, M.C. and Wands, J.R. (1979) Urticaria associated with acute viral hepatitis type B. Studies of pathogenesis. *Annals of Internal Medicine*, **89**, 34–40.
13. Dozois, R.R., Kempers, R.D., Dahlin, D.C. and Bartholomew, L.G. (1970) Ovarian tumors associated with the Peutz–Jeghers syndrome. *Annals of Surgery*, **172**, 233–238.
14. Dunlop, M.G., Wylie, A.H., Steel, C.M., Piris, J. and Evans, H.J. (1991) Linked DNA markers for presymptomatic diagnosis of familial adenomatous polyposis. *The Lancet*, **337**, 313–316.
15. Ely, P.H. (1980) The bowel bypass syndrome : a response to bacterial peptidoglycans. *Journal of the American Academy of Dermatology*, **2**, 473–487.
16. Flint, S.R., Keith, O. and Scully, C. (1988) Hereditary haemorrhagic telangiectasia : Family study and a review. *Oral Surgery*, **66**, 440–444.
17. Fryer, A.E. (1990) The management of neurofibromatosis. *Journal of Dermatological Treatment*, **1**, 137–141.
18. Gardner, E.J. (1951) A genetic and clinical study of intestinal polyposis, a predisposing factor for carcinoma of the colon and rectum. *American Journal of Clinical Genetics*, **3**, 167–176.
19. Gawkrodger, D.J., Ferguson, A. St C. and Barnetson, R. (1988) Nutritional status in patients with dermatitis herpetiformis. *American Journal of Clinical Nutrition*, **48**, 355–360.
20. Ghebrehiwet, B., Silverberg, M. and Kaplan, A.P. (1981) Activation of the classical pathway of compliment by the Hageman factor fragment. *Journal of Experimental Medicine*, **153** 665–676.
21. Giardelo, F.M., Welsh, F.B., Hamilton, S.R. *et al.* (1987) Increased risk of cancer in the Peutz–Jeghers syndrome. *New England Journal of Medicine*, **316**, 1511–1513.
22. Goodenberger, D.M., Lawley, T.J., Strober, W. *et al.* (1979) Necrolytic migratory erythema without glucagonoma. *Archives of Dermatology*, **115**, 1429–1432.
23. Graham-Brown, R.A., Sarkany, I. and Sherlock, S. (1982) Lichen planus and primary biliary cirrhosis. *British Journal of Dermatology*, **106**, 699–703.
24. Hurley, L. and Baly, D.L. (1982) The effects of zinc deficiency during pregnancy. In: *Clinical Biochemical and Nutritional Aspects of Trace Elements*, p. 145. (Ed.) Prasad, A.S. New York: Alan R. Liss.
25. Huson, S.M., Harper, P.S. and Compson, D.A.S. (1988) Von Recklinghausen neurofibromatosis : a clinical and population study in south east Wales. *Brain*, **111**, 1355–1381.
26. Jagelman, D.J. (1987) Extracolonic manifestations of familial polyposis coli. *Cancer Genetics and Cytogenetics*, **27**, 319–325.
27. Johnson, R.B. and Lazarus, G.S. (1982) Pulse therapy, therapeutic efficacy in the treatment of pyoderma gangrenosum. *Archives of Dermatology*, **118**, 76–84.
28. Lipkin, M., Scherf, S., Schecheter, L. and Brown, D. (1980) Memorial Hospital Registry of population groups at high risk for cancer of the large intestine: age onset of neoplasms. *Preventive Medicine*, **9**, 335–345.
29. Mack, D., Koletzko, B., Cunnane, S., Cutz, E. and Griffiths, A. (1989) Acrodermatitis enteropathica with normal serum zinc levels: diagnostic value to small bowel biopsy and essential fatty acid determination. *Gut*, **30**, 1426–1429.
30. Nelder, K.H. and Hambridge, K.M. (1975) Zinc therapy of acrodermatitis enteropathica. *New England Journal of Medicine*, **292**, 879–882.
31. Pope, F.M. (1974) Two types of autosomal recessive pseudoxanthoma elasticum. *Archives of Dermatology*, **110**, 209–210.
32. Pope, F.M., Narcisi, P., Nicholls, A.C., Liberman, M. and Oarthnys, J.W.E. (1988) Clinical presentations of Ehlers–Danlos syndrome type IV. *Archives of Disease in Childhood* **63**, 1016–1025.
33. Reunala, T., Blomquist, K., Tarpila, S., Halme, H. and Kangas, K. (1977) Gluten free diet in dermatitis herpetiformis. Clinical response of skin lesions in 81 patients. *British Journal of Dermatology*, **97**, 473–480.
34. Rigel, D.S. and Jacobs, M.I. (1980) Malignant acanthosis nigricans: a review. *Journal of Dermatologic Surgery and Oncology (New York)*, **6**, 923–927.
35. Shum, D.T. and Guenther, L. (1990) Metastatic Crohn's disease. *Archives of Dermatology*, **126**, 645–648.
36. Spigelman, A.D., Murday, V. and Phillips, R.K.S. (1989) Cancer and Peutz–Jeghers syndrome. *Gut*, **30**, 1588–1590.
37. Talaansky, A.L., Myers, S., Greenstein, A.J. and Janowitz, H.D. (1983) Does intestinal resection heal the pyoderma gangrenosum of inflammatory bowel disease? *Journal of Clinical Gastroenterology*, **5**, 207–210.
38. Talbot, S. and Wyatt, E.H. (1970) Blue rubber bleb naevi: a report of a family in which only males were affected. *British Journal of Dermatology*, **82**, 37–39.
39. Travis, W.D., Chin-Yang, L., Bergstralh, E.J., Yam, L.T. and Swee, R.G. (1988) Systemic Mast Cell Disease. Analysis of 58 cases and Literature Review. *Medicine (Baltimore)*, **67**, 345–368.
40. VanWouwe, J.P. (1989) Clinical and laboratory diagnosis of acrodermatitis enteropathica. *European Journal of Pediatrics*, **149**, 2–8.
41. Whelton, M.J. (1987) Personal communication to I. Sarkanay. In: *Dermatology in General Medicine* 3rd edn. vol. 2, p. 1956. (Ed.) Fitzpatrick, T.B., Eisen, A.Z., Wolff, K., Freedberg, I.M. and Austen, K.F. New York: McGraw-Hill.
42. Wilson, D.M., Pitts, W.C., Hintz, R.L. and Rosenfeld, R.G. (1986) Testicular tumors with Peutz–Jeghers syndrome. *Cancer*, **57**, 2238–2240.

CHAPTER 9

INFECTIONS AND INFESTATIONS OF THE GUT

CHOLERA

M.J.G. Farthing

INTRODUCTION

Cholera is one of the most devastating diarrhoeal diseases affecting the human race. It produces high-volume, watery diarrhoea which may exceed 20 l/day and which, without treatment, has a high mortality from dehydration and acidosis. Despite the clinical ravages of cholera epidemics through the centuries, this disease has taught us more than any other about the pathogenesis and treatment of secretory diarrhoea. It is the most well-studied model of a pure 'biochemical' diarrhoea, the intracellular sequence of events leading to this massive secretory state now being well characterized at a molecular level. The concepts generated by these studies have been applied to the study of other bacterial diarrhoeas. Cholera also acted as the model disease for the early studies of oral rehydration therapy with glucose–electrolyte solutions when it was evident that most patients with cholera, and indeed other watery diarrhoeas, could be safely managed without resorting to intravenous water and electrolyte replacement. It has been said that 'few major infectious diseases have moved with the times as successfully as cholera'.[26]

HISTORICAL ASPECTS

Severe epidemic diarrhoea has been written about since ancient times, notably in the works of Hippocrates (400 BC) and Galen. The modern history of cholera dates from 1817, which is the year when 'Asiatic' cholera previously restricted to India and beyond came to Europe and North America. Between 1817 and 1889 there were six cholera pandemics which resulted in approximately 100 000 deaths in the UK and 300 000 deaths in the USA. The sixth pandemic finally ended in 1923 and was the last epidemic to reach western Europe.[26]

During the third pandemic, John Snow in 1853 developed epidemiological methods sufficient to document the water-borne spread of cholera in England and made suggestions for its control and prevention. At this time, the Italian Philippo Pacini observed a highly motile bacterium in the intestinal effluent from cholera sufferers and named it *Vibrio cholerae*. However, discovery of the organism is generally attributed to Robert Koch in 1883, who called it the Kommabacillus (*Bacillus viglus*). Pacini's discovery was recognized in 1965 by the International Commission on Bacterial Nomenclature, which gave the official name of *Vibrio cholerae*, Pacini, 1854 to the organism.

In 1959, it was shown that *V. cholerae* produced an exotoxin that was liberated into culture filtrates; when introduced into a loop of mammalian ileum it caused profound intestinal secretion.[7] The toxin was rapidly purified and its mechanism of action through adenylate cyclase characterized.[9,10]

MICROBIOLOGY

Vibrios are gram-negative, curved, rod-shaped bacteria named because of their vibrating motility in aqueous media. They can be identified by direct dark-field examination of faeces, and confirmed by the inhibitory effect on vibrio motility of specific antibodies. The classic organism causing cholera is *V. cholerae* O1, which is divided into serotypes, Ogawa and Inaba, on the basis of agglutination tests with type-specific antisera for the lipopolysaccharide, heat-stable, somatic O antigen (*Table 9.1*). In addition, two biotypes have been identified. The classic biotype was responsible for the first six of the recent pandemics, whereas the El Tor biotype is responsible for the current, seventh pandemic. The El Tor vibrio takes its name from the quarantine station established in 1886 at El Tor on the Sinai peninsula where the organism was first discovered in dead pilgrims returning from Mecca. The El Tor biotype can be distinguished from the classic biotype on the basis of its resistance to polymyxin B and haemagglutination of chicken erythrocytes. The early isolates in 1961 possessed haemolytic activity, but subsequently vibrio El Tor lost its haemolytic properties. El Tor produces a milder disease and may be carried without causing symptoms. The ratio of infection to clinical disease is approximately 100:1 with the El Tor biotype compared with 10:1 for the classic vibrio.

Non-O-group 1 *V. cholerae* are found in the same geographical areas as *V. cholerae* O1. Non-O-group 1 vibrios may account for 3% of patients with diarrhoea in cholera areas.[25] *Vibrio parahaemolyticus* was first identified in Japan and is a common cause of food poisoning.

Table 9.1 Classification of cholera and non-cholera vibrios

	Group	*Serotypes*	*Biotypes*
Cholera vibrios			
Vibrio cholerae	O1	Ogawa	Classical
		Inaba	El Tor
	Non-O1	—	
Non-cholera vibrios			
Vibrio parahaemolyticus			
Vibrio fluvialis			
Vibrio mimicus			
Vibrio hollisae			
Vibrio furnissii			

EPIDEMIOLOGY

V. cholerae O1 is transmitted by contaminated water, shellfish and other seafood, and possibly by person-to-person contact.[8] The infective dose is usually around 10^9 vibrios but may be as low as 10^3 vibrios in situations of low gastric acidity. In endemic areas, children are at greatest risk, with age-specific prevalence falling with increasing age because of acquired immunity. Infants, however, have a smaller risk of infection, presumably as a result of less exposure to vibrios, combined with the protective effects of breast-feeding.[13] Individuals with blood group O have a higher risk of developing symptomatic cholera than blood groups A and B, and those with group AB are relatively protected.[14]

There is seasonality of cholera in endemic areas. This is complex in that it probably relates to conditions favouring multiplication of vibrios in its free-living cycle and also to seasonal changes in human contact with contaminated water. In Bangladesh, cholera increases with rising temperatures in April and May and reaches its peak at the end of the year.

Non-O-group 1 *V. cholerae* (*Table 9.1*) are also found in cholera regions and survive and multiply in brackish and salt water in the same way as *V. cholerae* O1. Infection most commonly occurs following consumption of raw seafood, particularly oysters.[25] *V. parahaemolyticus* is a common cause of food poisoning, usually associated with the consumption of raw or undercooked fish and seafood.

PATHOGENESIS

Following ingestion of *V. cholerae*, the highly motile vibrios colonize the proximal small intestine by penetrating the mucus coat and multiplying in close proximity to the intestinal epithelium. The organism causes no light microscopic or ultrastructural damage to the epithelial cells, but releases a secretory enterotoxin which causes massive secretion of sodium and chloride ions and water. Cholera toxin consists of one A and five B subunits (*Figure 9.1*). The B subunits bind multivalently to the oligosaccharide moieties of the monosialoganglioside GM1, which serves as the specific receptor for this toxin.[11] Following binding of the B subunits to their receptors, the A_1 subunit is released from A_2 following reduction of the disulphide bond, presumed to occur via cellular glutathione. The A_1 subunit then binds irreversibly to the stimulatory component (N_s of the enzyme adenylate cyclase which is situated in the basolateral membrane of the enterocyte (*Figure 9.2*). The A_1 subunit has both NAD glycohydrolase and ADP transferase activities and produces its effect on N_s by covalently modifying one of its subunits by ADP ribosylation of an arginine residue. This covalent modification of N_s continues throughout the life of the cell and, thus, leaves adenylate cyclase in a continuously active state.[24]

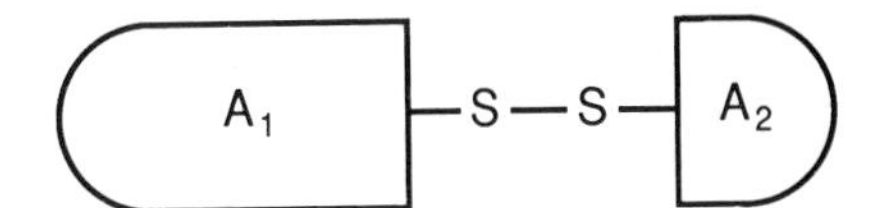

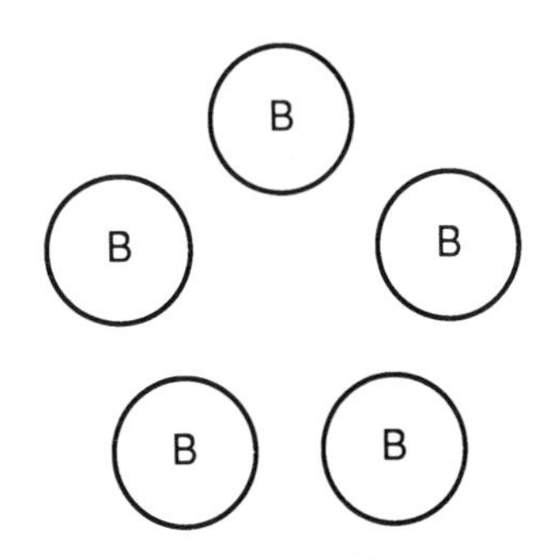

Figure 9.1 Structure of cholera toxin.

Second messenger–secretion coupling is achieved by cAMP-mediated phosphorylation of membrane proteins through the action of protein kinases.[24] In the case of cholera toxin this leads to a conformational change in proteins associated with the chloride channel in the apical membrane of the enterocyte, resulting in chloride ion secretion. Intracellular calcium also has modulatory effects on the activity of these protein kinases which may be calmodulin- or phospholipid-dependent. In addition to its chloride ion secretory effects, principally in crypt cells, cholera toxin also inhibits sodium and chloride ion absorption by villous cells. The net

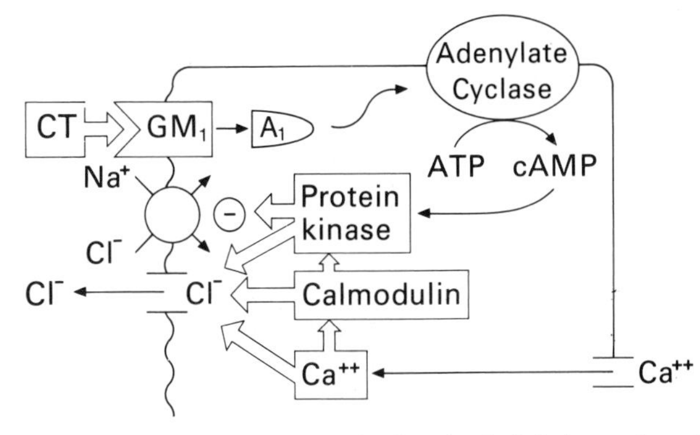

Figure 9.2 Interaction between the A_1 subunit of cholera toxin and adenylate cyclase.

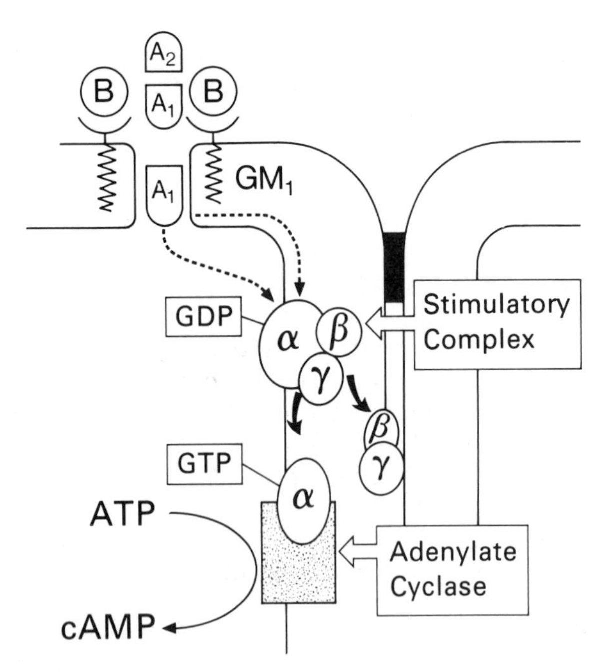

Figure 9.3 Second messenger–secretion coupling in intestinal secretion induced by cholera toxin.

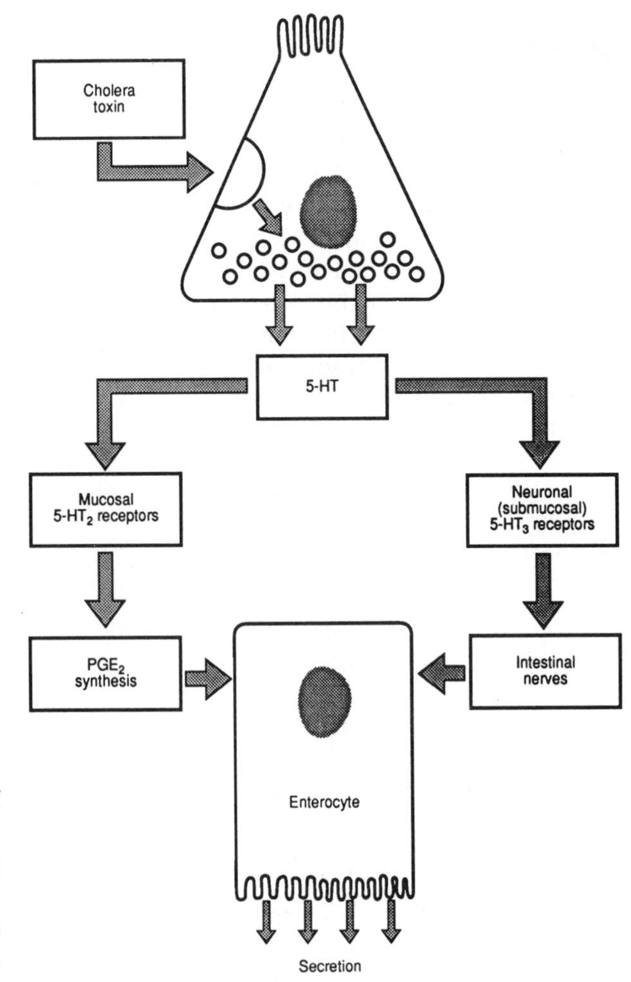

Figure 9.4 Possible role of 5-HT in cholera toxin-induced intestinal secretion.

result of these processes is the massive secretion of sodium and chloride ions and water (*Figure 9.3*). More recently, another toxin of *V. cholerae* has been described, namely, Zona Occludens Toxin (ZOT). This toxin affects the integrity of the tight junctions between enterocytes and is thought to increase fluid losses through the epithelium. Despite these secretory events, sodium absorption mediated by solute (glucose, amino acids) remains intact and can counteract the sodium and water losses caused by cholera toxin. This observation led to the rational design and implementation of oral rehydration therapy with glucose–electrolyte solutions, an intervention that has been considered the most important discovery of the century.[7]

Recent studies suggest that other neurohumoral pathways may be involved in cholera toxin-induced, intestinal fluid secretion.[22] There is evidence to suggest that cholera toxin is able to release serotonin (5-hydroxytryptamine or 5-HT) from enterochromaffin cells in the small intestine, possibly by activation of the adenylate cyclase–cAMP system in these cells (*Figure 9.4*). The release of 5-HT is then thought to activate prostaglandin E_2 formation via 5-HT_2 receptors which will enhance the secretory response. It has been proposed that 5-HT may also act on 5-HT_3 receptors on enteric nerves which could further enhance the secretory process.[2] These studies have been performed largely in animal models, but confirmation of these findings in humans might profoundly influence the future development of antisecretory drugs.

CLINICAL FEATURES

Mild cholera in adults and children may be indistinguishable from many other infective agents. This form of the disease occurs in the majority of infected individuals. However, severe cholera begins abruptly, often at night with severe diarrhoea up to 1 l/h in the first 24 hours. Fever is usually absent but vomiting is common at the onset of diarrhoea. Stools eventually take on the 'rice-water' character due to the presence of mucus in the iso-osmotic watery stool.

Dehydration, acidosis and hypotension rapidly follow. When the fluid deficit is more than 8%, there is usually evidence of cardiovascular collapse and oliguria. Ultimately, the patient loses consciousness and death usually follows when fluid losses exceed 12%. Untreated cholera has a mortality rate of 20–50% but no patient should die with adequate rehydration therapy early in the course of the illness.

INVESTIGATIONS

In endemic and epidemic cholera, diagnosis is usually made on clinical criteria, namely the extremely high-volume, watery diarrhoea with profound dehydration and acidosis. Microbiological diagnosis can be achieved by dark-field examination of the stool for the highly motile cholera vibrios, which is confirmed by the immobilizing effect of specific antisera. The presence of *V. cholerae* can be confirmed by culture.

IMMUNE RESPONSE AND HOST DEFENCE

Non-specific host defences, particularly low intragastric pH, are important for many intestinal infections including cholera. However, the high attack rate in children in endemic areas supports the view that the intestinal immune response is important for preventing and controlling infection. Epidemiological studies in endemic areas have shown that there is impressive resistance to challenge following an episode of clinical cholera.[16] In addition, the presence of vibriocidal antibody in serum increases with age, confirming the importance of acquired immunity. The immune response is directed towards a variety of *V. cholerae* antigens. Cholera toxin is a potent antigen, most of the immune response being directed towards the B subunit. Virtually all neutralizing activity of cholera antitoxin can be absorbed with purified B subunits. However, immune responses to other *V. cholerae* antigens are involved in the development of protective immunity following natural infection, and these include lipopolysaccharide and outer-membrane proteins.[16] Clearance of *V. cholerae* and protection against future infection depends on the development of specific secretory(s) IgA to the O-antigenic lipopolysaccharide of the outer-membrane protein and against cholera toxin. Specific sIgA has been found in breast milk from mothers in an endemic area and, when these antibodies are present, infants are protected from the development of diarrhoeal disease, although these antibodies do not prevent colonization with *V. cholerae* O1.[13]

TREATMENT

The most important aspects of the treatment of cholera are: (1) rapid rehydration and correction of acidosis, and (2) reduction of bacterial colonization and eradication of vibrios with antibiotics.

REHYDRATION

Cholera results in the loss of large volumes of fluid from the intestine containing relatively high concentrations of sodium (120 mmol/l), potassium (50 mmol/l) and bicarbonate (40 mmol/l). This results in marked dehydration and hypovolaemia with a low plasma bicarbonate level and, initially, plasma sodium and potassium concentrations within the normal range. Rehydration must take into account these losses and, in severely affected individuals (>10% dehydration), rehydration via the intravenous route is essential. Rehydration should commence early in the course of the illness and, providing there is no marked hypovolaemia, oral rehydration with the World Health Organization recommended oral rehydration solution (sodium 90, glucose 111, potassium 20, citrate 10 mmol/l) is usually effective.[15,21,23] Oral fluids may be given at rates of up to 15 ml/kg per hour with careful monitoring of haemodynamic parameters, urine and intestinal output. Simple glucose–electrolyte solutions, although effective for rehydration, do not reduce stool output. However, the use of complex carbohydrate oral rehydration solutions, particularly those containing rice powder, do reduce stool output and the total requirements for oral rehydration solutions.[20] In the developing world it is possible that these complex carbohydrate oral rehydration solutions may replace conventional oral rehydration solutions in the future.

ANTIBIOTICS

Tetracycline 250 mg four times daily for 3–5 days decreases the duration and severity of diarrhoea.[3] *V. cholerae* O1 is also sensitive to doxycycline, ampicillin, chloramphenicol, trimethoprim–sulphamethoxazole and furazolidone. A single dose of doxycycline (200–300 mg) is as effective as the standard multiple-dose tetracycline regimen.[1]

PREVENTION

Control of enteric infection, which is predominantly food- and water-borne can be achieved by provision of safe water supplies, adequate disposal of excreta and thorough cooking of seafood. Awareness of the risks of person-to-person spread in the home and the implementation of high standards of personal hygiene can reduce the secondary attack rates. Despite extensive knowledge of the mechanisms by which enteric pathogens are transmitted and the technical knowledge and skills to improve water quality and sanitation, much of the world continues to operate in less than ideal conditions. Additional preventive measures include (1) chemoprophylaxis and (2) vaccination.

CHEMOPROPHYLAXIS

The administration of tetracycline to family members of patients with cholera can substantially decrease the secondary attack rate.[18] Even mass treatment has been used to limit the spread during epidemics although this adds to the development of multiple antibiotic-resistant strains of *V. cholerae* O1.[19] However, mass treatment is probably not economically viable and should be restricted to immediate family members. Doxycycline is effective as a single dose (300 mg adults, 6 mg/kg children <15 years of age).

VACCINE

There is compelling evidence to suggest that, for non-invasive enteric infections, oral vaccination produces the most effective sIgA response in the intestine. Thus, although the classic, inactivated, whole-cell, parenteral cholera vaccine is still widely used and does provide modest protection in endemic areas for a few months, there is a need for more effective, longer-lasting, oral vaccines which could be used not only in travellers but in the population of endemic areas.

Non-living oral vaccines

An oral vaccine has been prepared consisting of a mixture of dead whole *V. cholerae* O1 including classic and El Tor biotypes and the two serotypes, Ogawa and Inaba. This vaccine was compared in a placebo-controlled field trial with the same killed whole-vibrio preparation but with the addition of purified B subunits of cholera toxin. The addition of pure B subunit substantially improved vaccine efficacy from 58 to 85% protection when assessed at 6 months.[4] However, long-term follow-up at 3 years showed that the efficacy of both vaccines had fallen to 50%, and there was no significant difference between the two approaches.[5] Although this represents an improvement over the parenteral vaccines, the effect was poor in young children, who have the highest incidence of cholera. In addition a multiple-dosage schedule was required to achieve protection, a drawback which makes it difficult to apply widely in the developing world.

Live oral cholera vaccines

Live oral enteric vaccines have been shown in animal models and in humans to be generally more effective than their inactivated parenteral or oral counterparts. Two main approaches are being used in cholera, namely (1) the expression of *V. cholerae* O1 antigens in an innocuous carrier organism such as attenuated *Salmonella typhi* Ty21a and (2) the development of attenuated forms of *V. cholerae* O1 by deleting genes encoding for virulence factors. Using recombinant techniques, O antigens of *V. cholerae* O1 have been expressed in *S. typhi* Ty21a and have been tested in experimental challenge studies in humans. Although its efficacy in protecting against cholera was poor (25% efficacy), excretion of the challenge strain was reduced as was stool volume.[12] Perhaps a more sophisticated vaccine strain might be produced if the gene encoding for the B subunit could be included in addition to that for the O antigens.

Deletion of the genes encoding the A subunit from *V. cholerae* O1 has been achieved but, unfortunately, early attempts produced strains which still produced a mild diarrhoeal illness, suggesting that other toxins might be involved. This approach was developed further by selecting *V. cholerae* strain 569B, which is known to be free of other toxins. Deleting the A subunit genes produced the vaccine strain CVD 103, which was relatively well tolerated and remarkably immunogenic.[17] A further modification was made by inserting a gene encoding for resistance to mercury so that the vaccine strain (CVD 103-HgR) could be distinguished from wild-type vibrios. Challenge studies with this vaccine have shown that it is relatively free from unwanted effects such as diarrhoea, while at the same time providing excellent protection against both biotypes and serotypes of *V. cholerae* O1.[17] Clinical trials are under way and it seems likely that this live oral vaccine strain will soon be introduced into clinical practice.

REFERENCES

1. Alam, A.M., Alam, N.H., Ahmed, T. and Sack, D.A. (1990) Randomised double-blind trial of single dose doxycycline for treating cholera in adults. *British Medical Journal*, **300**, 1619–1621.
2. Beubler, E. and Horina, G. (1990) 5-HT_2 and 5-HT_3 receptor subtypes mediate cholera toxin-induced intestinal fluid secretion. *Gastroenterology*, **99**, 83–89.
3. Carpenter, C.C.J., Barua, D. and Wallace, C.K. (1966) Chemical studies in Asiatic cholera. IV: antibiotic therapy in cholera. *Bulletin of Johns Hopkins Hospital*, **118**, 216–224.

4. Clemens, J.D., Sack, D.A., Harris, J.R. *et al.* (1986) Field trial of oral cholera vaccines in Bangladesh. *The Lancet*, **ii**, 124–127.
5. Clemens, J.D., Sack, D.A., Harris, J.R. *et al.* (1990) Field trial of oral cholera vaccines in Bangladesh: results from longterm follow-up. *The Lancet*, **335**, 270–273.
6. De, S.N. (1959) Enterotoxicity of bacteria-free culture filtrate of *Vibrio cholerae. Nature*, **183**, 1533.
7. Farthing, M.J.G. (1988) History and rationale of oral rehydration and recent developments in formulating an optimal solution. *Advances in Oral Rehydration. Drugs*, **36**(suppl.4), 80–90.
8. Feachem, R.G. (1982) Environmental aspects of cholera epidemiology: II. Transmission and control. *Tropical Diseases Bulletin*, **790**, 1–47.
9. Field, M. (1971) Intestinal secretions: effect of cyclic AMP and its role in cholera. *New England Journal of Medicine*, **284**, 1137–1144.
10. Finkelstein, R.D. and Lospalluto, J.J. (1969) Pathogenesis of experimental cholera. *Journal of Experimental Medicine*, **130**, 185–202.
11. Fishman P.H. (1982) Role of membrane gangliosides in the binding and action of bacterial toxins. *Journal of Membrane Biology*, **69**, 85–97.
12. Forrest, B.D., La Brooy, J., Attridge, S.R. *et al.* (1989) A candidate live oral typhoid/cholera hybrid vaccine is immunogenic in humans. *Journal of Infectious Diseases*, **159**, 145–146.
13. Glass, R.I., Svennerholm, A.-M., Stoll, B.J. *et al.* (1983) Protection against cholera in breast-fed children by antibodies in breast milk. *New England Journal of Medicine*, **308**, 1389–1392.
14. Glass, R.I., Holmgren, J., Haley, C.E. *et al.* (1985) Predisposition for cholera of individuals with O blood group: possible evolutionary significance. *American Journal of Epidemiology*, **121**, 791–796.
15. Hirschhorn, N., Kinzie, J.L., Sachar, D.B. *et al.* (1968) Decrease in net stool output in cholera during intestinal perfusion with glucose-containing solutions. *New England Journal of Medicine*, **279**, 176–181.
16. Levine, M.M., Kaper, J.B., Black, R.E. and Clements, M.L. (1983) New knowledge on pathogenesis of bacterial enteric infections as applied to vaccine development. *Microbiological Reviews*, **47**, 510–550.
17. Levine, M.M., Kaper, J.B., Herrington, D. *et al.* (1988) Safety, immunogenicity and efficacy in man of recombinant live oral cholera vaccines, CVD 103 and CVD 103-HgR. *The Lancet*, **ii**, 467–470.
18. MacCormack, W.M., Chowdhury, A.M., Jahangir, N. *et al.* (1968) Tetracycline prophylaxis of families of cholera patients. *Bulletin of the World Health Organisation*, **38**, 787–792.
19. Mhalu, F.S., Mtango, F.D.E. and Msengi, A.E. (1984) Hospital outbreaks of cholera transmitted through close person-to-person contact. *The Lancet*, **ii**, 80–84.
20. Molla, A.M., Molla, A., Nath, S.K. and Khatun, M. (1989) Food-based oral rehydration salt solution for acute childhood diarrhoea. *The Lancet*, **ii**, 429–431.
21. Nalin, D.R., Cash, R.A., Islam, R., Molla, M. and Phillips, R.A. (1968) Oral maintenance therapy for cholera in adults. *The Lancet*, **ii**, 370–373.
22. Nilsson, O., Cassuto, J., Larsson, P.A. *et al.* (1983) 5-Hydroxytryptamine and cholera secretion: a histochemical and physiological study in cats. *Gut*, **24**, 542–548.
23. Pierce, N.F., Banwell, J.G., Mitra, R.C. *et al.* (1968) Effect of intragastric glucose-electrolyte infusion upon water and electrolyte balance in Asiatic cholera. *Gastroenterology*, **55**, 333–343.
24. Rao, M.C. (1989) Molecular mechanisms of bacterial toxins. In *Enteric Infection* (Eds) Farthing, M.J.G. and Keusch, G.T. pp. 87–104. London: Chapman and Hall.
25. Stoll, B.J., Glass, R.I., Banu, H. *et al.* (1982) Surveillance of patients attending a diarrhoeal disease hospital in Bangladesh. *British Medical Journal*, **285**, 1185–1188.
26. Van Heyningen, W.E. and Seal, J.R. (1983) *Cholera. The American Scientific Experience 1947–1980.* Boulder: Westview Press.

SALMONELLA INFECTION

B.K. Mandal

BACTERIOLOGY

Salmonella organisms are Gram-negative, aerobic, generally motile bacilli which do not ferment lactose. There are more than 2000 serotypes identified on the basis of their somatic (O) and flagellar (H) antigens. These serotypes can be broadly separated into two categories according to their host predilection:

1. The causative organisms of typhoid and paratyphoid fevers – *Salmonella typhi, S. paratyphi* A, *S. paratyphi* B and *S. paratyphi* C – are primarily adapted to humans, although occasional animal infections with paratyphoid organisms have been encountered in nature.[22]

2. The other serotypes, which are primarily parasites of animals, generally produce a gastroenteritis type of illness in humans, often termed 'food-poisoning' because of the predominant source of infection. Although all are potentially pathogenic in humans, a small percentage of the many serotypes account for the vast majority of human infection in the world as a whole. Examples of commonly isolated serotypes are *S. typhimurium, S. hadar, S. enteritidis, S. virchow, S. heidelberg, S. agona, S. saint paul, S. montevideo, S. derby* and *S. bredeney*. Although *S. typhimurium* is the most common cause of salmonella gastroenteritis in most regions of the world, *S. enteritidis* has become the most prevalent strain in Britain in recent years[18] and a similar trend has become evident in the USA[11] and some areas of western Europe.[42]

S. typhi, S. paratyphi A, *S. paratyphin B* and some of the other common serotypes can be subdivided by bacteriophage typing, which is useful in epidemiological investigations.

TYPHOID AND PARATYPHOID

(synonym: enteric fever)

The term 'enteric fever' is frequently used to describe the prolonged febrile state caused by *S. typhi, S. paratyphi* A, *S. paratyphi* B and *S. paratyphi* C. Occasionally, other salmonella serotypes of the food poisoning variety may produce an invasive illness with prolonged bacteraemia, continued fever, enlargement of spleen and even the 'rose spots' that are characteristic of enteric fever.

EPIDEMIOLOGY

Typhoid and paratyphoid fevers occur throughout the world but are most prevalent in the Far East, Central and South America and Africa, reflecting the poor standards of sanitation and water supply in such areas. A low level of endemicity still persists in some areas of eastern and southern Europe but, in the rest of Europe, North America and Australasia, enteric fever is now largely an imported disease. The ultimate source of infection is invariably human, and transmission is via the alimentary tract through direct or indirect contact with the faeces or urine of a patient or a carrier. The principal vehicles of spread of typhoid infection are contaminated water and food: paratyphoid infection is less likely to be water-borne because of the necessity for a high infecting dose, which is unlikely to be found in drinking water unless there is heavy pollution. Raw fruit and vegetables are important vehicles in some tropical countries where use of human faeces for manuring vegetable crops is a common practice. Shellfish harvested in water polluted by sewage have caused outbreaks. Canned meat is generally very safe but outbreaks have occurred occasionally through faulty canning processes.

PATHOLOGY

Natural infection in enteric fever is by oral ingestion. The size of the infecting dose is important. A dose of 10^9 organisms will induce infection in most, whereas 10^3 organisms will rarely produce symptoms in otherwise healthy individuals.[28] Pathogenicity varies and host factors such as gastric hypoacidity may influence the infecting dose.[23]

Possession of Vi (virulence) antigen is probably linked with increased pathogenicity. Vi antigen is the capsular polysaccharide of *S. typhi*, so named because the strains with this antigen are highly pathogenic to experimental mice. The ability of Vi antigen-positive strains to cause clinical illness more common than the non-Vi variants[28] and the demonstrable efficacy of Vi antigen polysaccharide vaccine strongly[1,32] suggest the importance of Vi antigen in the pathogenesis of and immunity to typhoid fever.

After passing the acid barrier of the stomach, the organisms rapidly penetrate the small intestinal mucosa, reach the mesenteric glands via the lymphatics and, after a brief period of multiplication, spread to the spleen, liver and other reticuloendothelial tissues via the bloodstream. Here they multiply silently for the rest of the incubation period; they then enter the bloodstream in huge numbers, heralding the onset of the clinical illness. This secondary bacteraemia continues for the greater part of the febrile illness, and very few organs of the body escape involvement. However, from a clinical viewpoint the two most important sites affected are Peyer's patches in the small intestine and the gallbladder. Peyer's patches become hyperplastic, with infiltration of chronic inflammatory cells; later, necrosis of the superficial layer leads to formation of irregular, ovoid ulcers along the long axis of the gut, so stricture formation does not occur. Erosion into the blood vessels may produce severe intestinal haemorrhage or transmural perforation may lead to peritonitis. The lower ileum is the site most severely affected.

The gallbladder is probably affected via the liver; the resulting cholecystitis is usually subclinical. Pre-existing gallbladder disease predisposes to the chronic carrier state, which might explain the rarity of the carrier state in children and its frequency in middle-aged women. The organisms may be found in gallstones.

PATHOGENESIS OF FEVER

The pathogenesis of the prolonged fever and toxaemia of enteric fever is far from clear. A major role for endotoxaemia has been discounted after studies in volunteers who were rendered endotoxin-tolerant by repetitive intravenous endotoxin administration, but who nevertheless developed typical typhoid fever when challenged with viable organisms. Furthermore, it is impossible to produce a stage of prolonged fever by continuous infusion of endotoxin or to demonstrate endotoxaemia in natural typhoid fever by the *Limulus* lysate test, a sensitive indicator of endotoxaemia.[28]

Pyrogens released from the inflammatory response enhanced by local elaboration of endotoxin in the sites of *S. typhi* multiplication,[27] and production of macrophage-derived mediators and immunosuppressive factors, may both be responsible for the clinical manifestations.[17]

MECHANISM OF IMMUNITY

Cell-mediated immunity probably plays an important role in the recovery from infection, whilst humoral antibody formation has little relevance, because the patient continues to deteriorate even after the appearance of O, H and Vi antibodies. There is no correlation between these antibodies and relapse or reinfection in naturally acquired typhoid fever. Vaccine-induced resistance would seem to be humorally mediated but not related to O and H antibodies. Vi antibodies are clearly important in view of the demonstrable efficacy of Vi antigen polysaccharide vaccine, but the efficacy of the heat-killed typhoid vaccines (Vi antigen destroyed) suggests an additional protective role of antibodies to other, as yet undefined, antigens.

CLINICAL FEATURES

The duration of illness in a case of average severity is approximately 4 weeks but mild and inapparent cases are common. The incubation period of typhoid fever averages from 10 to 20 days but may be shorter when the infecting dose is large. Paratyphoid fever generally has a shorter incubation period (average 7–14 days).

In the *first week* there are few specific features. The onset is insidious, with mounting fever, headache, vague abdominal pain and constipation. There is often relative bradycardia and the spleen becomes palpable towards the end of the first week. During the *second week* the patient becomes dull and apathetic, with sustained fever and slightly distended abdomen. Crops of 2–4 mm maculopapules (rose spots) appear on the lower chest and upper abdomen between the seventh and 10th days of illness. The rose spots are often more numerous in paratyphoid fever. Cough is commonly present at this stage. During the *third week* the patient gradually lapses into the so-called 'typhoid state', characterized by prolonged apathy and toxaemia with delirium, disorientation or even coma. The abdomen becomes distended, with scanty bowel sounds, and greenish 'pea-soup' diarrhoea is common. Severe intestinal haemorrhage and perforation are prone to occur during this period. During the *fourth week* the temperature gradually returns to normal and the abdominal distension subsides, although the patient remains listless and anorexic for some time afterwards.

There is frequently variation in the clinical picture. Diarrhoea may be present from the onset, particularly in paratyphoid fever, which may behave as simple gastroenteritis. Chronic bacteraemia with fever of many months' duration can occur in association with urinary schistosomiasis, and is due to persistence of the organisms within the intestine of the parasites. In children, the onset may be abrupt, with vomiting, high fever and often convulsion, and they rarely have a relative bradycardia.

RELAPSE AND REINFECTION

In 10–15% of patients there may be a return to symptoms about 10 days after the cessation of antibiotic therapy and the blood culture is again positive, even in the presence of a high antibody titre. Such a relapse is usually mild and of short duration. Relapse occurs less frequently in paratyphoid fever. Natural immunity is generally long-lasting, and reinfection is rare. The relapse rate appears to be less after treatment with ciprofloxacin.

CARRIER STATE

During the immediate convalescence stool cultures are frequently positive but their frequency declines rapidly, so that after 3 months only 4–5% of patients excrete the organism. The 3% of patients who remain positive at the end of 1 year are regarded as chronic carriers and will remain so for the rest of their lives. Persistent urinary carriage is quite rare beyond the third month in the absence of urinary tract abnormalities, but urinary carriers are common in those countries where urinary tract schistosomiasis is endemic. With newer antimicrobial agents, such as the quinolones, the carriage rate appears to be much less.

COMPLICATIONS

Gastrointestinal tract

Haemorrhage

The introduction of chloramphenicol has strikingly reduced the incidence of this dreaded complication, and it is now seen only rarely in the Western world. Frank bleeding, as evidenced by the passage of red blood in the stools, is always serious and is most frequent during the third week when the slough in the intestinal ulcers separates. However, trivial bleeding as judged by positive occult blood is not uncommon.

Intestinal perforation

This remains one of the most frequently encountered complications of typhoid fever in countries where it is endemic. The diagnosis may be difficult because the perforation often occurs in a patient who is already severely ill, dehydrated and mentally apathetic with a vaguely tender, distended abdomen, so that the classic signs of perforation may not be present. Rigidity is encountered in less than half of the patients and bowel sounds may not disappear altogether. Free fluid in an already doughy and tender abdomen and gas under the diaphragm may be the only indications of perforation.

Rarely, the colon may be involved, giving rise to haemorrhage or toxic dilatation.[37]

These complications are less frequent in paratyphoid fevers.

Liver and gallbladder

Slight jaundice is not uncommon in typhoid fever and may be due to diffuse hepatitis, cholangitis, cholecystitis or haemolysis. Liver biopsy in typhoid hepatitis shows focal liver cell necrosis with associated mononuclear cell infiltration ('typhoid nodules'), sinusoidal congestion and dilatation, and portal tract infiltration with mononuclear cells.[43] Intact typhoid bacilli have been demonstrated in liver parenchyma in such cases.[10] Subclinical cholecystitis is a feature of the disease, but overt signs of gallbladder inflammation may infrequently appear either during the acute illness or some months later.

Central nervous system

A toxic confusional state characterized by severe disorientation, delirium and restlessness occurs during the second and third weeks of illness, but confusion may dominate the clinical picture from the onset and the patient may be admitted to a psychiatric unit.[29,41] Paranoid psychosis or catatonia may develop during convalescence and occasionally the features of acute parkinsonism or encephalomyelitis may complicate the clinical picture.

Haematological and renal

Subclinical disseminated intravascular coagulation is common in typhoid fever,[9] but there may be frank manifestations of the haemolytic–uraemic syndrome.[6] Immune complex glomerulitis with deposition of immunoglobin, C3 complement and salmonella Vi antigen in the glomerular capillary wall have been reported.[53] The nephrotic syndrome develops in some patients with chronic *S. typhi* bacteraemia when there is associated schistosomiasis.[20]

Other complications

Toxic myocarditis is a significant cause of death in countries where enteric fever is endemic. Frank pneumonic consolidation, pancreatitis and abscess formation in such diverse sites as spleen, ovary and bone are other rare complications.

INVESTIGATIONS

Definitive diagnosis requires isolation of the organism from blood, bone marrow, faeces or urine. Blood cultures are usually positive in 90% of patients during the first week and in a febrile patient the cultures may remain positive into the second or even third week. The frequency of positive blood culture is much less in patients already given antibiotics, but marrow cultures or clot cultures may remain positive. The organisms can also be cultured from a skin biopsy of the rose spot lesion. A polymorphonuclear leukopenia is characteristic, particularly during the first week.

With modern techniques, the stool cultures are often positive even during the first week, although the percentage positivity rises steadily as the illness progresses. In some patients the stool culture remains negative throughout the illness, particularly if they have received early antibiotic therapy. Urine culture is positive in 30% of patients during the third week.

Serological diagnosis

The Widal reaction measures titres of serum agglutinins against somatic (O) and flagellar (H) antigens; these agglutinins begin to appear during the second week. In acute infection, O antibody appears first and becomes negative after several months, whereas H antibody appears a little later but persists for a long time. O antibody generally signifies active infection; H antibody helps to identify the type of enteric infection. Positive O titres of 1/80 in non-immunized people living in non-endemic areas, and titres of 1/160 in people in endemic areas, are regarded as significant, but a rising titre has more significance. The Widal test has many limitations: significantly rising titres are often absent, false positives are common because of 'O' and 'H'-antigenic similarity among many members of the Enterobacteriaceae, and anamnestic reactions are common during may unrelated fibrile conditions. Prior immunization makes interpretation of serological tests difficult.

A number of other serodiagnostic tests are being evaluated and are probably superior to the traditional Widal test, e.g. Vi indirect immunofluorescent antibody test[16] and detection of IgM antibody to *S. typhi* lipopolysaccharide antigen by enzyme-linked immunosorbent assay;[52] however, further work is needed before such tests can be adopted for routine diagnostic use.

TREATMENT

The introduction of chloramphenicol in 1948 heralded the era of modern treatment for typhoid fever. The clinical response to the drug proved uniformly reliable throughout the world, with rapid improvement in the patients' general condition followed by defervescence within 2–5 days. The drug is given orally in a dose of 500 mg every 4 hours until defervescence, then 6-hourly for a total period of 14 days. Despite concern owing to occasional marrow toxicity, chloramphenicol remained the drug of choice for three decades, until the emergence of chloramphenicol-resistant *S. typhi* in Central and South America, Vietnam and India shifted attention to alternative drugs. Both amoxycillin in divided doses of 4 g/day[51] and co-trimoxazole (960–1920 mg twice daily),[25] for 14 days with either agents, have proved equal to chloramphenicol in terms of clinical efficacy and relapse rates, and became the drug of choice in areas having a high prevalence of chloramphenicol-resistant strains.

In Britain, where the majority of infections are acquired in the Indian subcontinent and West Africa, such strains were encountered rarely during the 1980s[47] and chloramphenicol was the most widely used drug.[19] Very recently, however, there has been a disturbingly rapid emergence of multiresistant *S. typhi* in India,[4] Pakistan,[3] China[57] and, no doubt, in other parts of the Far East where the organisms are frequently resistant to all three first-line drugs (chloramphenicol, amoxycillin and co-trimoxazole); this has led to urgent evaluation of the new quinolone group of drugs. Highly promising results have been obtained with ciprofloxacin in doses of 500 mg orally twice daily for 14 days, in treatment of typhoid and paratyphoid fevers, with an average defervescence period of around 5 days, and the convalescence carriage rate appears to be much less compared to the conventional drugs.[44,45] Other quinolones, such as ofloxacin, norfloxacin and pefloxacin, have been equally promising, and one of these agents should be regarded as the drug of choice in areas where multiresistant typhoid occurs and this includes Britain.

Treatment of children with multiresistant *S. typhi* presents a dilemma. Animal experiments have shown that quinolones can cause irreversible damage to cartilage in strained joints of young animals and, because a similar effect in humans cannot be excluded, the new quinolones are contraindicated in children and pregnant women. In such cases, clinicians have the option of using one of the third-generation cephalosporins, especially cefotaxime, ceftriaxone and cefoperazone, which have given a cure rate of about 90% with a defervescent period comparable to that seen with chloramphenicol.[54] The need to give these expensive drugs intravenously for 14 days (although shorter courses may be equally effective) is a major disadvantage, particularly in the economically poor endemic countries, and alternative oral regimens are urgently needed. The first quinolone drug, nalidixic acid, is also known to cause damage to young animal cartilage but is still licensed for paediatric use, and has been widely used in children with no reports of quinolone-associated arthropathy. Furthermore, paediatricians have used ciprofloxacin in children with cystic fibrosis without encountering any joint problems (T. David, personal communication), so use of ciprofloxacin in children with multiresistant *S. typhi* infections may thus be justifiable.

High-dose dexamethasone (initial dose 3 mg/kg body weight followed by eight doses of 1 mg/kg every 6 hours) reduces mortality in severely toxic patients with an abnormal state of consciousness or shock[26] and has a place in selected cases.

The management of haemorrhage is non-operative, using sedation and transfusion, unless there is evidence of perforation; then surgery is indicated. Early diagnosis, energetic resuscitation and rapid surgery are the key to successful outcome. Most surgeons prefer simple closure of perforation with drainage of the peritoneum and reserve small bowel resection for patients with multiple perforations.[30] Gentamicin and metronidazole should be added to the treatment regimen in these patients.

TREATMENT OF CHRONIC CARRIERS

Attempts to eradicate the chronic carrier state by giving prolonged courses of amoxycillin or co-trimoxazole have not been particularly successful. A cure rate of about 50% can be achieved provided the gallbladder is functioning but, as at least three-quarters of chronic carriers have diseased gallbladders, success can only be expected in a minority. The management of the carrier state has been considerably improved by the introduction of new quinolones, with reports of 78% and 83% cure rates using norfloxacin[24] (400 mg every 12 hours for 28 days) and ciprofloxacin[21] (750 mg every 12 hours for 28 days), respectively.

There is no guarantee that carriers will be cured by the removal of the gallbladder. It will eradicate the carrier state in 3 out of 4 cases but this is not an operation to be undertaken lightly. The operation should be advised only when the indications are similar to those in non-carriers, and not when the sole purpose is the eradication of the carrier state.

PREVENTION

Although mass immunization at regular intervals will reduce the incidence of typhoid fever considerably (there is no effective vaccine against paratyphoid in areas where the disease is endemic). The most cost-effective strategy is public health measures to ensure safe water supply and sanitary disposal of excreta to encourage high standards in personal hygiene, and in the handling/processing/storage of foodstuffs.

Heat-killed phenolized typhoid vaccines provide about 70% protection against water-borne infections, but a higher infecting dose which may be found in food-borne infections will break through this partial immunity. For primary immunization, two subcutaneous doses of 0.5 ml each are given 4 weeks apart. In cases of urgency this interval may be reduced to 10 days. Local and systemic reactions are common. Booster doses are necessary every 3 years. An intradermal dose of 0.1 ml is suitable for this purpose, giving much less reaction.

A single intramuscular dose of Vi capsular polysaccharide antigen vaccine prepared by the Merieux Institute has given promising results in field trials in Nepal[1] and South Africa,[32] with efficacy rate at least equal to the two dose-killed vaccine; side-effects are minimal. A live attenuated oral vaccine (Ty21a) using three doses given within a week has a useful 67% efficacy for at least 3 years and is free of side-effects.[33] Both are now available in Britain.

OTHER SALMONELLA INFECTIONS

Human salmonellosis has a world-wide distribution and is an increasing public health problem, especially in the economically advanced countries of western Europe and North America. Community and institutional outbreaks are common and much hospital, medical, laboratory and field time and expense are devoted to prevention and control measures. In the USA, an estimated 0.8–3.7 million cases of salmonella food poisoning occur annually[12] and, in England and Wales, where it accounts for 10–15% of all hospitalized cases of acute diarrhoea, there has been an alarming increase in the number of reported cases in recent years. This is largely due to a nationwide epidemic of *S. enteritidis* phage type (PT)4.[18]

EPIDEMIOLOGY

The organisms are widely distributed in the animal kingdom. Domestic species, notably cattle, pigs and poultry, are frequent excretors and the organisms can be found in many wild animals. Household pets, such as dogs, cats, birds and turtles, are all potential sources of infection. Human cases and convalescent carriers, especially those with mild or unrecognized disease, are other important sources.

TRANSMISSION

Transmission is almost always by the oral route following ingestion of food or drink contaminated either directly or indirectly with animal or human faeces. Food animals are the most important source; chicken and turkey are incriminated most frequently but other meats such as beef, pork and lamb, and animal offal, are important sources. The carcass of infected animals becomes contaminated during processing and contamination spreads to other meats during large-scale storage. Inadequately cooked meat is thus the main hazard. Salmonellae survive deep-freezing, and adequate thawing prior to cooking is essential otherwise temperature in the centre of the meat may not reach a sufficiently high level to kill salmonellae. The recent upsurge in the UK and the USA of *S. enteritidis* infection has been linked to poultry, meat and eggs.[11,18,34]

Numerous outbreaks have been traced to consumption of foods containing raw or undercooked eggs. Contamination of the contents of shell eggs is due either to faecal contamination through shell pores or cracks, or by vertical transmission following ovarian/oviduct infection. Transovarian infection of duck eggs has long been recognized but, until lately, this has seldom been a problem with hen eggs. Recent evidence suggests that such transovarian infection of hen eggs is now common with *S. enteritidis*, which has the ability to become host adapted to chickens and may colonize the ovaries and oviducts. Through vertical transmission, such adaptation also leads to infection of thousands of meat birds or egg-producing birds. The other factors that have contributed to the rising incidence of human salmonellosis include large-scale intensive farming methods which confine animals and fowls in close quarters, and use of bulk-imported, often infected, animal feedstuff. Infection in humans has been encouraged by the increasing number of people eating in community catering establishments, which has necessitated more bulk cooking of food of animal origin, and an increased sale of warmed-up precooked foods.

The rising incidence of drug-resistant salmonellae has been another major problem which is linked to the extensive and poorly controlled use of antimicrobials in farm animals.[46] Multiresistant *S. typhimurium* has been an important cause of morbidity and mortality in children in many developing countries for more than a decade. The source of such infections is often undetermined but hospitals may become involved in protracted nosocomial outbreaks and may act as reservoirs for maintaining the endemicity of multiresistant salmonellae in the community.[36] Person-to-person transmission does occur but convalescent excretors with an adequate standard of personal hygiene rarely transmit infection once they cease to have diarrhoea. In hospitals and residential institutions, most outbreaks are caused by contaminated food but outbreaks in maternity, children's and geriatric wards may follow admission of patients with undiagnosed salmonella infections.

Unpasteurized milk is a recognized source of infection in northern Britain. Unusual methods of transmission include the use of inadequately sterilized fibreoptic digestive endoscopes and administration of contaminated, commercially produced, pancreatic extract to children with cystic fibrosis.[35]

Salmonella infections are more common during the warmer months, when the organisms in the food have a better chance of multiplying and reaching an optimum infecting dose.

PATHOGENESIS

The outcome and the severity of illness after an exposure to infection depend on a number of factors.

Host factors

Salmonellosis is generally most severe in the very young and the elderly,[56] who are also more prone to develop bacteraemia, particularly those with an underlying debilitating disease or gastroduodenal conditions associated with low acidity.[38] Suppression of cell-mediated immunity increases susceptibility to bloodstream invasion as seen in patients with neoplastic diseases and acquired immune deficiency syndrome (AIDS).[37] Susceptibility of patients with sickle-cell anaemia to salmonella osteomyelitis is well recognized.

Virulence of the organism

There is a marked variability of disease-producing ability among the various serotypes and even among different strains within a given serotype. In general, salmonella infections remain confined to the bowels, but invasion of the bloodstream may occur, presenting either as a typhoidal illness or as septicaemia, with the bacteria being located in various organs. Most serotypes are capable of producing invasive illness, but this occurs more frequently with certain serotypes. Septicaemic illness is common in *S. choleraesuis* infection, which rarely produces gastroenteritis.[48] Other serotypes noted for their invasive potential are *S. virchow, S. dublin, S. panama* and *S. london*.[38,40,58] Multiresistant clones of *S. typhimurium* with enhanced virulence are currently causing problems in many developing countries in South America, the Middle East and the Far East, giving rise to a higher proportion of cases with septicaemia and meningitis.

Infecting dose

The size of the infecting dose is important in deciding the outcome of a particular infection. The frequency of food-borne outbreaks of salmonellosis, and the rarity of water-borne and person-to-person transmission, suggest a high infecting dose for salmonella infections. Limited experimental evidence in adult volunteers suggests that an infecting dose of 10^5 or more is necessary to produce clinical illness. Host factors such as gastric hypoacidity and the virulence of the strain probably influence the size of the infecting dose.

Mechanism of diarrhoea

The exact mechanism responsible for diarrhoea is not clear. Mucosal invasion/inflammation is clearly important but this does not adequately explain the copious watery diarrhoea often seen in salmonellosis, particularly in the early stages. Observation in experimental animals of non-invasive enteropathy with water and electrolyte transport defects[45] suggests the existence of a toxin-mediated mechanism. At least two mechanisms have been advanced to explain the 'secretory' type of diarrhoea in salmonellosis: the first through the action of endogenous secretagogues, and the second by the action of salmonella enterotoxins.[2] Salmonellae appear to produce at least two toxins: a cholera-like enterotoxin which activates adenylate cyclase and a cytotoxin which inhibits protein synthesis and causes detachment of cultured mononuclear leukocytes.[2]

CLINICAL FEATURES

Gastroenteritis

After an average incubation period of 12–48 hours the illness begins abruptly with colicky abdominal pain and large quantities of watery diarrhoea, which is often non-bloody to begin with and may remain so throughout the duration of the illness. However, the character of diarrhoea frequently changes to small-volume, bloody stools. Vomiting is not a predominant feature. Headache, malaise, fever and shivering are often present, particularly in the initial stages. The abdominal pain may become intense and more persistent, and there may be localized tenderness with some rebound over the sigmoid colon or in the right iliac fossa. Appendicitis may be misdiagnosed in the latter situation: should a laparotomy be undertaken the appendix is usually normal or only mildly abnormal, but the terminal ileum is acutely inflamed. Salmonellae are an important cause of acute ileitis, along with *Campylobacter* and *Yersinia* species.

There is much variation in the severity of the illness. Mild and inapparent infections are common. In extremes of age and in debilitated patients the diarrhoea may be pronounced and protracted, with rapid dehydration leading to renal failure. Those who have undergone gastric surgery previously are particularly prone to develop severe diarrhoea, which is often cholera-like in intensity.

The diarrhoea subsides within a few days in the average patient: persistent diarrhoea for more than 3 weeks is rare in salmonellosis, although some increased bowel frequency may be observed for a while due to the development of a postinfective irritable bowel state.

Carrier state

After recovery, patients usually continue to excrete salmonellae in stools for an average period of 4–8 weeks; the excretion period is longer in infants and the elderly. Chronic carriage is rare, occurring in far less than 1% of cases.[8]

Salmonella colitis

A mild degree of colorectal inflammation in not uncommon in salmonellosis, as judged by the frequency of inflammatory exudate in the stools. Sigmoidoscopic evidence of active proctocolitis can be found frequently in hospitalized patients, and this may dominate the clinical picture with frankly bloody stools.[7,39] Toxic dilatation may complicate the clinical picture.[50] A sigmoidoscopy reveals abnormalities ranging from mucosal oedema and hyperaemia, with or without petechial haemorrhages, to mucosal friability.[39] Gross ulceration and slough formation are rare. Barium enema shows diffuse loss of haustration, with fine irregularity of the bowel outline and a disturbance of the mucosal pattern usually confined to the distal colon, but occasionally there may be segmental involvement mimicking Crohn's disease (*Figure 9.5*).

The rectal biopsy histology is not specific and a similar pattern of inflammation may be seen in other infective colitides, including *Shigella* sp., *Entamoeba histolytica* and *Campylobacter* sp. The predominant features are those of acute inflammation

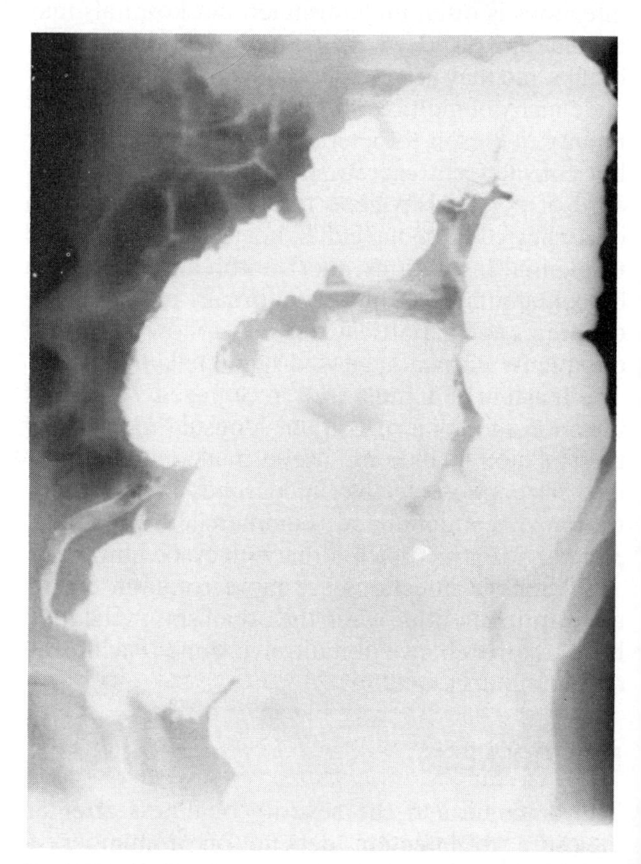

Figure 9.5 Barium in salmonella colitis, showing a right-sided segmental lesion.

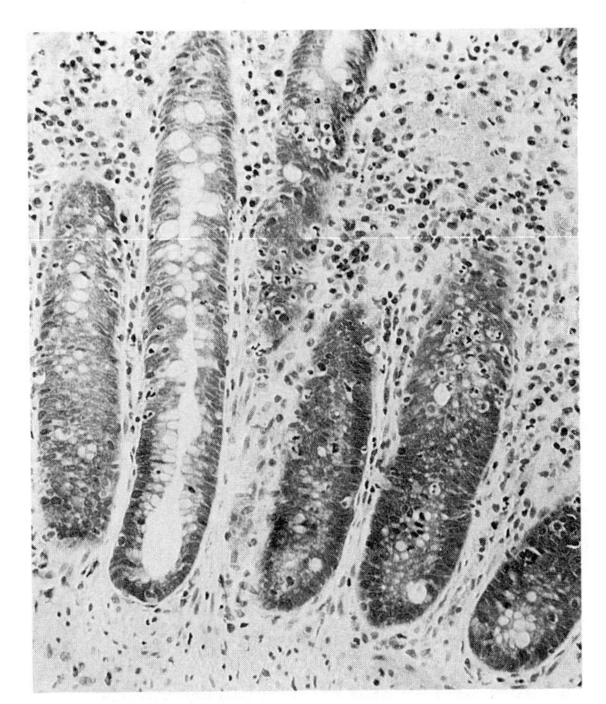

Figure 9.6 Rectal biopsy appearances in salmonella colitis, showing a polymorphonuclear infiltrate which is invading the crypts, but without any marked increase in chronic inflammatory cell content of the lamina propria. The goblet cell population is relatively well preserved as is the crypt architecture. Haematoxylin and eosin, × 500.

with oedema and focal collection of polymorphonuclear cells in the mucosa (*Figure 9.6*).[5,14] The rectal biopsies may show marked mucus depletion and crypt abscess formation in severe illness, and thus may mimic acute ulcerative colitis of short duration in which abnormalities of crypt architecture have not yet developed.

Invasive salmonellosis

Bacteraemia occurs not infrequently in non-typhi salmonellosis – particularly in infants and the elderly. Besides age, serotypes of the infecting organisms, as well as the presence of debilitating diseases and gastroduodenal conditions associated with hypoacidity, are often risk factors.[38] AIDS patients are particularly vulnerable to salmonella bacteraemia, often with repeated relapses.[37]

In previously healthy individuals, bacteraemia is usually a transient event but, in a minority of individuals, particularly those with the risk factors outlined, the bacteraemia may be clinically significant, presenting as (1) septicaemia, (2) typhoidal illness with sustained fever, splenomegaly and even rose spots, or (3) metastatic localization[13] in the meninges, bones and joints, lungs, endocardium, spleen or kidneys. Salmonellae are important causes of aortitis and other vascular infections in the elderly.[13] Infants are particularly prone to develop meningitis and bone involvement is more common in patients with sickle-cell disease.

Reactive arthritis

Sterile synovitis of a reactive nature may follow salmonella infection, particularly in HLA-B27-positive individuals. The symptoms of arthritis usually begin 1–2 weeks after the infection and any joint may be affected, although the knees and ankles are most frequently involved. Occasionally, there is migratory polyarthralgia, resembling acute rheumatic fever, or bilateral proximal interphalangeal joint involvement of rheumatoid type. Acute iridocyclitis may complicate the picture.

DIFFERENTIAL DIAGNOSIS

In food poisoning outbreaks the longer incubation period, fever and presence of inflammatory exudate in the stools may help to differentiate salmonella infection from 'toxin-type' poisoning caused by *Staphylococcus aureus, Clostridium perfringens (welchii)* or *Bacillus cereus*. However, definitive diagnosis depends on positive bacteriology because similar clinical features are seen also in *shigella*, *campylobacter* and *yersinia* infections.

The differentiation of severe salmonella colitis from the first episode of inflammatory bowel disease with coincident salmonella infection may pose problems because sigmoidoscopic, radiological and even histological features may be identical. In general, the duration of diarrhoea in salmonella colitis is short but, in more persistent infections, steroids and antibiotics are prescribed to cover both possibilities. In patients who respond promptly to this regimen, the diagnostic dilemma can only be resolved by further rectal biopsies and prolonged follow-up. In primary salmonella colitis, the rectal biopsy histology generally returns to normal after about a month, whereas this is uncommon in inflammatory bowel disease. Those patients who continue to show features of severe colitis for several weeks are usually suffering from underlying inflammatory bowel disease even if the stool cultures remain positive for salmonellae.

TREATMENT

Antimicrobial therapy is not generally necessary in the treatment of salmonella gastroenteritis which is brief and self-limiting, and such therapy may prolong the carrier state. Antimicrobials are indicated in invasive salmonellosis and should also be considered in the very young or the elderly, as well as in immunocompromised patients with severe symptoms even when there is no confirmation of bacteraemia. Patients with severe colitis should also receive antibiotics, although their value has not been established in controlled studies.

The choice of antimicrobials on such occasions is difficult because of the increasing resistance of non-typhi salmonellae to the commonly used antimicrobials, such as amoxycillin, co-trimoxazole and chloramphenical. The new quinolones, such as ciprofloxacin, are promising in these situations. Ciprofloxacin is also useful in eradication of the persistent carrier state.[15]

In children with invasive salmonellosis, one of the third-generation cephalosporins, such as ceftazidime, ceftriaxone and cefoperazone, would probably be the drug of choice.[31]

PROGNOSIS

The mortality is less than 1%. Most deaths are due to septicaemia or dehydration and renal failure in the elderly or the very young, often in patients who are already suffering from pre-existing disease.

PREVENTION

High standards of hygiene are essential in all food premises, including shops, factories, slaughterhouses, kitchens and restaurants. Raw and cooked meats must be handled and stored separately, food should be cooked or thoroughly reheated before use and frozen food should be completely thawed before cooking. Asymptomatic excretors who are handlers of unwrapped food, meant for consumption without further cooking, should have bacteriological clearance before returning to work, but others may do so, or return to school, so long as they have adequate standards of personal hygiene.

REFERENCES

1. Acharya, I.L., Lowe, C.U., Thapa, R. *et al.* (1987) Prevention of typhoid fever in Nepal with the Vi capsular polysaccharide of *Salmonella typhi*: a preliminary report. *New England Journal of Medicine*, **317**, 1101–1104.
2. Acheson, D. and Keusch, G.T. (1988) Invasive enteropathies. *Baillière's Clinical Tropical Medicine and Communicable Diseases*, **3**, 463–487.
3. Akhtar, M.A., Karamat, K.A., Malik, A.Z. *et al.* (1989) Efficacy of ofloxacin in typhoid fever, particularly in drug resistant cases. *Reviews of Infectious Diseases*, **2**(suppl. 5), S, 1193.
4. Anand, A.C., Kataria, V.K., Singh, W. and Chatterjee, S.K. (1990) Epidemic multiresistant enteric fever in eastern India. *The Lancet*, **i**, 352.
5. Appelbaum, P.C., Scragg, J. and Schonland, M.M. (1976) Colonic involvement in salmonellosis. *The Lancet*, **ii**, 102.
6. Baker, N.M., Mills, A. E. and Rachman, I. (1974) Haemolytic–uraemic syndrome in typhoid fever. *British Medical Journal*, **ii**, 84–87.
7. Boyd, J.F. (1976) Colonic involvement in salmonellosis. *The Lancet*, **i**, 1415.
8. Buchenwald, D.S. and Blaser, M.J. (1984) A review of human salmonellosis II. Duration of excretion following infection with non-typhi salmonella. *Reviews of Infectious Diseases*, **6**, 345–356.
9. Butler, T., Bell, W.R., Levin, J. *et al.* (1978) Typhoid fever: studies of blood coagulation, bacteraemia and endotoxaemia. *Archives of Internal Medicine*, **138**, 407–410.
10. Calva, J.J. and Ruiz-Palacios, G.M. (1986) Salmonella hepatitis: detection of salmonella antigens in the liver of patients with typhoid fever. *Journal of Infectious Diseases*, **154**, 373–374.
11. Centres for Diseases Control (1988) Update. Salmonella enteritidis infection and grade A shell eggs – United States. *Morbidity and Mortality Weekly Report*, **32**, 490–495.
12. Chalker, R.B. and Blaser, M.J. (1988) A Review of human salmonellosis III. Magnitude of salmonella infection in the United States. *Reviews of Infectious Diseases*, **10**, 111–124.
13. Cohen, J.I., Bartlett, J.A. and Corey, G.R. (1987) Extra intestinal manifestations of salmonella infections. *Medicine*, **66**, 349–388.
14. Day, D.W., Mandal, B.K. and Morson, B.C. (1978) The rectal biopsy appearances in salmonella colitis. *Histopathology*, **2**, 117–131.
15. Diridle, G., Pilcher, H. and Wolf, D. (1986) Treatment of chronic salmonella carriers with ciprofloxacin. *European Journal of Clinical Microbiology*, **5**, 260–261.
16. Doshi, N. and Taylor, A.G. (1984) Comparison of the Vi indirect fluorescent antibody test with the Widal agglutination method in the serodiagnosis of typhoid fever. *Journal of Clinical Pathology*, **37**, 805–808.
17. Edelman, R. and Levine, M.M. (1986) Summary of an international workshop on typhoid fever. *Reviews of Infectious Diseases*, **8**, 329–349.
18. Editorial (1988) Salmonella enteritidis phage type 4: chicken and egg. *The Lancet*, **ii**, 720–721.
19. Fallon, R.J., Mandal, B.K., Mayon-White, R.T. and Scott, A.C. (1988) Assessment of antimicrobial treatment of acute typhoid and paratyphoid fevers in Britain and the Netherlands 1971–1980. *Journal of Infection*, **16**, 129–134.
20. Farid, Z., Higashi, G.J., Bassily, S. and Miner, W.F. (1975) Immune-complex disease in typhoid and paratyphoid fevers. *Annals of Internal Medicine*, **83**, 432.
21. Ferreccio, C., Morris, J.G. Jr, Valdidieso, C. *et al.* (1988) Efficacy of ciprofloxacin in the treatment of

chronic typhoid carriers. *Journal of Infectious Diseases*, **157**, 1235–1239.
22. George, J.T.A., Wallace, J.G., Morrison, H.R. and Harbourne, J.F. (1972) Paratyphoid in man and cattle. *British Medical Journal*, **iii**, 208–211.
23. Gianella, R.A., Broitman, S.A. and Zamcheck, N. (1973) Influence of gastric acidity on bacterial and parasitic enteric infections. *Annals of Internal Medicine*, **78**, 271–276.
24. Gotuzzo, E., Guerra, J.G., Benavente, L. *et al.* (1988) Use of norfloxacin to treat chronic typhoid carriers. *Journal of Infectious Diseases*, **157**, 1221–1225.
25. Herzog, C. (1976) Chemotherapy of typhoid fever: a review of literature. *Infection*, **4**, 166–173.
26. Hoffman, S.L., Punjabi, N.H., Kumala, S. *et al.* (1984) Reduction of mortality in chloramphenical – treated severe typhoid fever by high dose dexamethasone. *New England Journal of Medicine*, **310**, 81–87.
27. Hornick, R.B. and Greiseman, S. (1978) On the pathogenesis of typhoid fever. *Archives of Internal Medicine*, **138**, 357–358.
28. Hornick, R.B., Greiseman, S.E., Woodward, T.E. *et al.* (1970) Typhoid fever: pathogenesis and immunological control. *New England Journal of Medicine*, **283**, 686–691, 736–746.
29. Khosla, S.M., Srivastava, S.C. and Gupta, S. (1977) Neuro-psychiatric manifestations of typhoid. *Journal of Tropical Medicine and Hygiene*, **80**, 95–98.
30. Kim, J.P., Oh, S.K. and Jarrett, F. (1975) Management of ileal perforation due to typhoid fever. *Annals of Surgery*, **181**, 88–91.
31. Kinsella, R.T., Yoger, R., Shulman, S.T. *et al.* (1987) Treatment of Salmonella meningitis and brain abscess with the new cephalosporins. *Paediatric Infectious Diseases*, **6**, 476–480.
32. Klugman, K.P., Gilberton, I.T., Koornof, H.J. *et al.* (1987) Protective activity of Vi capsular polysaccharide vaccine against typhoid fever. *The Lancet*, **ii**, 1165–1169.
33. Levine, M.M., Ferreccio, C., Black, R.M. and Germanier, R. (1987) Large scale field trial of Ty 21a oral typhoid vaccine in enteric coated capsule formulation. *The Lancet*, **i**, 1049–1057.
34. Lin, F.Y.C., Morris, J.G., Trump, D. *et al.* (1988) Investigation of an outbreak of *Salmonella enteritidis* gastroenteritis associated with consumption of eggs in a restaurant chain in Maryland. *American Journal of Epidemiology*, **128**, 839–844.
35. Lipson, A. and Meikle, H. (1977) Porcine pancreatin as a source of salmonella infection in children with cystic fibrosis. *Archives of Diseases in Childhood*, **52**, 569–572.
36. Mandal, B.K. (1986) Typhoid fever and other salmonella infections. *Current opinion in Gastroenterology*, **2**, 109–112.
37. Mandal, B.K. (1989) Typhoid fever and other salmonella infections. *Current opinion in Gastroenterology*, **5**, 121–125.
38. Mandal, B.K. and Brennand, J. (1988) Bacteraemia in salmonellosis: a 15 year retrospective study from a regional infectious diseases unit. *British Medical Journal*, **297**, 1242–1243.
39. Mandal, B.K. and Mani, V. (1976) Colonic involvement in salmonellosis. *The Lancet*, **i**, 887–888.
40. Mani, V., Brennand, J. and Mandal, B.K. (1974) Invasive illness with *Salmonella virchow* infection. *British Medical Journal*, **ii**, 143–144.
41. Osuntoken, B.O., Bademosi, O., Ogunremi, K. and Wright, S.G. (1972) Neuropsychiatric manifestations of typhoid fever in 959 patients. *Archives of Neurology*, **27**, 7–13.
42. Perales, I. and Andican, A. (1988) Salmonella enteritidis and eggs. *The Lancet*, **ii**, 1133.
43. Ramachandran, S., Godfrey, J.J. and Perera, M.F.V. (1974) Typhoid hepatitis. *Journal of the American Medical Association*, **230**, 236–240.
44. Ramirez, C.A., Bran, J.L., Mejia, C.R. *et al.* (1985) Open prospective study of the clinical efficacy of ciprofloxacin. *Antimicrobial Agents and Chemotherapy*, **28**, 128–132.
45. Rout, W.R., Formal, S.B., Dammin, G.J. and Gianella, R.A. (1974) Pathophysiology of salmonella diarrhoea in the rhesus monkey: intestinal transport, morphological and bacteriological studies. *Gastroenterology*, **67**, 59–70.
46. Rowe, B. and Threlfall, E.J. (1987) Antibiotic resistance in Salmonella. *Salmonella Special: March 1987 revision of the PHLS Microbiology Digest 1986*, **3**, 6–8.
47. Rowe, B., Threlfall, E.J. and Ward, L.R. (1987) Does chloroamphenical remain the drug of choice for typhoid? *Epidemiology and Infection*, **98**, 379–389.
48. Saphra, J. and Winter, J.W. (1957) Clinical manifestations of salmonellosis in man. An evaluation of 7779 human infections at New York Salmonella Centre. *New England Journal of Medicine*, **256**, 1128–1134.
49. Schofield, P.F. and Mandal, B.K. (1981) Acute ileitis. *British Medical Journal*, **283**, 1545.
50. Schofield, P.F., Mandal, B.K. and Ironside, A.G. (1979) Toxic dilatation of the colon in salmonella colitis and inflammatory bowel disease. *British Journal of Surgery*, **66**, 5–8.
51. Scragg, J. N. (1976) Further experience with amoxycillin in typhoid fever in children. *British Medical Journal*, **ii**, 1031–1033.
52. Sippel, J.E., Hanafy, H.M., Diab, A.S. *et al.* (1987) Serodiagnosis of typhoid fever in paediatric patients by anti-LPS ELISA. *Transactions of the Royal Society of Tropical Medicine and Hygiene*, **81**, 1022–1026.
53. Sitprija, V., Pipatanagul, V., Boonpucknavig, V. and Boonpucknavig, S. (1974) Glomerulitis in typhoid fever. *Annals of Internal Medicine*, **81**, 210–213.

54. Soe, G.B. and Overturf, G.D. (1987) Treatment of typhoid fever and other systemic salmonellosis with cefotaxime, ceftriaxone, cefoperazone and other newer cephalosporins. *Reviews of Infectious Diseases*, **9**, 719–736.
55. Stanley, P.J., Flegg, P.J., Mandal, B.K. and Geddes, A.M. (1989) Open study of ciprofloxacin in enteric fever. *Journal of Antimicrobial Chemotherapy*, **23**, 789–791.
56. Thuluvath, P.J. and McKendrick, M.W. (1988) Salmonella and complications related to age – Sheffield experience. *Quarterly Journal of Medicine*, **67**, 497–503.
57. Wang, F., Gu, X.-J., Zhang, M.-F. and Tai, T.-Y. (1989) Treatment of typhoid fever with ofloxacin. *Journal of Antimicrobial Chemotherapy*, **23**, 785–788.
58. Wilkins, E.G.L. and Roberts, C. (1988) Extraintestinal salmonellosis. *Epidemiology and Infection*, **100**, 361–368.

SHIGELLOSIS

D.W.K. Acheson, M.J.G. Farthing and G.T. Keusch

Bacillary dysentery due to organisms of the genus *Shigella*, initially described by Kioshi Shiga in 1898, continues to be an important cause of bacterial gastroenteritis worldwide. The four species of the genus *Shigella*, while sharing many biochemical, microbiological, clinical and epidemiological features, are capable of causing distinctive diseases and complications.

MICROBIOLOGY

The four species of genus *Shigella (S. dysenteriae, S. flexneri, S. boydii* and *S. sonnei)*, separable by group specific polysaccharide antigens designated A, B, C and D, share many characteristics and can be further categorized into several subtypes (*Table 9.2*). Shigellae are slender, non-motile Gram-negative rods closely related to *Escherichia coli*. Important differences, however, include the inability of shigellae to ferment lactose, their lack of flagella (and hence motility), failure to produce gas from glucose and inability to decarboxylate lysine (*Table 9.2*).

EPIDEMIOLOGY

Shigellosis occurs throughout the world and, although varying in incidence from place to place, has the same basic epidemiological characteristics everywhere. Shigellae are highly host adapted, naturally infect only humans and some non-human primates, and are usually transmitted by person-to-person contact, although point-source outbreaks can also occur.[24]

One striking feature of the spread of shigellosis is the extremely small inoculum of bacteria required to cause disease. As few as 10 organisms of *S. dysenteriae* type 1 may cause disease in healthy adults, and 500 or less of other *Shigella* species are also able to cause illness.[11] The precise reasons why humans are susceptible to such small doses of *Shigella* sp. are unknown. Theories regarding resistance to the gastric acid barrier in vivo have been proposed[17] and refuted.[14] Rapid invasion of gastric epithelial cells has also been suggested[23] to explain how these acid-labile organisms so readily pass through the stomach in such small numbers to cause disease.

Table 9.2 Usual laboratory characteristics of the genus *Shigella*, compared with those of enterotoxigenic *Escherichia coli*

Species	*Serological group*	*Serotypes (subtypes)*	*Mannitol utilization*	*Lactase utilization*	*Gas production*	*Lysine decarboxylase*	*Motility*
S. dysenteriae	A	10	–	–	–	–	–
S. flexneri	B	6	+	–	–	–	–
S. boydii	C	15	+	–	–	–	–
S. sonnei	D	1[a]	+	(Late+)	–	–	–
Enterotoxigenic *E. coli*			+	+	+	+	+(–)[b]

[a]Multiple subtypes can be identified by colicin typing.
[b]Ocassional *E. coli*, including enteroinvasive serotypes, are non-motile.

Historically, variations in the predominant *Shigella* species have been noted since the genus was first described. Before World War I, *S. dysenteriae* was the major isolate world-wide and was responsible for major epidemics. Subsequently, *S. flexneri* predominated, only to be replaced in industrialized nations by *S. sonnei* over the last three decades. *S. flexneri*, however, remains a major problem in less developed areas.[7] Although the reported overall incidence of *S. flexneri* decreased in the USA between 1975 and 1985, the median age of males from whom *S. flexneri* was isolated increased from 5 to 26 years. There was a five-fold increase in the isolation rate in men, but no change in women. This shift is thought to be due to increased homosexual transmission of *S. flexneri*,[43] although why this particular species is involved is unknown. Children in day-care centres are another high-risk population, with subsequent introduction of the infection into household contacts as a significant consequence.[36]

Since 1969, *S. dysenteriae* type 1 has re-emerged in sporadic epidemic outbreaks in Mexico and Central Africa.[25] The reasons for these epidemiological shifts and intermittent epidemics are unknown.

PATHOGENESIS

One of the most important steps in the pathogenesis of shigellosis is invasion of the colonic mucosa.[27,38,42] This involves entry of the organism into colonic epithelial cells followed by intracellular multiplication, intracellular spread and host cell death. This sequence of events results in amplification of the organisms, spread to the lamina propria and initiation of the inflammatory responses with resultant ulceration and abscess formation. The microbial genetic mechanisms involved are now more precisely understood and have been reviewed recently.[19,31,32,38]

A 220 kilobase plasmid found in virulent Shigella strains has been associated with the invasive phenotype.[3] At least four plasmid-encoded outer-membrane proteins have been identified, designated invasion plasmid antigens (ipa) A, B, C and D.[20] The precise role of these antigens in invasion is still not clear; however, ipaB, -C and -D appear to be required.[38]

Intracellular multiplication of *Shigella* sp. is an important aspect of pathogenesis for which plasmid genes are required. A critical event is early lysis of the membrane-bound phagocytotic vacuole and release of the organism into the cytoplasm.[40] A plasmid-encoded haemolysin is required. Direct interaction between the invading organisms and host cell microfilaments results in intracellular spread of bacteria. A plasmid gene, *icsA* (intracellular spread), coding for a 120 kDa outer-membrane protein[38] is essential for organisms to reach and infect adjacent cells. Contiguous spread leads to micro-ulcer formation.

Shigellae also produce potent cytotoxins, the best characterized of which is Shiga toxin from *S. dysenteriae* type 1, previously known as Shiga neurotoxin. The toxin is composed of one A subunit (molecular weight 32 000) and five B subunits (molecular weight 7700).[10] The A subunit is an *N*-glycohydrolase which cleaves a single base (adenine) in the 28-S component of the 60-S ribosomal subunit of mammalian cells.[13] This results in inhibition of protein synthesis with subsequent cytotoxicity of target cells, including human colonic mucosal epithelial cells.[34] The B subunit mediates toxin binding to a specific cell surface receptor (globotriaosylceramide) on the intestinal microvillous membrane. This receptor is selectively present on villous, but not crypt cells in rabbits[21] and is probably responsible for mediation of an enterotoxic effect in rabbit small bowel. There is also evidence, in rabbits at least, that this receptor in the gut is developmentally regulated and only appears as the animal matures.[33] Although toxin may be responsible for the watery diarrhoea phase of shigellosis, its precise role in human disease has not been fully elucidated. Experiments in primates, however, suggest that it may function principally as an endothelial cell-damaging agent, rather than acting solely on gut epithelial cells themselves.[15]

CLINICAL FEATURES

The symptoms and signs of shigellosis typically begin 1–5 days after ingestion of Shigella organisms, with fever, fatigue and anorexia. The initial presenting feature is usually fever and, in seizure-prone children, onset of fever is often rapid enough to provoke a febrile convulsion. The speed and extent of the progression of illness depends on the virulence of the infecting organism (*Table 9.3*), and the clinical epidemiological features of the host. Important host determinants are nutritional status and age, the most susceptible being formula-fed neonates or poorly nourished older infants, and the elderly.[5,26] Shortly after the onset of fever, a mild-to-moderate, not severely dehydrating, watery diarrhoea ensues. Nausea, vomiting and cramps are not usually prominent, and initially the stool is not bloody. When *S. sonnei* is the causal agent, the illness may not progress and is self-limiting, resolv-

Table 9.3 Clinical features of *Shigella* species

Species	Convalescent carriage	Frequency of symptoms		Frequency of haemolytic uraemic syndrome
		Diarrhoea	Dysentery	
S. dysenteriae	<4 weeks but prolonged in malnourished	+	+++	++
S. flexneri	<4 weeks but prolonged in malnourished	++	++	±
S. boydii	<3 weeks	+++	+	−
S. sonnei	<2 weeks	++++	Uncommon	−

ing in 3–7 days. Usually within 24 hours of the onset of diarrhoea, numerous pus cells and red cells can be detected in the stool (*Figure 9.7*), findings that are indicative of the invasive colitis phase of the disease. Stool frequency may number 15–20/day, even up to 100 times, although usually no more than 30 ml/kg per day of fluid is lost.[8]

Although the watery diarrhoea is probably, in part, small bowel in origin, the presence of pus and blood is evidence of extension of the disease to the colon, and some degree of colonic involvement is a consistent feature of shigellosis. Dysentery is generally least in *S. sonnei*, more in *S. boydii*, common in *S. flexeri* and the rule in *S. dysenteriae* type 1. Watery diarrhoea generally shows the reverse relationship (*Table 9.3*), although no absolute rules apply. With sufficient colonic involvement, a typical triad of signs and symptoms appears. These include intense cramps, tenesmus, and the frequent passage of small volumes of blood, pus and mucus.[30] With the most severe infection, such as that due to *S. dysenteriae*, the progression to dysentery may be very rapid and the initial symptoms overlooked. If colonic involvement is extensive, fatal necrotizing enterocolitis may occur, with toxic megacolon and Gram-negative sepsis as a consequence.

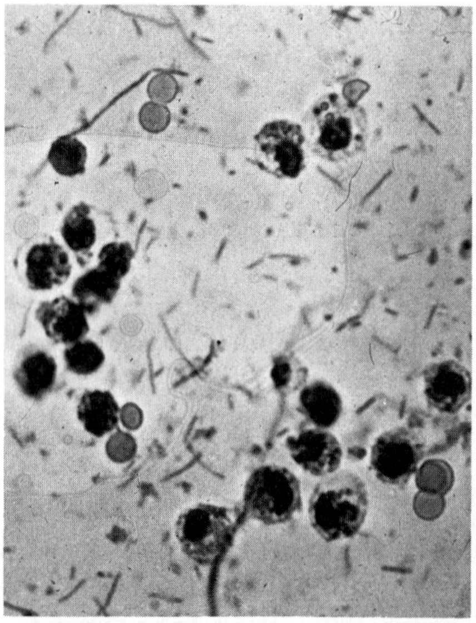

Figure 9.7 Wet mount of watery diarrhoea stool of patient with *S. sonnei* infection. Numerous pus and red cells are present. (Courtesy of M.M. Levine.)

Sigmoidoscopic examination of a patient with shigellosis may demonstrate mucosal hyperaemia, haemorrhage and mucosal friability. Microscopically, the specialized epithelial cells overlying lymphoid follicles are the first affected. There is epithelial cell damage and sloughing, with bleeding and inflammation in the lamina propria.[29] Stains with Giemsa or a tissue Gram stain reveal intraepithelial organisms (*Figure 9.8*). Barium enema examination may show segmental involvement of the rectum, sigmoid or descending colon with superficial ulcerations, collar-stud ulcers, oedema, spasm and skip areas, all of which may mimic Crohn's disease or ulcerative colitis.

COMPLICATIONS

Both intestinal and systemic complications are common in shigellosis.[4] Toxic megacolon is one of the more serious intestinal complications and has a high mortality if perforation occurs.[2] Protein-losing enteropathy due to the inflammatory enteritis contributes to the development of protein–energy malnutrition. Seizures are the most common neurological complication, and although resembling febrile convulsions they generally occur in children more than 5 years of age suggesting other important pathogenic mechanisms.[4] The most dramatic systemic complication is haemolytic uraemic syndrome (a triad of renal failure, haemolytic anaemia and thrombocytopenia) which is particularly associated with *S. dysenteriae* type 1 infection. This is probably due to the presence of Shiga toxin in this species, because haemolytic uraemic syndrome is also a well-recognized complication of haemorrhagic colitis in association with Shiga-like toxin producing *E.*

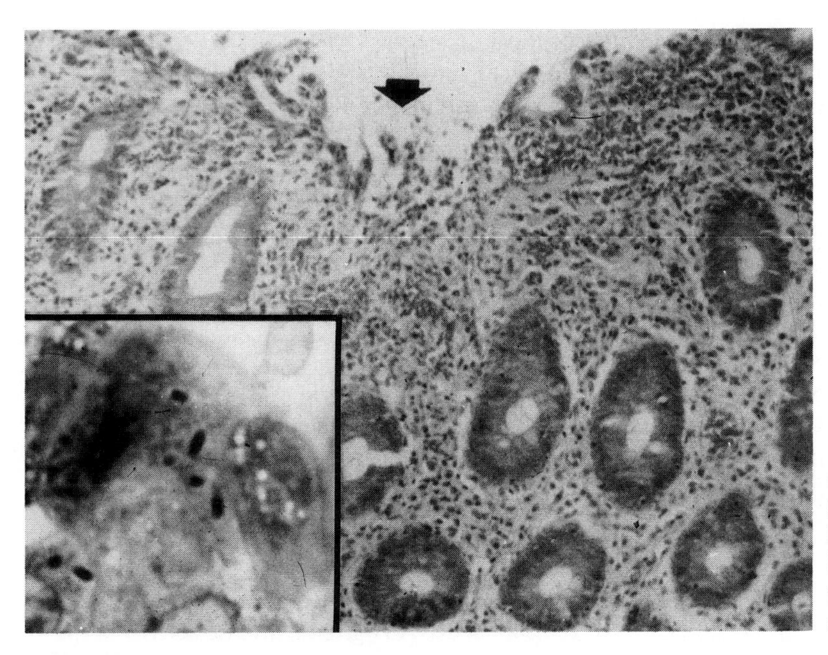

Figure 9.8 Colonic biopsy in shigellosis. Arrow points to a shallow ulceration. Note marked inflammatory response in the lamina propria. Insert shows an epithelial cell under higher magnification with intracellular micro-organisms stained with Giemsa.

coli.[22] Marked leukaemoid reactions with white counts in excess of 50 000 and mild thrombocytopenia with platelet counts of 30 000–100 000 are common. Bacteraemia with shigellae or Enterobacteriacae, previously thought to be rare, has been documented in 10% of severely ill, hospitalized patients in Bangladesh[40] with a high mortality in those less than 1 year old. Severe hyponatraemia and hypoglycaemia may also occur, the latter being a major cause of death in association with diarrhoea.[6] Other documented complications include respiratory symptoms, neurological complications, meningism and reactive arthritis.

INVESTIGATIONS

Shigellosis should be suspected in any patient who is febrile and has bloody diarrhoea, but the definitive diagnosis has to be microbiological. Culture of the organism from stool is not technically difficult but requires the use of a selective medium (e.g. MacConkey's agar plus another such as S-S, XLD, HE or Tergitol-7) and the plating of a specimen that is as fresh as possible. Rectal swabs are not a reliable way of obtaining adequate specimens to exclude the diagnosis. DNA probes have been used to identify shigellae but do not offer any advantage over standard techniques if a competent bacteriological laboratory with the appropriate antisera is available.[12]

TREATMENT

Shigellosis is not usually a severely dehydrating disease, and fluid replacement is readily accomplished by use of an oral rehydration solution. Watery diarrhoea secondary to infection with shigella is usually self-limiting and significantly improved by the time the diagnosis is confirmed. An appropriate antibiotic can shorten the course and severity of the illness and may be life-saving, especially in children who live in developing countries.[37] Antibiotic resistance is a problem in *shigella* infections and, depending on local conditions, resistance to ampicillin and trimethoprim–sulphamethoxazole may be common. These resistance patterns resulted in the use of nalidixic acid in developing countries, although some resistance has also been reported to this drug.[37] More recently, the 4-fluoroquinolone drugs (e.g. ciprofloxacin, norfloxacin, ofloxacin) have been reported as highly effective in the treatment of shigellosis. It is not yet known whether they are safe in young children. A significant advantage of the 4-fluoroquinolones may be the introduction of effective single-dose treatment as demonstrated in studies from Peru,[18] and in an outbreak of shigellosis in a home for the mentally handicapped in England.[44]

PREVENTION

Common-sense hygienic practices reduces person-to-person transmission of *shigella* infection. Handwashing with soap is effective in reducing the secondary case rate within families, even in rural settings in Bangladesh. Food preparation and eating should be separated from care for the patients and handling of objects potentially contaminated with faeces.

The development of an efficacious vaccine against

Shigellae spp. is a high priority, and it is generally accepted that oral live vaccines are the most likely candidates to be successful in generating significant immunity. Attempts to accomplish this have generally proceeded along two paths: first, by using a carrier strain approach in which certain genes from *Shigella* spp. known to encode specific antigens are transferred to non-pathogenic strains such as *Salmonella typhi* strain Ty21a or *E. coli* K12. Several such systems have been described[16,39] but have failed to provide consistent significant immunity in experimental systems. An alternative approach is genetically to attenuate the shigellae themselves, and use the attenuated strain as a vaccine. This approach is currently under investigation by several groups and early results are promising.[1,9,28]

REFERENCES

1. Ahmed, Z.U., Sarker, M.R. and Sack, D.A. (1990) Protection of adult rabbits and monkeys from lethal shigellosis by oral immunization with a thiamine-requiring and temperature-sensitive mutant of *Shigella flexeri* Y. *Vaccine*, **8**, 153–158.
2. Azad, M.A.K., Islam, M. and Butler, T. (1986) Colonic perforation in *Shigella dysenteriae* type 1 infection. *Pediatric Infectious Diseases*, **5**, 103–104.
3. Baudry, B., Maurelli, A.T., Clerc, P., Sadoff, J.C. and Sansonetti, P.J. (1987) Localization of plasmid loci necessary for the entry of *Shigella flexneri* into HeLa cells, and characterization of one locus encoding four immunogenic polypeptides. *Journal of General Microbiology*, **133**, 3409–3413.
4. Bennish, M.L. (1991) Potentially lethal complications of shigellosis. *Reviews of Infectious Diseases*, **13**, S319–S324.
5. Bennish, M.L. and Wojtyniak, B.J. (1991) Mortality due to shigellosis: community and hospital data. *Reviews of Infectious Diseases*, **13**, S245–S251.
6. Bennish, M.L., Azad, A.K., Rahman, O. and Phillips, R.E. (1990) Hypoglycaemia during diarrhea in childhood. *New England Journal of Medicine*, **322**, 1357–1363.
7. Bennish, M.L., Harris, J.R., Wojtyniak, B.J. and Strulens, M. (1990) Death in shigellosis: Incidence and risk factors in hospitalized patients. *Journal of Infectious Diseases*, **161**, 500–506.
8. Butler, T., Speelman, P., Kabir, I. and Banwell, J. (1986) Colonic dysfunction during shigellosis. *Journal of Infectious Diseases*, **154**, 817–824.
9. Dentchev, V., Marinova, S., Vassilev, T., Bratoyeva, M. and Linde, K. (1990) Live *Shigella flexneri* 2a and *Shigella sonnei* I vaccine candidate strains with two attenuating markers. II. Preliminary results of vaccination of adult volunteers and children aged 2–17 years. *Vaccine*, **8**, 30–34.
10. Donohue-Rolfe, A., Keusch, G.T., Edson, C., Thorley-Lawson, D. and Jacewicz, M. (1984) Pathogenesis of *Shigella* diarrhoea IX. Simplified high yield purification of *Shigella* toxin and characterization of subunit composition and function by the use of subunit-specific monoclonal and polyclonal antibodies. *Journal of Experimental Medicine*, **160**, 1767–1781.
11. Dupont, H.L., Levine, M.M., Hornick, R.B. and Formal, S.B. (1989) Inoculum size in shigellosis and implications for expected mode of transmission. *Journal of Infectious Diseases*, **159**, 1126–1128.
12. Echeverria, P., Sethabutr, O. and Pitarangsi, C. (1991) Microbiology and diagnosis of infections with *Shigella* and enteroinvasive *Escherichia coli*. *Reviews of Infectious Diseases*, **13**, S220–S225.
13. Endo, Y., Tsurugi, K., Yutsudo, T., Takeda, Y., Ogasawara, T. and Igarashi, K. (1988) Site of action of a Vero toxin (VTs) from *Escherichia coli* 0157:H7 and of Shiga toxin on eukaryotic ribosomes. RNA *N*-glycohydrolase activity of the toxins. *European Journal of Biochemistry*, **171**, 45–50.
14. Felson, J. and Osofsky, A. G. (1939) Gastric barrier in bacillary dysentery. *Archives of Internal Medicine*, **63**, 64–70.
15. Fontaine, A., Arondel, J. and Sansonetti, P.J. (1988) Role of Shiga toxin in the pathogenesis of bacillary dysentery studied by using a Tox-mutant of *Shigella dysenteriae* 1. *Infection and Immunity*, **56**, 3099–3109.
16. Formal, S.B., Baron, L.S., Kopecko, D.J., Washington, O., Powell, C. and Life, C.A. (1981) Construction of a potential bivalent vaccine strain: introduction of *Shigella sonnei* form 1 antigen genes into the galE *Salmonella typhi* Ty21a typhoid vaccine strain. *Infection and Immunity*, **34**, 746–750.
17. Garrod, L.P. (1937) The susceptibility of different bacteria to destruction in the stomach. *Journal of Pathological Bacteriology*, **45**, 473–474.
18. Gotuzzo, E., Oberhelman, R.A., Maguina, C. *et al.* (1989) Comparison of single dose treatment with norfloxacin and standard 5-day treatment with trimethoprim-sulfamethoxazole for acute shigellosis in adults. *Antimicrobial Agents and Chemotherapy*, **33**, 1101–1104.
19. Hale, T.L. and Formal, S.B. (1986) Genetics of virulence in *Shigella*. *Microbial Pathogenesis*, **1**, 511–518.
20. Hale, T.L., Oaks, E.V. and Formal, S.B. (1985) Identification and antigenic characterization of virulence-associated, plasmid-coded proteins of *Shigella* spp and enteroinvasive *Escherichia coli*. *Infection and Immunity*, **50**, 620–629.
21. Kandal, G., Donohue-Rolfe, A., Donowitz, M. and Keusch, G.T. (1989) Pathogenesis of *Shigella* diarrhoea. XIV. Selective targetting of Shiga toxin to villus cells on rabbit jejunum explains the effect of the toxin on intestinal electrolyte transport. *Journal of Clinical Investigation*, **84**, 1509–1517.
22. Karmali, M.A. (1989) Infection by verocytotoxin-

producing *Escherichia coli. Clinical Microbiological Reviews*, **2**, 15–38.
23. Kent, T.H., Formal, S.B., LaBrec, E.H., Sprinz, H. and Maenza, R.M. (1967) Gastric shigellosis in rhesus monkeys. *American Journal of Pathology*, **51**, 259–267.
24. Keusch, G.T. (1988) Antimicrobial therapy for enteric infections and typhoid fever: state of the art. *Reviews of Infectious Diseases*, **10**, S199–S205.
25. Keusch, G.T. and Bennish, M.L. (1989) Shigellosis. In *Bacterial Diseases of Humans* (Eds) Evans, A.S. and Brachman, P. pp. 593–620. New York: Plenum Press.
26. Keusch, G.T. and Bennish, M.L. (1989) *Shigella*. In *Enteric Infection* (Eds) Farthing, M.J.G. and Keusch, G.T. pp. 265–282. London: Chapman and Hall.
27. LaBrec, E.H., Schneider, H., Magnani, T.J. and Formal, S.B. (1964) Epithelial cell penetration as an essential step in the pathogenesis of bacillary dysentery. *Journal of Bacteriology*, **88**, 1503–1518.
28. Linde, K., Dentchev, V., Bondarenko, V. *et al.* (1990) Live *Shigella flexneri* 2a and *Shigella sonnei* I vaccine candidate strains with two attenuating markers. I construction of vaccine candidate strains with retained invasiveness but reduced intracellular multiplication. *Vaccine*, **8**, 25–29.
29. Mathan, M.M. and Mathan, V.I. (1991) Morphology of rectal mucosa of patients with shigellosis. *Reviews of Infectious Diseases*, **13**, S314–S318.
30. Mathan, V.I. and Mathan, M.M. (1991) Intestinal manifestations of invasive diarrheas and their diagnosis. *Reviews of Infectious Diseases*, **13**, S311–S313.
31. Maurelli, A.T. and Sansonetti, P.J. (1988) Genetic determinants of *Shigella* pathogenicity. *Annual Reviews of Microbiology*, **42**, 127–150.
32. Maurelli, A.T. and Sansonnetti, P.J. (1988) Identification of a chromosomal gene controlling temperature regulated expression of *Shigella* virulence. *Proceedings of the National Academy of Science USA*, **85**, 2820–2824.
33. Mobassaleh, M., Donohue-Rolfe, A., Jacewicz, M., Grand, R.J. and Keusch, G.T. (1988) Pathogenesis of *Shigella* diarrhoea: Evidence of a developmentally regulated glycolipid receptor for *Shigella* toxin involved in the fluid secretory response of rabbit small intestine. *Journal of Infectious Diseases*, **157**, 1023–1031.
34. Moyer, M.P., Dixon, P.S., Rothman, S.W. and Brown, J.E. (1987) Cytotoxicity of Shiga toxin for primary cultures of human colonic and ileal epithelial cells. *Infection and Immunity*, **55**, 1533–1535.
35. Munshi, M.H., Haider, K., Rahaman, M.M., Sack, D.A., Ahmed, Z.U. and Morshed, M.G. (1987) Plasmid-mediated resistance to nalidixic acid in *Shigella dysenteriae* type 1. *The Lancet*, **ii**, 419–421.
36. Pickering, L.K., Bartlett, A.V. and Woodward, W.E. (1986) Acute infectious diarrheas among children in day care: epidemiology and control. *Reviews of Infectious Diseases*, **8**, 539–547.
37. Salam, M.A. and Bennish, M.L. (1991) Antimicrobial therapy for shigellosis. *Reviews of Infectious Diseases*, **13**, S332–S341.
38. Sansonetti, P.J. (1991) Genetic and molecular basis of epithelial cell invasion of *Shigella* spp. *Reviews of Infectious Diseases*, **13**, S285–S292.
39. Sansonetti, P.J., Hale, T.L., Dammin, G.J., Kapfer, C., Collins, H.H. and Formal, S.B. (1983) Alteration of the pathogenecity of *Escherichia coli* K-12 after transfer of plasmid and chromosomal genes from *Shigella flexneri. Infection and Immunity*, **39**, 1392–1402.
40. Sansonetti, P.J., Ryter, A., Clerc, P., Maurelli, A.T. and Mounier, J. (1986) Multiplication of *Shigella flexneri* within HeLa cells: lysis of the phagocytic vacuole and plasmid mediated contact hemolysis. *Infection and Immunity*, **55**, 521–527.
41. Struelens, M.J., Pattre, D., Kabir, I., Salam, A., Nath, S.N. and Butler, T. (1985) *Shigella* septicemia: prevalence, presentation, risk factors and outcome. *Journal of Infectious Diseases*, **152**, 784–790.
42. Takeuchi, A., Formal, S.B. and Sprinz, H. (1968) Experimental acute colitis in the rhesus monkey following peroral infection with *Shigellla flexneri. American Journal of Pathology*, **52**, 503–519.
43. Tauxe, R.V., McDonald, R.C., Hargrett-Bean, N. and Blake, P.A. (1985) The persistence of *Shigella flexneri* in the United States: increasing role of adult males. *American Journal of Public Health*, **78**, 1432–1435.
44. Williams, H.M.S. and Richards, J. (1990) Single-dose ciprofloxacin for shigellosis. *The Lancet*, **335**, 1343–1344.

GIARDIASIS

M.J.G. Farthing

Giardiasis is the most common protozoal infection of the human intestinal tract and is found worldwide throughout temperate and tropical regions.[7] It is commonplace in the developing world but is also a common infection in Europe and North America. In the developing world, giardiasis probably has its most profound clinical effects on infants and preschool children.[13,14] Adult travellers from the developed world and immunodeficient individuals are also susceptible and may experience prolonged infection. Although the pathogenic potential of this parasite has been debated for almost a century, there is now no doubt that it can cause both acute and chronic diarrhoea with intestinal malabsorption. A substantial number of infected individuals (probably exceeding 50%) have no symptoms and appear to suffer no ill effects. The mechanisms by which this parasite produces gastrointestinal disease and the precise mechanisms by which the host often eradicates it from the intestine are still not fully understood.

HISTORICAL ASPECTS

Studies of prehistoric desiccated faecal material from the Middle East and North America indicate that *Giardia* sp. has been infecting humans for more than 2000 years.[17] The Dutch lens-maker Antoni van Leeuwenhoek was probably the first person to observe the organism in 1681, which he found in a specimen of his own diarrhoeal stool using one of his own lenses.[5] He described the organism as a 'pissabed', which in old Dutch means 'woodlouse'. He presumably mistook the vigorous movements of the flagella for a multitude of tiny legs. *Giardia* sp. was rediscovered by Vilem Lambl in 1859 and was named *Cercomonas intestinalis*. In 1882 Kunstler found a similar parasite in tadpoles and named it *Giardia agilis* after his teacher Professor Alfred Giard. Finally in 1915 Stiles introduced the binominal *Giardia lamblia* (taxonomically incorrect), by which the parasite is most commonly known.

THE PARASITE

Giardia sp. exists in two forms: the motile trophozoite and the thick-walled cyst. Three distinct morphological forms of giardia trophozoites have been described, namely *G. intestinalis* or *duodenalis* (otherwise known as *G. lamblia*), the parasite of humans and many mammals; *G. muris*, the mouse parasite; and *G. agilis*, which infects amphibia (*Figure 9.9*). The trophozoite is the form of the parasite that exists within the proximal small intestine and is responsible for the production of diarrhoeal disease. *Giardia* sp. has two oval nuclei and four pairs of flagella which give the trophozoite its mobility. The dorsal surface of the trophozoite is convex (*Figure 9.10*) whilst the ventral surface is concave, consisting of a spiral arrangement of microtubules (*Figure 9.11*). Several proteins have been identified in this ventral disc, including the contractile protein tubulin and a series of low-molecular-weight proteins called giardins.[1] These proteins modulate the shape of the disc and assist in attachment to the intestinal epithelium. Although trophozoites are excreted in the faeces they do not survive outside the human

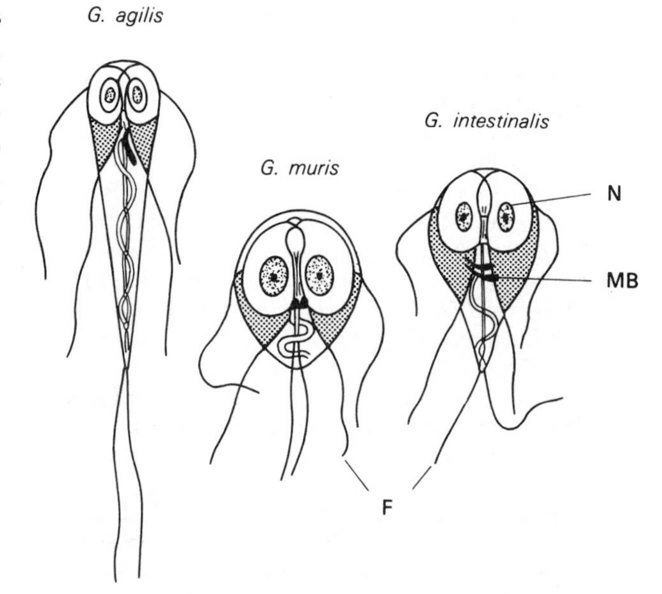

Figure 9.9 The three morphologically distinct forms of *Giardia*. N, nucleus; MB, median body; F, flagella.

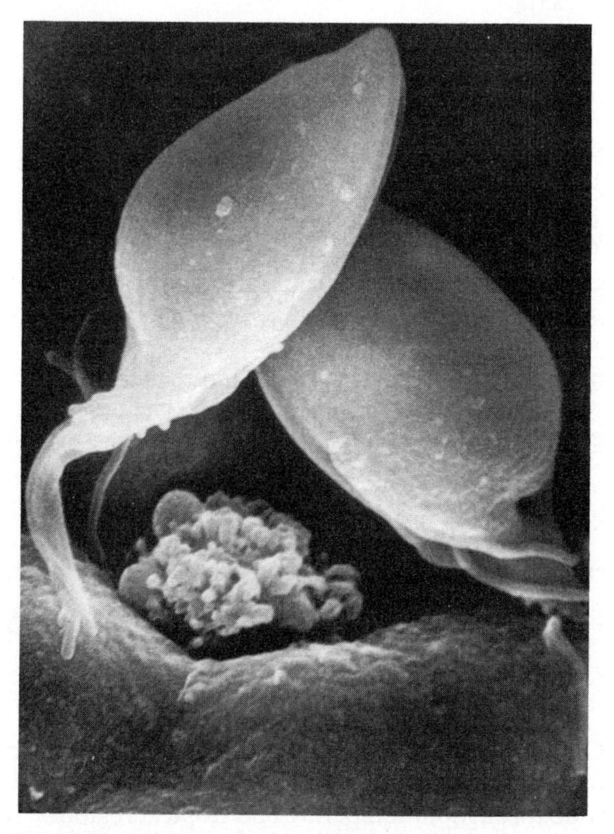

Figure 9.10 Scanning electron micrograph showing the dorsal surfaces of two *G. lamblia* trophozoites.

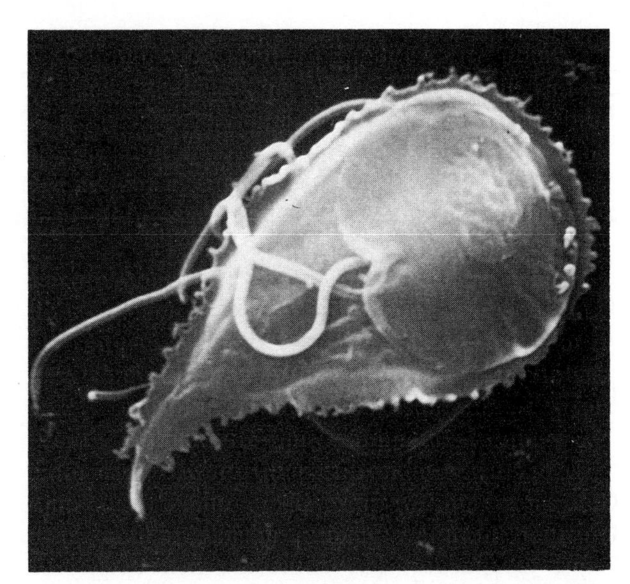

Figure 9.11 Scanning electron micrograph of the ventral surface of a *G. lamblia* trophozoite showing the spiral configuration of the ventral disc.

host. The infective form is the cyst, which is resistant to many environmental hazards outside the host and may survive for months in water or soil. The cyst wall is thought to contain the *N*-acetyl-D-glucosamine polymer chitin although recent evidence has disputed this, indicating that the major cyst wall sugar is *N*-acetyl-D-galactosamine.

Giardia lamblia is an aerotolerant anaerobe and respires in the presence of oxygen by a flavin, iron–sulphur, protein mediator, electron transport system.[25] Glucose is the major energy substrate being catabolized by the Embden–Meyerhof and hexose monophosphate pathways incompletely to carbon dioxide, ethanol and acetate. The organism is unable to initiate de novo purine or pyrimidine synthesis but has salvage pathways for both nucleotides. Similarly, *Giardia* sp. is unable to synthesize lipids, relying on uptake of preformed lipids from the small intestine.[25] Calcium transport in the parasite is mediated by a membrane-bound calmodulin-regulated Ca^{2+}-ATPase. The organism contains a variety of proteinases, although their role in the pathogenesis of intestinal disease is unknown. Growth of the parasite is stimulated by bile and pure bile salts, suggesting that their beneficial effect is mediated by facilitating uptake of preformed membrane lipids.[12] This may partly explain the parasite's predilection for the proximal small intestine where bile is plentiful.

Giardia isolates vary both in phenotype and genotype and several techniques, including identification of radiolabelled surface proteins, isoenzyme and chromosomal analysis, and restriction fragment length polymorphism analysis, have been used to demonstrate heterogeneity in *G. lamblia*.[4,8,30] There is preliminary evidence to suggest that human infection may consist of two or more isolates which could account for some treatment failures due to the emergence of a relatively drug-resistant strain. These differences between Giardia isolates could explain the broad clinical spectrum seen with this infection because isolates may vary in virulence.

EPIDEMIOLOGY

Prevalence rates for *G. lamblia* in the USA and Europe approach 10% in some areas, whereas in the developing world rates are higher and often reach 25%. A study in Guatemalan children showed that all members of a cohort followed from birth suffered at least one Giardia infection by the age of 3 years.[13] Giardiasis is now the most common water-borne disease in the USA, with a substantial number of outbreaks occurring each year. Large outbreaks are due to inadequate treatment of town water supplies which have been derived from surface-collecting grounds. Wild animals in North America often carry *Giardia lamblia* and thus provide a large reservoir of infection by which surface waters can be contaminated. Giardia cysts are relatively resistant to chlorination, so that it is essential that other aspects of water purification, notably flocculation, sedimentation and filtration, are adequate. A water-borne outbreak occurred in the Bristol area in 1985 involving more than 100 individuals.[26] Several outbreaks have been reported following contamination of swimming pool water with giardia cysts.[31] Giardiasis is a relatively common infection in travellers, in whom transmission occurs through contaminated food or water.[6]

Person-to-person transmission also occurs in nurseries, day-care centres and other residential institutions, within families and between sexually active male homosexuals. Studies in Australia and the UK have shown that pet cats and dogs may carry *Giardia* sp.[36] and thus act as a reservoir for infection in families, particularly young children.

CLINICAL FEATURES

Infection with *G. lamblia* presents in three ways: (1) an asymptomatic carrier state; (2) an acute self-limiting diarrhoeal illness and (3) chronic diarrhoea with or without evidence of intestinal malabsorption.[7] Asymptomatic carriage, meaning giardia cyst excretion without abdominal symptoms, is the most common form of infection particularly in the endemic areas of the developing countries. Whether

Table 9.4 Clinical features of giardiasis

Clinical features	*Cases (%)*
Diarrhoea	95
Weakness	76
Weight loss	68
Abdominal pain	69
Nausea	60
Steatorrhoea	56
Flatulence	35
Vomiting	29
Fever	17

From Butcher and Farthing[2] and Moore *et al.*[29]

Table 9.5 Diagnostic approaches in giardiasis

Microscopy	Faeces Duodenal fluid (aspirate/ string test) Mucosal biopsy/impression smear Endoscopic brushings
Immunodiagnosis	Faecal antigen ELISA Anti-giardia serum IgM
DNA probes	Faeces (under evaluation)

these individuals had a symptomatic initial illness is not clear and it is not known why immunologically competent persons should carry this parasite for many months or even years. Tolerance may develop to giardia antigens in the same way that most individuals tolerate the myriad of food antigens ingested daily.

The constellation of symptoms in acute giardiasis has been clearly documented from accounts in travellers moving from the developed to the developing world (*Table 9.4*).[2,29] Symptoms usually begin 1–3 weeks after ingestion of cysts, although in some instances the onset of symptoms may be delayed for up to 6 weeks. Diarrhoea is often watery initially and associated with nausea, anorexia, abdominal discomfort and bloating. Weight loss is common during this early phase of the illness. At least 50% of individuals will recover without antimicrobial chemotherapy and clear the infection. However, up to 30–50% of patients may develop subacute or chronic diarrhoea, approximately half of whom will have biochemical evidence of intestinal malabsorption. At this stage of the illness there may be profound anorexia with progressive weight loss.

Infants and children are particularly susceptible to infection and will probably experience the most serious clinical sequelae. Hospital- and community-based studies have confirmed that chronic infection in some children may lead to retardation of growth and development.[13,14] However, the majority of community-based studies have been conducted in the developing world where giardiasis is often associated with other enteric and respiratory infections. Despite acknowledgement of these difficulties, the precise role that *Giardia* sp. alone has to play is uncertain. A recent study of asymptomatic infants and children in Jerusalem failed to show that infection in this population has any deleterious effects on growth.[23] However, lactase deficiency detected by breath hydrogen testing was more common in infected children. Occasionally allergic manifestations occur during giardiasis with a symptom complex including arthralgia, myalgia, urticaria and eosinophilia.[11] Protein-losing enteropathy has been described.[27]

INVESTIGATIONS

The presence of *G. lamblia* is generally confirmed by the combination of a typical clinical history in symptomatic individuals and the presence of giardia forms (cysts and/or trophozoites) in faeces, small intestinal fluid or mucosal biopsy specimens. In recent years a variety of immunological approaches have been evaluated and the role of DNA probes is yet to be established (*Table 9.5*).

Microscopy

Giardia forms are detected in faeces either in direct saline mounts or following cyst concentration techniques. The precise sensitivity of faecal microscopy for diagnosing giardiasis in not known because there is no other 'gold standard' with which to compare this technique. However, published data suggest that three faecal specimens taken on different days will detect between 50 and 85% of cases.[20] The role of duodenal aspirate has been controversial, some studies suggesting that it should be regarded as the 'gold standard', detecting all infected individuals. A recent study from south India detected only 44% of cases; 15%, however, were only detected by microscopy of duodenal fluid, indicating that the two techniques are complementary.[20] Trophozoites in the small intestine can also be detected by the string test, brush cytology at endoscopy and mucosal biopsy impression smears.

Immunodiagnosis

Enzyme-linked immunosorbent analysis (ELISA) techniques are now available to detect giardia antigens in faeces.[24,33] Sensitivity and specificity data generally exceed 90% although sensitivity may fall when assays are rigorously tested under field conditions. A commercial ELISA kit is now available but its role in the routine diagnosis of giardiasis remains to be established.[33] Serological testing has not been highly rewarding.[16] IgG titres following giardiasis remain elevated for months or even years and are generally increased in all individuals resident in an endemic area. Thus, specific anti-giardia IgG titres are unable to distinguish current from past infection. Specific serum anti-giardia IgM responses, however, are relatively short lived and can detect current infection in both adults and children with *Giardia* sp.[19]

DNA probes

Cloned genomic DNA probes are now available, preliminary studies suggesting that they may detect up to 10^5 giardia cysts.[3] There are problems in releasing DNA from cysts without denaturation, although the sensitivity of detection can be increased substantially by use of the polymerase chain reaction. Further studies are required to determine whether this approach will have clinical application.

PATHOGENESIS OF DIARRHOEA AND MALABSORPTION

Giardia sp. must colonize the small intestine before it can produce diarrhoea and malabsorption. This occurs in a three-step process, namely (1) excystation (2) attachment to intestinal epithelium and (3) multiplication by binary fission. As few as 10 cysts are required to establish infection. Excystation occurs in the duodenum promoted by initial contact with gastric acid, followed by exposure to pancreatic hydrolytic enzymes particularly trypsin.[32] Once the motile trophozoites emerge from the cyst, attachment to the epithelium is desirable and probably essential to avoid clearance by mechanical peristaltic forces. Attachment is probably partially mechanical via the ventral disc[7] but may also be mediated by a mannose-binding surface lectin which binds to mannosyl residues on intestinal epithelial cells.[15,22] The lectin is present within the trophozoite as a prolectin which can be activated by trypsin.[28]

Giardia sp. is essentially a luminal parasite and therefore dependent on growth factors within the intestinal lumen. Growth of *Giardia* sp. requires exogenous lipid, the uptake of which is facilitated by the presence of bile salts.[13] High concentrations of bile salts, however, promote encystation[18] which probably occurs in the small and large intestine and is vital for the parasite to complete its life cycle and to survive outside its mammalian host.

The mechanism by which *Giardia* sp. causes diarrhoea and malabsorption has not been clearly established although mucosal injury and certain luminal factors may be involved.

Mucosal injury

Although many individuals infected with *Giardia* sp. have a normal jejunal mucosa by light microscopy, there is a wide spectrum of partial to subtotal villous atrophy.[8] Even when light microscopy is normal, shortening and distortion of microvilli may occur. Functional impairment has also been demonstrated, notably reduction in microvillous membrane disaccharidase activity and a preliminary description of a diffuse defect in sodium-mediated glucose transport. The mechanisms by which *Giardia* sp. produces these effects is poorly understood. Disruption of the microvilli occurs during the attachment process such that mirror image impressions of the ventral disc have been demonstrated in experimental *G. muris* infection in mouse intestine, with less impressive lesions in human infection. As yet, specific toxins or other toxic metabolic products have not been identified. A variety of proteases, however, have been demonstrated in *Giardia* which may act on proteins in the host microvillous membrane. Some plant lectins are toxic to the intestinal epithelium and, thus, the giardia lectin taglin may play a role in pathogenesis.

In the absence of a specific mucosal toxin, immunological mechanisms have been sought that might explain the disruption of epithelial structure and function. There is increasing evidence to support a primary role for mucosal inflammation.[8–10] The lymphocytic infiltrate in giardiasis occurs before villous shortening and there is a relationship between the intensity of lymphocytic infiltration and the severity of intestinal malabsorption.[9] Further compelling evidence comes from experimental infection with *G. muris* in athymic nude mice in which, despite prolongation of infection, villous architectural abnormalities are much less severe than those of immunocompetent animals. Further evidence comes from in vitro studies with human foetal small intestine which showed that T-cell activation can itself lead to increased proliferation of crypt cells and villous atrophy.[10] Thus, following sensitization to giardia antigens, T cells in the mucosa may become activated and produce architectural changes in villi and crypts. Other components of the mucosal inflammatory response may also be important in giardiasis, particularly the role of mast cells and local anaphylaxis.

Luminal factors

Bacterial overgrowth of the small intestine occurs in some patients with giardiasis although it is usually restricted to Indian patients or overland travellers to the Indian subcontinent.[34,35] A study in patients with giardiasis in the UK failed to show evidence of bacterial overgrowth.[21] However, in one study, deconjugated bile salts were found in the proximal small intestine, suggesting that bacterial overgrowth might be functionally important.[34] *Giardia* sp. itself is unable to deconjugate bile salts but does have an extraordinary capacity for taking up bile salts into its cytoplasm by what appears to be a carrier-mediated active transport process. Bile salt uptake by *Giardia* sp. could reduce intraluminal bile salt concentrations and possibly deplete the bile salt pool, particularly in infants and young children with chronic infection of 6 weeks or more. Bacterial overgrowth may have a part to play in contributing to the villous abnormalities in giardiasis. Abnormal pancreatic exocrine function has been reported in patients with symptomatic giardiasis, tryptic activity returning to normal following eradication of the parasite. Reduction in chymotrypsin activity has also been reported in symptomatic adults. However, it seems unlikely that the reductions in pancreatic enzyme activity are sufficient to account for intestinal malabsorption, although they may act in concert with other luminal and mucosal factors. Live giardia trophozoites and trophozoite sonicates are able to inhibit lipolysis by an as yet undefined mechanism.

IMMUNE RESPONSES AND HOST DEFENCE

Immune responses of the host play an important part in both clearing acute infection and in the development of protective immunity.[9,10] Epidemiological studies in giardiasis suggest however, that multiple exposures to the parasite are required before the development of protective immunity since age-specific prevalence only starts to decline in early adolescence. Increased susceptibility to infection in immunocompromised individuals particularly those with hypogammaglobulinaemia and HIV infection suggest a key role for the immune system in controlling infection.

Antibody

Specific anti-giardia IgG, IgM and IgA responses occur during the course of natural and experimental infections with *Giardia* sp.[8–10] In common with many other infections the initial response is an increase in specific anti-giardia IgM antibodies which usually decline after 2–3 weeks.[19] The IgG response appears later and IgG antibodies may persist for months or even years. Serum anti-giardia IgA responses can only be detected in up to 30% of patients with giardiasis, although this may be a sampling error reflecting selection of symptomatic patients who have been unable to clear the infection. There is some preliminary evidence to suggest that failure to switch specific anti-giardia IgM to secretory IgA production may be associated with prolonged infection. Occasionally, increased concentrations of total serum IgE have been reported in giardiasis but in one case this was due not to an increase in specific anti-giardia IgE but to an IgE antibody response to entry of other luminal antigens following an increase in intestinal permeability.[11] The presence of specific anti-giardia secretory IgA (sIgA) has been demonstrated in duodenal fluid of patients with giardiasis and also to be present on the surface of giardia trophozoites in human jejunal biopsies.[9] Specific sIgA and IgG can be detected in human milk and epidemiological studies suggest that these antibodies may protect breast-fed infants from giardiasis.

Surface antigens have been identified which serve as immune targets for antibody production.[9,10,30] Many high-molecular-weight giardia polypeptides are immunogenic, as are proteins of the cytoskeleton, particularly the giardin series of proteins with molecular masses of approximately 30 kDa. Several surface proteins are immunogenic in humans, including an 82–88 kDa protein and more recently a 57 kDa protein appears only to initiate antibody production in infected individuals. One surface antigen of 170 kDa has been shown to vary in the intensity of expression during the course of experimental infection in gerbils.[30] Antigen variation may be an important mechanism by which *Giardia* sp. evades the host immune response.

Cellular immune response

Mucosal lymphocytes are commonly increased in patients with giardiasis as are the number of intraepithelial lymphocytes which decline following treatment and clearance of the parasite.[9] Studies in the murine model of giardiasis indicate that lymphocyte numbers increase in Peyer's patches but return to normal following eradication. Importance of cell-mediated immunity is supported by the deleterious effect that corticosteroids, cyclosporin A and undernutrition have in increasing susceptibility and duration of experimental infection in animals.

Host defence

Non-immune mechanisms such as gastric acid, mucus and intestinal peristalsis almost certainly play a role in protecting the host against colonization with *Giardia*.[8] Normal, non-immune human milk kills giardia trophozoites in vitro, which is thought to be related to the release to free fatty acids and other lipolytic products. Normal human duodenal fluid is also toxic to trophozoites, possible via a similar mechanism involving the products of lipolysis. The precise immune mechanisms that are involved in eradication of the parasite from the intestine are not clearly understood; there is increasing evidence to suggest that the production of specific secretory antibody plays a major role either by agglutination of trophozoites and flagella immobilization or possibly by direct cytotoxic effects with or without the action of complement.[8,9] Current evidence suggests that *Giardia* sp. rarely invades the mucosa but there is compelling evidence to suggest that should this occur the parasite would be rapidly destroyed by antibody-dependent, cell-mediated cytotoxicity with subsequent destruction by tissue macrophages. Intraepithelial T lymphocytes may be directly cytotoxic to the parasite. Again, once in the intramucosal location *Giardia* sp. will activate the classic complement pathway which will lead to rapid death.[9]

TREATMENT

Nitroimidazole derivatives, metronidazole and tinidazole, are the most widely used class of drugs in treatment of giardiasis. Metronidazole may be given as a 2 g single dose on three successive days to adults with an expected efficacy of approximately 90%. Tinidazole has a similar efficacy given as a 2 g single dose on one day. In some individuals, several courses of treatment may be required and failure of the short treatment regimen should be followed by a more prolonged course of 1.2 g daily for 7–10 days. Many patients dislike nitroimidazole derivatives because of anorexia, nausea, vomiting, fatigue and a metallic taste in the mouth. Some individuals experience a disulfiram-like reaction with alcohol and prolonged use can result in peripheral neuropathy. Treatment failures with these drugs do occur which in some instances probably relate to drug resistance. However, some patients do have residual functional abdominal symptoms after clearance of the parasite and it is therefore wise to confirm continuing infection before considering second-line drugs such as mepacrine (100 mg three times daily for 7 days) or furazolidone (100 mg four times daily for 7–10 days).

PREVENTION

Giardia sp. is widely distributed in the environment in both human and animal reservoirs. Any attempt to reduce these reservoirs is likely to fail and therefore preventive measures should be targeted at reducing transmission, namely by ensuring high standards of water purification and to ensure that travellers to endemic areas take particular precautions such as avoiding tapwater, ice, and uncooked fruit and vegetables. Boiling water for 10 minutes is effective in destroying cysts although often impractical. Close attention to personal hygiene will reduce person-to-person transmission and when sporadic infection occurs in family members it may be worth scrutinizing pets and domestic animals to exclude these as a local reservoir.

The apparent delay in the development of protective immunity in individuals in the developing world is of great scientific interest but may indicate difficulties in the development of an effective vaccine strategy. However, further investigation should identify the antigenic determinants responsible for the development of protective immunity, which could form the basis of experimental vaccine studies.

Acknowledgements

The author gratefully acknowledges financial support by the Wellcome Trust and the Joint Research Board of St Bartholomew's Hospital. Special thanks are due to Ms Nicola Herrera for her assistance in the preparation of this manuscript.

REFERENCES

1. Aggarwal, A. and Nash, T.E. (1989) Characterization of a 33-kilodalton structural protein of *Giardia lamblia* and localization to the ventral disk. *Infection and Immunity*, **57**, 1305–1310.
2. Brodsky, R.E., Spencer, H.C. and Schultz, M.G. (1974) Giardiasis in American travellers to the Soviet Union. *Journal of Infectious Diseases*, **130**, 319–323.
3. Butcher, P.D. and Farthing, M.J.G. (1988) DNA probes for the faecal diagnosis of *Giardia lamblia* infections in man. *Biochemical Society Transactions*, **17**, 363–364.
4. Cevallos, A.M., Carnaby, S., McHugh, T.D. and Farthing, M.J.G. (1991) Phenotypic and genotypic variation in *Giardia lamblia*. *Saudi Medical Journal* (in press).
5. Dobell, C.A. (1920) The discovery of intestinal protozoa in man. *Proceedings of the Royal Society of Medicine*, **13**, 1–15.

6. Farthing, M.J.G. (1984) Giardiasis: a cause of traveller's diarrhoea. *Travel and Traffic Medicine International*, **2**, 3–10.
7. Farthing, M.J.G. (1987) Giardiasis. In *Advanced Medicine* (Eds) Pounder, R.E. and Chiodini, P. pp. 287–301. London: Baillière Tindall.
8. Farthing, M.J.G. (1989) Host-parasite interactions in human giardiasis. *Quarterly Journal of Medicine*, **70**, 191–204.
9. Farthing, M.J.G. (1990) Immunopathology of giardiasis. *Spinger Seminars in Immunopathology*, **12**, 269–282.
10. Farthing, M.J.G. and Goka, A.K.J. (1987) Immunology of giardiasis. In *Clinical Gastroenterology, Immunological aspects of the gut and liver* (Eds) Wright, R. and Hodgson, H.J. pp. 589–603. London: Baillière Tindall.
11. Farthing, M.J.G., Chong, S. and Walker-Smith, J.A. (1984) Acute allergic phenomena in giardiasis. *The Lancet*, **ii**, 1428.
12. Farthing, M.J.G., Keusch, G.T. and Carey, M.C. (1985) Effect of bile and bile salts on growth and membrane lipid uptake by *Giardia lamblia:* possible implications for pathogenesis of intestinal disease. *Journal of Clinical Investigation*, **76**, 1727–1732.
13. Farthing, M.J.G., Mata, L., Urrutia, J.J. and Kronmal, R.A. (1986) Natural history of *Giardia* infection of infants and children in rural Guatemala and its impact on physical growth. *American Journal of Clinical Nutrition*, **43**, 393–403.
14. Farthing, M.J.G., Mata, L.J., Urrutia, J.J. and Kronmal, R.A. (1986) Giardiasis: Impact on child growth. In *Diarrhoea and malnutrition in childhood* (Eds) Walker-Smith, J.A. and McNeish, A.S. pp. 68–78. London: Butterworth.
15. Farthing, M.J.G., Pereira, M.E.A. and Keusch, G.T. (1986) Description and characterisation of a surface lectin from *Giardia lamblia. Infection and Immunity*, **51**, 661–667.
16. Farthing, M.J.G., Goka, A.K.J., Butcher, P.D. and Arvind, A.S. (1987) Serodiagnosis of giardiasis. *Serodiagnosis and Immunotherapy*, **1**, 233–238.
17. Faulkner, C.T., Patton, S. and Johnson, S.S. (1989) Prehistoric parasitism in Tennessee: evidence from the analysis of desiccated fecal material collected from Big Bone Cave, Van Buren County, Tennessee. *Journal of Parasitology*, **75**, 461–463.
18. Gillin, F.D., Reiner, D.S. and Boucher, S.E. (1988) Small intestinal factors promote encystation of *Giardia lamblia in vitro. Infection and Immunity*, **56**, 705–707.
19. Goka, A.K.J., Rolston, D.D.K., Mathan, V.I. and Farthing, M.J.G. (1986) Diagnosis of giardiasis by specific IgM antibody enzyme-linked immunosorbent assay. *The Lancet*, **ii**, 184–186.
20. Goka, A.K.J., Rolston, D.D.K., Mathan, V.I. and Farthing, M.J.G. (1990) The relative merits of faecal and duodenal juice microscopy in the diagnosis of giardiasis. *Transactions of the Royal Society of Tropical Medicine and Hygiene*, **84**, 66–67.
21. Halliday, C.E.W., Inge, P.M.G. and Farthing, M.J.G. (1988) *Giardia*–bile salt interactions *in vitro* and *in vivo. Transactions of the Royal Society of Tropical Medicine and Hygiene*, **82**, 428–432.
22. Inge, P.M.G., Edson, C.M. and Farthing, M.J.G. (1988) Attachment of *Giardia lamblia* to mammalian intestinal cells. *Gut*, **29**, 795–801.
23. Ish-Horowicz, M., Korman, S.H., Shapiro, M. *et al.* (1989) Asymptomatic giardiasis in children. *Pediatric Infectious Disease Journal*, **8**, 773–779.
24. Janoff, E.N., Craft, J.C., Pickering, L.K. *et al.* (1989) Diagnosis of *Giardia lamblia* infections by detection of parasite-specific antigens. *Journal of Clinical Microbiology*, **27**, 431–435.
25. Jarroll, E.L., Manning, P., Berrada, A., Hare, D. and Lindmark, D.G. (1989) Biochemistry and metabolism of *Giardia. Journal of Protozoology*, **36**, 190–197.
26. Jephcott, A.E., Begg, N.T., Baker, I.A. (1986) Outbreak of giardiasis associated with mains water in the United Kingdom. *The Lancet*, **i**, 730–732.
27. Korman, S.H., Bar-Oz, R., Mandelberg, A. and Matoth, I. (1990) Giardiasis with protein-losing enteropathy: diagnosis by faecal 1-antitrypsin determination. *Journal of Pediatric Gastroenterology and Nutrition*, **10**, 249–252.
28. Lev, B., Ward, H., Keusch, G.T. and Pereira, M.E.A. (1986) Lectin activation in *Giardia lamblia* by host protease: a novel host-parasite interaction. *Science*, **232**, 71–73.
29. Moore, G.T., Cross, W.M., McGuire, D. *et al.* (1969) Epidemic giardiasis at a ski resort. *New England Journal of Medicine*, **281**, 402–407.
30. Nash, T.E. (1989) Antigenic variation in *Giardia lamblia. Experimental Parasitology*, **68**, 238–241.
31. Porter, J.D., Ragazzoni, H.P., Buchanon, J.D., Waskin, H.A., Juranek, D.D. and Parkin, W.E. (1988) *Giardia* transmission in a swimming pool. *American Journal of Public Health*, **78**, 659–662.
32. Rice, E.W. and Schaefer, F.W. (1981) Improved *in vitro* excystation procedure for *Giardia lamblia* cysts. *Journal of Clinical Microbiology*, **14**, 709–710.
33. Rosoff, J.D., Sanders, C.A., Sonnad, S.S. *et al.* (1989) Stool diagnosis of giardiasis using a commercially available enzyme immunoassay to detect *Giardia*-specific antigen 65 (GSA 65). *Journal of Clinical Microbiology*, **27**, 1997–2002.
34. Tandon, B.N., Tandon, R.K., Satpathy, B.K. and Shriniwas (1977) Mechanism of malabsorption in giardiasis: a study of bacterial flora and bile salt deconjugation in upper jejunum. *Gut*, **18**, 176–181.
35. Tomkins, A.M., Drasar, B.S., Bradley, A.K. and Williamson, W.A. (1978) Bacterial colonization of jejunal mucosa in giardiasis. *Transactions of the Royal Society of Tropical Medicine and Hygiene*, **72**, 33–36.
36. Winsland, J.K.D., Nimmo, S., Butcher, P.D. and Farthing, M.J.G. (1989) Prevalence of *Giardia* in dogs and cats in the United Kingdom: survey of an Essex veterinary clinic. *Transactions of the Royal Society of Tropical Medicine and Hygiene*, **83**, 791–792.

VIRUS INFECTIONS

I.L. Chrystie, W.D. Cubitt and J.E. Banatvala

Acute gastroenteritis is one of the leading causes of mortality and morbidity throughout the world. Among healthy adults, infection is usually mild and recovery occurs within a few days. Although not an appreciable cause of mortality among children in industrialized countries (gastroenteritis-associated deaths among children in the USA were of the order of 500 per annum between the years 1973 and 1983[100]) morbidity in such areas is high. For example, in the USA, over 210 000 children under the age of 5 years are admitted to hospital with gastroenteritis each year with an annual inpatient cost of nearly US$ 1000 million;[99] furthermore, 25 work/school days per 100 children are lost each year, and some 14% children are treated by a doctor for rotavirus-associated diarrhoea alone.[33]

The impact of diarrhoeal disease in developing countries is far greater, accounting for between 15 and 34% of all deaths in some countries, the majority among children.[230] In such developing countries as India, Indonesia and Guatemala, children were reported, in the early 1970s, to experience at least one or two episodes of acute gastroenteritis per year during the first 3 years of their lives, with mortality rates between 1 and 4%, representing a death rate of 20–55 per 1000 children. Combination of such data with contemporary demographic information suggested that in Asia, Africa and Latin America some 500 million episodes of diarrhoea occurred among children less than 5 years old, resulting in the deaths of 5–18 million.[176] Estimates for 1977–1978 suggested that in such developing regions there was an annual morbidity of 3000–5000 million cases with an associated mortality of 5–10 million.[219] World Health Organization estimates for 1989 for the global total number of diarrhoeal episodes among children less than 5 years old are more than 1500 million with a mean estimate of 3.0 episodes per child[232] Malnutrition and chronic debilitating disease are important contributing factors.[82]

Improvements in water supplies and sanitation would dramatically improve this situation, but limited resources preclude such improvements in those parts of the world where they are most needed.[219] Great emphasis has been placed on increased availability of oral rehydration therapy,[97] and on improved education. This approach has had considerable success[232] but is limited by available resources.

The development of vaccines against the major pathogens has been proposed.[59] However, those pathogens so far identified often manifest a rather complex antigenic variability. As yet, vaccines have been of only limited efficacy. However, even the development of truly effective vaccines would not solve the problem. An effective distribution strategy would be essential, and the lack of financial resources remains a major problem.

The data accumulated over many years have demonstrated that pathogenic bacteria or parasites can be implicated in only some 25–50% of episodes of acute diarrhoea.[185,193,206] Viruses were believed to be responsible for the remainder, but it was only recently that viruses were identified as causing gastroenteritis. The initial breakthrough occurred in 1972 with the identification, by negative staining electron microscopy of a 27 nm virus associated with an outbreak of winter vomiting disease in Norwalk, Ohio, USA.[113] Rotaviruses were first identified in 1973 by electron microscopy in thin sections of duodenal biopsies,[17] and, within a short time, they were also identified by negative staining electron microscopy.[72] The ease by which such viruses could be identified by the relatively simple technique of negative staining electron microscopy rekindled world-wide interest in viral gastroenteritis and further examples such as astroviruses, caliciviruses and adenoviruses, together with a variety of unidentified small round viruses, were identified world-wide. Those viruses associated with acute gastroenteritis are listed in *Table 9.6*.

This chapter considers the viruses associated with gastroenteritis in two parts. The first deals with the many small round viruses which have been identified ('small round structured' viruses, caliciviruses, astroviruses and, as yet, unidentified small round viruses); the second considers rotaviruses, adenoviruses and, briefly, coronaviruses, and toroviruses.

SMALL ROUND VIRUSES

'SMALL ROUND STRUCTURED' VIRUSES (SRSVs) (*Figure 9.12*)

Outbreaks of acute gastroenteritis have incubation periods which usually range from 4 to 48 hours. In general, a 4–6 hour incubation period is suggestive of an illness induced by bacterial toxins; illness with a longer incubation period is usually caused by bacterial or viral agents. There is now good evidence that many of these outbreaks are caused by small round viruses (*Table 9.6*). Investigation of out-

Table 9.6 Viruses associated with the majority of human viral gastroenteritis

Virus	*Classification*	*Size (nm)*	*Morphology*	*Buoyant density*	*Nucleic acid*	*Proteins*	*Serotypes*	*Diagnosis*
SRSV (e.g. Norwalk)	Candidate calicivirus	30–35	Amorphous, fuzzy	1.36–1.41	ssRNA 7.7kb	1 × major (60–70 kDa)	11 strains	EM, EIA, RIA, PCR
Calicivirus	Calicivirus	28–34	32 cups 2-fold axis = 4 hollows 3-fold axis = Star of David 5-fold axis = 10-pointed sphere	1.38–1.40	ssRNA	1 × major (62 kDa)	5	EM, EIA, RIA, PCR
Astrovirus	Unclassified	26–28	5 or 6-pointed star	1.36–1.38	ssRNA 7.2kb	See text	6	EM, EIA, RIA, culture
Small round viruses (Ditchling, Paramatta, Cockle)	Candidate parvovirus	22–26	Featureless, smooth outline	1.38–1.46	?ssDNA	Unknown	Unknown	EM
Rotavirus	Rotavirus	60–80	Complete particle 'wheel-like', smooth outline Incomplete spiky outline	1.36–1.38	dsRNA	6 (?7) structural	13 (see text)	EM, EIA, RIA, PCR, latex, culture
Adenovirus	Adenovirus	75–85	Distinct icosahedron	1.34	ssDNA	10–15 structural	41 (see text)	EM, EIA, latex, culture

EM, electronmicroscopy; EIA, enzyme immunoassay; RIA, radio-immunoassay; ssRNA, single-stranded RNA; dsRNA, double-stranded RNA; PCR, polymerate chain reaction.

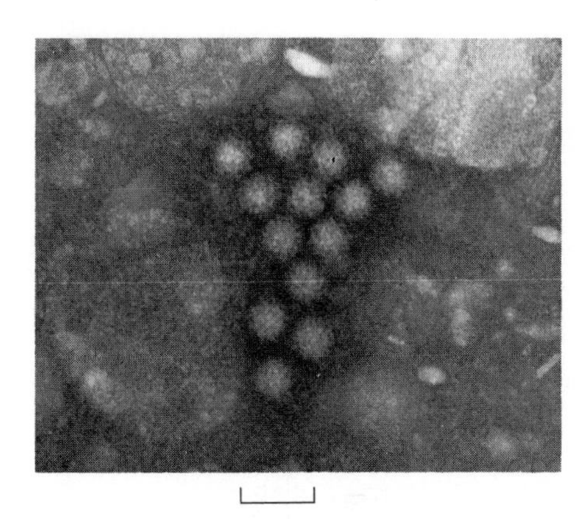

Figure 9.12 Electron micrograph of negatively stained faecal extract showing Norwalk-like (structured) virus particles (bar represents 50 nm).

breaks, particularly in the UK, the USA and Japan, have shown that SRSVs are the most frequent cause.[47,81,172,194] The clinical syndrome of acute, epidemic, non-bacterial gastroenteritis, also designated winter vomiting disease or, perhaps more appropriately, epidemic nausea and vomiting, as outbreaks occur throughout the year, is a self-limiting syndrome in which some or all of the following features occur: fever, nausea, vomiting, vertigo, myalgia, abdominal colic, diarrhoea and malaise. Diarrhoea and vomiting are the most common symptoms of illness, but, in some outbreaks, the symptoms are similar to those of influenza. Symptoms typically persist for 1–2 days, but a biphasic illness may occur with patients becoming ill again several days later. The disease is rarely severe enough to require hospital admission. Community-wide, family and hospital outbreaks, with high initial and secondary attack rates, are common and all age groups may be affected. Person-to-person spread is by the faecal–oral route, either by direct transmission or ingestion of food or water contaminated with virus particles, by contact with contaminated surfaces, or by inhalation of aerosols of vomitus or faecal material containing virus particles.[49,101,172,191]

The first SRSV to be described (the Norwalk agent) was detected in 1972 by immune electron microscopy of a faecal filtrate obtained from a patient involved in an outbreak in a primary school in Norwalk, Ohio, USA.[113] Since then, many morphologically indistinguishable, but antigenically distinct, strains of SRSVs have been described, e.g. Snow Mountain, Hawaii, and Taunton agents. Electron microscopy still remains the predominant method for diagnosing SRSV infections, other than in a few research laboratories which have developed radio-immunoassays, enzyme immune assays, or PCR. There are still no commercially available tests for detection of either antigen or antibody responses. The limitation of electron microscopy is the threshold of detection of approximately 10^6 particles/ml of faeces; it is known from human volunteer studies that the infectious dose may be as low as 10–100 particles. Diagnosis of infections is difficult, because excretion of detectable numbers of virus particles is transient (1–2 days) and samples are seldom available until the occurrence of an outbreak has come to the attention of the authorities. An alternative approach is to demonstrate significant serological responses, but this is dependent on sufficient stocks of antigen, and is not always successful because some individuals fail to serorespond, although they present with symptoms and shed virus in their stools.

Recently, the entire genome of Norwalk virus has been sequenced (Jiang, personal communication) and Norwalk virus recombinant protein, which self assembles into particles, has been expressed in baculovirus.[110] This has enabled high titred antisera to be raised and enabled the development of sensitive and specific enzyme immunoassays for the detection of Norwalk antigen and antibody.[162] The sequencing of another calicivirus/SRSV (Southampton strain) should lead to the development of other EIAs in the near future.[127]

HUMAN CALICIVIRUSES (HuCVs) (*Figure 9.13*)

HuCVs with the characteristic surface morphology of the Caliciviridae are the cause of outbreaks and sporadic cases of diarrhoea and vomiting, particularly among infants, schoolchildren and elderly patients in enclosed communities. Outbreaks have

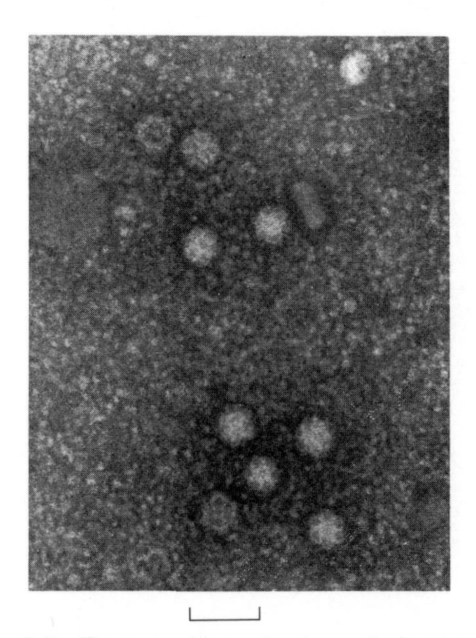

Figure 9.13 Electron micrograph of negatively stained faecal extract showing caliciviruses (bar represents 50 nm).

been reported in the UK, Canada, Japan and Australia.[37,52–54,85,91,158,200] The characteristics of the illness are indistinguishable from those described for SRSVs. At present diagnosis is dependent on electron microscopy, except in a few laboratories which have developed enzyme immune assays.

ASTROVIRUSES (*Figure 9.14*)

Astroviruses were first described as a cause of sporadic cases of diarrhoea and vomiting in 1975.[136] Since then they have been shown to cause symptoms in human volunteers,[126] and sporadic cases have been reported from countries throughout the world. In temperate regions of the world, astrovirus and rotavirus occur predominantly during the winter and spring, in contrast to enteric adenovirus, HuCV and SRSV infections, which show no significant seasonal distribution.[48] Outbreaks of infection have been recorded among infants and the elderly.[10,85,131,150] Recently, Marin County agent, the cause of an outbreak in a convalescent home for the elderly in the USA,[85] and which had previously been classified as an SRSV, is actually an astrovirus type 5.[95] The features of the illness are similar to those of SRSV and HuCV infections, other than that the incubation period is slightly longer at 3–4 days.

Diagnosis is generally made by electron-microscopy but several laboratories have propagated the virus in primary human embryonic kidney, LLCMK2 (Monkey kidney), and CaCO2 (continuous human colon) cell cultures.[128,225] This has enabled monoclonal antibodies to be raised and immune assays developed.

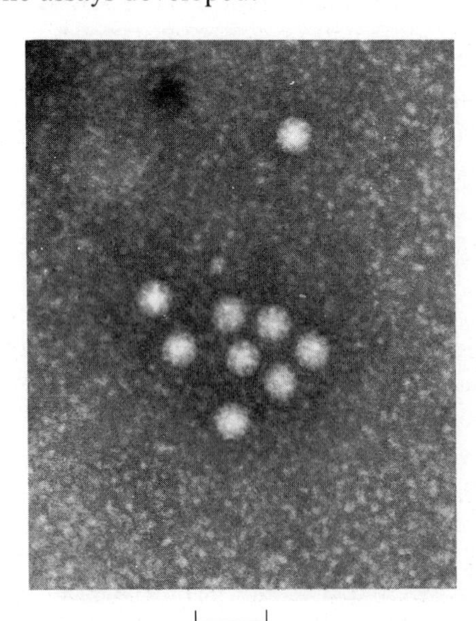

Figure 9.14 Electron micrograph of negatively stained faecal extract containing astroviruses (bar represents 50 nm).

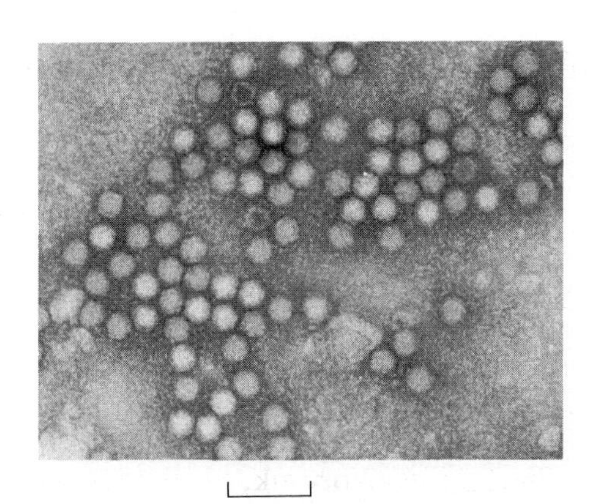

Figure 9.15 Electron micrograph of negatively stained faecal extract showing Ditchling-like (featureless) virus particles (bar represents 50 nm).

SMALL ROUND VIRUSES (*Figure 9.15*)

Small, round, featureless viruses (Wollan, Paramatta and cockle agents), which are considered as candidate parvoviruses, have been associated with several outbreaks of acute gastroenteritis following the consumption of raw or inadequately cooked shellfish.[9,39,165] In many outbreaks, small round viruses have been detected in the same samples as other agents – SRSV, HuCV or astrovirus.[39]

OUTBREAKS OF FOOD- AND WATER-BORNE INFECTION

Most outbreaks have been associated with SRSVs, but there are a few reports of astrovirus, calicivirus and small round virus infection, particularly following the consumption of shellfish.[7,49] Extensive outbreaks of diarrhoea and vomiting following the consumption of molluscan shellfish, caused by SRSVs and affecting thousands of people, have been recorded in Australia,[132,150] the UK,[80] the USA[148] and Japan.[77]

Contaminated drinking water and ice are the source of major outbreaks in the USA, involving over 5000 people in the community as a result of primary infections followed by secondary transmission, particularly within families.[147,170,205]

Swimming pools which have been inadequately chlorinated provide another potential source of infection.[116] SRSVs may survive chlorine treatment at concentrations as high as 10 mg/ml – three times the level known to be effective in inactivating poliovirus.[117]

Cold foods that undergo extensive handling, such as salads, sandwiches and fruit, have been identified as the source of outbreaks of SRSV infection in the USA and the UK.[69,109,222]

CLASSIFICATION OF SMALL ROUND VIRUSES

Until recently, most small round viruses have been classified on the basis of their size and morphology as observed by electron microscopy, according to the scheme proposed by Caul and Appleton.[30]

Attempts to establish SRSVs and HuCVs in cell culture or to transmit them to animals have been unsuccessful, and therefore only a few strains have been characterized. The results of studies in the UK, the USA and Japan are summarized in *Table 9.6*. Some of the SRSVs (Norwalk, Snow Mountain and SRSV9) should be considered as candidate caliciviruses, because they possess a single major structural polypeptide, of molecular mass 60–70 kDa, a feature unique to members of the Caliciviridae. Recently, two SRSVs (Norwalk virus and Southampton, which is antigenically related to Snow Mountain virus) have been sequenced and found to have a single strand RNA genome of about 7.7 kb.[127] The genomic organization consisting of three open reading frames is characteristic of the Caliciviridae. ORF1 codes for non-structural proteins and ORF2 for the capsid protein. The use of PCR has shown that Norwalk virus and some strains of HuCV are related. (Cubitt, W.D., Jiang, X, and Estes, M.K., unpublished data). It is, therefore, probable that the majority of SRSVs and HuCVs will eventually be classified within the Caliciviridae.

The astroviruses have yet to be fully characterized (*Table 9.6*). Preliminary data indicate that they may be members of the Picornaviridae, based on the finding of four polypeptides with molecular masses between 32 and 37 kDa.[125] However, recent evidence suggests that the major viral specific protein has a molecular mass of 90-kDa which is cleaved into one or more smaller proteins in the presence of trypsin.[146] The genome of human astrovirus is assumed to be positive sense since it possesses a poly A tract at the 3' end.[141,226] Immunofluorescence studies of the replication cycle of human and bovine astroviruses show nucleolar as well as cytoplasmic staining,[1,94] which also suggests that the replication cycle differs from that of the picornaviruses.

The characteristics of the small round viruses are uncertain but one report suggests that cockle agent contains single-stranded DNA, and that it may be a member of the Parvoviridae.[7]

PATHOGENESIS

'Small round structured' viruses

Jejunal biopsies obtained from volunteers infected with SRSVs (Norwalk and Hawaii agents) show histological abnormalities within 24–48 hours which persist for up to 2 weeks despite clinical recovery within a few days. Such changes also occur in asymptomatic individuals.[2,60,192] Although jejunal villi are blunted and broadened, and contain vacuolated cells, there is no break in the epithelial surface. The lamina propria is infiltrated with mononuclear cells and polymorphonuclear lymphocytes. No histological abnormalities are seen in rectal, colonic or gastric biopsies. Electron microscopic studies of ultrathin sections of the jejunum fail to reveal virus-like structures. The acute phase of infection is associated with a decrease in brush border enzymes and a transient impairment of fat and carbohydrate absorption which also occurs in the asymptomatic individual. There is also a leukopenia involving the lymphocyte subpopulations (T, B and null) which may be the result of a redistribution of cells to the site of virus infection.[60] The mechanism by which diarrhoea is induced has not been established, but, because jejunal adenylase activity is not increased, the mechanism is probably different from that induced by enterotoxic organisms.[129]

Human calicivirus

There have been no histopathological studies of HuCV in humans, other than a single report which showed the presence of virus particles in a sample of small bowel obtained from a child who had died of acute gastroenteritis.[71]

Human astrovirus

There are no studies concerning the pathogenesis of astrovirus other than a report that showed the presence of arrays of particles in a duodenal biopsy from a child with gastroenteritis.[169] Virus particles were found in epithelial cells of the lower part of the villi, similar to the situation found in calves infected with bovine astrovirus.[93]

IMMUNITY

It is now known that there are numerous antigenically distinct strains of SRSV, HuCV and astrovirus, and that infection with one strain does not confer immunity to subsequent infection with other strains.

'Small round structured' viruses

Human volunteer studies in the USA have shown that susceptibility to disease following administration of Norwalk agent correlates poorly with serum antibody levels. Some individuals become repeatedly ill when challenged, even though they have high levels of serum and gut antibodies, whereas others, with low levels of serum antibodies, remained asymptomatic.[164]

Human calicivirus and astrovirus

Laboratory reports of HuCV and astrovirus infections suggest that infections most commonly occur among infants and the elderly,[50,85,105,158] but this may be a reflection of the severity of the illness in these age groups rather than a true indication of the incidence. Some studies of outbreaks have shown that parents and nursing staff remained well and had high levels of antibodies to the infecting strains in their acute phase sera, indicating a degree of immunity to infection,[53] whereas, in other outbreaks, there was a high attack rate in all age groups. The reason for the differences between the various outbreaks probably reflects the degree of herd immunity to various strains circulating in the community.

SEROEPIDEMIOLOGICAL STUDIES

'Small round structured' viruses

Seroepidemiological studies suggest that most adults (57–77%) have experienced infections with Norwalk virus or antigenically related agents.[21,55,88] In the USA, antibody is acquired gradually and continually, beginning slowly in childhood until, in the fifth decade, about 50% have antibody.[88] In contrast, in Bangladesh, the majority of primary Norwalk infections occur before the age of 5 years.[19] In England, there is little evidence of infection with Norwalk virus until the age of 3 years, after which the prevalence of antibodies rises steadily throughout childhood to a level of 60% by the age of 18 years.[86,163]

Human caliciviruses

Studies using immune electron microscopy[51,188] and radio-immunoassay[153] have shown that infections with HCV are common throughout the world, acquisition of antibody rising rapidly between the ages of 6 months and 2 years; however, in an Australian aboriginal population, antibody levels were low until the age of 12 years, but increased rapidly in adults.

Astroviruses

There are only two small seroepidemiological studies of astrovirus which showed that in Oxford,[125] and north-west London, in the UK,[227] infections commonly occur in infants. Immune electron microscopic studies on batches of pooled immunoglobulin indicate that, in the UK and the USA, most adults have experienced infection with serotypes 1 and 2, and less with serotypes 3, 4 and 5; in China, infections with serotype 1 are rare and serotypes 2, 3, 4 and 5 common (W.D. Cubitt, unpublished data).

ROTAVIRUSES

CLASSIFICATION

Rotaviruses, together with reoviruses, orbiviruses, phytoreoviruses, fijiviruses, and the cytoplasmic polyhedrosis viruses, form the family Reoviridae.[142]

MORPHOLOGY

Intact rotavirus particles (*Figure 9.16*) have icosahedral symmetry, are some 70–75 nm in diameter, have a characteristic, well-defined outer margin, and an arrangement of capsomeres radiating from a 40 nm inner core, giving the virion a wheel-like appearance: hence the name (Latin, *rota* = wheel).[73] The outer capsid layer is often not present in faecal preparations, resulting in particles 55–60 nm in diameter which have a spiky margin. These variants are termed 'smooth' and 'rough', respectively.

The detailed structure of the virus particle is difficult to establish because of the problems associated with the interpretation of the two-sided images

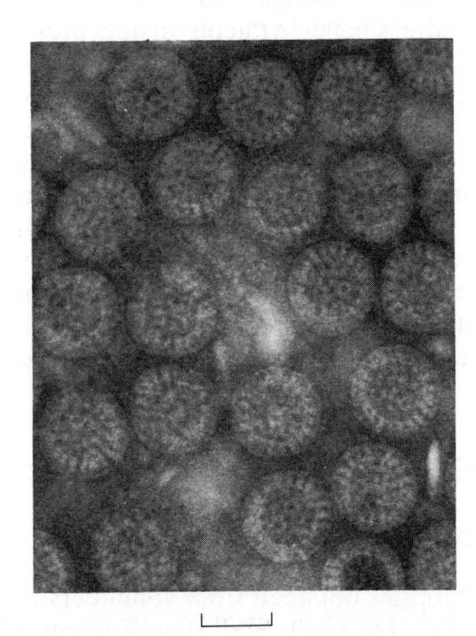

Figure 9.16 Electron micrograph of negatively stained faecal extract containing rotaviruses (bar represents 50 nm).

produced by basic negative staining. However, platinum shadowing has demonstrated that the inner capsid appears to consist of 132 capsomeres[134] arranged in a T = 13L configuration.[143,182] Further, cryoelectron microscopy coupled with image-averaging techniques have demonstrated that the outer shell is also arranged in a T = 13L symmetry.[171] In addition, the use of such cryoelectron microscopy and image-averaging techniques has demonstrated the presence of surface projections on the virus.[171] The presence of these spikes has been confirmed by low-dose negative staining electron microscopy: the spikes are composed of polypeptide VP4.[6]

The virus core contains the 11 RNA segments and three polypeptides, VP1, VP2, and VP3; the inner capsid layer consists of VP6, the major internal structural polypeptide, which exhibits group and subgroup specific antigens; the outer capsid layer contains two polypeptides, VP7 (major) and VP4 (minor), the serotype-specific antigens.[62] An additional polypeptide, VP9, has also been identified as a minor outer capsid component by some workers.[65]

GENOME

Rotaviruses have a segmented, double-stranded RNA genome. There are 11 segments, which may easily be resolved by polyacrylamide gel electrophoresis.[178] In group A rotaviruses, to which most human strains belong, the segments separate into four distinct size classes. From largest to smallest, these classes are: segments 1–4; segments 5 and 6; segments 7–9 (which often appear as only two or even one band); and segments 10 and 11. There are many small variations in the relative size, and therefore mobility, of segments; however, for the most part, these are only of use in pinpointing the point source of an outbreak because they do not relate to any antigenic variation. There is, however, one exception to this where the relative mobility of segments 10 and 11 produce what have become known as 'long' and 'short' patterns, and these almost always correlate with subgroup specificity (subgroups I and II, respectively).[179] However, in recent years the identification of a third subgroup,[151] coupled with the identification of subgroup I rotaviruses exhibiting 'long' electropherograms,[79,120] have reduced the usefulness of electropherotyping as a means of classifying group A rotaviruses.

Not all rotaviruses exhibit the classic 4, 2, 3, 2 electropherotype, and such atypical patterns were recognized as being indicative of non-group A rotaviruses.[155,180] However, even this means of classification has been confounded by the isolation of a group A rotavirus with an atypical electropherogram.[14]

The potential for genetic reassortment during multiple infections is great, and such reassortments have been observed between serogroup A rotaviruses, both in vitro and in vivo.[145] During the prolonged infection of immunodeficient patients with rotavirus, a further mechanism for genome change may occur. There is a partial duplication of genome segments which results in a variety of atypical electropherotypes in the same patient and electropherograms containing many more than the usual 12 bands.[166] Rotaviruses with such genome rearrangements reassort in vitro[5] and are likely to reassort in vivo.[106]

ANTIGENIC STRUCTURE

At least seven groups (serogroups) of rotaviruses have been recognized (designated A–G);[66,187] there is no antigenic cross-reactivity between these groups and there is no significant cross-hybridization of their genomes. Groups A, B, and C have been isolated from humans, with group A being, by far, the most common. Group B rotaviruses have, to date, been identified as human pathogens only in China[36] and the USA;[63] human group C rotaviruses have been reported in many other parts of the world.[24,32,159,167,199] Group A rotaviruses have been subdivided into three subgroups (I and II and III), based both on specific epitopes on VP6 and genetic homology by RNA–RNA hybridization assays.[151,152] Some isolates have been reported as exhibiting dual subgroup specificity.[214] In addition to the subgroup specificity, there is serotypic specificity involving the two outer capsid polypeptides which contain neutralization epitopes, VP4 and VP7. Group A rotaviruses can be classified into 14[25,26,87,103,184,198,213] serotypes, based on VP7 analysis, of which at least nine (1–4,6,8–10,12) have been detected in humans.[213] To date,[161] five human, three bovine and at least two porcine VP4s have been identified. With the demonstration of reassortments between VP7 and VP4 types, the need for a more complex antigenic classification system became evident. Such a system was devised at the VIIth International Congress of Virology, Edmonton, Canada, in 1987. Briefly, the VP7 polypeptide is defined as carrying the G (glycoprotein) serotype specificity, and the VP4 polypeptide as carrying the P (protease-sensitive) serotype specificity.[104]

VP4 may also be of major importance in determining rotavirus virulence.[157] This view is strengthened by the observation that asymptomatic infections endemic in some nurseries for newborns are associated with a VP4 gene of reduced virulence.[75]

Finally, the antigenic complexity of the rotaviruses is magnified by reports that serotypes can be classified into minor antigenic variants termed monotypes.[45] Such monotypes have, for example, been observed in serotypes 1–4.[121]

EPIDEMIOLOGY

Children

Throughout both the developing and the developed world, rotavirus-associated gastroenteritis is a disease mainly affecting the young. Thus, in many studies carried out in Asia, Central and South America, and Africa, rotaviruses were identified in 14–66% of faecal samples.[11] In Bangladesh, rotaviruses were associated with 46% of diarrhoea among children less than 1 year of age.[15] In a multicentre study performed in 42 developing countries, rotaviruses were more frequently associated with gastroenteritis in children aged 0–4 years than any other pathogen.[231] In both industrialized[9,92,236] and developing[20] regions of the world, there is almost universal acquisition of antibodies to rotavirus at a very early age.

In temperate regions, rotavirus infection has a marked seasonal distribution, infection occurring almost exclusively in the winter,[28,114] the highest attack rates being among children aged between 6 months and 2 years.

Thus, rotaviruses have been detected in about 25% of patients less than 1 year of age, in 60% of those aged between 1 and 3 years of age, and in 20–40% of children between the ages of 4 and 6 years.[70] During the winter, as many as 75% of children admitted with diarrhoea may excrete rotaviruses.[56]

Throughout the Tropics, the seasonal distribution of rotavirus-associated diarrhoea is more complex. Rotavirus infection is generally more common during the cooler seasons;[139] however, in countries with high ambient temperatures all the year round, rotavirus infection may be associated with either the dry or the rainy seasons.[11]

Adults

Although rotavirus infection is always considered a major pathogen of children, there is also a considerable amount of rotavirus-associated gastroenteritis in adults. Outbreaks have been reported among army recruits, staff in hospitals and playgroups, and in geriatric units. However, most community studies have demonstrated a preponderance of mild or asymptomatic infection,[112] although severe illness and fatalities have been recorded in elderly patients.

Such studies have been of group A rotaviruses, but recently group B rotaviruses have been implicated in very large outbreaks of severe gastroenteritis among adults in many parts of China.

During 1982 and 1983, nationwide epidemics of diarrhoea and vomiting, affecting over 1 million people, occurred throughout China. Although morphologically identical to rotaviruses, the viruses isolated from these outbreaks exhibited a non-standard electrophoretic pattern.[108] They did not react in immunological assays directed against group A rotaviruses and were identified as group B.[36] Morbidity ranged between 530 and 1305 per million and mortality was extremely low. All age groups were affected, although adults between the ages of 21 and 40 years seemed to be at highest risk. There was little seasonal variation. There was an apparent association of many outbreaks with contaminated water supplies, although others seemed to involve person-to-person transmission.[107]

Seroepidemiological studies have indicated that infection with viruses related to those detected in China is widespread. Thus, using the fairly insensitive technique of counterimmune electrophoresis, antibodies to the Chinese isolates have been detected in 9.5–20% of sera from Australia, Canada, the USA and Hong Kong.[107]

CLINICAL FEATURES

Infection with rotaviruses may be asymptomatic, cause mild diarrhoea and occasionally a severe, sometimes fatal, acute gastroenteritis.[28,34] After an incubation period of 24–48 hours, symptoms appear abruptly, usually with vomiting followed by diarrhoea; this diarrhoea is most profuse on the second and third days after infection. Very high concentrations of virus are excreted at this time – up to 10^{11} virus particles per gram of faeces. Fever is often present. Symptoms generally subside within 4–5 days, although in some patients they may persist for up to 14 days, as may virus excretion. Prolonged diarrhoea is uncommon.[98,181,196] However, protracted diarrhoea associated with rotavirus excretion, and rotavirus antigenaemia, occurs in many patients with immunodeficiency disorders.[190,228]

Children with immunodeficiency disorders may also excrete a number of different viruses. *Figure 9.17* shows some of the viruses being excreted simultaneously by an infant with severe combined immunodeficiency, failure to thrive and protracted diarrhoea, who, over a period of 2 months, excreted

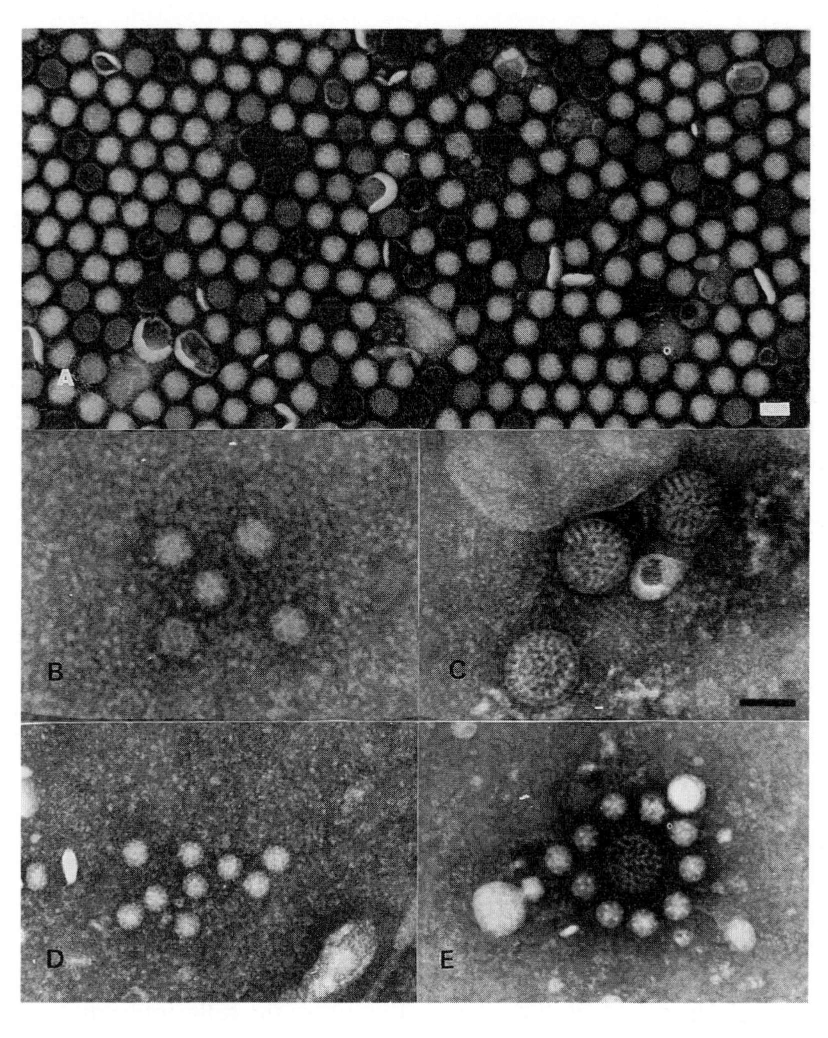

Figure 9.17 Electron micrographs of negatively stained faecal extracts showing viruses detected in a child with severe combined immunodeficiency: (A) adenovirus (bar represents 50 nm); (B) calicivirus; (C) rotavirus; (D) small round virus; (E) astrovirus + rotavirus (B–E to same scale: bar represents 50 nm). (Reproduced, with permission, from Chrystie *et al.*[42])

five different viruses.[43] In this patient, rotavirus was excreted for several months and was observed to undergo considerable genetic changes as manifest by abnormal electrophoretic patterns of the genomic RNA.[106,166] Persistent rotavirus excretion among children who fail to thrive should alert clinicians to the possibility of an underlying severe immunodeficiency disorder.

Respiratory symptoms and signs are common in patients with rotavirus-induced diarrhoea,[130] although whether this association is aetiological or temporal is not clear.[29] Rotavirus has been recovered from respiratory secretions of some,[189] but not all,[83] children studied. However, recent studies in China, in which rotavirus was detected by immunofluorescence and cell culture in oropharyngeal aspirates from children with respiratory disease, do suggest that rotavirus infection may involve the respiratory tract.[237]

Rotaviruses have also been associated with a variety of other conditions (e.g. intussusception, sudden infant death syndrome, aseptic meningitis and many others). The association of rotavirus infection with necrotizing enterocolitis in neonates has been reported.[183]

Life-threatening rotavirus infection is more common in developing countries but has been reported from time to time in industrialized regions. In one study of fatal rotavirus infection in Toronto, Canada, 21 cases were reported over a 5 year period.[28] Deaths usually resulted from profound dehydration, electrolyte imbalance, aspiration of vomitus and cardiac arrest.

Nosocomial infection

The stability of rotaviruses,[67] together with the high concentration of virus excreted, makes environmental contamination more or less inevitable. As the infective dose in a child can be as low as 10 particles,[220] in the absence of extremely stringent precautions cross-infection of susceptible contacts is likely. Thus, in the Hospital for Sick Children in Toronto, Canada, about one-fifth of rotavirus infections during 1 year were hospital acquired. Infant surgical wards were the most likely source of infection and there was strong evidence that infection was transmitted to patients by the staff.[61,144] A study in the UK in London showed that 43% of 51 cases of rotavirus infection were hospital acquired, and resulted in a total of 72 extra days spent in hospital.[156] Most infections were mild but sometimes associated with delayed healing of surgical wounds and secondary lactose intolerance. In a recent study, all children admitted to hospital for longer than 2 weeks during the rotavirus season shed the virus at some time, albeit often asymptomatically.[64]

The most probable mode of transmission is indirectly from patient to patient on the hands of medical and nursing staff, although fomites and aerosols may also contribute to nosocomial transmission.[33] An exhaustive survey of the efficacy of a wide range of commercially available chemical disinfectants on rotavirus viability, both in suspension and on a variety of surfaces, demonstrated that most were ineffective.[133,183] Proper handwashing procedures using antiseptic preparations such as chlorhexidine have no effect on rotavirus viability. Preparations containing ethanol may be of greater efficacy;[204] however, vigorous handwashing, with soap, performed consistently at appropriate intervals, is the preferred recommendation of the US Department of Health.[33]

Neonatal infection

Rotavirus infections have been extensively studied among neonates in maternity wards. First described in 1975 in the UK in London,[41] this phenomenon has now been observed in many other countries. Neonates are usually asymptomatic, although symptomatic infection has been reported.[124,149] Although circumstantial epidemiological evidence suggests that the virus was transmitted either by medical or nursing staff from the children's wards, or by visitors, probably children[138] electropherotypic analysis of the virus strains involved has, where performed, demonstrated that one or two strains only are involved in each neonatal outbreak, and that these strains differ from the contemporary ones circulating either in the children's wards or in the general community.[16,89,179,195]

Studies of rotavirus infection among neonates have shown that breast-fed babies are both less likely to become infected and, if infected, excrete less virus.[42] In other studies, a protective effect of breast-feeding was not observed.[46] In studies where breast-feeding appeared to confer some level of protection, conflicting results have been published. In one study, protection could be correlated with the level of lacteal antibody,[135] whereas in other studies protection could not be correlated with a variety of factors, including maternal and colostral antibody levels, antiviral factors, antitrypsin, and rotavirus-specific, cell-mediated immunity.[208,209] It is possible that such factors as infective dose of virus or serotype of both virus or serum or colostral antibody are of prime importance. Perhaps the protective effect of breast-feeding is passive in that it is bottle-feeding that potentiates infection.

Prospective studies of the possible protective effect of the, generally, asymptomatic infection of neonates has demonstrated that, over 3 years, children infected as neonates experience less severe gastroenteritis than those not infected.[18] Analysis of the rotavirus strains associated with asymptomatic infections in some nurseries for the newborn has shown that such strains possess the VP4 gene of reduced virulence.[75] Both of these observations may be of importance in vaccine design.

PATHOGENESIS

The histological features of infection are similar in children and other young animals.[229] The earliest lesions are present in the proximal end of the small intestine; in the severest cases its entire length may be involved. The features include loss of absorptive cells lining the small intestine. Villi are blunted; the columnar epithelium is desquamated and replaced by immature cuboidal cells which migrate rapidly from the crypts. Lymphocytic cells infiltrate the lamina propria; there are distended cisternae of the endoplasmic reticulum, and sparse, irregular microvilli. Vesicles in the villous epithelial cells can be seen, by electron microscopy, to contain rotavirus particles. Virus particles have also been seen in goblet cells and phagocytes in the lamina propria.[102,203]

The mechanism by which diarrhoea is produced differs from that in cholera and enterotoxic *Escherichia coli* infections in that adenylate cyclase and AMP levels remain constant. The immature cuboidal cells migrating from the crypts are deficient in intestinal disaccharides and have lowered sodium, potassium and ATPase activities.[68] Diarrhoeal symptoms result from water malabsorption coupled with intestinal hurry which persists until the villi are repopulated with columnar epithelial cells.

PROTECTION AGAINST INFECTION

The ubiquity of rotavirus-associated gastroenteritis among children, with the associated high mortality and morbidity, especially in the less developed areas of the world, demonstrates the need for prevention.

One means would be the development of an effective, and cheap, rotavirus vaccine, and determined efforts have been initiated by the World Health Organization to achieve this goal. Such a vaccine would, if administered to all infants under 6 months of age in the developing world, reduce diarrhoeal morbidity by 50 million cases and mortality by up to 800 000 deaths per annum.[59]

However, the problems associated with the development of such a vaccine are enormous. Reinfection with rotaviruses is common in all age groups,[90,140] although subsequent infections are often less severe, especially in older children and adults. Such reinfections may be due to different serotypes[78] but the same serotype as the original infection may also be responsible.[175] The degree of protection offered by rotavirus infection is the subject of some controversy. Some workers have suggested that even homotypic protection is unlikely to last longer than 12 months;[38] others have observed protection against reinfection lasting for at least 2 years. These workers also noted that asymptomatic primary infection was as effective a protector as symptomatic infection.[13] In addition, recent evidence has suggested that protection against rotavirus diarrhoea after natural infection is not dependant on neutralizing antibody,[221] However, protection from infection may not be necessary as neonates asymptomatically infected in hospital shortly after birth experienced fewer rotavirus-associated diarrhoeal episodes than did infants uninfected in nurseries. Follow-up studies for 3 years indicated that those children infected in the nurseries suffered fewer severe gastrointestinal episodes but not rotaviral infections than their uninfected contemporaries.[18]

Initial attempts to develop a rotavirus vaccine concentrated on the Jennerian approach of employing attenuated non-human virus.[115] A serotype 6 bovine rotavirus strain, attenuated by cold adaptation and high (147) passage has been extensively studied. In trials in Finland, this vaccine (RIT 4237) induced protection against diarrhoea in children from 8 to 12 months of age, as well as conferring protection against severe diarrhoea during a 16-month follow-up study.[217] However, when trials were carried out among children in developing countries, for example, The Gambia, it was less successful[57] and has now been discontinued.

Another bovine-derived vaccine, WC3, has also demonstrated its efficacy in the developed world.[44] Studies in the Central African Republic and China have also shown some protection, mostly to serotype 1 infection. Because of the inconsistent performance of this vaccine, a reassortment derivative, WI79-9, which produces the VP7 antigen of human rotavirus serotype 1, and which seems effective against both serotypes 1 and 3, has been developed. Initial trials in the USA have been promising.[232] Preliminary trials of a strain derived from a rhesus monkey, MMU 18006 or RRV-1, were encouraging, the vaccine offering protection against both severe (100%) and all (48–64%) rotavirus-associated diarrhoea.[75,83] However, other studies have not confirmed these findings.[39]

The inconsistency of such monovalent vaccines has prompted another approach, using the rotavirus's natural tendency to reassort to produce non-human virus strains carrying multiple human serotypic epitopes. Trials of such viruses using derivatives of MMU18006 are in progress, but initial results are not too promising, with only 40–80% seroconversion to the relevant serotypes and efficacy has been reduced in developing rather than developed countries.[77,232] The inability of human VP4 segments to reassort into rhesus rotavirus strains may also prove to be a limitation.

The observation that rotavirus strains implicated in outbreaks of mild or asymptomatic infection in neonatal nurseries have a modified VP4, and that such strains are partially protective against subsequent severe rotavirus infection,[18] have led to the development of a candidate vaccine M37. However, as this vaccine is less efficient than others currently on trial, no further studies are planned.[232]

Finally, it has been pointed out[186] that vaccines of only moderate efficacy can be most useful in reducing severe illness and mortality and that the decision to initiate a vaccine programme should be based on public health requirements rather than efficacy alone.

INVESTIGATIONS

In common with other viruses inducing acute gastroenteritis, rotaviruses will not grow in conventional cell cultures. Although trypsin pre-treatment of faecal samples, plus the incorporation of trypsin in the growth medium, resulted in a rotavirus isolation rate of 50% using a rhesus monkey kidney cell line, MA 104,[234] diagnosis required other techniques. However, the recent report that a human colon carcinoma cell line, HT-29, has provided an isolation rate of 100%[202] may permit the routine use of cell culture for rotavirus diagnosis.

The most widely used technique currently is negative staining electron microscopy of faecal suspensions. Such suspensions may be examined without pre-treatment; however, many workers recommend some degree of purification of the virus before electron microscopy. A brief clarification at 5000 × g for 10 minutes, followed by ultracentrifugation of the resultant supernatant at 100 000 × g for 60 minutes being sufficient. The electron micrographs illustrating this chapter result from staining such semi-purified virus with 3% sodium phosphotungstate pH 6.5. In the hands of an experienced electron microscopist, such a technique compares well with the more recently developed immunological techniques. It also has the advantage of being a 'catch-all' technique, whereas immunologically based assays can only identify those viruses to which their reagents are directed. The sensitivity of electron microscopy may be enhanced by the centrifugation of the sample on to the grid, using the Beckman Airfuge and electron microscope rotor. The use of solid phase immune electron microscopy, using specific antibodies or normal human immunoglobulin (as a 'catch-all' immune 'net'), has also been recommended.[154]

However, electron microscopy has two disadvantages: it is expensive, in that an electron microscope, and its associated equipment, are required, and it is also unsuitable for examining large numbers of specimens. The methods of choice in many laboratories are either enzyme immunoassay or latex assays, of which many commercial kits are now available for both group A and group B rotaviruses. Such assays do not require complex equipment and can cope with many hundreds of specimens per day. A polymerase chain reaction assay, an extremely sensitive means of detecting the virus genome, has recently been developed.[224]

ADENOVIRUSES

Adenoviruses are unenveloped, double-stranded DNA viruses exhibiting icosahedral symmetry (*Figure 9.18*). The capsid is composed of 252 capsomeres – 240 hexons and 12 pentons – and is some 75 nm in diameter. A projection, or fibre, projects from each penton.[216] Human adenoviruses form the *Mastadenovirus* genus within the Adenoviridae.

Adenoviruses have been recognized for some years as an established cause of respiratory infection, including pharyngoconjunctival fever, and have also been implicated in follicular conjunctivitis and keratoconjunctivitis. Throughout the 1960s many workers also isolated adenoviruses from faecal samples taken from patients with diarrhoea; however, a causative role could not be established because, in most studies, adenoviruses could be detected with equal frequency in both children with gastroenteritis and matched controls,[111] although in some studies a significant association was found.[173]

Such adenoviruses were detected by cell culture methods; the advent of the use of negative staining electron microscopy in the investigation of gastroenteritis identified adenoviruses from faecal samples which did not grow in conventional cell cultures.[74,137] Such viruses were termed 'uncultivable',[22] 'fastidious'[118] or 'enteric'[174] and were shown to be associated with episodes of diarrhoea.

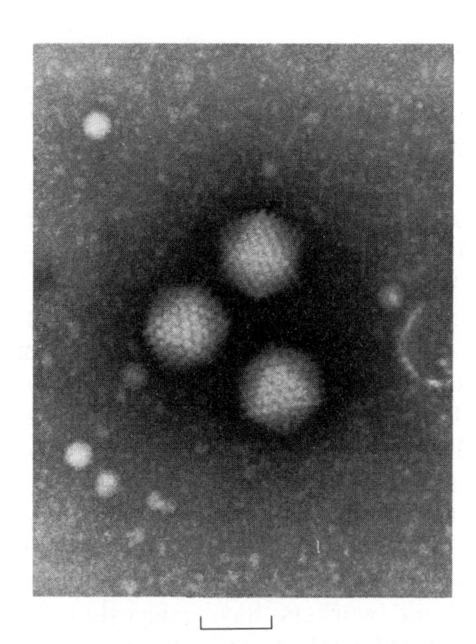

Figure 9.18 Electron micrograph of negatively stained faecal extract showing adenoviruses (bar represents 50 nm).

Conventional adenoviruses are divided into five subgroups: A, B, C, D and E.[210] The fastidious adenoviruses were shown to possess the group antigen common to all human adenoviruses[218] but were soon shown to belong to two new serotypes: 40 and 41.[57] Restriction endonuclease analysis of the viral DNA has subsequently placed these two serotypes in a new subgenus: F.[215] Although growth in conventional cell culture is not possible, these viruses will propagate in such cell lines as Chang's human conjunctival and Graham's 293 human embryo-kidney.[57]

EPIDEMIOLOGY

Fastidious adenoviruses have been detected in faecal samples from children with gastroenteritis worldwide.[3] Incidence varies from 4 to 17%, thus making fastidious adenoviruses second only to rotaviruses as a cause of diarrhoea in children. Seroepidemiological studies have demonstrated that fastidious adenoviruses are primarily pathogens of children.[119,197] Unlike rotaviruses, there seems to be no seasonal preponderance of fastidious adenovirus infection,[23] although a higher occurrence during the summer months was noted in Sweden[211] and Africa.[207]

CLINICAL FEATURES

Fastidious adenovirus infection causes diarrhoea with some vomiting and fever. The disease is usually mild or asymptomatic, although fatal infection has been reported.[223] The incubation period has been estimated as 8–10 days.[177]

The clinical characteristics of fastidious adenovirus infection have been investigated in detail.[211] The mean duration of diarrhoea was 8–12 days with prolonged diarrhoea being common, especially in adenovirus 41 infection. Fever and vomiting was mild and respiratory symptoms were rarely observed. Fastidious adenovirus infection has been reported to be milder but more protracted than that caused by rotaviruses,[212] although others have reported that fastidious adenovirus-associated diarrhoea is as severe as that caused by rotaviruses.[122] A recent Canadian study has suggested that adenovirus serotype 31 can produce a clinical picture indistinguishable from that produced by serotypes 40 and 41.[123] Further research is needed to establish the relevance of non-group F adenoviruses in gastroenteritis, particularly in immunodeficient and immunosuppressed patients.

INVESTIGATIONS

As with other viruses causing gastroenteritis, the most widely used technique is negative staining electron microscopy of faecal suspensions. However, as stated above, the fastidious adenoviruses will grow in such cell lines as Chang's human conjunctival and Graham's 293 human embryo kidney. Commercial enzyme immunoassays and latex assays are available. A polymerase chain reaction assay has been recently developed.[4]

OTHER VIRUSES

CORONAVIRUS-LIKE PARTICLES (*Figure 9.19*)

Although coronaviruses are established causes of diarrhoea in animals and respiratory diseases in humans, their role in enteric infections of humans is not clear. Coronavirus-like particles were first detected in 1975 in association with gastroenteritis in adults[31] or tropical sprue in both children and adults.[141] They have also been implicated in outbreaks of necrotizing enterocolitis in infants.[35] However, their detection in faecal samples of clinically well individuals has raised considerable doubt about their aetiological role.

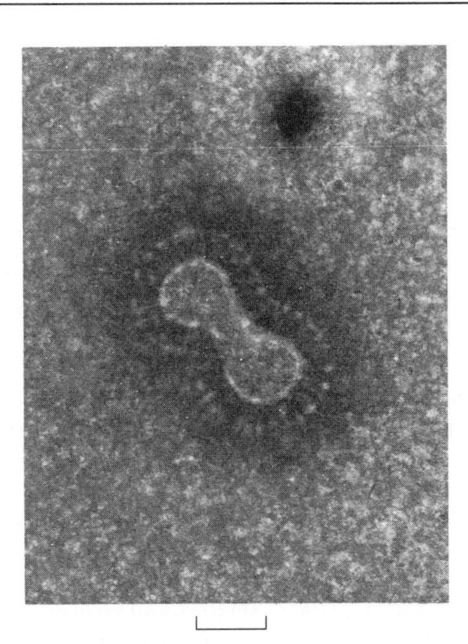

Figure 9.19 Electron micrograph of negatively stained faecal extract containing coronavirus-like particles (bar represents 50 nm).

PESTIVIRUSES

Pestiviruses – small (approximately 50 nm), pleomorphic RNA viruses – form a separate genus within the family Togaviridae. Viruses in this genus cause gastroenteritis in animals and include bovine diarrhoea virus, hog cholera virus and border disease virus. Recent studies in Arizona and Peru have suggested that an as yet unidentified pestivirus may be implicated in gastroenteritis in children.[234,235]

PICOBIRNAVIRUSES

There are reports from Brazil of the association between gastroenteritis in humans and a picobirnavirus.[168]

TOROVIRUSES

Since their discovery in 1972 in animals, toroviruses, fringed, pleomorphic RNA viruses, some 120–140 nm in diameter, have been associated with gastroenteritis in calves, pigs and horses. A single report of the visualization of a torovirus in human faeces has been published.[12]

REFERENCES

1. Aaroopraesert, D., Fagerland, J.A., Kelso, N. *et al.* (1989) Cultivation and partial characterisation of bovine astrovirus. *Veterinary Microbiology*, **19**, 151–160.
2. Agus, S.G., Dolin, R., Wyatt, R.G. *et al.* (1973)

Acute infectious nonbacterial gastroenteritis: intestinal histopathology. Histologic and enzymatic alterations during illness produced by the Norwalk agent in man. *Annals of Internal Medicine*, **79**, 18–25.

3. Albert, M.J. (1986) Enteric adenoviruses. *Archives of Virology*, **88**, 1–17.
4. Allard, A., Girones, R., Juto, P. and Wadell, G. (1990) Polymerase chain reaction for detection of adenoviruses in stool samples. *Journal of Clinical Microbiology*, **28**, 2659–2667.
5. Allen, A. M. and Desselberger, U. (1985) Reassortment of human rotaviruses carrying rearranged genes with bovine rotavirus. *Journal of General Virology*, **66**, 2703–2714.
6. Anthony, I.D., Bullivant, S., Dayal, S. *et al.* (1991) Rotavirus spike structure and polypeptide composition. *Journal of Virology*, **65**, 4334–4340.
7. Appleton, H. (1987) Small round viruses: classification and role in foodborne infections. In *Ciba Symposium 128. Novel Diarrhoea Viruses*, pp. 108–125. Chichester: Wiley.
8. Appleton, H. and Pereira, M.S. (1977) A possible virus aetiology in outbreaks of food poisoning from cockles. *The Lancet*, **i**, 780–781.
9. Appleton, H., Buckley, M., Thom, B.T. *et al.* (1977) Virus-like particles in winter vomiting disease. *The Lancet*, **i**, 409–411.
10. Ashley, C.R., Caul, E.O. and Paver, W.K. (1978) Astrovirus associated gastroenteritis in children. *Journal of Clinical Pathology*, **31**, 939–943.
11. Banatvala, J.E. (1979) The role of viruses in acute diarrhoeal disease. *Clinics in Gastroenterology*, **8**, 569–598.
12. Beards, G.M., Green, J., Hall, C. *et al.* (1984) An enveloped virus in stools of children and adults that resembles the Breda virus of calves. *The Lancet*, **i**, 1050–1052.
13. Bernstein, D.I., Sander, D.S., Smith, V.E. *et al.* (1991) Protection from rotavirus infection: a 2-year prospective study. *Journal of Infectious Diseases*, **164**, 277–283.
14. Besselaar, T.G., Rosenblatt, A. and Kidd, A.H. (1986) Atypical rotavirus from South African neonates. *Archives of Virology*, **87**, 327–330.
15. Bingnan, F., Unicomb, L., Rahim, Z. *et al.* (1991) Rotavirus-associated diarrhoea in rural Bangladesh: two-year study of incidence and serotype distribution. *Journal of Clinical Microbiology*, **29**, 1359–1363.
16. Bishop, R.F., Unicomb, L.E. and Barnes, G.L. (1991) Epidemiology of rotavirus serotypes in Melbourne, Australia, from 1973 to 1989. *Journal of Clinical Microbiology*, **29**, 862–868.
17. Bishop, R.F., Davidson, G.P., Holmes., I.H. and Ruck, B.J. (1973) Virus particles in epithelial cells of duodenal mucosa from children with non-bacterial gastroenteritis. *The Lancet*, **ii**, 1281–1283.
18. Bishop, R.F., Barnes, G.L., Cipriani, E. and Lund, J.S. (1983) Clinical immunity after neonatal rotavirus infection. A prospective longitudinal study in young children. *New England Journal of Medicine*, **309**, 72–76.
19. Black, R.E., Greenberg, H.B., Kapikian, A.Z. *et al.* (1982) Acquisition of serum antibody to Norwalk virus and rotavirus and relation to diarrhoea in a longitudinal study of young children in rural Bangladesh. *Journal of Infectious Diseases*, **145**, 483–489.
20. Blacklow, N.R., Echeverria, P. and Smith, P.H. (1976) Serological studies with reovirus-like agents. *Infection and Immunity*, **13**, 1563–1566.
21. Blacklow, N.R., Cukor, G., Bedigian, M.K. *et al.* (1979) Immune response and prevalence of antibody to Norwalk enteritis virus as determined by radioimmunoassay. *Journal of Clinical Microbiology*, **10**, 903–909.
22. Brandt, C.D., Kim, H.W., Yolken, R.H. *et al.* (1979) Comparative epidemiology of two rotavirus serotypes and other viral agents associated with pediatric gastroenteritis. *American Journal of Epidemiology*, **110**, 243–254.
23. Brandt, C.D., Kim, H.W., Rodriguez, W.J. *et al.* (1985) Adenoviruses and pediatric gastroenteritis. *Journal of Infectious Diseases*, **151**, 437–443.
24. Bridger, J.C., Pedley, S. and McCrae, M.A. (1986) Group C rotaviruses in humans. *Journal of Clinical Microbiology*, **23**, 760–763.
25. Browning, G.F., Chalmers, R.M., Fitzgerald, T.A. and Snodgrass D.R. (1991) Serological and genomic characterisation of L338, a novel equine group A rotavirus G serotype. *Journal of General Virology*, **72**, 1059–1064.
26. Browning, G.F., Fitzgerald, T.A., Chalmers, R.M. and Snodgrass, D.R. (1991) A novel group A rotavirus G serotype: serological and genomic characterization of equine isolate (F123). *Journal of Clinical Microbiology*, **29**,2043–2046.
27. Bryden, A.S., Davies, H.A., Hadley, R.E. *et al.* (1975) Rotavirus enteritis in the West Midlands during 1974. *The Lancet*, **ii**, 241–243.
28. Carlson, J.A.K., Middleton, P.J., Szymanski, M. *et al.* (1978) Fatal rotavirus gastroenteritis. An analysis of 21 cases. *American Journal of Diseases in Childhood*, **132**, 477–479.
29. Carr, M.E., Donald, G., McKendrick, W. and Spyridakis, T. (1976) *Scandinavian Journal of Infectious Diseases*, **8**, 241–243.
30. Caul, E.O. and Appleton, H. (1982) The electronmicroscopical and physical characteristics of small round human faecal viruses. An interim scheme for classification. *Journal of Medical Virology*, **9**, 257–265.
31. Caul, E.O., Paver, W.K. and Clarke, S.K.R. (1975) Coronavirus particles in faeces from patients with gastroenteritis. *The Lancet*, **i**, 1192.
32. Caul, E.O., Ashley, C.R., Darville, J:M. *et al.* (1990) Gp C rotavirus associated with fatal enteritis in a family outbreak. *Journal of Medical Virology*, **30**, 201–205.
33. Centers for Disease Control (1990) Viral agents of gastroenteritis: public health importance and

outbreak management. *Morbidity and Mortality Weekly Report*, **39**(RR-5): 1–24.
34. Champsaur, H.E., Questiaux, J., Prevot, M. *et al.* (1984) Rotavirus carriage, asymptomatic infection, and disease in the first two years of life. I. Virus shedding. *Journal of Infectious Diseases*, **149**, 667–674.
35. Chany, C., Moscovici, O., Lebon, P. and Rousset, S. (1982) Association of coronavirus infection with neonatal necrotizing enterocholitis. *Pediatrics*, **69**, 209–214.
36. Chen, G.M., Hung, T., Bridger, J.C. and McCrae, M.A. (1985) Chinese adult rotavirus is a group B rotavirus. *The Lancet*, **ii**, 1123–1124.
37. Chiba, S., Sakuma, Y., Kogasaka, R. *et al.* (1979) An outbreak of gastroenteritis associated with calicivirus in an infant home. *Journal of Medical Virology*, **4**, 249–254.
38. Chiba, S., Yokoyama, T., Nakata, S. *et al.* (1986) Protective effect of naturally acquired homotypic and heterotypic rotavirus antibodies. *The Lancet*, **ii**, 417–421.
39. Christopher, P.J., Grohmann, G.S., Milson, R.H. *et al.* (1978) Parvovirus gastroenteritis. A new entity for Australia. *Medical Journal of Australia*, **1**, 121–124.
40. Christy, C., Madore, H.P., Pichichero, M.E. *et al.* (1988) Field trial of rhesus rotavirus vaccine in infants. *Paediatric Infectious Diseases Journal*, **1**, 645–650.
41. Chrystie, I.L., Totterdell, B.M., Baker M.J. *et al.* (1975) Rotavirus infections in a maternity unit. *The Lancet*, **ii**, 79.
42. Chrystie, I.L., Totterdell, B.M. and Banatvala, J.E. (1978) Asymptomatic endemic rotavirus infections in the newborn. *The Lancet*, **i**, 1176–1178.
43. Chrystie, I.L., Booth, I.W., Kidd, A.H. *et al.* (1982) Multiple faecal virus excretion in immunodeficiency. *The Lancet*, **i**, 282.
44. Clark, H.F., Borian, F.E., Bell, L.M. *et al.* (1988) Protective effect of WC3 vaccine against rotavirus diarrhea in infants during a predominantly serotype 1 rotavirus season. *Journal of Infectious Diseases*, **158**, 570–586.
45. Coulsen, B.S. (1987) Variation in neutralisation epitopes of human rotaviruses in relation to genomic RNA polymorphism. *Virology*, **159**, 209–216.
46. Crewe, E. and Murphy, A.M. (1980) Further studies on neonatal rotavirus infections. *Medical Journal of Australia*, **1**, 61.
47. Cubitt, W.D. (1989) Diagnosis, occurrence and clinical significance of the human "candidate" caliciviruses. *Progress of Medical Virology*, **36**, 103–119.
48. Cubitt, W.D. (1990) Human SRSVs, Caliciviruses and Astroviruses. In *Clinical Gastroenterology, Virus Infections of the Gut and Liver* (Ed.) Farthing, M.J.G. pp. 643–656. London: Baillière Tindall.
49. Cubitt, W.D. (1991) A review of the epidemiology and diagnosis of waterborne viral infections. *Water Science Technology*, **24**, 197–203.
50. Cubitt, W.D. and McSwiggan, D.A. (1981) Calicivirus gastroenteritis in North West London. *The Lancet*, **ii**, 975–977.
51. Cubitt, W.D. and McSwiggan, D.A. (1987) A seroepidemiological survey of the prevalence of antibodies to a strain of human calicivirus. *Journal of Medical Virology*, **21**, 361–368.
52. Cubitt, W.D., McSwiggan, D.A. and Moore, W. (1979) Winter vomiting disease caused by a calicivirus. *Journal of Clinical Pathology*, **32**, 786–793.
53. Cubitt, W.D., McSwiggan, D.A. and Arstall, S.A. (1980) An outbreak of calicivirus infection in a mother and baby unit. *Journal of Clinical Pathology*, **33**, 1095–1098.
54. Cubitt, W.D., Pead, P.J. and Saeed, A.A. (1981) A new serotype of calicivirus associated with an outbreak of gastroenteritis in a residential home for the elderly. *Journal of Clinical Pathology*, **34**, 924–926.
55. Cukor, G., Blacklow, N.R., Echeverria, P. *et al.* (1980) Comparative study of the acquisition of antibody to Norwalk virus in pediatric populations. *Infection and Immunity*, **29**, 822–823.
56. Davidson, G.P., Bishop, R.F., Townely, R.R.W. *et al.* (1975) Importance of a new virus in acute sporadic enteritis in children. *The Lancet*, **i**, 242–246.
57. De Jong, J.C., Wigand, R., Kidd, A.H. *et al.* (1983) Candidate adenoviruses 40 and 41: fastidious adenoviruses from human stool. *Journal of Medical Virology*, **11**, 215–231.
58. De Mol, P., Zissis, G., Butzler, J.P. *et al.* (1986) Failure of live, attenuated oral rotavirus vaccine. *The Lancet*, **ii**, 108.
59. De Zoysa, I. and Feachem, R.G. (1985) Interventions for the control of diarrhoeal diseases among young children: rotavirus and cholera immunisation. *Bulletin of the World Health Organisation*, **63**, 569–583.
60. Dolin, R., Levy, A.G., Wyatt, R.G. *et al.* (1975) Viral gastroenteritis induced by Hawaii agent. Jejunal histopathology and seroresponse. *American Journal of Medicine*, **39**, 761–769.
61. Editorial (1976) Viral cross-infections in children's wards. *The Lancet*, **i**, 1391–1393.
62. Editorial (1990) Puzzling diversity of rotaviruses. *The Lancet*, **335**, 573–575.
63. Eiden, J., Vonderfecht, S. and Yolken, R. (1985) Evidence that a novel rotavirus-like agent of rats can cause gastroenteritis in man. *The Lancet*, **ii**, 8.
64. Eiden, J.J., Verleur, D.G., Vonderfecht, S.L. and Yolken, R.H. (1988) Duration and pattern of asymptomatic rotavirus shedding by hospitalized children. *Pediatric Infectious Diseases Journal*, **7**, 564–569.
65. Erickson, B.L., Graham, D.Y., Mason, B.B. and Estes, M.K. (1982) Identification, synthesis, and

modifications of simian rotavirus SA11 polypeptides in infected cells. *Journal of Virology*, **42**, 825–839.

66. Estes, M.K. and Cohen, J. (1989) Rotavirus gene structure and function. *Microbiological Reviews*, **53**, 410–499.
67. Estes, M.K., Graham, D.Y., Smith, E.M. and Gerba, C.P. (1979) Rotavirus stability and inactivation. *Journal of General Virology*, **43**, 403–409.
68. Eydelloth, R.S., Vonderfecht, S.L., Sheridan, J.F. *et al.* (1984) Kinetics of viral replication and local and systemic immune responses in experimental rotavirus infection. *Journal of Virology*, **50**, 947–950.
69. Fleissner, M.L., Herrmann, J.E. and Booth, J.W. (1989) Role of Norwalk virus in two foodborne outbreaks, definitive virus association. *American Journal of Epidemiology*, **129**, 168–173.
70. Flewett, T.H. Clinical features of rotavirus infection. In *Virus Infections of the Gastrointestinal Tract* (Ed.) Tyrrell, D.A. and Kapikian, A.Z. pp. 125–145. New York: Marcel Dekker.
71. Flewett, T.H. and Davies H. (1976) Caliciviruses in man. *The Lancet*, **i**, 311.
72. Flewett, T.H., Bryden, A.S. and Davies, H.A. (1973) Virus particles in gastroenteritis. *The Lancet*, **ii**, 1497.
73. Flewett, T.H., Bryden, A.S., Davies, H. *et al.* (1974) Relation between viruses from acute gastroenteritis of children and newborn calves. *The Lancet*, **ii**, 61.
74. Flewett, T.H., Bryden, A.S. and Davies, H. and Morris C.A. (1975) Epidemic viral enteritis in a long-stay children's ward. *The Lancet*, **i**, 530–533.
75. Flores, J., Midthun, K., Hoshino, Y. *et al.* (1986) Conservation of the fourth gene among rotaviruses recovered from asymptomatic newborn infants and its possible role in attenuation. *Journal of Virology*, **60**, 972–979.
76. Flores, J., Perez-Schael, I., Gonzalez, P. *et al.* (1987) Protection against severe rotavirus diarrhoea by rhesus rotavirus vaccine in Venezuelan infants. *The Lancet*, **i**, 882–884.
77. Flores, P., Perez-Schael, I., Blanco, M. *et al.* (1990) Comparison of reactogenicity and antigenicity of M37 rotavirus vaccine and rhesus-rotavirus-based quadrivalent vaccine. *The Lancet*, **336**, 330–333.
78. Friedman, M.G., Galil, A., Sarov, B. *et al.* (1988) Two sequential outbreaks of rotavirus gastroenteritis: evidence for symptomatic and asymptomatic reinfections. *Journal of Infectious Diseases*, **158**, 814–822.
79. Ghosh, S.K. and Naik, T.N. (1989) Detection of a large number of subgroup I human rotaviruses with a "long" RNA electropherotype. *Archives of Virology*, **105**, 119–127.
80. Gill, O.N., Cubitt, W.D., McSwiggan, D.A. *et al.* (1983) Epidemic of gastroenteritis caused by oysters contaminated with small round structured viruses. *British Medical Journal*, **287**, 1532–1534.
81. Glass, R.I., Monroe, S.S., Stine, S. *et al.* (1988) Small round structured viruses: the Norwalk family of agents. In *Viruses and the Gut. Proceedings of the Ninth BSG. Smith, Kline and French International Workshop*, pp. 87–90.
82. Gold, R. (1988) Overview of the world-wide problem of diarrhoea. *Drugs*, **36**(suppl. 4), 1–5.
83. Goldwater, P.N., Chrystie, I.L. and Banatvala, J.E. (1979) Rotaviruses and the respiratory tract. *British Medical Journal*, **ii**, 1551.
84. Gothefors, L., Wadell, G., Juto, P. *et al.* (1989) Prolonged efficacy of rhesus rotavirus vaccine in Swedish children. *Journal of Infectious Diseases*, **159**, 753–757.
85. Gray, J.J., Wreghitt, T.G. and Cubitt, W.D. (1987) An outbreak of astrovirus type 1 and calicivirus in a residential home for the elderly. *Journal of Medical Virology*, **23**, 377–381.
86. Gray, J.J., Jiang, X., Morgan-Capner, P., Desselberger, V. and Estes, M.K. (1993) The prevalence of antibody to Norwalk virus in England. Detection by indirect ELISA with baculovirus expressed Norwalk capsid protein. *Journal of Clinical Microbiology*, **31**, in press.
87. Green, K.Y., Hoshino, Y. and Ikegami, N. (1989) Sequence analysis of the gene encoding the serotype-specific glycoprotein (VP7) of two new human rotavirus serotypes. *Virology*, **168**, 429–433.
88. Greenberg, H.B., Valdesuso, J.R., Kalica, A.R. *et al.* (1979) Prevalence of antibody to Norwalk virus in various countries. *Infection and Immunity*, **26**, 270–273.
89. Grillner, L., Brobergei, U., Chrystie, I. and Raasfo, U. (1985) Rotavirus infection in newborns: an epidemiological and clinical study. *Scandinavian Journal of Infectious Diseases*, **17**, 349–355.
90. Grinstein, S., Gomez, J.A., Bercovich, J.A. and Biscotti, E.L. (1989) Epidemiology of rotavirus infection and gastroenteritis in prospectively monitored Argentine families with young children. *American Journal of Epidemiology*, **130**, 300–308.
91. Grohmann, G., Glass, R., Gold, J. *et al.* (1991) An outbreak of human calicivirus gastroenteritis in a daycare center in Sydney, Australia. *Journal of Clinical Microbiology*, **29**, 544–550.
92. Gust, I.D., Pringle, R.S., Barnes, G.L. *et al.* (1977) Complement-fixing antibody response to rotavirus infection. *Journal of Clinical Microbiology*, **5**, 125–130.
93. Hall, G.A. (1987) Comparative pathology of infection by novel diarrhoea viruses. In *Ciba Symposium 128. Novel Diarrhoea Viruses*. pp. 192–217. Chichester: John Wiley.
94. Herrmann, J.E., Hudson, R.W., Perron-Henry, D.M. *et al.* (1988) Antigenic characterisation of cell cultivated astrovirus serotypes and development of astrovirus specific monoclonal

antibodies. *Journal of Infectious Diseases*, **158**, 182–185.
95. Herrmann, J.E., Cubitt, W.D., Hudson, R.W. *et al.* (1990) Propagation and immunological characterisation of the Marin County strain of astrovirus and its detection by monoclonal antibody. *Archives of Virology*, **110**, 213–220.
96. Herrmann, J.E., Nowak, N.A., Perron-Henry, D.M. *et al.* (1990) Diagnosis of astrovirus gastroenteritis by antigen detection with monoclonal antibodies. *Journal of Infectious Diseases*, **161**, 226–229.
97. Hirschorn, N. (1980) The treatment of acute diarrhea in children: a historical and physiological perspective. *American Journal of Clinical Nutrition*, **33**, 637–663.
98. Hjelt, K., Krasilnikoff, P.A., Grauballe, P.C. and Rasmussen, S.W. (1985) Clinical features in hospitalised children with acute gastroenteritis. *Acta Paediatrica Scandinavica*, **74**, 89–95.
99. Ho, M., Glass, R.I., Pinsky, P.F. and Anderson, L. (1988) Rotavirus as a cause of diarrheal morbidity and mortality in the United States. *Journal of Infectious Diseases*, **158**, 1112–1116.
100. Ho, M.S., Glass, R.I., Pinsky, P.F. *et al.* (1988) Diarrheal diseases in American children. Are they preventable? *Journal of the American Medical Association*, **260**, 3281–3285.
101. Ho, M.S., Glass, R.I., Monroe, S.S. *et al.* (1989) Recurrent outbreaks of gastroenteritis aboard a cruise ship: environmental contamination as a mode of transmission of small round structured viruses. *The Lancet*, **ii**, 961–964.
102. Holmes, I.H., Ruck, B.J., Bishop, R.F. and Davidson, G.P. (1975) Infantile enteritis viruses: morphogenesis and morphology. *Journal of Virology*, **16**, 937–943.
103. Hoshino, Y., Wyatt, R.G., Greenberg, H.B. *et al.* (1984) Serotypic similarity and diversity of rotaviruses of mammalian and avian origin as studied by plaque-reduction neutralisation. *Journal of Infectious Diseases*, **49**, 694–702.
104. Hum, C.P., Dyall-Smith, M.L. and Holmes, I.H. (1989) The VP7 gene of a new G serotype of human rotavirus (B37) is similar to G3 proteins in the antigenic C region. *Virology*, **170**, 55–61.
105. Humphrey, T.J., Cruickshank, J.G. and Cubitt, W.D. (1984) An outbreak of calicivirus associated gastroenteritis in an old people's home. A possible zoonosis. *Journal of Hygiene*, **92**, 293–299.
106. Hundley, F., McIntyre, M., Clark, B. *et al.* (1987) Heterogeneity of genome rearrangements in rotaviruses isolated from a chronically infected immunodeficient child. *Journal of Virology*, **61**, 3365–3372.
107. Hung, T. (1988) Rotavirus adult diarrhea. *Advances in Viral Research*, **35**, 193–218.
108. Hung, T., Chen, G.M., Wang, C.A. *et al.* (1984) Waterborne outbreak of rotavirus diarrhoea in adults in China caused by a novel rotavirus. *The Lancet*, **i**, 1139–1142.
109. Iverson, A.M., Gill, M., Bartlett, C.L.R. *et al.* (1987) Two outbreaks of foodborne gastroenteritis caused by a small round structured virus. Evidence. *The Lancet*, **ii**, 556–558.
110. Jiang, X., Wang, M., Graham, D.Y. and Estes, M.K. (1992) Expression, self assembly, and antigenicity of the Norwalk virus capsid protein. *Journal of Virology*, **66**, 6527–6532.
111. Joncas, J. and Pavilanis, V. (1960) Diarrhoea and vomiting in infancy and childhood: viral studies. *Canadian Medical Association Journal*, **82**, 1108–1113.
112. Kapikian, A.Z. and Chanock, R.M. (1990) Rotaviruses. In *Virology* (Ed.) Fields, B.N. and Knipe, D.M. pp. 1353–1404. New York: Raven Press.
113. Kapikian, A.Z., Wyatt, R.G., Dolin, R. *et al.* (1972) Visualisation by immune electron microscopy of a 27 nm particle associated with acute infectious non-bacterial gastroenteritis. *Journal of Virology*, **10**, 1075–1081.
114. Kapikian, A.Z., Kim, H.W., Wyatt, R.G. *et al.* (1976) Human reovirus-like agent as a major pathogen associated with "winter" gastroenteritis in hospitalized infants and young children. *New England Journal of Medicine*, **294**, 965–972.
115. Kapikian, A.Z., Flores, J., Hoshino, Y. *et al.* (1986) Rotavirus: the major etiologic agent of severe infantile diarrhea may be controllable by a "Jennerian" approach to vaccination. *Journal of Infectious Diseases*, **153**, 815–822.
116. Kappus, K.D., Mark, J.S., Holman, R.C. *et al.* (1982) An outbreak of Norwalk gastroenteritis associated with swimming in a pool and secondary person to person spread. *American Journal of Epidemiology*, **116**, 834–839.
117. Keswick, B.H., Salterwhite, T.K., Johnson, P. *et al.* (1985) Inactivation of Norwalk virus in drinking water by chlorine. *Applied Environmental Microbiology*, **50**, 261–264.
118. Kidd, A.H. and Madeley, C.R. (1981) In vitro growth of some fastidious adenoviruses from stool specimens. *Journal of Clinical Pathology*, **34**, 213–216.
119. Kidd, A.H., Banatvala, J.E. and De Jong, J.C. (1983) Antibodies to fastidious faecal adenoviruses (species 40 and 41) in sera from children. *Journal of Medical Virology*, **11**, 333–341.
120. Kitaoka, S., Nakagomi, T., Fukuhara, N. *et al.* (1987) Serologic characteristics of a human rotavirus isolate, AU-1, which has a "long" RNA pattern and subgroup I specificity. *Journal of Medical Virology*, **23**, 351–357.
121. Kobayashi, N., Taniguchi, K., Urasawa, T. and Urasawa, S. (1991) Analysis of the neutralisation epitopes on human rotavirus VP7 recognised by monotype-specific monoclonal antibodies. *Journal of General Virology*, **72**, 1855–1861.
122. Kotloff K.L., Losonsky, G.A., Morris, J.G. *et al.* (1989) Enteric adenovirus infection and childhood

diarrhea: an epidemiologic study in three clinical settings. *Pediatrics*, **84**, 219–225.
123. Krajden, M., Brown, M., Petrasek, A. and Middleton, P.J. (1990) Clinical features of adenovirus enteritis: a review of 127 cases. *Pediatric Infectious Diseases Journal*, **9**, 636–641.
124. Kunz, J., Slongo, R., Schams, M. and Zbinden, R. (1990) An outbreak of rotavirus infections in newborns: new aspects? *Journal of Perinatal Medicine*, **18**, 357–362.
125. Kurtz, J.B. and Lee, T.W. (1987) Astroviruses: human and animal. In *Ciba symposium 128. Novel Diarrhoea Viruses*, pp. 92–107. Chichester: Wiley.
126. Kurtz, J.B., Lee, T.W., Craig, J.W. and Reed, S.E. (1979) Astrovirus infections in volunteers. *Journal of Medical Virology*, **3**, 221–230.
127. Lambden, P.R., Caul E.O., Ashley C.R. and Clarke, I.N. (1993) Sequence and genome organization of a human small round-structured virus (Norwalk-like virus). *Science*, **259**, 516–518.
128. Lee, T.W. and Kurtz, J.B. (1981) Serial propagation of astrovirus in tissue culture with the aid of trypsin. *Journal of General Virology*, **57**, 421–424.
129. Levy, A.G., Widerlite, L., Schwartz, P.R. *et al.* (1976) Jejunal adenylate nuclease activity in human subjects during viral gastroenteritis. *Gastroenterology*, 321–325.
130. Lewis, M.H., Parry, J.V., Davies, H.A. *et al.* (1979) A year's experience of the rotavirus syndrome and its association with respiratory illness. *Archives of Diseases in Childhood*, **54**, 339–346.
131. Lewis, D., Lightfoot, N.F., Cubitt, W.D. and Wilson, S.A. (1989) An outbreak of astrovirus type 1 and rotavirus in a geriatric inpatient population. *Journal of Medical Virology*, **23**, 377–381.
132. Linco, S.J. and Grohmann, G.S. (1980) The Darwin outbreak of oyster associated viral gastroenteritis. *Medical Journal of Australia*, **1**, 211–213.
133. Lloyd-Evans, N., Springthorpe, V.S. and Sattar, S.A. (1986) Chemical disinfection of human rotavirus-contaminated surfaces. *Journal of Hygiene*, **97**, 163–173.
134. Ludert, J.E., Gil, F., Liprandi, F. and Esparza, J. (1986) The structure of the rotavirus inner capsid studied by electron microscopy of chemically disrupted particles. *Journal of General Virology*, **67**, 1721–1725.
135. McLean, B. and Holmes, I.H. (1981) Effects of antibodies, trypsin, and trypsin inhibitors on susceptibility of neonates to rotavirus infection. *Journal of Clinical Microbiology*, **13**, 22–29.
136. Madeley, C.R. and Cosgrove, B.P. (1975) 28 nm particles in faeces in infantile diarrhoea. *The Lancet*, **i**, 451–452.
137. Madeley, C.R., Cosgrove, B.P., Bell, E.J. and Fallon, R.J. (1977) Stool viruses in babies in Glasgow. 1. Hospital admissions with diarrhoea. *Journal of Hygiene (Cambridge)*, **78**, 261–273.
138. Madeley, C.R., Cosgrove, B.P. and Bell, E.J. (1978) Stool viruses in babies in Glasgow, 2. Investigation of normal newborns in hospital. *Journal of Hygiene*, **81**, 285–294.
139. Maiya, P.P., Pereira, S.N., Mathan, M. *et al.* (1977) Aetiology of acute gastroenteritis in infancy and early childhood in southern India. *Archives of Disease in Childhood*, **52**, 482–485.
140. Mata, L., Simhon, A., Urrutia, R.A. *et al.* (1983) Epidemiology of rotaviruses in a cohort of 45 Guatemalan Mayan Indian children observed from birth to the age of three years. *Journal of Infectious Diseases*, **148**, 452–461.
141. Mathan, M., Mathan, V.I., Swaminathan, S.P. *et al.* (1975) Pleomorphic virus-like particles in human faeces. *The Lancet*, **i**, 1068.
142. Matthews, R.E.F. (1978) The classification and nomenclature of viruses: summary of results of meetings of the International Committee on Taxonomy of Viruses in The Hague, September 1978. *Intervirology*, **11**, 133–135.
143. Metcalf, P. (1982) The symmetry of reovirus. *Journal of Ultrastructural Research*, **78**, 292–301.
144. Middleton, P.J., Szymanski, M.T. and Petric, M. (1977) Viruses associated with acute gastroenteritis in young children. *American Journal of Diseases of Children*, **131**, 733–737.
145. Midthun, K., Valdesuso, K., Hoshino, Y. *et al.* (1987) Analysis of RNA–RNA hybridisation assay of intertypic rotaviruses suggests that gene reassortment occurs in vivo. *Journal of Clinical Microbiology*, **25**, 295–300.
146. Monroe, S.S., Stine, S.E., Gorelkin, L. *et al.* (1991) Temporal synthesis of proteins and RNAs during human astrovirus infection of cultured cells. *Journal of Virology*, **65**, 641–648.
147. Morens, D.M., Zweighraft, R.H., Vernon, R.H. *et al.* (1979) A waterborne outbreak of gastroenteritis with secondary person to person spread. *The Lancet*, **i**, 964–966.
148. Morse, D.G., Guzewick, J.J., Hanrahan, J.P. *et al.* (1986) Widespread outbreaks of clam and oyster associated gastroenteritis. Role of Norwalk virus. *New England Journal of Medicine*, **314**, 678–681.
149. Murphy, A.M., Albrey, M.B. and Crewe, E.G. (1977) Rotavirus infection of neonates. *The Lancet*, **ii**, 1149–1150.
150. Murphy, A.M., Grohmann, G.S., Christopher, P.J. *et al.*(1979) An Australia-wide outbreak of gastroenteritis from oysters caused by Norwalk virus. *Medical Journal of Australia*, **2**, 329–333.
151. Nakagomi, O., Nakagomi, T., Akatani, K. and Ikegami, N. (1989) Identification of rotavirus genogroups by RNA–RNA hybridization. *Molecular Cell Probes*, **3**, 251–261.
152. Nakagomi, T. and Nakagomi, O. (1989) RNA–RNA hybridization identifies a human rotavirus

that is genetically related to feline rotavirus. *Journal of Virology*, **63**, 1431–1434.

153. Nakata, S., Chiba, S., Terashima, H. *et al.* (1985) Prevalence of antibody to human calicivirus in Japan and Southeast Asia determined by radioimmunoassay. *Journal of Clinical Microbiology*, **22**, 519–521.
154. Nicolaieff, A., Obert, G. and van Regenmortel, M.H.V. (1980) Detection of rotavirus by serological trapping on antibody coated electron microscope grids. *Journal of Clinical Microbiology*, **12**, 101–104.
155. Nicolas, J.C., Cohen, J., Fortier, B. *et al.* (1983) Isolation of a human pararotavirus. *Virology*, **124**, 181–184.
156. Noone, C. and Banatvala, J.E. (1983) Hospital-acquired rotaviral gastroenteritis in a general paediatric unit. *Journal of Hospital Infection*, **4**, 297–299.
157. Offit, P.A., Blavat, G., Greenberg, H.B. and Clark, H.F. (1986) Molecular basis of rotavirus virulence: role of gene segment 4. *Journal of Virology*, **57**, 46–49.
158. Oishi, I., Maeda, A., Yamazaki, K. *et al.* (1980) Calicivirus detected in outbreaks of gastroenteritis in schoolchildren. *Biken Journal*, **23**, 163–168.
159. Oseto, M., Yamahita, Y., Takagi, K. *et al.* (1988) Four year survey of diarrhoea due to rotavirus in Matusuyana City (abstract) In *Proceedings of the Meeting of the US–Japan Panel on Viral Disease*, Tokyo.
160. Oshiro, L.S., Haley, C.E., Roberto, R.R. *et al.* (1981) A 27 nm virus isolated during an outbreak of acute nonbacterial gastroenteritis in a convalescent hospital: a possible new serotype. *Journal of Infectious Diseases*, **143**, 791–795.
161. Padilla-Noriega, L., Werner-Eckert, R., Mackau, E.R. *et al.* (1993) Serologic analysis of human rotavirus serotypes P1A and P2 by using monoclonal antibodies. *Journal of Clinical Microbiology*, **31**, 622–628.
162. Parker, S.P., Cubitt, W.D., Jiang, X. and Estes, M.K. (1993) A study of the efficacy of a recombinant Norwalk virus protein immunoassay for the diagnosis of infections with Norwalk virus and other human candidate caliciviruses. *Journal of Medical Virology*, **39**, in press.
163. Parker, S.P., Cubitt, W.D., Jiang, X. and Estes, M.K. (1993) Seroprevalence studies using a recombinant Norwalk virus protein immunoassay. *Journal of Medical Virology*, in press.
164. Parrino, T.A., Schreiber, T.S., Trier, J.S. *et al.* (1977) Clinical immunity in acute gastroenteritis caused by Norwalk agent. *New England Journal of Medicine*, **297**, 86–89.
165. Paver, W.K., Caul, E.O., Ashley, C.R. *et al.* (1973) A small virus in human faeces. *The Lancet*, **i**, 237–240.
166. Pedley, S., Hundley, F., Chrystie, I. *et al.* (1984) The genomes of rotaviruses isolated from chronically infected immunodeficient children. *Journal of General Virology*, **65**, 1141–1150.
167. Penaranda, M.E., Cubitt, W.D., Sinarchatant, P. *et al.* (1989) Group C rotavirus infections in patients in Thailand, Nepal and England. *Journal of Infectious Diseases*, **160**, 392–397.
168. Pereira, H.G., Fialho, A.M., Flewett, T.H. *et al.* (1988) Novel viruses in human faeces. *The Lancet*, **ii**, 103–104.
169. Phillips, A.D., Rice, S.J. and Walker-Smith, J.A. (1982) Astrovirus within human small intestine mucosa. *Gut*, **23**, A293–A294.
170. Poliner, J.R. and Canon, R.C. (1990) An outbreak of ice-related Norwalk gastroenteritis: Pennsylvania and Delaware. In *Workshop on Methods for Investigation of Waterborne Disease Outbreaks*, EPA/600/9-90/021. Washington, DC: US Environmental Protection Agency.
171. Prasad, B.V.V., Wang, G.J., Clerx, J.P.M. and Chui, W. (1988) Three dimensional structure of rotavirus. *Journal of Molecular Biology*, **199**, 269–275.
172. Public Health Laboratory Service Working Party on Viral Gastroenteritis. (1988) Foodborne viral gastroenteritis. *PHLS Microbiology Digest*, **5**, 69–75.
173. Ramos-Alvarez, M. and Olarte, J. (1964) Diarrheal diseases of children. *American Journal of Diseases of Children*, **107**, 218–231.
174. Retter, M., Middleton, P.J., Tam, J.S. and Petric, M. (1979) Enteric adenoviruses: detection, replication and significance. *Journal of Clinical Microbiology*, **10**, 574–578.
175. Reves, R.R., Hossain, M.M., Midthun, K. *et al.* (1989) An observational study of naturally acquired immunity to rotaviral diarrhea in a cohort of 363 Egyptian children. *American Journal of Epidemiology*, **130**, 981–988.
176. Rhode, J.E. and Northrup, R.S. (1976) Taking science where the diarrhoea is. In *Acute Diarrhoea (Ciba Foundation Symposium 42)* (Ed.) Elliott, K. and Knight, J. pp. 339–366. Amsterdam: Elsevier.
177. Richmond, S.J., Caul, E.O., Dunn, S.M. *et al.* (1979) An outbreak of gastroenteritis in young children caused by adenoviruses. *The Lancet*, **i**, 1178–1180.
178. Rodger, S.M., Schnagl, R.D. and Holmes, I.H. (1975) Biochemical and biophysical characteristics of diarrhea viruses of human and calf origin. *Journal of Virology*, **6**, 1229–1235.
179. Rodger, S.M., Bishop, R.F., Birch, C. *et al.* (1981) Molecular epidemiology of human rotaviruses in Melbourne, Australia, from 1973 to 1979, as determined by electrophoresis of genome ribonucleic acid. *Journal of Clinical Microbiology*, **13**, 272–278.
180. Rodger, S.M., Bishop, R.F. and Holmes, I.H. (1982) Detection of a rotavirus-like agent associated with diarrhea in an infant. *Journal of Clinical Microbiology*, **16**, 724–726.

181. Rodriguez, Q.J., Kim, H.W., Arrobio, J.O. *et al.* (1977) Clinical features of acute gastroenteritis associated with human reovirus-like agent in infants and young children. *Journal of Pediatrics*, **91**, 188–193.
182. Roseto, A., Escaig, J., Delain, E. *et al.* (1979) Structure of rotaviruses as studied by the freeze-drying technique. *Virology*, **98**, 471–475.
183. Rotbart, H.A., Nelson, W.L., Glode, M.P. *et al.* (1988) Neonatal rotavirus-associated necrotizing enterocolitis: case control study and prospective surveillance during an outbreak. *Journal of Pediatrics*, **112**, 87–93.
184. Ruiz, A.M., Lopez, I.V., Lopez, S. *et al.* (1988) Molecular and antigenic characterisation of porcine rotavirus YM, a possible new rotavirus serotype. *Journal of Virology*, **162**, 4331–4336.
185. Sack, R.B., Hirschorn, N., Brownlee, I. *et al.* (1975) Enterotoxigenic *Escherichia coli*-associated diarrheal disease in Apache children. *New England Journal of Medicine*, **292**, 1041–1045.
186. Sack, D.A., Freij, L. and Holmgren, J. (1991) Prospects for public health benefits in developing countries from new vaccines against enteric infections. *Journal of Infectious Diseases*, **163**, 503–506.
187. Saif, L.J. Nongroup A rotaviruses. In *Viral diarrheas of man and animals* (Ed.) Saif, L.J., Theil, K.W. pp. 73–95. Boca Raton: CRC Press.
188. Sakuma, Y., Chiba, S., Kogasaka, R. *et al.* (1981) Prevalence of antibody to human calicivirus in general population of northern Japan. *Journal of Medical Virology*, **7**, 221–225.
189. Santosham, M., Yolken, R.H., Quiroz, E. *et al.* (1977) Detection of rotavirus in respiratory secretions of children with pneumonia. *Journal of Pediatrics*, **103**, 583–585.
190. Saulsbury, F.T., Winkelstein, J.A. and Yolken, R.H. (1980) Chronic rotavirus excretion in immunodeficiency. *Journal of Pediatrics*, **97**, 61–65.
191. Sawyer, L.A., Murphy, J.J., Kaplan, J.E. *et al.* (1988) 25–30 nm particles associated with a hospital outbreak of acute gastroenteritis with evidence of airborne transmission. *Journal of Epidemiology*, **127**, 1261–1271.
192. Schreiber, D.S., Blacklow, N.R. and Trier, J.S. (1974) The small intestinal lesion induced by the Hawaii agent in infectious nonbacterial gastroenteritis. *Journal of Infectious Diseases*, **124**, 705–708.
193. Scrimshaw, D.S., Taylor, C.E. and Gordon, S.E. (1968) *Interactions of Nutrition and Infection*. Geneva: World Health Organization.
194. Sekine, S., Okada, S., Hayashi, Y. *et al.* (1989) Prevalence of small round structured virus infections in acute gastroenteritis in Tokyo. *Microbiology and Immunology*, **33,** 207–217.
195. Shahid, N.S., Banu, N.N., Bingnan, F. *et al.* (1991) Rotavirus infection detected in neonates from hospitals in urban Bangladesh. *Archives of Virology*, **119**, 135–140.
196. Shepherd, R.W., Truslow, S., Walker-Smith, J.A. *et al.* (1975) Infantile gastroenteritis: a clinical study of reovirus-like agent. *The Lancet*, **ii**, 1082–1084.
197. Shinozaki, T., Araki, K., Ushijima, H. and Fujii, R. (1987) Antibody response to enteric adenovirus types 40 and 41 in sera from various age groups. *Journal of Clinical Microbiology*, **25**, 1679–1682.
198. Snodgrass, D.R., Fitzgerald, T., Campbell, I. *et al.* (1990) Rotavirus serotypes 6 and 10 predominate in cattle. *Journal of Clinical Microbiology*, **28**, 504–507.
199. Sorrentino, A., Scodeller, E.A., Bellinzoni. *et al.* (1986) Detection of an atypical rotavirus associated with diarrhoea in Chaco, Argentina. *Transactions of the Royal Society of Tropical Medicine and Hygiene*, **80**, 120–122.
200. Spratt, H.C., Marks, M.I., Gomersall, M. *et al.* (1978) Nosocomial infantile gastroenteritis associated with minirotavirus and calicivirus. *Journal of Pediatrics*, **93**, 922–926.
201. Springthorpe, V.S., Grenier, J.L., Lloyd-Evans, N. and Sattar, S.A. (1986) Chemical disinfection of human rotaviruses: efficacy of commercially-available products in suspension tests. *Journal of Hygiene*, **97**, 139–161.
202. Superti, F., Tinari, A., Baldassarri, L. and Donelli, G. (1991) HT-29 cells: a new substrate for rotavirus growth. *Archives of Virology*, **116**, 159–173.
203. Suzuki, H. and Konno, T. (1975) Reovirus-like particles in jejunal mucosa of a Japanese infant with acute infectious non-bacterial gastroenteritis. *Tohoku Journal of Experimental Medicine*, **115**, 199–211.
204. Tan, J.A. and Schnagl, R.G. (1981) Inactivation of a rotavirus by disinfectants. *Medical Journal of Australia*, **1**, 19–23.
205. Taylor, J.W., Gary, G.W. and Greenberg, H.B. (1981) Norwalk related viral gastroenteritis due to contaminated drinking water. *American Journal of Epidemiology*, **114**, 584–592.
206. Thomas, M.E.H. and Tillet, H.E. (1975) Diarrhoea in general practice: a sixteen-year report of investigations in a microbiology laboratory, with epidemiological assessment. *Journal of Hygiene*, **74**, 183–194.
207. Tiemessen, C.T., Wegerhoff, F.O., Erasmus, M.J. and Kidd, A.H. (1989) Infection by enteric adenoviruses, rotaviruses and other agents in a rural African environment. *Journal of Medical Virology*, **28**, 176–182.
208. Totterdell, B.M., Chrystie, I.L. and Banatvala, J.E. (1980) Cord blood and breast milk antibodies in neonatal rotavirus infection. *British Medical Journal*, **i,** 828–830.
209. Totterdell, B.M., Nicholson, K.G., MacLeod, J. *et al.* (1982) Neonatal rotavirus infection: role of

lacteal neutralising activity, alpha 1 anti-trypsin and non-immunoglobulin antiviral activity in protection. *Journal of Medical Virology*, **10**, 37–44.

210. Uhnoo, I., Wadell, G., Svensson, L. and Johansson, M. (1983) Two new serotypes of enteric adenovirus causing infantile diarrhoea. *Developments in Biological Standardisation*, **53**, 311–318.
211. Uhnoo, I., Wadell, G., Svensson, L. and Johansson, M. (1984) Importance of enteric adenoviruses 40 and 41 in acute gastroenteritis in infants and young children. *Journal of Clinical Microbiology*, **20**, 365–372.
212. Uhnoo, I., Olding-Stenkvist, E. and Kreuger, A. (1986) Clinical features of acute gastroenteritis associated with rotavirus, enteric adenoviruses, and bacteria. *Archives of Diseases in Childhood*, **61**, 732–738.
213. Urasawa, S., Urasawa, T., Wakasugi, F. *et al.* (1990) Presumptive seventh serotype of human rotavirus. *Archives of Virology*, **113**, 279–282.
214. Urasawa, T., Taniguchi, K., Kobayashi, N. *et al.* (1990) Antigenic and genetic analyses of human rotavirus with dual subgroup specificity. *Journal of Clinical Microbiology*, **28**, 2837–2841.
215. van Loon, A.E., Rozijn, T.H., De Jong, J.C. and Sussenbach, J.S. (1985) Physicochemical properties of the DNAs of the fastidious adenovirus species 40 and 41. *Virology*, **140**, 197–200.
216. Valentine, R.C. and Pereira, H.G. (1965) Antigens and structure of the adenovirus. *Journal of Molecular Biology*, **13**, 13–20.
217. Vesikari, T., Isolauri, E., Delem, A. *et al.* (1985) Clinical efficacy of the RIT 4237 live attenuated bovine rotavirus vaccine in infants vaccinated before a rotavirus epidemic. *Journal of Pediatrics*, **107**, 189–194.
218. Wadell, G., Hammarskjold, M.L., Winberg, G. *et al.* (1980) Genetic ramability of adenoviruses. *Annals of the New York Academy of Science*, **354**, 16–42.
219. Walsh, J.A. and Warren, K.S. (1979) Selective primary health care. An interim strategy for disease control in developing countries. *New England Journal of Medicine*, **301**, 967–974.
220. Ward, R.L., Bernstein, D.I., Young, E.C. *et al.* (1986) Human rotavirus studies in volunteers: determination of infectious dose and serological response to infection. *Journal of Infectious Diseases*, **154**, 871–880.
221. Ward, R.L., Clemens, J.D., Knowlton, D.R., *et al.* (1992) Evidence that protection against rotavirus diarrhea after natural infection is not dependant on serotypic-specific neutralizing antibody. *Journal of Infectious Diseases*, **166**, 1251–1257.
222. White, K.E., Osterholm, M.T., Mariotti, J.A. *et al.* (1986) A foodborne outbreak of Norwalk virus. Evidence of post recovery transmission. *American Journal of Epidemiology*, **124**, 120–126.
223. Whitelaw, A., Davis, H. and Parry, J. (1977) Electronmicroscopy of fatal adenovirus gastroenteritis. *The Lancet*, **i**, 361.
224. Wilde, J., Yolken, R., Willoughby, R. and Eiden, J. (1991) Improved detection of rotavirus shedding by polymerase chain reaction. *The Lancet*, **337**, 323–326.
225. Willcocks, M.M., Carter, M.J., Laidler, F.R. and Madeley, C.R. (1990) Growth and characterization of human faecal astrovirus in a continuous cell line. *Archives of Virology*, **113**, 73–82.
226. Willcocks, M.M. and Carter, M.J. (1992) The 3' terminal sequence of human astrovirus. *Archives of Virology*, **124**, 279–289.
227. Wilson, S.A. and Cubitt, W.D. (1987) The development and evaluation of radioimmunoassays for the detection of immunoglobulins M and G against astrovirus. *Journal of Virological Methods*, **19**, 151–160.
228. Woode, D.J., David, T.J., Chrystie, I.L. and Totterdell, B. (1988) Chronic enteric virus infection in two T-cell immunodeficient children. *Journal of Medical Virology*, **24**, 435–444.
229. Woode, G.N. and Crouch, C.F. (1976) Isolation of small viruses resembling astroviruses and caliciviruses from acute enteritis of calves. *Journal of the American Veterinary Medical Association*. **173**, 522–526.
230. WHO (1973) Mortality due to diarrheal diseases in the world. *WHO Weekly Epidemiological Record*, **48**, 409–416.
231. WHO (1986) *Diarrhoeal Diseases Control Programme. Fifth Programme Report 1984–1985*. Geneva: World Health Organization.
232. WHO (1992) *WHO Programme for Control of Diarrhoeal Diseases. Eighth Programme Report 1990–1991.* Geneva: World Health Organization.
233. Wyatt, R.G., James, H.D. Jr, Pittman, A.L. *et al.* (1983) Direct isolation in cell culture of human rotaviruses and their characterisation into four serotypes. *Journal of Clinical Microbiology*, **18**, 310–317.
234. Yolken, R., Santosham, M., Reid, R. and Dubovi, E. (1988) Pestiviruses: major etiological agents of gastroenteritis in human infants and children? *Clinical Research*, **36**, 80A.
235. Yolken, R., Leister, F., Almeido-Hill, J. *et al.* (1989) Infantile gastroenteritis associated with excretion of pestivirus antigens. *The Lancet*, **i**, 517–519.
236. Yolken, R.H., Wyatt, R.G., Zissis, G. *et al.* (1978) Epidemiology of human rotavirus types 1 and 2 as studied by enzyme-linked immunosorbent assays. *New England Journal of Medicine*, **299**, 1156–1161.
237. Zheng, B.J., Chang, R.X., Zhang, G. *et al.* (1991) Rotavirus infection of the oropharynx and respiratory tract in young children. *Journal of Medical Virology*, **34**, 29–37.

PAEDIATRIC GASTROENTERITIS

D.C.A. Candy

While this textbook is predominantly directed towards adult gastroenterology, it is important to include a brief reference to a topic of world-wide importance – paediatric gastroenteritis. The reader is directed towards an excellent recent review for more detailed information.[8]

In spite of considerable advances in management, gastroenteritis remains the leading cause of death in childhood. An analysis of surveys and other sources carried out in 1988 revealed that over 1300 million episodes of diarrhoea occur each year in children under 5 years of age in Asia (excluding China), Africa and Latin America and that 4 million children in this age group die annually from diarrhoea.[12] A very different picture emerges from developed countries, where mortality rates continue to fall. Some European countries now report annual mortality rates of 0.[11] In England and Wales there has been a marked decrease from approximately 300 deaths per year in the late 1970s to around 25 in the late 1980s.[11] The statistics should be compared with mortality rates for England and Wales at the beginning of the century when 30 000–50 000 children died each year. None the less, gastroenteritis continues to be a significant cause of morbidity in children from developed countries.[6] The majority of children dying from watery diarrhoea do so from dehydration. It is now possible to virtually eliminate these deaths by oral rehydration therapy, and many thousands of lives have already been saved as a result. However, this measure will not prevent the morbidity associated with repeated attacks of acute diarrhoea, which, according to the majority of authors, results in malnutrition and growth faltering. Neither will oral rehydration therapy prevent the problem of persistent diarrhoea (defined as >14 days' duration), which in developing countries complicates up to 20% of attacks of acute diarrhoea and is associated with increased mortality.

EPIDEMIOLOGY

Most of the available data are derived from hospital-based studies, a few have included techniques to identify all known pathogens. There is an urgent need for extended, community-based studies in different parts of the world to identify the timing, frequency and effects of infections by the various agents capable of causing diarrhoeal disease.[2] Nevertheless, several general points can be made. Fifteen years ago, a microbiological cause for acute childhood diarrhoea could be ascertained in about 20% of cases; now, largely due to the description of certain viruses, bacteria and protozoa in humans (see elsewhere in this chapter) this figure has risen to nearer 80%, thus reinforcing the infectious nature of this syndrome.

ADVANCES IN THE TREATMENT OF PAEDIATRIC GASTROENTERITIS

Oral rehydration therapy remains the mainstay of the treatment of acute diarrhoea. Many inappropriate drugs are still given to infants and children with acute diarrhoea. Increasing pressure from the mass media and medical literature has forced the withdrawal of certain 'antidiarrhoeal' drugs and has brought others under careful scrutiny.[5] While oral rehydration therapy decreases morbidity and mortality, it is not expected to reduce stool output or duration of diarrhoea. However, there have been many reports that oral rehydration therapy solutions based on food, rather than glucose, do achieve all of these aims.[10] A number of hypotheses have been advanced to explain the improved efficacy. One possible factor is that a higher concentration of actively absorbed substrate can be included in food-based oral rehydration therapy, without causing osmotic diarrhoea. Additionally, the peptides released from the digestion of food can act in concert with hydrolysed starch in promoting water and electrolyte absorption via alternative active-transport systems. It remains to be established whether the same benefits will be conferred on children in developed countries with mild diarrhoea.

The need to continue feeding malnourished children with acute diarrhoea is self-evident. Children in industrialized countries with acute diarrhoea can also be offered free access to food, and dietary restrictions are unnecessary.

COMPLICATIONS OF ACUTE INFANTILE GASTROENTERITIS

DEHYDRATION

Fluid loss in diarrhoea stools varies from 5 to more than 200 ml/kg every 24 hours. Severe dehydration

Table 9.7 Solutions recommended for treatment of acute diarrhoea and vomiting

	Composition (mmol/l)					
	Sodium	*Potassium*	*Bicarbonate*	*Citrate*	*Chloride*	*Glucose*
Dioralyte (Rorer)	60	20	—	10	60	90
Electrolade (Nicholas)	50	20	30	—		111
Glucose electrolyte mixture (Martindale)	35	20	18	—		200
Oral rehydration solution (WHO/UNICEF)	90	20	—	10		110

is particularly likely in rotavirus and *Vibrio cholerae* O1-associated diarrhoea, producing total body deficits of sodium, potassium and chloride in the region of 70–110 mmol/l.[12] Signs of dehydration include thirst, restlessness or irritability, decreased skin turgor (assessed by lifting and releasing the skin of the abdomen and observing the rate of flattening), sunken eyes, sunken fontanelle (in infants) and suppression of tear and saliva formation. These signs become more pronounced in severe dehydration and are accompanied by hypovolaemic shock (absence of peripheral pulses, peripheral cyanosis and drowsiness). The child with some signs of dehydration has a fluid deficit of 50–100 ml/kg; severe dehydration is hence associated with a deficit of greater than 100 ml/kg.

Patients with some dehydration require 50–100 ml/kg of oral rehydration therapy (see *Table 9.7*) over 4–6 hours, followed by a return to the usual diet. Further oral rehydration therapy is administered if diarrhoea continues (50–100 ml oral rehydration therapy following each loose stool in children under 2 years of age, 100–200 ml if older than 2 years). Intravenous rehydration is required for severe dehydration, and for patients with coma, ileus or if other intra-abdominal pathology is suspected. Excess vomiting or stool output ($>$10 ml/kg per hour) can be managed by administration of oral rehydration therapy via a nasogastric tube. If hydration has not improved after 4–6 hours, intravenous fluids should be administered.

HYPERNATRAEMIC DEHYDRATION

Hypernatraemic dehydration (serum Na^+ concentration $>$150 mmol/l) is one of the most feared complications of acute diarrhoea, because of the association with cerebral hemorrhage, cerebral oedema during therapy, death, and brain damage in survivors. While this complication has virtually disappeared in developed countries, it is still a cause for serious concern in developing countries. Risk factors for hypernatraemic dehydration include severe dehydration, age less than 1 year, excess consumption of oral rehydration salts, the prescription of antibiotics and antidiarrhoeal drugs with consequent delay in starting oral rehydration therapy, and the use of traditional drinks containing sucrose.[13] Once the circulation has been restored, oral rehydration therapy is the treatment of choice. Extending the rehydration phase from 6–8 to 12–16 hours is recommended to allow slower re-equilibration of hyperosmolar dehydration.

HYPONATRAEMIA

Hyponatraemia (serum Na^+ concentration $<$130 mmol/l), which is associated with lethargy and convulsions, also responds to oral rehydration salts.

HYPOKALAEMIA

Although hypokalaemia (serum K^+ concentration $<$3 mmol/l) may be associated with weakness, ileus, impairment of renal concentrating ability and cardiac arrhythmias, in practice it is almost invariably asymptomatic. The amount of K^+ in oral rehydration salts (usually 20 mmol/l) is often inadequate to replace K^+ deficits during rehydration.

DYSENTERY

If there is blood in the stool, the diarrhoea is likely to be due to an invasive organism such as *Campylobacter, Shigella* or *Salmonella* sp. If the child is systemically unwell, antibiotic therapy should be considered (see previous chapters).

LACTOSE INTOLERANCE

Lactose intolerance is a declining problem in developed countries. Slow reintroduction of milk into the diets of children recovering from gastroenteritis is no longer necessary. This may reflect the decreased severity of the illness or because of improved adapted infant formulas which are less sensitizing. Cow's milk intolerance, whether due to lactose intolerance or cow's milk protein allergy, is now less likely to complicate gastroenteritis.[11] Lactose in breast milk is well tolerated during acute diarrhoea.[9] In developing countries, lactose intolerance may be a more common problem in infants who are not breast-fed, and dilution of milk with equal volumes of water for 2 days during gastroenteritis is recommended.[12]

PERSISTENT DIARRHOEA

If diarrhoea with or without blood lasts 14 days or more, the diarrhoea is said to be persistent. After 14 days, mortality rates begin to rise.

Investigations should include stool microscopy to detect pathogens such as enteropathogenic *Escherichia coli, Giardia lamblia* and *Cryptosporidium* spp.

Intravenous fluid and electrolytes may be required to maintain hydration if monosaccharide intolerance is present. The most essential intervention in such infants is to maintain nutrition. This is best achieved with a protein source such as comminuted chicken (Cow and Gate) to which is added starch, vegetable oil, vitamins and minerals.[4]

PREVENTION OF GASTROENTERITIS

Important alternative strategies for preventing diarrhoea exist, including promotion of hygiene and breast-feeding, nutritional supplementation and improving water supplies.[1,7] Nevertheless, the results of the recent vaccine trial in which cholera and non-cholera deaths were prevented by the expedient of administering cholera vaccine orally, rather than by injection, demonstrated the utility of immunization. In addition to cholera, development of vaccines against shigella dysentery, enterotoxigenic *E. coli* and rotavirus is a priority.[3] Reassortment attenuated rotavirus strains containing the genes for viral protein[13] (VP7) of serotypes 1, 2 and 4 have been constructed. If these prove protective, then it is to be hoped that the next edition of this book will contain reports of a safe, multivalent rotavirus vaccine, with the prospect of reducing attendances at hospitals with diarrhoea by 20%.

REFERENCES

1. Feacham, R.G., Hogan, R.C. and Merson, M.H. (1983) Diarrhoeal disease control: reviews of potential interventions. *Bulletin of the World Health Organization*, **61**, 637–640.
2. Bhan, M.K., Raj, P., Levine, M.M. *et al.* (1989) Enteroaggregative Escherichia coli associated with persistent diarrhea in a cohort of rural children in India. *Journal of Infectious Diseases*, **159,** 1061–1064.
3. Bishop, R. (1988) The present status of rotavirus vaccine development. *Southeast Asian Journal of Tropical Medicine and Public Health*, **19,** 429–435.
4. Booth, I.W. and Candy, D.C.A. (1987) Practical problems in protracted diarrhoea. *Journal of Tropical Paediatrics*, **33**, 69–74.
5. Costello, A.M.D. and Bhutta, T.I. (1992) Antidiarrhoeal drugs for acute diarrhoea in children. *British Medical Journal*, **304**, 1–2.
6. Conway, S.P., Phillips, R.R. and Panday, S. (1990) Admission to hospital with gastroenteritis. *Archives of Disease in Childhood*, **65,** 579–584.
7. Feacham, R.G. (1984) Interventions for the control of diarrhoeal diseases among young children: promotion of personal and domestic hygiene. *Bulletin of the World Health Organization*, **62**, 467–476.
8. Guerrant, R.L. and Bobak, D.A. (1991) Bacterial and protozoal gastroenteritis. *New England Journal of Medicine*, **325,** 327–340.
9. Khing-Maung-U, Nyunt-Nyunt-Wai, Myo-Khin, Mu-Mu-Khin and Tin-U, Thane-Toe (1985) Effect on clinical outcome of breast feeding during acute diarrhoea. *British Medical Journal*, **290,** 587–591.
10. Mahalanabis, D. (1990) Improved ORS formulations. *Journal of Diarrhoeal Diseases Research*, **1/2,** 1–11.
11. Walker-Smith, J.A. (1990) Management of infantile gastroenteritis. *Archives of Disease in Childhood*, **65,** 917–918.
12. WHO (1990) *A Manual for the Treatment of Diarrhoea. Programme for the Control of Diarroeal Diseases*, WHO/CDD/SER/80.2 Rev. 2. Geneva: World Health Organization.
13. Yousuf, A., Fayyad, I.M. and Ebrahim, G.J. (1988) The clinical epidemiology of hypernatraemia of diarrhoea during treatment with oral rehydration in Egypt. *Journal of Tropical Pediatrics*, **34**, 289–293.

CAMPYLOBACTER INFECTIONS

P. Katelaris and M.J.G. Farthing

The importance of infections caused by bacteria of the genus *Campylobacter* has only been recognized recently. The organism was isolated from blood in 1947 but the first isolation from stool was not made

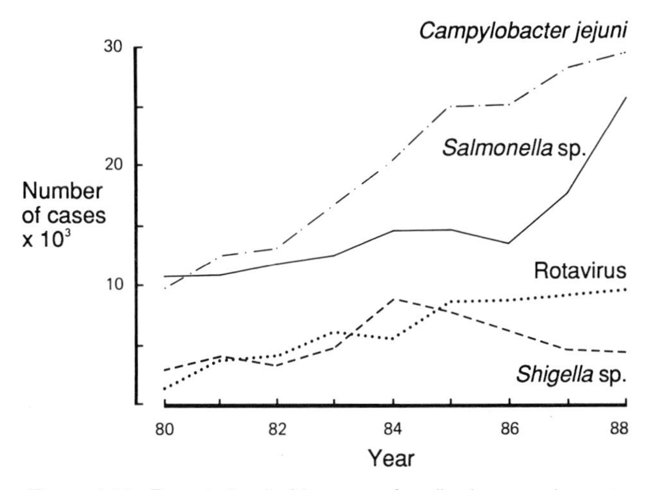

Figure 9.20 Reported incidence of diarrhoea due to *Campylobacter jejuni* and other common pathogens in England and Wales. (Data derived from the Communicable Diseases Surveillance Centre, Colindale.)

until 1972. This delay in identification was due to the fastidious growth requirements of the organism. Campylobacters have since been recognized as one of the commonest bacterial diarrhoeal pathogens of humans (*Figure 9.20*). Campylobacter infections may be divided into two broad categories. The commoner organism *Campylobacter fetus* ssp. *jejuni* (and the closely related organisms *C. coli* and *C. laridis*) predominantly cause enteric disease whereas *C. fetus* ssp. *fetus* is usually associated with systemic infection often in debilitated hosts. However, *C. jejuni* may cause systemic disease occasionally and *C. fetus* may cause enteric illness only. There are many less common *Campylobacter* strains and new strains are continually being identified. Recently, a catalase-negative or weakly positive organism, '*C. upsaliensis*' has been described and related to enteric and systemic infection.[16,33] This section focuses mainly on *C. jejuni* and related organisms. A campylobacter-like organism formerly called *C. pylori*, which infects the gastric epithelium and is closely associated with gastritis and peptic ulcer, has been re-classified into a new genus, *Helicobacter*, and is not considered here.

MICROBIOLOGY

Campylobacters are small ($0.2–0.5 \times 1.0–5.0\ \mu m$), spiral or curved non-sporulating Gram-negative rods (*Figure 9.21*). Light microscopy shows a characteristic morphology, the organisms appearing 'C' or 'S' shaped ('seagull' appearance). They have a single polar flagellum and are motile with a rapid, darting, corkscrew-like motion. Campylobacters may be isolated from stool by culture on selective media such as Skirrow's or Butzler's medium (modified blood agar containing a variety of antibiotics to inhibit the growth of other organisms). Blood-free selective media have been described recently.[52] Growth is best in microaerophilic conditions with enriched carbon dioxide (5% carbon dioxide, 5–10% oxygen) and incubation at 42°C for 24–48 hours. As campylobacters are relatively small in size, they may be isolated by selective filtration from stool specimens followed by culture, without the need for antibiotics.[48] Because a large stool sample can be used with this method, isolation rates may be increased.

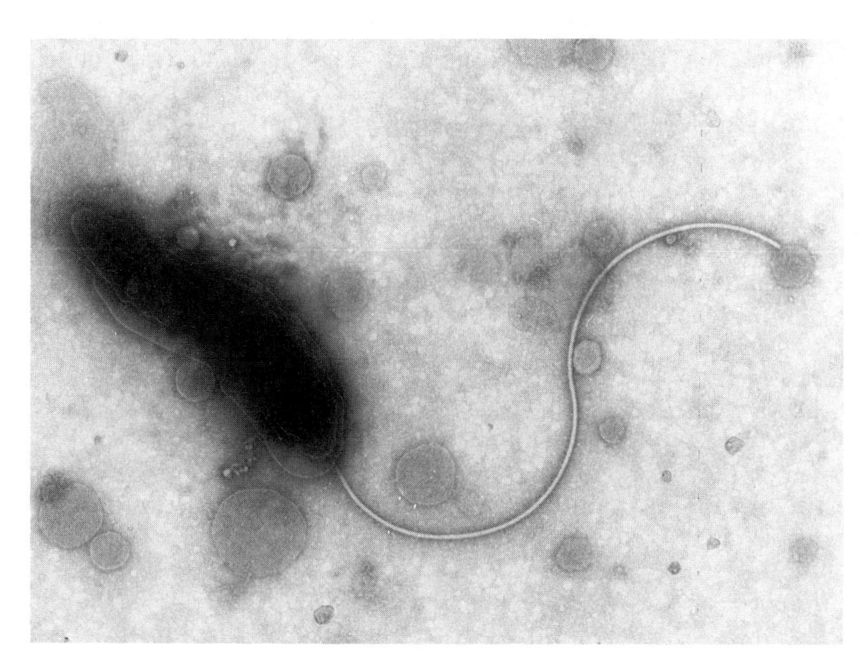

Figure 9.21 Electron micrograph of *C. jejuni* (×50 000). (Courtesy of A.D. Phillips, EM Department, Queen Elizabeth Hospital for Children.)

For *C. jejuni* and *C. coli*, antigenic diversity has been demonstrated by the description of multiple, different heat-stable and heat-labile antigens.[34,25] Serotyping may be used to distinguish strains when investigating outbreaks but little information is available regarding the virulence of different strains identified in this way. Whether all *C. jejuni* strains cause disease is unknown.

EPIDEMIOLOGY

C. jejuni occurs in the intestinal flora of many wild and domestic animals and these are the major reservoirs of human infection. Infections occur throughout the year but are commoner in the summer. Most cases occur sporadically although common source epidemics are well documented. Transmission to humans can occur in several ways. Infection has been reported following direct contact with infected animals, including pets.[49] Contamination of animal food sources is probably the major mode of transmission. Poultry is particularly implicated, but improperly handled meats may also result in infection. Contaminated animal products, especially unpasteurized or inadequately pasteurized milk, are another common source of infection and have been implicated in several epidemics.[40] Water-borne transmission also occurs, presumably following contamination of water by animal faeces.[51] *C. jejuni* can survive for 2–5 weeks in water at 4°C.

Only a small innocula is needed to cause infection. In volunteer studies, ingestion of as few as 800 organisms resulted in infection.[3] The incubation period is usually 2–5 days. Following resolution of diarrhoea in untreated immunocompetent subjects, organisms may be excreted for 2–12 weeks (median 2–3 weeks).[4] Infection with *C. jejuni* is found throughout the world but there are differences in the distribution of infection in different populations. In developed countries there is a peak of infection in children less than 1 year old and a second peak in adolescents and young adults. Asymptomatic carriage of the organism is rare sporadically but does occur during epidemics. In developing countries the disease predominates in young children and declines thereafter; asymptomatic excretion of the organism is commonplace. In India and Bangladesh more than a third of healthy children less than 5 years old may excrete *C. jejuni* at any one time.[5,39] These differences in the pattern of infection are probably due to the acquisition of immunity by people in the developing world rather than variation in the virulence of the organism, as no major differences between isolates from various geographical areas have been found. Furthermore, *C. jejuni* is a frequent cause of travellers' diarrhoea and results in a clinical picture indistinguishable from disease acquired by non-travellers in developed countries.[47]

PATHOLOGY

Enteric campylobacter infection may involve the jejunum, ileum and colon. Macroscopic changes include patchy or diffuse mucosal oedema and exudate sometimes with haemorrhagic ulceration. Inflammation is the feature of light microscopic examination of infected tissue. Small bowel mucosa may show villous damage with an inflammatory infiltrate.[12] In patients submitted to laparotomy, terminal ileitis and mesenteric adenitis have been observed. Rectal biopsy reveals colonic involvement in most cases.[37] Abundant neutrophils, mononuclear infiltration and eosinophilia in the lamina propria are observed and there may be crypt abscesses, mucus depletion and mucosal ulceration typical of acute colitis. These appearances are nonspecific.

PATHOPHYSIOLOGY

Three possible pathogenic mechanisms – tissue invasion, enterotoxin production and cytotoxin production – have been suggested for enterocolitis due to *C. jejuni*. Particular strains may display more than one of these mechanisms.[41] Invasiveness is consistent with the clinical feature of bloody diarrhoea with faecal leukocytes associated with mucosal inflammation and ulceration. Bacteraemia and mesenteric adenitis which may follow enteritis suggest preceding tissue invasion. Organisms have been demonstrated invading the mucosa in a few animal studies,[8,54] but are generally not easily shown even with immunofluorescent techniques, and Sereny tests have been negative. Some *C. jejuni* strains elaborate toxins. The best study is a heat-labile enterotoxin that stimulates cAMP and induces fluid accumulation in ligated rat ileal loops.[19,20] It is structurally and immunologically related to cholera toxin and *Escherichia coli* heat-labile toxin and has been identified in isolates from patients with secretory diarrhoea.[21,22] Some strains of *C. jejuni* have cytotoxic activity in tissue culture systems but the significance of this in relation to pathogenesis is uncertain.[56] The virulence of strains is variable. Lack of enterotoxicity or cytotoxicity has been demonstrated in isolates from asymptomatic individuals using in vitro and animal virulence assays.[22] However, no differences based on serotypes have been found.[18]

IMMUNITY

C. jejuni-specific serum IgA, IgM and IgG levels rise and remain elevated for several weeks following acute infection. The intestinal specific secretory IgA level also increases.[55] The increased severity and length of illness sometimes seen in hypogammaglobulinaemic hosts (especially those with IgA deficiency) suggest a primary role for humoral immunity in clearing the infection.[27] Continuous exposure results in persistently elevated serum immunoglobulin levels, particularly of IgG.[7] In Bangladesh where infection is hyperendemic, children have significantly higher titres of antibodies to *C. jejuni* than children from developed countries, and the rate of infection falls with increasing age, suggesting the development of protective immunity.[10] Following acute illness there is immunity to further illness (but not infection) with the same strain.[3] The non-specific bacteriocidal activity of serum mediated by complement and 'natural' antibody limits extraintestinal dissemination. *C. jejuni* is more serum 'sensitive' than *C. fetus* ssp. *fetus* and this may partially explain the frequency with which the latter disseminates.

CLINICAL FEATURES

ENTERIC DISEASE

Campylobacter enterocolitis has a broad clinical spectrum. Many subjects have mild self-limiting infection of short duration, while acute fulminating or relapsing colitis may occur occasionally. The disease tends to be milder in infected subjects in developing countries. A prodromal illness occurs in about half of the cases, characterized by fever, headache, myalgia and malaise, which precedes the onset of diarrhoea and sometimes overshadows the enteric symptoms. Abdominal pain is a prominent symptom (being reported in up to 80% of cases) and may precede the diarrhoea and be sufficiently severe to cause diagnostic confusion with acute abdominal problems, including appendicitis. The nature of the diarrhoea varies. In some cases it is profuse and watery diarrhoea. In one study, 15 or more stools were passed on the worst day of illness by 20% of patients.[9] In about half of the cases the stools contain blood. Other common symptoms include fever (74%), abdominal tenderness (50%) and nausea (43%). In the most severe cases, fulminant colitis with toxic megacolon has occurred and massive lower gastrointestinal haemorrhage has been reported.[28] In children and young adults, mesenteric adenitis and appendicitis due to *C. jejuni* have been described. In most cases the illness subsides spontaneously within a week but protracted or relapsing illness may occur. A post-infectious irritable bowel syndrome occurs in some patients. It is important in these patients to exclude recrudescent infection. Cholecystitis and pancreatitis occur occasionally.[13]

The infection cannot be distinguished on clinical grounds from illness caused by other enteric pathogens as no constellation of symptoms is specific for campylobacter infection. Furthermore, in a patient with fever, constitutional symptoms, abdominal pain and bloody diarrhoea, the diagnosis of acute inflammatory bowel disease must also be considered.[23] In patients with known inflammatory bowel disease, concurrent infection with *Campylobacter* sp. may cause an exacerbation of disease activity.[29]

In homosexual men, campylobacter-like organisms have been associated with proctitis, proctocolitis and enteritis although they can also often be identified from rectal swabs in asymptomatic homosexuals.[38] *C. cinneadi* is the most common such organism isolated. The culture requirements for these campylobacter-like organisms differ from those of other *Campylobacters* spp. and the organisms may be overlooked if standard techniques are used.

EXTRAINTESTINAL DISEASE

Campylobacter infection may disseminate. This is not common but, as the organism may be difficult to culture from blood, it may be overlooked. *C. jejuni* can cause transient bacteraemia and, rarely, more severe extraintestinal infection. Serious campylobacter septicaemia is usually due to *C. fetus* ssp. *fetus*. This occurs most commonly in compromised hosts, especially those with hypogammaglobulinaemia, malignancy, alcoholism, chronic renal failure, diabetes mellitus, malnutrition or extreme age. Septic phlebitis is a common complication. Systemic infection may localize, particularly in the meninges, heart valves, joints, and pre-existing aortic aneurysms.[44]

Extraintestinal complications associated with *C. jejuni* enteritis include aseptic reactive arthritis[17] and Reiter's syndrome, typically in a patient with HLA-B27.[43] Erythema nodosum has been described following campylobacter colitis[14] and cases of Guillain–Barré syndrome have also been reported.[46]

Campylobacter infection may be deleterious to pregnancy. Prolonged illness may cause fetal death in utero or premature labour.[45] In disseminated infection, septic abortion may result.

INVESTIGATIONS

Mild cases do not usually need investigation and many transient infections must occur without coming to medical attention. Enteric campylobacter infection may be suspected when a febrile prodrome precedes a diarrhoeal illness and abdominal pain is a prominent symptom. However, the manifestations of infection vary widely and it cannot be distinguished clinically from infection due to another pathogen such as *Shigella, Salmonella* or *Yersinia* sp. or from a non-infective illness.

On stool microscopy, leukocytes are usually seen, often with red blood cells. A rapid presumptive diagnosis may be made by identification of the organism in stool Gram stained and counter-stained with carbol–fuchsin or by demonstration of their characteristic motility using dark-field microscopy.[32] Although these techniques are specific, their sensitivity is low. The cornerstone of diagnosis is isolation of the organism from faeces by culture on selective media or by selective filtration. Campylobacters, especially *C. fetus*, may be recovered from blood cultures when systemic features are present. Serological diagnosis is not helpful as it is neither sensitive nor rapid. A variety of DNA probes to detect campylobacters have been developed in recent years. Most recently, the use of genomic DNA probes and synthetic oligonucleotide probes using non-radioactive labelling methods enables rapid identification of *C. jejuni* and distinction between a number of strains.[11,31]

TREATMENT

As most campylobacter infections are mild and self-limiting they do not require specific treatment. When fluid losses are significant, oral rehydration is usually effective. Anti-motility agents may make the illness worse[30] and are contraindicated when there is evidence of bloody diarrhoea or frank colitis. The decision to treat with antimicrobial agents is a clinical one. Antibiotics are recommended in patients with more severe infection, including the acutely ill with frequent bloody diarrhoea, fever or significant volume losses or in those who have prolonged symptoms or are immunocompromised.

Campylobacters are susceptible in vitro to a range of antibiotics. *C. jejuni* and *C. fetus* are usually sensitive to erythromycin, clindamycin and tetracycline unlike *C. coli*, which may be resistant.[53] Most organisms are sensitive to aminoglycosides, chloramphenicol and furazolidone whereas co-trimoxazole and ampicillin resistance is common. Studies have shown that antibiotic treatment of campylobacter enteritis does not hasten recovery from infection.[2,26] However, the numbers studied were small and patients were often not entered early in the course of the illness. There is some data in favour of a beneficial clinical effect of antibiotics.[5] Erythromycin within 4 days of the onset of diarrhoea decreases the duration of faecal shedding of the organism.[24,36] Erythromycin has generally been preferred because of its narrow antimicrobial spectrum, relatively low toxicity and low cost. Treatment is usually for 5–7 days in a dose of 15–30 mg/kg per day orally. Resistance to erythromycin is uncommon but does occur.[36,50] Hypogammaglobulinaemic patients may be predisposed to relapses and may require repeated treatment.[1] Extraintestinal infection with *C. jejuni* should be treated for at least 10 days while systemic infection with *C. fetus* warrants 2–3 weeks of treatment. Aminoglycosides and chloramphenicol have been used in systemic infection. Ciprofloxacin, one of a newer class of antibiotic, the fluoroquinolones, is active against *Campylobacter* spp. in vitro, reduces faecal excretion of the organisms and appears effective in reducing the duration of symptoms in infected patients.[15,35] The usual oral adult dose is 250–750 mg twice daily. The optimum duration of treatment may be as effective as a longer course for gastrointestinal infection. Another quinolone, norflaxin, also appears effective. These drugs are probably now the drugs of choice in intestinal campylobacter infection in adults. At present, they are not generally recommended for use in children because of the potential risk to developing cartilage.

PREVENTION

Transmission of infection can be minimized by appropriate handling of animal foodstuffs. Special care is needed when preparing poultry in the kitchen. Although the organism is usually destroyed when the meat is cooked, contaminated hands and utensils can transmit infection to salads and other uncooked vegetables. Pasteurization of milk and thorough cooking of meats are important. Water supplies should be protected from contamination by animals, and chlorination is bacteriocidal to *C. jejuni*. Personal hygiene, particularly following contact with animals, is also important. Isolation of infected individuals is not necessary as person-to-person spread is uncommon. Breast-feeding of infants reduces the incidence of diarrhoea caused by *C. jejuni* and is important in developing countries where attack rates are high.[42]

In the future, vaccination programmes may have a role in hyperendemic areas where young children bear the main burden of infection and illness. Vaccines raised from cellular components or possibly extracellular toxins may have a place in active immunization of young children. Alternatively, vaccination of mothers may increase passive transfer of immunity via the placenta or breast milk. Vaccination of animals to break the chain of infection is another possibility.

REFERENCES

1. Ahnen, D.J. and Brown, W.R. (1982) *Campylobacter* enteritis in immune-deficient patients. *Annals of Internal Medicine*, **96**, 187–188.
2. Anders, B.J., Laver, B.A., Paisley, J.W. and Reller, L.B. (1982) Double-blind placebo controlled trial of erythromycin for treatment of *Campylobacter* enteritis. *The Lancet*, **i**, 131–132.
3. Black, R.E., Levine, M.M., Clements, M.L., Hughes, T.P. and Blaser, M.J. (1988) Experimental *Campylobacter jejuni* infection in humans. *The Journal of Infectious Diseases*, **157**, 472–479.
4. Blaser, M.J. and Reller, L.B. (1981) *Campylobacter* enteritis. *New England Journal of Medicine*, **305**, 1444–1452.
5. Blaser, M.J., Berkowitz, I.D., LaForce, F.M., Cravens, J., Reller, L.B. and Wang, W.-L.L. (1979) *Campylobacter* enteritis: clinical and epidemiological features. *Annals of Internal Medicine*, **91**, 179–185.
6. Blaser, M.J., Glass, R.I., Huq, M.I., Stoll, B., Kibriya, G.M. and Alim, A.R.M.A. (1980) Isolation of *Campylobacter fetus* subsp. *jejuni* from Bangladeshi children. *Journal of Clinical Microbiology*, **12**, 744–747.
7. Blaser, M.J., Duncan, D.J., Osterholm, M.T., Istre, G.R. and Wang, W.L. (1983) Serologic study of two clusters of infection due to *Campylobacter jejuni*. *Journal of Infectious Diseases*, **147**, 820–823.
8. Blaser, M.J., Duncan, D.J., Warren, G.A. and Wang, W.L.L. (1983) Experimental *Campylobacter jejuni* infection of adult mice. *Infection and Immunity*, **39**, 908–916.
9. Blaser, M.J., Wells, J.G., Feldman, R.A., Pollard, R.A. and Allen, J.R. (1983) *Campylobacter* enteritis in the United States. *Annals of Internal Medicine*, **98**, 360–365.
10. Blaser, M.J., Black, R.E., Duncan, D.J. and Amer, J. (1985) *Campylobacter jejuni*-specific antibodies are elevated in healthy Bangladeshi children. *Journal of Clinical Microbiology*, **21**, 164–167.
11. Chevrier, D., Larzul, D., Megraud, F. and Guesdon, J.-L. (1989) Identification of classification of *Campylobacter* strains by using nonradioactive DNA probes. *Journal of Clinical Microbiology*, **27**, 321–326.
12. Conrad, S., Roderch, P. and Butzler, J.P. (1973) Enteritis due to "related vibrio" in children. *American Journal of Diseases of Children*, **126**, 152.
13. Darling, W.M., Peel, R.N. and Skirrow, M.B. (1979) *Campylobacter* cholecystitis. *The Lancet*, **i**, 1302.
14. Ellis, M.E., Pope, J., Mokaski, A. and Dunbar, E. (1982) *Campylobacter* colitis associated with erythema nodosum. *British Medical Journal*, **ii**, 937.
15. Goodman, L.J., Trenholme, G.M., Kaplan, R.L., Segneti, J. and Holmes, D. (1990) Empiric antimicrobial therapy of domestically acquired acute diarrhoea in urban adults. *Archives of Internal Medicine*, **150**, 541–546.
16. Goossens, H., Vlaes, L., De-Boeck, M. *et al.* (1990) Is "*Campylobacter upsaliensis*" an unrecognized cause of human diarrhoea? *The Lancet*, **335**, 584–586.
17. Gumpel, J.M., Martin, C. and Sanderson, P.J. (1981) Reactive arthritis associated with *Campylobacter* enteritis. *Annals of Rheumatic Diseases*, **40**, 64–65.
18. Kaijser, B. and Sjogren, E. (1985) Campylobacter strains in Sweden, serotyping and correlation to clinical symptoms. *Acta Pathologica, Microbioligica et Immunologica*, B, **93**, 315–319.
19. Klipstein, F.A. and Engert, R.F. (1984) Properties of crude *Campylobacter jejuni* heat-labile enterotoxin. *Infection and Immunity*, **45**, 314–319.
20. Klipstein, F.A. and Engert, R.F. (1984) Purification of *Campylobacter jejuni* enterotoxin. *The Lancet*, **i**, 1123–1124.
21. Klipstein, F.A. and Engert, R.F. (1988) Immunological relationship of the B subunits of *Campylobacter jejuni* and *Escherichia coli* heat-labile enterotoxins. *Infection and Immunity*, **48**, 629–633.
22. Klipstein, F.A., Engert, R.F., Short, H. and Schenk, E.A. (1985) Pathogenic properties of *Campylobacter jejuni*: assay and correlation with clinical manifestations. *Infection and Immunity*, **50**, 43–49.
23. Lambert, M.E., Schofield, P.F., Ironside, A.G. and Mandal, B.K. (1979) *Campylobacter* colitis. *British Medical Journal*, **i**, 857–859.
24. Levine, M. (1986) Antimicrobial therapy for infectious diarrhoea. *Reviews of Infectious Diseases*, **8**(suppl. 2), 107.
25. Lior, H., Woodward, D.L., Edgar, J.A., Laroche, L.J. and Gill, P. (1982) Serotyping of *Campylobacter jejuni* by slide agglutination based

on heat-labile antigenic factors. *Journal of Clinical Microbiology*, **15**, 761–768.
26. Mandal, B.K., Ellis, M.E., Dunbar, E.M. and Whale, K. (1984) Double-blind placebo-controlled trial of erythromycin in the treatment of clinical *Campylobacter* infection. *Journal of Antimicrobial Chemotherapy*, **13**, 619–623.
27. Melamed, I. (1983) *Campylobacter* enteritis in normal and immunodeficient children. *American Journal of Diseases of Children*, **137**, 752–754.
28. Michalak, D.M., Perrault, J., Gilchrist, M.J. *et al.* (1980) *Campylobacter fetus* ss *jejuni*: a case of massive lower gastrointestinal haemorrhage. *Gastroenterology*, **79**, 742–745.
29. Newman, A. and Lambert, J.R. (1980) *Campylobacter jejuni* causing flare-up in inflammatory bowel disease. *The Lancet*, **ii**, 919.
30. Nolan, C.M., Johnson, K.E., Coyle, M.B. and Faler, K. (1983) *Campylobacter jejuni* enteritis: efficacy of antimicrobial and antimotility drugs. *American Journal of Gastroenterology*, **78**, 621–626.
31. Olive, D.M., Johny, M. and Sethi, S.K. (1990) Use of an alkaline phosphatase-labeled synthetic oligonucleotide probe for detection of *Campylobacter jejuni* and *Campylobacter coli*. *Journal of Clinical Microbiology*, **28**, 1565–1569.
32. Paisley, J.W., Mirrett, S., Laver, B.A., Roe, M. and Reller, L.B. (1982) Darkfield microscopy of human faeces for presumptive diagnosis of *Campylobacter fetus* subsp. *jejuni* enteritis. *Journal of Clinical Microbiology*, **15**, 61–63.
33. Patton, C.M., Shaffer, N., Edmonds, P. *et al.* (1989) Human disease associated with "*Campylobacter upsaliensis*" (catalase-negative or weakly positive *Campylobacter* species) in the United States. *Journal of Clinical Microbiology*, **27**, 66–73.
34. Penner, J.L. and Hennessy, J.N. (1980) Passive hemagglutination technique for serotyping *Campylobacter fetus* subsp. *jejuni* on the basis of soluble heat-stable antigens. *Journal of Clinical Microbiology*, **12**, 732–737.
35. Pichler, H.E., Diridl, G., Stockler, K. and Wolf, D. (1987) Clinical efficacy of ciprofloxacin compared with placebo in bacterial diarrhoea. *American Journal of Medicine*, **82**, (suppl. 4A), 329–332.
36. Pitkänen, T., Pettersson, T. and Pönkä, A. (1982) Effect of erythromycin on the fecal excretion of *Campylobacter fetus* subspecies *jejuni*. *The Journal of Infectious Diseases*, **145**, 128.
37. Price, A.B., Jewkes, J. and Sanderson, P.J. (1979) Acute diarrhoea: *Campylobacter* colitis and the role of rectal biopsy. *Journal of Clinical Pathology*, **32**, 990–997.
38. Quinn, T.C., Goodell, S.E., Fennell, C. *et al.* (1984) Infection with *Campylobacter jejuni* and *Campylobacter*-like organisms of homosexual men. *Annals of Internal Medicine*, **101**, 187–192.
39. Rajan, D.P. and Mathan, V.I. (1982) Prevalence of *Campylobacter fetus* subsp. *jejuni* in healthy populations in Southern India. *Journal of Clinical Microbiology*, **15**, 749–757.
40. Robinson, D.A., Edgar, W.M., Gibson, G.L. *et al.* (1979) *Campylobacter* enteritis associated with the consumption of unpasteurised milk. *British Medical Journal*, **i**, 1171–1173.
41. Ruiz-Palacios, G.M., Escamilla, E. and Torres, E. (1981) Experimental *Campylobacter* diarrhoea in chickens. *Infection and Immunity*, **34**, 250–255.
42. Ruiz-Palacios, G.M., Calva, J.J., Pickering, J.K. *et al.* (1990) Protection of breast-fed infants against *Campylobacter* diarrhoea by antibodies in human milk. *Journal of Pediatrics*, **116,** 707–713.
43. Saari, K.M. and Kauranen, O. (1980) Ocular inflammation in Reiter's syndrome associated with *Campylobacter jejuni* enteritis. *American Journal of Ophthalmology*, **90**, 572–573.
44. Schmidt, U., Chmel, H., Kaminski, Z. and Sen, P. (1980) The clinical spectrum of *Campylobacter fetus* infections: report of five cases and review of the literature. *Quarterly Journal of Medicine*, **73,** 431–432.
45. Simor, A.E., Karmali, M.A., Jadavji, T. *et al.* (1986) Abortion and perinatal sepsis associated with *Campylobacter* infection. *Review of Infectious Diseases*, **8**, 397–402.
46. Sovilla, J.Y., Regli, F. and Francioli, P.B. (1988) Guillain-Barré syndrome following *Campylobacter jejuni* enteritis. Report of three cases and review of the literature. *Archives of Internal Medicine*, **148**, 739–741.
47. Speelman, P. and Struelens, M.J. (1983) Detection of *Campylobacter jejuni* and other potential pathogens in travellers' diarrhoea in Bangladesh. *Scandinavian Journal of Gastroenterology*, **18**(S84), 19–25.
48. Steele, T.W. and McDermott, S.N. (1984) Technical note: the use of membrane filters applied directly to the surface of agar plates for the isolation of *Campylobacter jejuni* from feces. *European Journal of Clinical Microbiology*, **20**, 636–640.
49. Svedham, A. and Kaijser, B. (1981) Isolation of *Campylobacter jejuni* from domestic animals and pets: probable origin of human infection. *Journal of Infection*, **3**, 37–409.
50. Taylor, D.N., Blaser, M.J., Echeverria, P., Pitarangsi, C., Bodhidatta, L. and Wang, W.L. (1987) Erythromycin-resistant *Campylobacter* infections in Thailand. *Antimicrobial Agents and Chemotherapy*, **31**, 438–442.
51. Vogt, R.L., Sours, H.E., Barrett, T., Feldman, R.A., Dickinson, R.J. and Witherell, L. (1982) Campylobacter enteritis associated with contaminated water. *Annals of Internal Medicine*, **96**, 292–296.
52. Walmsley, S.L. and Karmal, M.A. (1989) Direct isolation of atypical thermophilic *Campylobacter* species from human feces on selective agar medium. *Journal of Clinical Microbiology*, **27**, 668–670.
53. Wang, W.L.L., Reller, L.B. and Blaser, M.J. (1984) Comparison of anti-microbial susceptibility

patterns between *Campylobacter jejuni* and *Campylobacter coli*. *Antimicrobial Agents and Chemotherapy*, **26**, 351–353.
54. Welkos, S.L. (1984) Experimental gastroenteritis in newly-hatched chicks infected with *Campylobacter jejuni*. *Journal of Medical Microbiology*, **18**, 233–248.
55. Winsor, D.K., Matthewson, J.J. and DuPont, H.L. (1986) Western blot analysis of intestinal secretory immunoglobulin A response to *Campylobacter jejuni* antigens in patients with naturally acquired *Campylobacter* enteritis. *Gastroenterology*, **90**, 1217–1222.
56. Yeen, W.D., Puthucheary, S.D. and Pang, T. (1983) Demonstration of a cytotoxin from *Campylobacter jejuni*. *Journal of Clinical Pathology*, **36**, 1237–1240.

WORM INFESTATIONS

J.G. Banwell and E.P. Variyam

Worm infestations of the gastrointestinal tract are widely prevalent in the world and pose a major public health problem in many less-developed nations. In this section, intestinal infestation by nematodes (round worms) and cestodes (mostly long, segmented flat worms) is discussed.

FACTORS IN THE PATHOGENICITY OF WORM INFESTATIONS

HOST FACTORS

Environmental factors

The most important of these are factors that predispose to infection and reinfection such as the water supply, sanitation, defaecation habits and conditions of living in residential communities such as institutions for mentally retarded children.

Innate susceptibility

This can be of importance in animals but is less clearly demonstrable in humans. Hormonal influences may be important: strongyloidiasis may become invasive with steroid therapy. Changes in the environment (e.g. pH, short-chain fatty acids) of the intestinal lumen may condition the state of development of worms.

Nutrition

Protein–energy malnutrition depresses cellular immune responses, and this may predispose to infection. Most worm infections may not result in nutritional deficiencies in otherwise well persons with adequate dietary intake but infection may precipitate malnutrition when dietary intake is borderline. The status of a specific nutrient may be important: available iron stores in patients who are infected with hookworm will condition the rate of development of iron deficiency anaemia.

Coexistent diseases

It is generally believed that patients with other diseases are predisposed to parasitic infestation. For instance, megacolon may favour larval penetration in strongyloidiasis. Systemic diseases such as those that alter immune responses may favour parasitic invasion (for example, the acquired immune deficiency syndrome – AIDS).

Immune competence

Primary immune deficiency diseases are frequently associated with giardia infections, while secondary immunodeficiency resulting from drug therapy greatly influences the pathogenicity of strongyloidiasis.

PARASITE FACTORS[31]

Population density

Intestinal parasites require space for living. A population exceeding a threshold will be pathogenic in proportion to its size. For instance, with ascariasis a large worm load will cause greater symptoms than only one or two adult worms in the bowel lumen.

Lifespan of the worm

Since worms, in general, do not multiply within the definitive host, the duration of infestation is regulated by the worms' lifespan and by continued reinfection. However, *Strongyloides stercoralis* and *Capillaria philippinensis* amongst nematodes and

Hymenolepis nana amongst cestodes can persist by auto-infection. Prolonged periods of dormancy have been observed with *Ancylostoma duodenale*.

Pattern of entry

Hookworm disease is usually acquired through the skin; however, if larvae are ingested and enter via the oral cavity, they may cause more severe pulmonary symptoms.

Virulence

Virulence factors of specific parasitic strains are not clearly identified in metazoan parasites.

Location

The major site of colonization varies with different worms and leads to varied clinical manifestations. Worms generally invade by ingestion or by penetration of skin. They do not multiply within the host tissue.

Response to associated infections

Ascaris may be seen migrating from the mouth and nose during the course of intercurrent infestations in children. Combined infestations of ascaris with trichuris and hookworm are often encountered.

Response in the malnourished host

Several parasitic organisms (e.g. strongyloides) will overgrow in debilitated persons who are malnourished.

PREVALENCE AND INTENSITY OF INFESTATION[12,42]

The prevalence and intensity of intestinal helminthic infection show considerable variation in distribution and seasonal occurrence. Factors that control the level of endemicity of many infections are poorly understood. The factors influencing the infection pressure are best considered under two headings: environmental and socioeconomic.

ENVIRONMENTAL FACTORS

The environment has a major role in transmission of many infections. Excretion of large numbers of eggs as by ascaris, hookworm, and trichuris causes extensive contamination in the environment. This contamination is often uneven, occurring close to the house and in areas of defecation. The parasite distribution thus varies over the ground surface. Furthermore, the larvae may enter the soil to different degrees. Aspects of latency and survival under varying climatic conditions are of great importance in the persistence of the parasite: ascaris eggs are resistant and may survive many years in soil and yet remain infective.

SOCIOECONOMIC FACTORS

Socioeconomic factors greatly influence intestinal parasitic infestations. Many aspects of human behaviour influence their prevalence and intensity. Some age groups are more exposed than others to infestation: young children contract ascaris by playing on contaminated ground around houses and young adult agricultural workers contract hookworm by working in contaminated fields. Occupation may influence exposure: contact with faecal material may be more prevalent among sewage workers. Clustering of cases of parasitic infestation may be the result of secondary transmission from an index case or common risk factors (e.g. *Enterobius vermicularis*). Prevalence of soil-transmitted helminthic infestations is much higher among the lower socioeconomic classes. Nevertheless, most infested individuals harbour low worm burdens and only a few carry heavy loads. Improved general standards of living and sanitation reduce the intensity of infection in several populations in Japan, Poland and the USA.

PUBLIC HEALTH IMPORTANCE[13]

All intestinal parasitic infestations represent large and serious public health problems, particularly in developing countries. This is so, especially in tropical regions. Wherever a high prevalence of soil-transmitted infestations exists, living conditions are characteristically poor. Thus, the frequency of intestinal parasitic infestation has often been considered a general indicator of the level of economic and social development of these communities. Control has been achieved by improved sanitation and alteration in socioeconomic factors with repetitive drug therapy campaigns, but the effects of these interventions have been limited in rural areas of developing countries.

IMPACT OF PARASITIC INFESTATIONS

Intestinal parasitic infections can influence both social and economic aspects of living. Economic loss due to parasitic infestations is impossible to measure with any accuracy; however, the high prevalence of hookworm, ascaris and strongyloides infestations indicates major public health importance for these infestations. Their importance can be judged by their effects on young populations in causing weight loss, diarrhoea, blood and protein loss from the bowel and the complications that develop. Parasitic infestations are often prevalent in areas of the world where impaired nutrition makes life-support precarious.

DRUG THERAPY[8]

Important advances have been made in drug therapy. Intestinal helminths discussed here are more vulnerable to drug therapy than are some other parasitic organisms (e.g. schistosomiasis). In selecting a particular treatment it is important to determine (1) whether the infection is in an asymptomatic individual, (2) the likelihood of reinfection, (3) the cost of drug therapy to achieve eradication and (4) the consequences of treatment. In developed countries, most infestations, irrespective of intensity, should be treated unless specific contraindications exist. In contrast, in developing countries, and while planning mass treatment, intensity, economic considerations and the potential for reinfestation have to be taken into account. Frequently, a single agent may be used to eradicate several different helminthic infestations. Drug therapy for specific parasites will be discussed in relation to each infestation.

ASCARIASIS

Ascaris is the largest of the nematodes infesting the human intestinal tract; it is also the worm most frequently infesting humans, affecting more than a quarter of the world's population. Prevalence rates for ascariasis of 60–90% are common in many less developed parts of the world.[2,41]

Most cases of human ascariasis are due to *Ascaris lumbricoides*; a few are due to *A. suis*, the pig roundworm. The larval stages of the dog roundworm, *Toxocara canis*, and of the cat roundworm, *T. cati*, produce the syndrome of visceral larva migrans.

HELMINTHOLOGY[2,40]

Adult roundworms live in the upper small intestine. A gravid female produces 200 000 eggs per day. The eggs are passed unchanged in the stool. Under suitable environmental conditions the embryo in the egg transforms into an infective larva in 9–12 days. Ascaris eggs can survive 6–9 years in the soil. Human infection is usually acquired by the ingestion of infective eggs, although the eggs may be inhaled and then swallowed. Hatching of the egg is believed to occur by the action of gastric juice on the outer coat and that of the intestinal contents on the inner coat. The hatched larvae penetrate the intestinal mucosa and in 5–15 days are transported to the lungs by way of the portal vein and liver or the lymphatics. In the lung the larvae stay mostly in the capillaries and undergo further development. They then burrow into the alveoli, are coughed up and then swallowed. In the small intestine they develop into adult worms. Their lifespan is about 6 months to 1 year.

PATHOPHYSIOLOGY

Only minimal tissue reaction occurs when the hatched larvae penetrate the intestine or pass through the liver. Larvae in the lung elicit a predominantly eosinophilic response around the worm and in a perivascular fashion; the associated symptoms are proportional to the larval load. Adult worms rarely produce symptoms in mild infections, but large worm loads may be associated with abdominal symptoms and in patients with borderline nutritional status may be associated with nutritional deficiency states.[44,47] The in vivo effect, if any, of the trypsin inhibitor associated with the worm is not known.[37] The worms have a tendency to become tangled into a mass, which may produce intestinal obstruction, especially in children. Products of ascaris have been claimed to produce spasm of the host intestinal muscle, which may facilitate intestinal obstruction. Migration of the worms into sites such as the biliary tract may occur even in light infections and result in colic or bacterial infections. Worm migration is usually associated with the ingestion of a vermifuge administration of an anaesthetic agent or fever.[39] The worms return to the intestine with subsidence of symptoms or may stay in the bile duct for a variable period of time. If eggs are laid by a female worm they may migrate up the portal tracts and produce a granulomatous reaction and mild chronic liver disease; degeneration of the worm also have a similar outcome. Obstruction of the pancreatic duct or the appendix may lead to inflammation of the organ. Perforation of surgical stomas or even intact intestinal wall by worms has been reported.

CLINICAL FEATURES

During larval migration through the lungs patients may present with fever, cough, episodes of asthma and dyspnoea. Physical examination usually shows diffuse crepitation and rhonchi. The sputum is usually mucoid, but may be blood tinged. Chest radiographs show prominent bronchial markings and, rarely, a diffuse mottled infiltrate. Peripheral blood eosinophilia is common. The sputum usually shows abundant eosinophils but only rarely the nematode larvae. In heavy infections respiratory symptoms may be very severe. Symptoms usually subside in 1 week to 10 days.

Most patients with adult worms in the intestine are asymptomatic. Occasionally vague abdominal pain has been attributed to the presence of the worms even in light infection, but is more common in heavy infections. A heavy worm load may lead to nutritional deficiency states in patients with borderline dietary intake. Occasionally patients may present initially after vomiting the worms or passing them in the stool.

The most common intestinal complication of heavy ascaris infection is intestinal obstruction and this is seen mostly in children.[24] In endemic areas ascariasis accounts for 10–15% of the cases of intestinal obstruction and is second only to acute appendicitis as a cause of acute abdomen. The clinical presentation is similar to that of intestinal obstruction from other causes, with abdominal pain, distension, nausea and vomiting. A mass of tangled worms is palpable through the abdominal wall in about half the patients. The most frequent site of obstruction is the terminal ileum. A plain film of the abdomen may demonstrate the mass of worms. Other intestinal complications such as intussusception, volvulus and infarction are rare.

Biliary ascariasis presents, in decreasing order of frequency, with biliary colic, acute cholangitis, acute cholecystitis, hepatic abscess or with chronic granulomatous liver disease.[27,39]

Patients may rarely present with pancreatitis or appendicitis caused by an obstructing worm. Perforation of the intestine by the worm, mostly in the distal ileum, is very rare.

INVESTIGATIONS

Demonstration of the characteristic eggs in the faeces is the best method for diagnosis of ascaris infection. The fertilized eggs measure 45–75 × 35 μm, are golden brown in colour and mammillated with two distinct envelopes (*Figure 9.22A*). Unfertilized eggs are usually irregular and longer and have a thin shell (*Figure 9.22B*). Several concentration techniques for demonstration of eggs are available. The worm burden may be calculated from the egg output in faeces. Occasionally the worm may be detected on an abdominal radiograph,[14] or more often on a barium study (*Figure 9.23*). Examination of a worm vomited or passed would establish the diagnosis in some. Biliary ascariasis may be suspected from the demonstration of the characteristic shadow in an ultrasonographic or radiographic evaluation of the biliary tract.[10] Serological diagnosis remains unsatisfactory.

TREATMENT[8]

There are several effective drugs for the treatment of ascariasis. The choice depends on the clinical presentation and the presence of associated worm infestations.

Piperazine salts cause a flaccid paralysis of the ascaris worms and the worms are expelled by host intestinal motility. Several dosage regimes have been successful. A dose of 75 mg/kg (maximum 3.5 g) given as a single dose daily for two consecutive days is curative in almost 100% of patients. Piperazine is readily absorbed from the intestine. Toxic reactions are rare, and the drug has been safely used during pregnancy. Occasionally, gastrointestinal symptoms, transient neurological or urticarial symptoms have occurred. Piperazine in a longer course is effective against enterobiasis.

Pyrantel is also effective in ascariasis. It produces paralysis of the worm after initial spastic contractions. A single dose of 11 mg/kg (maximum 1.0 g) is curative in over 90% of cases of ascariasis. The drug is poorly absorbed from the intestine and toxicity is infrequent. Occasionally it causes transient gastrointestinal upset, headache and dizziness. Safe use in pregnancy has not been established.

Mebendazole is a broad-spectrum anthelmintic very effective in the treatment of ascariasis. It inhibits glucose uptake by the worm, leading to parasite immobilization and death. It is also ovicidal. The cure rate at a dose of 100 mg twice daily for three consecutive days is almost 100%. It is poorly absorbed from the gut and occasionally produces transient abdominal pain or diarrhoea. It is also effective against hookworm, pinworm, whipworm and strongyloides. It should not be used in pregnancy since embryotoxic and teratogenic effects have been seen in pregnant rats. Safety of its use in children below two years of age has not been established.

Thiabendazole is also a broad-spectrum anthelmintic slightly less effective then mebendazole. Thiabendazole inhibits the helminth-specific enzyme fumarate reductase. It is also ovicidal. At a

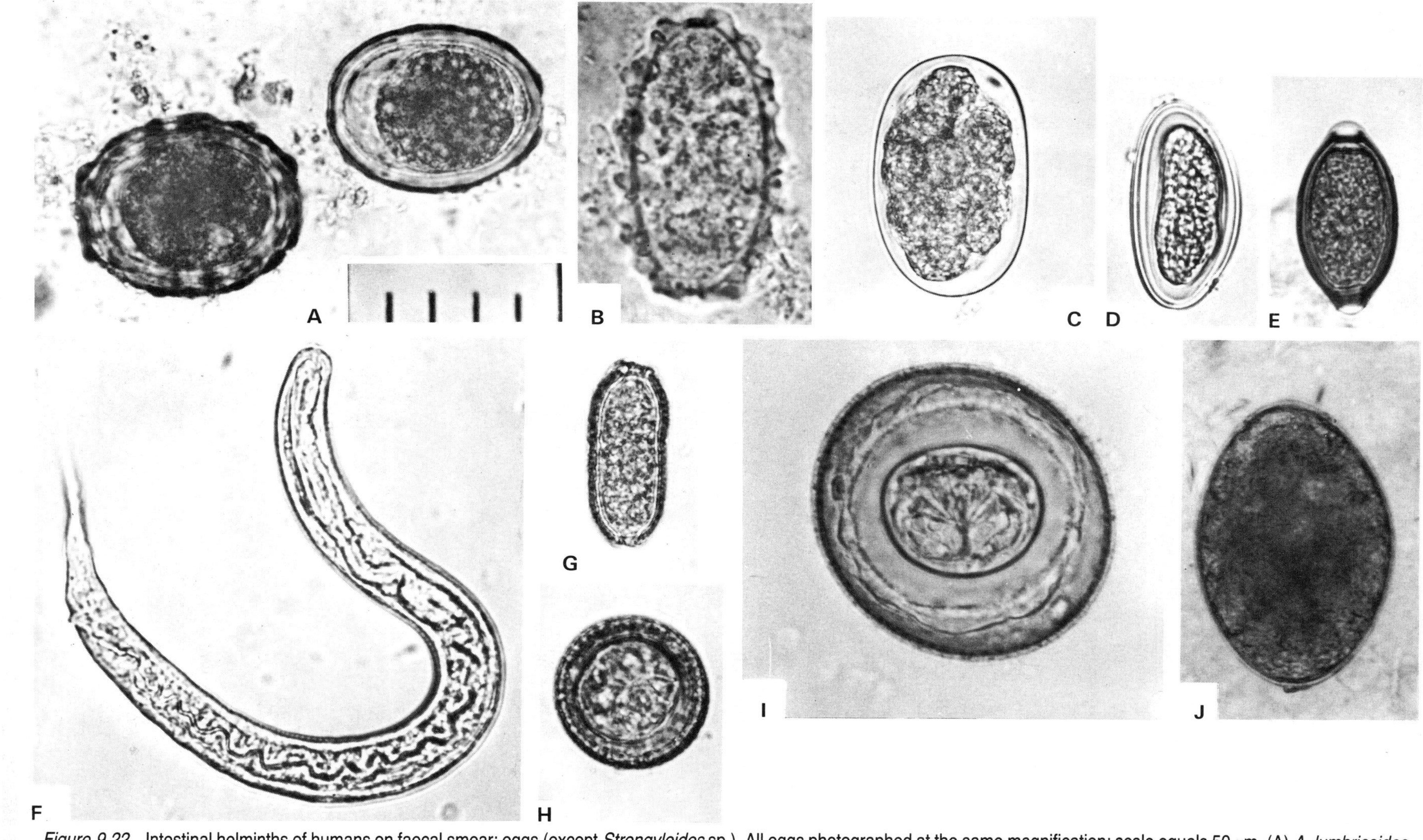

Figure 9.22 Intestinal helminths of humans on faecal smear: eggs (except *Strongyloides* sp.). All eggs photographed at the same magnification; scale equals 50 μm. (A) *A. lumbricoides* normal and decorticated; (B) *A. lumbricoides* unfertilized; (C) hookworm; (D) *Enterobius vermicularis*; (E) *Trichuris trichiura*; (F) *Strongyloides stercoralis* rhabditiform larva; (G) *Capillaria philippinensis*; (H) *T. saginata* and *T. solium*; (I) *Hymenolepsis nana*; (J) *Diphyllobothrium latum*. (Reproduced, with permission from Markell, E.K. and Voge, M. (1981) *Medical Parasitology*, 5th Edn, London: W.B. Saunders.)

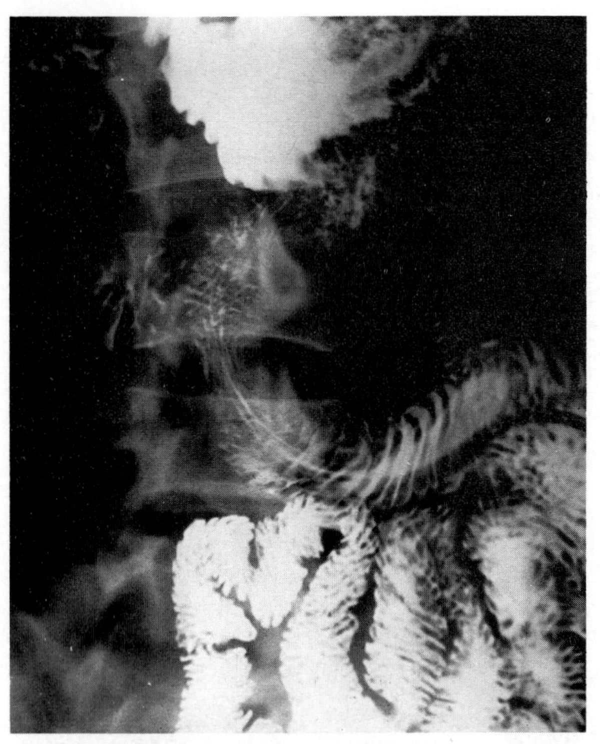

Figure 9.23 *A. lumbricoides* in the small intestine seen during barium examination as a long filling defect. A portion of the worm's intestine has also been filled with barium. (Produced, with permission, from Krause, G.R. (1949) In *Radiologic Examination of the Small Intestine* (Ed.) Golden, R. Philadelphia: Lippincott.

dose of 25 mg/kg (maximum 3.0 g daily) on two successive days it has a 70–80% cure rate in ascariasis.

Levamisole produces initial stimulation and subsequent paralysis of ascaris worms by ganglionic stimulation. At high concentrations it also inhibits the worm-specific enzyme fumarate reductase. A single dose of 5.0 mg/kg (maximum 150 mg) is over 90% curative. This agent is also an immunostimulant.

When coexisting hookworm infection is treated using tetrachloroethylene pretreatment of ascariasis is essential to avoid migratory complications due to ascaris.

Intestinal obstruction from ascariasis can be managed conservatively in most patients.[24] In addition to supportive therapy piperazine, 75–150 mg/kg, is administered using a nasogastric or intestinal tube. Drug-induced paralysis of the worms relieves the obstruction in most patients. Agents that stimulate worm activity (such as pyrantel, thiabendazole and levamisole) are contraindicated. If the obstruction is not relieved, gentle squeezing of the worms into the colon at surgical exploration may relieve the obstruction. Enterotomy or intestinal resection is rarely needed. During operation care should be taken to prevent migration of the worms into the peritoneal space, which may lead to peritonitis. Biliary colic often responds to conservative management with analgesics.[27,39] Worm removal by endoscopic or surgical approach is required if cholangitis ensues or if conservative management fails.

HOOKWORM INFESTATION

Worldwide, hookworm infestation is second in prevalence only to ascariasis. Several species of hookworm infect humans, but *Ancylostoma duodenale* and *Necator americanus* are the only common species which reach maturity in the human intestine. *A. ceylonicum* is usually a parasite of cats, dogs and other carnivores but may infect humans. *A. braziliense* is responsible for creeping eruption (cutaneous larva migrans) but the worm rarely matures in humans. *A. caninum*, the common hookworm of dogs and cats, is very rarely a parasite in humans.

HELMINTHOLOGY[34]

Adult hookworms are small cylindrical greyish white nematodes. The female worm is larger than the male. The chief morphological differences between species are in the shape of the mouthparts and permit distinction between *Necator* and *Ancylostoma* spp.

Adult hookworms attach themselves to the mucosa of the small intestine by their buccal capsules; the usual site is the upper intestine but may extend as far down as the lower ileum in heavy infections. Females are prolific egg layers and deposit their ova in the lumen of the intestine. Estimates of fecundity vary, but commonly cited figures are 10 000 eggs per female per day in the case of *N. americanus* and twice that number in the case of *A. duodenale*. Eggs have bluntly rounded ends; they are usually unsegmented but may have divided by the time of examination of fresh faeces.

Eggs leave the host in the faeces. When environmental conditions are favourable, eggs will embryonate and hatch within 24 hours. The larva which emerges from the egg is called a rhabditiform larva. By subsequent growth and moulting, this larva develops into a filariform larva which is infective. Larvae usually penetrate the skin at sites of contact with contaminated material. Infestation may also occur via the buccal mucosa: *N. americanus* infests more successfully via the skin than via the mouth, whereas *A. duodenale* is much more efficient in establishing itself via the stomach.[43] Larvae migrate through the circulation to the lungs where they enter the alveoli and move up the respiratory tree to the pharynx. Larvae are then swallowed and complete their development in the intestine. Prolonged dormancy of larvae in humans may occur with *A. duodenale*.[41] During these intervals the nematodes are drug resistant, and their metabolic rate remains low. Transmammary transmission to breast-fed babies has been reported with *A. duodenale* but not with *N. americanus*.

PATHOPHYSIOLOGY[34,41,51]

Hookworms attach to the mucosa of the upper intestine by their buccal capsules; in heavy infections they may be present as low as the ileum. This distribution has become clearer since the observations of Kalkofen in infected dogs.[26] Worms change their site of attachment to the mucosa every 4–6 hours to seek out new feeding sites. In addition less frequent movements occur for the purpose of mating. The buccal capsule of the worm is opposed to one or two villi or to the upper crypt region of the mucosal surface, and with attachment and suction a plug of the host tissue is drawn into the buccal capsule. Mucosal cells of the tissue plug are pulled free from the lamina propria, villous capillary loops burst and allow blood to flow out. Continuous or intermittent suction by the worm causes tissue and blood to be drawn into the worm's intestinal tract. Within the buccal cavity the mucosal cells show signs of increasing cytolysis as they migrate in a caudal direction; within 10 minutes the cells are frequently broken down and digested. Successive plugs of tissue are ingested and the areas of tissue destruction increase in size. The intensity of the inflammatory reaction in the surrounding mucosa is often greater than can be directly attributed to trauma inflicted by the worm. The muscularis mucosae defines the usual maximum depth of penetration of the worm prior to its detachment and fixation at another site. The maximally developed mucosal lesion usually involves about nine villi and an individual worm causes as many as six such lesions or numerous shallow ones each day. Blood loss occurs primarily by passage through the worm's intestinal tract, but bleeding from damaged mucosa external to the worm is also significant. In addition, the major source of nutrient loss to the host is thought to be the plugs of mucosal tissue ingested by the worm. Blood ingestion is only of secondary importance as a food source for the worm since intact erythrocytes are found at all levels in the worm's midgut surrounded by the remains of partially ingested mucosal tissue. After detachment of the worm, changes in the intestinal mucosa are often minimal and consist of general evidence of increased crypt mitotic activity. Repair of the intestinal mucosa is rapid.

It has been clearly shown that blood loss occurs from the mucosal injury. Recorded average blood losses are of the order of 0.03 (ml/day) per worm for *N. americanus*, reaching 0.15 (ml/day) per worm for *A. duodenale* infestations.[42] Some of the iron lost as haemoglobin into the intestine is reabsorbed. Patients with hookworm disease retain the ability to absorb orally administered iron. Variations in the rate of development of iron deficiency anaemia depend on available dietary iron sources and the duration and severity of the hookworm infection. Anaemia responds rapidly to treatment with iron salts. Gastric anacidity and associated vitamin B_{12} and folate deficiency are factors of only limited importance in the pathogenesis of hookworm anaemia.

Studies of infections with the hookworm-like *Nippostrongylus braziliensis* have demonstrated impairment of absorption of salt, water and glucose. A relationship between hookworm infection and impaired absorption in human subjects is however complicated by the fact that infection occurs (1) in association with features of malnutrition and hypoproteinaemia, and (2) with other diseases such as tropical sprue. Nevertheless, a variety of studies in Africa and India have demonstrated that no major generalized malabsorptive defect occurs in human hookworm infection.

Hypoproteinaemia with hypoalbuminaemia often accompanies anaemia in patients with hookworm infestation.[51] Intestinal protein loss may be severe in association with hookworm infection. Several studies have documented protein-losing enteropathy which responds to treatment of the worm load.[4] Others have suggested that inadequate dietary protein intake is often responsible for the hypoproteinaemia.

Many reports have suggested that infestation with hookworm is more severe in the host whose nutritional level is poor, but studies in which nutritional factors have been rigorously controlled have not clearly documented that there is a specific predisposition with malnutrition.[51] Studies with hookworms in dogs support the concept that heavier infestations occur in malnourished animals than in those that are well-fed. Balance studies in individuals with both hookworm and malnutrition have shown that nutritional repletion with high-protein diets does not alter either quantitative egg counts, intestinal blood loss or the number of spontaneously expelled worms.

CLINICAL FEATURES[43]

When the larvae penetrate the skin, maculopapules and localized erythema may occur; this has been termed 'ground itch' or 'dew itch'. Respiratory symptoms are uncommon although cough and wheezing may be associated with worm migration. Chest radiographs taken on these occasions may show fluffy infiltrates representing areas of pneumonitis. Occasionally, severe acute reactions may follow exposure to very large numbers of larvae. Such patients may develop allergic reactions associated with skin irritation, pharyngeal itching, cough, dyspnoea, wheezing, vomiting and abdominal pain. Small worm loads may be asymptomatic; however, most patients with significant worm loads will develop chronic symptoms associated with iron deficiency anaemia. Gastrointestinal symptoms of epigastric discomfort and tenderness occur with significant infestations and may be confused with peptic ulcer disease. Appetite is often increased, but in the later stages of anaemia and congestive heart failure it may be impaired. If serious disease develops during childhood, growth and development may be stunted. Alteration in bowel habit only occurs as a result of change in overall dietary intake. Symptoms of anaemia develop depending on the worm load and dietary intake of iron. Anaemia with haemoglobin values of 80 g/l or less is not uncommon. Cardiac and peripheral vascular manifestations of chronic anaemia are very common.

INVESTIGATIONS[53]

Accurate diagnosis is dependent on the identification of hookworm eggs in the faeces. A direct faecal film on a microscope slide mounted in saline or iodine solution is suitable for detection of moderate and severe infections. (*Figure 9.22C*), but light infections (less than 400 eggs per gram of faeces) usually require concentration techniques such as zinc sulphate flotation. Filariform larvae of *N. americanus* and *A. duodenale* can be reared on moist filter paper at 28–30°C. Larvae develop in 5–7 days and collect in a reservoir of water at the bottom of the tube. Their distinguishing features can then be defined microscopically.

The worm burden as determined by counting eggs in faecal samples gives only an approximation of the number of adult worms present. A measure of adult worm load can also be obtained after treatment with a vermifuge and the use of a purge, by sieving out the worms from the faecal specimen and directly counting the number of adult worms passed: 85–90% of adult worms can be recovered by this technique.

Antibodies can be detected to third and fourth stage larval antigens; however, they do not have sufficient specificity. Similarly, skin tests have no useful diagnostic purpose.

TREATMENT[8]

There are several effective drugs for the treatment of hookworm infestation and their selection is based on the presence of any associated worm infection and the general and haematological status of the patient.

Mebendazole and pyrantel embonate (pyrantel pamoate) are the drugs of choice in hookworm infestation. Mebendazole inhibits glucose uptake by worms, causing depletion of glycogen and ATP and leading to slow death of the worms. The recommended dose in adults and children over 2 years of age is 100 mg twice daily for 3 days. Because of its teratogenic effect in rats, mebendazole should not be used in early pregnancy. Pyrantel embonate produces spastic paralysis of the worms and can be administered as a single dose of 11 mg/kg (maximum 1.0 g); it is less effective against *N. americanus*.

Bephenium hydroxynaphthoate is an alternative drug, but is less effective against *N. americanus*. This drug is a cholinergic agonist and produces spastic paralysis of hookworm and roundworm. Thiabendazole, at a dose of 25 mg/kg (maximum 3.0 g) twice daily for 3 days is an alternative drug, but is less effective; it is useful against creeping eruption due to *A. braziliense*. Tetrachloroethylene continues to be used in less-developed countries; when treating with this agent, ascariasis, if present, should be treated first to prevent migratory complications of ascariasis.

Iron-deficiency anaemia of hookworm infection slowly resolves after worm removal but oral iron therapy is beneficial. Careful transfusion of blood or packed cells may be required prior to anthelmintic therapy in patients with severe anaemia. Prevention of reinfestation includes wearing of shoes and improvements in sanitation and personal hygiene. Iron supplementation or fortification is useful to prevent hookworm anaemia.

TRICHURIASIS

Infestation by *Trichuris trichiura* (whipworm) is worldwide in distribution and is estimated to be the third most prevalent intestinal worm infestation.

HELMINTHOLOGY[52,54,55]

The adult worms measure 25–50 mm in length and have a whip-like anterior three-fifths; they penetrate into and anchor to the lower bowel mucosa by a spear-like projection. The gravid female worm lays an average of 6000 eggs per day. The eggs are unsegmented on oviposition, are passed in the stool and become able to infest with fully developed larvae in approximately 3 weeks, preferring warm moist soil for their development. Humans become infested by ingesting eggs directly from contaminated soil; no secondary host is required. Young children are much more easily and continuously infected. Infestation rates are the greatest in the 5–15-year age group. Larvae are set free in the small intestine, where they penetrate the intestinal villi temporarily. There is no visceral phase in the life-cycle. The larvae pass down into their usual habitat in the caecal lumen, where they mature to adults in 30–90 days. Lifespan of adult worms is probably 3–5 years.[1] The parasite may occur in hogs, which may play a part in transmission.

PATHOPHYSIOLOGY[29,54,55]

The whip-like portion of the worm attaches to the mucosa of the caecum and ascending colon. Heavy infection may lead to localized superficial inflammation and subepithelial haemorrhages. The infiltration rarely extends deeper than the muscularis mucosae. A diffuse colitis and proctitis with diarrhoea may occur in heavy infections. Rectal prolapse may be a complication of heavy trichuris infection. Large numbers of worms together may occlude the appendiceal orifice and cause appendicitis.

Eosinophilia (range 5–15%) may occur. Generalized toxicity is uncommon. Blood loss into the colon occurs and may be significant, reaching 4 ml/day in heavy infections and it may lead to chronic anaemia in susceptible malnourished children.[2] Anaemia is unlikely in adults in whom heavy infestations are rare.

CLINICAL FEATURES

Few symptoms accompany light infestations. Moderate and heavy infestations may cause lower abdominal pain, diarrhoea, which may rarely be bloody, flatulence and distension. Appendicitis and rectal prolapse may occur.

INVESTIGATIONS

The diagnosis is confirmed by the presence of characteristic eggs on examination of a faecal smear or by using concentration techniques (*Figure 9.22D*). Numerous eggs, barrel shaped with bipolar translucent plugs, are usually seen. Adult worms may be visualized on proctoscopy or colonoscopy hanging freely from the mucosa.[15]

TREATMENT[8]

The majority of infestation are light: in non-endemic areas these should be treated. In endemic areas symptomatic individuals and those with heavy infestations should be treated. Mebendazole is the most useful and effective medication, providing egg reduction rates close to 100% and cure rates of about 70%. Patient tolerance to the medication is excellent. Good results have also been obtained with oxantel embonate (oxantel pamoate) but thiabendazole gives poor cure rates.

ENTEROBIASIS

Enterobiasis (oxyuriasis) is a widely prevalent intestinal worm infestation, more common in temperate than in tropical climates. It is caused by the small worm *Enterobius vermicularis* (oxyuris, pinworm, seat worm). It is the most prevalent nematode in North America and Europe, where as many as 40 million people may be infected.

HELMINTHOLOGY[35,54,55]

E. vermicularis is a small, yellowish spindle-shaped worm living in the caecum and adjacent portions of the large and small intestine. The worms attach to the intestinal mucosa. The male worm is smaller than the female and is rarely seen. The gravid female migrates to the perianal area, usually when the host is asleep, and deposits eggs in the perianal area; the worm most often dies thereafter. Only infrequently are eggs laid in the intestine. The eggs are oval and flattened on one side and have a well developed embryo. The commonest means of infection is by the anus–hand–mouth route, particularly in children, and it is aided by the perianal pruritus induced by the migrating female worm. Soiled clothing and sheets are good sources of contamination of the air or dust by ova. Transmission is favoured by overcrowding in institutions and poor hygiene. Rarely, auto-infestation by retrograde movement of newly hatched larvae into the colon occurs in adults. Commonly, the infestation is acquired by ingestion of eggs. The eggs hatch into mature larvae in the small intestine – within 6 hours at body temperature. The larvae moult during their passage into the caecum and develop into adult worms. Egg deposition usually begins 15–45 days after ingestion of the eggs causing infestation.

PATHOPHYSIOLOGY[35,54,55]

Worms attached to the mucosal surface of the caecum and proximal colon may cause mild inflammatory reactions associated with minute ulcerations. Eosinophilia (amounting to 6–12% of the total white cell count) can occur in patients with enterobiasis. Migration of the female worms at night with deposition of eggs in the perianal skin may cause severe irritation and lead to eczematous dermatitis and secondary bacterial infection. Obstruction of the lumen of the appendix by worms has been associated with acute appendicitis. Worm migration to other sites is uncommon; rarely, sites such as the vagina, uterus and the fallopian tubes have been involved, leading to vaginitis, endometritis and salpingitis. Granulomas on the peritoneum have been associated with migration of worms via the female genital tract. Occasional hepatic granulomas have been detected in males.[47]

CLINICAL FEATURES[35,54,55]

Light infestations may be asymptomatic. The most common and significant symptom is peri-anal pruritus, occurring at night. Scratching may lead to secondary skin changes and associated bacterial infection. Insomnia, restlessness and irritability may occur. Appendicitis and peritonitis may rarely be the presenting problem. Symptoms due to involvement of the genital tract are rare and urinary tract infections are rarely from this cause. Occasionally, thread-like worms may be identified in the perianal area or be seen on the surface of the bowel movements.

INVESTIGATIONS[35,54,55]

Infestation is suggested by symptoms of perianal itching and scratching in children. Diagnosis is dependent on examination of material taken from the perianal region, either at night or early in the morning before bathing. The simplest method to demonstrate the eggs is by applying a length of transparent tape to the perianal region and, after removal, placing the sticky side down in a drop of toluene on a clear microscope slide. Using a low-power objective the typical eggs, flattened on one side and containing an embryonated larva, can be identified (*Figure 9.22E*). Swabbing of the perianal area using other techniques is equally valuable. Five examinations are reported to yield a 99% detection rate. Examination of a faecal smear is not so sensitive. Other family members should be examined when one member is positive.[3]

TREATMENT[9]

A variety of drugs are effective in achieving cure rates greater than 90% in enterobiasis. Preferred treatment is with mebendazole. A single 100 mg tablet is usually effective at all ages. Pyrantel embonate is also very effective; dosage should be repeated in 2 weeks because mature worms seem more vulnerable than young worms to this drug. Viprynium embonate (pyrvinium pamoate) is another useful drug. However, it will cause discoloration of clothing due to excretion of the red dye. Local applications of petroleum jelly or zinc oxide cream to the perianal region may be necessary in addition to antibiotics.[1] Frequent reinfestations are likely unless hygienic measures are also carried out and repeated treatments instituted. Handwashing and finger-nail scrubbing should be performed frequently. Scrubbing and sterilization of the toilet area are necessary. Underwear should be changed regularly and frequent showers and washing performed. It is important, however, to avoid overzealous decontamination of all clothing in the houses since the ova are resistant to ordinary fumigants and disinfectants. It is often more practical to treat reinfestations and all likely susceptible subjects with appropriate drugs. An important component of therapy is appropriate reassurance and advice to the family to emphasize the pattern of transmission and the need for retreatment and that inferior hygiene has little role in its persistence.

STRONGYLOIDIASIS

Strongyloides stercoralis is a small nematode parasite infecting humans. It is present world-wide, although it is more prevalent in the tropics. The distribution of strongyloides generally follows that of hookworm. Prevalence rates for infection with *S. stercoralis* of over 80% have been found in low socioeconomic groups in warm humid regions. Because of the ability of the worm to survive by autoinfestation, it may persist for long periods; thus, 27.5% of Australian ex-prisoners-of-war were found to have the infection more than 30 years after their return from South-East Asia.[21] Occasionally, human infection with *S. fullerboni*, which is a common parasite in monkeys, has been noted.

HELMINTHOLOGY[6,30]

Adult female worms, measuring 2–3 × 0.1 mm, live in the crypts of the duodenum and jejunum. They burrow tunnels in the mucosa and lay 30–40 eggs each day. The male worm is not usually seen in the intestinal tract. Whether fertilization of the eggs takes place as a result of copulation during migration through the lungs or as a result of parthenogenesis is not clearly established. The eggs are similar in appearance to hookworm eggs, measure 50–60 × 30–35 μm and have a thin, transparent shell. They soon develop into rhabditiform larvae, which are passed in the stool. Under favourable conditions in the soil the rhabditiform larvae develop into free-living adults and can maintain a free-living cycle. Under unfavourable conditions the rhabditiform larvae transform into infective filariform larvae. The filariform larvae penetrate the skin or the mucosa on contact and are carried to the lungs through the veins. In the lungs they mature into adult worms; after burrowing their way into the respiratory passages, they are swallowed back into the intestine.

Occasionally the rhabditiform larvae, soon after being formed in the host, transform into filariform larvae. This process occurs more frequently when the host immunity is decreased as in malignancy or during glucocorticoid therapy. The larvae may invade the colon or perianal area or may disseminate widely in the body to the lung, liver, brain and meninges as a hyperinfestation syndrome.

PATHOPHYSIOLOGY[7,23,30]

When infestation is acquired, transient skin and lung symptoms occur as a response to larval migration; the host response is believed to be dependent on larval dose and prior exposure. In the majority of infested people, the adult worms produce no serious consequences to the host. In a few patients infiltration of the small intestine by larvae leads to malabsorption. In hyperinfestation, infiltration by larvae can produce colitis, pulmonary insufficiency and neurological findings. The larvae help disseminate enteric bacterial infestations, probably due to bacteria adhering to the surface or excreted by the larvae.[23]

CLINICAL FEATURES[21,30,33]

The skin manifestations at the time of infestation consist of urticarial lesions and petechiae, and are usually termed 'ground itch'. Lung manifestations ranging from mild cough to severe bronchopneumonia are noted in about half of the patients in one series.

The majority of patients with intestinal strongyloidiasis are asymptomatic. However, symptoms of diarrhoea (45%), urticaria (66%), 'indigestion' (73%), pruritus ani (59%) and weight loss (23%) were more common amongst those infested with *S. stercoralis* than amongst controls in a study of Australian ex-prisoners-of-war.[21] Diarrhoea, abdominal pain, nausea, vomiting and weight loss were the common presenting symptoms amongst those with strongyloidiasis seeking medical help.[34] The diarrhoea is often mild, but can be severe. It is usually watery, but in about a fifth of the patients it may be bloody. Abdominal pain is usually epigastric, sometimes cramping, but is often mistaken for peptic ulcer disease. Eosinophilic leukocytosis is common.

Hyperinfestation is usually seen in patients immunocompromised by neoplastic disease or glucocorticoid therapy. The commonest neoplastic disease associated with strongyloides hyperinfestation are leukaemias and lymphomas, but a few patients with oat-cell carcinoma of the bronchus have also developed this complication.[23] Symptoms usually depend on the major sites of larval migration. Colonic involvement with bloody diarrhoea is often seen in early hyperinfestation. Pulmonary and, less often, neurological manifestations usually predominate in the clinical picture. Bacterial sepsis, often with multiple enteric pathogens, is a frequent accompaniment of disseminated strongyloidiasis. Eosinophil counts in peripheral blood are often normal at this stage.

INVESTIGATIONS[52]

Careful examination of the stool or duodenal aspirate for larvae is the most important tool for the diagnosis of strongyloidiasis (*Figure 9.22F*). Routine examination of stools is only 27–37% sensitive and repeated examinations are necessary. Examination of larger stool specimens (1.0 g) detected the infestation in 84% of patients in one study.[21] Duodenal samples may be obtained by aspiration or by the use of a string held in a gelatin capsule; these have been claimed to be 90% sensitive in detecting strongyloidiasis, although in one study the string test was only 39% sensitive.[21]

Barium contrast studies are not sensitive; the findings are non-specific and unreliable. Increased or decreased motility, narrowing or dilatation of the lumen and mucosal thickening or ulcerations have been described on barium study. Mucosal biopsies of the affected areas may reveal the larvae in cross-section and a mild inflammatory response, often with large numbers of eosinophils (*Figure 9.24*), except in cases of hyperinfestation. With pulmonary involvement the larvae may be detected in the sputum or a lung biopsy specimen (*Figure 9.25*). When there is meningeal involvement, the larvae are seldom seen in the cerebrospinal fluid specimen obtained by lumbar puncture.

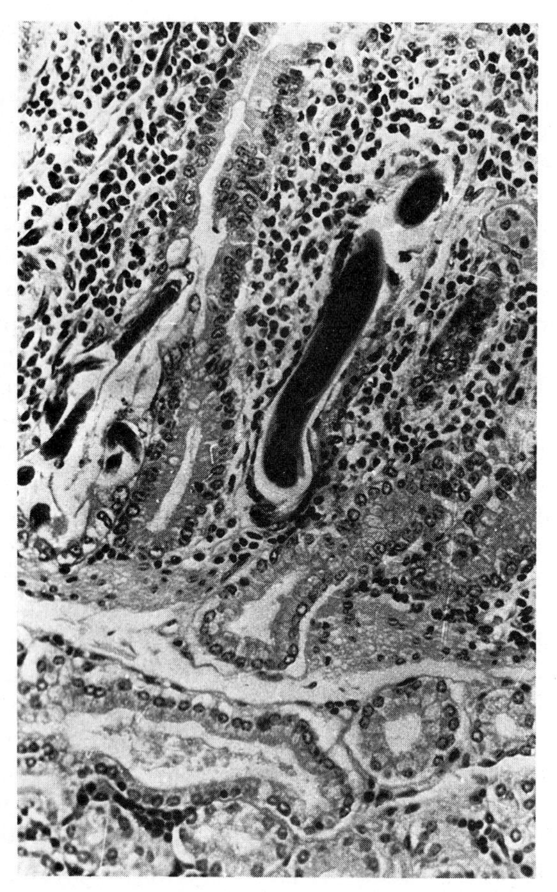

Figure 9.24 *S. stercoralis*: section of a mucosal biopsy of small intestine showing larvae invading the mucosa.

Serological testing by enzyme-linked immunosorbent assay (ELISA) using an antigen from the related species *S. ratti* has been found to be 84% sensitive in strongyloidiasis.[38] An indirect immuno-

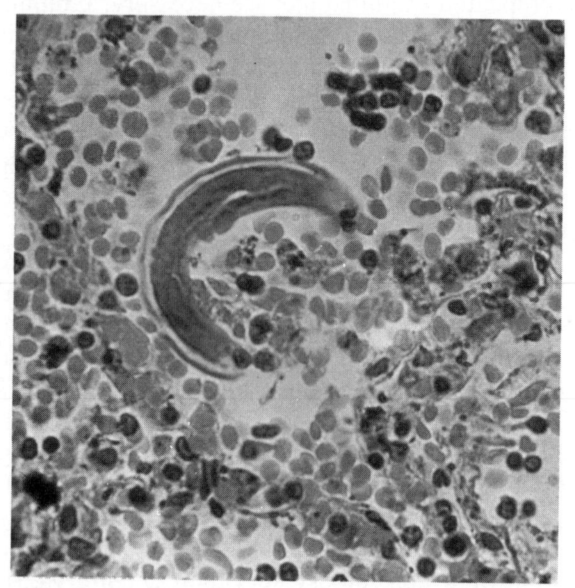

Figure 9.25 *S. stercoralis*: a stained touch preparation from cut surface of lung at autopsy showing a larva. Patient with chronic lymphocytic leukaemia who had overwhelming strongyloidiasis.

fluorescent test using the same antigen was reported to be 98% sensitive. These tests are not yet commercially available for routine use. Skin testing has not been found to be a sensitive method for diagnosis.

TREATMENT[6,9]

Thiabendazole is considered the drug of choice for the treatment of strongyloidiasis. It is usually administered at a dose of 25 mg/kg for 3–8 days. Although reduction or absence of larval excretion in stools is seen in 80% of patients soon after treatment it often recurs later; this is believed to be a result of the major action of the drug being the reduction of fecundity of the female and the drug being not sufficiently larvicidal. Ivermectin, at doses of ≥ 150 μg/kg effectively eradicated intestinal strongyloidiasis in 85% of treated patients in one recent study.[38] Both mebendazole and cambendazole were shown to be superior to thiabendazole against migrating *S. ratti* larvae in mice and *S. stercoralis* larvae in dogs,[22] but there are not sufficient data about their efficacy in treating human infestation to recommend their routine use.

INTESTINAL CAPILLARIASIS

Intestinal capillariasis is caused by the small roundworm *Capillaria philippinensis* and has been reported from the northern Phillippines and Thailand.[32,53] Adult worms live in the crypts of the jejunum. The female lays peanut-shaped bi-operculate eggs which are passed in the stools. The embryonated eggs cause infestation in fish. Human infestation is believed to result from the ingestion of raw fish containing larvae. Auto-infestation with infiltrations of the intestine by newly formed larvae can lead to the development of intestinal malabsorption. Clinical manifestations include watery diarrhoea, often profuse, steatorrhoea and weight loss. Malabsorption of vitamin B_{12} and luminal bile salt deconjugation have also been demonstrated in intestinal capillariasis. Diagnosis is made by the demonstration of the characteristic eggs in stools (*Figure 9.22G*) but eggs may be difficult to detect and be excreted in cycles. Therapy with mebendazole 300 mg daily for 10–30 days is very effective.[47]

VISCERAL LARVA MIGRANS

Visceral larva migrans was originally described as a syndrome consisting of tender hepatomegaly, marked eosinophilia and hypergammaglobulinaemia caused by larval nematodes that migrate in the tissues of a non-definitive host.[5] Some authors, however, have described similar manifestations in the definitive host as visceral larva migrans. Only those under the former definition are discussed here.

Most cases of visceral larva migrans in humans are caused by the larvae of the dog roundworm, *Toxocara canis*, and the cat roundworm, *T. cati*; rarely, larvae of other nematodes may also cause the same syndrome.[3,19] Visceral larva migrans is frequently seen even in developed countries, as shown by the high prevalence rates in the south-eastern USA.[18]

HELMINTHOLOGY[3,18,19]

Adult toxocara live in the upper intestinal tract of dogs and cats. The eggs laid by the female are passed on the stool. Humans acquire infestation by ingestion of eggs, which hatch in the upper intestine. The larvae penetrate the intestine and reach the lung by way of the portal vein and liver or lymphatics. Systemic spread from the lungs to other sites, including the central nervous system, may occur. The larvae do not develop into adult worms in humans.

PATHOPHYSIOLOGY[18,19]

Manifestations of visceral larva migrans are the result of the migration of toxocara larvae in tissues and the host immune response. The symptoms are related to the dose of the inoculum and prior exposure: in general, a large inoculum and prior exposure are associated with more severe features of visceral larva migrans. Larvae elicit IgM, IgG, and IgE antibody response; the inflammatory cell response to the larvae includes eosinophils, polymorphonuclear leukocytes and macrophages. A marked eosinophilic response often leads to destruction of the larvae but with other types of cellular response the larvae may persist in tissues and elicit a granulomatous inflammatory response. Visceral larva migrans is mostly a disease of infants and young children. Ocular larva migrans, by contrast, is believed to be associated with a smaller infesting dose, is more frequent in older children and adults and is only infrequently associated with visceral larva migrans. Titres of antibody against toxocara are much lower in ocular larva migrans than in visceral larva migrans.

CLINICAL FEATURES[3,5,19]

Young children, 1–5 years of age, in whom pica is common, most frequently develop visceral larva migrans. The illness manifests as fever (70%), asthmatic symptoms (66%), allergic skin manifestations, nausea, vomiting and abdominal pain (48%), hepatomegaly (70%) and eosinophilia (100%). The illness is generally self-limited. Ocular manifestations are rare in visceral larva migrans; when present, they consist of diminished visual acuity or a retinal mass which may be mistaken for retinoblastoma.

INVESTIGATIONS[19]

Definitive diagnosis of visceral larva migrans is not possible without the demonstration of the causative larvae in the tissues; this is almost impossible in biopsy specimens. The syndrome has to be suspected on the basis of clinical manifestations and epidemiology. Amongst patients so diagnosed, an ELISA test using an antigen from embryonated eggs of *T. cati* is 78% sensitive and 92% specific for the diagnosis of visceral larva migrans;[10] other serological tests are not clinically useful.

TREATMENT[3,19]

Visceral larva migrans usually runs a benign and self-limited course. Repeated reinfestations may cause persistent symptoms. Effective drug therapy regimens have not been established. Diethylcarbamazine has been claimed to be useful while thiabendazole and mebendazole are not thought to be beneficial. The use of glucocorticoids during the acute phase is controversial. Avoiding reinfestation by removal or treatment of the pet and controlling the pica are important aspects of therapy.

HELMINTHIC PSEUDOTUMOURS

The larval stages of several roundworms for whom man is not the definitive host, when ingested, may infiltrate or penetrate the intestinal wall and produce inflammatory masses. These pseudotumours may present with signs and symptoms of acute appendicitis or intestinal obstruction. It is often difficult to demonstrate the causative larvae in the resected tumours.[1,32]

ANISAKIASIS

Anisakiasis is caused by larval forms of the genera *Anisakis* and *Phocanema* and has been found mostly in Japan and the Netherlands.[33,51] Infestation is acquired by eating raw, undercooked or pickled fish. Symptoms suggesting acute gastritis may begin soon after ingestion of the larvae, when they reach the stomach. At this stage they have been demonstrated by barium contrast study and upper endoscopy. Removal of the larvae using fibre-optic endoscopes may relieve symptoms. The late result of larval ingestion is an eosinophilic phlegmon, most frequently seen in the ileocaecal region and usually presenting with signs and symptoms of appendicitis or intestinal obstruction. Operative treatment may be required for diagnosis and therapy.

ANGIOSTRONGYLIASIS

Abdominal angiostrongyliasis is caused by the larval stages of *Angiostrongylus costaricensis*.[29,32] The adult worm lives in the mesenteric vessels of a rodent and the eggs passed in the rodent's stools develop into larvae in a slug. Human infestation is acquired by the ingestion of the infected slug or its mucus secretions containing the larvae. The larvae penetrate the intestinal wall, most frequently in the ileocaecal region. The illness is common in children, usually begins 20–30 days after ingestion and is often confused with appendicitis or intestinal obstruction. Operative treatment is often performed for suspected appendicitis. Untreated, the illness lasts several weeks and may regress. No specific drug therapy regimen has so far been developed.

GNATHOSTOMIASIS

Gnathostomiasis is caused by the larval stages of *Gnathostoma spinigerum*, a roundworm of the dog and cat.[31] The eggs develop in fish and human infestation results from ingestion of raw or undercooked fish. Commonly, soon after ingestion, a visceral larva migrans syndrome develops, but later inflammatory pseudotumours form in the ileocaecal area. Drug treatment is ineffective and operative intervention is often needed for diagnosis and therapy.

OESOPHAGOSTOMIASIS

Oesophagostomiasis is caused by the larvae of the roundworms of the genus *Oesophagostomum*.[33] Adult worms infest non-human primates in Asia and Africa. The exact mode of human infestation is not known. The larvae penetrate the distal ileum or the colon and produce inflammatory masses. Operative treatment is often needed for diagnosis and therapy.

INTESTINAL TAPEWORM INFESTATIONS

Intestinal infestation by cestodes – long segmented intestinal flatworms or tapeworms – is widely prevalent throughout the world. The prevalence of the specific tapeworm infection is dependent on the dietary habits and the degree of sanitation. The common cestodes infecting the intestinal tract of humans are *Taenia saginata* (beef tapeworm), *T. solium* (pork tapeworm), *Hymenolepis nana* (dwarf tapeworm) and *Diphyllobothrium latum* (fish tapeworm). Occasionally, humans are infected with *Inermicapsifer madagascariensis, Dipylidium caninum, Hymenolepis diminuta* and *Echinococcus granulosus*. Infestation of humans by the larval stages of tapeworms other than those related to the common intestinal tapeworms is not discussed here.

HELMINTHOLOGY[8,53]

Adult tapeworms live in the intestinal tract of the definitive vertebrate host. The anatomical regions of a tapeworm are the head (scolex), the neck and the body, which consist of several segments (proglottides) (*Table 9.8*). The scolex enables the worm to attach to the intestinal mucosa with the aid of suckers and, in some, with hooklets in an area of the head (the rostellum). Each proglottid has male and female reproductive organs, a primitive nervous system, a muscular system and an excretory system. The surface of the proglottid has microvilli and is capable of absorbing nutrients. The size and branching of the uteri help to differentiate the species. Fertilized eggs accumulate in the gravid uterus. Intact proglottides or the eggs released from them after digestion of the proglottid are passed in the faeces of the definitive host. Larvae released from the eggs (called oncospheres or, in the case of *D. latum,* coracidia) penetrate the intestinal mucosa of the intermediate host and become encysted in the tissues, particularly the skeletal muscles. In the case of *T. solium* and *T. saginata* they develop into fluid-filled sacs called bladder worms (cysticerci), and in the case of *H. nana* they develop into cyst-like 'cysticercoids' that have little or no fluid.

There are two larval stages in the development of *D. latum*: the procercoid in *Cyclops* spp. and the

Table 9.8 Intestinal tapeworms of humans

	Taenia solium	Taenia saginata	Hymenolepis nana	Diphyllobothrium latum
Scolex	Four suckers + hooklets	Four suckers	Four suckers + hooklets	Two grooved suckers
Length of worm (metres)	3–10	15–25	0.025–0.040	10–20
Proglottid	Length > width	Length > width	Width > length	Width > length
Uterus	Central stem with 7–13 lateral projections	Central stem with 15–20 lateral projections	Central sac-like	Central, rosette-shaped
Larval stage/intermediate host	Cysticercus/pig (man)	Cysticercus/cattle	Cysticercoid/insect (human)	Procercoid in *Cyclops*; plerocercoid in fish
Mode of infestation	Pork with live larvae	Beef with live larvae	Ingestion of ova or insects with larvae/eggs	Fish with live larvae

plerocercoid in the fish. Scolices form as an invagination in the wall of the cyst. Human infestation is acquired by the ingestion of live encysted larvae. *H. nana* commonly develops also by internal autoinfestation.

PATHOPHYSIOLOGY[49]

Adult tapeworms do not produce any specific symptoms in the host. Whether in large numbers they produce nutritional deficits in the host is not well established. A trypsin inhibitor has been found on the surface of the rodent tapeworm, *H. diminuta*,[48] but whether such inhibitors are present in the major tapeworms infesting humans is not known. Absorption of proteins of the worm may lead to eosinophilia, allergic and neurological reactions and 'toxaemia', but these are not well established.

In the case of *T. solium*, larval development in humans leads to cysticercosis, which most frequently manifests itself in central nervous system findings.[6] Although eggs may be released from the adult tapeworm and develop in the same host, it is generally believed that human cysticercosis is more likely the result of ingestion of eggs.

D. latum, because of its ability to take up vitamin B_{12} from the intrinsic factor–vitamin B_{12} complex, can lead to deficiency of the vitamin, and thus cause megaloblastic anemia.

CLINICAL FEATURES[8]

Intestinal infection by adult tapeworms is mostly asymptomatic. They may be first discovered during radiological examination (plain X-ray film, barium studies)[20] or stool microscopy. Mild abdominal cramps, 'hunger pains' and dyspepsia have all been described in tapeworm infection, but their relationship to worm infection has not been clearly established. In the presence of marginal nutrition a large worm load may lead to nutritional deficiencies. Occasionally, the finding of a gravid proglottid in the perianal region or stool or the presence of pain and pruritus in the perianal region is the presenting symptom. Intestinal obstruction and appendiceal obstruction with appendicitis have been found with infection by the larger worms. On rare occasions, worms have been found in the gallbladder or perforating the intestine, leading to peritonitis. *T. solium* infestation may present with manifestation due to the larval stage, with neurological symptoms predominating. *D. latum* infestation may present with neurological or haematological manifestations of vitamin B_{12} deficiency.

INVESTIGATIONS[8,53]

The diagnosis of tapeworm infestation is usually made by microscopic examination of the stool, when the characteristic eggs are noted (*Figure 9.22H–J*). Stools may also show the gravid proglottides, and this allows identification of the species. Obtaining a sample from the perianal area using adhesive tape, as in the case of pinworm infection, may also be useful to demonstrate eggs or proglottides. Occasionally the tapeworms are seen on a plain radiographic film of the abdomen or a barium meal study.[20] Larval stages of *T. solium* (cysticercosis) may be demonstrated by appropriate imaging studies (e.g. computed tomography scan of head). The utility of several proposed immunological tests on the serum and cerebrospinal fluid in diagnosing neurocerebral cysticercosis must await further evaluation.

TREATMENT[9,53]

Niclosamide (Yomesan or Nicloside) is the drug of choice in the treatment of intestinal cestodiasis in humans. The drug inhibits glucose uptake by the worm and mitochondrial oxidative phosphorylation and anaerobic metabolism of the worm. It may partially digest the scolex and segments. The usual adult dose is 2 g given as a single dose or in two divided doses. The tablets have to be chewed well and taken with plenty of water and may be followed by a purgative. To confirm eradication of the worm the stool should be strained and examined for the scolex (or scolices, depending on number and type of worms), but if this is not possible follow-up stool microscopy a few months later is required. Associated vitamin and nutritional deficiency may also need to be treated.

Praziquantel, an isoquinolene derivative, is an effective drug in the treatment of intestinal taeniasis and diphyllobothriasis.[16,46] Early clinical trials indicate that this drug produces 100% cure rates in intestinal taeniasis and diphyllobothriasis with a single dose of 10 mg/kg and 80% cure rate for hymenolepiasis with a single does of 15–25 mg/kg. It is also one of the most effective agents against cerebral cysticercosis.

Mepacrine (quinacrine) is also an effective drug against intestinal tapeworm infestation, but side-effects may be prominent. The usual adult dose of 1.0 g is taken in five equal doses over 1 hour along with sodium bicarbonate and is followed by a saline purge if spontaneous evacuation does not occur. Mepacrine may also be administered using a duodenal tube. Screening of stool for scolex or scolices and follow-up stool microscopy are needed to confirm worm expulsion.

No drug with ovicidal properties has been identified so far. Neurocerebral cysticercosis may respond to praziquantel, but may need neurosurgical treatment in some patients.

REFERENCES

1. Anthony, P.P. and McAdam, W.J. (1972) Helminthic pseudotumours of the bowel. Thirty four cases of helminthoma. *Gut*, **13**, 8–16.
2. Arean, V.M. and Crandall, C.A. (1971) Ascariasis. In *Pathology of Protozoal and Heminthic Diseases with Clinical Correlation* (Ed.) Marcial-Rojas, R.A. pp. 769–807. Baltimore: Williams and Wilkins.
3. Arean, V.M. and Crandall, C.A. (1971) Toxocariasis. In *Pathology of Protozoal and Helminthic Diseases with Clinical Correlation* (Ed.) Marcial-Rojas, R.A. pp. 808–842. Baltimore: Williams and Wilkins.
4. Banwell, J.G., Marsden, P.D., Blackman, V. *et al.* (1976) Hookworm infection and intestinal absorption amongst Africans in Uganda. *American Journal of Tropical Medicine and Hygiene*, **16**, 304–308.
5. Beaver, P.C., Snyder, C.H., Carrera, G.M. *et al.* (1952) Chronic eosinophilia due to visceral larva migrans. Report of three cases. *Pediatrics*, **9**, 7–19.
6. Botero, D. and Castano, S. (1982) Treatment of cerebral cysticercosis with praziquantel in Columbia. *American Journal of Tropical Medicine and Hygiene*, **31**, 810–821.
7. Carvalho-Filho, E. (1978) Strongyloidiasis. *Clinics in Gastroenterology*, **7**, 179–200.
8. Castillo, M. (1971) Intestinal taeniasis. In *Pathology of Protozoal and Helminthic Infections with Clinical Correlation* (Ed.) Marcial-Rojas, R.A. pp. 618–626. Baltimore: Williams and Wilkins.
9. Cline, B.L. (1982) Current drug regimens for the treatment of intestinal helminth infections. *Medical Clinics of North America*, **66**, 721–742.
10. Cremin, B.J. (1982) Ultrasonic diagnosis of biliary ascariasis. *British Journal of Radiology*, **55**, 683–684.
11. Cypress, R.H., Karol, M.H., Zidian, J.L. *et al.* (1977) Larva-specific antibodies in patients with visceral larva migrans. *Journal of Infectious Diseases*, **135**, 633–640.
12. Dorozynski, A. (1976) The altered or tropical disease. *Nature*, **262**, 85–87.
13. Dunn, F.L. (1979) Behavioural aspects of the control of parasitic diseases. *Bulletin of the World Health Organization*, **57**, 499–512.
14. Ellman, B.A., Wynne, J.M. and Freeman, A. (1980) Intestinal ascariasis: new plain film features. *American Journal of Roentgenology*, **135**, 37–42.
15. Fisher, R.M. and Cremin, B.T. (1970) Rectal bleeding due to *Trichuris*. *British Journal of Radiology*, **43**, 214–215.
16. Gemmell, M.A. and Johnstone, P.D. (1981) Cestodes. *Antibiotics and Chemotherapy*, **30**, 54–114.
17. Gill, G.V. and Bell, D.R. (1979) *Strongyloides stercoralis* infection in former Far East prisoners of war. *British Medical Journal*, **iii**, 572–574.
18. Glickman, L.T. and Schantz, P.M. (1981) Epidemiology and pathogenesis of zoonotic toxacariasis. *Epidemiologic Reviews*, **3**, 230–250.
19. Glickman, L.T., Schantz, P.M. and Cypress, R.H. (1979) Canine and human toxocariasis: review of transmission, pathogenesis and clinical disease. *Journal of the American Veterinary Medical Association*, **175**, 1265–1269.
20. Gold, B.M. and Meyers, M.S. (1977) Radiologic manifestations of *Taenia saginata* infestation. *American Journal of Roentgenology*, **128**, 493–494.
21. Grove, D.I. (1980) Strongyloidiasis in Allied ex-prisoners-of-war in south-east Asia. *British Medical Journal*, **i**, 598–601.
22. Grove, J.I. and Blair, J. (1982) *Strongyloides ratti* and *S. stercoralis*. The effects of thiabendazole, mebendazole and cambendazole in infected mice. *American Journal of Tropical Medicine and Hygiene*, **31**, 469–476.
23. Igra-Siegman, Y., Kapila, R., Sen, P. *et al.* (1981) Syndrome of hyperinfection with *Strongyloides stercoralis*. *Reviews of Infectious Diseases*, **3**, 397–407.
24. Ihekwaba, F.N. (1980) Intestinal ascariasis and the acute abdomen in the tropics. *Journal of Royal College of Surgeons of Edinburgh*, **25**, 452–456.
25. Jones, T.C. (1978) Cestodes, *Clinics in Gastroenterology*, **7**, 105–128.
26. Kalkofen, U.P. (1974) Intestinal trauma resulting from feeding activities of *Ancylostoma caninum*. *American Journal of Tropical Medicine in Hygiene*, **16**, 613–619.
27. Khuroo, M.S., Zarger, S.A. and Mahajan, R. (1990) Hepatobiliary and pancreatic ascariasis in India. *The Lancet*, **i**, 1503–1506.
28. Layrisse, M., Apacedo, C.M. and Roche, M. (1967) Blood loss due to infection with *Trichuris trichiura*. *American Journal of Tropical Medicine and Hygiene*, **17**, 613–619.
29. Loia-Cortis, R. and Lobo-Sanahuja, F. (1980) Clinical abdominal angiostrongylosis. A study of 116 children with intestinal eosinophilic granuloma caused by *Angiostrongylus costaricensis*. *American Journal of Tropical Medicine and Hygiene*, **29**, 538–544.
30. Marcial-Rojas, R.A. (1971) Strongyloidiasis. In *Pathology of Protozoal and Helminthic Disease with Clinical Correlation* (Ed.) Marcial-Rojas, R.A. pp. 711–733. Baltimore: Williams and Wilkins.
31. Marsden, P.D. (Ed.) (1978) Intestinal parasites. *Clinics of Gastroenterology*, **7**(1) 1–243.
32. Marsden, P.D. (1978) Other nematodes. *Clinics in Gastroenterology*, **7**, 219–229.
33. Milder, J.E., Walzer, P.D., Kilgore, G. *et al.* (1981) Clinical features of *Strongyloides stercoralis*

infection in an endemic area of the United States. *Gastroenterology*, **80**, 1481–1488.
34. Miller, T.A. (1979) Hookworm infection in man. *Advances in Parasitology*, **17**, 315–384.
35. Msreno, E. (1971) Enterobiasis. In *Pathology of Protozoal and Helminthic Disease with Clinical Correlation* (Ed.) Marcial-Rojas, R.A. pp. 760–768. Baltimore: Williams and Wilkins.
36. Mukerji, K., Saxena, K.C., Ghatak, S. and Misra, P.K. (1976) Studies on human ascaris: purification of trypsin inhibitor. *Indian Journal of Medical Research*, **64**, 1611–1619.
37. Naquira, C., Jimemez, G., Guerra, J.G. *et al.* (1989) Ivermectin for human strongyloidiasis and other intestinal helminths. *American Journal of Tropical Medicine and Hygiene*, **40**, 304–307.
38. Neva, F.A., Gam, A.A. and Burke, J. (1981) Comparison of larval antigens in an enzyme-linked immunosorbent assay for strongyloidiasis in humans. *Journal of Infectious Diseases*, **144**, 427–432.
39. Ong, G.B. (1979) Helminthic diseases of the liver and biliary tract. In *Liver and Biliary Disease. Pathophysiology, Diagnosis, Management* (Ed.) Wright, R., Albert, K.G.M.M., Karran, S. and Millward-Sadler, G.H. pp. 1267–1303. London: Saunders.
40. Pawlowski, A.S. (1978) Ascariasis. *Clinics in Gastroenterology*, **7**, 157–178.
41. Roche, M. and Layrisse, M. (1966) The nature and causes of 'hookworm anemia'. *American Journal of Tropical Medicine and Hygiene*, **15**, 1040–1100.
42. Schad, G.A. (1973) Arrested development in human hookworm infection: an adaptation to seasonally unfavorable environment. *Science*, **180**, 502–504.
43. Schad, G.A. and Banwell, J.G. (1990) Hookworms. In *Tropical and Geographical Medicine*, 2nd edn, chap. 44 (Eds) Warren, K.S. and Mahmoud, A.F. pp. 379–393. New York: McGraw Hill.
44. Schultz, M.G. (1982) The effects of *Ascaris lumbricoides* infection on nutritional status. *Reviews of Infectious Disease*, **4**, 815–819.
45. Sharma, S., Dubey, S.K. and Iyer, R.N. (1980) Chemotherapy of cestode infections. *Progress in Drug Research*, **24**, 217–266.
46. Signson, C.N., Banson, T.C. and Cross, J.H. (1975) Mebendazole in the treatment of intestinal capillariasis. *American Journal of Tropical Medicine and Hygiene*, **24**, 932–934.
47. Stephenson, L.S. (1980) The contribution of *Ascaris lumbricoides* to malnutrition in children. *Parasitology*, **81**, 221–233.
48. Symmers, W.C. (1950) Pathology of oxyuriasis. *Archives of Pathology*, **50**, 465–516.
49. Uglem, G.L. and Just, J.J. (1983) Trypsin inhibition by tapeworms: Antienzyme secretion or pH adjustment? *Science*, **220**, 79–81.
50. van Thiel, P.H. (1976) The present state of anisakiasis and its causative worms. *Tropical and Geographic Medicine*, **28**, 75–85.
51. Variyam, E.P. and Banwell, J.G. (1982) Hookworm disease: nutritional implications. *Reviews of Infectious Diseases*, **4**, 830–835.
52. Whalen, G.E., Strickland, G.T., Cross, J.H. *et al.* (1969) Intestinal capillariasis. A new disease in man. *The Lancet*, **i**, 13–16.
53. WHO (1981) *Intestinal Protozoan and Helminthic Infections. WHO Technical Report Series 666*. Geneva: World Health Organisation.
54. WHO (1987) Public health significance of intestinal parasitic infections. *Bulletin of the WHO*, **65**, 575–588.
55. Wolfe, M. (1978) *Oxyuris, Trichostrongylus* and *Trichuris. Clinics in Gastroenterology*, **7**, 201–217.

PSEUDOMEMBRANOUS COLITIS AND ANTIBIOTIC-ASSOCIATED COLITIS

J. Webberley

Diarrhoea is a well-recognized adverse effect of antimicrobial therapy. The diarrhoea is usually benign and responds to withdrawal of the offending antibiotic. Some individuals, however, experience overt antibiotic-associated or pseudomembranous colitis, with a few progressing to serious complications, even death. A toxigenic organism, *Clostridium difficile*, is now recognized as the major aetiological agent in antibiotic-associated diarrhoea and colitis.

CLINICAL FEATURES

Antibiotic-associated colitis is described as inflammation of the colon which occurs in association with the use of antimicrobial agents and is otherwise unexplained. Nearly all agents with a spectrum of activity against bacteria have been implicated, whereas drugs with activity restricted to mycobacteria, parasites or fungi do not appear to cause this complication. The most frequent offending agents are the lincomycins, ampicillin and the cephalosporins.[2] With these drugs, the incidence and severity of symptoms does not correlate with the route of administration, dose or duration of treatment.

Most patients with antibiotic-associated colitis have diarrhoea as the initial and most prominent complaint. The stool in these cases is usually watery or mucoid; gross blood is relatively uncommon except in the haemorrhagic colitis which has been noted most frequently with ampicillin. The diarrhoea usually occurs in the first 4–10 days of antibiotic administration. However, at least one-third of patients note the initial change in bowel habit up to 4–6 weeks after the implicated agent has been discontinued.[46] The spectrum of symptoms ranges from 'simple' self-limiting diarrhoea with no systemic complaints to severe colitis which may mimic an acute abdomen. Characteristic findings include abdominal cramps, abdominal tenderness and leukocytosis. Late and serious complications include severe dehydration, electrolyte imbalance, hypotension, hypoalbuminaemia with anasarca, toxic megacolon or colonic perforation. Extraintestinal symptoms are rare, although occasional patients have polyarthritis. The natural course of the disease in different studies shows mortality rates which vary from nil[46] to 20%.[33]

DIAGNOSIS

The preferred methods of diagnosis are endoscopy and stool examination to detect the cytopathic toxin of *C. difficile*. The most characteristic lesion is pseudomembranous colitis, with multiple elevated yellowish white plaques which vary in size from a few millimetres to 15–20 mm in diameter.[41] The intervening mucosa may appear normal or show hyperaemia and oedema. Occasionally, the pseudomembranes coalesce to involve large segments of the colonic mucosa; these may slough to leave large denuded areas of mucosa. Histological studies show that pseudomembranes arise from a point of superficial ulceration on the intact mucosa. Lesions have been classified into three categories.[36] The earliest or most mild form consists of focal necrosis with polymorphonuclear cells and an eosinophilic exudate in the lamina propria. Splaying out from the necrotic focus is a collection of fibrin and acute inflammatory cells which form the characteristic 'summit lesion'. The second category shows disrupted glands containing mucin and polymorphonuclear cells surmounted by typical pseudomembranes. Both types of lesion show areas of intervening normal mucosa, and the inflammatory changes are limited to the superficial portion of the lamina propria, predominantly subepithelial in location. The third and most advanced form of the disease shows complete structural necrosis with extensive involvement of the lamina propria, which is overlaid by a thick confluent pseudomembrane. Pseudomembranous colitis is the most severe form of colitis noted with antibiotic-associated diarrhoea. Patients without demonstrable pseudomembranes may also have granularity and friability of the intestinal mucosa visible on gross inspection, and histological changes may resemble those noted with idiopathic ulcerative colitis.

The distal colon is involved in the majority of patients, so that sigmoidoscopy is generally adequate. However, about 20% have typical lesions restricted to the right colon, necessitating the use of colonoscopy. Care must be exercised in endoscopic technique in order to detect and biopsy appropriate lesions.[41] Copious amounts of mucus must often be removed with caution in order to avoid separation of pseudomembranes from the typical stalk attachment which is necessary for histological confirmation of pseudomembranous colitis. Radiological studies, especially air contrast examinations, may show typical lesions of pseudomembranous colitis.[39] However, this procedure must be performed with caution because of the potential complication of colonic perforation; it is not considered to be as sensitive or specific as endoscopy.

The differential diagnosis of pseudomembranous colitis is wide and includes Crohn's colitis, ulcerative colitis and infection with other intestinal pathogens (*Salmonella* spp, *Shigella* spp, verotoxin-producing strains of *Escherichia coli*, *Entamoeba histolytica*, *Campylobacter* spp and *Yersinia* spp).

MICROBIOLOGY

Studies from the 1950s suggested that *Staphylococcus aureus* was responsible for most cases of antibiotic-associated colitis.[3] The diagnosis at that time was usually based on the detection of this organism with direct stains and culture of stool specimens. Many now regard this work as rather inconclusive because of the frequency with which staphylococci may be found in the stools of healthy persons, especially those who have received antibiotics. It is not possible in retrospect to know if 'staphylococcal enterocolitis' was a valid diagnosis or simply a reflection of the attention devoted to the organism of that time.[3] At any rate, this organism is not now an important cause of antibiotic-associated colitis according to more recent reviews.[24]

C. difficile, an obligate anaerobic Gram-positive rod, was originally described in 1935 as a component of the normal faecal flora of newborn infants.[21] Studies at that time showed that the isolates produced a toxin which proved lethal to a variety of experimental animals. Nevertheless, the role of *C. difficile* as a clinically significant pathogen was not recognized until 1977, when Koch's postulates were satisfied for this as the agent of antibiotic-associated colitis.[4,5] The organism produces at least two toxins, an enterotoxin, toxin A and a cytotoxin, toxin B.[40,44]

The preferred method to implicate *C. difficile* as a cause of colitis is a tissue culture assay on stool to detect the cytopathic toxin which is neutralized by *Clostridium sordellii* or *C. difficile* antitoxin.[5,11,23,27] This is a highly sensitive and specific test which is preferred to stool cultures because of its relative simplicity and improved specificity according to clinical correlations.[49] The cytopathic toxin produced by this organism shows highly characteristic actinomorphic changes in cell lines containing fibroblast cells;[12] the quantity necessary to elicit these changes is only 0.2–5 pg.[40] The cytotoxin is thermolabile, showing decreases in titre which correlate directly with time and temperature.[11,20] Many clinical laboratories have no tissue culture facilities, which necessitates referral of specimens to distant laboratories. The thermolability of the toxin dictates that specimens be delivered within 24 hours of sampling, or be maintained in a frozen state prior to processing. Results of the assay are available in 24 hours. Titres may be determined using serial dilutions, but these do not correlate with the severity of clinical symptoms.[9] Alternative methods for toxin detection include counter-immunoelectrophoresis (CIE), enzyme-linked immunosorbent assay (ELISA) and latex particle agglutination. None of these is likely to match the sensitivity of tissue culture assay, although the ELISA technique (able to detect toxin A or B, depending on the specific antibody used) may be promising.[28] Stool cultures are not required in the diagnosis of *C. difficile* disease, although they may be useful in the investigation of possible outbreaks in order to permit strain typing. Several typing schemes have been described, based on various epidemiological markers of *C. difficile*.[42]

The clinical experience with *C. difficile* toxin assays indicates that nearly all patients with antibiotic-associated pseudomembranous colitis have positive tests (*Table 9.9*). The incidence among patients with other forms of colitis associated with antibiotic usage is 50–70%. Approximately 10–20% of patients with 'simple' diarrhoea complicating a course of antibiotic exposure will have this toxin. These data indicate that *C. difficile* has been implicated in the entire specrum of clinical and pathological changes noted in patients with antibiotic-associated diarrhoea and colitis. However, the incidence of the toxin seems to increase with the severity of the disease process. Nevertheless, it is necessary to emphasize that some patients with antibiotic exposure will have positive assays with no change in bowel habits and many have very trivial bouts of self-limiting diarrhoeal disease. The only other patient population in which this toxin has been detected with any frequency is infants.[25,31,37,49] The incidence in this population is between 14 and 43% and it is not associated with overt symptoms in the vast majority. Carriage rates for the organism and the toxin decrease during the first year of life so that virtually all children over 2 years old have negative toxin assays unless there is antibiotic exposure. Although most cases of pseudomembranous colitis occur in association with antibiotic usage, it has also been described independently in conditions such as chronic colonic obstruction, colonic cancer, leukaemia and uraemia. Limited experience in those patients with pseudomembranous colitis which does occur independently of antibiotic exposure shows that *C. difficile* is usually implicated. Some investigators have noted high rates of positive assays in patients with inflammatory bowel disease and

Table 9.9 Incidence of *C. difficile* toxin assay in various patient populations

Patient category	*Literature experience*[a]
Antibiotic-associated pseudomembranous colitis	83–100%
Antibiotic-associated diarrhoea or colitis without pseudomembranous colitis	17–34%
Gastrointestinal diseases unrelated to antibiotic usage	2%
Antibiotic exposure without diarrhoea	2–8%
Healthy adults	0–0.5%
Healthy neonates	14–43%

[a] Incidence range based on reported experience.[5,17,20,23,25,27,30,31,33,37]

severe relapse,[48] but this has not been a consistent observation.[32]

PATHOGENESIS

The pathogenesis of antibiotic-associated colitis involving *C. difficile* appears to require antibiotic exposure, a source of the organism and toxin production.

The organism is a component of the normal flora of approximately 3% of healthy adults who are presumed to be at risk when given an appropriate inducing agent.[29] Most cases of antibiotic-associated diarrhoea are sporadic, although outbreaks have been reported in hospitals, suggesting exogenous sources of the organism.[33] Colonization rates are higher in hospitalized patients, although prevalence varies widely between institutions.[38] Environmental cultures show excessive recovery rates in case-associated areas compared to control sites, the most common sources being toilets, bedpans and floors, as well as the hands and stools of asymptomatic hospital personnel caring for these patients.[18,34] The spores of *C. difficile* may persist on fomites and inanimate surfaces for long periods. Another potential source is endoscopy equipment, which has been implicated in at least one major outbreak.[33] Certainly, hospital patients are more susceptible to pseudomembranous colitis than individuals receiving antibiotics in the community. This increased vulnerability may reflect underlying disease states of hospital patients, use of broad-spectrum antibiotics and nosocomial acquisition.[38]

An impressive feature of *C. difficile*-induced enteric disease is that it occurs almost exclusively in the presence of antibiotic exposure. An attractive thesis is that this represents a superinfection involving the selection of resistant strains which are allowed to flourish when the competing flora is inhibited. In vitro susceptibility tests do not support this concept in either experimental animals or patients, since the organisms recovered are often susceptible to the agent implicated in causing the disease.[50] For example, ampicillin represents one of the most frequent offending agents despite the fact that this antibiotic is almost uniformly active against *C. difficile.* Similarly, approximately half of the strains recovered in patients with clindamycin-induced colitis are highly susceptible to this antibiotic. The organism presumably survives by sporulation, with regeneration of vegetative forms when antibiotic levels are low in the colonic lumen. The implication is that sensitivity profiles of *C. difficile* isolates are not particularly useful in determining drugs which are likely to cause the complication, although they may prove useful in determining potential therapeutic agents. The role of antimicrobial agents in altering the normal colonic flora with the elimination of colonization resistance is a critical factor in pathogenesis. Animal studies have shown that as few as 1 colony forming unit (cfu) of *C. difficile* may produce fatal enterocolitis when given to antibiotic-treated hamsters, whereas normal control hamsters given large numbers of the organism remain well.[27]

C. difficile-induced colitis is a toxin-mediated enteric disease in which typical pathological changes are noted after intraluminal challenge using the cell-free supernatant of *C. difficile* or its partially purified toxins.[4,44] Mucosal invasion by the organism has not been observed. Studies of the two major toxins (toxin A and toxin B), indicate they are high-molecular-weight proteins with somewhat different biological activities. Both toxins are cytopathic, and produce identical changes in tissue cultures. However, toxin B is much more potent, and is generally regarded as the marker in the cell culture assay, with as little as 0.2 pg producing typical cytopathic changes.[40] Toxin A is more active in animal models of enteric disease such as the rabbit ileal loop assay; this enterotoxin, which binds to intestinal brush border membranes, may be more important in clinical expression and pathological changes associated with *C. difficile*-induced disease. Both toxins A and B would appear to have some importance in pseudomembranous colitis, however, because hamsters immunized with toxoids prepared from both toxins, but not either alone, can be protected from the disease.[29] The organism produces both toxins at the termination of log phase growth, suggesting release with lysis of replicating strains. Most strains of *C. difficile* are toxigenic, although there is considerable variation in the amount of toxin produced in vitro.[49] This work suggests that the central role of antibiotics is a reflection of their impact on the normal flora, resulting in deregulated growth of *C. difficile* which is present either as a component of the normal flora or acquired from an environmental source.

An additional factor to emphasize in pathogenesis concerns the apparent age-related risk. As previously noted, infants often harbour *C. difficile* and its toxins with no deleterious consequences. Lower prevalence rates are found as the adult gut flora becomes established during the first year of life. *C. difficile* has been clearly implicated in antibiotic-associated diarrhoea and colitis in older children, but the incidence is low considering the frequent exposure to antibiotics such as ampicillin. For reasons as yet unclear, adults are far more susceptible to antibiotic-associated enteric disease. Studies in the pre-antibiotic era indicated that the patients most vulnerable to pseudomembranous colitis were those with intestinal neoplasms, ischaemia or surgery.[23] The implication is that age and physiological disturbances of the colon may enhance susceptiblity to *C. difficile* toxin.

TREATMENT

Colitis should be suspected in any patient who develops diarrhoea which is otherwise unexplained and occurs during or up to 6 weeks following antibiotic exposure. This complication has been most frequently seen in patients given ampicillin, lincomycins or cephalosporins, although almost any drug with antibacterial activity may be responsible. These include some cancer-chemotherapeutic agents as well.[16] Stool examination may show leukocytes, especially with pancolitis, but this is an inconsistent non-specific observation. The preferred method to establish the diagnosis of colitis or pseudomembranous colitis is endoscopy. However, the decision to treat is often based on clinical symptoms and detection of *C. difficile* toxin in faeces. This organism has been implicated in the entire spectrum of anatomical changes found in the colon of patients with antibiotic-associated diarrhoea ranging from an entirely normal mucosa to the most serious and characteristic form of colitis, pseudomembranous colitis. Thus, a distinction is made between studies done to establish the anatomical diagnosis and those used for an aetiological diagnosis. Indications for endoscopy include severe or debilitating diarrhoea, diagnostic evaluation of other gastrointestinal disease, and prolonged diarrhoea following withdrawal of the implicated antimicrobial agent. Previous studies indicate that most patients with antibiotic-associated diarrhoea have resolution of their bowel complaints within 1–2 weeks without specific therapy other than discontinuation of the implicated agent.

Patients with severe disease should be treated with appropriate supportive measures including intravenous fluids to correct fluid and electrolyte disturbances. Antiperistaltic drugs should be avoided.[35] The use of corticosteroids is controversial, although some recommend these drugs for severely ill individuals. Patients with *C. difficile*-induced disease pose an epidemiological hazard to susceptible hosts within the hospital setting, especially if they are incontinent. Specific guidelines to reduce environmental contamination and nosocomial spread are limited, but enteric isolation precautions are generally recommended.[18] Thorough handwashing after patient contact is particularly important. Such measures have proved useful in curtailing hospital outbreaks,[9] although have not been universally successful.[7]

The withdrawal of the inducing antibiotic, although desirable, is probably not essential if specific therapy is given. Such treatment utilizes antibiotics directed against *C. difficile* or anion exchange resins to bind toxin (*Table 9.10*). Vancomycin is the most frequently advocated antibiotic for several reasons. This drug is active against virtually all strains of *C. difficile*, and it is not absorbed when given orally so that levels within the colonic lumen are extremely high while systemic absorption is nil.[23,47] The clinical experience with this drug indicates that most patients have a prompt resolution of fever and other systemic complaints within 24–48 hours and a gradual resolution of diarrhoea over 2–14 days. Nearly all patients respond. The major problems are the high cost of the drug, its unpalatable taste and a relatively high incidence of relapses. The incidence of relapses in one series was 14% among 79 patients with *C. difficile*-induced

Table 9.10 Treatment of *C. difficile*-induced colitis

1. Seriously ill patients
   (a) Oral regimen (preferred): vancomycin 125 mg orally, 4 times daily, 7–14 days
   (b) Parenteral regimen: metronidazole 500 mg intravenously every 6 hours until patient will tolerate oral medications
2. Moderately ill patients
   (a) Vancomycin, 125 mg orally, 4 times daily, 7–14 days
   (b) Bacitracin, 500 mg (25 000 units) orally, 4 times daily, 7–14 days
   (c) Metronidazole, 250–500 mg orally, 3 times daily, 7–14 days
   (d) Cholestyramine, 4 g packet orally, 4 times daily, 7–14 days
3. Relapses following treatment
   (a) Repeat any of above regimens
   (b) Vancomycin, 125 mg orally, 4 times daily, 7–14 days; followed by cholestyramine, 4 g orally, 4 times daily, 2–3 weeks. Or vancomycin pulses (125 mg every other day)

disease,[61] and some of these individuals suffered repeated relapses with sequential courses. Other investigators have noted the incidence of relapse to vary from nil[23] to 35%.[19] Relapses are characterized by the recurrence of diarrhoeal symptoms with positive toxin assays for *C. difficile* at 2–30 days following discontinuation of oral vancomycin treatment.[6] Cultures at this time indicate that the implicated strains remain susceptible to vancomycin. Two postulated mechanisms for relapse are (1) that the organism is incompletely eliminated from the intestinal tract because of sporulation or (2) that a new strain is acquired from environmental sources in a host who is susceptible owing to reduced colonization resistance following vancomycin treatment. The frequency of relapse is not influenced by the choice of antibiotic for treatment, dose or duration of therapy. Many regimens have been suggested for preventing relapse, including prolonged low-dose vancomycin, or repeated 'pulse doses' of the drug, the aim being to eradicate vegetative organisms as they emerge from spores.[45]

Alternative antibiotics include bacitracin, fusidic acid and metronidazole.[13–15] Bacitracin has the same potential advantages as vancomycin in that it is active against most strains of *C. difficile* and it is poorly absorbed when given by the oral route so that levels in the colonic lumen are exceptionally high.[13] However, clinical response is slower and less certain than with vancomycin. Metronidazole is extremely active against *C. difficile* in vitro and is considerably cheaper than vancomycin. However, because the drug is well absorbed after oral administration, colonic lumen levels are modest; and it has been implicated in causing *C. difficile* disease in occasional patients. Parenteral metronidazole has been suggested for patients who are too seriously ill to receive oral medication, but it must be stressed that no form of parenteral therapy has proved reliable and effective.[14,31] Oral therapy should be used if at all possible. Vancomycin can be given via a nasogastric tube, and direct instillation into the colon using a caecostomy tube has also been attempted in patients unable to tolerate oral medication.

The anion exchange resin most frequently used is cholestyramine but the clinical experience with these resins is highly variable, ranging from universal success[26] to almost no detectable response.[22] In view of this erratic track record, cholestyramine is generally reserved for patients who are less seriously ill or have contraindications to vancomycin. This drug should not be given concurrently with vancomycin since it binds the antibiotic to produce a marked reduction in stool levels of biologically active drug.[43]

The loss of colonization resistance is a fundamental factor in the pathophysiology of *C. difficile*-induced enteric disease, so attempts to re-establish the normal flora are a theoretically attractive approach to treatment. Recolonization with lactobacilli has not been extensively studied, although previous experience with this approach shows that repopulation may be difficult to achieve, possibly reflecting the fact that these organisms are not prevalent components of the normal flora. A more physiological approach is use of faecal enemas; this has proved modestly successful in animal models as well as in patients with antibiotic-associated colitis.[8] Despite theoretical advantages, this approach is unlikely to gain wide acceptance owing to its lack of aesthetic appeal as well as the possibility of transmitting an enteric pathogen. In patients who have recovered from pseudomembranous colitis, there is little evidence to suggest that repeat exposure to the inducing antibiotic leads to recurrence.

REFERENCES

1. Aronsson, B., Mollby, R. and Nord, C.E. (1981) Occurrence of toxin-producing *Clostridium difficile* in antibiotic-associated diarrhea in Sweden. *Medical Microbiology and Immunology*, **170**, 27–35.
2. Bartlett, J.G. (1981) Antimicrobial agents implicated in *Clostridium difficile* toxin-associated diarrhea or colitis. *John Hopkins Medical Journal*, **149**, 6–9.
3. Bartlett, J.G. and Gorbach, S.L. (1977) Pseudomembranous colitis. In *Advances in Internal Medicine* (Ed.) Stollerman, G.H. pp. 455–476. Chicago: Year Book.
4. Bartlett, J.G., Onderdonk, A.B., Cisneros, A.B. and Kasper, D.L. (1977) Clindamycin-associated colitis due to toxin-producing species of clostridium in hamsters. *Journal of Infectious Disease*, **136**, 701–705.
5. Bartlett, J.G., Chang, T.W., Gurwith, M. *et al.* (1978) Antibiotic associated pseudomembranous colitis due to toxin-producing clostridia. *New England Journal of Medicine*, **198**, 531–534.
6. Bartlett, J.G., Tedesco, F.J., Shull, S., Lowe, B. and Chang, T. (1980) Symptomatic relapse after oral vancomycin therapy of antibiotic-associated pseudomembranous colitis. *Gastroenterology*, **78**, 421–434.
7. Bender, B.S., Bennett, R., Laughon, B.E. *et al.* (1986) Is *Clostridium difficile* endemic in chronic care facilities? *The Lancet*, **ii**, 11–13.
8. Bowden, T.A. Jr, Mansberger, A.R. Jr and Lykins, L.E. (1981) Pseudomembranous enterocolitis: mechanism for restoring floral homeostasis. *American Surgery*, **47**, 178–183.
9. Burdon, D.W. (1982) *Clostridium difficile*: the epidemiology and prevention of hospital acquired infection. *Infection*, **10**, 203–204.

10. Burdon, D.W., George, R.H. and Mogg, G. (1981) Faecal toxin and severity of antibiotic-associated pseudomembranous colitis. *Journal of Clinical Pathology*, **34**, 548–551.
11. Chang, T.W., Lauermann, M. and Bartlett, J.G. (1979) Cytotoxicity assay in antibiotic-associated colitis. *Journal of Infectious Disease*, **140**, 765–770.
12. Chang, T.W., Lin, P.S., Gorbach, S.L. and Bartlett, J.G. (1979) Ultrastructural changes of cultures human amnion cells by *Clostridium difficile* toxin. *Infection and Immunity*, **23**, 795–798.
13. Chang, T.W., Gorbach, S.L., Bartlett, J.G. and Saginur, R. (1980) Bacitracin treatment of antibiotic-associated colitis and diarrhea caused by *Clostridium difficile. Gastroenterology,* **78**, 1584–1586.
14. Cherry, R.D., Portnoy, D., Jabbari, M. *et al.* (1982) Metronidazole: an alternate therapy for antibiotic-associated colitis. *Gastroenterology*, **82**, 849–851.
15. Cronberg, S., Castor, B. and Thorn, A. (1984) Fusidic acid for the treatment of antibiotic-associated colitis induced by *Clostridium difficile. Infection*, **12**, 276–279.
16. Cudmore, M.A., Silva, J. Jr, Fekety, R. *et al.* (1982) *Clostridium difficile* colitis associated with cancer chemotherapy. *Archives of Internal Medicine*, **142**, 333–335.
17. Delmee, M. and Wauters, G. (1981) Rôle de *Clostridium difficile* dans les diarrhées survenant après antibiothérapie: étude de 87 cas. *Acta Clinica Belgica*, **36**, 178–184.
18. Fekety, R., Kim, K.-H., Brown, D. *et al.* (1981) Epidemiology of antibiotic-associated colitis. *American Journal of Medicine*, **70**, 906–908.
19. George, W.L., Rolfe, R.D., Harding, G.K.M. *et al.* (1982) *Clostridium difficile* and cytotoxin in feces of patients with antimicrobial agent-associated pseudomembranous colitis. *Infection*, **10**, 205–207.
20. Gilligan, P.H., McCarthy, L.R. and Genta, V.M. (1981) Relative frequency of *Clostridium difficile* in patients with diarrheal disease. *Journal of Clinical Microbiology*, **14**, 26–31.
21. Hall, I.C. and O'Toole, E. (1935) Intestinal flora in newborn infants with description of a new pathogenic anaerobe. *Bacillus difficilis. American Journal of Diseases of Children*, **49**, 390–402.
22. Keighley, M.R.B. (1980) Antibiotic-associated pseudomembranous colitis. Pathogenesis and management. *Drugs*, **20**, 49–56.
23. Keighley, M.R.B., Burdon, D.W., Arabi, Y. *et al.* (1978) Randomized controlled trial of vancomycin for pseudomembranous colitis and postoperative diarrhoea. *British Medical Journal*, **ii**, 1667–1669.
24. Keusch, G.T. and Present, D.H. (1976) Summary of workshop on clindamycin colitis. *Journal of Infectious Disease*, **133**, 578–587.
25. Kim, K.-H., Fekety, R., Botts, D.H. *et al.* (1981) Isolation of *Clostridium difficile* from the environment and contacts of patients with antibiotic-associated colitis. *Journal of Infectious Disease*, **143**, 42–50.
26. Kreutzer, E.W. and Milligan, F.D. (1978) Treatment of antibiotic-associated pseudomembranous colitis with cholestyramine resin. *Johns Hopkins Medical Journal*, **143**, 67–72.
27. Larson, H.E., Price, A.B., Honour, P. and Borriello, S.P. (1978) *Clostridium difficile* and the aetiology of pseudomembranous colitis. *The Lancet*, **i**, 1062–1066.
28. Laughon, B.E., Viscidi, R.P., Gdovin, S.L., Yolken, R.H. and Bartlett, J.G. (1984) Enzyme immunoassays for detection of *Clostridium difficile* toxins A and B in fecal specimens. *Journal of Infectious Disease*, **149**, 781–788.
29. Libby, J.M., Jortner, B.S. and Wilkins, T.D. (1982) Effect of the two toxins of *Clostridium difficile* in antibiotic-associated cecitis in hamsters. *Infection and Immunity*, **36**, 822–829.
30. Lishman, A.H., Al-Jumaili, I.J. and Record, C.O. (1981) Spectrum of antibiotic-associated diarrhea. *Gut*, **22**, 34–37.
31. Meuwissen, S.G.M. and Rietra, P.J.G.M. (1980) Antibiotic-associated pseudomembranous colitis. *Acta Gastro-enterologica Belgica*, **43**, 377–385.
32. Meyers, S., Mayer, L., Bottone, E. *et al.* (1981) Occurrence of *Clostridium difficile* toxin during the course of inflammatory bowel disease. *Gastroenterololgy*, **80**, 697–700.
33. Mogg, G.M., Keighley, M., Burdon, D. *et al.* (1979) Antibiotic-associated colitis – a review of 66 cases. *British Journal of Surgery*, **66**, 738.
34. Mollby, R., Nord, C.E. and Aronsson, B. (1980) Diagnosis of *Clostridium difficile* associated enterocolitis in Sweden. Laboratory and epidemiological aspects. *Scandinavian Journal of Infectious Disease*, **22**, 30–36.
35. Novak, E., Lee, J.G., Seckman, C.E. *et al.* (1976) Unfavorable effect of atropinediphenoxylate (Lomotil) therapy in clindamycin-caused diarrhea. *Journal of the American Medical Associations*, **235**, 1451–1454.
36. Price, A.B. and Davies, D.R. (1977) Pseudomembranous colitis. *Journal of Clinical Pathology*, **30**, 1–12.
37. Sheretz, R.J. and Sarubbi, F.A. (1982) The prevalence of *Clostridium difficile* and toxin in a nursery population: a comparison between patients with necrotizing enterocolitis and an asymptomatic group. *Journal of Pediatrics*, **100**, 435–439.
38. Silva, J. and Iezzi, C. (1988) *Clostridium difficile* as a nosocomial pathogen. *Journal of Hospital Infection*, **11**(supp. A), 378–385.
39. Stanley, R.J., Melson, G.L. and Tedesco, F.J. (1974) The spectrum of radiographic findings in antibiotic-related pseudomembranous colitis. *Radiology*, **111**, 519–524.
40. Sullivan, N.M., Pellett, S. and Wilkins, T.D. (1982) Purification and characterization of toxins A and B of *Clostridium difficile. Infection and Immunity*, **35**, 1032–1040.

41. Sumner, H.W. and Tedesco, F.J. (1975) Rectal Biopsy in clindamycin-associated colitis. *Archives of Pathology*, **9**, 237.
42. Tabaqchali, S. (1990) Epidemiologic markers of *Clostridium difficile. Reviews of Infectious Diseases*, **12**(suppl. 2), 192–199.
43. Taylor, N.S. and Bartlett, J.G. (1980) Binding of *Clostridium difficile* cytotoxin and vancomycin by anion exchange resins. *Journal of Infectious Disease*, **141**, 92–97.
44. Taylor, N.S., Thorne, G.M. and Bartlett, J.G. (1981) Comparison of two toxins produced by *Clostridium difficile. Infection and Immunity*, **34**, 1036–1043.
45. Tedesco, F.J. (1982) Treatment of recurrent antibiotic-associated pseudomembranous colitis. *American Journal of Gastroenterology*, **77**, 220–221.
46. Tedesco, F.J., Barton, R.W. and Alpers, H.D. (1974) Clindamycin-associated colitis. *Annals of Internal Medicine*, **81**, 429–433.
47. Tedesco, F.J., Markham, R., Gurwith, M. *et al.* (1978) Oral vancomycin therapy of antibiotic-associated pseudomembranous colitis. *The Lancet*, **ii**, 226–228.
48. Trnka, Y.M. and LaMont, J.T. (1981) Association of *Clostridium difficile* toxin with symptomatic relapse of chronic inflammatory bowel disease. *Gastroenterology*, **80**, 693–696.
49. Viscidi, R., Willey, S. and Bartlett, J.G. (1981) Isolation rates and toxigenic potential of *Clostridium difficile* isolates from various patient populations. *Gastroenterology*, **81**, 5–9.
50. Willey, S.H. and Bartlett, J.G. (1979) Cultures for *Clostridium difficile* in stools containing a cytotoxin neutralized by *Clostridium sordellii* antitoxin. *Journal of Clinical Microbiology*, **10**, 880–884.

TRAVELLERS' DIARRHOEA

J. Webberley

With the considerable increase in international travel during the last two decades there has been an explosive increase in the number of acute attacks of diarrhoea among visitors (on holiday or on business) and temporary residents (volunteers or contract workers) in areas where sanitation and hygiene are poor. The attacks are most frequent in tropical areas,[21] where up to 50% of travellers may be affected, and instructive eponyms such as 'Delhi belly', 'the Aztec two-step' and 'Basrah belly' are used to describe the illness. However, there have also been epidemics of acute diarrhoea amongst travellers in southern Europe (particularly the Mediterranean), some areas of Russia and parts of the USA.

MICROBIOLOGY

Traveller's diarrhoea may be caused by a variety of bacteria (*Escherichia coli*, salmonella, shigella, *Campylobacter* spp., *Vibrio* spp.), viruses (rotavirus, Norwalk agent) and parasites (*Giardia lamblia*, *Entamoeba histolytica*, cryptosporidia), with geographical and epidemiological factors dictating which of the various agents may be responsible. Mixed infections are not uncommon.

Enteropathogens such as shigella, salmonella and *Campylobacter* spp. can be readily identified by the use of appropriate culture media and incubation conditions.[1,2] However, the commonest bacterial pathogens, enterotoxigenic *E. coli* (ETEC), first implicated as a cause of traveller's diarrhoea in 1970, can only be recognized by toxin detection.[9,15] This poses diagnostic problems for routine microbiology laboratories. ETEC may produce one, or more usually both, of two types of enterotoxin: heat-labile (LT) and heat-stable (ST). The ability to produce toxins is determined by possession of a bacterial plasmid, many serotypes of *E. coli* being capable of acquiring such plasmids by genetic transfer. Thus, although a limited number of *E. coli* serotypes account for the majority of ETEC strains, serotyping alone cannot identify toxigenic strains. LT, a high-molecular-weight protein related to the toxin of *Vibrio cholerae*, may be detected by measuring fluid secretion in the rabbit ileal loop assay, or by observing characteristic effects on certain tissue culture cells. Immunological methods, such as enzyme-linked immunosorbent assay (ELISA) and gel precipitation have also been used; ST is rather small in comparison for satisfactory immunological tests and has no effect on tissue culture cells. More recently, DNA probes have been developed that are capable of recognizing the plasmids encoding enterotoxin production. Such methods can detect ETEC in crude faeces without the need for culture.

Enterotoxins are produced in the proximal small intestine, where ETEC attaches itself to enterocytes by means of specific fimbrial colonization factors. LT and ST activate intracellular adenylate and guanylate cyclase, respectively, increasing the concentrations of the cyclic nucleotides (cAMP and cGMP). This stimulates secretion of fluid and electrolytes from the enterocytes into the intestinal lumen, so producing watery diarrhoea.[7]

ETEC should be differentiated from three other types of *E. coli*, which caused diarrhoea by other mechanisms: enteroinvasive *E. coli* (EIEC), enteropathogenic *E. coli* (EPEC) and verotoxin-producing *E. coli* (VTEC).[10] EIEC invades and proliferates within the mucosal epithelium (especially in the colon) to produce a typical shigella-like dysentery syndrome of blood and mucus. EPEC causes destruction of intestinal microvilli, and causes outbreaks of diarrhoea in infants, young children and, less commonly, in adults. It is traditionally identified by serotyping. VTEC produces a clinical picture of crampy abdominal pain, bloody diarrhoea with little or no fever; it has been cited as the commonest cause of diarrhoea in some geographical settings.[13] Life-threatening complications such as haemorrhagic colitis and haemolytic–uraemic syndrome may occur. VTEC produces one or both of two Shiga-like cytotoxins, VT1 and VT2, recognized by their cytopathic effect in Vero cell cultures.[18] Free verotoxin may be detected by specific DNA probes. The most commonly associated *E. coli* serotype is O157:H7, although other serotypes may also produce verotoxins.

Rotavirus and Norwalk agent are recognized as important causes of traveller's diarrhoea.[19] Both cause tissue destruction of the jejunal mucosa and there is acute watery diarrhoea without blood or mucus. Although the viruses are most reliably detected by electron microscopy, recent ELISA techniques applied to whole faecal homogenates have been successful. A rising titre of serum antibodies may be used to confirm a diagnosis retrospectively.

Parasitic infections are diagnosed microscopically on appropriately prepared samples. It is important to recognize that cysts and trophozoites of *G. lamblia* are intermittently excreted and a single microscopic examination may miss the diagnosis.[22] Trophozoites of *Ent. histolytica* may be identified microscopically if fresh specimens are examined.

CLINICAL FEATURES

Diarrhoea often occurs within a few days of arriving in a contaminated area. The attack may be brief, lasting less than 24 hours, but often lasts for three to five days.[6] There are several forms of clinical presentation, which vary according to the nature of the infecting organism:

1. Watery diarrhoea, up to 10–20 times a day, with normally coloured stools. This is the most frequent presentation, commonly due to ETEC, rotavirus, Norwalk agent or *Campylobacter* spp.
2. Initial watery diarrhoea progressing to malabsorption. This suggests the presence of *G. lamblia*.
3. Dysentery (blood and mucus). This suggests the presence of EIEC, *Shigella* spp., *Salmonella* spp., *Ent. histolytica*, *Campylobacter* spp. or VTEC.

Nausea and abdominal pain may be common, and vomiting (especially with Norwalk agent) also occurs. Pyrexia, headache and rigors are often experienced in the first few days. A few patients have severe fluid and electrolyte loss, with hypokalaemia in severe illness. The combination of nausea, anorexia and vomiting causes some weight loss in most patients but this is usually regained quickly.

PROGNOSIS

Most sufferers from traveller's diarrhoea, particularly those with the acute watery diarrhoea syndrome, recover within the first week. In others, for example those with *G. lamblia* or *Ent. histolytica*, symptoms can persist for many weeks. A further group recovers from the initial watery diarrhoea, but protracted diarrhoea with symptoms of malabsorption occurs. This postinfective malabsorption syndrome appears to be related to bacterial colonization of the upper intestine which develops at the time of, or soon after, the acute diarrhoea.

INVESTIGATIONS

These should be considered in relation to treatment, because the bacteriological findings do not influence management in the majority of patients who have a brief, self-limiting disease. When there is acute watery diarrhoea the diagnosis of ETEC, rotavirus and Norwalk agent can be made on single faecal specimens. Most laboratories can offer routine diagnosis of rotavirus by ELISA or latex agglutination, and Norwalk agent can be recognized by ELISA or immune electron microscopy. Documentation of ETEC, however, requires referral to a specialist laboratory. In dysenteric diarrhoea it is essential to culture on specific media for *Salmonella* spp. and *Shigella* spp. and to use specific culture media and incubation conditions for *Campylobacter* spp., which are microaerophilic. EPEC may be identified by serotyping; so also may VTEC, with referral made to a specialist laboratory for verotoxin detection. It is important to subject the stools to light microscopy for the detection of trophozoites and cysts of *Ent. histolytica* and *G. lamblia* in traveller's diarrhoea that persists for more than 1 week.

DIFFERENTIAL DIAGNOSIS

There are several groups of diseases which should be considered: first, other diarrhoeal diseases that are endemic in a particular area (e.g. *V. cholerae*, *Aeromonas* spp., *Yersinia enterocolitica*, *Vibrio parahaemolyticus*); secondly, diarrhoea which presents as part of a food poisoning syndrome, in which nausea and vomiting are classically the dominant symptoms (e.g. *Staphylococcus aureus*, *Bacillus cereus*, *Clostridium perfringens*); thirdly, diarrhoea which is the presenting symptom in the first attack of inflammatory bowel disease.

The enteric fevers, typhoid and paratyphoid, must not be forgotten, although diarrhoea is a late feature of these diseases.

TREATMENT

The majority of patients require an explanation of the expected natural history and cause of the disease together with symptomatic therapy and reassurance. Antibiotics are rarely indicated.

SYMPTOMATIC TREATMENT

Complete rest and a liquid diet for 48 hours will often improve the diarrhoea. It is best to replace fluid and electrolyte losses at an early stage. This may be achieved using the World Health Organization formula oral rehydration solution glucose–electrolyte packets, which are made up in water to give a fluid concentration of glucose 110 mmol/l, sodium 90 mmol/l and potassium 20 mmol/l.[16] These concentrations ensure that the glucose stimulates the absorption of sodium and water, even in the presence of a damaged mucosa. If the packets are not available, travellers can make a sugar and salt solution themselves, using a small soft-drink bottle (300 ml) and its cap as a measure (one level capful of salt plus eight level capfuls of sugar in three bottles of water gives a sodium concentration of about 90 mmol/l). Lucozade (a soft drink containing glucose) is a good source of sugar and water but it requires the addition of salt. A cup of yeast extract (constituted using one level teaspoon of yeast extract in 150 ml of water) is another useful source of sodium – this recipe provides 60 mmol/l of sodium. However, it requires glucose or sugar to stimulate the sodium absorption.

ANTIDIARRHOEAL AGENTS

In the majority of patients, symptomatic therapy alone is sufficient, but if abdominal discomfort is severe it is advisable to use drugs which reduce intestinal motility, such as loperamide, diphenoxylate or codeine phosphate. Their use should be restricted to adults because in young children they tend to permit some enteropathogens to proliferate to dangerous levels in the intestine. Drugs which make the stool more formed by increasing its bulk, such as kaolin, have a good reputation for reducing the explosive watery stools. They are generally safe but they do nothing to reduce the electrolyte or water loss. Bismuth salicylate (subsalicylate) reduces the fluid loss and abdominal pain. So far, unfortunately, it is effective only in traveller's diarrhoea due to ETEC; it does not improve the diarrhoea caused by EIEC or *Shigella* sp. Lactobacilli have been prescribed for diarrhoea, usually in the form of live yoghurt or in dried bacterial form. The rationale is sound in that lactobacilli may produce an intestinal milieu which is inhibitory to several enteropathogens but, unfortunately, several trials have failed to show any significant benefit in traveller's diarrhoea.

ANTIBIOTICS

There are only a few indications for antibiotic administration and it is essential to consider the local pattern of drug resistance. This may be a severe problem and recently there has been a striking increase in the numbers of strains of *Shigella* spp. and *Salmonella* spp. with multiple antibiotic resistance patterns among travellers returning to the UK from abroad, especially the subcontinent of India. The most appropriate antibiotic will be indicated by the drug sensitivity pattern but ampicillin, tetracycline and co-trimoxazole (trimethoprim plus sulphamethoxazole) may be useful. The new quinolones, ciprofloxacin and norfloxacin, have also proved effective.[8] Antibiotics should be reserved for patients with moderate or severe dysentery; those in whom diarrhoea is improving spontaneously and those who are asymptomatic carriers should not receive antibiotics.

Similar indications apply in those with *Salmonella* spp. infections. Mild dysentery or watery diarrhoea is best left untreated. Indeed, antibiotic therapy may actually prolong excretion in asymptomatic carriers.

Ciprofloxacin, ampicillin, chloramphenicol and co-trimoxazole are the most useful for those with severe dysentery.

G. lamblia is treated with metronidazole or tinidazole.

Ent. histolytica is treated with a combination of metronidazole, which is active against trophozoites, and diloxanide furoate, active against cysts.

PROPHYLAXIS

The best way to avoid diarrhoea is by avoiding those foods or drinks which are faecally contaminated.[5] The traveller should be made aware of the high-risk areas. Among British travellers, most cases of diarrhoea occur in those who visit the Mediterranean, North Africa, the Middle East, the Far East, the Indian subcontinent or Central America. Any food, however well presented, can be bacteriologically contaminated, but salads, fresh fruits and fruit juices, especially those bought from street vendors, are all hazardous. It is often valuable to use local knowledge about which restaurants and cafes have reliable reputations. If the visitor is self-catering, then salads, vegetables and fruit can be soaked in solutions of potassium permanganate or sodium hypochlorite. Although most enteropathogens are contracted from food rather than water it is important to caution against drinking any tap-water. Bottled drinks and boiled beverages are usually safe. If it is essential to drink local water, purifying tablets can be used, and lightweight portable water filters suitable for packing in a small suitcase are available.

Chemoprophylaxis is becoming more popular but not all drugs are effective. Of the antimicrobial agents there is some evidence that sulphathiazole, clioquinol,[14] Streptotriad (sulphadiazine, sulphadimidine, sulphathiazole and streptomycin), neomycin, trimethoprim,[4] co-trimoxazole,[4] doxycycline,[17] and the new quinolones[8] protect against diarrhoea. However, side-effects are important: these include optic nerve damage (clioquinol), mucosal damage (neomycin), skin rashes (co-trimoxazole) and increased excretion rates of *Salmonella* spp.[11] Many authorities believe that clioquinol (Entero-Vioform) should not be used, because of its capacity to cause serious toxic reactions. Furthermore, there is evidence that drug resistance is increased by the indiscriminate use of antimicrobial agents.[12] Recent studies show that bismuth subsalicylate can be used to prevent travellers' diarrhoea and is also effective in controlling the disease once it is established.[3] In general it is best to limit the use of chemoprophylaxis to certain groups of patients: first, those whose mission is very important (travellers on business, politicians, athletes and others who are on a brief visit); secondly, individuals whose resistance to infection is low (for example those with achlorhydria, whether idiopathic or due to cimetidine, those with previous gastric surgery and the elderly); thirdly, those who seem to experience diarrhoea particularly frequently when they go abroad.

IMMUNIZATION

Travellers should be protected by immunization against typhoid, polio, cholera and hepatitis A as appropriate. ETEC-associated traveller's diarrhoea invokes antitoxin responses in the intestine, mainly directed against the immunogenic LT. It has been shown that passive administration of cow's milk immunoglobulin concentrate, containing high levels of antibody to fimbrial colonization factors and LT, may provide protection against challenge with ETEC.[20] Although this is not yet of practical public health value, it may encourage the future development of an oral vaccine against travellers' diarrhoea.

REFERENCES

1. Butzler, J.P. and Skirrow, M.B. (1979) *Campylobacter* enteritis. *Clinics in Gastroenterology*, **8**, 737–765.
2. DuPont, H.L., Olarte, J., Evans, D.G. *et al.* (1976) Comparative susceptibility of Latin American and United States students to enteric pathogens. *New England Journal of Medicine*, **295**, 1520–1521.
3. DuPont, H.L., Sullivan, P., Evans, D.G. *et al.* (1980) Prevention of travellers' diarrhoea (emporiatric enteritis): prophylactic administration of subsalicylate bismuth. *Journal of American Medical Association*, **243**, 237–241.
4. DuPont, H.L., Galindo, E., Evans, D.G. *et al.* (1983) Prevention of travellers' diarrhoea with trimethoprim–sulfamethoxazole and trimethoprim alone. *Gastroenterology*, **84**, 75–80.
5. Ericsson, C.D., Pickering, L.K., Sullivan, P. and DuPont, H.L. (1980) The role of location of food consumption in the prevention of traveler's diarrhoea in Mexico. *Gastroenterology*, **79**, 812–816.
6. Farmer, R.G., Gulya, A.J. and Whelan, G. (1981) Travellers' diarrhoea: clinical observations. *Journal of Clinical Gastroenterology*, **3**(1), 27–29.
7. Gemmell, C.G. (1984) Comparative study of the nature and biological activities of bacterial enterotoxins. *Journal of Medical Microbiology*, **17**, 217–235.
8. Gorbach, S.L. (1987) Bacterial diarrhoea and its treatment. *The Lancet*, **ii**, 1378–1382.

9. Gorbach, S.L., Kean, B.H., Evans, D.G. *et al.* (1975) Travellers' diarrhoea and toxigenic. *Escherichia coli. New England Journal of Medicine*, **292**, 933–936.
10. Levine, M.M. (1987) *Escherichia coli* that cause diarrhea: enterotoxigenic, enteropathogenic, enteroinvasive, enterohaemorrhagic, and enteroadherent. *Journal of Infectious Disease*, **155**, 377–389.
11. Mentzing, L.O. and Ringertz, O. (1968) Salmonella infection in tourists. 2. Prophylaxis against salmonellosis. *Acta Patholigica et Microbiologica Scandinavica*, **74**, 405–413.
12. Murray, B.E., Rensimer, E.R. and DuPont, H.L. (1982) Emergence of high-level trimethoprim resistance in fecal *Escherichia coli* during oral administration of trimethoprim or trimethoprim–sulfamethoxazole. *New England Journal of Medicine*, **306**, 130–135.
13. Pai, C.H., Ahmed, N., Lior, H., Johnson, W.M., Sims, H.V. and Woods, D.E. (1988) Epidemiology of sporadic diarrhea due to verocytotoxin-producing *Escherichia coli*: a two year prospective study. *Journal of Infectious Disease*, **157**, 1054–1057.
14. Richards, D.A. (1970) A controlled trial in travellers' diarrhoea. *Practitioner*, **204**, 822–824.
15. Rowe, B., Taylor, J. and Bettelheim, K.A. (1970) An investigation of travellers' diarrhoea. *The Lancet*, **i**, 1–5.
16. Sack, R.B., Pierce, N.F. and Hirschhorn, N. (1978) The current status of oral therapy in the treatment of acute diarrhoeal illness. *American Journal of Clinical Nutrition*, **31**, 2251–2257.
17. Santosham, M., Sack, R.B., Froehlich, J. *et al.* (1981) Biweekly prophylactic doxycycline for travellers' diarrhoea. *Journal of Infectious Disease*, **143**, 598–608.
18. Scotland, S.M., Willshaw, G.A., Smith, H.R. and Rowe, B. (1987) Properties of strains of *Escherichia coli* belonging to serogroup O157 with special reference to production of Vero cytotoxins VT1 and VT2. *Epidemiology and Infection*, **99**, 613–624.
19. Sheridan, J.F., Aurelian, L., Barbour, G. *et al.* (1981) Travellers' diarrhoea associated with rotavirus infection: analysis of virus-specific immunoglobulin classes. An enzyme-linked immunosorbent assay for the detection of rotavirus-specific immunoglobulin G (IgG). *Infection and Immunity*, **31**(1), 419–429.
20. Tacket, C.O., Losonsky, G., Link, H. *et al.* (1988) Protection by milk immunoglobulin concentrate against oral challenge with enterotoxigenic *Escherichia coli. New England Journal of Medicine*, **318**, 1240–1243.
21. Turner, A.C. (1967) Travellers' diarrhoea: a survey of symptoms, occurrence and possible prophylaxis. *British Medical Journal*, iv, 653–654.
22. Wright, S.G., Tomkins, A.M. and Ridley, D.S. (1977) Giardiasis: clinical and therapeutic aspects. *Gut*, **18**, 343–350.

YERSINIA INFECTIONS

J. Webberley

The genus *Yersina* includes eight species, although the term 'yersiniosis' usually refers to infection with *Y. enterocolitica* and *Y. pseudotuberculosis*. The other species are *Y. pestis*, the plague bacillus; *Y. ruckeri*, a fish pathogen; and four *Y. enterocolitica*-like organisms (*Y. intermedia, Y. frederiksenii, Y. kristensenii* and *Y. aldovae*), differentiated by DNA and other biochemical studies.[5] These last four species, although often isolated from clinical specimens, the environment and food, have not been established as human pathogens.

Y. enterocolitica and *Y. pseudotuberculosis* produce a variety of predominantly gastrointestinal disorders, with severity ranging from benign self-limiting to life-threatening. The very young, the elderly and the immunocompromised are particularly susceptible and secondary immunological complications are not uncommon.

PATHOGENESIS

YERSINIA ENTEROCOLITICA

The pathogenesis of *Y. enterocolitica* infection usually involves ingestion of the organism. The only successful human infection experiment recorded involved ingestion of 3.5×10^9 organisms.[6] Similar large numbers of organisms via the oral route have been required to produce infection in animal models. Infection is usually via the faecal–oral route or by contaminated food, water or milk. The incubation period appears to range from 4 to 10 days. The organisms invade the epithelial lining of the ileum and colon, creating small focal ulcerations associated with neutrophils and a pyroninophilic response with numerous mitotic figures in regional lymph nodes. At the same time a systemic inflammatory response is manifested by an elevated erythrocyte sedimentation rate, a leukocytosis and an increase in immature polymorphonuclear leukocytes in peripheral blood. When invasion proceeds beyond the gastrointestinal tract the involved systems (liver, joints and, rarely, the central nervous system) also manifest a polymorphonuclear leukocyte invasion with micro- or gross abscess formation. During the gastrointestinal illness, blood and pus can often be found in the stool, as befits an invasive pathogen.[2,3,13]

Much recent work has centred about differences in the virulence properties characterizing the environmental strains which rarely cause human disease and the four serotypes known to be pathogenic to humans (0:3, 0:8, 0:9 and 0:5,27). It appears that the ability of strains to invade HeLa cells, resist the lethal effect of fresh serum, and possibly replicate within macrophages correlates well with their in vivo virulence as judged by presence in fresh human isolates and isolates which are virulent in animal models. The production of virulence-associated V and W antigens by *Y. enterocolitica*, a nutritional requirement for calcium, the property of autoagglutination, and alteration in outer-membrane proteins have been linked to the presence of one or more 42–48 MDa plasmids.[9,16] Loss of these plasmids results in transition to avirulent strains. Similar plasmids are present in *Y. pestis* and *Y. pseudotuberculosis*, but have not as yet been found in other *Yersinia* spp.

Most strains of *Y. enterocolitica* produce a 10 kDa heat-stable enterotoxin antigenically similar to that produced by some enterotoxigenic *Escherichia coli.* The presence of this toxin in nearly all strains of *Y. enterocolitica*, including environmental strains, the report of the toxin-negative isolates causing illness in animals and man, the inability to detect the toxin in the stools of infected animals, and the ability of the bacteria to produce the toxin at 25°C but not at 37°C, have cast doubt on its role in the pathogenesis of enteric disease.[9,16]

Unlike most other aerobic bacteria, yersinia do not produce iron binding compounds, or siderophores, so that they are dependent on iron bound by other bacteria, or compete with host iron-binding proteins within body tissues. In iron-overloaded patients, such as those receiving frequent blood transfusions (e.g. for thalassaemia), or in haemachromatosis, there is a ready supply of iron and the organisms can thrive. Desferrioxamine therapy has been particularly associated with yersinia sepsis, acting as a bacterial iron-binding protein and possibly inhibiting the polymorphonuclear defence against infection.[17] Even patients with accidental iron overdose treated with desferrioxamine have died from yersinia septicaemia.

Recovery from illness in humans and animals has been associated with antibody production. Protection from an intravenous challenge with *Y. enterocolitica* in mice is mediated by antibody but not by immune cells. Immunodeficient animals (cytotoxin-treated, nude or irradiated mice) and humans (neonates, diabetics, alcoholics, patients with liver cirrhosis or malignancy and those receiving immunosuppressive therapy) have increased susceptibility to unusually severe life-threatening yersiniosis, often complicated by sepsis. This suggests an important role for lymphocyte or macrophage function as well as antibody in recovery from this infection.[2,3]

YERSINIA PSEUDOTUBERCULOSIS

The pathogenesis of *Y. pseudotuberculosis* is much like that of *Y. enterocolitica* except that it appears to be more invasive in animals and humans, usually causing impressive purulent mesenteric adenitis and, less commonly, pyogenic extension to other organs. The pathological hallmark is the epithelioid granuloma with microabscesses in the affected mesenteric nodes, appendix and terminal ileum.[12]

EPIDEMIOLOGY

YERSINIA ENTEROCOLITICA

There has been a rapid increase in the number of cases of *Y. enterocolitica* reported in the past two decades. Whether this is due to improved recognition or a change in incidence is difficult to ascertain, although a serological study performed in Finland demonstrated a 10-fold increase in the prevalence of high levels of anti-*Y. enterocolitica* antibody in donors in 1973 as compared with 1969.

By 1979, over 8000 isolates of *Y. enterocolitica* had been reported worldwide and in several countries (The Netherlands, Belgium, Canada and Australia) the organism now surpasses *Shigella* spp., and rivals *Salmonella* spp. and *Campylobacter* spp. as a cause of acute gastroenteritis. *Y. enterocolitica* has been reported from every continent except Antarctica, with the majority from Western Europe and Canada. In general, serotypes 0:3 (80%) and 0:9 (10–15%) account for most European cases, 0:3 for most Japanese and Canadian cases, and 0:8, 0:5,27 and, more recently, 0:3 for most US cases. Worldwide, 0:3 and 0:9 account for the majority of isolates.[2,3,6] Serotype 0:5,27 has been particularly associated with systemic disease in immunocompromised hosts.

There is a wide geographic variation, with an apparent predilection for colder temperate-climate regions, including Scandinavia, Canada and the northern USA. In most series, except for that from Montreal, Canada, there is an increased incidence of illness in the late autumn and winter months. In prospective studies, 2.8% of ill Canadian children and 5% of Swedish, 1.5% of German and 1.3% of Belgium patients with apparent appendicitis had yersiniosis. In the USA, 0.7–2% of stool cultures from northern states and almost none from southern states have contained yersinia in large prospective studies employing techniques of cold enrichment. In most series, asymptomatic carriage is unusual except in family outbreaks. There does not appear to be a sex predilection for the gastrointestinal syndromes of *Y. enterocolitica*.[2,3,6]

While many non-human serotypes of *Y. enterocolitica* have been isolated from such environmental sources as water, wild and domestic animals and animal products (milk and cheese), there is convincing evidence to implicate contaminated water, milk, pork and family dogs in the spread of *Y. enterocolitica* to humans. Pigs in particular are regarded as important reservoirs of human disease, since they regularly harbour the human pathogenic serotype 0:3. The ability of yersiniae to grow at temperatures at or below 4°C indicates that prolonged refrigeration of certain foodstuffs may provide a source of infection. Family studies have revealed a considerable risk of intrafamily spread. Nearly 30% of families in one large study had multiple cases.[15] More extensive family outbreaks, hospital outbreaks in Finland and Canada, and very large outbreaks in Japan and the USA, including two in the USA linked to contaminated milk, have occurred. There are several reports implicating drinking water as a source of this organism for human infection in single cases and outbreaks.

Although ingestion of the organism accounts for the majority of yersinia infection, transfusion of infected blood products has also been associated with *Y. enterocolitica* sepsis of high mortality. Blood storage temperatures, and the availability of free iron through haemolysis, promotes multiplication of *Yersinia* spp. so that only a small initial inoculum is required from a donor with recent yersinia infection.[1]

YERSINIA PSEUDOTUBERCULOSIS

There are at least six pathogenic serotypes (I–VI) of *Y. pseudotuberculosis* but their relative pathogenicity has not yet been fully investigated. 70% of European strains are group I.

The reservoir of *Y. pseudotuberculosis* is similar to that for *Y. enterocolitica*. It is commonly found in domestic and wild animals, and small family outbreaks have been linked to disease in dogs, cats, chickens and canaries. The cold weather predominance for human disease mirrors that seen in animals. Males are much more frequently infected than females, and the peak age is 5–15 years.

FEATURES

YERSINIA ENTEROCOLITICA

The major clinical syndromes associated with *Y. enterocolitica* include acute febrile gastroenteritis, terminal ileitis and mesenteric adenitis. Less common syndromes include a typhoid-like septicaemic syndrome, extraintestinal pyogenic localized syndromes such as arthritis, meningitis, cellulitis, liver abscess and a host of reactive syndromes such as erythema nodosum, reactive arthritis and, possibly, autoimmune thyroiditis.[2,3,6,8,13]

The most common syndrome (75–80% of cases) is a self-limiting acute febrile gastroenteritis, with nearly 80% of patients being under 5 years of age.[13] This resembles that seen with other invasive bacterial pathogens such as shigella, campylobacter, salmonella, enteroinvasive *E. coli* and *Entamoeba histolytica*. The clinical features include fever of a few days' duration (in 50–90%), vomiting (in 20–40%), abdominal pain (in 20–65%) and diarrhoea (five to ten stools per day) of 2–3 weeks' duration. There may be an associated pharyngitis, with *Y. enterocolitica* isolated from throat swabs. There are case reports of more chronic illness lasting several months which simulates chronic inflammatory bowel disease. Radiographs reveal a patchy mucosal inflammation, ulcerations and 'cobblestoning' of the mucosa, nodular filling defects and occasionally polyp-like structures. Lesions are usually confined to 10–20 cm of the distal ileum or less commonly the ascending colon. Fistulas and strictures are not seen. Sigmoidoscopy reveals ulceration or swollen friable mucosa.[7,18] In a quarter of patients the stool contains blood, and 80% of the time it contains polymorphonuclear leukocytes. Rarely, cases of intestinal ulceration, massive bleeding, perforation and peritonitis have been reported. In most patients, blood cultures are negative and diagnosis is established by recovery of the organism from the stool.

In older children or adults, or possibly in association with more invasive organisms, a pseudo-appendicitis syndrome is encountered in addition to gastroenteritis. This accounts for 10–15% of *Y. enterocolitica* cases and is clinically identical to classical appendicitis, with right lower quadrant tenderness and fever. Radiological examination reveals coarse, irregular nodularity of the intestinal mucosa and ulcerations which resolve over several months. Endoscopy shows colitis, aphthoid ulcers and rarely pseudomembranes.[7,18] The findings at surgery are usually terminal ileitis or mesenteric lymphadenitis. Occasionally, true acute appendicitis or colitis may occur; and, in the USA, the 0:8 serotype may cause severe gangrenous enterocolitis. Diagnosis can be established by culture of the stool and also the involved mesenteric nodes or peritoneal fluid. All cases of mesenteric adenitis should have the involved nodes cultured for *Yersinia* spp.; as well, all cases of acute febrile enteritis and chronic inflammatory bowel disease should have stool cultures performed to exclude yersiniosis.

Cutaneous manifestations including erythematous maculopapular rashes, ulcerative skin lesions, wound infections and erysipelas-like rashes have been reported either in association with the gastrointestinal manifestations or alone. Erythema nodosum, especially in older European women, is not an uncommon finding with or following yersiniosis. Arthritis, usually of the culture-negative reactive variety involving multiple joints, is the most frequent complication of yersiniosis. From 10 to 30% of adults may be affected, with symptoms occurring a few days to a month after the onset of acute diarrhoea. Of those suffering from yersinia arthritis, 90% are of tissue type HLA-B27. Focal signs such as iritis are also more common in HLA-B27-positive patients, whereas erythema nodosum has no correlation with this antigen. This manifestation is much more common in Europe (one-third of cases) than the USA, giving rise to the hypothesis that certain strains, such as 0:3, are more arthritogenic than others. Carditis, haemolytic anaemia, thyroiditis, glomerulonephritis and Reiter's syndrome are less commonly reported non-suppurative sequelae of infection.[2,3,6,8,13]

Septicaemia is unusual and most often reported in children or adults compromised by aplastic anaemia, malnutrition, haemoglobinopathy (especially thalassaemia), malignant disease, liver disease, haemochromatosis or immunosuppressive therapy. Septicaemia in apparently otherwise healthy childen and adults has also been reported. Typical manifestations include fever, headache, malaise and depressed sensorium. Hepatic involvement, with hepatomegaly and abscess, may also occur. The most serious manifestation of yersinia infection, a severe typhoid-like illness, is associated with a case:fatality ratio of approximately 50% despite antibiotic treatment.

Focal pyogenic infections, which are probably secondary to sepsis and which usually occur in similarly immunocompromised individuals, have been reported infrequently. These manifestations, more common in adults than in children, include intra-abdominal abscess, suppurative arthritis, hepatitis, urethritis, meningitis, cholangitis, ophthalmitis, osteomyelitis, endocarditis and lung abscess.

YERSINIA PSEUDOTUBERCULOSIS

The clinical manifestations of *Y. pseudotuberculosis* infection, much rarer than *Y. enterocolitica* disease, are nearly identical to those of the latter agent except for the relative rarity of the typical febrile gastroenteritis syndrome. Instead, the mesenteric and adenitis–pseudoappendicitis syndrome is the most common clinical manifestation of infection with *Y. pseudotuberculosis*, followed by the reactive syndrome (arthritis, erythema nodosum) and sepsis in the categories of patients also susceptible to *Y. enterocolitica* sepsis.[12] Far-eastern scarlatiniform fever is an unusual form of *Y. pseudotuberculosis* infection seen in the USSR, where large outbreaks have occurred. Diagnosis is by appropriate cultures of blood and tissue, especially mesenteric lymph nodes and peritoneal fluid at the time of appendicectomy. Laparoscopy has been utilized to obtain culture material.

INVESTIGATIONS

Yersinia spp. belong to the family Enterobacteriaceae and are Gram-negative coccobacillary rods. *Y. enterocolitica*, originally isolated from humans and first described in the 1930s, has been previously referred to as *Bacterium enterocoliticum*, 'Germe X', *Pasteurella* X, *Pasteurella pseudotuberculosis* B and *Pasteurella pseudotuberculosis rodentium. Y. pseudotuberculosis* was first described as an animal pathogen in 1883, with the first human case reported 75 years later.

YERSINIA ENTEROCOLITICA

Like other Enterobacteriaceae, *Y. enterocolitica* ferments glucose and is oxidase-negative. Lactose is not generally fermented, so that typical pale colonies are produced on lactose-containing media. Cellobiose is fermented, giving rise to a distinctive burgundy pigmentation when the organism is grown on cellobiose–arginine–lysine agar. Urease is produced and, when triple-sugar iron agar is used, both slant and butt reactions are acid, with little or no gas produced.[2,14]

The diagnosis of yersinia infection should ideally combine a positive culture and demonstration of a rise and fall of specific serum antibodies correlated with the clinical course of disease.[4,14] The mere presence of *Yersinia* spp. in faeces may reflect transient passage of non-pathogenic bacteria, while absence of the organism does not exclude infection within mesenteric nodes or other site from which no excretion is occurring.

Y. enterocolitica is relatively easy to isolate from otherwise uncontaminated specimens although strains are remarkable for their physiological diversity, some growing well on media inhibitory for others. It grows well on blood agar and Enterobacteriaceae differential plating media such as MacConkey, desoxycholate-citrate (DCA), and, in most cases, shigella–salmonella agar. Since *Y. enterocolitica* grows slower at 37°C than most enteric pathogens it may be somewhat difficult to isolate from heavily contaminated specimens such as stool. During the acute enteric phase of the illness, especially in children infected with the 0:3 serotype, shedding is so heavy that the organism is relatively easily isolated on the above media in laboratories familiar with the morphology of the 0.5–1.0 mm colonies. For optimal isolation of the organism from heavily contaminated clinical specimens or environmental sources, a good selective medium (such as cefsulodin–irgasan–novobiocin medium) and cold enrichment utilizing the ability of yersinia to grow at a temperature as low as 4°C has proven valuable. Phosphate-buffered saline (5 ml, pH 7.6, 0.067 mol/l) or Rappaport broth is generally inoculated with 0.5 g of faeces and incubated at 4°C for 3–4 weeks with weekly or biweekly subculturing of three separate specimens. Because these techniques are not routine, they require specific communication between the clinician and the microbiology laboratory. Stool cultures positive only after prolonged cold enrichment should be interpreted with caution. Biotyping and serotyping such isolates help in the assessment of clinical relevance.

Subsequent identification by biochemical reactions and motility is performed by standard methods. Presumptive virulence of *Y. enterocolitica* strains is usually indicated by serotyping. Other tests (e.g. detection of V and W antigens) are unsuitable for routine diagnostic use, although use can be made of the nutritional requirement for calcium of virulent strains. *Y. enterocolitica* bearing virulence-associated plasmids produces pin-point colonies on calcium-deficient media, whilst avirulent plasmid-less strains produce much larger colonies (0.5–1 mm diameter).[14] Recently, enzyme-linked immunosorbent assay (ELISA) has been used to detect temperature-dependent proteins released by plasmid-bearing strains of *Yersinia* spp.[11] Antibiotic susceptibility tests by disc and agar diffusion methods have demonstrated susceptibility to co-trimoxazole (trimethoprim–sulphamethoxazole), aminoglycosides (gentamicin, kanamycin, amikacin), chloramphenicol, tetracycline and the new quinolones (e.g. ciprofloxacin). By virtue of β-lactamase activity, *Y. enterocolitica* is resistant to penicillins and the first-generation cephalosporins. The more β-lactamase-stable cephalosporins such as cefotaxime and ceftazidime are active in vitro, but few reports support their use in systemic disease.

Antibodies in animals and humans to various serotypes of *Y. enterocolitica* have been measured by direct tube agglutination, ELISA and differential detection of IgA and IgM by specific techniques. These techniques have been primarily utilized for epidemiological studies or diagnosis of the extraintestinal manifestations of yersinia. The specificity of these methods is generally high, although cross-reactions occur, particularly with *Y. enterocolitica* serotype 0:9 and *Brucella* spp. (rarely of practical importance unless brucellosis is endemic), and serotype 0:5,27 and *E. coli*. Other cross-reactions with *Salmonella* spp. can be largely overcome by absorbing serum with the cross-reacting antigens before measuring agglutinating titres. False negative results may also occur, especially in young children. Agglutinating antibodies to *Y. enterocolitica* appear soon after onset of illness, but generally disappear within 2–6 months, although titres remain higher for longer in patients with arthritis or erythema nodosum. A four-fold rise in antibody titre (samples taken 10 days apart), or a significantly high titre with subsequent fall is compatible with invasive disease. A titre of 1/160 for *Y. enterocolitica* is regarded as significantly elevated.[4,14]

YERSINIA PSEUDOTUBERCULOSIS

Y. pseudotuberculosis shares many of the biochemical and motility characteristics of *Y. enterocolitica* but is cellobiose-negative. Isolation techniques for its growth are similar to those for *Y. enterocolitica.*

Laboratory diagnosis of *Y. pseudotuberculosis* infection is established by isolation of the organism from biopsy material, histological examination of lymph nodes, and by demonstration of specific antibodies in serum.[14] A titre of 1/320 is regarded as significantly elevated on direct tube agglutination. A retrospective diagnosis of *Y. pseudotuberculosis* infection can be made by a positive response to a specific skin test antigen. This skin sensitivity may persist for 5–6 years, and so does not necessarily indicate active infection.

Unlike *Y. enterocolitica*, *Y. pseudotuberculosis* does not produce β-lactamase, and so most strains are sensitive to penicillins.

DIFFERENTIAL DIAGNOSIS

The differential diagnosis of yersinia gastroenteritis and mesenteric adenitis includes infection by shigella, salmonella, campylobacter, *Ent. hystolytica*, enteroinvasive *E. coli*, antibiotic-associated colitis, chronic inflammatory bowel disease and rarely tuberculosis, tularaemia, brucellosis, sarcoid and Epstein–Barr virus infection. The typhoidal-sepsis syndrome can be simulated by any organism causing septicaemia, but especially salmonella.

TREATMENT

Therapy for the milder yersinia syndromes such as gastroenteritis and mesenteric adenitis and for the reactive syndromes such as erythema nodosum and arthritis remains controversial. There is no evidence that antimicrobial treatment either modifies the clinical syndrome or the duration of shedding of the organism. Supportive therapy with fluids and electrolytes as well as anti-inflammatory agents in the reactive syndromes are indicated.[3,6,13]

Specific antimicrobial therapy is indicated in the *Y. enterocolitica*-caused typhoidal-sepsis syndrome and the rare pyogenic complications (wound infections, hepatic abscess, meningitis and septic arthritis). In these settings chloramphenicol (50–75 mg/kg per day), aminoglycosides (gentamicin, 5–7.5 mg/kg per day) and tetracycline (20–30 mg/kg per day) have had apparently beneficial effects. It would be anticipated from in vitro susceptibility testing and experiences with shigellosis and salmonellosis that trimethoprim–sulphamethoxazole (trimethoprim 10–20 mg/kg per day orally or intravenously) would be efficacious. The new quinolones (e.g. ciprofloxacin) are also effective, and may prove to be the future drugs of choice.[10] In gastroenteritis in a highly susceptible host, such as a neonate or a patient with malnutrition, cancer, haemochromatosis or haemoglobinopathy or receiving immunosuppresive therapy, specific antimicrobial therapy is probably indicated to treat 'incipient' sepsis.[3,13]

Similar principles probably hold true for therapy of *Y. pseudotuberculosis*, with therapy including ampicillin (100–200 mg/kg per day), tetracycline (20–30 mg/kg per day orally) or streptomycin (20–30 mg/kg per day intramuscularly).

CONTROL, PREVENTION AND PROGNOSIS

Basic control measures rely on appropriate personal and food hygiene to prevent spread from animals to humans and from person to person. This is especially important in families with an index case and in hospitals. Patients with yersiniosis must be cared for with enteric isolation strictly enforced. The normal period of shedding of *Y. enterocolitica* in stools of convalescing humans varies from 2 weeks to as long as 4 months, with a mean of 42 days in one large prospective series. There is no vaccine for this illness or any data regarding the value of prophylactic antimicrobial therapy. In a common-source outbreak, rapid identification of the source will help to curtail the spread of illness as well as possibly prevent unnecessary operations for the pseudoappendicitis syndrome. Unfortunately, it may be necessary to perform an appendicectomy to exclude true appendicitis.

Nearly all the syndromes caused by *Y. enterocolitica* and *Y. pseudotuberculosis* are self-limiting with full recovery. The exceptions are those cases of sepsis with a 50–75% mortality rate, and septic complications, which may require prolonged antimicrobial therapy as well as drainage of areas of purulence.[2,3,6,13,15]

The ability of the organism to grow at 4°C, and the probability of meats (especially pork) being a source of infection, indicate that at-risk foodstuffs should not be refrigerated for prolonged periods before consumption. If milk-borne outbreaks are to be prevented, then care must be taken in dairies to prevent contamination of milk after pasteurization. Screening potential blood donors for gastrointestinal symptoms in the month prior to donation, and minimizing periods of blood product storage, may reduce the risk of tranfusion-associated yersiniosis.[1]

Further understanding of the virulence factors and basic immunity should allow the development of an efficacious vaccine for use in high-risk settings. At present, a high index of suspicion in the appropriate setting and communication between the clinician and the microbiology laboratory will facilitate diagnosis and our further understanding of these fascinating organisms.

REFERENCES

1. Aber, R.C. (1990) Transfusion-associated *Yersinia enterocolitica*. *Transfusion*, **30**, 193–195.

2. Bottone, E.J. (1977) *Yersinia enterocolitica*: a panoramic view of a charismatic microorganism. *CRC Critical Reviews in Microbiology*, **5**, 211–241.
3. Bottone, E.J. (1981) *Yersinia enterocolitica*. Boca Raton: CRC Press.
4. Bottone, E.J. and Sheehan, D.J. (1983) *Yersinia enterocolitica*: guidelines for serologic diagnosis of human infection. *Reviews of Infectious Disease*, **5**, 898–906.
5. Brenner, D.J., Ursing, J., Benovier, H. *et al.* (1980) Deoxyribonucleic acid relatedness in *Yersinia enterocolitica* and *Yersinia enterocolitica*-like organisms. *Current Microbiology*, **4**, 195–200.
6. Carter, P.B., LaFleur, L. and Toma, S. (1979) *Yersinia enterocolitica*. Biology, epidemiology and pathology. In *Microbiology and Immunology*, Vol. 5. Basel: Karger.
7. El-Maraghi, N.R.H. and Main, N.S. (1979) The histopathology of enteric infection with *Yersinia pseudotuberculosis*. *American Journal of Clinical Pathology*, **71**, 631–639.
8. Friedberg, M., Larsen, S. and Denneberg, T. (1978) *Yersinia enterocolitica* and glomerulonephritis. *The Lancet*, **i**, 499.
9. Gemski, P., Lazere, J.R. and Casey, T. (1980) Plasmid associated with pathogenicity and calcium dependency of *Yersinia enterocolitica*. *Infection and Immunity*, **27**, 682–685.
10. Hoogkamp-Korstanje, J.A. (1987) Antibiotics in *Yersinia enterocolitica* infections. *Journal of Antimicrobial Chemotherapy*, **20**, 123–131.
11. Kaneko, S. and Maruyama, T. (1989) Evaluation of enzyme immunoassay for the detection of pathogenic *Yersinia enterocolitica* and *Yersinia pseudotuberculosis* strains. *Journal of Clinical Microbiology*, **27**, 748–751.
12. Knapp, W. (1958) Mesenteric adenitis due to *Pasteurella pseudotuberculosis* in young people. *New England Journal of Medicine*, **259**, 776–778.
13. Kohl, S. (1979) *Yersinia enterocolitica* infections. *Pediatric Clinics of North America*, **26**, 433–444.
14. Mair, N.S. and Fox, E.J. (1986) *Yersiniosis*. London: Public Health Laboratory Service.
15. Marks, M.I., Pai, C.H., LaFleur, L. *et al.* (1980) *Yersinia enterocolitica* gastroenteritis. A prospective study of clinical, bacteriologic, and epidemiologic features. *Journal of Pediatrics,* **96**, 26–31.
16. Portney, D.A., Moseley, S.L. and Falkow, S. (1981) Characterization of plasmids and plasmid-associated determinants of *Yersinia enterocolitis* pathogenesis. *Infection and Immunity*, **31**, 775–782.
17. Robins-Browne, R.M. and Prpic, J.K. (1983) Desferrioxamine and systemic yersiniosis. *The Lancet*, **i**, 1372.
18. Vantrappen, G., Agg, H.O., Ponette, E. *et al.* (1977) Yersinia enteritis and enterocolitis: gastroenterological aspects. *Gastroenterology*, **72**, 220–227.

SCHISTOSOMIASIS

G. Webbe

Some 200 million people are probably infested with schistosomiasis – also termed bilharziasis – and 500 million to 600 million exposed to the risk of infestation in 76 countries.[85] Three main species of schistosomes or 'blood flukes' cause human infections, *Schistosoma haematobium*, *S. mansoni* and *S. japonicum* (*Table 9.11*).

Cercariae of other mammalian schistosomes, such as *S. margrebowiei* (Le Roux, 1933) and *S. rodhaini* (Brumpt, 1931) also penetrate humans, as do schistosomes of birds, and may cause cercarial dermatitis ('swimmer's itch').[86]

PARASITOLOGY

The species of human schistosomes are similar in their basic life-cycles, but they exhibit pronounced differences in their ability to infest the particular groups of snails which they utilize as intermediate hosts and in their ability to infest other mammalian hosts.

The adult schistosomes are approximately 10–20 mm in length and superficially resemble roundworms: an adaptation to their habitat inside blood vessels. The filiform female worm is held within the 'schist' or gynaecophoric canal of the shorter male worm. The integument of the schistosome is a living tissue rather than a chitinous protective sheath and is an important site for host antigen attachment. The worms ingest red blood cells and possess a protease that breaks down globin and haemoglobin, releasing tyrosine. The black, haematin-like pigment, which is regurgitated by the adult worms, is taken up by the mononuclear phagocytic system in the liver and spleen. The adult worms may live for 20–30 years, but the mean life-span is probably much shorter (3–8 years). Each worm pair, according to the species of schistosome, produces 300–3000 or more eggs per day. The schistosomes do not multiply in the definitive hosts, and the infestation process produces, or

Table 9.11 Important schistosomes, their geographical distribution and some characteristics

	Distribution	*Molluscs*	*Location*	*Eggs*	*Infection*
Schistosoma haematobium (Bilharz, 1852)	Most African and some Middle Eastern countries.	Genus *Bulinus* (aquatic)	Veins of vesical plexus.	Terminal spine, passed in urine and sometimes faeces. 20–300 per worm pair daily	Urinary or vesical schistosomiasis
Schistosoma mansoni (Sambon, 1907)	Most African countries, parts of Arabia, northern and eastern parts of South America, some Caribbean islands	Genus *Biomphalaria* (aquatic)[11,64]	Inferior mesenteric vein and tributaries	Lateral spine, passed in faeces and sometimes urine. 100–300 per worm pair daily	Intestinal schistosomiasis
Schistosoma japonicum (Katsurada, 1904)	Mainland China, Philippines, Japan (very small extent), Celebes, Malaysia	Genus *Oncomelania* (amphibians)[25]	Superior and inferior mesenteric veins and tributaries	Vestigial spine, passed in faeces. >3000 per worm pair daily	Intestinal schistosomiasis
Schistosoma mekongi[77] (Voge, Buckner and Brucer, 1978)	Laos, Cambodia, Thailand, Central African Republic	Genus *Tricula*[25]	Superior and inferior mesenteric veins and tributaries	Vestigial spine – smaller than *S. japonicum*	Intestinal schistosomiasis[77]
Schistosoma intercalatum (Fisher, 1934)	Zaire, Cameroon, Gabon, Central African Republic	Genus *Bulinus*	Inferior mesenteric vein and tributaries	Large terminal spine, passed in faeces	Intestinal schistosomiasis[98]
Schistosoma mattheei (Veglia and LeRoux, 1929)	Southern Africa, where it replaces *S. bovis*	Genus *Bulinus* (parasite of cattle, infections in humans together with *S. haematobium or S. mansoni*	Probably veins of vesical plexus and inferior mesenteric vein and tributaries	Terminal spine, passed in urine and faeces	Urinary and intestinal symptoms[67]

tends to produce, an overdispersed distribution of parasites within the host population, in which most individuals carry few parasites and a small proportion are heavily infested. Thus, in schistosomiasis, although the proportion of those with infestations of high intensity is relatively low, morbidity may be appreciable.

The complex life-cycle involves alternating parasitic and free-living stages: the egg, miracidium, first-stage (mother) sporocyst, second-stage (daughter) sporocyst, cercaria, schistosomulum, and adult schistosome. The sexual generation of adult schistosomes is present in the definitive vertebrate host and the multiplicative asexual phase in a molluscan host (see *Figure 9.26*).

The non-operculate yellowish eggs contain the embryo (miracidium), which develops inside over a period of 6 days. If the egg remains in the tissues, it lives for a further 15 days, secreting histiolytic antigenic material. The egg dies some 21 days after oviposition, releasing products of autolysis. The eggshell is destroyed over a period of weeks or months, depending upon whether or not calcification has taken place. The ova which pass through the bladder or intestinal wall (probably less than 50% of total egg production) contain embryos which are usually visibly motile and ready to hatch when the eggs are passed. When urine or faeces is diluted by fresh water, and usually under the influence of warmth (10–30°C) and light, the miracidia become active and emerge from the eggshells.

The miracidia of the schistosomes that infest humans differ in size but are similar in their behaviour and morphology. Penetration of the miracidium occurs when the larva becomes attached to the body surface of the snail by a secretion from the apical gland cells. The cycle within the snail intermediate hosts (sporocysts) between the penetration of the miracidium larva and the production of mature cercariae lasts approximately 4–5 weeks for *S. mansoni*, 5–6 weeks for *S. haematobium* and 7 weeks or more for *S. japonicum*.

Daily output of cercariae from the snail may vary from one or two to several thousand. The penetration process of the cercaria is quite rapid and may penetrate the stratuum corneum within a few minutes, and at the same time the larva changes in appearance to become a worm-like schistosomulum (*Figure 9.27a*). Within a few hours of penetration, the trilaminate membrane of the cercaria is replaced by the multilaminate integument of the schistosomulum and adult. The passage through the subcutaneous tissue may be effected within 48 hours, and peripheral lymphatic and venous vessels are penetrated, from which transportation to the right heart and the lungs is achieved. Available evidence suggests that worms leave the lungs via the pulmonary veins and pass through the heart to the systemic circulation, and that an individual worm may make several circuits of the pulmonary and systemic circulation before entering a blood vessel which leads to the hepatic–portal system. Most sexually mature worms leave the liver when they have mated and, depending on the species, migrate to the different egg-laying sites. A period of some 30–40 days may elapse between successful cercarial penetration and the appearance of eggs in the urine or stools of the definite host, but it may be much longer.[87]

PATHOLOGY

Three disease syndromes are associated with schistosome infestation: dermatitis, which results from cercarial penetration of the skin; acute schistosomiasis, or Katayama fever, which occurs in intense initial infestation and usually coincides with the onset of egg-laying by the worms; and chronic schistosomiasis, in which lesions in different organs are dependent on main egg-laying sites of the adult worms. Approximately 4–12% of patients in endemic areas show advanced disease, but most patients are asymptomatic carriers of the parasite, or show a mild non-specific symptomatology, the pathology of the schistosome infestation being represented by a few scattered granulomas around eggs in different organs (see *Table 9.12*).

The major parasite factor responsible for the occurrence of chronic disease is the egg. The host granulomatous response to the egg plays an essential part in the pathogenesis of the various disease syndromes[81] (see *Table 9.13*).

An exaggerated fibroblastic reaction to focally accumulated eggs may give rise to a pseudoneoplastic lesion and patients may be falsely diagnosed as having malignancy, especially if they develop intestinal masses. The cause of such a pseudoneoplastic lesion is apparently local, since host reaction to the schistosome eggs in other areas may be focal and limited.[4] In tissue sections, live schistosome worms may be identified inside blood vessels unaccompanied by any local reaction (*Figure 9.27b*). When the worm dies and disintegrates it may produce vascular thrombosis and inflammation.

INFESTATION WITH *S. MANSONI*

Several factors contribute to pathogenesis, including intensity of infestation. The worm burden in the

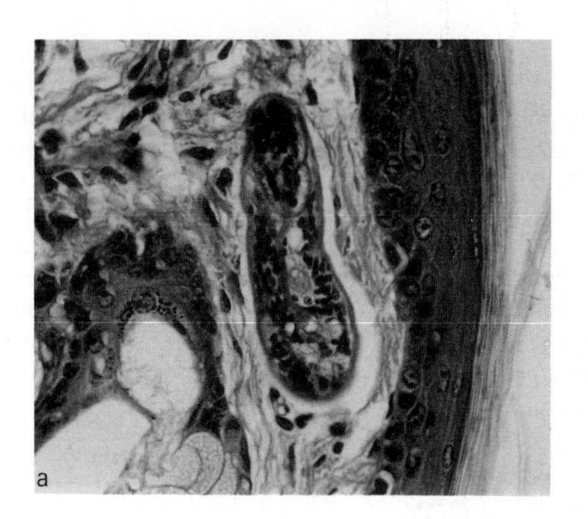

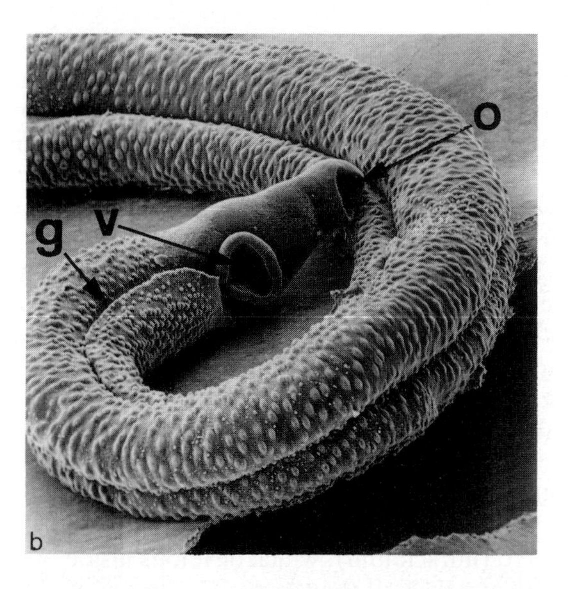

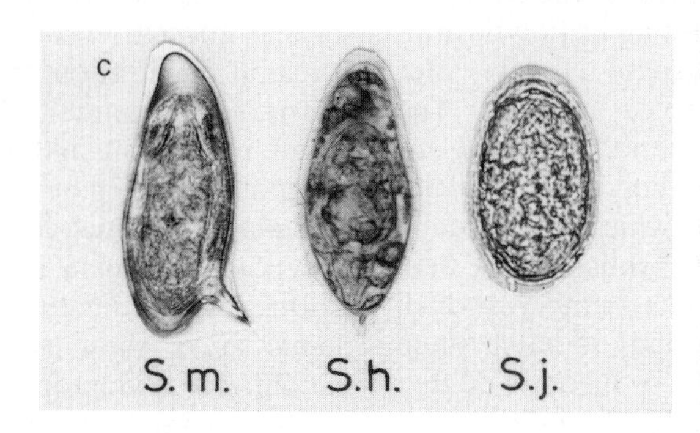

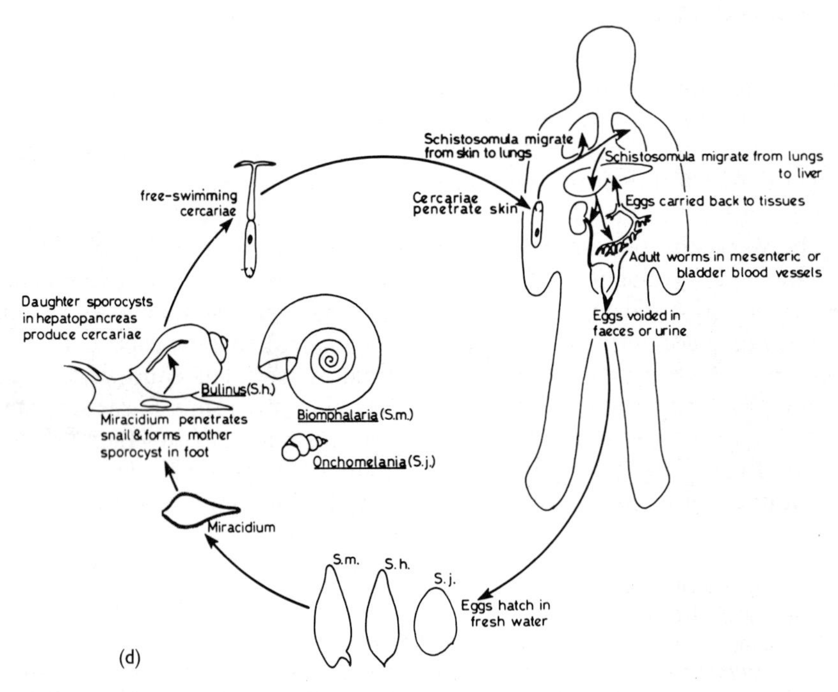

Figure 9.26 (a) Schistosomulum (*S. haematobium*, section 6 μm, stained with haematoxylin and eosin) in the dermis of a mouse 2 days post-infestation. (Photomicrograph courtesy of M. Nilsson.) (b) Adult male *S. haematobium* showing oral (o) and ventral (v) suckers, integument with tubercles and gynaecophoric canal (g). (Scanning electron micrograph courtesy of M. Hicks.) (c) Eggs of *S. mansoni* (S.m.), *S. haematobium* (S.h.) and *S. japonicum* (S.j.). (d) Schistosome life-cycle (*S. mansoni*, S.m.; *S. haematobium*, S.h.; *S. japonicum*, S.j.). (Diagram courtesy of E. James.)

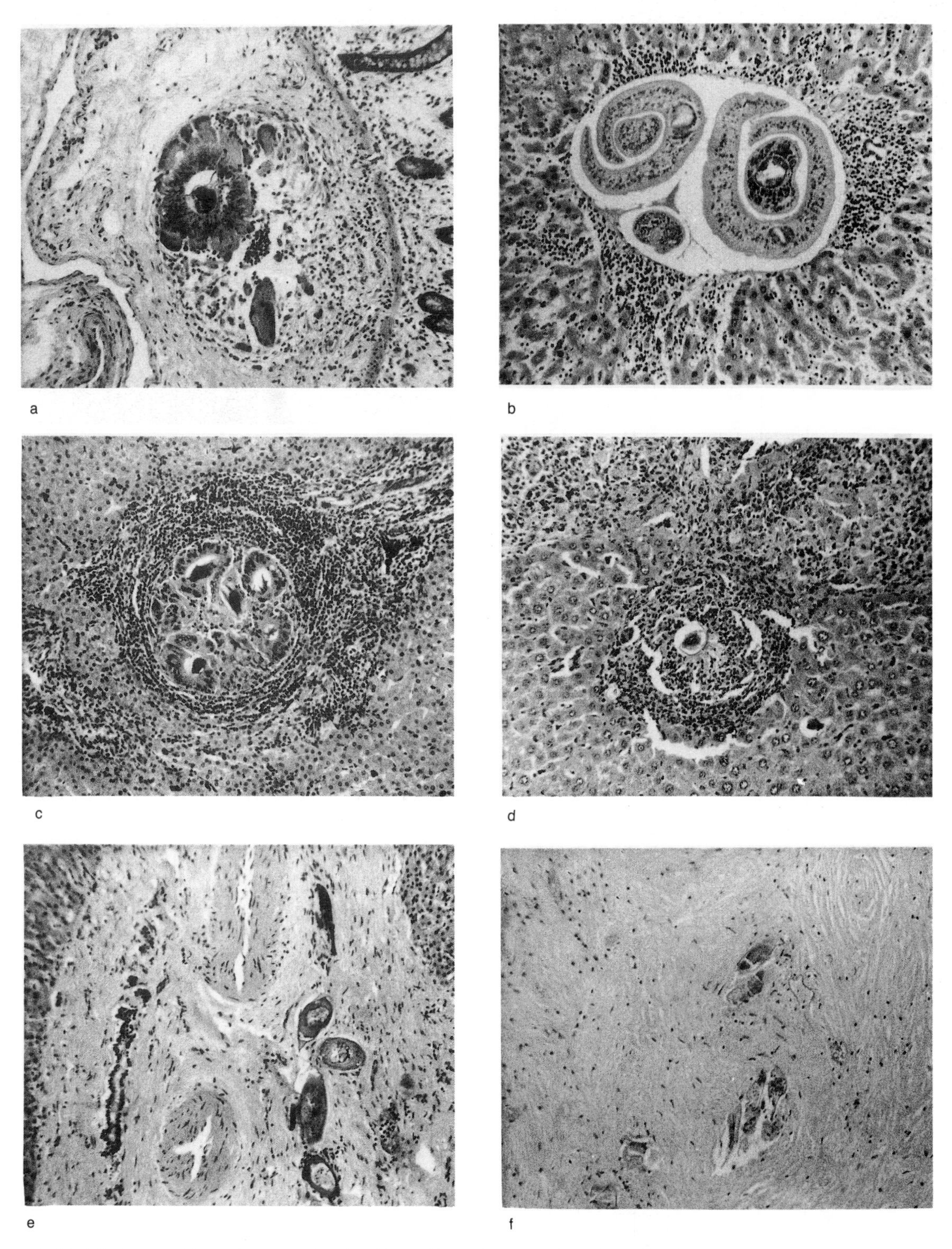

Figure 9.27 (a) Section of large intestine showing 'Hoeppli' reaction around an *S. mansoni* egg; surrounding cellular infiltrate contains giant cells. (b) Transverse section of a blood vessel showing two pairs of adult schistosomes, the females lying in the gypaecophoric canal of the male worms. (c) Schistosome granuloma in liver; a clump of eggs and surrounding giant cells with an intense cellular infiltrate. (d) Granuloma around an *S. japonicum* egg in liver section. (e) Symmers' fibrosis: increased periportal connective tissue and bundles of fibrous tissue surrounding a large clump of eggs. (f) *S. haematobium* eggs surrounded by concentric rings of loose fibrous tissue in a peritoneal mass. (Sections 5 μm, stained with haematoxylin and eosin, kindly provided by H. Furse.)

Table 9.12 Pathology and clinical features[82,91]

Stage	*Parasitological*	*Clinical*	*Pathological*
1. Invasive	Penetration – cercariae	Hypersensitivity reaction – immediate and delayed types	Papular dermatitis
	Migration – schistosomula	Fever and cough	Inflammatory reactions in lungs and liver
2. Maturation	Maturation – adult worms, migration to egg-laying sites, early oviposition	Acute febrile illness, Katayama fever – form of serum sickness or immune complex disease	Intense reactions (general and local) to products of eggs and/or young schistosomes
3. Established infection	Intense oviposition: high levels of egg excretion	Early chronic disease, digestive symptoms, haematuria. Severity of disease related to worm burden and intensity of host response. Initial massive infection produces more severe clinical symptoms	Reaction around viable eggs is destructive. Periovular area of necrosis with or without deposition of hyaline eosinophilic band (Hoeppli phemomenon), surrounded by exudative cellular reaction with many eosinophils. New eggs produced as infection progresses, but reaction around them becomes smaller (modulates), more discrete, and purely proliferative. Granuloma formation with little fibrosis in early stages
4. Chronic	Prolonged duration often with reduced egg excretion	Chronic diseases, portal hypertension, pulmonary hypertension, cor pulmonale, obstruction of gastrointestinal tract, obstructive uropathy	Development of fibrous tissue in different sites according to species of schistosome with lesions in different organs

Table 9.13 The schistosome egg granuloma or pseudotubercle

	Mechanisms of formation	*Cellular constituents*
S. mansoni *S. haematobium*	A cell-mediated immune reaction dependent on thymus-derived lymphocytes and formed independently of humoral antibody	Ovum engulfed by multinucleated giant cells surrounded by macrophages, eosinophils, polymorphonuclear and mononuclear leukocytes, round cells and plasma cells – in contrast to tubercle granulomas which consist almost entirely of macrophages. Fibroblasts replace some cells as healing takes place
S. japonicum	Possibly an immediate hypersensitivity (antibody-mediated) response or 'foreign body' type of reaction	In *S. japonicum* infestation, granulomas contain more neutrophils and plasma cells, necrosis and exudation occur with Hoeppli phenomenon frequently present – also less frequently seen in *S. mansoni* and *S. haematobium* infestations. Hoeppli phenomenon is an eosinophilic corona around usually viable *S. japonicum* ova within about 10% of granulomas in heavy infestations. Precipitate is an antigen–antibody complex with gradient to antibody excess at periphery

human population (best represented indirectly by faecal egg counts) increases with age, and usually reaches a maximum between 10 and 20 years and declines thereafter. According to De Cock,[26] clinical, epidemiological and pathological studies support the relationship between intensity of *S. mansoni* infestation and severity of the disease but may not be reliable for evaluating individuals. Heavy *S. mansoni* infestation is probably the most important factor in the development of fibrosis. *S. mansoni* is a complex of parasites and ten polymorphic gene loci have been reported in *S. mansoni*.[51] Studies in Brazil have shown a greater resistance in black people to the development of severe forms of *S. mansoni*, while intensity of infestation and prevalence rates were similar in the three racial groups (whites, mulattos and blacks) studied.[8] In St Lucia, a higher proportion of East Indian patients had hepatosplenomegaly than black persons.[43] Among patients in Brazil, with untreated *S. mansoni* infestation, those with blood group A had a higher frequency of hepatosplenic disease than those with blood group O, who tended to have a milder form of the disease.[13] No difference could be established in a study from the Sudan.[29] Genetic factors relating to HLA haplotype may influence the pathogenesis of disease and susceptibility to infestation in human schistosomiasis.[1] Thirty-two antigens of the HLA series were studied from Egyptian children, with asymptomatic *S. mansoni* infestation, colonic polyposis and schistosomal hepatosplenomegaly. The results showed that the hepatosplenomegaly was associated with the presence of two HLA antigens, HLA-A1 and -B5, and colonic polyposis with a presence of HLA-B5 and -B8. A significant association was found with antigen HLA-CW2 in patients with asymptomatic infections. Other genetic predisposition has been considered in the development of hepatic schistosomiasis. α-1-Antitrypsin deficiency was not associated with hepatosplenic schistosomiasis.[37]

ACUTE SCHISTOSOMIASIS

Pathology

There is evidence of hepatitis on needle biopsy of the liver and the spleen signs of acute infectious splenitis, with intense eosinophilic infiltrates. The intestinal mucosa, including the jejenum and ileum, may show superficial necrotic and haemorrhagic ulcers. The acute phase is characterized by large granulomata which are found mainly in the liver and intestine and less frequently in other organs. Intralobular foci of necrosis and destruction of hepatocytes occur in the enlarged liver, with portal infiltration of histiocytes, eosinophils, lymphocytes, and hyperplasia and hypertrophy of the Kupffer cells.[10] The spleen enlarges with intensive eosinophilia and congestion of the sinuses. In severe cases a necrotizing arteritis may occur in the lungs with miliary dissemination of eggs and granulomas with exudate and necrosis in the liver, intestines, peritoneum, abdominal and pulmonary lymphatic glands, pleura, lungs and pancreas. Severe eodema, erythema, haemorrhages, petechiae, small ulcerations and punctate elevations are found in the rectum and sigmoid.

Clinical features

The acute form of *S. mansoni* infestation (the Katayama syndrome) is rarely observed in endemic populations; however, visitors to endemic areas are susceptible to developing the acute symptoms.[32,35] The incubation period of the Katayama syndrome varies between 2 and 8 weeks. Severity is usually related to intensity of infestation. In a small proportion of infestations, acute symptoms can start before egg deposition by the female worms. Symptoms last from a few weeks to several months, and gradually abate without therapeutic intervention. The main clinical manifestations of acute infestations include fever (intermittent or remittent, with breaks in the late evening), rigors, sweating, headache, general muscular pain, unproductive cough, abdominal pain, diarrhoea, urticaria, focal oedema, lymphadenopathy and loss of weight. The liver is usually tender and enlarged, with or without a slightly enlarged and soft spleen. During the acute phase of *S. mansoni* infestation death is exceptional.[68]

Investigations

There is commonly a leukocytosis, with a high percentage of eosinophils (10–75%). Serum concentrations of IgM, IgE and IgG are elevated, whereas IgA is normal.[32] The titres of species-specific anti-schistosome antibody in serum are also markedly elevated.[35] Serological responses to schistosome-specific antigens may differentiate patients in the acute phase from those in the chronic phase.[59] In acute cases, comparatively higher IgM antibody and lower IgG levels were seen; in chronic cases, comparatively lower IgM antibody and higher IgG concentrations were observed compared with healthy individuals. Faecal egg counts which depend on the time of examination after infestation are often high, although low faecal egg counts in the acute syndrome are frequently observed.

CHRONIC SCHISTOSOMIASIS

Following the acute phase of infestation, patients may be symptom-free or progress to the chronic phase. The chronic intestinal form produces vague, poorly defined symptoms. Patients lack pronounced hypersensitivity to *S. mansoni* and do not develop an acute clinical syndrome following chronic re-exposure. *S. mansoni* eggs are present in the stool, and the egg excretion pattern is relatively stable. Asymptomatic infestation may become symptomatic after recurrent exposure and reinfestation, or with continuous, long-term egg deposition without treatment. The typical population distribution of *S. mansoni* infestations shows heavy infestations (more than 100–800 eggs per gram of faeces, depending on the endemic area) being seen only in a small proportion of the infested population, i.e. an example of a truncated form of the negative binomial.[12,38,68] Whether the number of eggs in faeces per worm pair decreases as the number of worm pairs in a person increases, as observed in some other intestinal helminth infestations (i.e. egg production of *S. mansoni* is influenced by a density-dependent factor), has led to some disagreement.[17,56,89] While morbidity is related to the intensity of the infestation, there are variations between geographical areas.[85] Patients with hepatosplenic schistosomiasis usually have fewer eggs per gram of faeces per worm pair than persons with earlier-stage chronic disease. Involvement of the small intestine involving two cases of duodenal disease, diagnosed by gastroscopy and biopsy and following jejunal biopsy have been reported.[33,73]

It is uncertain whether *S. mansoni* infestation plays a role in the pathogensis of hepatocellular carcinoma.[57] No geographical association of liver carcinoma and *S. mansoni* infestation has been documented, and in autopsy series from Brazil, Puerto Rico, Egypt and Mozambique hepatomas were almost equally distributed in patients not infested and infested with *S. mansoni*.[15,90] Also, patients with inflammatory bowel disease have an increased risk of developing colorectal cancer and chronic colitis, with or without polyposis, which is common in *S. mansoni* infestation. The association of *S. mansoni* infestation with colon cancer is coincidental in Egypt, elsewhere in Africa and in the Western hemisphere.[16]

Pathology

Variable degrees of fibrosis are seen in the portal tracts of the liver, with eggs, granulomata and cellular infiltrates (*Figure 9.27c,d*). These changes are found in the intestines (*Figure 9.27a*) and, less often, in the lungs and other organs. Eggs are trapped in the mucosa and submucosa of the large intestines, where they produce granulomatous reactions and are eventually destroyed. Bilharziomas are localized masses of fibrous and inflammatory tissue containing numerous eggs. They develop most frequently in the intestinal serosa or in the mesentery. *S. mansoni* eggs become much less frequently calcified, however, than those of *S. japonicum* and severe changes are rarely seen. Increased vascularity of the mucosa of the large intestine is common and small papillomatous growths may occur.[28] Extreme fibrosis and oedema of the intestinal wall and of the retroperitoneal tissues have been reported. Granulomatous tumours on the ante-mesenteric surface of the small intestine with intestinal obstruction has been reported from Africa.[99] Schistosomal stenosis has been recorded in Brazil.[14]

Symmers' fibrosis is an irreversible but not necessarily inevitable lesion of chronic *S. mansoni* and *S. japonicum* infestation. Portal tracts become surrounded by broad bands of fibrotic (collagen-rich) tissue, with a macroscopic appearance similar to clay pipe stems.[14] Diffuse bilharzial fibrosis also occurs when ova are deposited in small numbers over a period of time.[39]

Unlike cirrhosis, when fibrosis follows degeneration of the liver cells, it is interstitial and invasive, being unique to schistosomiasis.[39] Granulomata around ova are numerous in the portal spaces and smaller than in the early stages of infestation, and may disappear completely. The liver parenchyma remains intact except in focal areas of necrosis.[18]

In many cases of Symmers' fibrosis, the spleen increases in size due to congestion caused by portal hypertension, and hyperplasia of the reticuloendothelial elements results. In some patients with hepatosplenic schistosomiasis in Brazil, progressive glomerulosclerotic changes have been noted leading to glomerulonephritis. IgG and IgM complexes have been found in kidney biopsy specimens of patients with *S. mansoni* infestations with or without nephrosis.[5,69]

Liver changes in *S. mansoni, S. japonicum* and *S. haematobium* infestations are similar but differ in degree. In addition to granuloma formation, portal inflammation is seen, with possible invasion of the parenchymal border by lymphocytes and histiocytes. Portal inflammation is probably due to toxins from ova, being a delayed hypersensitivity reaction due to schistosome antigen.

Clinical features

Despite the almost universal involvement of the intestine in *S. mansoni* infestation, malabsorption is rare.[81] Protein-losing enteropathy is uncommon, but has been recorded in patients in Egypt with intestinal polyposis[49] where colonic polyposis is a common complication of schistosomiasis. It is rare in other parts of Africa, including the endemic countries neighbouring Egypt such as the Sudan.[30,95] Patients in Egypt with colonic polyposis are men less than 30 years of age.

The fibrotic changes in the liver lead to portal hypertension with enlargement of the spleen and specifically in most children with more than 800 *S. mansoni* eggs per gram of faeces. In persistent infestation and an evolving pathological process hepatic enlargement occurs in the second or third decades of life.[31]

Symmers' 'clay pipe stem' fibrosis occurs in the 6–20 year age group some 5–15 years after the onset of infection (*Figure 9.27e*). The liver and spleen are palpable, the liver eventually becomes hard and nodular.[9] The portal hypertension produces oesophageal varices, a common site of haematemesis.

Hepatic encephalopathy is unusual in hepatic schistosomiasis and death from hepatic failure in *S. mansoni* infestation is rare, with the exception of cases complicated with hepatitis B infection, which may lead to decompensated hepatosplenic disease.[31] Splenectomy with splenorenal anastomosis has been used in the treatment of portal hypertension in Brazil and Egypt, but portacaval anastomosis has lead to encephalopathy in 35–40% of cases. Many patients with hepatosplenomegaly have massive oesophageal varices but they carry a better prognosis than patients with non-schistosomal cirrhoses.[79] Haematemesis, although difficult to treat, is rarely fatal and few patients develop hepatic coma. As portal hypertension increases, so does the chance of developing pulmonary hypertension and cor pulmonale. A cyanotic syndrome with clubbing of the fingers has been reported in patients with portal hypertension and hepatosplenomegaly.[3]

Ultrasonography is used in the investigation, diagnosis and study of hepatic schistosomiasis and the sonographic features of schistosomal periportal fibrosis have been described by Abdel-Wahab *et al.*[2]

INFESTATION WITH *S. JAPONICUM*

Peak prevalence and intensity of infestation are generally observed in the 15–20 year age groups, but may occur in older persons.[92]

EPIDEMIOLOGY

The epidemiology and control of *S. japonicum* infestations are greatly influenced by zoonotic infestation, and in endemic areas in China some 31 mammalian species have been found naturally infested with *S. japonicum*. Cattle are the most important reservoirs of contamination of the environment[7] and, in the Philippines, animal reservoirs were considered responsible for about 25% of the total potential environmental contamination.[58] In Sulawesi, Indonesia, at least 13 species of wild and domestic animals have been found to be infested with *S. japonicum*.[48]

Several different factors act independently or synergistically to influence pathological changes due to *S. japonicum* infestations in humans. These include: intensity of infestation;[94] strains of *S. japonicum* (there are at least four geographical strains from China, the Philippines, Japan and Indonesia that may infest humans[20]) host genetic factors,[78] and the immune status of the host.[60] Thus, some degree of protective immunity does occur in *S. japonicum* infestations, irrespective of race, sex and age but is only incomplete or partial.[55]

PATHOLOGY

Changes in the liver are similar to those in *A. mansoni* infestations. The left lobe of the liver is usually disproportionately enlarged in *S. japonicum* infestation. In addition to the pipe stem portal fibrosis, extensive intralobular fibrosis may be present. The gastrointestinal tract lesions tend to be focal and isolated compared with *S. mansoni* infestation.[75,76]

The pathogenesis of the brain lesions is not clearly understood. An intense granulomatous reaction is caused in the central vessels and in the brain or there may be diffuse involvement with scattered lesions.[46]

CLINICAL FEATURES

Advanced hepatosplenic disease is usually associated with abdominal collateral vein dilatation and oeosophagogastric varices. Haematemesis, melena and ascites are frequent. Ascites associated with the late stage of schistosomiasis has a more protracted natural evolution than liver cirrhosis, and it may persist for as long as 10–20 years with a variable clinical course.[62] Blood loss due to bleeding of the oeosophagogastric varices is the major cause of death in *S. japonicum* infestation.[26]

ACUTE INFESTATION

Clinical features

There is little evidence that *S. japonicum* cercariae produce swimmer's itch. The 'Kabure' syndrome of

Japan is probably due to non-human cercariae.[80] There may be early skin manifestations following cercarial penetration, which with the accompanying pruritis, has been ascribed to anaphylaxis. The acute stage or 'Katayama fever' most commonly found in *S. japonicum* infestation is characterized by fever, eosinophilia (30–80%), splenomegaly, lymphadenopathy, urticaria and frequently diarrhoea or dysentery. It is usually seen in heavy primary infestations and may result in death.[80] The incubation period usually lasts some 40 days with a range of 14–84 days.[19,60,74]

Pathology

Granulomatous disease of the rectum and sigmoid colon with mucosal hyperplasia, pseudopolyposis, ulceration, thickening of the bowel wall and stenosis may occur and may be followed by malignant transformation. In a large autopsy series in Japan, the rate of carcinoma of the colon in infested persons was 25 times greater than that of non-infested persons and is usually a well-differentiated adenocarcinoma with pseudopolyps, calcified eggs being identified in the tissues.[58]

Clinical features

The early chronic stages of the disease are usually asymptomatic as in *S. mansoni* but diarrhoea and abdominal pain related to intensity of infestation are common. Hepatic coma is frequently observed as a terminal event in China; however, in the Philippines the main terminal episode is massive bleeding in the upper gastrointestinal tract.[72]

The frequency of severe portal hypertension, associated with shunting of eggs to the pulmonary circulation and cor pulmonale, depends upon the intensity of infestation. The brain is principally involved in *S. japonicum* infestation in contrast to the spinal cord in *S. mansoni* and *S. haematobium* infestations. Clinically, the latter infestations are manifested by the occurrence of transverse myelitis. Clinical manifestations of cerebral schistosomiasis differ greatly between those seen in the acute phase and those in the chronic phase of the infestation.[47] The first clinical manifestations of cerebral schistosomiasis are Jacksonian-type paroxysmal seizures, usually in persons over 20 years of age, followed by grand mal seizures in many fatal cases.[6,46]

Schistosomal dwarfism has been reported in China and Brazil. It is accompanied by impairment of gonad formation and sexual immaturity, and is thought to be due to depressed activity of the anterior lobe of the pituitary gland.[41]

INFESTATION WITH *S. HAEMATOBIUM*

EPIDEMIOLOGY

The peak prevalence and intensity of *S. haematobium* infestation occurs among children who are 10–14 years of age. In general, 60–70% of all infested persons are between 5 and 14 years of age and approximately 75–80% of all persons with more than 50 eggs per 10 ml of urine are in this age group.[96]

PATHOLOGY

Kidneys, ureters, urinary bladder, urethra, and genital tissues may be involved, but eggs are most numerous in the bladder, ureters and seminal vesicles (*Figure 9.28*). Lung, colon and appendix also contains *S. haematobium* ova in almost all infestations. The worms tend to remain in one location for prolonged periods laying large numbers of eggs which accumulate at one site, thus causing focal lesions.[52] The eggs calcify and produce granulomata which are generally smaller than those of *S. mansoni* but have the same cellular composition.[83,97]

CLINICAL FEATURES

Cercarial dermatitis may occur some 24 hours after infestation and last approximately 48 hours. The acute or toxaemic state usually begins 8 weeks after infestation (range 5–12 weeks). Haematuria is seen in 50% of cases. Although there is evidence of urinary tract disease with kidney involvement no hypertension occurs and, in East Africa, low blood pressures are recorded. Pulmonary changes due to *S. haematobium* may lead to cor pulmonale. Cutaneous manifestations are reported with lesions in the genital and perigenital areas and severe urinary schistosomiasis may be associated with osteoporosis.[36,44]

In the bladder, polypoid, fibrous and sandy patches, ulceration, stricture, leukoplakia and cystitis glandularis, fibrosis and calcification of the bladder wall and bladder neck may occur.[28] Secondary bacterial infection sometimes occurs, but not usually related to the infestation, with consequent pyelonephritis. In Egypt, *S. haematobium* infestation is associated with a high prevalence of cancer of the bladder, particularly squamous cell carcinomas[54] (*Figure 9.28d*). Obstructive uropathy is clearly demonstrated by intravenous pyelography,[34] and the development of hydronephrosis and hydroureter is commonly seen in children and adoles-

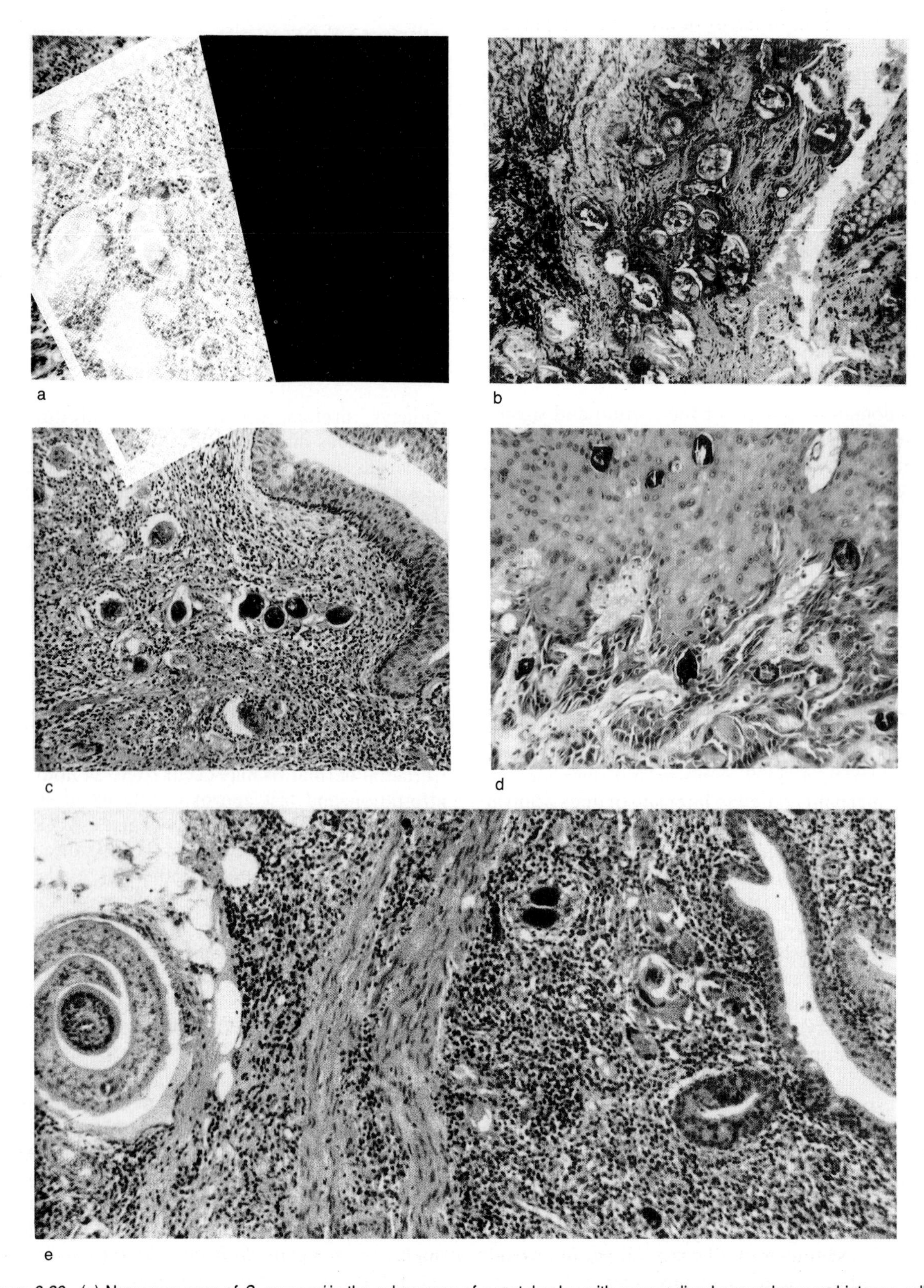

Figure 9.28 (a) Numerous eggs of *S. mansoni* in the submucosa of a rectal polyp with surrounding haemorrhage and intense cellular infiltrate. (b) Nests of *S. mansoni* eggs in the mucosa of a rectal polyp. (c) Nest of *S. haematobium* eggs in the bladder wall; acute stage with cellular reaction around the eggs. (d) Section of bladder wall showing squamous cell carcinoma with *S. haematobium* ova. (e) Section across ureter showing adult worms in a vessel and eggs surrounded by intense cellular reaction in the ureteric wall. (Sections 5 μm, stained with haematoxylin and eosin, kindly provided by H. Furse.)

cents. Associated bacteriuria and hydronephrosis may impair urine-concentrating ability.[50] Children with a high level of infestation may have abnormal pyelograms, and renographic abnormalities are also common.[40,63] Ultrasonography has been validated in identifying structural changes of the urinary tract due to schistosomiasis.[27] Computed tomography has been used in detecting calcification of the urinary tract and delineating its location.[45]

Involvement of the rectum occurs in 70% of *S. haematobium* infestations, and the remainder of the large intestine and appendix may also be involved. Large granulomata may cause acute obstruction in the large intestine.[28,96]

SYNERGISTIC AND ANTAGONISTIC EFFECTS

Synergistic and antagonistic interrelations between schistosomiasis and salmonellosis may explain the association of these diseases in China, Brazil and Egypt. There is experimental evidence for an association between hepatitis, malaria and *Entamoeba histolytica*.[81] Further investigations are required to define the importance of other infections and malnutrition in the pathogenesis of human schistosomiasis.[70]

INVESTIGATIONS

The definitive diagnosis of an active infestation is made by detecting schistosomes' ova in concentrated urine, faeces or biopsy material. Eggs may be found in excreta as early as 5–6 weeks after infestation with *S. mansoni* or *S. japonicum*, and some 10–12 weeks with *S. haematobium*. Longer delays between exposure and patency are common and, in the case of *S. japonicum*, repeated stool examinations may be necessary because, in light infestations, ova are laid in clusters in the faeces and tend to be aggregated.[58] Qualitative techniques for detection of ova are used in clinical practice, but quantitative techniques are mainly used for research in the fields of epidemiology, control, and drug trials.[42] The semiquantitative measurement of haematuria and proteinuria by reagent strips has been widely used for morbidity surveys of *S. haematobium* infestations in recent years.[71]

Quantitative techniques to examine stools now include modifications of the Kato method – that is, the quick Kato method and the Kato/Katz method – and nucleopore filtration of urine specimens has been developed.[66]

Special stains are sometimes useful. The eggshells of *S. mansoni* are acid-fast, while those of *S. haematobium* are not. The shells of *S. intercalatum*, which are very similar to *S. haematobium* are acid-fast after Bouin's fixation. In patients with light or inactive infestations, rectal biopsy is particularly effective in detecting eggs. They are best seen by crushing the biopsy between glass slides. Eggs may also be recovered by hydrolysis of tissues in 4% potassium hydroxide for 18 hours, incubating at 37°C for fresh tissues and 56°C for fixed tissues.[52]

Promising immunodiagnostic tests are now available, including radio-immunoassay and enzyme-linked immunosorbent assay (ELISA), as well as detection of circulating antigens.[65,81]

TREATMENT

A number of highly effective drugs are available for the treatment of schistosomiasis and these have now largely displaced the tri-antimonials and the later generation of non-antimonial compounds such as lucanthone, hycanthone and niridazole.[21] *Metrifonate* (Bilarcil)®, although only effective against *S. haematobium*, is very cheap and of low toxicity; a widely used schedule of 7.5 mg/kg, given in three oral doses at intervals of 14 days, is the standard treatment regimen.[23] Cholinergic symptoms may be expected during treatment, but tolerance is extremely good, and such symptoms, if they occur, are mild and disappear spontaneously in a few hours. High cure rates and substantial reductions in egg output are reported in selective population chemotherapy programmes. The drug is extensively used in Egypt and elsewhere.

Oxamniquine (Mansil, Vansil)®, which is highly effective against *S. mansoni* only, being administered as a single oral dose with few side-effects, is used clinically in the treatment of acute, subacute, chronic and complicated cases of *S. mansoni* infestation with excellent results. In the Western hemisphere, a single oral dose of 15 mg/kg bodyweight in adults produces high cure rates but, in children under 30 g in weight, the optimum regimen is a total dose of 20 mg/kg given in two divided doses of 10 mg/kg at a 4–6 hour interval; in Africa, total doses of 40 and 60 mg/kg administered over 2 or 3 days are necessary to obtain good therapeutic response – even if parasitological cure is not achieved, egg output is appreciably reduced by 80–90%. The drug is very suitable for population-based chemotherapy and is widely used in South America.[21]

Praziquantel (Biltricide)®, is highly effective against all human schistosomes species and is a major advance in the chemotherapy of the diseases. The drug is highly effective when given in a single oral dose of 40 mg/kg bodyweight for *S. haematobium*; a single dose of 40 mg/kg or 2 × 20 mg/kg at an interval of 4 hours in 1 day is effective against *S. mansoni*; and 2 × 30 mg/kg at an interval of 4 hours in 1 day, or 3 × 20 mg/kg in 1 day is the present recommended regimen for *S. japonicum*. The available evidence shows that patients with advanced disease from infestation with *S. japonicum* or *S. mansoni*, with ascites or portal hypertension, tolerate the drug well. An optimistic outlook for the future treatment of advanced cases is justified.[24]

Following chemotherapy, haematuria, dysuria and suprapubic pain resolve. Bladder granulomata decrease in size with relief of obstruction and resolution of hydroureter and hydronephrosis.[61] Schistosomal polyposis has been successfully treated solely with oxamniquine, but hepatic schistosomiasis with splenomegaly can be safely treated with oxamniquine or praziquantel.

Glomerulonephritis associated with *S. mansoni* may resolve with clinical improvement after treatment with both oxamniquine and praziquantel. Cerebral lesions due to *S. japonicum* have been successfully treated with praziquantel, while central nervous system lesions in the acute phase of *S. japonicum* infestation may resolve spontaneously.[84] Prolonged salmonella infections associated with *S. mansoni* infestation have been successfully treated with oxamniquine and praziquantel.[88,93]

PROGNOSIS

The prognosis of uncomplicated cases of the schistosome infestation is good provided that specific treatment is given. Improvement in the function and structure of damaged organ systems can be expected.[22]

REFERENCES

1. Abdel-Salam, E., Khalik, A.A., Abdel-Meguid, A., Abrakat, W. and Mahmoud, A.A.F. (1986) Association of HLA class I antigens (A1, B5, B8 and CW2) with disease manifestations and infection in human schistosomiasis mansoni in Egypt. *Tissue Antigens*, **27**, 142–146.
2. Abdel-Wahab, M.F., Esmat, G., Narooz, S.I., Yosery, A., Struewing, T.P. and Strickland, G.T. (1990) Sonographic studies of school children in a village endemic for *Schistosoma mansoni*. *Transactions of the Royal Society of Tropical Medicine and Hygiene*, **84**, 69–73.
3. Andrade, Z.A. and Andrade, S.G. (1970) Pathogenesis of schistosoma pulmonary arteritis. *American Journal of Tropical Medicine and Hygiene*, **19**(2), 305–310.
4. Andrade, Z.A. and Rodrigues, G. (1954) Pseudoneoplastic manifestations of intestinal schistosomiasis. *Archives of Brazilian Medicine*, **44**, 437–444.
5. Andrade, Z.A., Andrade, S.G. and Sadigursky, M. (1971) Renal changes in patients with hepatosplenic schistosomiasis. *American Journal of Tropical Medicine and Hygiene*, **20**(1), 77–83.
6. Ariizumi, M. (1963) Cerebral *Schistosomiasis japonica*: report of one operated case and fifty clinical cases. *American Journal of Tropical Medicine and Hygiene*, **12**, 40–45.
7. Basch, P.F. (1986) Schistosomiasis in China. *American Journal of Chinese Medicine*, **14**, 17–25.
8. Bina, J.C., Tavares-Neto, J., Prata, A. and Azevedo, E.S. (1978) Greater resistance to development of severe schistosomiasis in Brazilian negroes. *Human Biology*, **50**, 41–49.
9. Bogliolo, L. (1957) Anatomical picture of the liver in hepato-splenic *Schistosomiasis mansoni*. *Annals of Tropical Medicine and Parasitology*, **51**, 1–14.
10. Bogliolo, L. (1967) The pathogenesis of *Schistosomiasis mansoni*. In *Bilharziasis* (Ed.) Mostofi, F.K. pp. 184–196. Berlin: Springer-Verlag.
11. Brown, D.S. (1980) *Freshwater Snails of Africa and their Medical Importance*. London: Taylor and Francis.
12. Bukenya, G. and Andama, S. (1986) Circumstantial epidemiology of *Schistosoma mansoni* in the West-Nile district of Uganda: results of a cross-sectional study in the Rhino Camp area. *Journal of Tropical Medicine and Hygiene*, **89**, 243–248.
13. Camus, D., Bina, J.C., Carlier, Y. and Santoro, F. (1977) A, B, O blood groups and clinical forms of schistosomiasis mansoni. *Transactions of the Royal Society of Tropical Medicine and Hygiene*, **71**, 182.
14. Cheever, A.W. (1972) Pipe-stem fibrosis of the liver (correspondence). *Transactions of the Royal Society of Tropical Medicine and Hygiene*, **66**, 946–948.
15. Cheever, A.W. (1978) Schistosomiasis and neoplasia. *Journal of the National Cancer Institute*, **61**, 13–18.
16. Cheever, A.W. (1981) Schistosomiasis and colon cancer. *The Lancet*, **i**, 1369–1370.
17. Cheever, A.W. (1986) Density-dependent fecundity in *Schistosoma mansoni* infection in man: a reply. *Transactions of the Royal Society of Tropical Medicine and Hygiene*, **80**, 991–992.
18. Cheever, A.W. and Andrade, Z.A. (1967) Clinical and pathological aspects of Schistosomiasis in Brazil. In *Bilharziasis* (Ed.) Mostofi, F.K. pp. 157–166. Berlin: Springer-Verlag.
19. Chen, W.C., Lui, H., Hu, S.Y., Lu, K.H., Kao, C.F. and Lu, S.T. (1964) Clinical analysis of 580

cases of acute Schistosomiasis (Chinese). *Chinese Journal of Internal Medicine*, **12**, 259–262.
20. Cross, J.H. (1984) *Schistosoma japonicum*-complex. *Southeast Asian Journal of Tropical Medicine and Public Health*, **15**, 523.
21. Davis, A. (1982) Management of the patient. In: *Schistosomiasis: Treatment, Epidemiology and Control* (Ed.) Jordan, P. and Webbe, G. pp. 184–226. London: Heinemann.
22. Davis, A. (1986) Recent advances in schistosomiasis. *Quarterly Journal of Medicine, New Series*, **58**, 95–110.
23. Davis, A. and Bailey, D.R. (1969) Metrifonate in urinary schistosomiasis. *Bulletin of the World Health Organization*, **41**, 209–224.
24. Davis, A. and Wegner, D.H.G. (1979) Multicentre trials of praziquantel in human schistosomiasis: design and techniques. *Bulletin of the World Health Organization*, **57**, 761–771.
25. Davis, G.M. (1979) The origin and evolution of the gastropod family *Pomatiopsidae*, with emphasis on the Mekong River Triculinae. *Monograph of the Academy of Natural Sciences of Philadelphia*, **20**, 1–120.
26. De Cock, K.M. (1986) Hepatosplenic schistosomiasis: a clinical review. *Gut*, **27**, 734–745.
27. Degremont, A., Burki, A., Burnier, E., Schweizer, W., Meudt, B. and Tanner, M. (1985) Value of ultrasonography in investingating morbidity due to *Schistosoma haematobium* infection. *The Lancet*, **i**, 662–665.
28. Edington, G.M. and Gilles, H.M. (1969) *Pathology in the Tropics*. Baltimore: Williams and Wilkins.
29. El-Masri, S.H. and Sharfi, A.R.M. (1982) A, B, O blood group in hepato-splenic schistosomiasis. *Journal of Tropical Medicine and Hygiene*, **85**, 223–224.
30. El-Masry, N.A., Farid, Z., Bassily, S., Kilpatrick, M.E. and Watten, R.H. (1986) Schistosomal colonic polyposis: clinical, radiological and parasitological study. *Journal of Tropical Medicine and Hygiene*, **89**, 13–17.
31. El-Rooby, A. (1985) Management of hepatic schistosomiasis. *Seminars in liver disease*, **5**, 263–276.
32. Farid, Z., Trabolsi, B. and Hafez, A. (1986) Acute schistosomiasis (Katayama syndrome). *Annals of Tropical Medicine and Parasitology*, **5**, 563–564.
33. Fedail, S.S. and Gardir, A.F.M.A. (1985) The pathology of the small intestine in human schistosomiasis mansoni in the Sudan. *Tropical Medicine and Parasitology*, **36**, 94–96.
34. Forsyth, D.M. and Bradley, D.J. (1964) Irreversible damage by *Schistosoma haematobium* in schoolchildren. *The Lancet*, **ii**, 169–171.
35. Gazzinelli, G., Lambertucci, J.R., Katz, N., Rocha, R.S., Lima, M.S. and Colley, D.G. (1985) Immune response during human schistosomiasis mansoni XI. Immunological status of patients with acute infections and after treatment. *Journal of Immunology*, **135**, 2121–2127.
36. Gilles, H.M. (1982) Infection with *S. haematobium*. In *Schistosomiasis: Treatment, Epidemiology and Control* (Ed.) Jordan, P. and Webbe, G. pp. 79–104. London: Heinemann.
37. Goodgame, R.W. and Bartholomew, R.K. (1978) Lack of association of hepatosplenic schistosomiasis and alpha-1-antitrysin deficiency. *American Journal of Tropical Medicine and Hygiene*, **27**, 779–781.
38. Harries, A.D., Fryatt, R., Walker, J., Chiodini, P.L. and Bryceson, A.D.M. (1986) Schistosomiasis in expatriates returning to Britain from the tropics: a controlled study. *The Lancet*, **i**, 86–88.
39. Hashem, M. (1947) The etiology and pathogenesis of the endemic form of splenomegaly: Egyptian splenomegaly. *Journal of the Egyptian Medical Association*, **30**, 48–79.
40. Higashi, G.I., Abdel-Salam, E., Soliman, M., Abdel-Meguid, A.E. and El-Ghadban, H. (1984) Immunofluorescent analysis of renal biopsies in uncomplicated *Schistosoma haematobium* infections in children. *Journal of Tropical Medicine and Hygiene*, **87**, 123–129.
41. Hsueh, C.H. and Wu, Y.H. (1963) Endocrine disturbances in late schistosomiasis: a clinical study of 17 cases. *Chinese Medical Journal*, **82**, 519–527.
42. Jordan, P. (1982) Diagnostic and laboratory techniques. In *Schistosomiasis: Treatment, Epidemiology and Control* (Ed.) Jordan, P. and Webbe, G. pp. 165–183. London: Heinemann.
43. Jordan, P. (1985) *Schistosomiasis: The St Lucia Project*. pp. 1–442. London: Cambridge University Press.
44. Jordan, P. and Webbe, G. (1969) *Human Schistosomiasis*. London: Heinemann.
45. Jourlif, H. and Lindstedt, E. (1985) Urogenital schistosomiasis: CT evaluation. *Radiology*, **157**, 745–749.
46. Kane, C.A. and Most, H. (1948) Schistosomiasis of the central nervous system. Experiences in World War II and a review of the literature. *Archives of Neurological Psychiatry (Chicago)*, **59**(2), 141–183.
47. Kirchhoff, L.V. and Nash, T.E. (1984) A case of schistosomiasis japonica: resolution of CAT-scan detected cerebral abnormalities without specific therapy. *American journal of Tropical Medicine and Hygiene*, **33**, 1155–1158.
48. Kumar, V. and de Burbare, G. (1986) Schistosomes of animals and man in Asia. *Helminthological abstracts (Series A)*, **55**, 469–480.
49. Lehman, J.S., Farid, Z., Bassily, S., Haxton, J., Abdel Wahab, M.F. and Kent, D.C. (1970) Intestinal protein loss in schistosomal polyposis of the colon. *Gastroenterology*, **59**(30), 433–436.
50. Lehman, J.S., Farid, Z., Bassily, S. and Kent, D.C. (1971) Hydronephrosis, bacteriuria and maximal urine concentration in urinary bilharziasis. *Annals of Internal Medicine*, **75**(1), 49–55.
51. LoVerde, P.T., deWald, J. and Minchella, D.J. (1985) Further studies of genetic variation in *Schistosoma mansoni*. *Journal of Parasitology*, **71**, 732–734.

52. McCully, R.M., Barron, C.H. and Cheever, A.W. (1976) Schistosomiasis: Diseases caused by trematodes. In *Pathology of Tropical and Extra-ordinary Diseases*, Vol. II. (Ed.) Bindford, C.H. and Connor, D.H. pp. 482–508. Washington, DC: Armed Forces Institute of Pathology.
53. McLaren, M.L., Lilleywhite, J.E., Dunne, D.W. and Doenhoff, M.J. (1981) Serodiagnosis of human *Schistosoma mansoni* infections: enhanced sensitivity and specificity in ELISA using a fraction containing *S. mansoni* egg antigens ω_1 and α_1. *Transactions of the Royal Society of Tropical Medicine and Hygiene*, **75**, 72–79.
54. Makar, M. (1967) Some clinopathological aspects of urinary bilharziasis. In *Bilharziasis* (Ed.) Mostofi, F.K. pp. 45–47. Berlin: Springer-Verlag.
55. Mao, S.P. and Chen, M.G. (1984) *Schistosoma* and schistosomiasis. In *Chinese Medical Encyclopaedia, Parasitology and Parasitic Diseases* (Ed.) Wu, Z.J., Mao, S.P. and Wang, J.W. pp. 41–43. Shanghai: Shanghai Publishing House for Sciences and Technology (in Chinese).
56. Medley, G. and Anderson, R.M. (1985) Density-dependent fecundity in *Schistosoma mansoni* infections in man. *Transactions of the Royal Society of Tropical Medicine and Hygiene*, **79**, 532–534.
57. Miyasato, M. (1984) Experimental study of the influence of *Schistosoma japonicum* infection on carcinogenesis of mice liver treated with *N*-2-fluorenylacetamide (2-FAA). *Japanese Journal of Parasitology*, **33**, 41–48.
58. Mott, K.S. (1982) *S. japonicum* and *S. japonicum*-like infections. In *Schistosomiasis: Treatment, Epidemiology and Control* (Ed.) Jordan, P. and Webbe, G. pp. 128–149. London: Heinemann.
59. Nash, T.E., Garcia-Coyco, C., Ruiz-Tiben, E., Nazario-Lopez, H.A., Vazquez, G. and Torres-Borges, A. (1983) Differentiation of acute and chronic schistosomiasis by antibody responses to specific schistosome antigens. *American Journal of Tropical Medicine and Hygiene*, **32**, 776–784.
60. National Schistosomiasis Research Committee (1985) *Summaries of Research on Schistosomiasis in China between 1961 and 1979*. pp. 1–577. Wuxi: People's Printing House (in Chinese).
61. Naude, J.H. (1984) The natural history of ureteric bilharzia. *British Journal of Urology*, **56**, 599–601.
62. Okuyama, T., Imai, S. and Tsubara, Y. (1985) Egg of *Schistosoma japonicum* in ascitic fluid. *Acta Cytologica*, **29**, 651–652.
63. Oyediran, A.B.O.O. (1979) Renal disease due to schistosomiasis of the lower urinary tract. *Kidney International*, **16**, 15–22.
64. PAHO/WHO (1968) *An introductory Guide for Intermediate Hosts of Schistosomiasis in the Americas*. Washington, DC: World Health Organization.
65. Pelley, R.P., Warren, K.S. and Jordan, P. (1977) Purified antigen radio-immunoassay in serological diagnosis of *Schistosomiasis mansoni*. *The Lancet*, **11**, 781–786.
66. Peters, P.A., Warren, K.S. and Mahmoud, A.A.F. (1980) Rapid, accurate quantification of schistosome eggs in nucleopore filters. *Journal of Parasitology*, **62**, 145–155.
67. Pitchford, R.J. (1959) Cattle schistosomiasis in man in the eastern Transvaal. *Transactions of the Royal Society of Tropical Medicine and Hygiene*, **54**(3), 285–290.
68. Prata, A. (1982) Infection with *S. mansoni*. In *Schistosomiasis: Treatment, Epidemiology and Control* (Ed.) Jordan, P. and Webbe, G. pp. 105–127. London: Heinemann.
69. Silva, L.C. da, Brito, T. de, Camargo, M.E., Boni, D.R. de, Lopes, L.D. and Gunji, J. (1970) Kidney biopsy in the hepatosplenic form of infection with *Schistosoma mansoni* in man. *Bulletin of the World Health Organization*, **42**(6), 907–910.
70. Stephenson, L.S. (1986) Schistosomiasis and human nutrition. *Cornell International Nutrition Monograph Series*, **16**, 1–21.
71. Stephenson, L.S., Latham, M.C., Kinoti, S.N. and Oduori, M.L. (1984) Sensitivity and specificity of reagent strip in screening of Kenyan children for *Schistosoma haematobium* infection. *American Journal of Tropical Medicine and Hygiene*, **33**, 862–871.
72. Sulit, Y.S.M., Domingo, E.O., Dalmucio-Cruz, A.E., Perueta, D.S. de and Imperial, E.S. (1964) Parasitic cirrhosis among Filipinos. *Journal Philippine Medicine Association*, **40**(12,11), 1021–1038.
73. Thatcher, B.S., Fleischer, D., Rankin, G.B. and Petras, R. (1984) Duodenal schistosomiasis diagnosed by endoscopic biopsy of an isolated polyp. *American Journal of Gastroenterology*, **79**, 927–929.
74. Tsai, C.Y. and Yu, W. (1966) Investigation in incubation period of acute schistosomiasis. *Chinese Medical Journal*, **85**, 183–185.
75. Tsutsumi, H. and Hasada, A. (1964) Studies in liver fibrosis (cirrhosis) due to *Schistosomiasis japonica*. III: the state of intervention of ova in the digestive tract. *Kurume Medical Journal*, **11**, 80–87.
76. Tsutsumi, H., Watanabe, A. and Nakashima, T. (1963) Studies on fibrosis (cirrhosis) due to *Schistosomiasis japonica*. Morphology of liver: part 1. *Kurume Medical Journal*, **10**, 51–59.
77. Voge, M., Bruckner, D. and Bruce, J.I. (1978) *Schistosoma mekongi* sp. n. from man and animals, compared with four geographic strains of *Schistosoma japonicum*. *Journal of Parasitology*, **64**, 577–584.
78. Wang, C.G., Zhu, Q.Y., Hang, P.Y. *et al.* (1984) HLA and schistosomiasis japonica. *Chinese Medical Journal*, **97**, 603–605.
79. Warren, K.S. (1968) Pathophysiology and pathogenesis of hepatosplenic schistosomiasis mansoni. *Bulletin of the New York Academy of Medicine*, **44**(3), 280–294.
80. Warren, K.S. (1971) Worms. In *Cecil-Loeb Textbook of Medicine*, 13th edn. (Ed.) Beeson,

P.B. and McDermott, W. pp. 745–752. Philadelphia: W.B. Saunders.
81. Warren, K.S. (1973) The pathology of schistosome infections. *Helminthological Abstracts, Series A. Animal and Human Helminthology*, **42**, 592–633.
82. Warren, K.S. (1977) Modulation of immunopathology and disease in schistosomiasis. *American Journal of Tropical Medicine and Hygiene*, **26**, 113–119.
83. Warren, K.S. and Domingo, E.O. (1970) Granuloma formation around *Schistosoma mansoni, S. haematobium* and *S. japonicum* eggs. Size and rate of development, cellular composition, cross-sensitivity and rate of egg destruction. *American Journal of Tropical Medicine and Hygiene*, **29**(2), 292–304.
84. Watt, G., Adapon, B., Long, G.W., Fernando, M.T., Ranoa, C.P. and Cross, J.H. (1986) Praziquantel in treatment of cerebral schistosomiasis. *The Lancet*, **ii**, 529–532.
85. Webbe, G. (1981) Schistosomiasis: some advances. *British Medical Journal*, **283**, 1104–1106.
86. Webbe, G. (1982) The Parasites. In *Schistosomiasis: Treatment, Epidemiology and Control* (Ed.) Jordan, P. and Webbe, G. pp. 1–15. London: Heinemann.
87. Webbe, G. (1982) The life-cycle of the parasites. In *Schistosomiasis: Treatment, Epidemiology and Control* (Ed.) Jordan, P. and Webbe, G. pp. 50–77. London: Heinemann.
88. Webbe, G. (1987) Treatment of Schistosomiasis. *European Journal of Clinical Pharmacology*, **32**, 433–436.
89. Wertheimer, S.P., Vermund, S.H., Lumay, L.H. and Singer, B. (1987) Lack of demonstrable density-dependent fecundity of schistosomiasis mansoni: analysis of Egyptian quantitative human autopsies. *American Journal of Tropical Medicine and Hygiene*, **37**, 79–84.
90. Winawer, S.J. and Miller, D. (1987) Screening for colorectal cancer. *Bulletin of the World Health Organisation*, **65**, 105–111.
91. WHO (1974) Memoranda. Immunology of schistosomiasis. *Bulletin of the World Health Organization*, **51**, 553–595.
92. WHO (1980) Workshop. Quantitative aspects of the epidemiology of *Schistosoma japonicum* infection in a rural community in Luzon, Philippines. *Bulletin of the World Health Organization*, **58**, 629–638.
93. WHO (1983) The role of chemotherapy in schistosomiasis control WHO/SCHISTO/83.70 (unpublished report).
94. WHO (1984) World Health Organization new strategy on schistosomiasis. *Southeast Asian Journal of Tropical Medicine and Public Health*, **15**, 469–470.
95. WHO (1985) The control of schistosomiasis. Report of a WHO Expert Committee. *WHO Technical Report Series*, **728**.
96. WHO (1987) Progress in assessment of morbidity due to *Schistosoma haematobium* infection: a review of recent literature, WHO/SCHISTO/87.91 (unpublished report).
97. Winslow, D.J. (1967) Histopathology of schistosomiasis. In *Bilharziasis* (Ed.) Mostofi, F.K. pp. 230–241. Berlin: Springer-Verlag.
98. Wright, C.A., Southgate, V.R. and Knowles, R.J. (1972) What is *Schistosoma intercalatum* Fisher 1934? *Transactions of the Royal Society of Tropical Medicine and Hygiene*, **66**, 28–64.
99. Wydell, S.H. (1958) Some abdominal complications of *S. mansoni* as seen on Ukerewe island. *East African Medical Journal*, **35**(8), 413–426.

INTESTINAL AMOEBIASIS

I. Zaidman

Since Fedor Losch first described amoebic dysentery in 1875,[21] much progress has been made in the understanding of this disease. Amoebiasis may be acute or chronic and either a symptomatic or asymptomatic infestation of the bowel. Extraintestinal disease is quite common, particularly amoebic liver abscess and pulmonary, skin, genital and neurological disease.

Originally it was thought to be a tropical disease peculiar to underdeveloped countries, but the parasite can exist in temperate climates.

INCIDENCE AND EPIDEMIOLOGY

Until recently, amoebiasis was considered a disease transmitted through the ingestion of contaminated food and water and occurring in underdeveloped countries, where poor sanitary conditions prevail.[38] While this is generally true, and the highest incidence is still found in tropical regions – South America and southern Asia – of the so-called Third World, a dramatic change has occurred in the incidence of amoebic infestation within the last decade: there has been an alarming spread of the disease in the northern hemisphere, now that amoebiasis is regarded as a venereal disease transmitted through homosexual practices.

Numerous epidemiological studies have been carried out using serological diagnosis. One such survey[24] found a 12% positive response to indirect hemagglutination in the general population of San Jose, Costa Rica, 30% in Medellin, Colombia, 58% in Bangkok and 76% in Calcutta.

In Mexico City, 4–6% positive response is reported[19] and amoebic liver abscess has been found in 2% of patients hospitalized in the National Medical Centre of Mexico City and in 3.2–4% of autopsies practised. In a study carried out in Maracaibo, Venezuela,[5] it is reported that seropositivity ranged from 4.4 to 6.5% depending on the population studied, and amoebic liver abscess is found in 0.3–0.8% of hospitalized patients.[47]

In New York and San Francisco, several studies of the homosexual community have revealed a high incidence of amoebiasis. Thus, Phillips,[37] in a venereal disease clinic in Manhattan, found an incidence of *Entamoeba histolytica* in 25.5% of homosexual men, 6.2% of bisexual men and 0% of heterosexual men and women.

Pomerantz *et al.*[38] recently reported a sharp increase in the number of cases of amoebiasis reported, noting that 'the incidence of amoebiasis in New York City exceeded totals for most other major infectious diseases of public health importance such as tuberculosis and hepatitis'.[23] Between 1958 and 1970, 47.8% of the cases were reported in males, and this figure increased to 65% of all cases between 1977 and 1978. Similar data have been reported from other cities in the USA and UK.[10,26,31] This is a new era for amoebiasis; it is no longer a disease transmitted by contamination, but has incorporated a whole new transmission mechanism.[23]

PATHOLOGY AND PATHOGENESIS

Classically, amoebiasis is contracted through the ingestion of contaminated food and water containing cysts of *Ent. histolytica*. These cysts have a considerable capacity for survival in most conditions. The route is faecal–oral. Ingested trophozoites are destroyed by gastric juices. In the small intestine, the cysts develop into trophozoites which invade the tissues, mainly in the colon.

The increased frequency of amoebiasis in homosexuals is probably due to the transmission of parasitic and other infections through frequent oral–anal sexual contact, and the promiscuity of these contacts could result in severe disease due to frequent reinfestation. There are other questions which have yet to be solved[13] concerning the transmission of amoebiasis in non-tropical areas and in the developed world. Frequent international travel may be responsible for the infestation of tourists and further spread of the disease, as reported from Sweden.[35] The contamination of public facilities, the role of food handlers and of immigrants, and the presence of the parasite in asymptomatic carriers are yet to be defined.

Ent. histolytica in the intestine first produces necrosis of the microvilli, followed by degeneration of the cells and infiltration of the surrounding tissues by polymorphonuclear leukocytes. The organism separates the intercellular junctions, penetrates the lamina propria and invades all layers of the intestinal wall. Further necrosis is followed by the formation of an amoebic ulcer surrounded by a dense inflammatory infiltrate. Occasionally, a desmoplastic inflammatory reaction occurs, leading to the formation of a pseudotumour known as an amoeboma.

In vitro studies have demonstrated that *Ent. histolytica* is capable of killing and phagocytosing cells exclusively on direct contact.[41] Neighbouring cells not in contact with amoebae remain intact. Although microfilaments are apparently required for a contact-dependent extracellular cytopathic effect, the exact mechanism has yet to be identified. Phagocytosis is important, but apparently not essential.

Host factors including intestinal bacterial flora, nutritional conditions and general immunological status are all important.

It is uncertain why a number of infected individuals never develop invasive disease and remain asymptomatic carriers. Brumpt[4] suggested that the virulence of amoebae varied, and described two types of morphologically indistinguishable amoebas, of which one was pathogenic. Amoebae in asymptomatic carriers may be less virulent than those present in acute clinical cases[51] and virulence may follow a changing pattern which is related to the parasite itself and/or to immune factors present in the host.

Sargeaunt[43,44] studied lysates from different strains of amoebae, by thin-layer starch electrophoresis, for isoenzyme patterns, and was able to identify and differentiate the unique patterns associated with 11 different types of amoebae. Those taken from asymptomatic carriers are clearly different from those originating from individuals with clinical disease. If these findings are confirmed, the implications could be of major importance;[11] however, this line of investigation is not, as yet, reflected in the practical approach to the clinical management of patients.

IMMUNE RESPONSE TO *E. HISTOLYTICA*

Amoebae are recognised by the immune system,[45] and antibodies form in response to amoebic antigens. Their effectiveness as a mechanism of host resistance is not clear. Cellular immune mechanisms seem to be an important factor in the control of amoebiasis.[29] There is evidence[8] that patients cured of amoebic liver abscess will not be reinfested. There is also experimental evidence[48] that, in animals, amoebic antigens can produce antibodies and in turn protect the animals when challenged with large doses of pathological parasites. Antibodies may produce passive immunization in suckling hamsters[7] although this finding was not confirmed in another study.[15]

CLINICAL FEATURES

The manifestations of amoebiasis encompass a broad spectrum of disease, ranging from the asymptomatic carrier to acute dysentery, chronic bowel disease, liver abscess and extradigestive diseases.

ACUTE AMOEBIC DYSENTERY

Patients present with non-specific diarrhoea and subsequently develop a more severe picture, with abdominal pain, cramps and severe tenesmus. The stools are liquid with an abundance of mucus and bright red blood. Fever is uncommon and, as the disease develops, the patient can become seriously ill.

The diarrhoea may stop spontaneously, or following non-specific treatment, but recurs within weeks or months.

Prolonged dysenteric disease is also seen in the young and elderly with bloody diarrhoea and deterioration in the patient's general health. These cases are clinically and even endoscopically indistinguishable from chronic ulcerative colitis. In endemic areas it is extremely difficult to distinguish between the two diseases because, not infrequently, they may coexist. Patients with ulcerative colitis may be more susceptible to invasive amoebiasis and, consequently, in every new case of ulcerative colitis, care is taken in endemic areas to rule out amoebiasis.

Patients may present with recurrent attacks, which are evidence of repeated reinfestation. Occasionally, severe disease ensues with dehydration, toxic shock, peritonitis and a clinical picture of toxic megacolon due to transmural ulceration. The colon may perforate, or a tender abdominal mass may be palpable due to sealed perforation covered with omentum. Abdominal rigidity is usually absent. Leukocytosis is present. Disassociated fever has been observed, just as in typhoid fever,[28] and liver abscess is a frequent complication.

Amoebomas are pseudotumours which follow either a chronic or acute course. They are usually located in the caecum and occasionally in the sigmoid. Differential diagnosis includes carcinoma of the bowel, and Crohn's disease. The distinction from carcinoma is most important since amoebomas can be cured with simple medical treatment, whereas surgery is associated with significant mortality. A positive diagnosis can only be established by serological tests and by biopsy of the lesion to exclude carcinoma.

CHRONIC AMOEBIASIS

The clinical picture is one of irritable bowel syndrome with or without pain, constipation and/or diarrhoea, with cysts present in the stools. It is difficult to determine whether or not the cysts are responsible for the symptoms. Caution must be exercised in attributing the symptoms to amoebae, because quite often they persist after successful treatment. The persistence of a clinical irritable bowel following successful treatment of acute dysenteric disease has been attributed to residual damage to the bowel wall. However, there is no evidence to support this assumption.

In view of the growing awareness of the disease and the emphasis placed on its severe complications, it is good practice to refrain from attaching excessive importance to the diagnosis of chronic amoebic colitis, although cyst shedders, even when asymptomatic, should be treated because of potential cross-infestation.

AMOEBIC LIVER ABSCESS

This is a frequent complication in the severe forms of amoebic colitis, or it may present as a primary disease without previous intestinal symptoms. The clinical picture is usually pain in the right upper quadrant, tender hepatomegaly, fever, malaise and loss of weight.

The white cell count is elevated, together with an increased sedimentation rate. Jaundice is rare and the aminotransferase levels are normal. The alkaline phosphatase level is increased.

The diagnosis is established by ultrasonography, which is the most useful imaging method.[39] The abscess is seen as a single hypoechoic mass, depending on the degree of liquefaction of the parenchyma, in the right or left lobe of the liver. The abscesses may be large or small and usually single. In endemic areas the diagnosis is established on an epidemiological basis. Serological tests are useful and nearly always positive in extraintestinal disease. In case of doubt, diagnostic liver aspiration can be performed. The characteristic 'chocolate-coloured' sterile pus is obtained. Amoebae are visible in the pus, but are difficult to find in a single small diagnostic aspirate.

Differential diagnosis includes pyogenic abscess; the most important distinguishing feature is the sterile nature of the amoebic pus, which only becomes secondarily infected through frequent invasive manipulation.[14]

Therapeutic percutaneous drainage of amoebic liver abscess is only necessary occasionally[40] and is only undertaken to decompress large abscesses which may rupture into the peritoneal cavity, particularly if they are located in the left lobe of the liver where they may perforate into the pleura or pericardium.

Computed axial tomography and magnetic resonance imaging[12] have been used in the diagnosis but do not add much to the findings of ultrasonography. In case of doubt, repeat examinations after treatment are usually diagnostic.

Rare manifestations of amoebiasis include skin infections, either perianal, genital or at the opening of a sinus tract from a draining abscess. They may imitate squamous cell carcinoma and present as an ulcer or fungating mass.

In non-tropical countries[16] the disease may present in three clinical settings:

1. Amoebiasis in groups of middle-aged people who contracted the disease whilst abroad. Often initially interpreted as a case of traveller's diarrhoea.
2. Amoebiasis in immigrants from tropical countries who have brought the disease with them.
3. Male homosexuals who develop intestinal disease which may be due to amoebae alone, or in combination with a number of bacterial and parasitic infections. Association with *Giardia* sp. is not infrequent in this clinical setting.

AMOEBIASIS IN HOMOSEXUAL MEN

In clinics for the treatment of sexually transmitted disease in the USA,[22] Italy[1] and the UK,[6] 20–30% of the subjects examined harbour amoebae and are considered to be asymptomatic carriers.[2] Whether it is necessary to treat every case is uncertain, as is the role of the frequent association with other intestinal parasites in this clinical picture in the homosexual male. Non-pathogenic amoebae can change when subjected to different bacterial environments.[25] It may be[18] that *Ent. histolytica* produces a lectin that is mutagenic for lymphocytes and may stimulate viral replication of HTLV-III virus in the infected lymphocyte, and the ensuing viral replication can shorten the latency period and lead to an earlier appearance of clinical manifestations of acquired immune deficiency syndrome (AIDS).[34,36]

INVESTIGATIONS

ENDOSCOPIC DIAGNOSIS

Proctoscopic examination provides the most important evidence of acute amoebic colitis. Ulcers are usually 1–5 mm in diameter, randomly distributed in the mucosa and located adjacent to normal mucosa (*Figure 9.29*). In the more severe cases there is diffuse inflammation of the mucosa with large ulcers, which are extremely difficult to distinguish

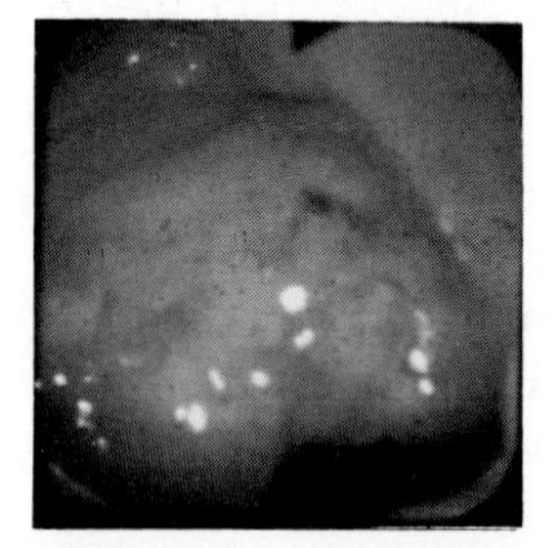
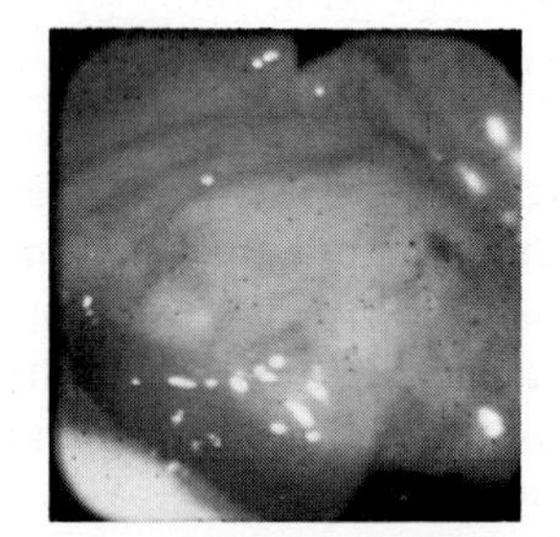
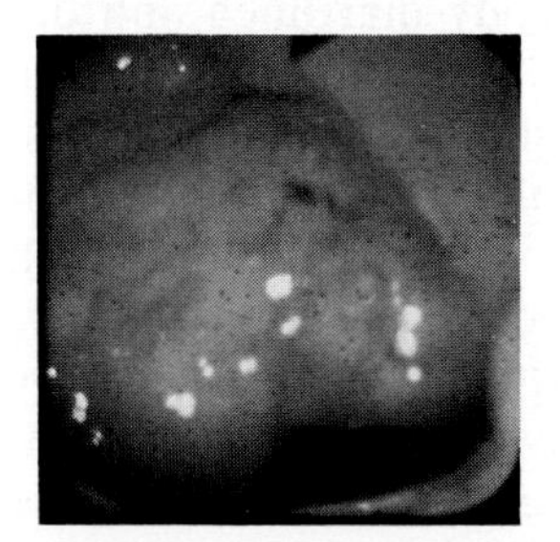
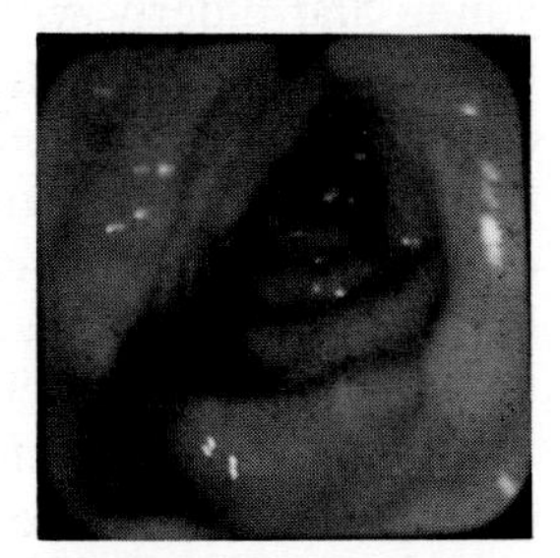

Figure 9.29 The rectal mucosa appears to be oedematous and there is a scattering of shallow, bleeding ulcers in the mucosa in the typical case of amoebic dysentery. Usually the sigmoid and the more proximal colon are normal, or there is only slight oedema.

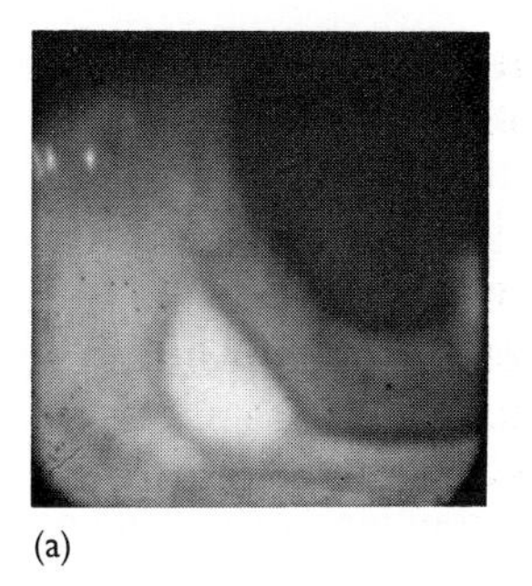
(a)

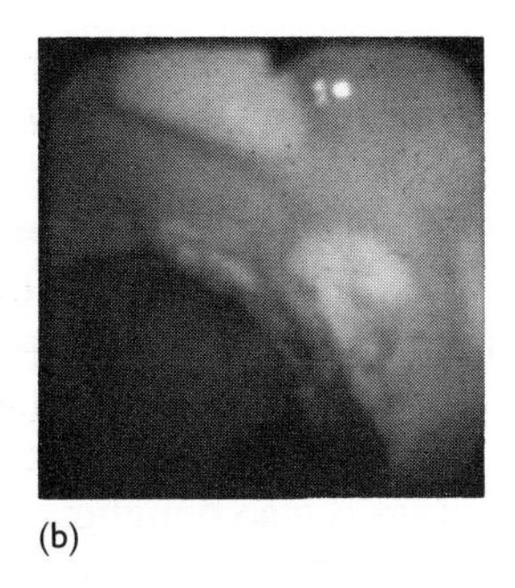
(b)

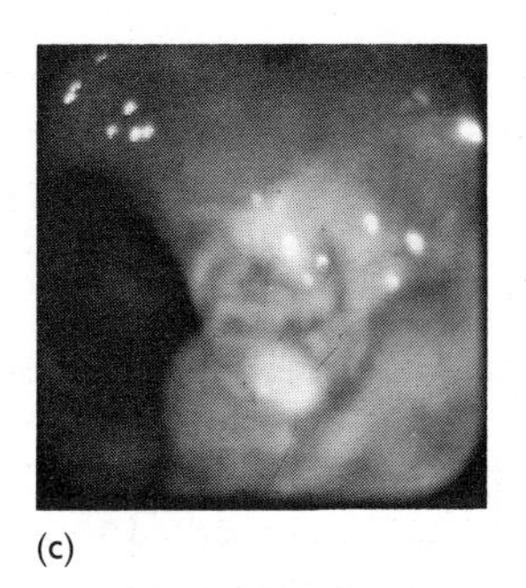
(c)

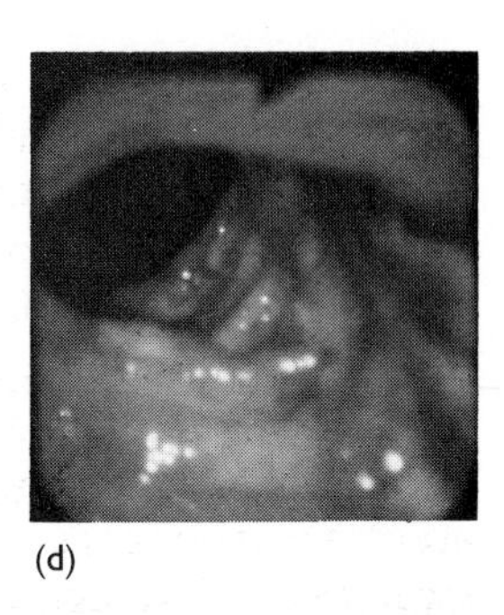
(d)

Figure 9.30 In very severe infections the ulcers become very deep and large (a,b), but the mucosa between has a fairly normal appearance. Some ulcers (c) have an irregular base and swollen border. There are deep, bleeding ulcers in the sigmoid and descending colon. *Entamoeba histolytica* was found in the stools and in the mucosal biopsy of this patient.

from ulcerative colitis (*Figure 9.30*). Colonoscopic examination reveals lesions confined to the descending colon, but in some cases the whole colon is involved. Colonoscopic examination is essential for the diagnosis of amoeboma of the caecum. A large ulcerated mass is seen, often fungating, with freely bleeding ulcers suggestive of adenocarcinoma. Biopsy and the presence of parasites in the fibrous tissue indicate a diagnosis of amoeboma.

Scrapings of the ulcers should always be taken and freshly examined. If biopsies are taken, amoebae can be identified with the aid of ferric haemotoxylin or periodic acid–Schiff staining (*Figure 9.31*).

RADIOLOGY

Barium enema is contraindicated in acute amoebic dysentery. In chronic cases, or in the event of any diagnostic doubt, the radiograph will show ulcerations along the edge of the gut, either in the form of fine serrations or larger ulcers which, when present, may extend throughout the whole length of the colon, but are more marked in the sigmoid and descending colon. Thumb-printing is occasionally seen and the mucosa has a cobblestone appearance.

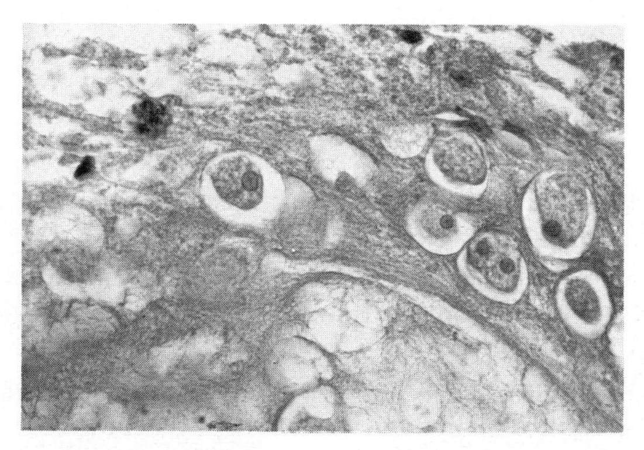

Figure 9.31 Multiple trophozoites are present in the exudate and necrotic material on the surface of the ulcer. Haematoxylin and eosin, ×900.

The differential diagnosis of these severe atypical cases by radiography is not easy and it is often difficult to exclude ulcerative colitis. Once the disease responds to treatment, the lesions heal completely and the colon returns to normal.

In toxic dilatation of the colon, plain films of the abdomen[52] resemble those seen in ulcerative colitis. The colon is dilated with loss of haustral pattern. Amoeboma is seen as an irregular filling defect with ulceration located in the caecum or the left colon. The diagnosis of amoeboma is suspected from the clinical picture and epidemiological situation; endoscopic and histological confirmation is always necessary.

MICROSCOPIC DIAGNOSIS

Amoebiasis is best diagnosed by stool examination, when the specimen is studied by an able and experienced technician. Stools must be examined within an hour of passing because, at room temperature, trophozoites lyse and become unrecognizable.

The stool specimen must be free of contaminants such as barium, castor oil or mineral oil, or magnesium hydroxide, because these substances interfere with parasite identification.

Pretreatment with tetracyclines, sulphonamides, bismuth and kaolin compounds will prevent an adequate diagnosis.

Trophozoites may be confused with polymorphonuclear leukocytes and macrophages, and the innocuous trophozoites of *Entamoeba coli* can be mistaken for *Ent. histolytica*. Likewise, the cysts of *Entamoeba hartmani* should be differentiated from the cysts of *Ent. histolytica*.

If, for technical or geographical reasons, fresh stools are not available for examination, then specimens fixed or preserved in 10% formalin for cysts, or in polyvinyl alcohol for trophozoites, must be used.[9] The formalin–ether method should be used for concentration of the fixed specimen. The specimen preserved in polyvinyl alcohol should be smeared on cover slides and stained with iron hematoxylin or Gomori's trichrome stain.

The examination of three to six samples, if carried out adequately, establishes the diagnosis in 80–90% of cases.

SEROLOGICAL DIAGNOSIS

Ent. histolytica is antigenic and produces an immune response in the host. Antibodies usually persist for a long time, making it difficult to differentiate between past infection and existing disease.

Positive reactions always indicate invasive amoebiasis and are most useful in the diagnosis of extraintestinal disease. Nevertheless, epidemiological studies can best be done by serological methods, although they will not distinguish between active disease, postinfection and asymptomatic carriers.

Indirect hemagglutination,[30,33] latex agglutination,[30] cellulose acetate precipitation,[30,33] counter immunoelectrophoresis,[46,50] complement fixation,[17] the gel diffusion precipitin test[33] and fluorescent immunoassay[49] have all been used with variable degrees of sensitivity and specificity. They have a 90–98% positivity in extraintestinal disease and 80–90% in intestinal infection.[17,33,46,50]

The enzyme-linked immunosorbent assay (ELISA) method for the detection of amoebic antigens in stools deserves special attention.[32,42] It is a very simple and highly sensitive method, but has not yet been completely evaluated. It could become a most useful diagnostic test.

TREATMENT

Ipecacuanha was used in the treatment of dysentery in the 19th century and its alkaloid, emetine, was isolated in 1912. It is effective in the treatment of intestinal and invasive amoebiasis, but its side-effects prompted the investigation of different drugs.

Oxyquinolines, arsenicals and antibiotics such as paromomycin, erythromycin and tetracyclines have been used. Chloroquine also possesses amoebicidal properties, but only in extraintestinal disease. Dehydroemetine was synthesized and found to have the same properties as emetine, without its neuromuscular and cardiac side-effects.

In 1966, Powel and Elsdon Dew demonstrated that metronidazole was highly effective in intestinal as well as tissue invasion. Although some resistance has been reported occasionally, most of the cases respond very well, with prompt resolution of symptoms. A number of metronidazole derivatives, such as ornidazole and tinidazole, are in common use and are better tolerated orally than the parent drug metronidazole. For severe cases of intestinal amoebiasis and liver abscess, or when the drug cannot be administered orally, parenteral metronidazole and ornidazole are also available.

The effect of metronidazole on anaerobic intestinal flora is also beneficial and is currently the drug of choice in the treatment of intestinal and extraintestinal disease. In the rare cases of severe amoebic colitis which do not respond to metronidazole, dehydroemetine should be administered parenterally at a dose of 1 mg/kg per day for 10 days, with monitoring of the electrocardiogram.

Another problem is the treatment of the asymptomatic cyst shedder. Iodochlorhydroxyquinoline is a highly effective drug, but it can cause subacute myelo-optic neuropathy and thus is no longer used.

Consequently, the choice now lies between metronidazole (750mg three times a day for 7–10 days), diloxamide furoate[53] (500 mg three times a day for 10 days) and the antibiotic paromomycin three times a day (500 mg for 10–12 days). They can be administered serially if necessary.

The asymptomatic homosexual should be treated, although the problem of treating large series of patients in the setting of clinics for sexually transmitted disease has been acknowledged, and it is more effective and important to educate them in the dangers of promiscuous homosexual activities and oral–anal sexual practices.

In liver abscess, metronidazole or tinidazole is highly effective. It has been reported[20] that one single does of 2 g of ornidazole or tinidazole will cure over 95% of patients. The present chemotherapy of amoebiasis is quite effective and resistance is not a problem.[27] *Table 9.14* summarizes the most useful drugs and their dosage for the management of intestinal and extraintestinal infections.

In cases of toxic megacolon, or when perforation occurs, if the diagnosis can be established, treatment should be initiated as soon as possible, together with general support. Surgery is required on an emergency basis and partial or total colonic resection is necessary. Primary anastomosis is not usually indicated.[3,28] The death rate is extremely high in this form of amoebic colitis if left untreated. With aggressive medical and surgical treatment, the death rate has been reduced to somewhere between 45 and 55%.

When an amoeboma is diagnosed, medical treatment should be given, preferably parenteral dehydroemetine and metronidazole, because the drug has to penetrate the fibrous tissue to kill the parasite. Usually these patients will heal medically. Occasion-

Table 9.14 Drugs used in intestinal and extraintestinal amoebic infections

Form of infection	*Dosage*	*Route*
Intestinal		
Trophozoites in stool		
Metronidazole, Ornidazole, Tinidazole	500–750 mg t.i.d. for 5–10 days	Oral
Dehydroemetine	1 mg · kg^{-1} · day^{-1} for 10 days	Subcutaneous
Cysts		
Metronidazole, Ornidazole, Tinidazole	500–750 mg t.i.d. for 5–10 days	Oral
Diloxanide furoate	500 mg t.i.d. for 10 days	Oral
Paromomycin sulphate	500 mg t.i.d. for 5–10 days	Oral
Di-iodohydroxyquinoline (iodoquinol)	650 mg t.i.d. for 20 days	Oral
Extraintestinal		
Metronidazole, Ornidazole, Tinidazole	500–750 mg t.i.d. for 5–10 days	Oral
Dehydroemetine	1 mg · kg^{-1} · day^{-1} for 10 days	Subcutaneous
Dehydroemetine +	1 mg · kg^{-1} · day^{-1} for 10 days +	Subcutaneous
metronidazole	500 mg t.i.d. for 5–10 days	Oral
Tetracycline	500 mg every 6 hours for 10 days	Oral
Metronidazole, Ornidazole	500 mg every 6–8 hours for 5 days	Intravenous

t.i.d. = three times a day.

ally they will perforate and emergency surgery is required. Not infrequently, amoebomas and acute fulminant colitis coincide with liver abscesses, and these should be sought out and treated as indicated.

REFERENCES

1. Aceti, A., Pennica, A., Ippolito, G. *et al.* (1987) Antiamebic antibodies in homosexual men. *New England Journal of Medicine*, **316**(11), 692.
2. Allason-Jones, E., Mindel, A., Sargeaunt, P. and Williams, P. (1986) *Entamoeba histolytica* as a commensal intestinal parasite in homosexual men. *New England Journal of Medicine*, **315**, 353–356.
3. Bautista, J. (1978) Tratamiento quirurgico de las complicaciones de la amibiasis invasora. *Archivos de Investigacion Medica (Mexico)*, **9**, 411–415.
4. Brumpt, E. (1925) *Bulletin de L'Academie Nationale de Medecine (Paris)*, **94**, 943 (cit. (1979) *The Lancet*, **i**, 303).
5. Chacin-Bonilla, L. and Bonpart, D. (1981) A seroepidemiological study of amebiasis in adults in Maracaibo, Venezuela. *American Journal of Tropical Medicine and Hygiene*, **30**, 1201–1205.
6. Chin, A.T.L. and Gerken, A. (1984) Carriage of interstinal protozoal cysts in homosexuals. *British Journal of Venereal Disease*, **60**, 193–195.
7. De La Torre, M., Ortiz-Ortiz, L., De La Hoz, R. and Sepulveda, B. (1973) Accion del suero humano inmune de la gammaglobulina antiamibiana sobre los cultivos de *E. histolytica*. *Archivos de Investigacion Medica (Mexico)*, **4**, 155.
8. De Leon, A. (1970) Pronostico tardio en el absceso hepatico amibiano. *Archivos de Investigacion Medica (Mexico)*, **1**, 205.
9. Despommier, D.D. (1981) The laboratory diagnosis of *Entamoeba histolytica*. *Bulletin of the New York Academy of Medicine*, **57**, 212–216.
10. Dritz, S.K., Ainsworth, T.E., Back, A. *et al.* (1977) Patterns of sexually transmitted enteric diseases in a city. *The Lancet*, **ii**, 3–4.
11. Editorial (1979) Pathogenic *Entamoeba histolytica*. *The Lancet*, **i**, 303.
12. Elizondo, G., Weissleder, R., Stark, D.D., Todd, L.E., Compton, C., Wittenberg, J. *et al.* (1987) Amebic liver abscess: diagnosis and treatment evaluation with MR imaging. *Radiology*, **165**(3).
13. Fodor, T. (1981) Unanswered questions about the transmission of amebiasis. *Bulletin of the New York Academy of Medicine*, **57**, 224–226.
14. Gathiram, V., Simjee, A.E., Bhamjee, A., Jackson, T.F.H.G., Pillay, L.V. and Anderson, C.B. (1984) Concomitant and secondary bacterial infection of the pus in hepatic amoebiasis. *South African Medical Journal*, **65**(24), 51–53.

15. Gold, B., Diamantstein, T. and Hahn, H. (1982) Attempts to immunize golden hamsters against *Entamoeba histolytica*. *Annals of Tropical Medicine and Parasitology*, **76**(3), 367–369.
16. Kean, B.H. (1981) Clinical amebiasis in New York city: symptoms, signs and treatment. *Bulletin of the New York Academy of Medicine*, **57**, 207–211.
17. Kim, H. and Finkelstein, S. (1978) Serologic responses in amebiasis. *Archivos de Investigacion Medica (Mexico)*, **9**, 357–361.
18. Kobiler, D. and Mirelman, D. (1980) A lectin activity in *Entamoeba histolytica* trophozoites. *Archivos de Investigacion Medica (Mexico)*, **11**(suppl.), 101.
19. Landa, L., Audanel, M., Segovid, E. and Sepulveda, B. (1972) Seroepidemiologia de la amibiasis en adultos. *Archivos de Investigacion Medica (Mexico)*, **3**, 377–380.
20. Lassere, R., Jaroonvesama, N., Kurathong, S. and Soh, C.T. (1985) Single day drug treatment of amebic liver abscess. *American Journal of Tropical Medicine and Hygiene*, **32**(4), **721**, 23.
21. Losch, F. (1875) Massenhafte Entwickelung von Amoeben in Dickdarm. *Arch. F. Path. Anat.*, **211**, 65, 196.
22. Markell, E.K., Havens, R.F., Kuritsubo, R.A. and Wingerd, J. (1984) Intestinal protozoa in homosexual men of the San Francisco Bay area: prevalence and correlates of infection. *American Journal of Tropical Medicine and Hygiene*, **33**, 239, 45.
23. Marr, J.S. (1981) Amebiasis in New York city: a changing pattern of transmission. *Bulletin of the New York Academy of Medicine*, **57**, 224–226.
24. Meerovitch, E., Healy, G.R. and Ambroise-Thomas, P. (1978) *Canadian Journal of Public Health*, **69**, 286–288.
25. Mirelman, D., Bracha, R., Chayen, A., Aust-Kettis, A. and Diamond, L.S. (1986) *Entamoeba histolytica*: effect of growth conditions and bacterial associates on isoenzyme patterns and virulence. *Experimental Parasitology*, **62**, 142–148.
26. Monillan, A. and Robertson, D.H. (1977) Sexually transmitted diseases in homosexual males in Edinburgh. *Health Bulletin (Edinburgh)*, **35**, 266–271.
27. Neal, R.A. (1983) Experimental amoebiasis and the development of anti-amoebic compounds. *Parasitology*, **86**, 175–191.
28. Nicholls, J.C. (1981) Amoebiasis: a surgeon's view. *Annals of the Royal College of Surgery of England*, **63**, 25–27.
29. Ortiz-Ortiz, L., Garmilla, C., Tanimoto-Weki, M. and Zamacona-Ravelo, G. (1973) Hipersensibilidad celular en amibiasis. I. Reacciones en hamsters inoculados con *E. histolytica*. *Archivos de Investigacion Medica (Mexico)*, **4**, 141.
30. Ortiz-Ortiz, L., Capin, N.R., Capin, R. and Zamacona, G. (1978) Un nuevo metodo de hemaglutinacion para determinar anticuerpos contra *Entamoeba histolytica*. *Archivos de Investigacion Medica (Mexico)*, **9**, 351–356.
31. Ostrow, D.G. and Shaskey, G.M. (1977) The experience of the Howard Brown Memorial Clinic in Chicago with sexually transmitted diseases. *Sexually Transmitted Diseases*, 4R53–55.
32. Palacios, O. and De La Hoz, R. (1978) Determinacion del antigeno amibiano en heces por el methodo ELISA. *Archivos de Investigacion Medica (Mexico)*, **9**, 339–348.
33. Patterson, M., Healy, G.R. and Shabot, J.M. (1980) Serologic testing for amoebiasis. *Gastroenterology*, **78**, 136–141.
34. Pearce, R.B., Abrams, D.I. *New England Journal of Medicine*, **316**, 690.
35. Pehrson, P.O. (1983) Amoebiasis in a non-endemic country. *Scandinavian Journal of Infectious Diseases*, **15**, 207–214.
36. Petri, W.A. Jr and Ravdin, J. (1986) Treatment of homosexual men infected with *Entamoeba histolytica*. *New England Journal of Medicine*, **315**, 393.
37. Phillips, S.C., Mildram, D. and William, D.C. (1981) Sexual transmission of enteric protozoa and helminths in a venereal disease clinic population. *New England Journal of Medicine*, **305**, 603–606.
38. Pomerantz, B.M., Marr, J.S. and Goldman, W.D. (1981) Amebioasis in New York city. 1958–1978: identification of the male homosexual high risk population. *Bulletin of the New York Academy of Medicine*, **56**, 232–244.
39. Ralls, P.W., Colletti, P.M., Quinn, M.F. and Halls, J. (1982) Sonographic findings in hepatic amebic abscess. *Radiology*, **145**, 123–126.
40. Ralls, P.W., Barnes, P.F., Johnson, M.B., De Cock, K.M., Randall Radin, D. and Halls, J. (1987) Medical treatment of hepatic amebic abscess: rare need for percutaneous drainage. *Radiology*, **165**(3).
41. Ravdin, J.I., Croft, B.Y. and Guerrant, R.L. (1980) Cytopathogenic mechanisms of *Entamoeba histolytica*. *Journal of Experimental Medicine*, **152**, 377–390.
42. Root, D.M., Cole, F.X. and Williamson, J.A. (1978) The development and standardization of an ELISA method for the detection of *Entamoeba histolytica* antigens in stool samples. *Archivos de Investigacion Medica (Mexico)*, **9**, 203–210.
43. Sargeaunt, P.G. and Williams, J.E. (1978) The differentiation of invasive and non-invasive *Entamoeba histolytica* by isoenzyme electrophoresis. *Transactions of the Royal Society of Tropical Medicine and Hygiene*, **72**, 519–521.
44. Sargeaunt, P.G., Williams, J.E., Kumate, S. and Jimenez, E. (1980) The epidemiology of *Entamoeba histolytica* in Mexico City. *Transactions of the Royal Society of Tropical Medicine and Hygiene*, **74**, 653–656.
45. Sepulveda, B., Tanimoto, M., Vazquez-Saavedra, J.A., Calderon-Lara, P. and Landa, L. (1971) Induccion de inmunidad antiamibiana en el hamster con antigeno obtenido de cultivos axenicos de

Entamoeba histolytica. *Archivos de Investigacion Medica (Mexico)*, **2**, 289.
46. Sharma, P., Das, P. and Dutta, G.P. (1981) Rapid diagnosis of amoebic liver abscess using *Entamoeba histolytica* antigen. *Archivos de Investigacion Medica (Mexico)*, **12**, 553–557.
47. Sociedad Venezolana de Gastroenterologia (1972) Amibiasis en Venezuela. *Rev. Ven. San. Asist. Social*, **37**, 716–763.
48. Tanimoto-Weki, M., Vazquez-Saavedra, J.A., Calderon-Lara, P. and Aguiree-Garcia, J. (1973) Inmunidad consecutiva a la inyeccion de antigeno amibiano axenico en el hamster. *Archivos de Investigacion Medica (Mexico)*, **4**, 147.
49. Taylor, R.G. and Perez, T.R. (1978) Serology of amebiasis using the Fiax™ system. *Archivos de Investigacion Medica (Mexico)*, **9**, 363–366.
50. Tosswill, J.H.C., Ridley, D.S. and Warhurst, D.C. (1980) Counter immuno-electrophoresis as a rapid screening test for amoebic liver abscess. *Journal of Clinical Pathology*, **33**, 33–35.
51. Vinayak, V.K., Naik, S.R., Sawhney, S., Sehmi, N. and Chhuttani, P.N. (1977) Pathogenicity of *Entamoeba histolytica* – virulence of strains of amoeba from symptomatic and asymptomatic cases of amoebiasis. *Indian Journal of Medical Research*, **66**, 935–941.
52. Wig, J.D., Talwar, B.L. and Bushnurmath, S.R. (1981) Toxic dilatation complicating amoebic colitis. *British Journal of Surgery*, **68**, 135–136.
53. Wolfe, M.S. (1973) Non-dysenteric intestinal amebiasis: treatment with diloxamide furoate. *Journal of the American Medical Association*, **224**, 1601–1604.

ABDOMINAL TUBERCULOSIS

R.K. Tandon

HISTORICAL PERSPECTIVE

Tuberculosis has been known since ancient times but the relationship between pulmonary and enteric tuberculosis was only clarified by John Hunter in 1835.[10] The discovery of the causative organism (*Mycobacterium tuberculosis*) and subsequently of potent chemotherapeutic agents brought a better understanding of the disease and relief from a long-standing scourge.

EPIDEMIOLOGY

The prevalence of abdominal tuberculosis is not known. Its incidence in patients with pulmonary tuberculosis has been steadily decreasing since the advent of antituberculous drugs and is estimated by autopsy studies to be present in 10–30% of patients with active pulmonary tuberculosis.[32] The incidence is much higher in populations where pasteurization of milk is not routinely practised.

Although tuberculosis had almost disappeared from the affluent Western countries, the appearance of the acquired immune deficiency syndrome (AIDS) led to a resurgence of the disease, particularly of its extrapulmonary and disseminated forms.[28,33]

PATHOGENESIS

M. tuberculosis and not atypical mycobacterium is the causative agent. The routes of infection include direct invasion by micro-organisms, haematogenous spread and extension from contiguous organs.

DIRECT INVASION

Primary gut tuberculosis is rare owing to the extensive practice of pasteurization of milk. Gut infection when it occurs is mostly by the human strain of mycobacterium secondary to ingestion of contaminated chyme or swallowing of infected sputum. After ingestion the bacillus passes into the small bowel, as its fatty capsule cannot be digested in the stomach. Intestinal involvement is determined by the number and virulence of ingested organisms and the individual's resistance. The terminal ileum is the most commonly affected site, perhaps because of the rate of water and electrolyte absorption, the abundance of lymphoid tissue and prolonged contact time of bacteria with the mucosa. Other sites of involvement in decreasing order of frequency include the colon, jejunum, rectum and duodenum.[9] Stomach and oesophagus[3,17] are the rarest sites of involvement by tubercle bacilli.

Once within the intestine the organism penetrates

the crypts of mucosal glands and causes submucosal invasion, leading to the formation of a caseating granuloma which ultimately ruptures and results in formation of a typical shallow tuberculous ulcer with undermined edges.

HAEMATOGENOUS SPREAD

Localization of the disease in the submucosa with overlying normal mucosa suggests that silent bacteraemia may have occurred during the active phase of pulmonary tuberculosis.

CONTIGUOUS EXTENSION

The gut may also be involved by direct extension from infected organs, e.g. female adnexa or mesenteric lymph nodes.

PATHOLOGY

The predominant involvement in the abdomen is of the intestinal tract (43–69% of patients). Involvement of lymph nodes occurs in about 30% and the peritoneum in 24–30%.[5] Of those with peritoneal involvement, 60% have the ascitic form and 40% have the dry form of peritonitis. One-quarter of patients present with adhesions.[5]

INTESTINAL TUBERCULOSIS

The intestinal lesion can be of three types: ulcerative, hypertrophic or combined. The ulcers result from ischaemia secondary to endarteritis caused by a large load of mycobacteria of high virulence. They may be single or multiple, usually less than 1 cm in diameter with shaggy margins and overhanging edges. In the acute stage, ulcers cause intestinal obstruction due to associated spasm. In the chronic phase the ulcers may develop into circumferential ('napkin ring') strictures, thus resulting in constrictive lesions in 59% of patients (94% in the small intestine and 6% in the right side of the colon).[12] The hypertrophic form results from fibroblastic reaction to a small load of bacilli of low virulence and is seen most commonly in the ileocaecal region.[30] The palpable mass in the right iliac fossa usually comprises thickened indurated bowel wall with mesenteric fat, lymph nodes and peritoneal adhesions with adherent bowel loops. The third variety combines the features of both ulcerative and hypertrophic forms of tuberculosis.[43]

MICROSCOPIC APPEARANCE

The most characteristic histological feature of tuberculosis is caseating granuloma with acid-fast bacilli. These granulomata are multiple, large and confluent compared to the discrete granulomata of sarcoidosis. Granulomata heal by hyalinization occasionally with calcification.

CLINICAL FEATURES

The symptoms of gut tuberculosis are not specific and depend on the region involved. The average age of affected individuals is 31 years (26 years in India and 46 years in the rest of the world).[18] Similarly, whereas in the Western world 60% of the patients are male, in India females outnumber males (37%) with an overall world figure for males of 42%.

SYMPTOMS

The disease is frequently asymptomatic. Emaciation, weight loss, easy fatiguability and generalized weakness are common symptoms (45–74%).[5] The commonest abdominal symptom is pain (93%), (umbilical in 35%, generalized in 32% and localized to the right iliac fossa in 21%).[12] The character of the pain is non-specific and diffuse in 50% of patients and cramping in the rest (occurring either in the epigastrium, periumbilical region or right lower quadrant). About half of the patients complain of vomiting (primarily those with obstructive lesions). Anorexia and fever are present in 40% of patients. Diarrhoea alone occurs in 19% alternating with constipation in 3–9%.[5] Frank blood in the stool, jaundice and steatorrhoea are uncommon symptoms.

DURATION OF SYMPTOMS

The average duration ranges from 4.7 months to 1 year.[18] An occasional patient may be symptomatic for several years; for example, Louis XIII (1601–1643) is thought to have suffered for 16 years.[15]

PHYSICAL EXAMINATION

The most frequent finding on clinical examination is abdominal tenderness present in two-thirds of patients.[5] Ascites occurs in a varying proportion of patients, depending upon the form of abdominal tuberculosis. A palpable mass can be found in the abdomen in 35–50% of patients, mostly in the right iliac fossa with an average size of 5–8 cm. A right iliac region mass is generally due to hypertrophic ileocaecal tuberculosis. Tuberculous lymphadenitis occurs in 18% and rolled up omentum in 3%.[5] Associated visible peristalsis occurs in about a third of patients. Doughy feel of the abdomen, though thought to be characteristic of abdominal tuberculosis, is rare and is typically a manifestation of a diffuse intra-abdominal inflammatory process.[25]

ABDOMINAL TUBERCULOSIS IN CHILDHOOD

The clinical manifestations of abdominal tuberculosis in childhood are variable and non-specific and therefore an early diagnosis is seldom possible. As in adults, the presentation depends on the site and extent of the disease process. The most common variety is the adhesive type with symptoms of intestinal obstruction. However, (unlike in adults) stricture formation and hypertrophic tuberculosis are rarely encountered in childhood. Similarly, ascitic variety of peritoneal tuberculosis is distinctly uncommon in children.[36]

COMPLICATIONS

Obstruction of the small or large bowel occurs in 10–60% of patients and is classically chronic and intermittent. Factors responsible for obstruction include contraction of collagenous tissue following healing of the circumferential intestinal tubercular ulcers, hypertrophy of the bowel wall leading to narrowing of the lumen, kinking of intestines due to intraperitoneal adhesions and retraction of mesentery and shortening of the right colon by scar tissue.

Fistulas develop in 1–13% of patients, which is much less common than in regional enteritis.[12] The most frequent variety is spontaneous faecal fistula. Free perforations occur in 2.7% (1–26%) of patients; the majority are located in the distal 100 cm of ileum or in the appendix. Unfortunately, the incidence of perforations has increased since the advent of chemotherapy.

Perianal complications including fissures and perianal abscesses are prominent, especially in the presence of diarrhoea. Massive haemorrhage is rare. Enterolithiasis and traction diverticula are other rare complications.

Malnutrition is common and a consequence of anorexia, poor energy intake and malabsorption.

DIFFERENTIAL DIAGNOSIS

The diagnosis of abdominal tuberculosis is difficult, especially when there is no concomitant pulmonary tuberculosis. Symptoms are often non-specific so that the preoperative diagnosis is made in less than half the cases.[37] The frequent use of therapeutic trials further modifies the picture by making the clinical course of abdominal tuberculosis more protracted.[40] Antitubercular therapy not only alters the characteristic findings of caseating granuloma but also inhibits the culture of tubercle bacilli.

The problem of establishing a correct diagnosis of abdominal tuberculosis is compounded in Western countries, where it has to be distinguished from Crohn's disease with overlap even in histopathology.[39] The similarities between the two diseases include symptoms, recurrent intestinal obstruction, fistulas, abdominal masses and granulomata. Even the prolonged course of illness characteristic of Crohn's disease may be seen in some patients with abdominal tuberculosis. Features which help to distinguish the two are listed in *Table 9.15*.

The differential diagnosis includes abdominal lymphoma, fungal infections of the bowel, ulcerative colitis, colonic malignancy, sarcoidosis, amoeboma, ischaemic colitis, lymphogranuloma venereum, diverticulitis and endometriosis.

The specific criteria (Paustian criteria)[30] for diagnosis include fulfilling at least one of the following:

1. Animal inoculation or culture of suspected enteric, mesenteric or regional lymph node tissue, resulting in the growth of tubercle bacilli.
2. Histological demonstration of the typical acid-fast bacilli of *M. tuberculosis* in the lesion.
3. Histological evidence of tubercles with caseation necrosis.
4. The typical gross changes at operation with biopsies from mesenteric lymph nodes showing histological evidence consistent with tuberculosis.

A further category of 'probable tuberculosis' has been suggested where there is a clear cut response to antituberculous therapy for concurrent tuberculosis elsewhere providing there is no recurrence of disease after chemotherapy has been completed.[27] This category is used especially in developing countries, such as India, where the disease is prevalent and diagnostic facilities are not widely available.

Table 9.15 Differences between abdominal tuberculosis and Crohn's disease

Characteristic	*Tuberculosis*	*Crohn's disease*
Aetiology	*Mycobacterium tuberculosis*	Not known
Incidence	Decreasing or same	Increasing
Main populations affected	Third World countries	Europe and America
Clinical features		
Age at peak occurrence	Any age	15–35 years
Sex ratio	M > F (Western countries) F > M (India)	M = F
Familial incidence	Very rare	2–5%
Internal fistulae	Rare	Common
Anal lesion	Rare	Common
Risk of malignancy	None	Increased
Investigations		
Chest radiograph	Pulmonary tuberculosis (30%)	Normal
Mantoux Test	Positive	Negative
Skin lesions	Rare	Common
Gross pathology	1. Miliary nodules on serosa 2. Strictures (<3 cm) are transverse and circumferential	1. Perianal fistula 2. Longitudinal strictures on anterior mesenteric border
Histopathology		
Granuloma	Large, confluent caseating with surrounding fibrosis in all	Small, discrete non-caseating in 25%
Culture for tuberculosis	Positive	Negative
Response to antitubercular drugs	Good	Nil/poor
Follow-up	No relapses after cure	Remission and relapses

M, male; F, female.

INVESTIGATIONS

ABDOMINAL TUBERCULOSIS

The investigations for establishing the diagnosis of abdominal tuberculosis include (1) laboratory tests, (2) radiological studies, (3) serological tests, (4) culture of body fluids and tissue and (5) histological examination of biopsy material.

Laboratory tests

Mild anaemia, leukocytosis with relative lymphocytosis and a raised erythrocyte sedimentation rate are common. About 20% of patients are hypoproteinaemic. The serum alkaline phosphatase level is often raised, possibly because of hepatic or body involvement.

The Mantoux test is positive in 70–90% of patients but it has severe diagnostic limitations, particularly in developing countries where exposure to tubercle bacilli is common in childhood. Thus, a positive response does not establish the presence of active disease, nor does a negative response exclude the disease because severe disease and malnutrition may produce immunological hyporesponsiveness. A strongly positive Mantoux test (>20 mm diameter) in an appropriate clinical setting is highly suggestive of tuberculosis.

Radiological investigations

Radiological signs may be suggestive although not commonly diagnostic of abdominal tuberculosis.

Chest and abdominal films

Chest radiographs are suggestive of tuberculosis in 30–50% of patients with abdominal tuberculosis. Erect and supine abdominal films are helpful in 60% of patients when air–fluid levels are present suggesting subacute intestinal obstruction (*Figure 9.32*). Other useful findings include calcification of mesenteric lymph nodes and the presence of a diffuse haze

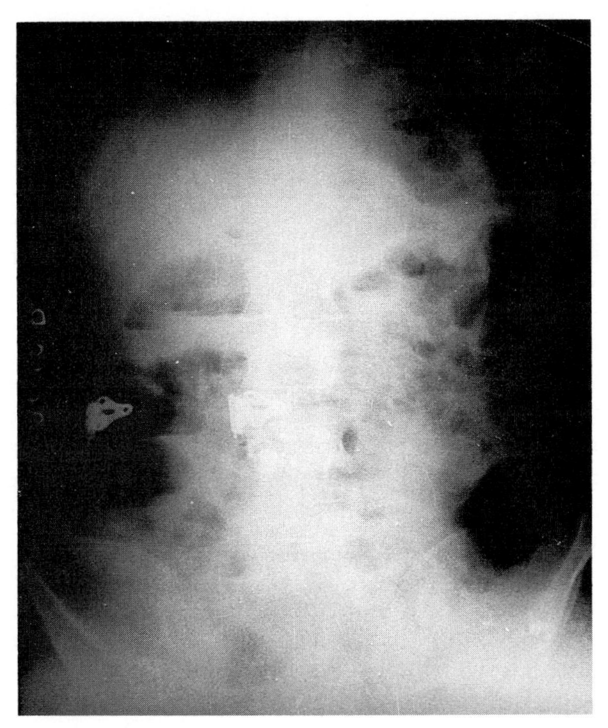

Figure 9.32 Plain radiograph of the abdomen showing air–fluid levels in the small bowel.

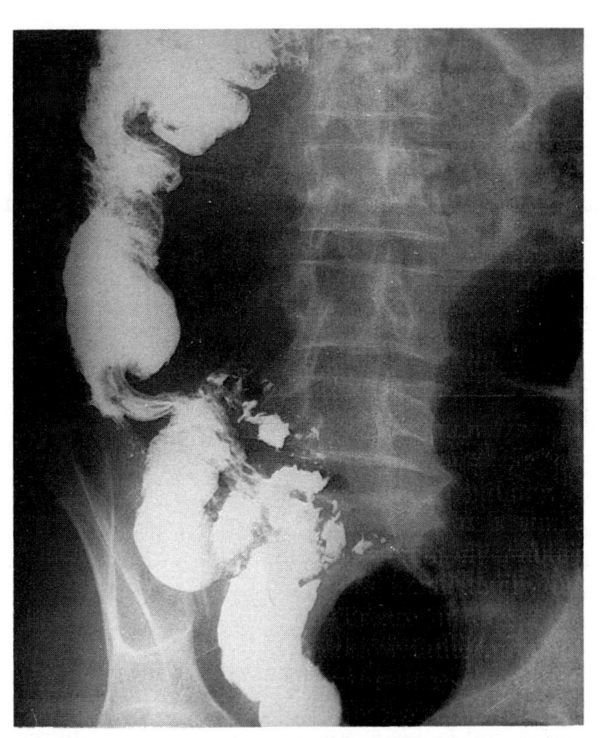

Figure 9.33 Barium meal follow-through study showing contraction and irregularity of the terminal ileum, increase in the ileocaecal angle and retraction of the caecum.

and obliteration of psoas shadows in the presence of ascites.

Contrast studies of the small and large bowels

Barium meal and follow-through studies are abnormal in 50–80% of patients. The earliest finding is of delayed transit accompanied by hypersegmentation and flocculation of barium. The resulting appearance may mimic malabsorption syndrome. Linear or stellate ulcers may be identified in the advanced stage. Stricture of the small bowel, obliteration of the ileocaecal valve and deformity of the caecum and ascending colon are characteristic (*Figure 9.33*). A variety of radiological signs suggestive of abdominal tuberculosis have been described but none of them is diagnostic. Poor filling of barium seen in the diseased segment of small bowel with adequate filling of both the proximal and distal intestine is referred to as 'Sterlin's sign'. Barium in a segment of bowel which has become stenotic due to hypertonicity or fibrosis is known as the 'string sign' but is equally common in Crohn's disease. The ulceration, granulation and fibrosis in the ileocaecal region is manifest by a broad triangular base of the caecum (Fleischner's sign). 'Goose neck' deformity of the colon results from widening of the ileocaecal angle.[12,22] Hyperplastic lesions in the colon may produce a 'pipe stem' or 'apple core' sign indistinguishable from colonic cancer.[14] Typically colonic involvement is segmental with masses, annular constriction and ulceration. Diffuse ulcerative lesions mimicking lymphoma or ulcerative colitis are rare.

Angiography and lymphangiography

Both these invasive investigations provide non-specific findings of enlarged mesenteric lymph nodes with central filling defects and lymphatic obstruction. Similar findings occur in patients with abdominal lymphoma.

Ultrasonography

The presence of a hypoechoic non-homogeneous mass lesion suggests tuberculous lymphadenitis and a highly echogenic mass may suggest tuberculous pathology on abdominal ultrasonography.[44]

Computed tomography (CT) scanning

CT scan manifestations of abdominal tuberculosis vary from slight and symmetrical thickening of gut wall with a few small regional lymph nodal enlargements (changes indistinguishable from those of Crohn's disease or ileocaecal lymphoma) to thickening of the ileocaecal valve and medial wall of the caecum surrounded by soft tissue, low-density regional lymph node masses of heterogeneous appearance (characteristic of tuberculosis). Such abnormalities are seen in 67% of patients with abdominal tuberculosis.[20]

Serological tests

Antigen complexity and cross-reactivity and the variability in antibody response make it difficult to produce a reliable serological test which will clearly distinguish healthy individuals from those with tuberculosis. The following tests are helpful.

Soluble antigen fluorescent antibody (SAFA) test

This is an indirect fluorescent antibody detection procedure employing soluble antigen fixed on an artificial matrix; the test results are read on a fluorometer. A positive result is indicative of current or very recent active tuberculosis and often is positive even before the conventional intradermal tests have become reactive. Its diagnostic value has been demonstrated in pulmonary and abdominal tuberculosis.[6]

Enzyme-linked immunosorbent assay (ELISA)

This test detects IgG antibody to purified protein antigen and yields a positive result only if tuberculous infection is chronic or extensive. The use of a mycobacterial saline extract antigen has a sensitivity of 81% and a specificity of 88% in diagnosing abdominal tuberculosis. Further purification of the antigen results in an even better sensitivity and specificity.[11]

Monoclonal antibodies

Detection of specific antigens of *M. tuberculosis* by monoclonal antibodies may not be very specific, as its antigens are shared by *Mycobacterium leprae* and *Legionella* ssp. Hence, for the development of specific serological tests, specific epitomes need to be selected.[16]

DNA probes and the polymerase chain reaction

DNA probes have been used for the rapid detection of mycobacterial infection but the low sensitivity of the technique limits its use. The polymerase chain reaction has been used to amplify the target DNA and to greatly enhance the sensitivity of diagnosing mycobacterial infection with a rapid result (1–2 days).[29] This test may eventually provide a rapid and simple method of diagnosing tuberculosis in peripheral blood.

Other serological tests

These include latex particle agglutination, radioimmunoassay, nitrocellulose dot-ELISA, and improved ELISA with immunosorbent purified antigens. However, they have not yet been applied to the diagnosis of abdominal tuberculosis.

Histopathology and bacteriological culture

Demonstration of the acid-fast bacilli in the affected tissue or fluid can be achieved through any of the following techniques.

Sputum or gastric washings

These obviously only yield positive results in patients with associated pulmonary tuberculosis.

Fine needle aspiration

This may be rewarding from intra-abdominal or peripheral lymph nodes. Ultrasound or CT guidance may be helpful for aspirating the material from intra-abdominal lymph nodes. These methods are helpful in distinguishing tuberculous lymph nodes from lymphoma.[31]

Endoscopy

The colonoscopic features in patients with ileocaecal tuberculosis include a deformed, oedematous ileocaecal valve, mucosal nodules 2–6 mm in size, hypertrophied caecal valve and pseudopolypoid folds; transverse ulcers may be present between the nodules. Although highly suggestive in the appropriate clinical setting, none of these changes is diagnostic of a tuberculous lesion. Biopsies may show caseating granulomata or acid-fast bacilli on histopathological examination or appropriate culture or guinea-pig inoculation in 30–50% of cases.[34]

Laparotomy

Laparotomy may be necessary in a few patients to establish the diagnosis of tuberculosis.

PERITONEAL TUBERCULOSIS

Further tests may be helpful to establish the diagnosis of peritoneal tuberculosis.

Ascitic fluid examination

The ascitic fluid protein content varies between 2.5 and 7.5 g/l and the cell count between 100 and 2200 cells/ml (92% lymphocytes). A cell count of more than 250/ml and a protein content of more than 2.5 g/l suggest an exudate compatible with the diagnosis of tuberculous ascites. About 30% of ascitic fluid aspirates yield positive culture for acid-fast bacilli.

Adenosine deaminase

Adenosine deaminase is a T-cell lymphokine which is released by lymphocytes and macrophages during the cellular immune response. Concentrations in serous fluids are increased in mycobacterial infection and may be of diagnostic value in patients with tuberculous meningitis and pleural effusion. A value of 32.3 units/l or more of adenosine deaminase in ascitic fluid has a sensitivity of 95% and specificity of 98% in diagnosing tuberculous ascites.[7] However, false positive results do occur in ascites due to fungal infections and malignant diseases, including T-cell abdominal lymphoma.

Abdominal ultrasonography and CT scanning

The presence of ascites with generalized echogenicity (turbidity) and multiple thread-like interlacing septa (possibly because of a high protein content) are suggestive of tuberculous ascites.

Peritoneal biopsy

In patients with exudative ascites, peritoneal biopsy can be obtained percutaneously using either an Abraham's or a Cope's needle with a positive yield of nearly 100%.[24] Das and Shukla utilized a simple, small grid-iron incision in the right iliac fossa to obtain adequate tissue yielding positive results in 11 of 12 patients with peritoneal tuberculosis.[12] Peritoneoscopy provides a good view of the abdominal viscera and peritoneum, which is studded with tubercles in such cases.

TREATMENT

A nutritious high-energy diet with adequate vitamin supplements is part of the treatment of abdominal tuberculosis, and treatment of tuberculosis before chemotherapy comprised long-term supportive care and heliotherapy in a sanatorium. Antituberculous drugs now play the major role in treatment.

MEDICAL

The basic principles guiding the use of antituberculous drugs for abdominal tuberculosis are the same as for pulmonary tuberculosis, i.e. a combination of two or three drugs given for 6–12 months.

A recent publication by the American College of Chest Physicians[38] suggested that optimal medical chemotherapy should comprise 9 months of isoniazid (5–10 mg/kg up to 300 mg orally or intramuscularly) and rifampicin (10–20 mg/kg up to 600 mg orally) with pyrazinamide, streptomycin or ethambutol for the first 3 months of therapy. Such a regimen produces cure rates of 78%.

Shorter courses are now being recommended to improve compliance. Thus, Dutt *et al.*[13] treated newly diagnosed and drug-susceptible cases of extrapulmonary tuberculosis with daily isoniazid (300 mg) and rifampicin (600 mg) for 1 month, followed by twice weekly isoniazid (900 mg) and rifampicin (600 mg) for a further 8 months and obtained good results. Such treatment not only reduces cost but also minimizes the risks of drug toxicity.

In a randomized trial of even shorter courses of therapy,[4] 104 patients with abdominal tuberculosis were treated either with a 6 month regimen comprising rifampicin, isoniazid and pyrazinamide daily for 2 months and rifampicin and isoniazid daily for the next 4 months ($n=51$) or a 12-month regimen of streptomycin, ethambutol and isoniazid daily for 2 months, followed by ethambutol and isoniazid for 10 months ($n=53$). The cure rates achieved by the two regimens were similar, suggesting that the 6-month regimen is sufficient for patients with abdominal tuberculosis.

The role of corticosteroids, if any, in the treatment of abdominal tuberculosis to try and prevent fibrosis and stricture formation is controversial.[23] However, in patients with severe toxaemia and continuing fever the addition of a small dose of steroids for short periods of time is often beneficial (personal observation).

Response

The response to medical therapy is evident within days with resolution of fever and improved well-being. The abdominal pain decreases significantly within 7 days – a much faster response than observed with pulmonary tuberculosis which is attributed to the smaller load of tubercle bacilli in abdominal tuberculosis – and the fact that isoniazid and rifampicin penetrate extrapulmonary sites better.[26] A recent study has shown complete resolution of strictures following standard antituberculous treatment.[1]

Thus, there should be considerable improvement in patients with abdominal tuberculosis within 2 weeks of therapy. This response justifies therapeutic trials in areas where the disease is common and diagnostic capabilities limited.

Side-effects

Common side-effects of antituberculous drugs include:

- Isoniazid – hepatitis, peripheral neuritis and hypersensitivity.

- Rifampicin – hepatitis, thrombocytopenia, fever, orange-coloured urine, tears and saliva.
- Pyrazinamide – hyperuricaemia and hepatotoxicity.
- Ethambutol – optic neuritis and skin rash.
- Streptomycin – ototoxicity, nephrotoxicity and hypersensitivity.

However, drug-induced hepatitis is the most common complication. This is directly related to increasing age and high alcohol intake.[42] Furthermore, rifampicin and isoniazid have synergistic effect in respect of hepatotoxicity.

Newer antituberculous drugs

Several new drugs have been developed although most have not yet been widely tested. They include mycolic acid, arabinogalactan, peptidoglyctan and mycobactins, all of which inhibit biosynthesis of mycobacteria. Spiropiperdyl, rifamycin (Rifabutin), fluoroquinolones and β-lactam agents are other drugs under trial for the treatment of mycobacterial infections. Rifabutin is long-acting (a weekly dose can be given) and has fewer side-effects.[35] Ofloxacin is another new drug with moderately effective antituberculous activity and few side-effects.[41]

Compliance

The problem of compliance may be solved by implantation of biodegradable polymeric systems (polylactic and polyglycolic acid polymers) which contain antituberculous drugs. However, the need for implants of large size (containing large amounts of antituberculous drugs) and their high cost make such a proposition impractical at the present.

Drug resistance

Fortunately, drug resistance is not very common. An incidence of 6% has been reported in the USA.[19] The drugs available for use in this situation include cycloserine, vancomycin, ethionamide, kanamycin, capreomycin and pyrazinamide.

SURGICAL

Surgical intervention was the mainstay of treatment before chemotherapy but is now only required for treating complications. Treatment includes bowel resection (33%), bypass of diseased bowel (24%) and suturing of perforation with or without bypass (5%). The preferred option is right hemicolectomy, as the disease occurs mostly in the ileocaecal region. However, when other areas are involved the treatment of choice is resection of the stenosed segment and tuberculous mass. Strictureplasty produces good results for resolution of strictures.[21]

Treatment with isoniazid, ethambutol and rifampicin is recommended for 6 weeks before surgery. Postoperative chemotherapy is only advocated for active disease.

The common postoperative complications include adhesions (4%), faecal fistulas (2%) and incisional hernia (2%).[2]

Prevention

To eradicate tuberculosis, new infections and progression of latent infection must be prevented. Unfortunately, these objectives are not being achieved because of the limitations of the current methods of diagnosis and treatment and the inability to utilize them fully in Third World countries. Existing resources must be utilized by making them available only to the people in real need. Also, the major advances in molecular biology should be exploited to develop rapid methods for diagnosis and treatment.

The presently available vaccine – bacille Calmette–Guérin (BCG) – neither prevents infection nor reactivation of latent infection; it only prevents dissemination of the initial infection. Efforts are therefore being made to develop a new more effective vaccine. One approach is to mark out virulence factors to identify the antigens that are important for protection. Using recombinant DNA technology these immunogenic antigens might then be incorporated in the production of a vaccine to provide effective protection.[8]

REFERENCES

1. Anand, B.S., Nanda, R. and Sachdev, G.K. (1988) Response of tuberculous stricture to antitubercular treatment. *Gut*, **29**, 62–69.
2. Anand, S.S. (1956) Hypertrophic ileocaecal tuberculosis in India with a record of fifty hemicolectomies. *Annals of the Royal College of Surgeons of England*, **19**, 205–222.
3. Annamalai, A. and Shree Kumar, S. (1972) Tuberculosis of the oesophagus. *American Journal of Gastroenterology*, **57**, 166–168.
4. Balasubramanium, R., Rajasambandam, P., Madanagopalan, N., Thiruvengadam, K.V., Rangabashyam, N. and Prabhakar, R. (1989) Drug treatment of abdominal tuberculosis (abstract). *Indian Journal of Gastroenterology*, **8**, A17.
5. Bhansali, S.K. (1977) Abdominal tuberculosis:

experience with 300 cases. *American Journal of Gastroenterology*, **67**, 324–337.
6. Bhargava, D.K., Shriniwas, Tandon, B.N., Kiran, U., Chawla, T.C. and Kapur, B.M.L. (1986) Serodiagnosis of intestinal tuberculosis by soluble antigen fluoroscent antibody test (SAFA test). *Journal of Tropical Medical Hygiene*, **89**, 61–65.
7. Bhargava, D.K., Nijhawan, S. and Gupta, M. (1989) Adenosine deaminase and tubercular peritonitis. *The Lancet*, **i**, 1260–1261.
8. Bloom, B.R. (1989) New approaches to vaccine development. *Review of Infectious Diseases, II*, **2**, 5460–5465.
9. Bruckstein, A.H. (1988) Abdominal tuberculosis. *New York State Journal of Medicine*, **88**, 18–21.
10. Cohen, S. (1835) Works of John Hunter. *Lectures on Surgery*, **1**, 567.
11. Daniel, T.M. and Debanne, S.M. (1987) The serodiagnosis of tuberculosis and other mycobacterial diseases by enzyme-linked immunosorbent assay. *American Review of Respiratory diseases*, **135**, 1137–1151.
12. Das, P. and Shukla, H.S. (1976) Clinical diagnosis of abdominal tuberculosis. *British Journal of Surgery*, **63**, 941–946.
13. Dutt, A.K., Mores, D. and Stead, W.W. (1986) Short course chemotherapy for extrapulmonary tuberculosis. *Annals of Internal Medicine*, **104**, 7–12.
14. Gadwood, K.A., Bedetti, C.D. and Herbert, D.L. (1981) Colonic tuberculosis mimicking annular carcinoma: report of a case. *Diseases of the Colon and Rectum*, **24**, 395–398.
15. Goldfischer, S. and Janis, M. (1981) A 42-year old king with cavitary pulmonary lesion and intestinal perforation. *New York Academy of Medicine*, **57**, 139–143.
16. Good, R.C. (1989) Serologic methods for diagnosing tuberculosis (editorial). *Annals of Internal Medicine*, **110**, 97–98.
17. Gordon, A.H. and Marshall, J.B. (1990) Oesophageal tuberculosis. Definite diagnosis by endoscopy. *American Journal of Gastroenterology*, **85**, 174–177.
18. Haddad, F.S., Ghossain, A., Sawaya, E. and Nelson, A.R. (1987) Abdominal tuberculosis. *Diseases of the Colon and Rectum*, **30**, 724–735.
19. Hobby, G.L., Johnson, P.M. and Boy-tar-papirnyik, V. (1974) Primary drug resistance: a continuing study of drug resistance in a veteran population within the United States. *American Review of Respiratory Diseases*, **110**, 95–101.
20. Hulnick, D.H., Megibow, A.J., Naidich, D.P., Hilton, S., Cho, K.C. and Balthazar, E.A. (1985) Abdominal tuberculosis. CT evaluation. *Radiology*, **157**, 199–204.
21. Kataria, R.N., Sood, S., Rao, P.G. and Rao, L. (1977) Strictureplasty for tubercular strictures of the gastrointestinal tract. *British Journal of Surgery*, **64**, 496–498.
22. Kausulke, R.J., Andersons, W.J., Gupta, S.K. and Gliedman, M.L. (1981) Primary tuberculous enterocolitis: report of three cases and review of the literature. *Archives of Surgery*, **116**, 110–113.
23. Klimach, O.E. and Ormerod, L.P. (1985) Gastrointestinal tuberculosis: a retrospective review of 109 cases in a district general hospital. *Quarterly Journal of Medicine, New Series*, **56**, 569–678.
24. Levine, H. (1968) Needle biopsy diagnosis of tuberculous peritonitis. *American Journal of Respiratory Diseases*, **97**, 889–894.
25. Lewis, E.A. and Kolawole, T.M. (1972) Tuberculous ileo-colitis in Ibadan: a clinico-radiological review. *Gut*, **13**, 646–653.
26. Mandell, G.L. and Sande, M.A. (1985) Drugs used in the chemotherapy of tuberculosis and leprosy. In *The Pharmacological Basis of Therapeutics* (Ed.) Gilman, A.G., Goodman, L.S., Rall, T.W. and Murad, F. pp. 1199–1218. New York: Macmillan.
27. Moss, J.D. and Kanuer, C.M. (1973) Tuberculous enteritis. *Gastroenterology*, **65**, 959–966.
28. Murray, C.J. (1990) World tuberculosis burden (letter). *The Lancet*, **335**, 1043–1044.
29. Noel, A.B., Gicquel, B., Lecossier, D., Frebault, V.L., Nassif, X. and Hance, A.J. (1989) Rapid diagnosis of tuberculosis by amplification of mycobacterial DNA in clinical samples. *The Lancet*, **ii**, 1069–1071.
30. Paustian, F.F. and Monto, G.L. (1976) Tuberculosis of the intestine. In: *Gastroenterology*, 3rd end, Vol. 2 (Ed.) Bockus, H.L. pp. 750–777. Philadelphia: W.B. Saunders.
31. Radhika, S., Gupta, S.K., Chakrawarty, A., Rajwanshi, A. and Josho, K. (1989) Role of culture for mycobacteria in fine-needle aspiration diagnosis of tubercular lymphadenitis. *Diagnostic Cytopathology*, **5**, 260–262.
32. Riggins, H.M. (1942) Tuberculosis of the alimentary tract. *Medical Clinics of North America*, **1**, 819–829.
33. Rosengart, T.K. and Coppa, G.F. (1990) Abdominal mycobacterial infections in immunocompromised patients. *American Journal of Surgery*, **159**, 125–131.
34. Sakai, Y. (1979) Colonoscopic diagnosis of intestinal tuberculosis. *Materia Medica Poland*, **11**, 275–278.
35. Sensi, P. (1989) Approach to the development of new antitubercular drugs. *Review of Infectious Diseases*, **II**(suppl.), s467–470.
36. Sharma, A.K., Agarwal, L.D. and Sharma, C.S. (1990) Abdominal tuberculosis in childhood. *Tropical Gastroenterology*, **11**, 140–143.
37. Sherman, S., Rohwedder, J.J., Ravi Krishnan, K.P. and Weg, J.G. (1980) Tuberculous enteritis and peritonitis: report of 36 general hospital cases. *Archives of Internal Medicine*, **140**, 506–508.
38. Snider, D.E. Jr, Cohn, D.L., Davidson, P.T. *et al.* (1985) Standard therapy for tuberculosis. *Chest*, **87**(suppl.), 117S–124S.
39. Tandon, H.D. and Prakash, A. (1972) Pathology of

intestinal tuberculosis and its distinction from Crohn's disease. *Gut*, **13**, 260–269.
40. Tandon, R.K., Sarin, S.K., Bose, R.L., Berry, M. and Tandon, B.N. (1986) A clinico-radiological reappraisal of intestinal tuberculosis – changing profile? *Gastroenterologica Japonica*, **21**, 17–22.
41. Tsukumara, M. (1986) Chemotherapy of lung tuberculosis by a new antibacterial substance ofloxacin (DL 8280). In *Mycobacteria of Clinical Interest* (Ed.) Casal, M. *et al*. pp. 234–240. Amsterdam: Excerpta Medica.
42. Tuberculosis Advisory Committee (1974) Special consultants to the director of the centre for disease control. Isoniazid hepatitis. *Journal of the American Medical Association*, **23**, 97–99.
43. Vasantha, V.C., Habibullah, C.M. and Kumar, A. (1975) Abdominal tuberculosis with special reference to pathological aspects. *Journal of the Indian Medical Association*, **65**, 302–303.
44. Zirinsky, K., Auh, Y.H., Kneeland, J.B., Ruben Stein, W.A. and Kazam, E. (1985) Computed tomography, sonography and MR imaging of abdominal tuberculosis. *Journal of Computer Assisted Tomography*, **9**, 961–963.

CHAGAS' DISEASE

A. Habr-Gama

EPIDEMIOLOGY

Chagas' disease – the name commonly given to American trypanosomiasis – is of enormous medical and social significance because, in some countries, it is the main cause of heart disease among young adults and causes severe damage to the digestive system, mainly to the oesophagus and colon, resulting in inability to work and social incapacity.

Chagas' disease was first described and researched by Carlos Chagas between 1907 and 1909.[3] It is a tissue and blood disease transmitted to humans by *Trypanosoma cruzi,* a haemoflagellate which is inoculated in humans by an insect, a bug belonging to the subfamily Triatomidae.

Chagas' disease has existed on the American continent since ancient times: prehistoric communities that settled along the northern most part of Chile over 200 years ago suffered from it. Chagasic megacolon and, very probably, cardiomyopathy has been identified in mummies excavated from an archaeological site 1100 m above sea level in the province of Taracapá (now Bolivia). Initially the parasite spread among mammal and forest vectors; later it adapted to the domestic cycle of transmission as a result of the development of permanent settlements by the pre-Columbian tribes that constructed dwellings and domesticated animals.

Currently, Chagas' disease predominates in the region from Mexico to Patagonia because of the contact between humans and the invertebrate vectors of the parasite. While the parasitic infestation is present over this wide area, the most important foci are in South America. There are approximately 15 million to 20 million individuals affected by the disease on the South American continent: 7 million in Brazil, 3 million in Argentina and 20 000 in Venezuela.[33]

In Brazil, the areas most affected are the rural central and north-eastern regions. The disease is becoming endemic in the cities because of the migratory waves and changes in the country's social structure. There are over 300 000 chagasic patients living in São Paulo city and over 200 000 in Rio de Janeiro. As a result, the risk of transmission of *T. cruzi* by other means has increased. An important 'non-vectorial' route is blood transfusion. Serological tests for Chagas' disease are positive in 0.5–2% of blood donors in the large Brazilian cities. This figure may reach 10–15% in medium-sized cities in endemic regions. Transmission is also possible via breast milk, organ transplants and laboratory accidents.

T. cruzi is inoculated in humans through the bite of an infected blood-sucking insect, a bug that lives in the mud walls or roof of thatched huts and known by the local population as 'barbeiro' (barber). It usually bites the face, and contaminates the skin wound or conjunctiva with infected faeces containing numerous parasites. The reservoir of infection extends not only to humans but also to dogs and cats living in the huts and to many surrounding wild animals.

The inoculated *T. cruzi* enters macrophages in the skin and produces a local inflammatory swelling (chagoma). Trypomastigotes then convert to amastigotes (leishmania) and invade smooth muscle and myocardium. As leishmanias they multiply in these tissues and cause destruction with the formation of cyst-like cavities. These pseudocysts then rupture and most of the leishmanias are destroyed by the natural defences of the body, but some reappear in the blood circulation. This cycle is repeated many times during the first week. During this acute phase, the diagnosis of Chagas' disease can be confirmed by direct examination of blood smears.

PATHOPHYSIOLOGY

T. cruzi is a parasite of muscle tissue, but it damages nerve cells of the autonomic nervous system and reduces their number considerably; these lesions are the most important consequence of the disease. The entire autonomic nervous system may be invaded, but some areas are more commonly affected, particularly the distal segments of the oesophagus, colon and rectum and intramural plexus of the heart. Other hollow muscular organs such as the pylorus, duodenum, ileum and ureter may be involved occasionally.[23] The two most frequent digestive forms are megaoesophagus and megacolon. In most patients a single manifestation occurs, although lesions in the nervous plexus are usually present elsewhere but do not produce symptoms. Occasionally, more extensive lesions occur together.[5,22,32]

The exact pathophysiological mechanism by which the neuronal destruction causes visceral dilatation has been the subject of much discussion. Neuronal lesions could primarily alter motility, producing motor dysfunction followed by stasis and dilatation because the myoenteric plexus is important in maintaining tone, coordination of movement and control of peristalsis.[12] Denervated smooth muscle is abnormally sensitive to stimuli and tends to contract permanently;[2] a small stimulus will then provoke strong, irregular and often complex contractions. In the colon, the first effect of denervation is loss of muscular coordination, the degree of functional disturbance varying according to its extent.

Most authors accepted that neuronal lesions of the enteric nervous plexuses were the sole explanation for the pathophysiology of chagasic megacolon. However, recent research has shown the ultrastructural complexity of the neurons of Auerbach's nervous plexuses: up to nine morphologically distinct neurons have been identified and about 10 substances have been claimed as neurotransmitters. As a consequence, the pathophysiology of chagasic megacolon cannot be explained simply by the reduction of the number of neurons of the enteric nervous system, detected by studies with the light microscope. The smooth muscle cell has not been adequately considered, mainly because it does not exhibit conspicuous alterations under the light microscope. Ultrastructural lesions, however, were detected with the electron microscope, showing an increase in the number of points of close contact between neighbouring cells, cytoplasmatic vacuolization, dilatation of the endoplasmic reticulum and disorganization of myofilaments.[20]

Cellular physiology studies have shown that the longitudinal muscle coat receives only excitatory innervation. The circular coat, on the other hand, behaves as an electrical syncytium; the basis for control of the circular muscle layer appears to be neuronal inhibition of the inherent excitable myogenic system, located in the longitudinal muscle layer.[8]

Cell-mediated immunity plays an important role in Chagas' disease. Recent research has revealed the participation of T lymphocytes cytotoxic to the myoenteric nervous plexus and to cardiac muscle cells, cross-reacting with *T. cruzi*'s antigens.[38] Antibodies against myocardium, smooth muscle, efferent vessel invasion factor, antineurons, antiperipheral nerves and deposition of immune complexes on the walls of heart arteries in the perivascular and interstitial areas have been described.[19,29] Strong evidence, therefore, points to autoimmunity phenomena participating in the pathophysiology of Chagas' disease.

Motility of the bowel has been studied by electromanometry in normal subjects and in patients with Chagas' megacolon, at rest and after the injection of methacholine chloride.[14,26,28,41] Hypermotility and incoordination of waves, characterized by synchronous activity of the sigmoid and rectum, were found. These changes were present in the whole colon. Methacholine significantly increased the number, amplitude and duration of the waves. The hypersensitivity of the muscle to this drug is a functional demonstration of the parasympathetic block due to degeneration of the myoenteric plexus.

Studies of the physiology of the internal anal sphincter in chagasic megacolon were repeated by Habr-Gama *et al.*[15] Basal activity of this muscle was normal; however, immediate relaxation following transient distension of the rectum with air does not occur. Muscular hypertrophy of the bowel is the final result of alterations in motor function. The muscular wall, although hypertrophied, has no propulsive power and stasis of intestinal contents occurs with progressive dilatation. Although destruction of ganglion cells is observed in the whole bowel, it is more prominent in the rectum. The distal segment of bowel, with its impaired function, acts as an obstacle to the passage of faeces; the higher intraluminal pressures and hard faecal content usually seen in the sigmoid colon may explain why this segment is more dilated.

CLINICAL FEATURES

Acute Chagas' disease usually occurs in children but is clinically recognized in only 1% or less. About 1–2 weeks following development of the chagoma, a febrile illness begins, lasting for several weeks, often associated with hepatosplenomegaly, generalized lymphadenopathy and, occasionally, myocarditis and meningoencephalitis. Mortality in the acute form of the disease is about 10%.[21]

Patients who survive progress to a chronic persistent phase. This phase is usually not clinically apparent for at least 10–15 years. In Brazil it is usually characterized by heart block, megaoesophagus in 3% of patients and megacolon in 1%.[32] In Argentina and Chile, however, megacolon appears to be commoner than megaoesophagus. Colonic symptoms generally only begin in patients at least 20 years old because of the long interval between the infection and the presentation of clinical illness.

Chagasic megacolon may be seen at any age but is more frequent from 30 to 50 years. It occurs equally in both sexes and in any race. Most patients come from rural areas and belong to the poorer and lower social classes. The main symptom is chronic constipation. This is initially relieved by laxatives or rectal enemas but becomes progressively more severe, bowel movements occurring with intervals of days or even months. Anorexia and malnutrition are often seen due to chronic constipation or to dysphagia. Palpitations, dizziness and transitory loss of consciousness are manifestations of chronic cardiomyopathy. *Faecal impaction* and *sigmoid volvulus* are the most common complications of megacolon.

Faecal impaction occurs commonly. The bolus of faeces is usually located in the rectum or rectosigmoid and, exceptionally, is not reached by digital examination. It is managed by repeated rectal enemas helped sometimes by manual emptying under light anaesthesia. Occasionally, when it is high in the sigmoid or descending colon, laparotomy may be required.

Sigmoid volvulus is very common and is responsible for 20% of all cases of intestinal obstruction.[16] Volvulus is due to torsion or twisting of the sigmoid colon over its mesenteric axis, with partial or total obstruction of the lumen. Patients tolerate the torsion well and maintain good health, providing gangrene does not occur. Medical care is not sought usually until some hours or even days after the onset of symptoms. Constipation, abdominal distension and pain are the usual complaints.

INVESTIGATIONS

Diagnosis may be confirmed by the complement fixation test (the Machado–Guerreiro test) which, when positive, remains so throughout life and is thus a good indicator of previous infection.

Diagnosis of megacolon is made by the clinical history, origin of patients from endemic areas of the country, and by physical examination. The chagasic aetiology in this chronic phase is confirmed by serological tests. The complement fixation test as described by Machado–Guerreiro in 1913 and improved by many authors, among them Pedreiras de Freitas, is still the most used and valuable method; it is positive in 90% of the patients.[32] Other serological tests are the immunofluorescence and immunoenzymatic (enzyme-linked immunosorbent assay, ELISA) tests.

Plain abdominal radiographs may show a gross amount of faeces (*Figure 9.34*), or large air-filled loops of bowel with loss of haustrations and pelvic

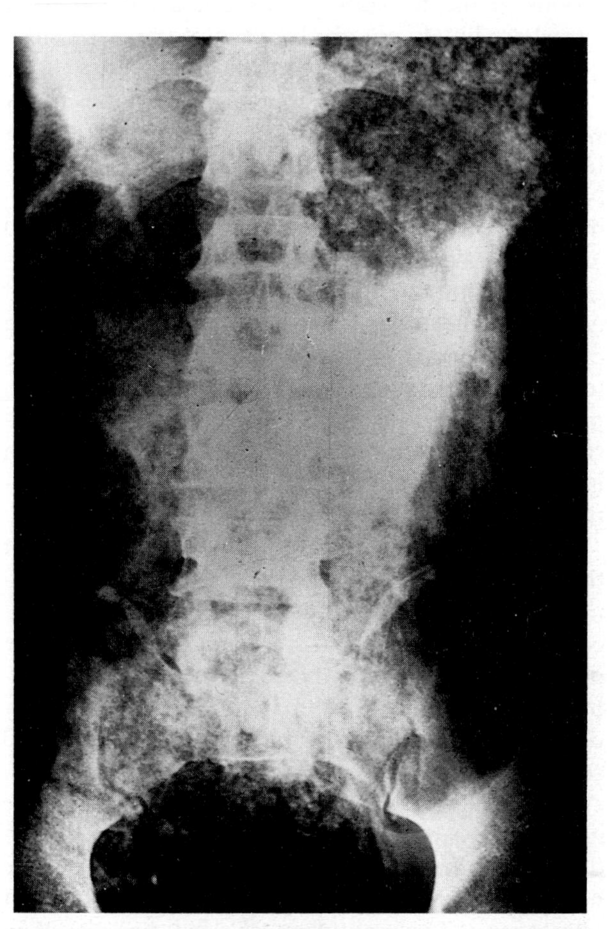

Figure 9.34 Plain abdominal radiograph showing a voluminous faecaloma: megacolon with faecaloma.

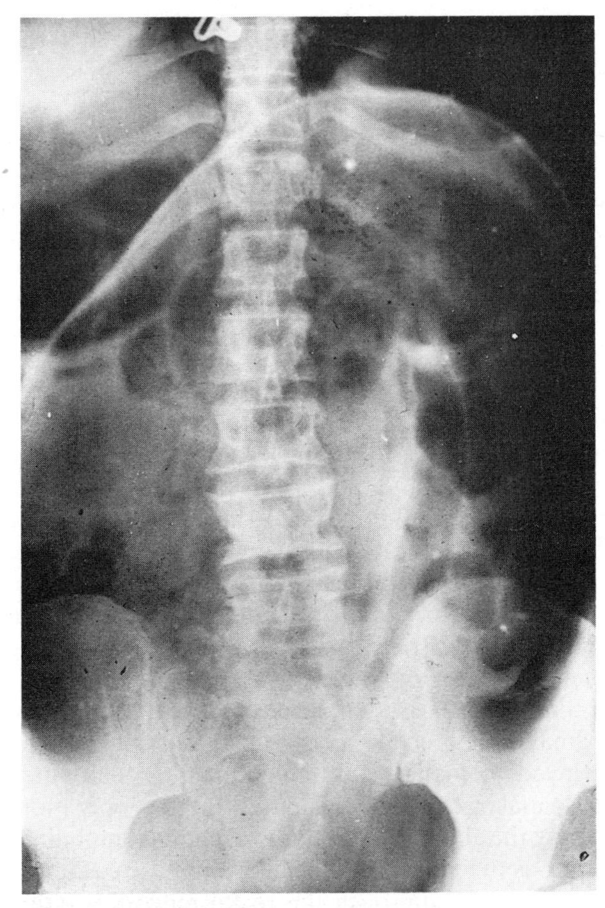

fluid levels in sigmoid volvulus (*Figure 9.35*). Barium enema radiography is essential to confirm the diagnosis of megacolon: it shows dilatation and elongation mainly of the sigmoid colon and rectum to different degrees (*Figure 9.36*). In sigmoid volvulus it shows the typical bird-beak configuration (*Figure 9.37*).

TREATMENT

Treatment of Chagas' megacolon is surgical. Conservative measures are indicated only in patients with mild degrees of constipation who can evacuate their bowel with moderate doses of laxative or periodic rectal enemas and without previous history of frequent faecal impaction or recurrent sigmoid volvulus. It is also indicated in the high-risk group which includes the elderly and those with other severe diseases.

Figure 9.35 (left) Plain abdominal radiograph showing a dilated air-filled loop of bowel with loss of haustration in a patient with sigmoid volvulus.

Figure 9.36 (below) Barium enema radiographs showing dilatation and elongation of sigmoid colon and rectum in chagasic megacolon.

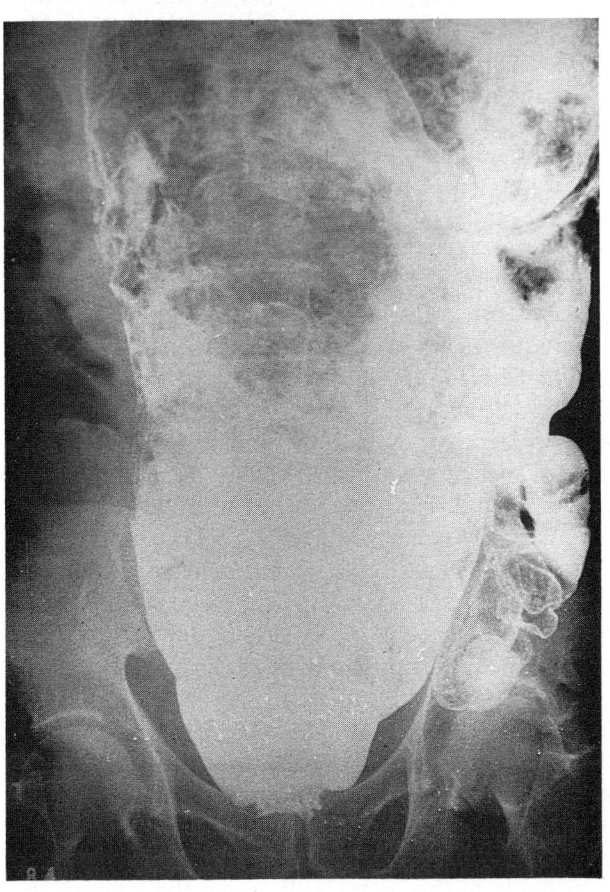

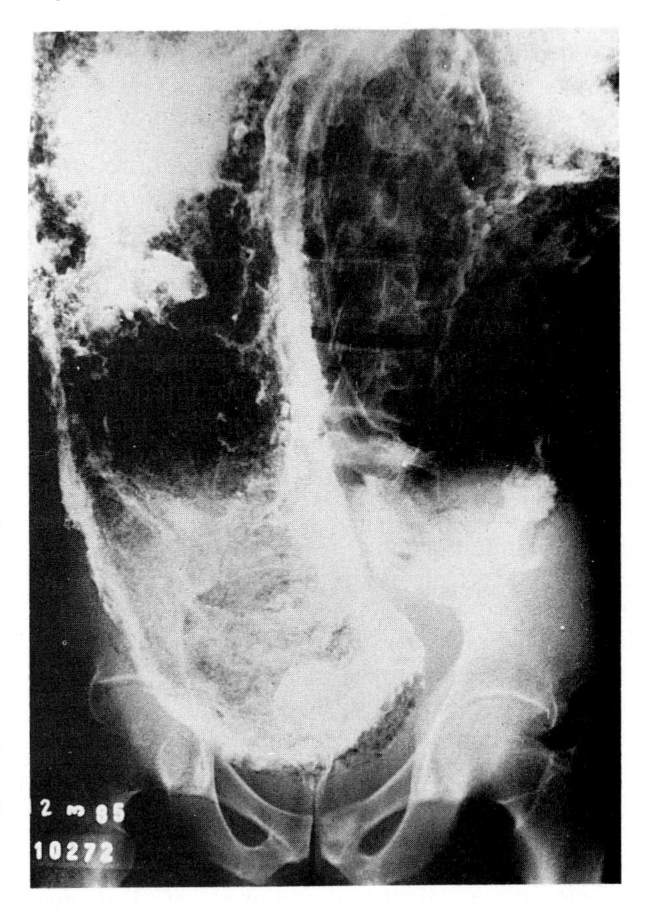

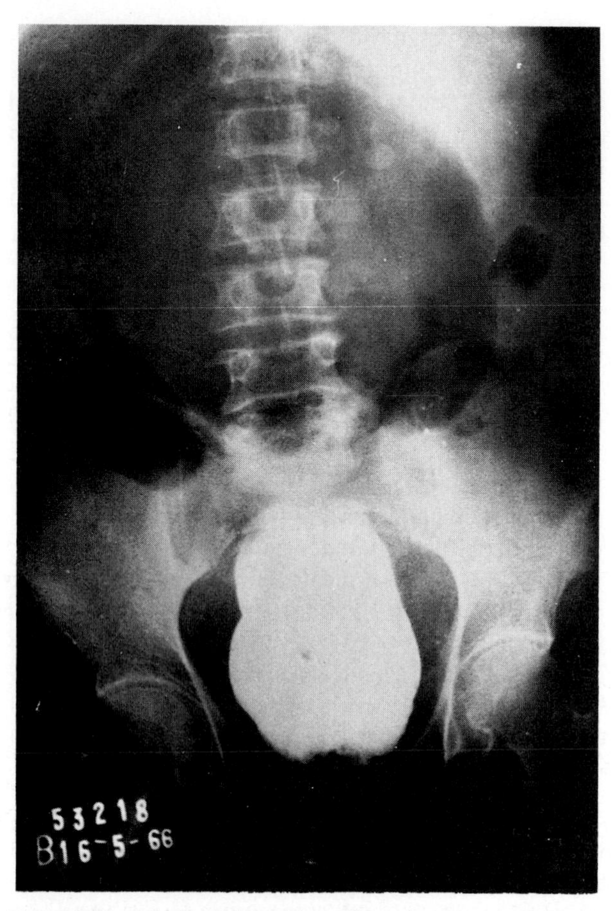

Figure 9.37 A typical bird-beak configuration in a patient with sigmoid volvulus.

Many operative techniques have been used in Brazil. In 1934, Corrêa Netto and Etzel proposed sphincterotomy of the pelvirectal and internal anal sphincters, believing that achalasia of these sphincters was the most important functional disorder.[5] For many years this operation was performed, but recurrence was the rule.

Colectomy was formerly employed by many surgeons in the belief that only resection of the most dilated segment of the colon would cure the patient. Recurrences with this technique were also seen frequently.[11,30]

Corrêa Netto in 1940 called attention to the failure of limited colonic resection and advocated abdominal rectosigmoidectomy with low colorectal anastomosis.[4] Considering the high incidence of leakage and postoperative sepsis, he advocated the use of abdominoperineal rectosigmoidectomy performed as popularized by Swenson and Bill in 1948 for treating congenital megacolon.[37] The aim of this technique was to resect the dilated sigmoid colon and a greater part of the rectum, making possible a very low colorectal anastomosis. However, at that time, even with the protection of a transverse loop colostomy, a significant number of leakages occurred: the mortality rate in 217 patients was 7.3% and leakage to different degrees was observed in 42.4%.[6] To prevent this leakage, Cutait and Figliolini in 1962[7] advocated the technique of delayed colorectal anastomosis following the abdominoperineal rectosigmoidectomy. This procedure was first described by Toupet in 1950[39] for treating selected cases of rectal cancer and was also employed by Turnbull and Cuthbertson in 1961[40] for congenital megacolon. In this procedure the colon is pulled through to the perineum and is left exteriorized as a perineal colostomy. The colorectal anastomosis is performed at least 7 days later when adhesion between the muscular surface of the everted rectum and the serosal surface of the colon has occurred, thus reinforcing the anastomosis. The results of this operation were good and the incidence of serious complications was significantly reduced compared with previous techniques; it has been employed in Brazil by several surgeons, among them Brenner[1] and Silveira,[34] with good results.

Simonsen *et al.*[35] avoided the complications of primary colorectal anastomosis by performing delayed coloanal anastomosis after abdominal endoanal rectosigmoidectomy. In this operation, during the abdominal phase, the rectum is mobilized as far as the level of the levator ani muscle. During the endoanal approach the rectal mucosa is circularly incised 0.5 cm above the pectinate line. The rectal mucosa is dissected in the submucosal plane until the levator ani muscle is passed, when the rectal muscle wall is then divided. The internal and external sphincter and the levator ani are left intact. The colon is pulled through the distal rectal muscle and anal canal, and a segment is kept exteriorized as a perineal colostomy. After at least 15 days this segment is resected at the level of the pectinate line, thus restoring the normal bowel continuity. This technique was used in 200 patients from 1961 to 1968 at the Clinical Hospital of the University of São Paulo. The mortality rate was 4%. Necrosis of the exteriorized colon was the most serious complication and occurred in 4.5% of patients. Recurrences of the disease were not seen during a long follow-up. However, although good operations for the cure of chagasic megacolon, these two types of operations – delayed colorectal and coloanal anastomosis – were progressively abandoned due to the potential complication of sexual dysfunction.

Duhamel's operation[9] was used and gained popularity in Brazil in the mid-1960s. In this technique the diseased colon is resected, the retrorectal space is opened and the rectum is divided and closed at the level of peritoneal reflection; the descending colon is pulled down behind the rectum through an incision made in the rectal wall above the level of the

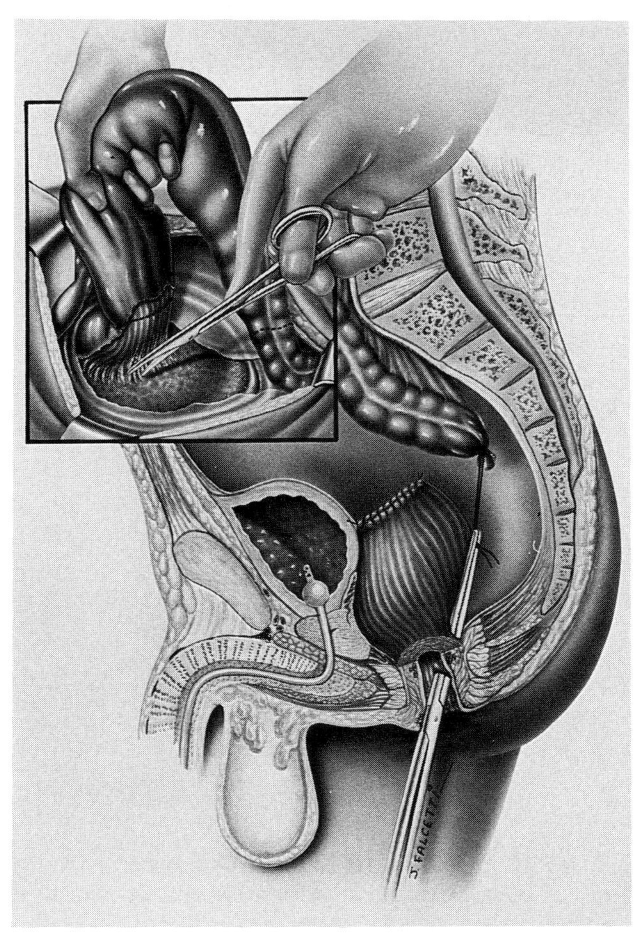

Figure 9.38 Duhamel's operation: the dilated colon is resected; the descending colon is being pulled through the rectal wall behind the rectum.

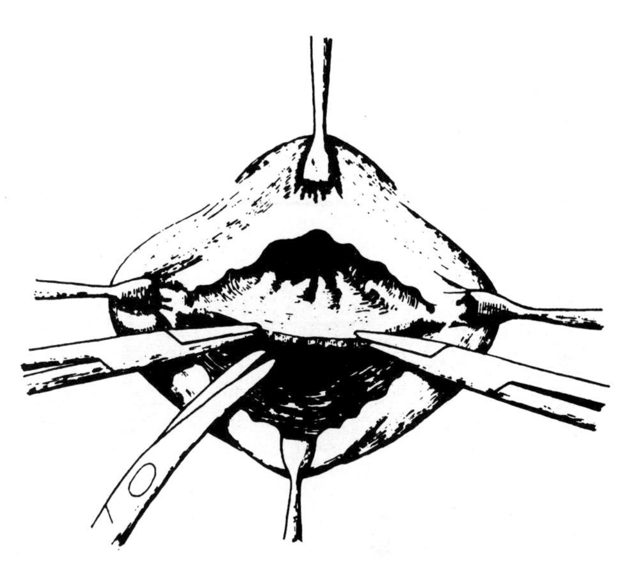

Figure 9.39 The posterior half of the rectal mucosa is incised and, by submucosal dissection, the posterior wall of the rectum is reached and sectioned.

puborectalis muscle; the posterior wall of the colon is then sutured to the external anal sphincter with a single layer of interrupted sutures; the septum formed by the posterior wall of the rectum together with the anterior wall of the lowered colon is crushed with two clamps placed in an inverted 'V' position; ischaemia of the septum causes the clamps to fall off on about the fifth day.

Duhamel's operation[9] has several advantages: it is easier to perform and avoids the complications which may follow the dissection of the rectum such as disturbed urinary and sexual function and prolonged faecal incontinence. The major criticisms of the technique have been the unpredictability of completing the side-to-side colorectal anastomosis, which is a potential source of faecal collection, and some degree of faecal incontinence in children. Some variations have been introduced by different surgeons to solve these problems. Grob,[13] to prevent faecal incontinence, advised that the anastomosis should be performed above the pectinate line, a procedure which others, including Duhamel himself,[10] have adopted. Martin and Cardill,[24] to eliminate the blind rectal pouch, suggested that the rectal pouch should be anastomosed to the side of the adjacent descending colon below the peritoneal floor.

Steichen *et al.*[36] introduced the technique of primary side-to-side colorectal anastomosis using the GIA stapling instrument, thus avoiding the incomplete spur problem; also, the immediate primary anastomosis eliminated the possibility of accidental clamp dislodgement, the patient's discomfort and difficulties in nursing care.

Haddad *et al.*[18] modified the Duhamel technique: during the first part of a two-stage procedure the dilated colon is resected, the presacral space opened and the rectum sectioned and sutured above the peritoneal reflection (*Figure 9.38*). By perineal access, the posterior half of the rectal mucosa is incised 0.5 cm above the pectinate line by submucosal dissection, and the posterior muscular wall of the rectum is sectioned above the anorectal ring (*Figure 9.39*). The colon is pulled to the perineum behind the posterior half of the rectal mucosa and a 5 cm segment is kept exteriorized as a perineal colostomy (*Figure 9.40*). The posterior rectal mucosa is then sutured to the anterior seromuscular coats of the colon. The second stage is performed after 7 days; the colonic stump is cut into halves and two clamps are placed in the rectocolonic septum in an inverted 'V' position; the anterior half of the colonic stump and the rectocolonic septum are resected; the natural anastomosis is reinforced with some interrupted chronic catgut sutures. The posterior half of the stump is resected and the posterior surface of the

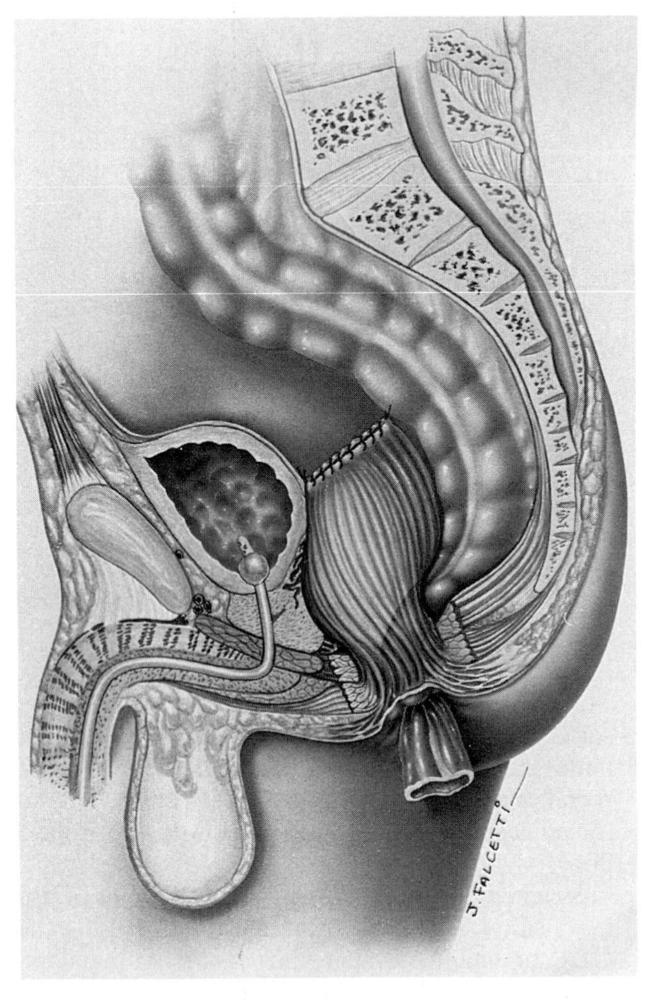

Figure 9.40 Haddad's modification of Duhamel's operation: the descending colon is pulled to the perineum through the posterior half of the rectal mucosa and 4–5 cm is kept exteriorized as a perineal colostomy.

colon is sutured to the internal sphincter of the anus (*Figures 9.41* and *9.42*).

Haddad's modification of the Duhamel technique has proved valuable for treating acquired megacolon and has certain advantages. It avoids problems from the use of crushing clamps. The colon stump causes no pain and does not interfere with ambulation. If some leakage of the excluded rectum occurs, pelvic infection of the colon stumps is avoided, since it acts as a temporary perineal colostomy, evacuations taking place outside the anal canal.

Many surgeons in Brazil use Haddad's modification of Duhamel's operation as the technique of choice for the majority of patients;[17,25,27,31] exceptions are the elderly, in whom minor operations such as sigmoidectomy or left colectomy are preferable because the expected life-span of chagasic patients is short.

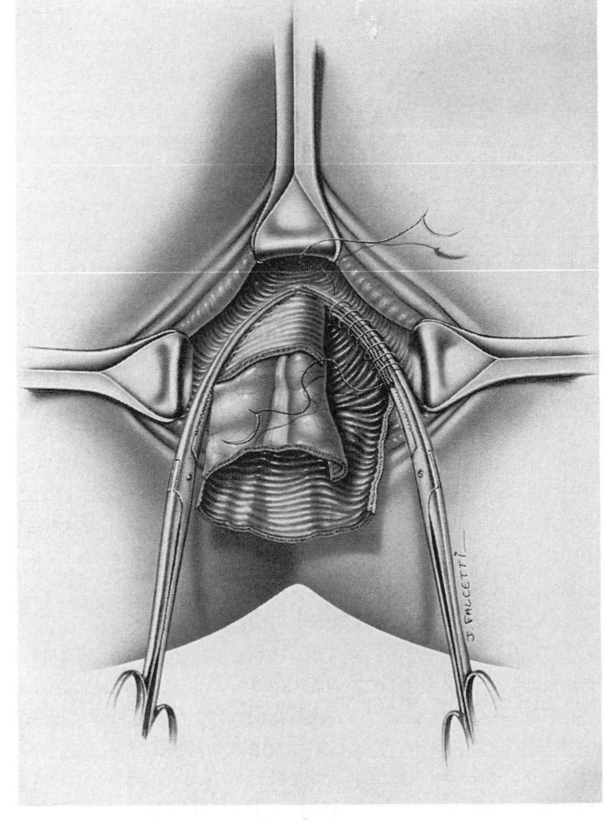

Figure 9.41 Second stage of the Duhamel–Haddad operation: the exteriorized colon is cut; the rectocolonic septum is resected and the anastomosis is performed.

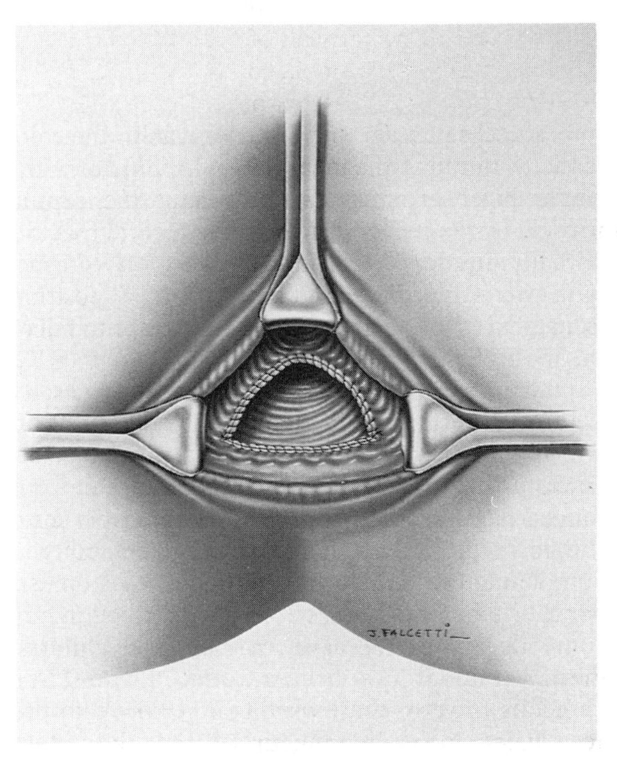

Figure 9.42 Frontal view of the colorectal anastomosis.

In a recent review of the results of the Duhamel–Haddad operation for treatment of chagasic megacolon at the Surgical Department of the Clinical Hospital, São Paulo, from 1968 to 1990, a mortality rate of 2.0% was found. Complications common to all types of pull-through operations, and mainly represented by necrosis of the lowered colon or pelvic infection, were seen in 5.2% of the patients. Complications directly related to the Duhamel–Haddad procedure, and mainly represented by leakage of the rectal stump, rectal faecaloma or stricture of the anastomosis, occurred in 11.3% of the patients. Bowel function became normal in 90% of patients investigated with a minimum follow-up of 2 years, the others requiring mild laxatives. No recurrence of the disease was seen. Normal peristalsis and propulsion of barium were seen in radiological examinations performed in 70 patients. Loss of ejaculation was seen in one male.

Although the Duhamel–Haddad technique is an adequate procedure for treatment of chagasic megacolon and the author's results are satisfactory, the author considers that this is a procedure which should not be used indiscriminately, because unacceptable complication rates may occur when it is performed by surgeons unfamiliar with pull-through techniques. Recently, the author has used a new procedure whose final result is similar to that obtained by Duhamel's operation, and end-to-end low colorectal anastomosis; however, this is performed only by the abdominal approach, using staplers applied to the posterior wall of the rectum. In this technique the dilated sigmoid colon is resected and a purse-string suture is passed around the distal end of the descending colon. The rectum is sutured below the level of the peritoneal reflection. A circular stapler with the anvil removed is inserted through the anus and its rod perforates the posterior wall of the rectum, just above the anorectal ring. The anvil is replaced on the centre rod and is inserted in to the lumen of the colon. The purse-string suture is tied around the centre rod and, after aligning the rectum and colon, the stapler is closed and fired. The instrument is removed and the accomplished end-to-side colorectal anastomosis is checked for safety (*Figure 9.43*).

To date, the author has performed this technique in 30 patients. All had an uneventful postoperative recovery. No leakages, infection or other major complications were seen. The average follow-up period is 1 year and all have a normal bowel transit time.

Although the results with this procedure are encouraging, a larger number of patients and a longer period of follow-up is needed to judge the real value of this procedure for treatment of chagasic megacolon.

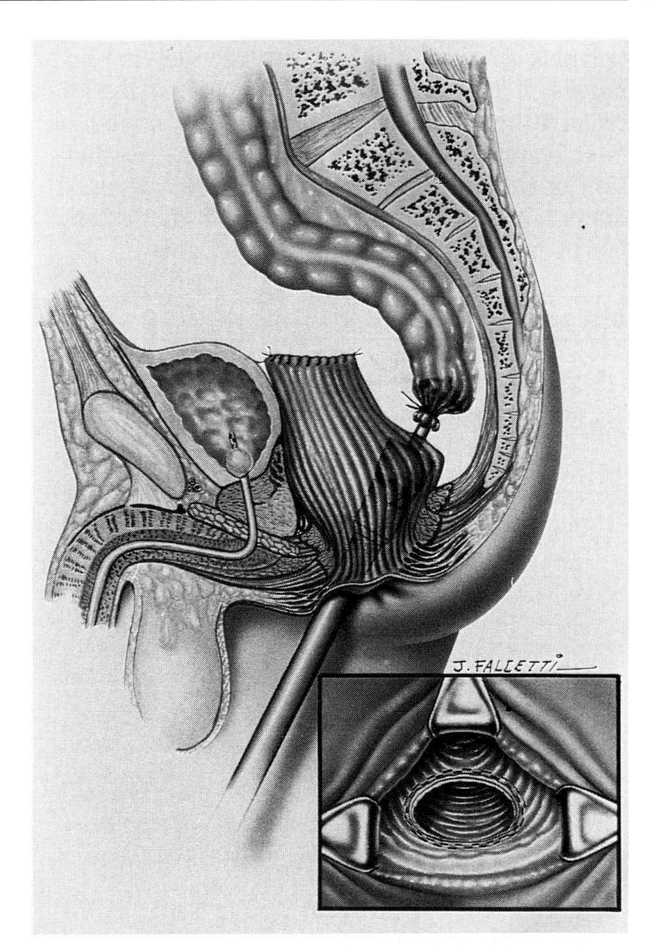

Figure 9.43 Low end-to-side stapled posterior low colorectal anastomosis.

TREATMENT OF SIGMOID VOLVULUS

Sigmoid volvulus as seen in Brazil is an acute complication of Chagas' disease. Its treatment is usually in two stages. During the acute phase, the main purpose is relief of obstruction; this should be done in such a manner so as to make the second stage easier which is the definitive treatment of the megacolon.

Treatment has undergone successive modifications. From the review of 230 cases treated at the Surgical Department of the Clinical Hospital, University of São Paulo School of Medicine, Habr-Gama *et al.*[16] recommended the following management: endoscopic emptying in cases without clinical, roentgenographic or endoscopic signs of intestinal ischaemia: laparotomy should be performed when a complicated volvulus is suspected or when it is not possible to empty the sigmoid loop. When a simple volvulus is found at laparotomy, the loop should be untwisted and the gaseous content siphoned off by a rectal catheter. The megacolon must be treated soon after endoscopic emptying or surgical decompression of the volvulus, because recurrences are frequent. When there is necrosis of the colon, a Hartman's operation should be performed.

REFERENCES

1. Brenner, S. (1974) Retocolectomia abdominoperineal com anastomose retardada no tratamento do megacólon do adulto. Thesis, Federal University of Paraná.
2. Cannon, W.B. (1930) A law of denervation. *American Journal of the Medical Sciences*, **198**, 737–750.
3. Chagas, C. (1909) Nova tripanosomiase humana. *Memórias do Instituto Oswaldo Cruz*, **1**, 159–218.
4. Corrêa Netto, A. (1940) Um caso de megacólon curado pela amputação perineal intra esfincteriana do reto. *Boletim da Sociedade de Medicina e Cirurgia de São Paulo*, **24**, 29–39.
5. Corrêa Netto, A. and Etzel, E. (1934) Le megaesophage et le megacolon devant la theorie de l'achalasie. Étude clinique et anatomopathologie. *Revista Sudamericana de Medicina y Cirugia*, **5**, 395–421.
6. Corrêa Netto, A., Haddad, J., Azevedo, P.A.V. and Raia, A. (1962) Etiology, pathogenesis and treatment of acquired megacolon. *Surgery, Gynecology and Obstetrics*, **114**, 602–608.
7. Cutait, D.E. and Figliolini, F.J. (1962) Megacólon adquirido. Nova técnica de anastomose colorretal na retossigmoidectomia abdomino-perineal. *Revista Paulista de Medicina*, **60**, 447–458.
8. Daniel, E.E., Taylor, G.S., Daniel, V.P. and Holman, M.E. (1977) Can nonadrenergic inhibitory varicosities be identified structurally? *Canadian Journal of Physiology and Pharmacology*, **55**, 243–250.
9. Duhamel, B. (1956) Une nouvelle operation de megacolon congenital. *Presse Médicale*, **64**, 2249–2250.
10. Duhamel, B. (1960) A new operation for the treatment of Hirschsprung's disease. *Archives of Disease in Childhood*, **35**, 38–39.
11. Ferreira-Santos, R. (1961) Discussions on megacolon and megarectum with the emphasis on conditions other than Hirschsprung's disease. *Proceedings of the Royal Society of Medicine*, **54**, 1035–1056.
12. Garry, R.C. (1957) Innervation of abdominal viscera. *British Medical Bulletin*, **13**, 202–206.
13. Grob, M. (1960) Intestinal obstruction in the newborn infant. *Archives of Disease in Childhood*, **35**, 40–50.
14. Habr-Gama, A., Raia, A. and Corrêa Netto, A. (1971) Motility of the sigmoid colon and rectum. Contribution to the physiopathology of megacolon in Chagas' disease. *Diseases of the Colon and Rectum*, **14**, 291–304.
15. Habr-Gama, A., Haberkorn, S., Gama-Rodrigues, J.J., Raia, A. and Bettarello, A. (1974) Manometria ano-reto-cólica. Comportamento motor normal e patológico. *Arquivos de Gastroenterologia de São Paulo*, **11**, 201–216.
16. Habr-Gama, A., Haddad, J., Simonsen, O. *et al.* (1976) Volvulus of the sigmoid colon in Brazil. A report of 230 cases. *Diseases of the Colon and Rectum*, **19**, 314–320.
17. Habr-Gama, A., Goffi, F.S., Raia, A., Ferrão, S.O.T. and Yamagushi, N. (1982) Tratamento cirúrgico do megacolo. Operação de Duhamel-Haddad. *Revista do Colégio Brasileiro de Cirurgiões*, **9**, 25–31.
18. Haddad, J., Raia, A. and Corrêa Netto, A. (1965) Abaixamento retro-retal do cólon com colostomia perineal no tratamento do megacólon adquirido. Operação de Duhamel modificada. *Revista da Associação Médica Brasileira*, **11**, 83–88.
19. Khoury, E.L., Ritacco, V., Cossio, P.M. *et al.* (1979) Circulating antibodies to peripheral nerve in American trypanosomiasis (Chagas' disease). *Clinical and Experimental Immunology*, **36**, 8–15.
20. Kiss, D.R., Habr-Gama, A. and Pinotti, H.W. (1986) Megacólon chagásico: considerações sobre novas perspectivas fisiopatológicas. *Revista Paulista de Medicina*, **104**, 145–155.
21. Koeberle, F. (1956) Die Chagaskrankheit, eine Erkrankung der neurovegetativen peripherie. *Weiner Klinische Wochenschrift*, **68**, 333–339.
22. Koeberle, F. (1963) Pathogenesis of Brazilian and European mega-esophagus. *Revista Goiana de Medicina*, **9**, 79–116.
23. Koeberle, F. and Alcântara, F.G. (1960) Mecanismo de destruição neuronal do sistema nervoso periférico na moléstia de Chagas. *O Hospital*, **57**, 1057–1062.
24. Martin, L.W. and Cardill, D.R. (1967) A method for elimination of the blind rectal pouch in the Duhamel operation for Hirschsprung's disease. *Surgery*, **62**, 951.
25. Medeiros, R.R., Reis Neto, J.A., Leonardi, L.S., Pires, A.M. and Accorroni, M.E. (1980) Estudo comparativo entre as técnicas de Duhamel e Duhamel–Haddad na cirurgia do megacólon chagásico. *Revista Paulista de Medicina*, **96**, 61–65.
26. Meneghelli, U.G. (1968) Estudos farmacológicos no megacólon chagásico. *Revista Goiana de Medicina*, **14**, 61–67.
27. Moreira, H. (1971) Tratamento do megacolo chagásico pela técnica de Duhamel–Haddad. Experiência pessoal. *Arquivos de Gastroenterologia*, **8**, 185–190.
28. Moreira, H., Rezende, M.J. and Rassi, L. (1970) Estudo da motilidade do colo transverso nas esofagocoloplastias. *Revista Goiana de Medicina*, **16**, 5–22.
29. Peralta, J.M., Manigot, D.A., Muscelli, E.O.A., Magalhães, T.C.R., Almeida, E.A. and Bastos, A.

(1982) Anticorpos EVI e NP na infecção chagásica crônica. Estudo em pacientes com diferentes formas clínicas. *Revista do Instituto de Medicina Tropical de São Paulo*, **24**, 6–10.
30. Raia, A. and Campos, O.M. (1948) O tratamento do megacólon. Estudo de follow-up de várias técnicas adotadas. *Revista de Medicina e Cirurgia de São Paulo*, **8**, 287–291.
31. Reis Neto, J.A. (1975) Duhamel procedure in the treatment of acquired megacolon. *International Surgery*, **60**, 399–401.
32. Rezende, J.M. (1969) Chagas' disease of the gastrointestinal tract: megaesophagus, megacolon and dennervation. *Medizinische Monatsschrift*, **23**, 344–350.
33. Sherlock, J. (1979) Vetores. In *Trypanosoma cruzi e Doença de Chagas* (Eds) Brener, Z. and Andrade, Z. pp. 42–88. Rio de Janeiro: Guanabara Koogan.
34. Silveira, G.M. (1976) Chagas' disease of the colon. *British Journal of Surgery*, **63**, 831–835.
35. Simonsen, O., Habr-Gama, A. and Gazal, P. (1960) Retossigmoidectomia endoanal com ressecção da mucosa retal. *Revista Paulista de Medicina*, **57**, 116–118.
36. Steichen, F.M., Talbert, J.L. and Ravitch, M.M. (1968) Primary side-to-side anastomosis in Duhamel operation for Hirschsprung's disease. *Surgery*, **64**, 475–483.
37. Swenson, O. and Bill, H. (1948) Resection of rectum and rectosigmoid with preservation of the sphincter for benign spartic lesions producing megacolon. An experimental study. *Surgery*, **24**, 213–220.
38. Teixeira, A.R.L., Junqueira, L.F. Jr, Solorzano, E. and Zappala, M. (1983) *Trypanosoma cruzi*-sensitized T-lymphocyte mediated 51 Cr release from human heart cells in Chagas' disease. *American Journal of Tropical Medicine and Hygiene*, **27**, 1097–1107.
39. Toupet, A. (1950) Techniques de reséction du rectum abdominotransanale par retournement sans anus preable avec abaissement systématique du côlon transverse. *Journal de Chirurgie*, **66**, 37–55.
40. Turnbull, R.B. Jr and Cuthbertson, A.M. (1961) Abdominorectal pull-through resection for cancer and Hirschsprung's disease. *Cleveland Clinic Quarterly*, **28**, 109–115.
41. Vieira, C.B., Godoy, R.A. and Carril, C.F. (1964) Hypersensitivity of the large intestine to cholinergic agents in patients with Chagas' disease and megacolon. *Revista Brasileira de Gastroenterologia*, **16**, 41.

SEXUALLY TRANSMITTED DISEASES RELEVANT TO GASTROENTEROLOGY

B.G. Gazzard

Many organisms infecting the gastrointestinal tract may be acquired by sexual activity. Perhaps the best known of these are the hepatitis B and C viruses, the human immunodeficiency virus (HIV) and organisms producing diarrhoea which have become grouped together as causes of the gay bowel syndrome.

This section summarizes recent knowledge on the sexual acquisition of these infections and the gastrointestinal manifestations of the acquired immune deficiency syndrome (AIDS).

HEPATITIS VIRUSES

Probably all the common viruses responsible for hepatitis can be acquired sexually.

HEPATITIS A

The hepatitis A virus is spread mainly by the faeco-oral route but homosexuals are also at risk of hepatitis A, probably via oral-anal sexual contact.[32]

HEPATITIS B

This infection is spread parenterally and vertically. However, sexual transmission is also important. The hepatitis B virus is found in body secretions, including semen and cervical mucus. Most seroprevalence studies indicated that hepatitis B infection is commoner in homosexual men, although most of these studies were done in sexually transmitted disease clinics where men tend to have a large number of sexual partners. Up to 74% of gay men have markers for present or past hepatitis B infection with 3–11% being carriers of the surface antigen.[13] Prospective studies in the early 1980s indicated that the annual incidence of hepatitis B infection was of the order of 27%, although the prevalence has fallen considerably following changes in the pattern of sexual behaviour accompanying the AIDS epidemic and the increased use of hepatitis B vaccination.[48]

Risk factors for the acquisition of hepatitis B in homosexual men include large numbers of partners, the length of homosexual activity and a history of other sexually transmitted diseases. As with other sexually transmitted diseases the major risk factors are sexual practices involving the rectal mucosa, in particular receptive anal intercourse. Orogenital sex and oro-anal sex have also been implicated in transmission.

Heterosexual transmission of hepatitis B undoubtedly occurs and, in the sentinel surveillance programme in the USA, at least 25% of all cases of hepatitis B were acquired heterosexually.[20] Female partners of hepatitis B-positive individuals, prostitutes and heterosexuals attending sexually transmitted disease clinics all have higher HIV seroprevalence rates than a control population, such as age-matched blood donors.[109] Between one-third and a half of female or male heterosexual partners of hepatitis B surface carriers show evidence of past or present hepatitis B infection.[11] Heterosexual transmission of hepatitis B is increased with an increasing number of lifetime sex partners and a history of sexually transmitted disease.[4] The status of the infecting person is important as the transmission of hepatitis B is more likely in those patients who are also positive for hepatitis B e antigen or who were hepatitis B DNA polymerase positive. In one study, evidence of hepatitis B infection was found in nearly 80% of the spouses or sexual partners of individuals who were hepatitis B e antigen (HB_eAg) and DNA polymerase positive compared with 25% of spouses of partners who were anti-HB_eAg-positive and did not have DNA polymerase. This contrasts with an incidence of less than 20% for household contacts of the same individuals.[91]

HEPATITIS C

The hepatitis C virus is likely to be transmitted by sexual activity but only very inefficiently. Previous exposure to hepatitis C can now be detected using antibody techniques, although the kits have deficiencies, in particular hypergammaglobulinaemia may be associated with non-specific positive results.[76] It is possible that some of the present data about prevalence and risk of acquisition of hepatitis C will be modified as more sophisticated tests, and in particular confirmatory tests, become available. Two to six months may be required for hepatitis C antibody to develop, so that it is difficult at present to identify events likely to be associated with transmission. There is evidence that hepatitis C is the predominant cause of transfusion hepatitis in most countries where blood is screened for hepatitis B. There is probably a close parallel between hepatitis C transmission and the modes of acquisition of hepatitis B. Sporadic hepatitis C seems to be common and an early community study of non-A, non-B hepatitis in London (hepatitis A and B were excluded by serological testing) showed that infection occurred amongst close family members and sexual contacts, and was also commoner in single women.[43] So far, there has been a surprisingly low incidence of hepatitis C infection in the homosexual community, both in those infected with HIV and those not.[97]

HEPATITIS D

It is also likely that the δ agent can be sexually transmitted, either in conjunction with hepatitis B or subsequently to a hepatitis B-positive carrier.

THE GAY BOWEL SYNDROME

The term 'gay bowel syndrome' was coined by Sohn and Ribilotti in 1977 to described a group of colonic and rectal diseases occurring with higher frequency in homosexual men. Most but not all these conditions are caused by sexually transmitted infection but anal fissures, trauma and foreign bodies were also included under this broad category. Some of the infecting agents were recognized venereal organisms but others, such as *Giardia* and *Shigella* spp., were common enteric pathogens. The symptomatic importance of these organisms is sometimes difficult to establish as multiple infections are common and asymptomatic carriage is frequent. Two major series[8,94] assessed the frequency of these infections prior to the AIDS epidemic. Studies carried out since the recognition of the importance of sexual activity in the spread of AIDS showed a marked reduction in the incidence of gay bowel pathogens;[73] it is difficult to decide whether HIV infection increases susceptibility to these organisms. The spread of these infections among the homosexual community is likely to be encouraged by asymptomatic carriage, and by sexual activity with large numbers of partners, particularly if they are anonymous, as under these circumstances contact tracing and breaking the cycle of transmission by early treatment is impossible. Acquisition of these infections is not confined to homosexuals but also occurs in bisexuals and heterosexuals indulging in anal intercourse. Oro-anal sex (rimming) appears to be particularly important in transmission.

Rectal gonorrhoea

Infection of the rectum by *Neisseria gonorrhoeae* is not confined to homosexual men because between

20 and 60% of women with genital gonorrhoea also have rectal infection.[67] Seventy five per cent of these women in one study also had anal intercourse[90] but other studies have failed to show any relationship. It is possible that vaginal secretions autoinfect the rectal mucosa.

In men, rectal gonorrhoea is mainly found in homosexuals practising passive anal intercourse. The incidence of rectal gonorrhoea has fallen in recent years but still accounts for approximately half the patients with gonorrhoea in a sexually transmitted disease clinic.[90]

At least two-thirds of the patients are asymptomatic. Some patients report excessive mucus in the stool and rectal discomfort but these symptoms occur commonly in uninfected patients who have had anal sex.[74] Severe symptoms such as blood in the stool, ischiorectal abscesses or copious mucopurulent discharge, and complications such as rectal strictures, septicaemia and infection in distant sites probably affect less than 5% of patients. Symptoms subside rapidly, although asymptomatic carriage of the organism may persist.

Sigmoidoscopy is normal in a fifth of the patients, the others having mild or severe erythema with some degree of mucopurulent discharge. Inflammation may be confined to the proximal anal canal or extend into the lower rectum.[74] The mainstay of the diagnosis is culture rather than staining of rectal smears, which is only positive in 30% of cases.[12]

Other *Neisseria* spp. particularly *Neisseria meningitidis*, also occur in the rectum. As these are commensals in the throat, oro-anal sex is a likely route of transmission. These may produce no symptoms or symptoms which are indistinguishable from rectal gonorrhoea.

Treponema pallidum *infection*

Homosexual men have a much increased risk of a primary chancre developing in the anal region, which usually occurs within 10–90 days of exposure, either on the anal verge or within the canal, rather than in the rectum (*Figure 9.44*). The ulceration may be single or multiple and indistinguishable from multiple fissures. Occasionally, rectal polyps, masses and mucosal friability have been reported, associated with early syphilis.[105] A primary chancre may be asymptomatic or produce mild non-specific proctitis, or very occasionally constipation, bleeding or tenesmus. The ulcer usually heals spontaneously in 2–4 weeks and diagnosis is made by dark-field examination.

The lesions of secondary syphilis are condyloma lata, which are multiple hypertrophic papules, often associated with a typical rash on the body, and general lymphadenopathy. Although usually asymptomatic, minor anal rectal irritation may occur. Dark-field illumination is the diagnosis of choice, although by this stage syphilitic serology is nearly always positive.

Tertiary syphilis is rare with gummata of the rectum now a curiosity.

Chlamydial infections

Both lymphogranuloma venereum (LGV) and non-LGV serotypes are capable of causing mild proctitis and appear to be commoner in homosexual men. In one study, Quinn *et al.*[93] found *Chlamydia trachomatis* in 11 of 96 homosexual men with diarrhoea and in 3 of 75 asymptomatic patients. Most non-

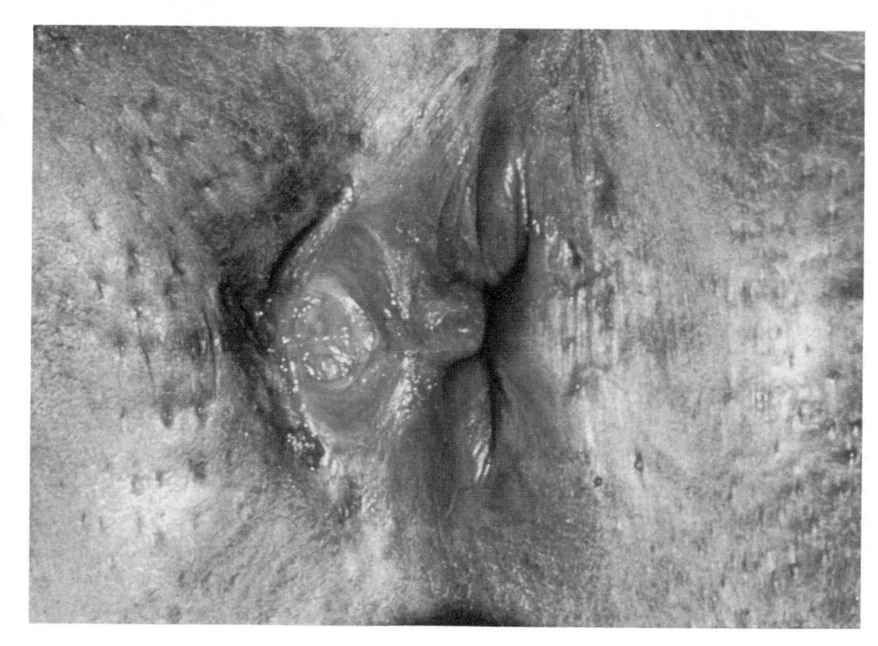

Figure 9.44 Primary chancre at the anal margin.

LGV chlamydial strains produced either no symptoms or only mild proctitis.

Infection with LGV strains has been recognized for 50 years but is still rare. Primary infections usually go unnoticed as they cause single or multiple painless vesicular lesions. However, 3–6 weeks later, tender inguinal adenopathy occurs, often associated with systemic symptoms. Chronic inflammation of the rectum may be followed by lymphatic blockage, oedema and fistula formation with rectal stricturing. These changes are seen in both men and women and, when fully developed, the symptoms and macroscopic and microscopic appearances may be difficult to distinguish from Crohn's disease, although the prominent inguinal adenopathy may give a clue to the diagnosis.

The diagnosis of chlamydial infection depends primarily on culture. Antibodies to chlamydiae do develop during infection but there are cross-reactions between LGV and non-LGV strains, and once antibodies have developed they remain positive for life.

Herpes infections

Herpes simplex genitalis is the second commonest cause of proctitis in homosexual men[93] and occurs in about 30% of symptomatic gay individuals. It is commoner in AIDS, and mucocutaneous infection for more than a month is one of the criteria for the diagnosis of fully developed disease by the US Centers for Disease Control in Atlanta, Georgia.[19] There is a strong correlation between anal herpes and passive anal sex. Oro-anal sex may also be important in some cases, particularly those caused by herpes type 1 virus, which normally causes conjunctivitis, blisters and encephalitis. Type 2 infections are much more commonly spread by sexual activity.

Itching and soreness around the anus develop between 2 and 7 days after infection and the pain rapidly increases in severity and can radiate to the groin, buttocks and thighs. Constipation, tenesmus and rectal discharge also occur and there is sometimes fever and headache. Urinary frequency and acute urinary retention may be due to herpetic infection of the sacral ganglia or due to reflex spasm of bladder muscles.

The appearance of the perianal area and anal canal are usually typical with clusters of small vesicles which rapidly ulcerate, producing superficial aphthous ulcers, which may become confluent (*Figure 9.45*). Inflammation may extend up into the distal rectum with either non-specific inflammation or severe haemorrhagic friability. In patients who are not immunocompromised the infection usually settles spontaneously over 1–3 weeks although recurrence occurs in up to two-thirds of patients within the first year.

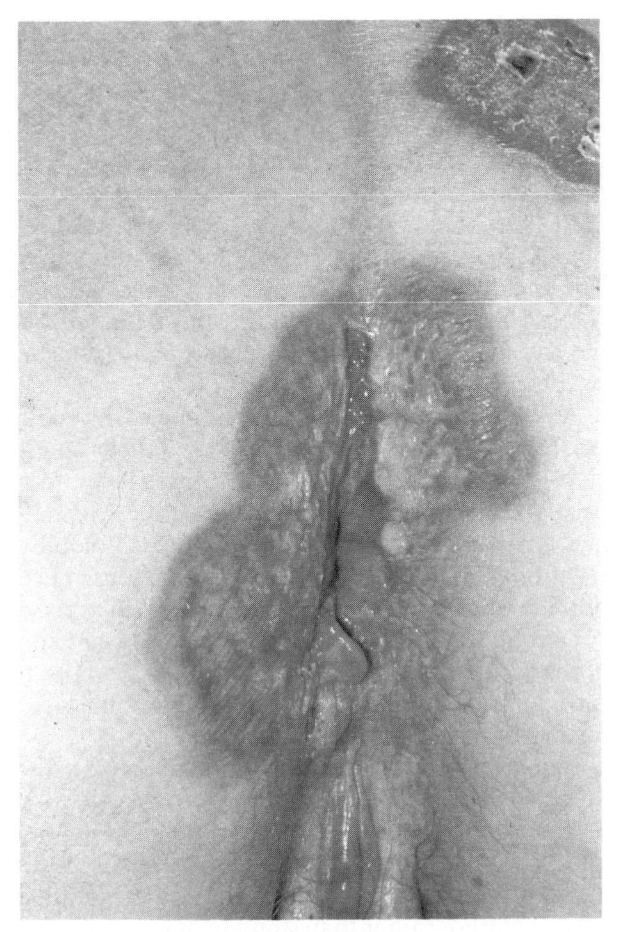

Figure 9.45 Genital herpes.

Papilloma virus infection

The papilloma virus produces condylomata acuminata, which are cauliflower-like lesions encircling the anus and extending into the anal canal (*Figure 9.46*). Both men and women with anal warts have usually had anal intercourse and 15% have warts elsewhere on the body. Both trauma and the presence of the papilloma virus are probably necessary to produce these lesions. The papilloma virus is likely to be associated with an increased risk of the development of cloacal carcinoma, which is more common in homosexual men.

Shigellosis

An increase in the frequency of shigellosis and a change in the incidence of the common species from *Shigella sonnei* to *S. flexneri* in the mid-1970s was

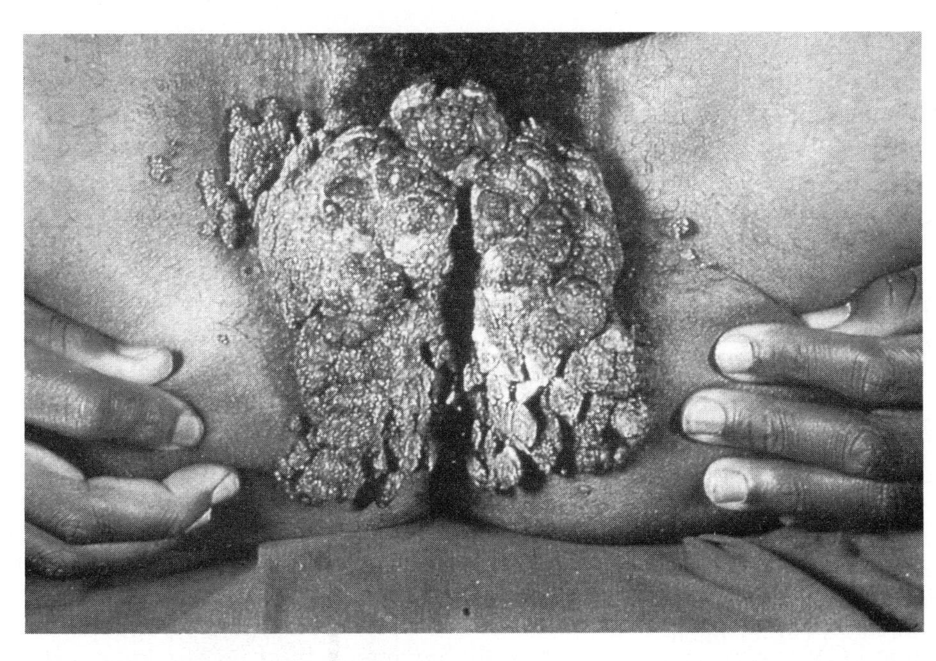

Figure 9.46 Anal warts.

associated with an increased antibiotic resistance and the recognition that this organism was transmitted venereally among gay men.[7] Shigellosis has also been described in HIV-positive gay men, possibly with an increased incidence of septicaemia and an associated high mortality rate. Shigellosis is an uncommon cause of pseudomembranous colitis and bloody diarrhoea.

Campylobacter infection

Campylobacter jejuni infection is one of the commonest enteric illnesses in the UK. As well as a common cause of food poisoning, campylobacter infections are probably venereally transmitted and a number of unusual species have been found in gay men, including *Campylobacter laridis, C. fetus* and *C. sinaedi*.[22,39] Five per cent of symptomatic gay men and 3% of asymptomatic patients had evidence of campylobacter infection in one study. Although the number of case reports in HIV-positive individuals is small it is probably a common cause of diarrhoea with a frequently relapsing course and sometimes an associated septicaemia.

Giardiasis

Giardiasis lamblia is thought to be sexually transmitted and in the 1970s giardiasis was found in 4–18% of homosexual men some of whom were asymptomatic. The incidence of infection in the gay community has decreased,[95] perhaps because of changing sexual practices. Giardia infection has been documented in HIV-positive individuals[23] but co-infection of other pathogens is frequent, as is asymptomatic carriage.[73] In patients previously exposed to *G. lamblia* the presence of secretory IgA antibodies reduces the chances of subsequent reinfection.[60] Classic giardiasis produces watery diarrhoea or steatorrhoea with abdominal bloating and excessive wind. Diagnosis is difficult as stool examination for cysts is negative in up to one-third of cases. *G. lamblia* can be identified by histological examination of jejunal biopsy material or analysis of aspirated duodenal fluid.

Amoebiasis

The capacity of the protozoan *Entamoeba histolytica* and other species of this genus to produce diarrhoea in gay men is subject to debate; Allason-Jones *et al*.[2] showed that gay men had similar symptoms with and without infection. Zymedene analysis has indicated that most strains isolated are non-pathogenic,[51] and invasive amoebiasis has not been observed.[60] Although the treatment of amoebiasis in gay men with diarrhoea does not have a secure scientific basis[108] a pragmatic clinical view would be to treat amoebic organisms but to continue the search for other infections. Resolution of symptoms associated with eradication of the organism suggests that the amoebas were pathogenic.

Spirochaetosis

Spirochaetes are found in up to 25% of gay men undergoing rectal biopsy, equally divided between symptomatic and asymptomatic individuals.[62] The incidence of this infection is lower in HIV antibody-positive individuals (about 10%; B.G. Gazzard, personal observation) and is similar to that seen in the general population. Treatment with penicillin, although eradicating the organisms, does not seem to produce symptomatic improvement.

Pudendal lice infestation

Lice can be transmitted during sexual activity and are an unusual cause of pruritus ani.

HIV INFECTION

INTRODUCTION

In 1981 the Centers for Disease Control received reports of five cases of *Pneumocystis carinii* pneumonia in homosexual men.[18] At the same time it received increasing notification of cases of Kaposi's sarcoma also in homosexual men. This had previously been regarded as an indolent vascular tumour occurring mainly in elderly Mediterranean males. It was known that Kaposi's sarcoma and *P. carinii* pneumonia were associated with immunosuppression and thus the increased incidence of these two diseases was likely to represent a new syndrome of obscure aetiology, associated with severe immune deficiency. By 1983 the causative organism of this new epidemic – the human immunodeficiency virus (HIV) – had been identified and shown to infect cells containing CD4 receptors on their surface, primarily activated lymphocytes and macrophages.[9]

Perhaps the best evidence that HIV is the primary cause of AIDS comes from the transmission by blood transfusion to individuals who are otherwise not at risk. The donors of the blood in these cases have AIDS, or else HIV can be cultured from their blood.

Different risk groups, e.g. homosexuals, heterosexuals, intravenous drug users and haemophiliacs, all progress to the fully developed syndrome at similar rates. The two factors known to influence progression are age and whether the virus was acquired from an asymptomatic individual (a possibly less virulent strain) or from a patient with AIDS (possibly a more virulent strain).

SEXUAL TRANSMISSION

The transmission of HIV is similar in some ways to that of the hepatitis B virus. A multicentre AIDS cohort analysis study[65] investigated the seroconversion rate in large groups of homosexual patients who practised exclusively one form of sexual activity. This study showed that passive anal intercourse with more than two partners a month was associated with a high seroconversion rate whereas that associated with active anal intercourse or fellatio was much lower. The high risk in receptive anal intercourse is probably due to the frequency of mucosal damage causing rectal bleeding.

HIV can also be transmitted heterosexually. This is the major route of transmission in Africa,[92] where the disease affects patients in the most sexually active age groups, and the male-to-female ratio is approximately 1. Several cases of male-to-female, female-to-male transmission chains have been documented. The risk of heterosexual transmission in Africa is strongly correlated with genital ulcer disease and consorting with prostitutes.[16]

The frequency of heterosexual transmission in the Western world is more difficult to ascertain, partly because of the reluctance to engage in large-scale screening of healthy individuals. Nevertheless, heterosexual sex is the commonest route of transmission in western Europe and is the fastest growing category of AIDS patients in the USA, particularly amongst poor ethnic minorities in whom intravenous drug use is common.

Male-to-female transmission

A recent European study showed that the risks of male-to-female transmission were increased by a history of sexually transmitted disease in the female, the stage of HIV infection in the male and the practice of anal intercourse.[41] This data can be misinterpreted; the number of women practising anal intercourse was small and the majority of women became infected through 'normal' vaginal intercourse with men who were apparently fit and well. Other studies have shown that the risks of transmission to the female are increased with chlamydial infection, which increases the number of lymphocytes present in the cervical mucus, and also with the use of oral contraceptives, which may induce cervical ectropion where the fragile endocervix is exposed to trauma during sexual intercourse.

Female-to-male transmission

The factors involved in female-to-male transmission of HIV have been studied in a group of known HIV-negative men who visited a prostitute in a region where 85% of such individuals were known to be HIV-positive. Nine per cent of these men seroconverted within a few weeks. Men who had active genital ulcer disease, or who were uncircumcised had a much increased risk with a seroconversion rate of 53% when both factors were present.[16] Other genitally acquired infections are also commoner in the uncircumcised and the reasons that genital ulcer disease might be associated with increased risk of infection are obvious. The frequency of chancroid infection in Africa may be one of the underlying reasons for the major outbreak of heterosexually acquired AIDS.

Although long-term studies are limited, it is becoming clear that, like all other venereally acquired infections, the risk of female acquisition of HIV from a male is greater than female-to-male transmission.[89] One of the surprising features of the epidemiology of HIV infection is the lack of correlation between the risk of heterosexual transmission and the number of contacts with one partner or the duration of a sexual relationship with an HIV-positive individual. Such data may indicate the importance of innate biological resistance to the acquisition of infection in some individuals, or differential infectivities of various strains of HIV virus.

GASTROINTESTINAL MANIFESTATIONS OF HIV DISEASE

A high proportion of patients with HIV infection develop gastroenterological manifestations during the course of the disease. At first presentation with the fully developed AIDS syndrome a high proportion of patients have diarrhoea and/or weight loss and smaller number have oesophageal symptoms. These symptoms become commoner as the disease progresses.

The mouth

Oral manifestations may be the first indication of HIV infection and are often a sign of mucocutaneous immune deficiency, with a high predictive value for the development of AIDS.

Buccal candidosis

Buccal candidosis is a common manifestation of HIV disease, and fully developed AIDS emerged in 59% of such patients within 3 months.[68] Some of these patients, however, may have had an AIDS-defining illness (oesophageal candidiasis) at the time of the initial diagnosis. Buccal candidiasis is usually associated with a considerable reduction in the circulating T-helper cell count and follows a relapsing course. Although topical agents such as nystatin or amphotericin are often effective, usually the newer systemic antifungal agents, such as ketoconazole, itraconazole or fluconazole are now used.

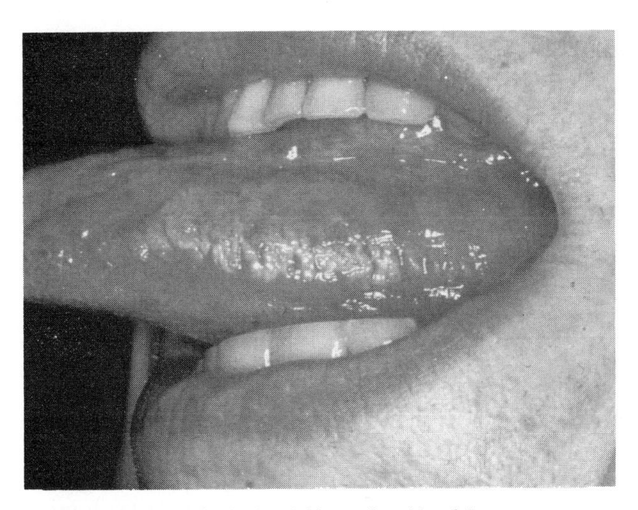

Figure 9.47 Hairy leukoplakia on the side of the tongue.

Hairy leukoplakia

This condition was first recognized as a complication of HIV infection but has since been diagnosed occasionally in other patients with immune deficiency. An opportunistic infection with the Epstein–Barr virus produces characteristic rugose white plaques, most commonly on the side of the tongue, but occasionally elsewhere in the buccal cavity. Eighty per cent of patients will develop fully developed AIDS within a 2 year period (*Figure 9.47*).[54] Treatment is not required as the condition is usually asymptomatic.

Mouth ulcers

Non-specific ulcers occur in the buccal cavity and often repeated biopsy fails to reveal an underlying cause. Occasionally, multiple cytomegalovirus (CMV) inclusions are found and the ulcers respond to appropriate therapy. Sometimes ulceration is associated with lymphoma, particularly over the tonsil.

Aphthous ulcers of the Bechet type are no commoner than in the general population (up to 10% of patients,[5]), but they can be painful and difficult to treat. Thalidomide treatment produces rapid healing.[117]

In some ulcers, evidence of HIV infection has been found and reports have appeared of improvement with oral or intralesional injections of steroids.[71]

Other dental conditions

Poor dental hygiene, gum retraction and dental abscesses are all common. Necrotizing gingivitis is a dental emergency as prompt improvement can be obtained with appropriate antibiotic therapy.

Kaposi's sarcoma

Kaposi's sarcoma is frequently found on the hard palate where it may be asymptomatic or interfere with eating and bleed profusely. In one small study, 75% of patients with Kaposi's sarcoma of the palate had lesions elsewhere in the gastrointestinal tract.

Oesophageal conditions

Oesophageal symptoms presenting in HIV disease are different to those seen in general gastroenterological practice. Thus, of 48 patients prospectively studied, all had pain on swallowing, particularly hot liquids or solids and two-thirds had dysphagia. Weight loss is not a prominent feature. The commonest cause of oesophageal disease is candidiasis, either alone or accompanied by other pathology.[25]

Oesophageal candidiasis

The appearance of oesophageal candidiasis with either isolated plaques or confluent fungal masses is sufficient to fulfil the Centers for Disease Control criteria for AIDS.[19] In a person who is HIV antibody-positive, confirmation of the endoscopic diagnosis is not required.

Despite the frequency of this condition, candida septicaemia is rare in AIDS, although common in other immunosuppressed states. A relatively intact humoral immune system may be important in preventing widespread candida sepsis. IgG antibodies to the 47 kDa antigen of candida are usually present in high titre in HIV-positive patients[79] but are often absent in patients with candidial septicaemia.

Conditions causing ulceration of the gullet

One-third of HIV-positive patients with oesophageal symptoms have ulceration related to CMV infection, herpes simplex infection, aphthous ulceration of the mouth or ulcerating hairy leukoplakia. Necrotic ulcers associated with seroconversion, possibly due to direct HIV infection, have also been described.[96]

CMV ulcers are usually linear or serpiginous with raised edges, and can be confused with carcinoma.[25] Widespread oesophagitis without ulceration has also been described. Confirmation that the diagnosis of CMV causes disease can be difficult as serological evidence of past CMV infection is common, particularly in homosexuals. The normal immunological markers of reactivation of infection with the production of IgM antibody do not occur in AIDS patients and so the diagnosis can only be suggested pathologically by large numbers of CMV inclusion bodies with surrounding inflammation. A careful search of histopathological specimens often yields an occasional CMV cytomegalovirus inclusion body in otherwise normal mucosa, where the organism is unlikely to be causing disease. The best evidence for the importance of this virus is provided by effective treatment. Ganciclovir – an analogue of acyclovir – has recently been licensed for use against life-threatening CMV infections and heals CMV infection of the oesophagus,[21] as has foscarnet, a pyrophosphate analogue with activity against viral DNA kinases and a broad spectrum of activity against herpes virus. Foscarnet is also a reverse transcriptase inhibitor. Both these drugs have to be administered intravenously and have serious toxic profiles –agranulocytosis and bone marrow suppression being the main problem with ganciclovir while foscarnet is toxic to the kidneys. Both agents are virostatic and require a competent immune system for complete elimination of CMV. Thus, in AIDS patients treatment of CMV may require repeated courses of therapy. This is particularly true of CMV retinitis, which always seems to progress without maintenance therapy. However, both ganciclovir and foscarnet may result in prolonged remission of oesophageal ulceration after a single course of treatment.[25]

Herpes simplex infection of the oesophagus is accompanied by pharyngeal or peri-oral herpes. The lesions in the oesophagus are fluid-filled vesicles but the roof of the vesicles may be removed by trauma, producing the appearance of a haemorrhagic distal oesophagitis. The diagnosis may be confirmed by brush cytology showing giant cells, but more reliably by finding nuclear inclusion bodies on histopathological specimens.

Ulcerating hairy leukoplakia, which is often painful, tends to occur in the mid-gullet and treatment with high-dose acyclovir may improve the symptoms.[66]

Diagnosis of oesophageal symptoms

There is controversy about the need to confirm the diagnosis of HIV antibody-positive patients who present with oesophageal symptoms. This is usually due to oesophageal candidosis, and buccal candidosis is almost always present. One view is that a systemic antifungal agent should be given to all patients with oesophageal symptoms and buccal candidosis and further investigations should be reserved for those patients who fail to respond. A definite diagnosis, however, is beneficial for prognosis and because treatment will be delayed in patients with mixed pathology or ulcerating conditions of the gullet. The confirmation of the diagnosis of oesophageal pathology requires endoscopy. If a pathological diagnosis is used as the 'gold standard' the sensitivity and specificity of a barium swallow is 25 and 100%, compared with 97.5 and 100% for gastroscopy.[26]

WEIGHT LOSS

Weight loss is an important feature of HIV infection not least because of deterioration in the quality of life as a result of poor cognitive and locomotor function as well as a distorted body image. Virtually all AIDS patients lose significant amounts of weight, and death follows rapidly when this falls below a critical level.[69]

Weight loss may be an important intermediary disease mechanism in the immunological deterioration which follows HIV infection. Direct HIV infection of gut epithelial cells[84] may lead to micronutrient malabsorption which may produce suppression of the immune system or a failure of free radical scavenging mechanisms. An excess of free radicals will interfere with many body functions including the immune system and may be responsible for a vicious circle of further weight loss.

Causes of weight loss

Poor food intake

Lesions of the oropharynx lead to poor food intake and various systemic diseases are associated with anorexia, perhaps secondary to cytokine release. Malabsorption may cause anorexia because nutrients in the distal ileum stimulate appetite-suppressant hormones.

A number of patients may be persuaded to take hypocaloric 'healthy diets' as a way of controlling their disease. The standard 'health diet' which encourages a reduction in saturated fats and sugar with limitation of protein intake and extra roughage is not applicable to HIV-positive patients with a limited prognosis. However, dietary intake is not the major cause of weight loss in most AIDS patients. There are two small studies which show that, in clinically stable AIDS patients, food intake over short periods was similar to a control group.[69] This, however, may not apply to the subgroup of AIDS patients who have lost more than 10% of their total body weight with no obvious cause now included in the Centers for Disease Control definition of the fully developed syndrome. This wasting syndrome was originally described in Uganda and called 'slim disease' but closer investigation of many of these patients reveals cryptosporidiosis or oesophageal candidiasis.[103] However, there is a group of patients who do lose weight at a fairly early stage of HIV infection without any obvious opportunistic pathogen but no studies have yet been performed on dietary intake in this group.

Malabsorption and weight loss

Malabsorption is well documented in AIDS patients, including abnormal xylose tolerance tests and steatorrhoea. A specific ileal defect is suggested by vitamin B_{12} malabsorption and excess bile salt deconjugation. Activation of a retrovirus infection has been associated with small bowel injury in a cat model of immunodeficiency and suggests that direct HIV infection may also produce small bowel damage. Early studies of small intestinal structure showed partial villus atrophy and crypt hyperplasia.[50] Recent studies in which other parasites, particularly *Cryptosporidium* spp. and species of the class Microsporidea, have been more rigorously excluded, either show no evidence of villus atrophy or only low-grade mucosal changes and evidence of individual cell cytopathic effects.[49] Crypt hyperplasia may be present and reflect more rapid cellular turnover, perhaps producing a functional immaturity of epithelial cells. The quantitative significance of malabsorption as a cause of weight loss in patients with no identifiable pathogen other than HIV infection itself has not been directly investigated but is unlikely to be of major importance.

Severe malabsorption is usually related to secondary infection of the gut by such organisms as *Cryptosporidium* spp., microsporidia, *Giardia lamblia* and *Isospora belli*.

Metabolic changes and weight loss

In patients with a normal dietary intake, and no diarrhoea or significant malabsorption, weight loss must be caused by increased metabolic requirements. This can occur in patients with any infection but has also been described in some AIDS patients with no other known pathogen. However, a lower basal metabolic rate has also been described in such groups.[36]

A possible cause of increased metabolic rate in AIDS patients is the release of tissue cytokines, perhaps as a direct result of HIV infection of macrophages and OKT-4 cells. Thus, blood levels of tumour necrosis factor are slightly elevated in AIDS patients.[100] This cytokine may provoke weight loss by reduction in appetite, by increasing the metabolic rate or by diverting liver protein synthesis to synthesis of acute phase reactants.

Micronutrient malabsorption

Zinc, selenium and vitamin B_{12} deficiency may occur in HIV-infected patients.[40,42] As serum folate is an acute phase reactant, the variable levels described in patients may not be an accurate reflection of folate stores in the body.

Treatment

The appetite of some HIV-infected individuals may be stimulated by megestrol acetate, which is a synthetic progestogen used as adjuvant therapy for breast cancer, where an appetite-stimulant effect was demonstrated. This has also been shown in an uncontrolled study of AIDS patients, and various placebo-controlled trials are now under way.[114]

Dietary advice is important at an early stage of HIV infection to encourage a high-energy intake.

Increases in lean body mass can be induced by enteral or parenteral feeding in some patients. Small pilot studies indicate that lean body mass will increase in those patients with a gastrointestinal cause of weight loss but not those with systemic disease.[44]

DIARRHOEA AND ITS CAUSES

Diarrhoea results from an interaction between the virulence of the organism, the resistance of the host and the dose of infection. The difference between opportunistic infections which cause disease only in an immunosuppressed host and non-opportunist organisms is not always clear. The opportunist cryptosporidia cause a self-limiting diarrhoeal illness in normal individuals.[3] Likewise, although species of the genera *Salmonella* and *Campylobacter* are regarded as non-opportunists, in immunosuppressed hosts they are likely to cause a more severe illness, more frequent relapses and recurrent septicaemia. The Centers for Disease Control now include two or more episodes of salmonella septicaemia as part of the diagnosis of fully developed AIDS.[19] Similarly, although herpes simplex virus causes disease in immunocompetent individuals, mucocutaneous disease persisting for more than 1 month is diagnostic of fully developed AIDS.

Host resistance in HIV infection

Non-specific mechanisms of host resistance may be impaired in some HIV-infected individuals, e.g. reduced gastric secretion. Antibody-mediated immune function in the gut is also reduced as HIV-infected patients have reduced numbers of plasma IgA-secreting cells in the lamina propria.[70] Although serum levels of IgA increase as HIV disease progresses, this is not true of secretory IgA, which is mostly in particulate form, perhaps because it is complexed with antigen.[72] In addition, a specific reduction in IgA2 has recently been demonstrated. Secretory IgA is likely to prevent adherence of potential pathogens to the gut lining.

The cellular immune system of the gut (gut-associated lymphoid tissue) forms part of the common mucosal immune defence system, which is of major importance in the development of AIDS. Many of the premonitory features (buccal candidosis and hairy leukoplakia) and opportunistic infections (*Pneumocystis carinii* pneumonia, oesophageal candidosis, cryptosporidiosis) are due to failure of this system. Other opportunists gain access to the body via a breakdown in this barrier. Little is known about changes in this system during HIV infection. There is a reduction in the number of lymphocytes bearing CD4 receptors in the lamina propria in AIDS patients, but the extent of this change is controversial.[99,113]

The numbers of activated T cells (CD25) are also decreased.[113] What influence these changes have on the resistance to enteric infection is unknown.

Non-opportunistic pathogens

Most non-opportunistic pathogens have been considered in the earlier subsection on the gay bowel syndrome.

Salmonella infection

There is a 20-fold increase in the incidence of salmonella infections associated with any cause of cellular immune suppression, including AIDS.[15] Although *Salmonella typhimurium* is probably the most frequent organism, *Salmonella enteritidis* is also common in the UK, associated with ingestion of infected eggs or poultry. A high incidence of salmonella septicaemia and recurrent infection despite adequate courses of antimicrobial chemotherapy have been reported in HIV antibody-positive patients.[58,83]

Opportunistic infection

Protozoa

CRYPTOSPORIDIA

Cryptosporidium spp., notably *C. parvum*, the cause of diarrhoea in up to 50% of patients with AIDS,[24] must persist for at least a month for a diagnosis of AIDS to be confirmed.

Cryptosporidium spp. were first described early this century[111] but the first human example was reported in 1976.[85] Cryptosporidiosis remained an esoteric rarity until the development of the AIDS epidemic. Cryptosporidia are unusual members of the subphylum Sporozoa because they undergo a complete life-cycle within one host and autoreinfection can therefore occur without the need for an intermediary host.[34] In addition, the sporozoites are immediately infective. Although a variety of species have been described in different animals, biochemical and cultural evidence now suggests that they are identical.

The routes of transmission of cryptosporidiosis vary. Faeco-oral transmission is responsible for nosocomial outbreaks[17] and outbreaks in day-care centres.[3] Although animal handlers in rural environments are at increased risk,[17] in the urban environment human-to-human transmission, possibly including venereal spread, is more important. Transmission by water supplies is possible. Outbreaks of this condition in immunocompetent people have occurred from contaminated water. The seasonal variation in cryptosporidiosis in HIV-infected people which follows a similar pattern to that seen in cattle may be due to contaminated drinking water.[24] Immunocompromised patients should therefore boil the water they use for drinking and for washing vegetables.

The pathogenesis of diarrhoea in patients with cryptosporidiosis is uncertain. On light microscopy there are mild inflammatory changes of the gut associated with infection. Although electron microscopy reveals some stripping of the microvillus structure adjacent to cryptosporidial attachment, there is no extensive damage (*Figure 9.48*). The diarrhoea must be secretory in part because of the high stool volumes and the continued diarrhoea during parenteral feeding. No toxin has yet been identified.

The clinical symptoms of cryptosporidiosis are watery diarrhoea and massive weight loss and, in severe cases, dehydration. Although daily stool volumes may reach 17 litres, 1–3 litres are more commonplace.[24] The diarrhoea is watery and not bloody. Abdominal pain is not a major feature. Vomiting tends to occur in the terminal phases. When abdominal pain does occur, it is commonest in the right upper quadrant, and associated with changes on cholangiography suggestive of sclerosing cholangitis.

Although there are no prospective studies, it is likely that stool microscopy is the most sensitive test to detect cryptosporidia. Stools are concentrated by stool flotation. The Ziehl–Neelsen stain colours the organisms red and fungi green. *Isospora belli* can also be stained by the same method,[10] but the cysts are much larger. Cryptosporidia are detected on rectal and small intestinal biopsies in about half the cases identified by stool analysis. In asymptomatic individuals, they may only be identified histologically.

No therapy has convincingly eradicated cryptosporidia from the stools. Macrolide antibiotics, in particular spiromycin, will reduce stool volumes and in one study the oocytes were eradicated from the stools in a third of patients.[82] However, clinical experience indicates that diarrhoea usually recurs.[24] As infection of the bile duct may act as a reservoir for infection, systemic therapy may be necessary rather than local bowel disinfection. Initial results of a study to determine whether intravenous spiromycin is valuable have been disappointing (R. Soave, personal communication). Reports have appeared that zidovudine therapy may eradicate oocysts but diarrhoea usually recurs during therapy.[53] Recombinant interleukin-2 has been administered intravenously to some patients with cryptosporidiosis and has produced improvement in the diarrhoea associated with disappearance of oocysts from the stool. The way in which such treatment works is unclear and side-effects are common.[27] A veterinary product, diclazuril, is effective against infection by *Eimeria* spp. in poultry[6] and has been suggested as a treatment for human disease. It is ineffective in a dose of 200 mg/day[31] but in larger doses there was

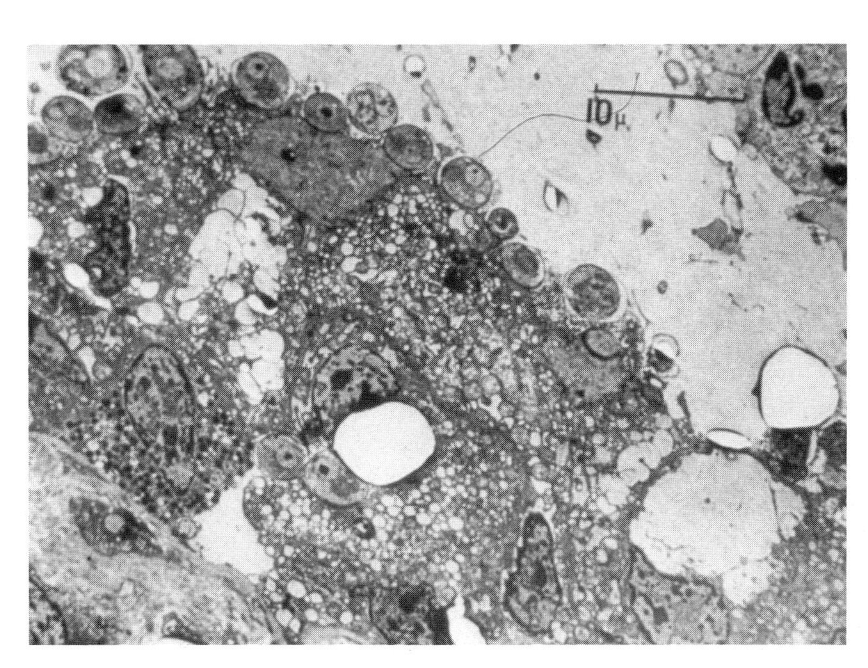

Figure 9.48 Electron microscopy demonstrating cryptosporidia on the surface of rectal epithelial cells. There is no underlying major damage.

some improvement in stool volumes with a quantitative reduction of the shedding of oocytes but the organisms were not eliminated.[107]

In patients with cryptosporidiosis, long-term survival is possible with careful attention to fluid balance including oral rehydration therapy if necessary.[24] Antidiarrhoeal agents may also have a major impact on the number of stools passed per day.

ISOSPORA

I. belli produces self-limited diarrhoea in immunocompetent patients[106] and a protracted illness with watery stools, similar to cryptosporidiosis in HIV antibody-positive individuals. Although isospora infection is rare in the UK, it accounts for 1% of AIDS patients with diarrhoea in the USA and up to 15% of patients with diarrhoea in the developing world, e.g. Haiti. The diagnosis is confirmed using the Ziehl–Nielsen stain on concentrated stool samples. The organism may be recovered from fluid obtained during duodenal aspiration or identified on small intestinal biopsy although electron microscopy may be required for precise identification.

MICROSPORIDIA

More than 500 species of the genus *Microsporidium* have been described. Human disease is rare although myocytis and encephalitis have been recorded. Occasional reports of microsporidial involvement in the small intestine of HIV-infected patients occurred in the mid-1980s[37,80] but Orenstein *et al.*[87] presented a study in Montreal where organisms were found in a third of patients with apparently pathogen-negative diarrhoea. The association with diarrhoea is not proven but is strongly suggested by the presence of microsporidia only in symptomatic HIV-positive patients with associated abnormalities of villus architecture. Little is known about the life-cycle or means of acquisition of microsporidia, although serological studies in Scandinavia indicate that a particular species of this protozoan is commoner in gay men, particularly among those who have visited the tropics.[116]

Oocytes are shed within the epithelial cells in the small intestine but they have only recently been identified in the stool. Initial reports suggested that electron microscopy of jejunal biopsy material was necessary for diagnosis[37,88] but recent experience, particularly with the use of thin plastic sections, indicate that light microscopic examination does uncover the organisms. All stages of the life-cycle, except the infecting sporoplast, are visible on light microscopy, although the highly refractile spores (5 μm in diameter) are most easily identified.

A case of peritonitis and another of granulomatous hepatitis in HIV-positive individuals have been attributed to microsporidium infection.[110,117] Recently disseminated infection with a new *Sp.* of microsporidia (*Septata intestinales*) has been described causing sinusitis.

BLASTOCYSTIS

The pathogenicity of *Blastocystis hominis* infection in immunocompromised individuals is controversial. In some studies, infection is associated with diarrhoea and a high mortality whereas, in others, treatment is associated with rapid resolution of symptoms.[64,102] The organisms are readily identified in stool samples if Field's stain is employed.[81]

Viruses

CYTOMEGALOVIRUS

CMV infection is becoming commoner in HIV-positive patients, particularly those with a low OKT-4 cell count (less than 0.05/litre).

The symptoms of CMV infection of the colon vary from symptoms of proctitis and low-volume diarrhoea to high-volume bloody stools, associated with prostration and shock. Some patients pursue an indolent course with continuing diarrhoea while others have a fulminating illness associated with toxic dilatation and perforation.[59] Abdominal pain and tenderness is a frequent feature of CMV-related diarrhoea and increases the difficulty in diagnosis of both toxic dilatation and perforation.

The diagnosis of CMV infection is dependent upon rectal biopsy samples obtained during sigmoidoscopy. The uniformity of CMV involvement of the colon is unknown. Although early case reports indicated that radiological abnormalities may be limited to the right side of the colon and terminal ileum, in one prospective study sigmoidoscopic abnormalities with histological confirmation were present in all cases of CMV colitis except one who had large ulcers in the transverse colon.[30] A post-mortem study found infection in the rectum in all but one patient.[98]

Both ganciclovir and foscarnet will slowly bring the symptoms of CMV colitis under control although relapse is frequent immediately after stopping treatment.

HERPES SIMPLEX VIRUS

Herpes simplex virus is defined as an opportunistic infection if mucocutaneous lesions persist for longer than 1 month. Usually infection produces low-volume bloody proctitic stools, and extension of inflammation to the sigmoid colon with large volume diarrhoea is rare.[52]

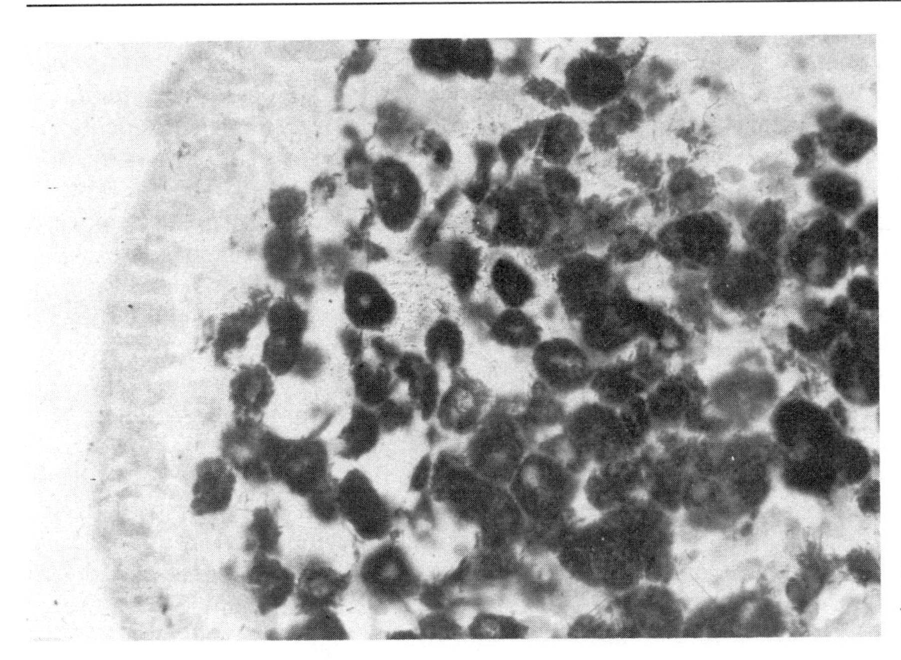

Figure 9.49 Massive infiltration of jejunal biopsy with *M. avium-intracellulare* infection.

Bacteria

MYCOBACTERIUM AVIUM-INTRACELLULARE

Infection with *M. avium-intracellulare* occurs in non-AIDS patients who are immunosuppressed but diarrhoea is not a feature. Although *M. avium-intracellulare* is cultured from up to 10% of AIDS patients with diarrhoea its pathogenicity is unclear. Colonization of body fluids such as sputum or faeces by this organism may occur without disease but active infection is more likely in the presence of systemic symptoms such as fever or anaemia and if the organism can be cultured from more than one site.[57] Infiltration of *M. avium-intracellulare* in intestinal tissue provides a diagnosis of AIDS but culture from these tissues is difficult (*Figure 9.49*). The diagnosis of *M. avium-intracellulare* is often suspected from histological examination of tissue as the organisms are slightly more curved than *Mycobacterium tuberculosis*. Infiltration may also be seen on jejunal biopsy, where characteristic foamy macrophages reminiscent of Whipple's disease can be seen.[101] Treatment is difficult, but recently combinations of rifabutin and clofazimine have been associated with defervescence of fever in patients with *M. avium-intercellulare* infection and a new agent, clarithromycin inhibited the growth of the organism in the bloodstream.

Investigations to detect pathogens causing diarrhoea

The investigations available include stool culture, rectal biopsy, microbiological analysis of fluid obtained by duodenal aspiration, histology of jejunal biopsy material, double-contrast barium enema studies and flexible fibre-optic examination of both the upper and lower gastrointestinal tract. Analysis of which tests should be used in HIV antibody-positive patients with diarrhoea is complicated as between 10 and 20% of patients have no demonstrable pathogen, despite exhaustive investigation.

The sensitivity and specificity of the various investigations are the most important determinants of which tests to use in the diagnosis of diarrhoea in HIV-positive patients. Stool microbiological analysis or histological examination of rectal biopsy material alone are unsatisfactory but in combination they provide a sensitivity and specificity for the diagnosis of diarrhoea in excess of 95%.[30] The sensitivity for double-contrast barium enema and fibre-optic colonoscopy in the same study was low. Rene *et al.*[98] also found microbiological analysis of stool samples the single most useful investigation and sigmoidoscopy and rectal biopsy increased the likelihood of diagnosis of CMV colitis. If these preliminary investigations are negative, the clinician is faced with a dilemma as to whether to do more stool analyses or pursue alternative investigations such as duodenal aspiration. One study showed that simple clinical features were a useful guide to determine whether subsequent stool samples were likely to yield a positive diagnosis. Thus, macroscopic abnormality on sigmoidoscopy or microscopic evidence of severe inflammation of the rectal biopsy indicated infection with an identifiable pathogen, particularly CMV or a bacterial infection. Patients with stool volumes in excess of 500 ml/day or those who had lost more than 5 kg in weight nearly always had a pathogen uncovered eventually, particularly cryptosporidia. Similarly, an abnormally low

Schilling test indicated terminal ileal disease due to cryptosporidiosis.[46]

Rene has stressed the value of duodenal intubation in patients in whom stool analysis yields no pathogen.[98] This is a valuable investigation in patients living in the tropics. In one study from Burundi the cause of diarrhoea was established in virtually all patients by analysis of duodenal aspiration fluid, which showed the presence of isospora, cryptosporidia or helminthic species.[45] In the developed world, analysis of fluid obtained by duodenal aspiration is less likely to increase the yield of pathogens, except for giardia. Although cryptosporidial organisms may be seen either in duodenal fluid or histologically on jejunal biopsies they are nearly always found in the stools as well.

Examination of jejunal histology is the only means at present to detect microsporidial infection. It is not clear whether such material needs to be obtained by Crosby capsule or whether infection can also be detected in duodenal pinch biopsies taken routinely during upper gastrointestinal endoscopy. It is likely in the future that the detection of spores in the stools using fluorescent antibody techniques will be straightforward and highly sensitive and specific.

In summary, all patients should initially be investigated by six stool samples sent for microbiological assessment and sigmoidoscopy coupled with rectal biopsy. If these preliminary investigations are negative and there are no suggestive clinical features, a pathogen-negative diarrhoea can be assumed. Occasionally, pathogens may be uncovered by performing upper gastrointestinal fibre-optic endoscopy coupled with duodenal aspiration and jejunal biopsy. Double-contrast barium enema or fibre-optic colonoscopy are rarely useful.[28]

HIV enteropathy

The possibility of a specific HIV-related enteropathy was suggested early in the AIDS epidemic because pathogens were not always found in patients with the wasting syndrome or diarrhoea.[68] Although improved investigation techniques and the recognition of additional organisms has reduced the frequency of undetermined causes for wasting or diarrhoea, it is of interest that HIV infection has been identified in gut epithelial cells.[84] The presence of viral particles such as of HIV in ulceration of the gullet seen at the time of seroconversion had already suggested this possibility.[96] Enterochromaffin cells, enterocytes and goblet cells have all been identified as being infected with HIV by argentaffin staining.[75,84] The findings have been confirmed by some workers[78] but not others,[47,61,112] who only found evidence of HIV infection in the mononuclear cells of the lamina propria or intraepithelial lymphocytes.

Some support for the hypothesis that enterocytes are infected with HIV has come from studies of colonic cancer cell lines where only those cultures containing messenger RNA for CD4 receptor protein were infectable with HIV.[1] CD4 receptors, however, have not been demonstrated on normal gut epithelial cells and it may be that alternative mechanisms for HIV entry to cells which have been suggested for other cell types, particularly in the brain, may be important. Recent evidence using fetal intestine implanted in athymic mice has also failed to show infection of epithelial cells where cell-free HIV was injected into the lumen.

Whether HIV infection of epithelial cells is responsible for a functional defect is not yet clear because no associated cytopathic alterations have been documented[1,63] although aptotic bodies due to individual cell necrosis are a common feature of intestinal biopsies in HIV-infected individuals. However, alterations of the structure of the small intestine have been demonstrated in HIV-positive patients and linked to a possible HIV enteropathy. Initial studies reported severe gross villous atrophy in some patients with diarrhoea[68,77] although more recent studies using refined techniques and more rigorous exclusion of potential pathogens have demonstrated much more limited abnormalities. Using three-dimensional morphometry of microdissected specimens, villous atrophy and crypt hyperplasia was confined to patients with intestinal pathogens and, when no infection was found, only slight villous atrophy was seen with normal crypt depth and a reduced mitotic rate.[112] Broadly similar findings were observed by Cummins *et al.*[32] These findings imply a reduced regenerative capacity of the villus which is associated with abnormal maturation of the epithelial cells with a reduced or absent lactase activity in one study.[112] These changes may be secondary to the HIV infection of epithelial cells or infection of immunologically active monocytes within the lamina propria, as it is known that villous regeneration is under T-cell control.

ABDOMINAL PAIN

Abdominal pain is a common gastrointestinal complaint of many patients with AIDS. The causes of abdominal pain are conveniently divided according to the site at which it occurs.

Upper abdominal pain

CMV infection of the stomach may produce a gastritis and upper abdominal discomfort. Rarely, lymphoma of the upper gastrointestinal tract or Kaposi's sarcoma (which is usually asymptomatic) produces similar symptoms.

The precise incidence of pancreatitis in HIV-positive individuals is unclear but it is certainly a major side-effect of the nucleoside analogue, dideoxyinosine, which is used as an antiretroviral therapeutic agent. Post-mortem reports in AIDS patients indicate that more than 5% of patients have evidence of pancreatitis. CMV infection, toxoplasmosis and HIV infection itself have all been implicated as possible causes.[104]

Right upper quadrant pain

There is a high incidence of right upper quadrant pain in HIV-positive patients. This pain is nonspecific and waxes and wanes over several months. Although a number of lesions in the stomach or in the lymph nodes surrounding the porta hepatis may be responsible, the commonest explanation is a form of sclerosing cholangitis known as AIDS-related sclerosing cholangitis. These patients usually have abnormal liver function tests with a marked elevation of the serum alkaline phosphatase level, although liver function tests were normal in up to a third of cases in one series. Ultrasound examination of the upper abdomen is frequently abnormal, showing dilatation of the common bile duct without obvious changes in the intrahepatic ducts.[38] However, the diagnosis is usually confirmed by endoscopic retrograde cannulation of the bile duct, which shows both beading and stricturing. The common bile duct may be prominently dilated and in some patients there is delayed emptying with stricturing of the sphincter of Oddi. AIDS-related sclerosing cholangitis is probably caused by a variety of infections. In some patients there is evidence of CMV infection elsewhere and, in a minority, biopsy of the ampulla reveals numerous CMV inclusions. More patients have evidence of cryptosporidial infection. Even asymptomatic patients with cryptosporidiosis may have beading of the common bile duct. Up to one-third of patients have no evidence of infection with either cryptosporidia or CMV.

Unlike idiopathic sclerosing cholangitis, recurrent episodes of jaundice and progression to liver failure are very uncommon in AIDS-related sclerosing cholangitis. Treatment is difficult; a few patients seem to respond to treatment for CMV disease and, in some, sphincteroplasty may produce improvement.

Lower abdominal pain

Lower abdominal pain is most commonly associated with constipation, because of administration of opiates for other conditions.

Right iliac fossa pain

The commonest cause of right iliac fossa pain is appendicitis, sometimes caused by CMV infection.

Diffuse abdominal pain

Diffuse abdominal pain in AIDS patients is most commonly associated with diarrhoea due to CMV infection.[59] CMV colitis is often associated with rebound abdominal tenderness and diffuse abdominal pain. As the two major complications of CMV infection are perforation (probably due to an associated arteritis) and toxic dilatation of the colon,[29] these patients represent a difficult diagnostic challenge, particularly as treatment of CMV only produces slow improvement.

In patients with abdominal pain, particularly when diffuse, abdominal ultrasound or computed axial tomography (CAT) scanning may demonstrate intra-abdominal lymphadenopathy.[86] The commonest causes for this are lymphoma, infection with *M. avium-intracellulare*, or Kaposi's sarcoma. Diagnosis can be confirmed by a needle biopsy under CAT scan control, and the need for laparotomy is now rare.

ENDOSCOPIC DECONTAMINATION

HIV infection can be found by the polymerase chain reaction on endoscopes used in routine procedures in HIV-positive patients. HIV transmission during endoscopy has, however, not been demonstrated either to other patients or to health workers. All evidence of HIV infection is removed by standard cleaning and washing techniques[55] and it should be emphasized that this is the most important part of decontaminating endoscopes. To facilitate washing, endoscopes should be of the totally immersible type and automatic washing machines may have advantages.

The best disinfectant for routine use in endoscopy units remains a matter of dispute. HIV is not the major problem as it is readily destroyed by contact with 2% glutaraldehyde for 4 minutes.[115] However, both tuberculosis and cryptosporidial species are more resistant, which may be important because of the possibility of transferring opportunistic infection from one immunocompromised individual to another. In the UK, endoscopy units dealing with mycobacterial contamination of endoscopes are advised to leave the instrument in contact with glutaraldehyde for a minimum of 60 minutes. The oocytes of cryptosporidium are destroyed by 10% (v/v) hydrogen peroxide.[14]

The major risk to health workers associated with

endoscopy is not handling of contaminated instruments but 'sharp' injuries. This is particularly important with biopsy forceps and needles used to administer drugs during endoscopy. 'Sharp' precautions are essential and ultrasonic cleaners should be used to clean biopsy forceps.

REFERENCES

1. Adachi, A., Koenig, S., Gendelman, H.E. *et al.* (1987) Productive, persistent infection of human colorectal cell lines with human immunodeficiency virus. *Journal of Virology*, **61**, 209–213.
2. Allason-Jones, E., Mindel, A., Sargeaunt, P. *et al.* (1986) *Entamoeba histolytica* as a commensal internal parasite in homosexual men. *New England Journal of Medicine*, **315**, 353–356.
3. Alpert, G., Bell, L.M. and Kirkpatrick, C.E. (1986) Outbreak of cryptosporidiosis in a day-care center. *Paediatrics*, **77**, 152–157.
4. Alter, M.J., Ahtone, J., Weisfuse, I. *et al.* (1986) Hepatitis B virus transmission between homosexuals. *Journal of the American Medical Association*, **256**, 1307.
5. Andriolo, M., Wolff, J.N. and Rosenberg, J.S. (1986) AIDS and AIDS-related complex: oral manifestations and treatment. *Journal of the American Dental Association*, **113**, 586–589.
6. Anon. (1987) *Basic Veterinary Information Brochure.* Beerse: Janssen Research Foundation.
7. Bader, M., Pedersen, A.H.B., Williams, R. *et al.* (1977) Venereal transmission of shigellosis in Seattle, King County. *Sexually Transmitted Diseases*, **4**, 89.
8. Baker, R.W. and Peppercorn, M.A. (1982) Gastrointestinal ailments of homosexual men. *Medicine*, **61**: 390–405.
9. Barre-Sinoussi, F., Chermann, C., Rey, F. *et al.* (1983) Isolation of a T lymphotropic retrovirus from a patient at risk for acquired immunodeficiency syndrome (AIDS). *Science*, **220**, 868–871.
10. Baxby, D., Blundell, N. and Hart, C.A. (1984) The development and performance of a simple, sensitive method for the detection of cryptosporidium oocysts in faeces. *Journal of Hygiene*, **92**, 317–323.
11. Bernier, R.H., Sampliner, R., Gerety, R., Tabor, E., Hamilton, F. and Nathanson, N. (1982) Hepatitis B infection: households of chronic carriers of hepatitis B service antigen: factors associated with prevalence of infection. *American Journal of Epidemiology*, **116**, 119.
12. Bhattacharyya, M.N. and Jephcott, A.E. (1974) Diagnosis of gonorrhoea in women; role of the rectal sample. *British Journal of Venereal Diseases*, **50**, 109–112.
13. Bleeker, A., Coutinhor, A., Bakkerkok, J., Tio, D. and Dekoning, G.A.J. (1981) Prevalence of syphilis and hepatitis B amongst homosexual men in two saunas in Amsterdam. *British Journal of Venereal Diseases*, **57**, 196.
14. Blewett, D.A. (1989) Disinfection in oocytes – cryptosporidiosis. In *Proceedings of the First International Workshop* (Eds) Angus, K.W. and Blewett, D.A. p. 107. Edinburgh: Moredun Research Institute.
15. Bodey, G.P., Feinstein, V. and Guerrant, R. (1986) Infections of the gastrointestinal tract in the immunocompromised patients. *Annual Review of Medicine*, **37**, 271–281.
16. Cameron, D.W., Simonsen, J.N., D'Costa, L.J. *et al.* (1989) Female to male transmission of HIV1: risk factors for seroconversion. *The Lancet*, **ii**, 403–40406.
17. Casemore, D.P. (1990) Epidemiological aspects of human cryptosporidiosis (review). *Journal of Epidemiology and Infection*, **104**, 1–28.
18. Centers for Disease Control (1981) Pneumocystis pneumonia. *Morbidity and Mortality Weekly Report*, **30**, 250–252.
19. Centers for Disease Control (1987) Revision of the CDC surveillance case definition for acquired immunodeficiency syndrome. *Morbidity and Mortality Weekly Report*, **36**(suppl.), 1S.
20. Centers for Disease Control (1988) Changing patterns of groups at high risk for hepatitis B in the United States. *Morbidity and Mortality Weekly Report*, **37**, 429.
21. Chachoua, A., Dietrich, D. and Krasinski, D. (1987) 9-(1,3-Dihydroxy-2-propoxymethyl) guanine (ganciclovir) in the treatment of cytomegalovirus gastrointestinal disease with the acquired immunodeficiency syndrome. *Annals of Internal Medicine*, **107**, 133–137.
22. Cimolai, N., Gill, M.J., Jones, A. *et al.* (1987) Campylobacter sinaedi bacteraemia: case report and laboratory findings. *Journal of Clinical Microbiology*, **25**, 942–943.
23. Colebunders, R., Lusakumuni, K., Nelson, A.M. *et al.* (1988) Persistent diarrhoea in Zairian AIDS patients: an endoscopic and histological study. *Gut*, **29**, 1687–1691.
24. Connolly, G.M., Dryden, M.S., Shanson, D.C. *et al.* (1988) Cryptosporidial diarrhoea in AIDS and its treatment. *Gut*, **29**, 593–597.
25. Connolly, G.M., Hawkins, D., Harcourt-Webster, J.N., Parsons, P.A., Hussain, O.A.N. and Gazzard, B.G. (1989) Oesophageal symptoms, their causes, treatment and prognosis in patients with the acquired immunodeficiency syndrome. *Gut*, **30**, 1033–1039.
26. Connolly, G.M., Forbes, A., Gleeson, J. and Gazzard, B.G. (1989) The investigation of upper gastrointestinal symptoms in patients with AIDS. *AIDS*, **3**, 453–456.
27. Connolly, G.M., Owen, S.L., Hawkins, D.A. *et al.* (1989) Treatment of cryptosporidial infection with recombinant interleukin-2 (rIL-2). *5th International Conference on AIDS, Montreal*, WBP 47, p. 359.

28. Connolly, G.M., Forbes, A., Gleeson, J. and Gazzard, B.G. (1989) The value of barium enema and colonoscopy in patients infected with human immunodeficiency virus. *Gut*, **30**, 721.
29. Connolly, G.M., Shanson, D., Hawkins, D.A. *et al.* (1989) Non-cryptosporidial diarrhoea in human immunodeficiency virus (HIV) infected patients. *Gut*, **30**, 195–200.
30. Connolly, G.M., Forbes, A., Gazzard, B.G. *et al.* (1990) The investigation of seemingly pathogen-negative diarrhoea in patients infected with HIV-1. *Gut*, **31**, 886–889.
31. Connolly, G.M., Youle, M. and Gazzard, B.G. (1990) Diclazuril in the treatment of severe cryptosporidial diarrhoea in AIDS patients. *AIDS*, **4**, 700–701.
32. Corey, L. and Holmes, K.K. (1980) Sexual transmission of hepatitis A in homosexual men: incidence and mechanisms. *New England Journal of Medicine*, **302**, 435–438.
33. Cummins, A.G., LaBrooy, J.T., Stanley, D.P. *et al.* (1990) Quantitative histological study of enteropathy associated with HIV infection. *Gut*, **31**, 317–321.
34. Current, W.L. and Reese, N.C. (1986) A comparison of endogenous development of three isolates of cryptosporidium in suckling mice. *Journal of Protozoology*, **33**, 98–108.
35. D'Antonio, R.G., Winn, R.E., Taylor, J.P. *et al.* (1985) A waterborne outbreak of cryptosporidiosis in normal hosts. *Annals of Internal Medicine*, **103**, 886–888.
36. DeHovitz, J.A., Pape, J.W., Boncy, M. *et al.* (1986) Clinical manifestations and therapy of *Isospora belli* infection patients with the acquired immunodeficiency syndrome. *New England Journal of Medicine*, **315**, 87–90.
37. Dobbins, W.O. and Weinstein, W.M. (1985) Electron microscopy of the intestine and rectum in acquired immunodeficiency syndrome. *Gastroenterology*, **88**, 738–749.
38. Dowsett, J.F., Miller, R., Davidson, R. *et al.* (1988) Sclerosing cholangitis in acquired immunodeficiency syndrome: case reports and review of the literature. *Scandinavian Journal of Gastroenterology*, **23**, 1267–1274.
39. Dworkin, B., Wormser, G.P., Rosenthal, W.S. *et al.* (1985) Gastrointestinal manifestations of the acquired immunodeficiency syndrome: a review of 22 cases. *American Journal of Gastroenterology*, **80**, 774–778.
40. Dworkin, B.M., Rosenthal, W.S., Wormser, G.W. *et al.* (1986) Selenium deficiency in the acquired immunodeficiency syndrome. *JPEN. Journal of Parenteral and Enteral Nutrition*, **10**, 405–407.
41. European Study Group (1989) Risk factors for male to female transmission of HIV. *British Medical Journal*, **298**, 411–415.
42. Faluta, J., Tsoukas, C. and Deutsch, G. (1989) The role of zinc in HIV induced immunosuppression. *5th International Congress on AIDS, Montreal*, ThBP 315.
43. Farrow, L.J., Stewart, J.S., Stern, H., Clifford, R.E., Smith, H.G. and Zuckerman, A.J. (1981) Non-A, non-B hepatitis in west London. *The Lancet*, **i**, 982–984.
44. Ferraro, R., Kotler, D.P., Cuff, P., Tierney, A.R., Smith, R. and Heymsfield, S. (1989) Effect of enteral nutritional therapy on body cell mass in AIDS *5th International Conference on AIDS, Montreal*, ThBP 37.
45. Floch, J.J., Laroche, R., Kadende, P. *et al.* (1989) Parasites, etiological agents of diarrhoea in AIDS patients in Burundi. Interest of the aspirated duodenal liquid examination. *Bulletin de la Societé de Pathologie Exotique et de ses Filiales*, **82**, 316–320.
46. Forbes, A., Connolly, G.M., Smithson, J., Russell, J. and Gazzard B.G. (1989) Evaluation of a simple scoring system to assist diagnosis of diarrhoea in patients with AIDS. *Gut*, **30**(10), 1478.
47. Fox, C.H., Kotler, D., Tierney, A. *et al.* (1989) Detection of HIV-1 RNA in the lamina propria of patients with AIDS and gastrointestinal disease. *Journal of Infectious Diseases*, **159**, 467–471.
48. Francis, D.P., Hadler, S.C., Thompson, S.E. *et al.* (1982) The prevention of hepatitis B with vaccine: report of the Centers for Disease Control; multicentre efficacy trial among homosexual men. *Annals of Internal Medicine*, **97**, 362.
49. Francisco, A.N. and Kotler, D.P. (1988) Jejunal histopathology in AIDS. *Gastroenterology*, **94**(suppl.) A134.
50. Gillin, J.S., Shike, M., Alcock, B. *et al.* (1985) Malabsorption and mucosal abnormalities of the small intestine in the acquired immune deficiency syndrome. *Annals of Internal Medicine*, **102**, 619–622.
51. Goldmeier, D., Price, A.B., Billington, O. *et al.* (1986) Is *Entamoeba histolytica* in homosexual men a pathogen? *The Lancet*, **i**, 641–644.
52. Goodel, S.E., Quinn, T.C., Mkrtichian, E. *et al.* (1983) Herpes simplex virus proctitis in homosexual men. Clinical, sigmoidoscopic and histopathological features. *New England Journal of Medicine*, **308**, 868–871.
53. Greenberg, E., Bank, M.I.R. and Siegal, P. (1989) Resolution of intestinal cryptosporidiosis after treatment of AIDS with AZT. *Gastroenterology*, **97**, 1327–1330.
54. Greenspan, D., Greenspan, J.S., Conant, M. *et al.* (1987) Relation of oral hairy leukoplakia to infection with the Human immunodeficiency virus and the risk of developing AIDS. *Journal of Infectious Diseases*, **155**, 475–481.
55. Hanson, P.J.V., Gor, D., Clarke, J.R. *et al.* (1989) Contamination of fibreoptic endoscopes in AIDS. *The Lancet*, **ii**, 86–88.
56. Hommes, M., Romijn, J.A., Godfried, M.H., Endert, E., Danner, S.A. and Sauerwein, H.P.

(1989) Increased resting energy expenditure in HIV infected men. *5th International Conference on AIDS, Montreal*, ThBO 38, p. 218.

57. Horsburgh, C.R. Jr, Mason, U.G. III, Farhi, D.C. *et al.* (1983) Disseminated infection with mycobacterium avium intracellulare – a report of 13 cases and a review of the literature. *Medicine*, **64**, 36–48.
58. Jacobs, J.L., Gold, J.W.M., Murray, H.W. *et al.* (1985) Salmonella infections in patients with the acquired immunodeficiency syndrome. *Annals of Internal Medicine*, **102**, 186–188.
59. Jacobsen, M.A., O'Donnell, J.J., Porteous, D., Brodie, H.R., Fiegal, D. and Mills, J. (1988) Retinal and gastrointestinal disease due to cytomegalovirus in patients with the acquired immunodeficiency syndrome: prevalence, natural history and response to ganciclovir therapy. *Quarterly Journal of Medicine*, **67**, 473–486.
60. Janoff, E.N. and Smith, P.D. (1988) Perspectives on gastrointestinal infections in AIDS. *Gastroenterology Clinics of North America*, **17**, 451–463.
61. Jary, A., Brousse, N., Rene, E. *et al.* (1988) Infected cells and immune cells in the gastrointestinal tract of AIDS patients (abstract). *Gastroenterology*, **94**, A207.
62. Jones, J.M., Miller, J.N. and Georges, W.L. (1986) Microbiological and chemical characterization of spirochetes isolated from the feces of homosexual males. *Journal of Clinical Microbiology*, **24**, 1071–1074.
63. Kagnoff, M.F., Bish, R., Omary, M. *et al.* (1989) HIV-infection of intestinal epithelium (abstract). *International Congress of Mucosal Immunology*.
64. Kain, K.C., Noble, M.A., Freeman, H.J. *et al.* (1987) Epidemiology and clinical features associated with *Blastocystis hominis* infection. *Diagnostic Microbiology and Infectious Disease*, **8**, 235–244.
65. Kingsley, L.A., Kaslow, R., Rinaldo, C.R. Jr *et al.* (1987) Risk factors for seroconversion to human immunodeficiency virus among male homosexuals. *The Lancet*, **i**, 345–349.
66. Kitchen, V., Helbert, M., Francis, N., Logan, R., Lewis, F., Pinching, A. *et al.* (1989) Ulcerating pharyngo-oesophageal leukoplakia in advanced HIV disease. *5th International Conference on AIDS, Montreal*, MBP 224, p. 262.
67. Klein, E.J., Fisher, L.S., Chow, A.W. and Guz, L.B. (1977) Anorectal gonococcal infection. *Annals of Internal Medicine*, **86**, 340–346.
68. Klein, R.S., Harris, C.A., Small, C.B. *et al.* (1984) Oral candidiasis in high risk patients as the initial manifestation of the acquired immunodeficiency syndrome. *New England Journal of Medicine*, **311**, 354–358.
69. Kotler, D.P. (1989) Malnutrition in HIV infection and AIDS. *AIDS*, S175–180.
70. Kotler, D.P., Scholes, J.V. and Tierney, A.R. (1987) Intestinal plasma cell alterations in acquired immunodeficiency syndrome. *Digestive Diseases and Sciences*, **32**, 129–138.
71. Kotler, D.P., Wilson, C.S., Haroutiounian, G. and Fox, C.H. (1989) Detection of human immunodeficiency virus 1 by 35S-RNA in situ hybridisation in solitary oesophageal ulcers in two patients with the acquired immune deficiency syndrome. *American Journal of Gastroenterology*, **84**, 313–317.
72. Kotler, D.T., Gaetz, H.P. and Lang, M. (1984) Enteropathy associated with the acquired immune deficiency syndrome. *Annals of Internal Medicine*, **101**, 421.
73. Laughon, B.E., Druckman, D.A., Vernon, A. *et al.* (1989) Prevalence of enteric pathogens in homosexual men with and without acquired immunodeficiency syndrome. *Gastroenterology*, **94**, 984–993.
74. Lebedeff, D.A. and Hochman, E.B. (1980) Rectal Gonorrhoea in men: diagnosis and treatment. *Annals of Internal Medicine*, **92**, 463–466.
75. Levy, J.A., Margaretten, W. and Nelson, J. (1989) Detection of HIV in enterochromaffin cells in the rectal mucosa of an AIDS patient. *American Journal of Gastroenterology*, **84**, 787–789.
76. MacFarlane, I.G., Smith, H.M., Johnson, P.J., Bray, G.P., Vergani, D. and Williams, R. (1990) Hepatitis C virus antibodies in chronic active hepatitis: pathogenetic factor or false-positive result? *The Lancet*, **335**, 754–757.
77. Malebranche, R., Guerin, J.M., Laroche, A.C. *et al.* (1983) Acquired immunodeficiency syndrome with severe gastrointestinal manifestations in Haiti. *The Lancet*, **ii**, 873–877.
78. Mathijs, J.M., Hing, M., Gierson, J. *et al.* (1988) HIV infection of rectal mucosa. *The Lancet*, **i**, 1111.
79. Matthews, R., Burnie, J., Smith, D. *et al.* (1988) Candida and AIDS – evidence for protective antibody. *The Lancet*, **ii**, 263–266.
80. Modigliani, R., Bories, C., le Charpentier, Y. *et al.* (1985) Diarrhoea and malabsorption in acquired immune deficiency syndrome: a study of four cases with special emphasis on opportunistic protozoan infestations. *Gut*, **26**, 179–187.
81. Moody, A.H. and Fleck, S.L. (1985) Versatile Field's stain. *Journal of Clinical Pathology*, **38**, 842–843.
82. Moskovitz, B.L., Stanton, T.L. and Kusmierek, J.J.E. (1988) Spiramycin therapy for cryptosporidial diarrhoea in immunocompromised patients. *Journal of Antimicrobial Chemotherapy*, **2**, 189–191.
83. Nadelmann, R.B., Mathur-Wagh, U., Yancovitz, S.R. *et al.* (1985) Salmonella bacteremia associated with the acquired immunodeficiency syndrome (AIDS). *Annals of Internal Medicine*, **145**, 1968–1971.
84. Nelson, J.A., Reynolds-Kohler, C., Margaretten, W. *et al.* (1988) Human immunodeficiency virus

detected in bowel epithelium from patients with gastrointestinal symptoms. *The Lancet*, **i**, 259–261.
85. Nime, F.A., Burek, J.D., Page, D.L. *et al.* (1976) Acute enterocolitis in a human being infected with the protozoon *Cryptosporidium*. *Gastroenterology*, **70**, 591–598.
86. Nyberg, D.A., Federle, M.P., Jeffery, R.B., Bottles, J. and Woofsy, C. (1985) Abdominal CT findings of disseminated Mycobacterium avium-intracellulare in AIDS. *American Journal of Radiology*, **145**, 297–299.
87. Orenstein, J., Steinberg, W., Chiang, J. *et al.* (1989) Intestinal microsporidiosis as a cause of diarrhoea in AIDS. *5th International Conference on AIDS, Montreal*, WBO 38, p. 209.
88. Owen, R.L. (1989) In *Parasitic Disease in Gastrointestinal Disease –Pathophysiology, Diagnosis, Management,* 4th edn (Eds) Sleisenger, M.H. and Fordtran, J.S. pp. 1153–1155. Philadelphia: W.B. Saunders.
89. Padian, N.S. (1987) Heterosexual transmission of acquired immunodeficiency syndrome: international perspectives and national projections. *Revue of Infectious Diseases*, **9**, 947–960.
90. Pariser, H. and Marino, A.F. (1970) Gonorrhoea – frequently unrecognised reservoirs. *Southern Medical Journal*, **63**, 198–201.
91. Perrillo, R.B., Gelb, L., Campbell, C. *et al.* (1979) Hepatitis B e antigen DNA polymerase activity, and infection of household contacts with hepatitis B virus. *Gastroenterology*, **76**(6), 1319–1325.
92. Piot, P., Plummer, F.A., Mhalu, F.S., Lamboray, L., Chin, J. and Mann, J.M. (1988) AIDS: an international perspective. *Science*, **239**, 573–579.
93. Quinn, T.C., Corey, L., Chavee, R.G. *et al.* (1981) The etiology of anorectal infection in homosexual men. *American Journal of Medicine*, **71**, 395–406.
94. Quinn, T.C., Mann, J.M., Curren, J.W. *et al.* (1986) AIDS in Africa and epidemiological paradigm. *Science*, **234**, 955–963.
95. Quinn, T.C., Stamm, W.E., Goodell, S.E. *et al.* (1983) The polymicrobial origin of intestinal infections in homosexual men. *New England Journal of Medicine*, **309**, 576–582.
96. Rabeneck, L., Boyko, W.J., McLean, D.M. *et al.* (1986) Unusual oesophageal ulcers containing enveloped virus-like particles in homosexual men. *Gastroenterology*, **90**, 1882–1889.
97. Ranger, S., Weinbreck, P., Loustaud, V., Mounier, M., Delpeyroux, C. and Dennis, F. (1990) Sero problems of hepatitis C virus antibodies in HIV European seropositive patients. *International Conference on AIDS, San Francisco*, ThB 452, Vol. 2, p. 235.
98. Rene, E., Marche, C., Chevalier, T. *et al.* (1988) Cytomegalovirus colitis in patients with acquired immunodeficiency syndrome. *Digestive Disease and Sciences*, **33**, 741–750.
99. Rogers, V.D., Fasset, R. and Kagnof, M.F. (1986) Abnormalities in intestinal mucosa T cells in homosexual populations including those with lymphadenopathy syndrome and acquired immunodeficiency syndrome. *Gastroenterology*, **90**, 552–558.
100. Rossol, S., Voth, R. Brunner, S. *et al.* (1989) Enhanced endogenous TNF-a production in peripheral blood mononuclear cells of HIV-1 infected patients. *5th International Conference on AIDS, Montreal*, ThBP 98, p. 432.
101. Roth, R.I., Owen, R.L. and Keren, D.F. (1985) Intestinal infection with mycobacterium avium in acquired immunodeficiency syndrome (AIDS). Histological and clinical comparison with Whipples disease. *Digestive Diseases and Sciences*, **30**, 497–504.
102. Russo, A.R., Stone, S.L., Taplin, M.E. *et al.* (1988) Presumptive evidence for blastocystis hominis as a cause of colitis. *Archives of Internal Medicine*, **148**, 1064.
103. Sewadda, D., Mugera, R.D., Sewankambo, N.K. *et al.* (1985) Slim disease: a new disease in Uganda associated with HTLVIII infection. *The Lancet*, **ii**, 849–852.
104. Silver, M.A., Silver, M.C., Lema, T.S., Lemos, O., Correa-Lema, C.E.B. (1990) Pancreatitis in AIDS patients. *International Conference on AIDS, San Francisco*, abstract 2021, V2, p. 359.
105. Smith, D. (1965) Infectious syphilis of the rectum. *Diseases of the Colon and Rectum*, **8**, 57–58.
106. Soave, R. and Johnson, W.D. (1988) Cryptosporidium and *Isospora belli* infections. *Journal of Infectious Diseases*, **157**, 225–229.
107. Soave, R., Dieterich, D. and Kotler, D. (1990) Oral diclazuril therapy for cryptosporidiosis. *Abstracts of the 6th International Conference on AIDS, San Francisco*, ThB 250, V2, p. 25.
108. Sullam, P.M. (1987) *Entamoeba histolytica* in homosexual men. *New England Journal of Medicine*, **315**, 690.
109. Szmuness, W., Much, M.I., Prince, A.M. *et al.* (1975) The role of sexual behaviour in the spread of hepatitis B infection. *Annals of Internal Medicine*, **83**, 489.
110. Terada, S., Reddy, R., Jeffers, L.J. *et al.* (1987) Microsporidian hepatitis in the acquired immunodeficiency syndrome. *Annals of Internal Medicine*, **107**, 61–62.
111. Tyzzer, E.E. (1907) A sporozoan found in the peptic glands of the common mouse. *Proceedings of the Society for Experimental Biology and Medicine*, **5**, 12–13.
112. Ullrich, R., Zeitz, M., Heise, W. *et al.* (1989) Small intestinal structure and function in patients infected with human immunodeficiency virus (HIV): evidence for HIV-induced enteropathy. *Annals of Internal Medicine*, **111**, 15–21.
113. Ullrich, R., Zeitz, M., Heise, W. *et al.* (1990) Mucosal atrophy is associated with loss of activated T cells in the duodenal mucosa of human

immunodeficiency virus (HIV)-infected patients. *Digestion*, **46**, Suppl. 2, 302–307.

114. Van Roenn, J.H., Murphy, R.L., Wever, K.M., Williams, L.M. and Weitzman, S.A. (1988) Megestrol acetate for treatment of cachexia associated with human immunodeficiency virus infection. *Annals of Internal Medicine*, **109**, 840–841.
115. Working Party of the British Society of Gastroenterology (1988) Cleaning and disinfection of equipment for gastrointestinal flexible endoscopy: interim recommendations. *Gut*, **29**, 1134–1151.
116. WHO (1983) Parasitic diseases surveillance antibody to *Encephalitozoon cuniculi* in man. *WHO Weekly Epidemiology Record*, **58**, 30–32.
117. Youle, M., Clarbour, J., Farthing, C. *et al.* (1989) Treatment of resistant aphthous ulceration with thalidomide in patients positive for HIV antibody. *British Medical Journal*, **298**, 432.
118. Zender, H.O., Arrigoni, E., Eckert, J. *et al.* (1989) A case of *Encephalitozoon cuniculi* peritonitis in a patient with AIDS. *American Journal of Clinical Pathology*, **92**, 352–356.

ENDOSCOPIC AND SURGICAL INTERVENTION IN HIV-POSITIVE INDIVIDUALS

B.G. Gazzard

Endoscopy and operations in human immunodeficiency virus (HIV)-positive individuals still arouses controversy and raises moral and ethical dilemmas, some of which are considered in this section.

The ethical issues involved in refusing to treat HIV-positive patients are complex. Although most doctors feel that their profession has an honourable history, investigation of previous epidemics like the black plague indicate that, not surprisingly, individual standards of behaviour amongst doctors have not always been heroic.[9] The general public usually regard doctors as having a 'contractual ethic' to provide good health for all members of society and reports suggest that they would not be too concerned if individual doctors refused to treat particular patients.[4] Others would regard such a refusal as a serious offence, unless there was a clear risk to the physician which outweighed the risk to the patient.

Although the fears of HIV infection among health care workers remain great the real risk is extremely low.[3] No surgeon has been shown to seroconvert as a result of his or her profession, although there is circumstantial evidence that this might have occurred in a handful of individuals. In the one case where a 'sharp' injury with a colonoscopy forceps was associated with seroconversion, there were other possible routes of transmission and there are no other cases associated with endoscopic procedures. Needlestick injury is associated with a small but definite risk of seroconversion of less than 0.5%. Although there were only five cases where contamination of the intact skin with massive amounts of blood led to seroconversion, these episodes led to a major reappraisal of precautions taken in some hospitals dealing with large numbers of HIV-positive patients.[3] Unfortunately, there is little scientific evidence to demonstrate that these precautions are beneficial, in particular to the surgeon. The benefits of waterproof gowns and eye protection are not established but double or triple gloving does reduce the risk of needlestick injury and exposure to infected blood.

Preoperative screening for HIV antibodies has become an important issue because most surgeons feel that if they know the status of their patients this will increase the care taken during operation and therefore reduce the risk. The one study which has addressed this issue showed that knowledge of the status of the patient had no effect on the risks of injury. The study was criticised because it took place in a centre (San Francisco) where maximum precautions were already being taken because of the high seroprevalence rate.[5] The issues surrounding HIV antibody testing prior to surgery have been made more complex because it has been appreciated that the treatment of asymptomatic HIV-positive patients may prolong life.[8] Unfortunately, counselling and discussion is often not optimal immediately prior to surgery or endoscopy. In this situation an HIV test is often requested, not primarily for the benefit of the patient, but in order to provide theoretical protection for health care staff. As always, these issues are best resolved by detailed discussion with the patient but this requires knowledge of the issues surrounding HIV testing, particularly counselling, support and treatment.

SURGERY IN HIV-POSITIVE INDIVIDUALS

Initial anecdotal evidence suggested that HIV-positive individuals and in particular those with the acquired immune deficiency syndrome (AIDS) fared badly after surgery but this is not the case. Most people who are HIV-positive, and indeed some patients with AIDS, will have a better prognosis than large numbers of individuals routinely subjected to surgery for example for cancer of the gastrointestinal tract. Infection is commonly the underlying cause of disease in AIDS patients requiring surgery. The commonest cause of disease in a recent series of patients coming to emergency laparotomy in large central London units dealing with HIV-positive patients was cytomegalovirus infection and the short-term results of operating on these patients were good, with the majority surviving to leave hospital.

ENDOSCOPY IN AIDS PATIENTS

The problems surrounding endoscopy in HIV-positive patients are three-fold: first, transmission of HIV infection to staff, which has already been considered; secondly, HIV transmission from patient to patient; and, thirdly, the problems of endoscopy in the immunocompromised individual.

Although hepatitis B transmission from one patient to another has been described during endoscopy, a similar example has not yet arisen in HIV infection.[1] Experiments have been conducted which show that the virus (detected by the polymerase chain reaction) does contaminate endoscopes during endoscopy.[6] However, this virus was not able to infect tissue cultures and, most importantly, was completely removed by thorough washing, which must remain the mainstay of prevention of transmission. Glutaraldehyde inhibits the virus after 4 minutes of exposure, providing washing has removed any significant amounts of serum.[7] Glutaraldehyde remains the safest disinfectant to use in an endoscopy unit following washing. Endoscopy is easier and safer with the newer totally immersible endoscopes and automatic washing machines.

It is only possible to give pragmatic advice about the risks of transmission of opportunistic infections from one immunocompromised individual to another. The main theoretical risks would appear to be *Cryptosporidium* spp. and *Mycobacterium avium intracellulare*. These organisms *may* be present in tap water as an additional source of contamination of endoscopes. They are both likely to be relatively resistant to disinfection and, thus, the British Society of Gastroenterology[2] has recommended at least 1 hour of immersion in glutaraldehyde before and between endoscopy of one immunocompromised individual and another. Again, thorough washing of the equipment prior to sterilization is vital.

REFERENCES

1. Birnie, G.G., Quigley, E.M., Clements, G.B., Follett, E.A.C. and Walkinson, G. (1983) Endoscopic transmission of hepatitis B virus. *Gut*, **24**, 171–174.
2. British Society of Gastroenterology (1988) Cleaning and disinfection of equipment for gastrointestinal flexible endoscopy, interim recommendations of a working party of the British Society of Gastroenterology. *Gut*, **29**, 1134–1151.
3. Centre for Disease Control (1989) Guidelines for prevention of transmission of human immunodeficiency virus and hepatitis B virus to health care and public safely worker. *Morbidity and Mortality Weekly Report* (Suppl. 86).
4. Cook, M. (1990) Occupational transmission of HIV. The ethics of physician risk and responsibility. In *AIDS Clinical Review 1990* (Eds) Volberding, P. and Jacobson, M.A. New York: Marcel Dekker.
5. Gerberding, J.L., Littell, C., Tarkington, A., Brown, A. and Schecter, W.P. (1990) Risk of exposure of surgical personnel to patients' blood during surgery at San Francisco General Hospital. *New England Journal of Medicine*, **322**, 1788–1793.
6. Hanson, P.J.V., Gor, D. and Clark, J.L. (1989) Contamination of fibreoptic endoscopes in AIDS. *The Lancet*, **ii**, 86–88.
7. Hanson, P.J.V., Gor, D., Jefferies, D.J. and Collins, J.V. (1989b) Chemical inactivation of HIV on surfaces. *British Medical Journal*, **298**, 862–864.
8. Volberding, P.A., Lagakos, S.W., Koch, M.A. *et al.* (1990) Zidovudine in asymptomatic human immunodeficiency infection – a controlled trial in persons with fewer than 500 CD4-positive cells per cubic millimeter. *New England Journal of Medicine*, **322**, 941–949.
9. Zuger, A. and Miles, S.H. (1987) Physicians, AIDS and occupational risk. *Journal of the American Medical Association*, **258**, 1924–1928.

CHAPTER 10

FUNCTIONAL DISORDERS OF THE GUT

APPETITE AND SATIETY

R.T. Jung

Anorexia is common in many gastrointestinal diseases. Many reasons for this have been suggested, such as pain and gastric distension in obstructive lesions, pyrexia in inflammatory conditions and some enigmatic anorectic factor released by cancerous tissue.[7] However, is it only recently that some progress has been made in the understanding of appetite control, especially in the linkage of psychological factors with physiological and metabolic events, and the influence of peptide and monoamine neurotransmitters on the control of food intake.

PSYCHOLOGICAL FACTORS

Four factors influence eating in animals and humans:

1. Incentive properties of food: this refers to a preference for one food over another.
2. Level of arousal: it is possible to induce eating in satiated animals by a mild stress such as tail pinching. Stress can also result in over-eating in satiated people, as can be shown by the excess consumption of food by students during examinations and by some women suffering loneliness or depression.
3. Environmental stimuli: this is best illustrated by the classic experiment of making food especially noticeable by directing light on it; obese subjects then will eat more than when the food is poorly lit.[19]
4. Learning: this is intertwined with all the other factors.

PHYSIOLOGICAL DEVELOPMENTS

Traditionally, the hypothalamus has been considered to contain both the 'satiety' and 'feeding' centres. As bilateral lesions in the ventromedial hypothalamus result in hyperphagia and electrical stimulation induces satiety, this area has been known as the 'satiety' centre. The lateral hypothalamus has been known as the 'feeding' centre because lesions in this area stop eating and electrical stimulation induces feeding.[6] However, problems have arisen with this 'dual centre' hypothesis.

LATERAL HYPOTHALAMUS – FEEDING CENTRE

It has been shown that the lateral hypothalamus lesions which were particularly effective in producing aphagia were situated far lateral and were actually damaging pallidofugal fibre pathways, including a dopaminergic nigrostriatal bundle; if the latter was damaged outside the hypothalamus, aphagia was also produced.[13] This dopaminergic pathway appears important in tail-pinch arousal: such arousal does not produce eating in the presence of dopaminergic blockade.[18]

Neurophysiological studies in rat, cat and monkey have shown that the firing rate of lateral hypothalamus neurons can alter both before and during feeding, and this has indicated a physiological basis for the psychological factors.[17] Those neurons involved appear to extend out lateral to the lateral hypothalamus into the substantia innominata. Some of the neurons are associated with just the sight of food, these neurons firing only when the monkey actually sees food and responding most to the animal's preferred food. These sight-responsive neurons only fire if the animal has learnt that the object visualized is actually food. Other neurons respond to the taste of food, again with greater firing in response to preferred tastes already learnt. Such neurons only respond to the sight or taste of food if the animal is hungry, and the response diminishes as the intensity of satiety increases. Interestingly, a specific neuron that has ceased to respond to the sight of food on which the monkey has been fed to satiety can still respond to the sight of a different food. This is the physiological explanation of 'sensory-specific satiety' where the desire for the particular food being eaten decreases more than for foods that have not been eaten.

The importance of the hypothalamus in feeding is its close relationship to the forebrain, through which it receives learning-related, visualized, olfactory inputs, and its ability to modulate autonomic, endocrine and feeding responses in the hungry animal when food is sighted or scented.

VENTROMEDIAL HYPOTHALAMUS – SATIETY CENTRE

It is now thought that the real effects of neurosurgical destruction of the ventromedial hypothalamus are slight and that hyperphagia may only be induced if the adjacent *ventral* noradrenergic bundle, which courses in the region of the ventromedial hypothalamus, is damaged.[5] This bundle, after arising from the lateral tegmental cell groups (A1–A5), ascends to join the medial forebrain bundle in the mesencephalon and courses through the periventricular region of the diencephalon, providing a few fibres to the ventromedial hypothalamus nucleus. These fibres may exert a dual effect depending on whether α- or β-adrenergic receptors are involved; an α stimulus produces feeding, whereas eating is inhibited by a β stimulus.[10] Lesions of this bundle produce behavioural changes similar to those described in ventromedial hypothalamus-lesioned animals, suggesting that they may result from depletion of hypothalamic noradrenaline. These behavioural changes involve an exaggeration of those psychological factors (incentive properties, arousal, cue stimulus) which are important in the control of feeding, and result in the animal overreacting to environmental stimuli. It is now thought that this overreaction is a primary effect of the lesion and not secondary to metabolic changes such as the hyperinsulinaemia seen in such lesioned animals. This can be demonstrated by a unilateral ventromedial hypothalamic lesion, which produces hyperactivity to environmental stimuli and excessive eating only on the side opposite to the lesion, despite the general presence of mild hyperinsulinaemia and gastric acid hypersecretion.[12] This has led Powley to propose that in such lesioned animals the exaggerated sensory reaction to stimuli results in exaggerated food-related reflexes (cephalic reflexes) such as insulin and gastric acid secretion, which then make the animal 'feel' more hungry than it really is, resulting in the consumption of more food.[15]

Nevertheless, even when pair-fed, the animal lesioned in the ventromedial hypothalamus gains more weight than the sham-lesioned control, indicating enhanced metabolic efficiency, which may be a consequence of a decrease in brown fat activity.[24] A close link has been shown to exist between the area of the ventromedial hypothalamus and brown fat; electrical stimulation of this area specifically enhances lipogenesis and heat production in brown fat, but not in liver or white fat.[14,21] This has led to the view that satiety may be associated with a stimulation of brown fat thermogenesis to burn off excess energy consumed.

How is this related to humans? Quaade has electrically stimulated the lateral hypothalamus in (obese) humans and reported 'convincing hunger responses' whereas damage to the ventromedial hypothalamus area in humans can result in hyperphagia, obesity and hyperinsulinaemia.[16] Obese people have also been shown to have a significantly greater rise of insulin in response to food presentation than non-obese controls, and there may be a relationship between the degree of obesity and the size of cephalic insulin secretion.[22]

NEUROTRANSMITTER DEVELOPMENTS

In 1972 Smith and his colleagues clearly demonstrated that a decrease in glucose utilization was not the dominant mechanism for the initiation of eating an ordinary meal (the 'glucostatic control theory').[23] In the same year Yaksh and Myers showed that when a monkey was fed, the ventromedial hypothalamus released a substance which, on cross-perfusion into this area of a hungry monkey, inhibited feeding.[26] These reports stimulated further research into the role that monoamines, hormones and peptides play in the modulation of food intake. Serotonin (5-hydroxytryptamine, 5-HT) agonists produce satiety whereas chemical selective inhibition of serotoninergic cells results in hyperphagia and obesity.[1] In animals that feed nocturnally, noradrenaline and serotonin appear to interact antagonistically to control carbohydrate and protein ingestion.[11] Noradrenaline is thought to stimulate the first meal of the nocturnal cycle which is usually rich in carbohydrate. As a consequence, serotonin actively increases inducing carbohydrate satiety and switches the animal's preference towards protein, which is the nutrient chosen by such animals for the second meal. In humans, the clinically used drugs, fenfluramine and fluoxetine which enhance serotonin availability, inhibit appetite possibly via cental 5-HT_{1B} and 5-HT_{1C} receptors.[19] Neuropeptide Y (*Table 10.1*) also appears to increase carbohydrate intake preferentially and may also be important in nocturnal feeding animals, in association with noradrenaline, in stimulating the intake of the first carbohydrate meal.[11] Neuropeptide Y is found in association with noradrenaline in the food-related hypothalamic areas where intense high-frequency stimulation favours neuropeptide Y release. It has, therefore, been suggested that neuropeptide Y exerts its effect physiologically on food intake specifically during conditions that evoke high-frequency stimulation such as those in severe food deprivation.[11]

Table 10.1 Food intake regulation by peptides

Decreased food intake	*Increased food intake*
Bombesin	γ-Aminobutyric acid
Calcitonin	Diazepam
Calcitonin gene-related peptide	Galanin
Cholecystokinin	Neuropeptide Y
Corticotrophin-releasing factor	Opioids
	Pancreatic polypeptide
Glucagon	Peptide YY
Insulin	
Neurotensin	
Serotonin	
Somatostatin	
Thyrotrophin-releasing hormone	

Systemic infusion of cholecystokinin produces satiety in both animals and humans, whereas highly selective cholecystokinin antagonists increase the feeding behaviour of rats.[25] This latter fact and the finding that L-phenylalanine, a potent releaser of cholecystokinin, can reduce food intake, whereas D-phenylalanine (which does not release cholecystokinin) does not, suggests that endogenous cholecystokinin reduces meal size in animal experiments, although its satiety effect appears dependent on an intact serotoninergic system and is enhanced by insulin. The finding of low circulatory endogenous cholecystokinin levels in response to a standard test meal in patients with bulimia nervosa, and the return of the cholecystokinin response to normal upon successful treatment, has suggested that pathological alterations in cholecystokinin may underlie eating disorders.[3] Nevertheless, other peptide disturbances are also involved in bulimia nervosa, e.g. neuropeptide Y and peptide YY.[11] *Table 10.1* shows the many other peptides that are known to alter food intake. Much interest has been centred on corticotrophin-releasing factor which if antagonized by α-helical corticotrophin-releasing factor (9-41) causes weight gain, whereas if increased by the antiglucocorticoid RU486, hypophysectomy or adrenalectomy, produces weight loss.[8,9] Corticotrophin-releasing factor not only reduces food intake but also markedly increases brown fat thermogenesis in rodents via stimulation of specific pathways in the sympathetic nervous system.[8]

There is evidence to suggest that food intake is also influenced by the size of the body's fat mass. Following lipectomy, animals given an adequate diet eat more and replace precisely the amount of fat lost.[2,25] The signal for this would appear to be insulin that interacts with other satiety factors such as cholecystokinin.[25] It is known that systemic insulin can cross the blood–brain barrier and is found in those specific areas of the brain that control food intake and body weight. Injection of insulin antibodies into the ventromedial hypothalamic area activates feeding behaviour and insulin-sensitive neurons have been detected in this precise area. Central serotoninergic pathways are also involved because insulin does increase hypothalamic serotonin levels and the action of insulin on thermogenesis (which insulin stimulates) is inhibited by the serotonin antagonist metergoline.[25] It is to be noted that some of the peptides that decrease food intake (e.g. corticotrophin-releasing factor, insulin, thyrotrophin-releasing hormone, bombesin) also increase brown fat thermogenesis in rodents suggesting a linkage between satiety and thermogenic stimulation.[8] The interaction of so many agents in appetite control is complex but it is hoped that, with increasing knowledge, new agents for the control of appetite will become available for clinical use.

REFERENCES

1. Dourish, C.T., Hutson, P.H. and Curzon, G. (1985) Characteristics of feeding induced by the serotonergic agonist 8-hydroxy-2 (di-*n*-propylamine) tetralin (8OHDPAT). *Brain Research Bulletin*, **15**, 377–384.
2. Faust, I.M., Johnson, P.R. and Hirsch, J. (1988) Adipose tissue regeneration following lipectomy. *Science*, **197**, 391–393.
3. Geracioti, T.D. and Liddle, R.A. (1988) Impaired cholecystokinin secretion in bulimia nervosa. *New England Journal of Medicine*, **319**, 683–688.
4. Gibbs, J., Falasco, J.D. and McHugh, P.R. (1976) Cholecystokinin-decreased food intake in rhesus monkeys. *American Journal of Physiology*, **230**, 15–18.
5. Gold, R.M. (1973) Hypothalamic obesity: the myth of the ventromedial nucleus. *Science*, **182**, 488–490.
6. Grossman, S.P. (1976) Neuroanatomy of food and water intake. In *Hunger: Basic Mechanisms and Clinical Implications*, pp. 51–59. (Ed.) Novin, D., Wyrwicka, W. and Bray, G. New York: Raven Press.
7. Hall, R.J. (1975) Progress report: normal and abnormal food intake. *Gut*, **16**, 744–752.
8. Hardwick, A.J., Linton, E.A. and Rothwell, N.J. (1989) Thermogenic effects of the antiglucocorticoid RU-486 in the rat; involvement of corticotrophin releasing factor and sympathetic activation of brown adipose tissue. *Endocrinology*, **124**, 1644–1648.
9. Le Feuvre, R.A., Rothwell, J.N. and Stock, M.J. (1987) Activation of brown fat thermogenesis in response to central injection of corticotrophin releasing hormone in the rat. *Neuropharmacology*, **26**, 1217–1221.
10. Liebowitz, S.F. (1976) Brain catecholaminergic mechanisms for control of hunger. In *Hunger: Basic Mechanisms and Clinical Implications*, pp 1–18. (Ed.) Novin, D., Wyrwicka, W. and Bray, G. New York: Raven Press.
11. Leibowitz, S.F. (1990) Hypothalamic neuropeptide Y, Galanin and Amines. *Annals of the New York Academy of Sciences*, **575**, 221–233.
12. Marshall, J.F. (1975) Increased orientation to sensory stimuli following medical hypothalamic damage in rats. *Brain Research*, **86**, 373–387.
13. Marshall, J.F., Richardson, J.S. and Teitelbaum, P. (1974) Nigro-striatal bundle damage and the lateral hypothalamic syndrome. *Journal of Comparative Physiology and Psychology*, **87**, 808–830.
14. Perkins, M.N., Rothwell, N.J., Stock, M.J. and Stone, T.W. (1981) Activation of brown adipose tissue thermogenesis by the ventromedial hypothalamus. *Nature*, **289**, 401–402.
15. Powley, T.L. (1977) The ventromedial hypothalamic syndrome, satiety and a cephalic phase hypothesis. *Psychological Review*, **84**, 89–126.
16. Quaade, F. (1974) Stereotaxy for obesity. *The Lancet*, **1**, 267.
17. Rolls, E.T. (1981) Central nervous mechanisms related to feeding and appetite. *British Medical Bulletin*, **37**, 131–134.
18. Rowland, N.E. and Antelman, S.M. (1976) Stress-induced hyperphagia and obesity in rats: a possible model for understanding human obesity. *Science*, **191**, 310–311.
19. Samanin, R. and Garattini, S. (1990) Serotonin and the pharmacology of eating disorders. *Annals of the New York Academy of Sciences*, **575**, 194–207.
20. Schacter, S. and Rodin, J. (1974) *Obese Humans and Rats.* Potomac, MA: Lawrence Erlbaum Associates.
21. Shimazu, T. and Takahashi, A. (1980) Stimulation of hypothalamic nuclei has different effects on lipid synthesis in brown and white adipose tissue. *Nature*, **284**, 62–63.
22. Sjostrom, L., Garellick, G., Krotkiewski, M. and Luyskx, A. (1980) Peripheral insulin in response to the sight and smell of food. *Metabolism*, **29**, 901–909.
23. Smith, G.P., Gibbs, J., Strohmayer, A.J. and Stokes, P.E. (1972) Threshold doses of 2-deoxy-D-glucose for hyperglycaemia and feeding in rats and monkeys. *American Journal of Physiology*, **222**, 77–81.
24. Trayhurn, P. and James, W.P. (1981) Thermogenesis: dietary and non-shivering aspects. In *The Body Weight Regulatory System: Normal and Disturbed Mechanisms* (Ed.) Oioffi, L.A., James, W.P.T. and Van Itallie, T.B. New York: Raven Press.
25. Woods, S.C. and Gibbs, J. (1990) The regulation of food intake by peptides. *Annals of the New York Academy of Sciences*, **575**, 236–243.
26. Yaksh, T.L. and Myers, R.D. (1972) Neurohumoral substances released from the hypothalamus of the monkey during hunger and satiety. *American Journal of Physiology*, **222**, 503–515.

OBESITY

R.T. Jung

DEFINITION

Obesity is an excessive accumulation of adipose tissue. The term 'overweight' is now used to describe a body weight of 110–119% above an ideal reference weight (equivalent to 100%) for height and sex, and the term 'obesity' is used when the body weight is 120% or more above this reference (*Table 10.2*).

In their report on obesity, the Royal College of Physicians of London used body mass index (BMI – weight divided by the square of the height).[21] Obesity is defined as a body mass index of 30 or above in males and 28.6 or above in females. Another grading system defines obesity grade I as a body mass index of 25–29.9, grade II as 30–40 and grade III as over 40.[8] Using the latter system, 40% of men and 39% of women in the UK (in 1980) are within obesity grades I–III.[8] The corresponding figures for the USA are 43% of males and 36% of females and, for Australia, 41% of males and 31% of females.[8] The latest census in the UK indicates that 8% of males and 12% of females have a body mass index of 30 or above. The importance of the abdominal distribution of fat must be emphasized because this is associated with an increased risk of hyperinsulinaemia, glucose intolerance, hyperlipidaemia, hypertension, ischaemic heart disease, cerebrovascular events and death.[8,17] Comparison of the circumference of waist and hip is measured with a ratio of over 0.8 in females and 0.95 in males being considered hazardous to health.

AETIOLOGY

Obesity is only rarely associated with a clear genetic defect. The Laurence–Moon–Biedl syndrome is inherited as a recessive trait and is characterized by

Table 10.2 Appropriate body weight and the lower limits for defining overweight and obesity

	Men				*Women*			
Height (cm)	*Average (kg)*	*Acceptable range (kg)*	*Overweight (kg)*	*Obese (kg)*	*Average (kg)*	*Acceptable range (kg)*	*Overweight (kg)*	*Obese (kg)*
145					46.0	37–53	58	64
148					46.5	37–54	59	65
150					47.0	38–55	61	66
152					48.5	39–57	63	68
156					49.5	39–58	64	70
158	55.8	44–64	70	77	50.4	40–58	64	70
160	57.6	45–65	72	78	51.3	41–59	65	71
162	58.6	46–66	73	79	52.6	42–61	67	73
164	59.6	47–67	74	80	54.0	43–62	68	74
166	60.6	48–69	76	83	55.4	44–64	70	77
168	61.7	49–71	78	85	56.8	45–65	72	78
170	63.5	51–73	80	88	58.1	45–66	73	79
172	65.0	52–74	81	89	60.0	46–67	74	80
174	66.5	53–75	83	90	61.3	48–69	76	83
176	68.0	54–77	85	92	62.6	49–70	77	84
178	69.4	55–79	87	95	64.0	51–72	79	86
180	71.0	58–80	88	96	65.3	52–74	81	89
182	72.6	59–82	90	98				
184	74.2	60–84	92	101				
186	75.8	62–86	95	103				
188	77.6	64–88	97	106				
190	79.3	66–90	99	108				
192	81.0	68–93	102	112				

Figures adjusted to take account of extended lower range suggested by the society of Actuaries 1979 Build Study. Limits of overweight taken to be 110–119% of upper limit, with obesity present when weight is 120% or more.

obesity, mental handicap, retinitis pigmentosa and hypogonadism.[13] In the Prader–Willi syndrome the obesity is associated with diabetes mellitus, hypotonia, mental handicap and hypogonadism.[13] The Morgagni–Stewart–Morel syndrome appears mainly in women and is inherited as a dominant trait. It is characterized by obesity, hypertension, hirsutism, hyperostosis of the frontal bones, hypogonadism and mental abnormalities. In all three syndromes the obesity is associated with hyperphagia, although a temperature-regulating defect has been discovered in some individuals with the Prader–Willi syndrome.[13]

Hypothalamic damage due to trauma, inflammation or neoplasm is also a rare cause of obesity in humans. An endocrine basis for obesity has long been sought but in only a few cases can a hormonal defect, for example occurring in Cushing's syndrome, myxoedema, insulinoma and steroid medication, be identified.[13] In most cases the aetiology of the obesity has eluded investigators. Recent interest has centred on studies of genetically obese mice especially the *ob/ob* mouse, where the obesity appears to be mainly related to a defect in non-shivering thermogenesis due to an abnormality in the thermogenic activity of brown fat.[12]

Whether a similar mechanism could account for obesity in humans is still disputed. Although anatomical studies have indicated the presence of brown fat in adults its energetic significance appears to be slight.[4]

Accurate metabolic ward studies have suggested that the obese eat on average 20% more than the lean to maintain their obese state. This has recently been supported by the measurement of free living energy expenditure using doubly labelled stable isotopic water ($^2H_2{}^{18}O$) where the obese expend 28% more energy on average than the lean.[22] Nevertheless, thermogenic abnormalities to food and noradrenaline have been reported in those who have returned to normal weight after being obese (i.e. post-obese).[15,26] Also studies in infants suggest that a reduced energy expenditure may be an important factor in the rapid weight gain observed during the first year of life in infants born to overweight mothers.[25] Such work suggests that some may have a predisposition to obesity by having a lower energy expenditure. Such heterogeneity has been reported in a survey of south-western American Indian families where those with a 24-hour energy expenditure 200 kcal (0.8 MJ) below average had a fourfold increased risk of gaining more than 7.5 kg than others whose energy expenditure was 200 kcal above average.[23] In this study energy expenditure levels appeared to be aggregated within families, suggesting a familial predisposition. Genetic studies of Danish adoptees has emphasized that this genetic leak for weight of adoptees was closely associated with biological parents, especially mothers.[27] In contrast there was no apparent relationship between the body mass index of the adoptive parents and the weight of the adoptees.

MORTALITY AND MORBIDITY FROM DIGESTIVE DISEASES

In a recent analysis of mortality by weight in 750 000 men and women in the USA, the mortality rates for weights (relative to the ideal reference weights) of 120–129%, 130–139% and 140% or more were, respectively, 28%, 46% and 88% higher than for the optimal-weight group.[19] Although coronary heart disease was the major factor in the weight mortality of obese individuals, the highest relative mortality for both sexes was from diabetes mellitus and the next highest from digestive diseases. In those with a weight of 140% or more, the mortality from digestive diseases for males was four times as great, and that for females 2.25 times as great as in those of optimal weight. The Build and Blood Pressure Study of 1959, covering 4500 000 people, also showed high mortality rates from digestive diseases in obese individuals.[28] Cancer mortality was elevated only among those weighing 140% or more, being 1.33 and 1.55 times as great in males and females respectively. Colorectal cancer was the principal site of excess cancer mortality in males (relative rates: 1.73 in males, 1.22 in females), whereas in females the highest incidence was from cancer of the gallbladder and biliary passages (relative mortality of 3.6). The relative mortality rates for cancer of the stomach and pancreas were higher in males (1.88 and 1.62 respectively) than in females, where the relative mortality rate for stomach cancer (1.03) was similar to that in the optimal weight group and that for pancreatic cancer (0.61) was significantly lower. Abdominal obesity in both males and females is a better predictor of cardiovascular disease, diabetes and death than the degree of overall adiposity.[17] Weight loss reduces mortality as has been shown by life assurance data and also recently in obese diabetics. In the latter study a 10-kg weight loss was predicted to restore one-third of the reduced life expectancy.[18]

Obese women also have a high incidence of gallbladder disease. Rimm *et al.* in a study of over 70 000 obese women reported a 2.7-fold increased incidence of gallbladder disease.[24] There was an increased incidence of diabetes mellitus (4.5-fold), hypertension (3.3-fold), gout (2.6-fold) and jaundice of all types (1.4-fold). Gallbladder disease in obese women has been subject to particular scrutiny recently. As obesity develops there is an increase in the endogenous synthesis of cholesterol by the liver and other tissues. The body pool of cholesterol expands with an increase in the rate at which cholesterol is excreted into the bile.[20] The catabolism of cholesterol to bile salts, the other major route for cholesterol excretion, does not seem to compensate, so biliary cholesterol increases disproportionately, exceeding the capacity of bile salts to solubilize cholesterol. The bile, therefore, becomes supersaturated with respect to cholesterol, which precipitates out.

The high incidence of gallstones in young obese females may also be associated with other factors. The contraceptive pill both increases biliary cholesterol saturation and, by eliminating ovulation, reduces the usual surge in metabolism which occurs at this time. The latter effect could result in as much as a 5% reduction in the monthly energy expenditure, which if unaccompanied by a reduction in food intake, or compensatory thermogenesis, could result in weight gain. Many women attempt to slim by specifically limiting those foods containing carbohydrates such as potatoes and bread. This lowers their intake of fibre, so altering the composition of the bile salt pool,[11] decreasing the solubilization of excreted cholesterol and thus increasing the tendency to gallstone formation. It may be that the low intake of cereal fibre in most slimming diets could increase the incidence of diverticular disease.

TREATMENT

DIET

The treatment of obesity consists of a suitable reduction in energy intake with the maintenance of an adequate intake of protein, fibre and electrolytes. Diets that only involve reducing carbohydrate intake are not to be recommended because they foster an excess intake of fat-enriched foods. Such regimens can also produce postural hypotension, which may be a consequence of a reduction in sympathetic outflow; starch will relieve or prevent this postural hypotension. Protein-only diets should also be avoided because they have been associated with an increased incidence of arrhythmias and sudden death, possibly due to an associated low potassium intake.[16] Similarly, total starvation is never justified because it can cause large losses in electrolytes, especially potassium, and result in sudden death. Very-low-calorie diets have been subject to a recent specialist review.[10] It is now recommended that such diets contain a minimum 400 kcal (1.65 MJ) per day for women under 173 cm in height and 500 kcal (2.1 MJ) per day for all men and also women over 173 cm in height. Such diets must contain sufficient protein of good biological value (minimum 50 g for males and 40 g for females), have adequate minerals, vitamins and carbohydrates, the last being essential to prevent excessive muscular protein breakdown to glucose.

In designing a diet, consideration must be given to individual energy needs, personal idiosyncracies and home circumstances. Also, the individual must be provided with more than just an outline of the diet: in practice, such cursory dietary advice can result in the individual ingesting up to 70% more calories than expected.

Restriction of energy intake results in a fall in the basal metabolic rate by as much as 15% early in the dieting period. With substantial weight loss there is also less metabolically active lean tissue, which further reduces the basal metabolic rate. Hence weight loss can be arrested despite strict adherence to the diet because the energy intake of the diet is balanced by the reduction in the basal metabolic rate. There should be an aim of achieving a 4.2 MJ (1000 kcal) energy deficit each day, but in short individuals with limited mobility (e.g. the elderly) this may not be possible without developing a special low-energy regimen with additional vitamins and electrolytes. All dietary regimens should be supported by patient monitoring which seems to be most effectively carried out by group therapy with the incorporation of behaviour modification into the diet schedule.

Special care is required for those who achieve the desired weight loss. It can be estimated that with every 10 kg loss in weight the individual loses about 420 kJ (100 kcal) of basal metabolic activity per day because of a decline in lean tissue. The individual who loses 30 kg and reaches the ideal weight may consider dieting is finished and neglect the fact that there is a permanent loss of about 1.05 MJ (300 kcal) of metabolizing lean tissue and hence dietary intake must be restricted accordingly. Long-term dietary changes are, therefore, essential if the individual is not to regain the lost weight.

DRUGS

Anorectic drugs should not be used as the sole method for treating obesity and are best used as an adjunct to appropriate dietary therapy if hunger is a problem after some weeks of strict dietary perseverance. Intermittent therapy is not recommended, especially if fenfluramine is prescribed because depression may occur if the drug is suddenly stopped.[14] The recent discovery on brown adipocytes of a unique β_3-agonist receptor which activates thermogenesis, has resulted in the emergence of a new class of selective β_3-agonist drugs (e.g. BRL 26830A). Although still experimental, such drugs acutely raise the metabolic rate in humans and have been shown to enhance weight loss appreciably.[3] Loss of lean body mass, which is a problem with thyroid hormone, does not appear to be hastened with these novel β_3-agonist drugs. Severe depression occurs in up to 30% of very obese women and can severely limit attempts at weight loss.[13] Conventional therapy with tricyclic antidepressants causes weight gain but the introduction of serotonin-uptake inhibitors for the treatment of depression (e.g. fluoxetine) has advanced the management of such patients because weight loss is promoted.[7]

SURGERY

Jaw wiring is sometimes used as a temporary measure to limit food intake. It should only be used in selected patients, e.g. those needing rapid weight loss prior to surgery. Careful dental hygiene is required. The patient relies on liquid nutrients such as milk with vitamin supplements. The patients can still gain weight if they desire by ingesting large volumes of energy-rich fluid and they often rapidly gain weight once the wires are removed despite a suitable dietary regimen. The use of a welded cord around the waist, which reminds the subject of minor degrees of weight gain, also reduces weight regain.[9]

Jejunoileal bypass, in which the first 14 inches of jejunum are anastomosed to the last 4 inches of the ileum, has been used with success. The operation is very successful in achieving rapid early weight loss by a permanent reduction in appetite. Although malabsorption is responsible for much of the early loss of weight, absorption improves after 6–12 months as the intestine adapts.[6] The operative mortality (5%) and high morbidity (up to 70%) after this operation has greatly reduced its role in management. The operation is associated with serious metabolic sequelae: hypoproteinaemia, hypocalcaemia, alkalosis and deficiency of certain trace elements. There is also a high incidence of hepatocellular change; ultimately this may progress to cirrhosis which is not always reversible by restoring intestinal continuity.

Gastric plication has the advantage that it has a much lower morbidity than jejunoileal bypass. Staples are used to fashion an upper pouch with a volume of 0–20 ml. The aperture from the upper pouch is limited to a 12 mm ring, which should be reinforced to prevent later dilatation.[13] Weight loss in a series of 50 patients has been reported to average 26 kg after 1 year with no further weight loss thereafter. Although overall mortality is 4% and morbidity 33%, surgical experience can reduce both figures substantially.[1]

Gastric balloon

This is inserted into the stomach by gastroscopy in a deflated state and then inflated with warm sterile water to a capacity of up to 500 ml volume. Latex balloons have a tendency to deflate and may be irritant, features said to be less of a problem with silicone rubber balloons. Trials comparing balloon with diet alone indicate weight losses of 1 kg compared to 0.6 kg/week respectively. With the latex balloon, 5% develop gastric ulceration and vomiting, heartburn and intestinal obstruction may also be a problem.[5]

REFERENCES

1. Anderson, T., Backer, O.G., Stokholm, K.H. and Quaade, F. (1984) Randomised trial of diet and gastroplasty for morbid obesity. *New England Journal of Medicine*, **310**, 352–356.
2. Arch, J.R.S., Ainsworth, A.T., Cawthorne, M.A. *et al.* (1984) A typical β adrenoceptor on brown adipocytes as target for anti obesity drugs. *Nature*, **309**, 163–165.
3. Connacher, A.A., Jung, R.T. and Mitchell, P.E.G. (1988) Increased weight loss in diet restricted obese subjects given BRL 26830A – a new atypical β agonist. *British Medical Journal*, **296**, 1217–1220.
4. Cunningham, S., Leslie, P., Hopwood, D. *et al.* (1985) The characterization and energetic potential of brown adipose tissue in man. *Clinal Science*, **69**, 343–348.
5. Durrans, D., Taylor, T.V., Pullar, B.R. and Rose, P. (1985) Intragastric balloons. *Journal of the Royal College of Surgeons of Edinburgh*, **30**, 369–371.
6. Faloon, W.W. (1977) Symposium on jejunoileostomy for obesity. *American Journal of Clinical Nutrition*, **30**, 1–128.
7. Ferguson, J.M. and Feighner, J.P. (1987) Fluoxetine induced weight loss in overweight non-depressed humans. *International Journal of Obesity*, **11** (suppl. 3), 163–169.
8. Garrow, J.S. (1988) *Obesity and Related Diseases.* Edinburgh: Churchill Livingstone.
9. Garrow, J.S. and Gardiner, G.T. (1981) Maintenance of weight loss in obese patients after jaw wiring. *British Medical Journal*, **282**, 858–860.
10. Great Britain Working Group on Very Low Calorie Diets (1987) The use of very low calorie diets in

obesity. Committee on Medical Aspects of Food Policy. *Report on Health and Social Subjects 31.* London: HMSO.
11. Heaton, K.W. (1975) Bile salts and fibre. In *Fiber Deficiency and Colonic Disorders* (Ed.) Reilly, R.W. and Kirsner, J.P. New York and London: Plenum Medical Books.
12. James, W.P.T. and Trayhurn, P. (1981) Thermogenesis and obesity. *British Medical Bulletin*, **37**, 43–46.
13. Jung, R.T. (1990) *A Colour Atlas of Obesity.* London: Wolfe Medical.
14. Jung, R.T. and Connacher, A.A. (1990) New approaches to the treatment of obesity. *Hospital Update*, **16**, 521–534.
15. Jung, R.T., Shetty, P.S., James, W.P.T. *et al.* (1979) Reduced thermogenesis in obesity. *Nature*, **279**, 322–323.
16. Lantigua, R.A., Amatruda, J.M., Biddle, T.L. *et al.* (1980) Cardiac arrhythmias associated with a liquid protein diet for the treatment of obesity. *New England Journal of Medicine*, **303**, 735–738.
17. Larsson, B., Svardsudd, K., Welin, L., Wilhelmsen, L., Bjorntorp, P. and Tibblin, G. (1984) Abdominal adipose tissue distribution, obesity and risk of cardiovascular disease and death: 13 year follow up of participants in the study of men born in 1913. *British Medical Journal*, **288**, 1401–1404.
18. Lean, M.E.J., Powrie, J.K., Anderson, A.S. and Garthwaite, P.H. (1990) Obesity, weight loss and prognosis in type 2 Diabetes. *Diabetic Medicine*, **7**, 228–233.
19. Lew, E.A. and Garfinkel, L. (1979) Variations in mortality by weight among 750,000 men and women. *Journal of Chronic Diseases*, **32**, 563–576.
20. Mabee, T.M., Meyer, P., Den Besten, L. and Mason, E.E. (1976) The mechanism of increased gallstone formation in obese human subjects. *Surgery*, **79**, 460–468.
21. Royal College of Physicians of London (1983) Obesity; a report. *Journal of the Royal College of Physicians*, **17**, 5–65.
22. Prentice, A.M., Black, A.E., Coward, W.A. *et al.* (1986) High levels of energy expenditure in obese women. *British Medical Journal* **292**, 983–987.
23. Ravussen, E., Lillioja, S. Knowler, W.C. *et al.* (1988) Reduced rate of energy expenditure as a risk factor for body weight gain. *New England Journal of Medicine*, **318**, 467–472.
24. Rimm, A.A., Werner, L.H., Yserloo, B. van and Bernstein, R.A. (1975) Relationship of obesity and disease in 73,532 weight-conscious women. *Public Health Reports*, **90**, 44–51.
25. Roberts, S.B., Savage, J., Coward, W.A., Chew, B. and Lucas, A. (1988) Energy expenditure and intake in infants born to lean and overweight mothers. *New England Journal of Medicine*, **318**, 461–466.
26. Shetty, P.S., Jung R.T., James, W.P.T. *et al.* (1981) Postprandial thermogenesis in obesity. *Clinical Science*, **60**, 519–525.
27. Stunkard, A.J., Sorensen, T.I.A., Hanis, C. *et al.* (1986) An adoption study of human obesity. *New England Journal of Medicine*, **314**, 193–198.
28. Society of Actuaries (1959) *Build and Blood Pressure Study 1959*, Vol. 1. Chicago: The Society of Actuaries.
29. Society of Actuaries (1979) *Build Study 1979.* Association of Life Insurance Medical Directors of America.

CHRONIC FUNCTIONAL ABDOMINAL PAIN

K.W. Heaton and J.I. Alexander

DEFINITION

Chronic functional abdominal pain is the term proposed by an international working party[5] to describe a group of patients whose persistent abdominal pain has no discernible organic cause and is unaccompanied by the symptoms of a recognized functional gut disorder such as functional dyspepsia or irritable bowel syndrome. Indeed, there are no clues to the organ of origin on history-taking, physical examination or investigation. Obviously pain from the abdominal wall is excluded, as is pain of gynaecological origin including venous congestion of the ovaries.[1]

To deserve the label chronic the pain must have been present for at least 3 months, some would say 6,[5] and must be continuous or present most of the time.

EPIDEMIOLOGY

Chronic functional abdominal pain is much less common than typical irritable bowel syndrome in the gastroenterology clinic. Appropriately designed surveys to determine its prevalence in the community have not been carried out. In the gastrointestinal clinic the great majority of patients are women.[4]

PATHOGENESIS[2,3]

Pain is a sensory experience but it is also an emotional and cognitive one. Everyday speech testifies to this: we may refer to someone we dislike as 'a pain in the neck'. All pains are modulated by psychological factors; in the heat of battle a soldier may not even notice that he has been wounded.

Afferent pathway from the viscera are relatively few – less than 10% of those from the equivalent somatic parts of the body, i.e. abdomen, chest and back, even though the latter are relatively insensitive. This scarce innervation from the internal organs, despite their large surface area, probably accounts for the diffuse nature of visceral pain.

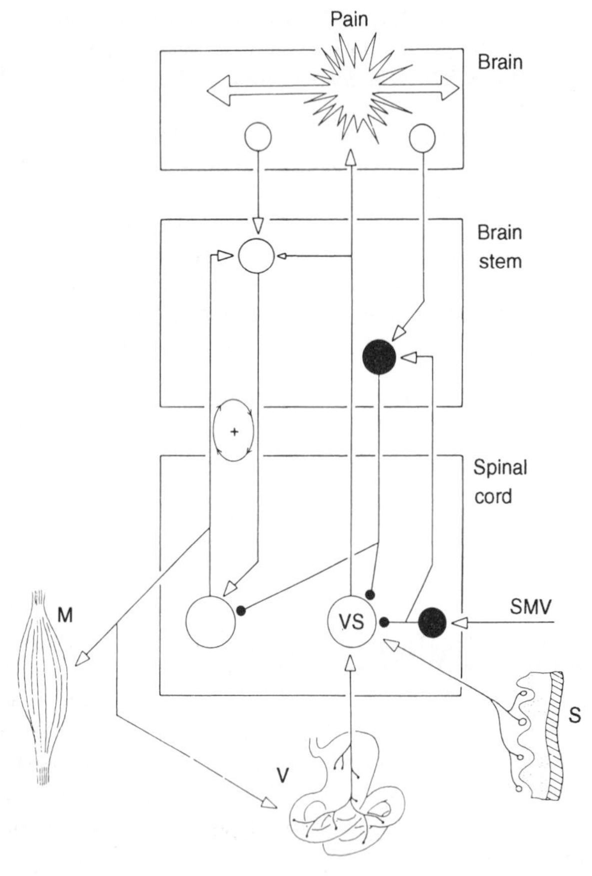

Figure 10.1 Model of the way in which visceral nociceptive signals are processed by the central nervous system. The perception of visceral pain depends on the activation of pathways shared with somatic afferents (viscerosomatic convergent pathways) (VS). The activity of these pathways is modulated by interaction with segmental inputs from the skin (S), muscle (M) or other viscera (V) and by suprasegmental inhibitory influences. These higher *inhibitory* systems are represented by the black neurons. Opposing forces consist of *excitatory* loops between the spinal cord and the brain stem. These maintain activity within the system, enhancing motor and autonomic reflexes and encouraging pain to persist. (Reproduced from Cervero[3] with kind permission.)

Visceral afferent information does not travel on pathways empty of other neuronal traffic. It enters the same system as is used by the numerous somatic organs at the same segmental level, and these have their own afferents and reflexes. The sensory pathway is subject to inhibitory and facilitatory influences within the spinal cord. (*Figure 10.1*). These influences occur at segmental level (predominantly in the fifth lamina of the dorsal horn) and at suprasegmental sites, chiefly the nucleus raphé magnus in the medulla, which contains serotoninergic cells. Tonic inhibition is enhanced at a supraspinal level by mental activity, sleep and rest, and at segmental and supraspinal levels by physical exercise. However, painful afferent stimuli can activate reflexes involving skin, muscle and the autonomic system that generate muscular spasm and further pain and sensitivity. Spinobulbospinal positive-feedback loops have been described which maintain excitability within the sensory channel. The balance between this excitatory system and inhibitory influences is believed to determine the intensity and persistence of visceral pain and of accompanying muscular spasm and autonomic phenomena such as sweating and tachycardia.[3]

Thus mechanisms exist to explain how the perception of pain is affected by memory, attention and emotion. Indeed, there is evidence that, in people with chronic pain, the neuronal circuitry receives more signals from the brain than from the periphery. The patient may perceive the pain as coming from the abdomen but in fact there is little or no peripheral nociceptive input.

PSYCHOPATHOLOGY*

Psychologically, patients with chronic functional pain fit into one of four categories, which can overlap:[6]

1. The emotionally fit person who is under exceptional stress.
2. The patient with an emotional illness – anxiety or especially depression – which lowers the pain threshold. Some such people and some who are exceptionally stressed have difficulty articulating their feelings ('alexithymia') and refer their distress to their body rather than to their mind. They complain to their doctor about a physical symptom rather than an emotional one. To use the jargon, they somatize their feelings.

* See also under 'Anorexia nervosa and other psychological disorders of the gastro intestinal tract', p. 1526.

3. The patient with a personality disorder. This may be a lifelong hypochondriacal tendency in which the person responds to the upsets of daily life by complaining of pain. The severe form is now called somatization disorder. There is also a late-onset type, now called somatoform pain disorder, in which the pain begins after a mid-life crisis such as re-marriage or husband's retirement. In both forms the pain is unconsciously reinforced by its seemingly beneficial consequences (secondary gains). Being in pain can legitimize otherwise unacceptable behaviour, such as not going to work or ceasing unwanted sexual relations. And, of course, it elicits sympathetic attention from relatives, neighbours and colleagues. A spouse who is normally undemonstrative (or even alexithymic) may be stimulated into unwonted care and attention so that, in an odd way, the relationship is strengthened and feelings of self-worth increased on both sides.
4. Rarely pain represents a somatic delusion as part of a psychosis or is part of a hysterical conversion disorder.

CLINICAL FEATURES

Although the definition suggests that the diagnosis is made by exclusion of other disorders, and to some extent this is true, there are some positive pointers to the diagnosis. It is important for the gastroenterologist to know these in order to have confidence in the diagnosis and so avoid unnecessary investigation. In fact, the worst dangers faced by a patient with chronic functional abdominal pain arise from inappropriate tests and treatments. These stem from medical anxiety as much as from medical ignorance, and this anxiety can be alleviated only by familiarity with the features of chronic functional pain.

Six positive pointers have been identified:[9]

1. Pain is constant, poorly localized and vividly described.
2. Discrepancy between symptoms and signs.
3. Preoccupation with the pain.
4. Conviction of organic disease.
5. Dissatisfaction with previous medical care.
6. Association with stress factors.

They are common to patients with any chronic non-organic pain, be it abdominal, facial or in the back.

The pattern of symptoms

The location and timing of the pain do not fit a recognizable organic disease or a recognized functional disorder of the gut, and the pain is present all or most of the time. It is often poorly localized and its site may change with repeated history-telling. Vivid adjectives are used, such as 'stabbing' or 'twisting', and emotive ones such as 'horrible' or 'torturing'.

Discrepancy between symptoms and signs

Despite describing severe pain the patients is calm, and appears to be comfortable in the chair or bed.

Preoccupation with the pain

The patient keeps talking about the pain. If she (or he) is diverted to another topic she soon comes back to the pain and to the way it rules her life.

Conviction of organic disease

The patient insists that the pain has an organic cause 'if only it could be found'. Disconcertingly, she may even name the tests she wants done. Often there is an accompanying relative who is similarly convinced and deeply concerned. The pair of them may be so persuasive that the doctor's own convictions are shaken and he or she begins to wonder about rare organic causes, even when instincts and all the evidence are to the contrary.

Dissatisfaction with previous medical care

Patients may list their past medical history in great detail and emphasize how previous treatments have failed to help. Operations such as cholecystectomy, hysterectomy, appendicectomy and division of adhesions have been in vain except, perhaps, for a brief remission postoperatively. Prescribed drugs have been useless or have caused intolerable side effects with the result that only a few of the tablets have been taken. The litany of failures by previous doctors to find a cause or a tolerable remedy can sound – to the beleaguered physician – like a veiled attack on the whole medical profession or even an attack on him or her personally, especially when the patient also hints at lack of understanding and sympathy by previous doctors. It is easy for the doctor to let his or her hackles rise but he or she must at all costs remain calm. Some doctors feel so frustrated and helpless that they start to wonder if 'some patients make a career of suffering' or even if 'in the game of painsmanship, the patient's aim is to produce undiagnosable pain and unrelievable suffering'.[8] But such ideas insult the patients. Their pain is genuine. Very few are malingerers.

Association with stress factors

The onset of pain often coincides with a crisis such as bereavement, divorce, a child leaving home or even remarriage ('to a wonderful husband'). The patient may deny the linkage. There may be evidence of chronic friction at home – a difficult relationship with someone who shares bed or board. Again this may not be admitted at first. Another buried factor may be sexual abuse in childhood. In one study this was uncovered in no less than 74% of women with chronic 'pelvic' pain.[10]

A further feature of patients with chronic pain is *physical inactivity*. Professionals who run pain clinics believe that the amount of exercise taken by patients with chronic pain and their 'pain behaviour' are inversely related, suggesting that physical inactivity and chronic pain exacerbate each other.[7]

TREATMENT

Organic causes of constant abdominal pain are rare and usually easy to diagnose whilst patients with chronic functional abdominal pain continue to consult doctors and are hard to manage. The objectives of the physician should be threefold: to avoid unproductive investigations and inappropriate treatments, to understand what motivates the patient to keep consulting doctors, and to encourage the patients to live as normally as possible with their pain, rather than to attempt a 'cure'. All three activities demand much of the doctor's patience, restraint and benevolence, and to abandon 'cure' may even be repugnant – doctors like to believe they can always relieve pain. Once the diagnosis is made, the physician must resist the temptation to do one more test or to seek one more opinion and must, like U.S. President Harry S. Truman, accept that 'the buck stops here'. One danger of multiple investigations is that they often throw up red herrings in the form of asymptomatic pathology such as gallstones, gastritis, hiatus hernia and diverticular disease of the colon.

It is particularly difficult for doctors to accept that a pain cannot be abolished. They must constantly remind themselves that this particular pain is minimally, if at all, due to peripheral nociceptive input. They should aim their efforts at educating the patient to reduce pain behaviour and at limiting reinforcing factors. This requires better understanding, relaxation and diversionary tactics. The help of a clinical psychologist is valuable.

An international panel of doctors interested in functional gut disorders has made a number of practical suggestions (*Table 10.3*) on which the following are based:

Table 10.3 Aspects of the management of chronic functional abdominal pain[9]

1.	Focus history on patient's circumstances, attitudes, mood and experiences
2.	Notice illness behaviour
3.	Say 'there is nothing *seriously* wrong'
4.	Explain how pain is perpetuated
5.	Discourage pain behaviour, encourage activity
6.	Consider antidepressant drugs, especially tricyclics
7	Avoid other drugs including analgesics and benzodiazepines
8.	Follow-up with the same doctor each visit
9.	Consider referral to a pain clinic
10.	Accept allies, even if unconventional

1. In initial history-taking ask when the patient was last well. Find out what tests have been done and what treatments have been tried. Ask about the degree of disability. Move into the psychological mode by asking about the patient's circumstances of life at the onset of pain and sound out her or his attitude to the illness and to doctors. Ask about symptoms of anxiety and, especially, of depression (early waking, poor appetite, loss of enjoyment generally, sadness, hopelessness). Enquire about unpleasant childhood experiences such as parental deprivation, violence or mental illness. Consider enquiring about sexual abuse and current sexual problems but this is often best left to a later interview.
2. In examining the patient assess her or his mood and notice abnormal illness behaviour, such as exaggeration when a relative is present.
3. Do not tell the patient that there is nothing wrong; rather say that there is nothing seriously wrong.
4. Adopt a confident, positive approach. Say you accept that there was an organic cause initially, but that the pain has been perpetuated by the circuitry of the nervous system. Explain how pain circuits in the spinal cord are under control of higher centres. Explain the harm of repeated investigations, which can raise hopes only for them to be dashed again. Disappointment is itself a pain.
5. If there is frank depressive illness use full doses of antidepressants. In lesser degrees of depression a low initial dose is advisable to minimize side effects. A moderate dose of tricyclic, e.g. amitryptyline 75 mg/day, seems to have an

analgesic effect in its own right, possibly by raising serotonin levels in the brain.

6. Discourage pain behaviour by reducing inertia and inactivity and encouraging the patient to lead as normal a life as possible *in spite of the pain*. Sitting and brooding on the pain increases awareness of it whereas activity in the outside world reduces it. The pain should not be used as an excuse for putting off tasks or holidays.
7. Prescribe as few drugs as possible, including analgesics which usually work poorly with chronic functional pain. Avoid opiates altogether – also non-steroidal anti-inflammatory drugs and benzodiazepines (which can even exacerbate pain). If there is constipation treat it with bulking agents.
8. Accept that follow-up is usually necessary and may need to be frequent at first. Make sure that the patient *always sees the same doctor*, preferably a senior one. Each interview can start with a discussion of the pain but should move on to psychosocial aspects. This policy has a flavour of collusion about it, but is a realistic compromise where secondary gains are so strong that the patient cannot survive without them.
9. Refer to a psychiatrist only if there is severe depression with suicidal ideas, a delusional element or a gross personality defect that the physician cannot manage. Hypnotherapy has not been shown to help as it does in irritable bowel syndrome.
10. Consider referral to a pain clinic. Guidelines for doing this have not been established and must vary with the expertise available. Pain clinics offer a wide range of conventional and unconventional techniques for pain relief but not all are relevant to abdominal pain. Most clinics have the services of a clinical psychologist.
11. Do not be offended if the patient wants to see an alternative practitioner such as an acupuncturist or aromatherapist. You need allies as long as they are unlikely to do harm! But be wary of 'herbal' remedies because they can contain potent drugs in unpredictable amounts.

CONCLUSION

Doctors find chronic functional abdominal pain difficult to handle because its management requires unfamiliar attitudes and superhuman restraint. It is less difficult if the doctor forms a close relationship with the patient, getting to know 'what makes her or him tick', showing interest in her or his social and emotional problems rather than her or his pain. From being a 'heartsink case' the patient becomes even a friend of sorts. Of course, as the years go by, the doctor's antennae must be out for any intercurrent organic disease. The shepherd boy in the story may have cried wolf too often but, in the end, the wolf did come!

REFERENCES

1. Beard, R.W., Reginald, P.W. and Pearce, S. (1986) Pelvic pain in women. *British Medical Journal*, **293**, 1160–1162.
2. Buccini, R.V. and Drossman, D.A. (1988) Chronic idiopathic abdominal pain. *Current Concepts of Gastroenterology*, **12**, 3–11.
3. Cervero, F. (1988) Visceral pain. In *Pain Research and Clinical Management*, vol. 3, *Proceedings of the Vth World Congress on Pain*, pp. 216–226 (Ed.) Dubner, R., Gebhart, G.F. and Bond, M.R. Amsterdam: Elsevier.
4. Drossman, D.A. (1982) Patients with psychogenic abdominal pain: six years observation in the medical setting. *American Journal of Psychiatry*, **139**, 1549–1557.
5. Drossman, D.A., Thompson, W.G., Talley, N.J., Funch-Jensen, P., Janssens, J. and Whitehead, W.E. (1990) Identification of sub-groups of functional gastrointestinal disorders. *Gastroenterology International*, **3**, 159–172.
6. Feinmann, C. (1990) Psychogenic regional pain. *British Journal of Hospital Medicine*, **43**, 123–127.
7. Hardy, P.A.J. and Hill, P. (1990) A multidisciplinary approach to pain management. *British Journal of Hospital Medicine*, **43**, 45–47.
8. Hawkins, C. (1984) An approach to the patient with chronic abdominal pain. In *Textbook of Gastroenterology*, pp. 867–875. (Ed.) Bouchier, I.A.D., Allan, R.N., Hodgson, H.J.F. and Keighley, M.R.B. London: Baillière Tindall.
9. Thompson, W.G., Creed, F., Drossman, D.A., Heaton, K.W. and Mazzacca, G. (1992) Working Team Report: Functional bowel disease and functional abdominal pain. *Gastroenterology International*, **5**, 75–91.
10. Walker, E., Katon, W., Harrop-Griffiths, J., Holm, L., Russo, J. and Hickok, L.R. (1988) Relationship of chronic pelvic pain to psychiatric diagnoses and childhood sexual abuse. *American Journal of Psychiatry*, **145**, 75–80.

IRRITABLE BOWEL SYNDROME

K.W. Heaton

Much has been learnt about irritable bowel syndrome in the years that have passed since the first edition of this book and a more rational approach is possible to this, the most common disorder in gastroenterology clinics.

DEFINITION AND TERMINOLOGY

When a person keeps having intestinal symptoms but has no apparent disease in the intestine he, or more often she, can be said to have the irritable bowel syndrome. An international working party has stated firmly the irritable bowel syndrome should be defined positively by the pattern of symptoms.[60] This is logical because a syndrome is defined as a characteristic collection of symptoms. The working party saw irritable bowel syndrome as a functional intestinal disorder characterized by abdominal pain, bloatedness (distension) and symptoms of disturbed defaecation, namely urgency, straining, feelings of incomplete evacuation, altered stool form (consistency) and altered frequency of defaecation. Two conditions that overlap with irritable bowel syndrome, but that are usually considered separately, are idiopathic or functional constipation and functional abdominal pain (see page 1535). Some experts separate functional or painless diarrhoea from irritable bowel syndrome but this is arbitrary. Many regard constipation-predominant irritable bowel syndrome as different from the diarrhoea-predominant form. However, the distinction can be spurious because there is much pseudo-constipation and pseudo-diarrhoea in patients with irritable bowel syndrome. Because the terms 'diarrhoea' and 'constipation' are liable to be misleading, it is better to avoid them unless there is proven fast transit with unformed stools or slow transit with lumpy, hard stools. The term 'spastic colon' should be discontinued, as should old names such as mucous colitis.

IS IRRITABLE BOWEL SYNDROME A REAL ENTITY?

A few gastroenterologists deny the existence of irritable bowel syndrome as a real entity on the grounds that there are no consistent pathophysiological abnormalities and the symptoms are all experienced from time to time by healthy people. Such sceptics view their patients as being unduly aware of and worried by normal gut phenomena. There is a grain of truth in all these statements but each is also misleading. All the symptoms of irritable bowel syndrome are experienced occasionally by many if not most healthy people, but they are experienced more often by patients and in a more severe form.[19] There is no single test which is specific to irritable bowel syndrome but there are measurable disturbances of intestinal transit,[4] intestinal sensitivity,[47,50] defaecation rhythm and faecal form[19] which correlate with and explain patients' symptoms. It is true that patients with irritable bowel syndrome – at least those who are sent to specialists and are studied – tend as a group to be more anxious and depressed than the general population[7,66] but many individuals are not neurotic and those who are have a readily recognizable reason for being upset. Such individuals can certainly not be dismissed simply as people with a low symptom threshold because careful studies have shown that their threshold to somatic pain is not lower but higher than normal.[5,69]

Perhaps the most convincing evidence that irritable bowel syndrome is an entity is that on mathematical analysis the symptoms known as irritable bowel syndrome do cluster together, both in the general population[61,68] and in gastroenterology clinic attenders.[59]

The essence of diagnosing and managing irritable bowel syndrome is to be familiar with these symptoms and the way they cluster together, and to take the symptoms seriously.

EPIDEMIOLOGY

The prevalence of irritable bowel syndrome depends on its definition. A commonly used definition for survey purposes is abdominal pain occurring on more than 6 days in the last year and relieved by defaecation on more than 25% of occasions. By this definition 10–20% of apparently healthy people seem to have irritable bowel syndrome in Western countries.[17] A large random sample of the population is necessary to obtain reliable figures. In the one such study known to the author, recurrent defaecation-relieved pain was admitted to by 10.4% of women and 5.7% of men in Bristol, England.[20] Another definition is three or more of the recognized symptoms of irritable bowel syndrome. By this definition the Bristol survey found 13% of women and 5% of men to have the syndrome, of whom less than half had consulted a doctor. There was no clear trend with age but subjects under 25 years were excluded and other data suggest that this is the age group, of women at least, most prone to irritable bowel syndrome.[12,61]

The true prevalence of intermittent symptoms is underestimated by a point prevalence survey, if only because many people forget their symptoms or discount them as normal phenomena. When young women in Bristol had all symptoms of irritable bowel syndrome recorded prospectively for a month, every single women had one or more symptoms occasionally, especially bloating (93%), abdominal pain (81%) and incomplete evacuation (100%).[19] These findings imply that to some extent symptoms of intestinal dysfunction are practically universal, at least in women.

Most people who admit to symptoms of irritable bowel syndrome have not consulted a doctor. This does not mean that those who do consult a doctor are just introspective worriers or hypochondriacs. They often have worse symptoms and more disturbed bowel function than non-consulters.[19,52]

Data are not available to allow statements on the precise prevalence of irritable bowel syndrome in different countries, communities or races. The disorder is common in the USA where, according to a national survey, 1 in 50 people have been told by a doctor that they have 'spastic colon or mucous colitis'.[51] This is three times more often true for women than for men, and five times more often true for whites than for blacks. Irritable bowel syndrome is apparently common in the Indian subcontinent[24] where, in contrast to Western countries, most of the patients are male.

PATHOPHYSIOLOGICAL BASIS OF SYMPTOMS OF IRRITABLE BOWEL SYNDROME

Despite much research, a physiological abnormality consistent in and unique to irritable bowel syndrome has not been discovered.[3,53] Perhaps it is too much to expect if, as the epidemiology suggests, most people suffer some intestinal dysfunction at one time or another and there is a continuum from occasional mild symptoms to those that are frequent and severe. Furthermore, as the symptoms are intermittent it is likely that any pathophysiological marker will be inconstant.

Notwithstanding, when groups of irritable bowel syndrome patients are compared with symptom-free controls they can be shown to have a supersensitive intestine. Patients have abnormal discomfort with normal events such as the discharge of ileal contents into the caecum[4] and with artificial stimuli such as infusion of gas into the small intestine[31] or inflation of a balloon in the colon or rectum.[39,50] Being readily accessible, the rectum is the most studied part of the gut and there is good evidence for rectal supersensitivity, at least in patients with 'diarrhoea'[47,69] (*Figure 10.2*). However, rectal tolerance to balloon distension is so variable in normal subjects[26] that this test is not a practical diagnostic tool. All the same, rectal sensitivity or irritability is an attractive concept because it explains two characteristic symptoms of irritable bowel syndrome – urgency and frequent passage of small stools. It might also explain the sensation of incomplete evacuation or rectal dissatisfaction (and, hence, straining to complete defaecation), but this has proved hard to demonstrate.[44] Rectal irritability might also explain unproductive calls to stool.

Abnormal motility has long been considered to be the basis of irritable bowel syndrome. However, this

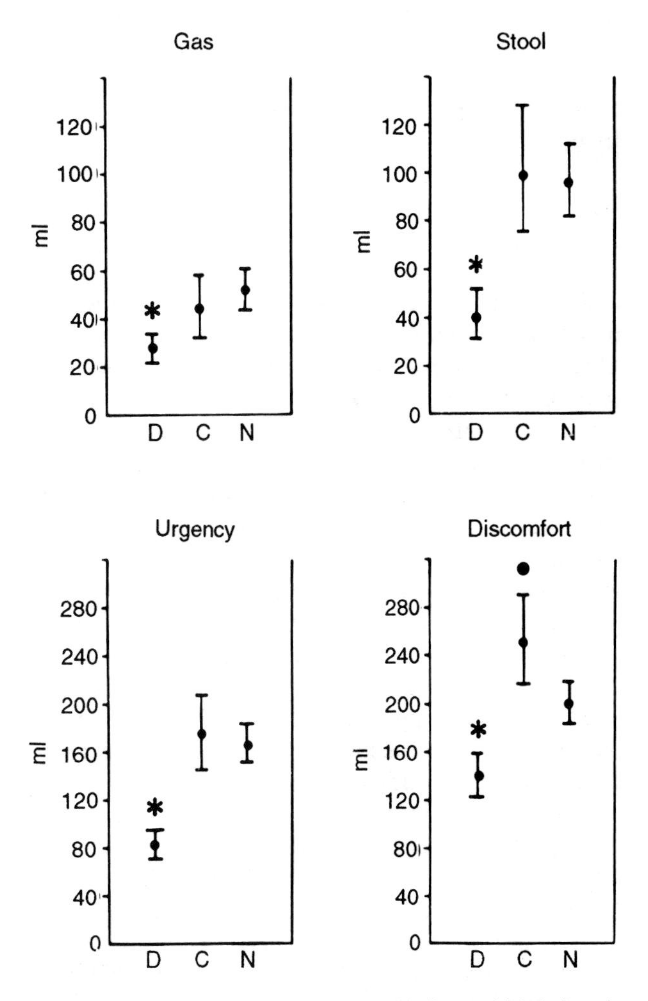

Figure 10.2 Volume of air within a rectal balloon which induced sensations of increasing intensity – awareness of gas, awareness of stool, urgent desire to defaecate, and discomfort or pain – in patients with diarrhoea-predominant irritable bowel syndrome (D), constipation-predominant irritable bowel syndrome (C) and normal subjects (N). (Reproduced from Prior *et al.*[47] with kind permission.)

has been even more difficult to document conclusively than abnormal sensitivity. Episodes of pain do tend to coincide with contractions of the intestine, and several studies have shown excessive segmenting movements in the sigmoid colon in response to food, cholinergic agents and balloon distension. However, other studies have failed to observe this which may be partly due to methodological difficulties.[53,63] Myoelectric abnormalities have been claimed and disputed. Recent attention has focused on the small intestine and ileocaecal area where a number of motility abnormalities have been claimed.[25,30] One problem with nearly all studies of gut motility in the irritable bowel syndrome is that the controls are not matched for emotional state which is known to affect motility. Furthermore, little or no allowance is made for the highly intermittent nature of symptoms of irritable bowel syndrome which, presumably, implies that there are variations in the physiological state of the intestine, including its reactivity.

PSYCHOLOGICAL PROFILE

For many years, it has been axiomatic that many, if not most, irritable bowel syndrome patients are excessively anxious and/or depressed and some commentators even consider the syndrome as primarily a behavioural disorder.[13] Certainly surveys of hospital patients find a high proportion with psychopathology.[7,66] However, hospital patients are a minority. Most people with symptoms of irritable bowel syndrome do not consult a doctor and, of those who do, only half at most are sent to consultants in hospitals.[17] Non-consulters have psychological profiles similar to those of people without symptoms.[10,67] Moreover, when patients who have consulted a family doctor and been referred to hospital have been compared to patients with organic gastrointestinal disease similarly referred, they have been found to have similar psychological profiles – *both* groups having more psychopathology than the general population and less psychopathology than patients with somatoform disorder or hypochondriasis.[54,58] The conclusion must be that psychological distress is one of the factors that make people consult a GP, whether their symptoms are organic or functional in origin.

Another factor is the severity of the symptoms. In those with irritable bowel syndrome it has been shown that consulters have more pain,[10,52] indeed, more of every type of symptom,[19] than non-consulters, and that the consultation rate is directly related to the number of symptoms.[20] The same could well be true of organic disease.

CHILDHOOD ANTECEDENTS

Many patients with irritable bowel syndrome admit to having experienced abdominal pains as children and it is claimed that often 'little bellyachers become big bellyachers'.[2] Illness behaviour can be learnt in childhood.[32] Children with recurrent abdominal pain usually come from a family with a history of psychiatric disturbance[64] and adults with irritable bowel syndrome are likely to have experienced disruption of the family in their childhood.[32] A history of sexual abuse is common in women with irritable bowel syndrome[9] which may explain why a high proportion of women with the syndrome have sexual problems, especially dyspareunia.[14]

STRESS AND LIFE EVENTS

We all have 'gut reactions' to events, some more than others. The sigmoid colon contracts in response to a stressful interview or a standardized stress test in normal people as well as in patients with irritable bowel syndrome.[1,41] The same may be true for all parts of the gut. The question is this: Do patients with irritable bowel syndrome react more strongly than normal people or react differently, for example, in a more prolonged way, or are they just more aware of their reaction? Such patients certainly endure pain as well as other people,[5,69] but is this at the expense of more autonomic disturbance, more distress, which translates into more disturbance of intestinal function? These questions are hard to answer but data on life events preceding the onset of abdominal pain suggest that irritable bowel syndrome can represent a reaction to stress. Creed and colleagues[6] studied the frequency of life events in the 9 months before the onset of symptoms and found that patients with 'functional abdominal pain' were three times more exposed to a severely threatening life event, usually the break-up of a close relationship, or to extreme interpersonal tensions in the home, than patients with organic gastrointestinal disorders or healthy controls.

Mechanism of the mind–gut link

The neural mechanisms determining the sensory and motor functions of the gut are still being unravelled. Much sensory information from the gut is relayed to the brain which transmits impulses to the spinal cord, thereby influencing the processing of afferent (sensory) signals. Theoretically, these impulses could lead to increased motor activity of the gut by enhancing local spinal reflexes. It has been proposed that patients with irritable bowel syndrome have up-regulation of visceral afferents due to modulating influences from the central nervous system. Consequently there is inappropriate transmission of afferent signals to the central nervous system and enhanced awareness of intestinal events.[37] The frequent co-existence of somatic symptoms such as headache and backache may be explained by the spinal pathways used to convey visceral sensations to the brain being used to convey somatic sensations as well, including pain.[37]

DIETARY FACTORS

The onset of irritable bowel syndrome sometimes follows a sudden change in diet. This can be a slimming diet; such a diet is prone to cause constipation which may be the root of the trouble because artificially inducing constipation in normal volunteers leads to most of the symptoms of irritable bowel syndrome and, conversely, people with spontaneous constipation lose at least some of their irritable bowel syndrome symptoms if they take a laxative.[34] Therefore, a low-fibre intake may be the cause of irritable bowel syndrome in such patients. However, in general, patients with irritable bowels do not consume less dietary fibre than average. Some individuals develop bowel symptoms when they take a high-fibre diet.

Food intolerance is much debated as a cause of irritable bowel syndrome. Gastroenterologists in Oxford/Cambridge find that 50–70% of patients are relieved by a diet excluding cereals (except rice), dairy products, eggs, citrus fruits, onions, tea, coffee, nuts, alcohol and any food containing additives or preservatives.[23,40] However, several other groups have not found this.[17] Moreover, in nearly all reported cases, the diagnosis of food intolerance has rested on open re-introduction of a previously banned food (about which the patient may have preconceived ideas) rather than on a series of double-blind challenges. Such challenges are very difficult and time-consuming but they are essential if food intolerance is to rest on a firm scientific footing. Meanwhile, sceptics believe that the problem is often food aversion or pseudo-food allergy.[46] A balanced view might be as follows: in patients who have diarrhoea as their main symptom, a certain but undefined proportion will have a food intolerance. Most commonly this intolerance is to wheat.

CLINICAL FEATURES

The taking of a precise and detailed history is time-consuming but is essential to avoid misunderstanding and unnecessary investigation. Patients may be embarrassed to talk about their bowel function in down-to-earth terms and often they use euphemisms or circumlocutions such as 'I can't go properly' or 'it's a job to go' or 'I don't know where I am with my stomach'. It is good practice to record patients' complaints in their own words, using inverted commas, but this must be followed by a detailed analysis of exactly what they mean.

PAIN

The pain is usually abdominal but can be elsewhere – at the rib margins, in the flanks or lumbar regions, in the rectum or down the thigh. Inflating a balloon in the ascending and transverse colon evokes pain in the mid or upper abdomen as often as in the lower abdomen.[57] The pain of irritable bowel syndrome has many features that distinguish it from pain of organic origin. Sometimes it is in multiple sites or at varying sites,[45] whereas the pain of organic disease usually remains in one particular place. Often pain is intermittent, but lacks the regular timing of peptic ulcer pain; it is seldom in clear-cut, easily remembered episodes such as biliary or ureteric pain. Close enquiry sometimes reveals that the pain is very short-lived, even momentary. Constant pain is more characteristic of functional abdominal pain (see page 1535) than of irritable bowel syndrome.

The severity of the pain varies from person to person and from time to time. It can be mild discomfort or pain severe enough to induce fainting or addiction to opiates. Vivid adjectives such as 'terrible', 'burning' or 'cutting' are used more often than they are by patients with organic disease.[28]

In most patients the pain bears some relationship to defaecation. It is often eased or abolished by a bowel movement but can become worse. The development of pain is often accompanied by a change in bowel habit, usually towards looser and/or more frequent stools but sometimes the reverse. This diagnostically helpful point will often be missed unless the patient is asked about his or her bowel habit before the pains began. Other diagnostically helpful symptoms include the following:[19,24,33,59]

Relief of pain with defaecation
Defaecation more frequent since pains began
Stools looser since pains began
Distension or bloated feelings in the abdomen
Urgency of defaecation
Feelings of incomplete evacuation
Straining to finish evacuating
Passage of mucus per rectum

The pain of irritable bowel syndrome is often made worse by eating, especially large or rich meals.

Some patients notice that specific foods induce pain. To avoid pain, patients may reduce their food consumption and lose weight but this is unusual. More often patients gain weight even if they have less appetite (an odd and unexplained phenomenon).

In some women the symptoms worsen before or during the menstrual flow. Regrettably, women with lower abdominal pain are often sent to a gynaecologist before a proper history is taken.[49]

BOWEL DISTURBANCE

True diarrhoea occurs but is usually intermittent, often lasting only a few hours.[19] Pseudo-diarrhoea also occurs, i.e. frequent urgent passage of small *solid* stools.[43,45] True constipation occurs but, again, this is usually episodic. Pseudo-constipation is common, i.e. straining to get rid of the feeling of incomplete evacuation even though the stool is of normal or loose consistency.[19] There is much scope for diagnostic confusion and inappropriate prescription of laxatives or antidiarrhoeal drugs unless careful enquiry is made into the form of the stools. This is easier and less embarrassing if the doctor shows the patient a list of recognized stool types (*Table 10.4*).

All of the stool types listed in *Table 10.4* are passed from time to time by healthy people, but extreme types are passed more often by irritable bowel syndrome patients.[19] Defaecation is also more erratic in timing.

Defaecation should be a simple, matter-of-fact business, easily done and quickly forgotten. In people with irritable bowel syndrome it is obtrusive and disconcertingly unpredictable. It often begins suddenly with a violent urge to empty the bowel, perhaps at a most inconvenient time. Despite this there may be pathetically little to evacuate – perhaps nothing except wind, or wind and slime – or an explosive discharge may spatter the toilet bowl. Afterwards there still seems to be something in the rectum, so the sufferer sits and waits for the feeling to pass, or strains uselessly, wondering when it is safe to leave the toilet. The whole affair is frustrating, confusing and unpleasant, especially if the race to the toilet is lost and the underclothes are soiled. It is not surprising that some patients become demoralized or obsessed with their bowels. To make matters worse, the burden is hard to share with friends or relatives, or even the family doctor because, for many, defaecation is a taboo subject. If the sufferer does pluck up courage and go to the doctor he or she will often be lost for words and fail to communicate the real problem; the vocabulary in this area is rudimentary. And always there is the fear – could it be serious? So the seeds are sown of social isolation, anxiety and depression.

Table 10.4 The Bristol stool form scale

Type	*Form of stool*
1	Separate hard lumps, like nuts
2	Sausage-shaped but lumpy
3	Like a sausage or snake but with cracks on its surface
4	Like a sausage or snake, smooth and soft
5	Soft blobs with clear-cut edges
6	Fluffy pieces with ragged edges, mushy
7	Watery, no solid pieces

FUNCTIONAL DIARRHOEA (PAINLESS DIARRHOEA)

True diarrhoea with daily stool weight consistently more than 250 g/day can be functional, but this is relatively uncommon,[4] especially if idiopathic bile acid malabsorption, food intolerance and laxative abuse are excluded. The underlying problem is probably rapid transit through the small and large intestine.[4] Unlike typical irritable bowel syndrome, continuous diarrhoea deserves extensive investigation to exclude an organic cause. There may be a morning rush of several defaecations in the first hour or two of the day, or a defaecation after any food or drink is taken, or an urgent call to stool whenever the patient has to go out of the home. The last type most clearly deserves the old title of nervous diarrhoea.

DISTENSION

Feelings of distension or abdominal bloating are admitted to by most patients with irritable bowel syndrome. They occur occasionally in nearly all normal women, especially premenstrually, but they are more frequent and severe in irritable bowel syndrome.[19] Sometimes they are the main complaint. Often the distension is visible; clothes have to be loosened or changed, women may even be accused of being pregnant. Distension is usually worse in the evening. It is never constant as with organic causes of increased girth. Girth does increase measurably but why is unknown – it is not due to increased gas in the intestines.[35] In the past, distension has been blamed on unconscious hyperextension of the lumbar spine but this has been challenged.[35]

DYSPEPTIC SYMPTOMS

Many patients with irritable bowel syndrome complain of gastro-oesophageal symptoms such as anorexia, nausea, belching and epigastric fullness after meals and, less often, heartburn and acid regurgitation. There is considerable overlap between irritable bowel syndrome and functional dyspepsia.

NON-GASTROINTESTINAL SYMPTOMS

In hospital patients lassitude is often a leading complaint; backache is also prominent.[36] It is tempting but usually incorrect to label these patients as unduly anxious or depressed. Frequency and urgency of micturition are common and are associated with objective evidence of bladder irritability.[70] In women dyspareunia is not uncommon.[14,71] The origin of all these symptoms is obscure but they may indicate a diffuse disorder of smooth muscle function.

PHYSICAL EXAMINATION

The patient is usually well nourished and may be tense, anxious or resentful (of perceived poor management by previous doctors). There are no proven discriminating physical signs of irritable bowel syndrome but bitten nails, cold hands and excessive perspiration are said to be common. The colon may be palpable or tender. Digital examination of the rectum may reveal hard or scybalous stools (type 1) in a patient who claims a normal bowel habit, or soft faeces in someone who thinks he or she is constipated. A negative stool occult blood finding is an important observation.

SIGMOIDOSCOPY

Examination by sigmoidoscopy is essential to exclude organic disease of the rectum but it must be performed with great gentleness. It is usually normal. Mucosal hyperaemia with loss of visible vessels may be observed when there is excessive diarrhoea. Excess mucus may make the rectal wall shiny or the mucus may appear as discrete strands. Actual spasm or hypermotility may also be seen. Insufflating air may reproduce the patient's pain which is valuable because it convinces the patient as well as the doctor that the pain comes from the bowel.

INVESTIGATIONS

The diagnosis should be made firmly and confidently at the first visit if the history, physical examination and sigmoidoscopy are characteristic and there are no pointers to organic colonic disease such as weight loss, anaemia or rectal bleeding. The only exceptions might be individuals over 40 years old with recent onset of symptoms when a barium enema or colonoscopy is a sensible precaution to exclude cancer of the colon, although the chances of finding it are minimal.[11,16,62] Inevitably many older patients will have diverticula or small polyps on barium enema, but these should be disregarded as an incidental finding. Diverticular disease does not cause symptoms unless there is marked narrowing of the lumen or, of course, perforation and pericolic infection ('diverticulitis'). Occasionally, a patient is so convinced that there is an organic lesion that a barium enema or colonoscopy is necessary to convince them otherwise.

Functional diarrhoea and pseudo-diarrhoea are usually intermittent whilst organic diarrhoea is mostly continuous. Only patients with continuous diarrhoea (or showing other pointers to organic disease) need screening for malabsorption and Crohn's disease, with full blood count, serum or red cell folate and an acute phase protein measurement. If a continuous diarrhoea had started after recent travel abroad the stools should be cultured to exclude amoebiasis, giardiasis and other possible infestations. A therapeutic trial of a milk-free diet (for lactose intolerance) or of cholestyramine (for bile acid diarrhoea) may be helpful to establish a diagnosis.

Food intolerance seems to be a common cause or, at least, an association of irritable bowel syndrome in some centres.[23,40] It can be diagnosed only by demonstrating that symptoms disappear on an elimination diet and recur on re-introduction of particular foods. Unfortunately, it is difficult to separate organic food reactions from psychological ones except by double-blind challenges. These are difficult to perform and very few successful studies have been reported. Even without blind challenges, diagnosing food intolerance is time-consuming for the doctor and especially for the dietitian, and difficult for the patient. It is only feasible with intelligent, highly motivated patients and even they can become confused. Introspective patients are liable to diagnose themselves as having multiple food intolerances which may result in their eating very restricted diets that are nutritionally inadequate.

TREATMENT (*Table 10.5*)

It is remarkably difficult to carry out controlled therapeutic trials in irritable bowel syndrome which

Table 10.5 Treatment possibilities in the irritable bowel syndrome

First line
- Explanation
- Reassurance
- Treatment of obvious constipation
- Avoidance of obvious precipitants (dietary, psychosocial)

Second line
- Stress-management counselling, relaxation classes
- Bulking agents, especially ispaghula, high-fibre diet

Third line
- Musculotrophic drugs (mebeverine)
- Anticholinergic drugs
- Elimination diet (if diarrhoea prominent)
- Antidiarrhoeal drugs
- Hypnotherapy

are immune to criticism[27] and most of the statements that follow are based on clinical experience rather than on rigorous science.

Management begins with the taking of a careful, detailed history because, among other features, this creates the essential atmosphere of trust. By the time patients reach a gastroenterologist they are likely to have seen several doctors and may wonder if anyone will be able to understand their condition or be able to help them. The gastroenterologist must cloak his or her scientific ignorance and give the impression that he or she understands the patient's complaint and can deal with it confidently, even if he or she cannot necessarily cure it. To do this, the gastroenterologist must be seen to take the patient's complaints seriously. Pain is pain and urgency is urgency, whatever the causes.

The patients should be told the probable diagnosis at their first visit if at all possible. If tests are undertaken they should be 'just to be 100% certain'. The patient should not be told that there is nothing wrong but that 'there is nothing *seriously* wrong'.

The diagnosis should be explained, in detail, as a genuine disorder or 'misbehaviour' of the intestines. A diagram of the intestines may help. Some experts emphasize that the bowel has its own (enteric) nervous system or 'little brain' and that this is where the trouble lies, explaining that the 'little brain' is greatly influenced by the big brain, thus introducing the role of emotions.

Reassurance begins with such explanations but it should proceed to include an enquiry of whether the patient fears she or he has cancer or some other serious condition. It may be the first time that this had been brought into the open and the patient's relief when it is dispelled can be gratifying. Death of a relative from bowel cancer can cause an awareness or fear of a gut symptom that had been ignored. In such a situation reassurance may be all the treatment that is needed.

An enquiry into threatening life events or relationship difficulties is often necessary and their role in causing gut symptoms should be discussed. Sometimes this is best left to a second visit when the results of tests or diary-keeping are available. However, if the patient is obviously tense and anxious, it is best to launch straight into a discussion of the emotional problems and ways of dealing with them such as relaxation classes, stress-management counselling, yoga, meditation or, simply, regular vigorous aerobic exercise (which aids relaxation). Stopping regular exercise can precipitate irritable bowel syndrome. The physician should, if possible, obtain the services of psychologist colleagues to whom patients can be referred but, increasingly, general practices and health centres provide counselling services.

If enquiry about dietary precipitants reveals a possible cause this should be attended to before any other treatment is advised, for example, by restoring missed breakfasts, cutting down on excessive coffee or beer, avoiding onions or curries. It is often helpful to have the patient record his or her dietary intake for several days from which it may be obvious he or she is taking an unbalanced diet such as too much fried food, or too much sugar, or too little fruit and vegetables. Rectifying this can help.

Before treating diarrhoea or constipation symptomatically it is important to exclude pseudodiarrhoea. To do this, it is helpful to give the patient a booklet in which to record the date and time of each defaecation, the form of the stool on a 7-point scale (see *Table 10.4*), and whether or not there is urgency or a feeling of incomplete evacuation.[19,43] Inspection of this booklet can be very revealing.

Where there is obvious constipation, i.e. most stools are type 1 or 2, it is logical to prescribe a bulking agent. It is always worth trying a high-fibre diet, with or without wheat bran. The dose of bran should be increased gradually from one tablespoonful a day until the stools become type 3 or preferably type 4. Bran is cheap and effective but has several disadvantages; it is impossible to monitor the dose, palatability is often a problem and, in elderly people or others with small appetites, there are concerns about inducing mineral deficiencies. A useful alternative without these limitations is testa triticum tricum or Trifyba – a powdery concentrate of bran (80% dietary fibre) which is virtually free of phytate and is conveniently packaged in sachets. It is prescribable on the NHS (*Table 10.6*).

Ispaghula or psyllium seed preparations (Isogel, Fybogel, Regulan, Metamucil) have been popular in

Table 10.6 Doses of the pharmaceutical preparations useful in treating irritable bowel syndrome

Testa triticum tricum (Trifyba) powder (3.5 g sachets)	Two sachets daily, increasing as necessary
Granulated or powdery preparations of ispaghula husk (Isogel, Metamucil) or in 3.5 g sachets (Fybogel, Regulan)	One teaspoon or one sachet two or three times daily
Senna tablets (Senokot) 7.5 mg	One to four tablets at night
Mebeverine hydrochloride (Colofac) 135 mg tablets	One tablet three times daily (increase to two tablets if necessary) 20 min before meals
Peppermint oil 0.2 ml capsules	One or two capsules three times daily before meals
Antimuscarinics	See *British National Formulary*
Loperamide 2 mg tablets	One to four tablets once to four times daily according to need

treating irritable bowel syndrome for many years and their effectiveness is fairly well supported by clinical trials.[29,48] At worst, they are a safe and inexpensive placebo and, at best, they help both diarrhoea and constipation. Trials of other bulking agents (sterculia, methylcellulose) are lacking. Some constipated patients do not tolerate bulking agents, because of increased bloating, and may require a regular dose of a chemical laxative such as senna. Before introducing these agents, it is desirable to confirm that the stools are hard and lumpy or that whole-gut transit time is slow using a simple abdominal radiological method with radio-opaque pellets.[38] Some patients have obstructed defaecation or anismus, and in these investigation and treatment should be discussed with a specialized colorectal surgeon.

No drug is of proven benefit in irritable bowel syndrome[27] and drug therapy should be minimized in a disorder that is intermittent, is totally benign and may last a lifetime. Smooth muscle relaxants (mebeverine and peppermint oil) and antimuscarinic drugs are widely used, are safe and relatively cheap. But they are no substitute for the measures outlined above and should be used in short courses, if at all. Patients who are overtly depressed should receive appropriate treatment. Antidiarrhoeal drugs such as loperamide are useful when there is true diarrhoea. They are best taken prophylactically or regularly rather than after the event.

As described above, elimination diets may help some patients with diarrhoea-predominant irritable bowel syndrome but they are safe and feasible only when the patient is intelligent and well motivated and there is close supervision by a dietitian.

The treatments that seem to work best in controlled trials are intensive psychotherapy and hypnotherapy.[55,72] Unfortunately these are only available at very few centres. Group hypnotherapy may be more feasible and seems to be effective.[15] In a careful analysis of psychological treatments for irritable bowel syndrome, Creed and Guthrie[8] concluded that the most important element was a close doctor–patient relationship. In most patients this is the responsibility of the physician, and ultimately the family doctor, not of the psychiatrist.

SOME SPECIAL PROBLEMS

SEVERE PAIN

The pain can be so severe as to mimic an acute abdomen or renal colic and lead to emergency admission to hospital. Patients with irritable bowel syndrome are often to be found in surgical wards with a label of 'non-specific abdominal pain'.

HYPOCHONDRIASIS AND SECONDARY GAINS

When an individual with a hypochondriacal personality develops irritable bowel syndrome more reassurance than usual is necessary. The doctor must be patient and firm, especially in resisting requests for further investigations. The occasional patient may be allowed to become a chronic attender at the clinic but only if the same doctor is seen each time. The occasional patient 'needs' to be ill to obtain the care and concern that they crave, perhaps from a spouse. This is more often a problem with chronic functional abdominal pain (see page 1535).

HEALTH-CARE SEEKING BEHAVIOUR

If an individual has been brought up in a family that takes every ailment seriously, they can be bewildered and quite disabled by the multiplicity of symptoms that make up the irritable bowel syndrome. Education and reassurance must be the doctor's first response but sometimes a placebo helps to satisfy the patient. However, it is better in the long run to try and direct the patient towards more self-management. In this regard, it may help to recommend one of the books written for the public.[42,65]

ASSOCIATION WITH ORGANIC BOWEL DISEASE

Many older patients will have *diverticula* visible on a barium enema. These should usually be disregarded as an incidental finding, although the doctor may exploit the finding as demonstrating that 'the colon has ruptured itself by struggling to process small, firm stools' (Painter's hypothesis), which is why the patient needs a bulking agent or high-fibre diet. The occasional patient with severe, left iliac fossa pain and tenderness, and advanced diverticular disease in the sigmoid colon, deserves to be considered for surgery.

Being so common, irritable bowel syndrome is bound to afflict some patients with *Crohn's disease* with the danger that there will be over-investigation and over-treatment. If inflammatory indices (perhaps including a radioactively labelled leukocyte scan) are normal and there is no stricture – and even in some cases where these conditions are not fulfilled – the doctor should always bear in mind the possibility that the irritable bowel syndrome is the cause of a patient's pain and bowel irregularities. This is especially so if the symptoms are intermittent or associated with stress. *Ulcerative colitis* is the only organic disease that can produce the whole range of symptoms of irritable bowel syndrome. It is easily distinguished. The symptoms are more constant, there is usually blood in the stool or on rectal examination, and sigmoidoscopy is diagnostic. When the colitis is in remission, a third of patients still have symptoms of irritable bowel syndrome,[22] possibly because inflammation sensitizes the colon.

PROGNOSIS

The outlook for patients is good in the sense that it is not known to lead on to any other disease. It is also good because it is very seldom that the diagnosis has to be revised. During a 5–10 year follow-up of 603 patients, only 2 were found to have cancer of the large bowel, which is not more than would be expected by chance.[17]

The prognosis in terms of symptoms is less good. Most patients continue to have symptoms[56] but they tend to be less troublesome[16,21] partly, perhaps, because patients have come to terms with them. Patients in whom symptoms seem to be induced by stress should be warned to expect a recurrence at times of upheaval.

Data are scanty on the factors affecting prognosis but there is some evidence that loss of symptoms is associated with male sex, a short history, predominant constipation, an acute illness (not necessarily diarrhoeal) preceding symptoms and absence of previous abdominal surgery.[16,56]

REFERENCES

1. Almy, T.P. (1951) Experimental studies on the irritable colon. *American Journal of Medicine*, **10**, 60–67.
2. Apley, J. (1975) *The Child with Abdominal Pain.* Oxford: Blackwell.
3. Camilleri, M. and Neri, N. (1989) Motility disorders and stress. *Digestive Diseases and Sciences*, **34**, 1777–1786.
4. Cann, P.A., Read, N.W., Brown, C., Hobson, N. and Holdsworth, C.D. (1983) Irritable bowel syndrome: relationship of disorders in the transit of a single solid meal to symptom patterns. *Gut*, **24**, 405–411.
5. Cook, I.J., van Eeden, A. and Collins, S.M. (1987) Patients with irritable bowel syndrome have greater pain tolerance than normal subjects. *Gastroenterology*, **93**, 727–733.
6. Creed, F., Craig, T. and Farmer, R. (1988) Functional abdominal pain, psychiatric illness, and life events. *Gut*, **29**, 235–242.
7. Creed, F. and Guthrie, E. (1987) Psychological factors in the irritable bowel. *Gut*, **28**, 1307–1318.
8. Creed, F. and Guthrie, E. (1989) Psychological treatments of the irritable bowel syndrome. *Gut*, **30**, 1601–1609.
9. Drossman, D.A., Leserman, J., Nachman, G. *et al.* (1990) Sexual and physical abuse in women with functional or organic gastrointestinal disorders. *Annals of Internal Medicine*, **113**, 828–833.
10. Drossman, D.A., McKee, D.C., Sandler, R.S. *et al.* (1988) Psychosocial factors in the irritable bowel syndrome. A multivariate study of patients and non-patients with irritable bowel syndrome. *Gastroenterology*, **95**, 701–708.
11. Farrands, P.A. and Hardcastle, J.D. (1984) Colorectal screening by self-completion questionnaire. *Gut*, **25**, 445–447.
12. Fielding, J.F. (1977) The irritable bowel syndrome Part I: Clinical spectrum. *Clinics in Gastroenterology*, **6**, 607–622.
13. Ford, M.J. (1986) Invited review: the irritable bowel syndrome. *Journal of Psychosomatic Research*, **30**, 399–410.

14. Guthrie, E., Creed, F.H. and Whorwell, P.J. (1987) Severe sexual dysfunction in women with the irritable bowel syndrome: comparison with inflammatory bowel disease and duodenal ulceration. *British Medical Journal*, **295**, 577–578.
15. Harvey, R.F., Hinton, R.A., Gunary, R.M. and Barry, R.E. (1989) Individual and group hypnotherapy in treatment of refractory irritable bowel syndrome. *The Lancet*, **1**, 424–425.
16. Harvey, R.F., Mauad, E.C. and Brown, A.M. (1987) Prognosis in the irritable bowel syndrome: a 5-year prospective study. *The Lancet*, **1**, 963–965.
17. Heaton, K.W. (1988) Functional bowel disease. In *Recent Advances in Gastroenterology 7*, (Ed.) Pounder, R.E. pp. 291–312. Edinburgh: Churchill Livingstone.
18. Heaton, K.W. (1991) IBS in the community. In *Towards Confident Management of the Irritable Bowel Syndrome* (Ed.) Creed, F. and Heaton, K.W., Southampton: Duphar.
19. Heaton, K.W., Ghosh, S. and Braddon, F.E.M. (1991) How bad are the symptoms and bowel dysfunction of patients with the irritable bowel syndrome? A prospective controlled study with emphasis on stool form. *Gut*, **32**, 73–79.
20. Heaton, K.W., O'Donnell, L.J.D., Braddon, F.E.M., Mountford, R.A., Hughes, A.O. and Cripps, P.J. (1992) Symptoms of irritable bowel syndrome in a British Urban Community: Consulters and non-consulters. *Gastroenterology*, **102**, 1962–1967.
21. Hillman, L.C., Stace, N.H. and Pomare, E.W. (1984) Irritable bowel patients and their long-term response to a high fiber diet. *American Journal of Gastroenterology*, **79**, 1–7.
22. Isgar, B., Harman, M., Kaye, M.D. and Whorwell, P.J. (1983) Symptoms of irritable bowel syndrome in ulcerative colitis in remission. *Gut*, **24**, 190–192.
23. Jones, V.A., McLaughlan, P., Shorthouse, M., Workman, E. and Hunter, J.O. (1982) Food intolerance: a major factor in the pathogenesis of irritable bowel syndrome. *The Lancet*, **2**, 1115–1117.
24. Kapoor, K.K., Nigam, P., Rastogi, C.K., Kumar, A. and Gupta, A.K. (1985) Clinical profile of irritable bowel syndrome. *Indian Journal of Gastroenterology*, **4**, 15–16.
25. Kellow, J.E., Gill, R.C. and Wingate, D.L. (1990) Prolonged ambulant recordings of small bowel motility demonstrate abnormalities in the irritable bowel syndrome. *Gastroenterology*, **98**, 1208–1218.
26. Kendall, G.P.N., Thompson, D.G., Day, S.J. and Lennard-Jones, J.E. (1990) Inter- and intraindividual variations in pressure–volume relations of the rectum in normal subjects and patients with the irritable bowel syndrome. *Gut*, **31**, 1062–1068.
27. Klein, K.B. (1988) Controlled treatment trials in the irritable bowel syndrome: a critique. *Gastroenterology*, **95**, 232–241.
28. Kruis, W., Thieme, Ch., Weinzierl, M., Schussler, P., Holl, J. and Paulus, W. (1984) A diagnostic score for the irritable bowel syndrome. Its value in the exclusion of organic disease. *Gastroenterology*, **87**, 1–7.
29. Kumar, A., Kumar, N., Vij, J.C., Sarin, S.K. and Anand, B.B. (1987) Optimum dosage of ispaghula husk in patients with irritable bowel syndrome: correlation of symptom relief with whole gut transit time and stool weight. *Gut*, **28**, 150–155.
30. Kumar, D. and Wingate, D. (1985) The irritable bowel syndrome: a paroxysmal motor disorder. *The Lancet*, **2**, 973–977.
31. Lasser, R.B., Bond, J.H. and Levitt, M.D. (1975) The role of intestinal gas in functional abdominal pain. *New England Journal of Medicine*, **293**, 524–526.
32. Lowman, B.C., Drossman, D.A., Cramer, E.M. and McKee, D.C. (1987) Recollection of childhood events in adults with irritable bowel syndrome. *Journal of Clinical Gastroenterology*, **9**, 324–330.
33. Manning, A.P., Thompson, W.G., Heaton, K.W. and Morris, A.F. (1978) Towards positive diagnosis of the irritable bowel. *British Medical Journal*, **2**, 653–654.
34. Marcus, S.N. and Heaton, K.W. (1987) Irritable bowel type symptoms in spontaneous and induced constipation. *Gut*, **28**, 156–159.
35. Maxton, D.G., Martin, D.F., Whorwell, P.J. and Godfrey, M. (1991) Abdominal distension in female patients with irritable bowel syndrome: exploration of possible mechanisms. *Gut*, **32**, 662–664.
36. Maxton, D.G., Morris, J.A. and Whorwell, P.J. (1989) Ranking of symptoms by patients with the irritable bowel syndrome. *British Medical Journal*, **229**, 1138.
37. Mayer, E.A. and Raybould, H.E. (1990) Role of visceral afferent mechanisms in functional bowel disorders. *Gastroenterology*, **99**, 1688–1704.
38. Metcalf, A.M., Phillips, S.F., Zinsmeister, A.R., MacCarty, R.L., Beart, R.W. and Wolff, B.G. (1987) Simplified assessment of segmental colonic transit. *Gastroenterology*, **92**, 40–47.
39. Moriarty, K.J. and Dawson, A.M. (1982) Functional abdominal pain: further evidence that whole gut is affected. *British Medical Journal*, **284**, 1670–1672.
40. Nanda, R., James, R., Smith, H., Dudley, C.R.K. and Jewell, D.P. (1989) Food intolerance and the irritable bowel syndrome. *Gut*, **30**, 1099–1104.
41. Narducci, F., Snape, W.J., Battle, W.M., London, R.L. and Cohen, S. (1985) Increased colonic motility during exposure to a stressful situation. *Digestive Diseases and Sciences*, **30**, 40–44.
42. Nicol, R. (1989) *Coping Successfully with Your Irritable Bowel*. London: Sheldon Press.
43. O'Donnell, L.J.D., Virjee, J. and Heaton, K.W. (1990) Detection of pseudodiarrhoea by simple clinical assessment of intestinal transit rate. *British Medical Journal*, **300**, 439–440.
44. Oettlé, G.J. and Heaton, K.W. (1986) 'Rectal dissatisfaction' in the irritable bowel syndrome. A

manometric and radiological study. *International Journal of Colorectal Disease*, **1**, 183–185.

45. Oettlé, G.J. and Heaton, K.W. (1987) Is there a relationship between symptoms of the irritable bowel syndrome and objective measurements of large bowel function? A longitudinal study. *Gut*, **28**, 146–149.
46. Pearson, D.J. (1985) Food allergy, hypersensitivity and intolerance. *Journal of the Royal College Physicians of London*, **19**, 154–162.
47. Prior, A., Maxton, D.G. and Whorwell, P.J. (1990) Anorectal manometry in irritable bowel syndrome: differences between diarrhoea and constipation predominant subjects. *Gut*, **31**, 458–462.
48. Prior, A. and Whorwell, P.J. (1987) Double blind study of ispaghula in irritable bowel syndrome. *Gut*, **28**, 1510–1513.
49. Prior, A. and Whorwell, P.J. (1989) Gynaecological consultation in patients with the irritable bowel syndrome. *Gut*, **30**, 996–998.
50. Ritchie, J. (1973) Pain from distension of the pelvic colon by inflating a balloon in the irritable bowel syndrome. *Gut*, **14**, 125–132.
51. Sandler, R.S. (1990) Epidemiology of irritable bowel syndrome in the United States. *Gastroenterology*, **99**, 409–415.
52. Sandler, R.S., Drossman, D.A., Nathan, H.P. and McKee, D.C. (1984) Symptom complaints and health care seeking behavior in subjects with bowel dysfunction. *Gastroenterology*, **87**, 314–318.
53. Schuster, M.M. and Whitehead, W.E. (1986) Physiologic insights into irritable bowel syndrome. *Clinics in Gastroenterology*, **15**, 839–853.
54. Smith, R.C., Greenbaum, D.S., Vancouver, J.B. *et al.* (1990) Pyschosocial factors are associated with health care seeking rather than diagnosis in irritable bowel syndrome. *Gastroenterology*, **98**, 293–301.
55. Svedlund, J., Sjodin, I., Ottosson, J-O. and Dotevall, G. (1983) Controlled study of psychotherapy in irritable bowel syndrome. *The Lancet*, **2**, 589–592.
56. Svendsen, J.H., Munck, L.K. and Andersen, J.R. (1985) Irritable bowel syndrome – prognosis and diagnostic safety. A 5-year follow-up study. *Scandinavian Journal of Gastroenterology*, **20**, 415–418.
57. Swarbrick, E.T., Hegarty, J.E., Bat, L., Williams, C.B. and Dawson, A.M. (1980) Site of pain from the irritable bowel. *The Lancet*, **2**, 443–446.
58. Talley, N.J., Phillips, S.F., Bruce, B., Twomey, C.K., Zinsmeister, A.R. and Melton, L.J. (1990) Relation among personality and symptoms in nonulcer dyspepsia and the irritable bowel syndrome. *Gastroenterology*, **99**, 327–333.
59. Talley, N.J., Phillips, S.F., Melton, L.J., Willgen, C. and Zinsmeister, A.R. (1989) A patient questionnaire to identify bowel disease. *Annals of Internal Medicine*, **111**, 671–674.
60. Thompson, W.G., Dotevall, G., Drossman, D.A., Heaton, K.W. and Kruis, W. (1989) Irritable bowel syndrome: guidelines for the diagnosis. *Gastroenterology International*, **2**, 92–95.
61. Thompson, W.G. and Heaton, K.W. (1980) Functional bowel disorders in apparently healthy people. *Gastroenterology*, **79**, 283–288.
62. Treacher, D.F., Chapman, J.R., Nolan, D.J. and Jewell, D.P. (1986) Irritable bowel syndrome: is a barium enema necessary? *Clinical Radiology*, **37**, 87–88.
63. Trotman, I.F. and Misiewicz, J.J. (1988) Sigmoid motility in diverticular disease and the irritable bowel syndrome. *Gut*, **29**, 218–222.
64. Turner, R.M. (1978) Recurrent abdominal pain in childhood. *Journal of the Royal College of General Practice*, **28**, 729–734.
65. Watts, G. (1990) *Irritable Bowel Syndrome: a Practical Guide.* London: Mandarin Paperbacks.
66. Whitehead, W.E. (1989) Effects of psychological factors on gastrointestinal function. In *Pathogenesis of Functional Bowel Disease*, pp. 37–53 (Ed.) Snape, W.J. New York: Plenum.
67. Whitehead, W.E., Bosmajian, L., Zonderman, A.B., Costa, P.T. and Schuster, M.M. (1988) Symptoms of psychologic distress associated with irritable bowel syndrome. Comparison of community and medical clinic samples. *Gastroenterology*, **95**, 709–714.
68. Whitehead, W.E., Crowell, M.D., Bosmajian, L. *et al.* (1980) Existence of irritable bowel syndrome supported by factor analysis of symptoms in two community samples. *Gastroenterology*, **98**, 336–340.
69. Whitehead, W.E., Holtkotter, B., Enck, P. *et al.* (1990) Tolerance for rectosigmoid distention in irritable bowel syndrome. *Gastroenterology*, **98**, 1187–1192.
70. Whorwell, P.J., Lupton, E.W., Erduran, D. and Wilson, K. (1986) Bladder smooth muscle dysfunction in patients with irritable bowel syndrome. *Gut*, **27**, 1014–1017.
71. Whorwell, P.J., McCallum, M., Creed, F.H. and Roberts, C.T. (1986) Non-colonic features of irritable bowel syndrome. *Gut*, **27**, 37–40.
72. Whorwell, P.J., Prior, A. and Colgan, S.M. (1987) Hypnotherapy in severe irritable bowel syndrome: further experience. *Gut*, **28**, 423–425.

FLATULENCE

I.A.D. Bouchier

Flatulence is defined as the awareness of intestinal gas in the form of either belching, abdominal distension and discomfort, or the passage of excess flatus. It is generally perceived as a common complaint, although there are no firm data on its frequency in the general population. Flatulence may present as a complaint in its own right or as part of a conglomerate of symptoms called dyspepsia which includes additionally epigastric discomfort or pain, fullness, burning, nausea, vomiting, fatty food intolerance or difficulty in completing a meal. Prevalence studies on dyspepsia suggest that anywhere between 25% and 30% of people experienced dyspepsia[6] of which the majority are likely to include excess wind among their complaints.

COMPOSITION OF INTESTINAL GAS

More than 99% of the gas passed per rectum is made up of five gases: nitrogen, oxygen, carbon dioxide, hydrogen and methane. The range is wide: nitrogen, 23–80%; carbon dioxide 5–29%; hydrogen 0–47%; oxygen 0–23%; and methane 0–26%.[2,8] Hydrogen concentrations are associated with periods of rapid flatus excretion. Flatus also contains traces of the more odiferous gases which can be detected by the human nose in concentrations of less than 1 part per million, including ammonia, hydrogen sulphide, indole, skatole, volatile amines, short-chain fatty acids, methanethiol and dimethylsulphide, the latter two gases being principally responsible for the unpleasant odour of human faeces.

ORIGIN OF INTESTINAL GAS

The composition of intestinal gas varies throughout the gastrointestinal tract depending on the site of origin of the gas. Normally the fasting intestinal gas volume is about 100 ml with a range of 30–200 ml, of which not more than 50 ml is present in the stomach. The quantity of flatus is much more variable – between 200 ml and 2 litres daily, with a mean of 600 ml. There are three sources of intestinal gas: swallowed air, intraluminal gas production and diffusion in the gut lumen.

SWALLOWED AIR

Swallowed air is the major source of gas in the stomach and is responsible for the 'gastric bubble' which is absent in patients who cannot swallow air, e.g. in achalasia of the cardia. All of the oxygen in the gut is derived from swallowed air but it is absorbed rapidly and significant volumes are found only in the upper gastrointestinal tract. Much of the nitrogen also originates from swallowed air.

Approximately 2–3 ml air enters the stomach with each swallow, probably more during rapid eating or drinking. Most swallowed air probably never enters the duodenum and the amount that passes into the small bowel is determined by posture. Air can be trapped in the stomach when the individual is in the supine position because the oesophagus enters the posterosuperior aspect of the stomach. In this position, air can be trapped above the fluid overlying the gastro-oesophageal junction.

INTRALUMINAL GAS PRODUCTION

Intestinal gas production is responsible for the presence of hydrogen, carbon dioxide, methane, volatile fatty acids, indoles, skatoles, methanethiol and dimethylsulphide. Carbon dioxide is produced in the upper small intestine from the interaction between carbonate and hydrogen ions but most of the gas is absorbed. Carbon dioxide in flatus is produced by the metabolism of colonic bacteria either directly or following the production of acids which interact with bicarbonate to produce carbon dioxide.

Bacterial metabolism is the sole source of gut hydrogen and methane. These gases are absorbed in part and excreted in the breath. This phenomenon is exploited in the various breath tests for malabsorption and intestinal transit. The hydrogen-liberating organisms are mainly in the colon but a small amount also originates in the caecum[4] and hydrogen production is inhibited by an acid pH. The main source of these gases is the intestinal fermentation of carbohydrates such as lactose (and lactulose), wheat, corn, oats, potatoes and a variety of vegetables that contain polysaccharides and oligosaccharides which cannot be digested by human small intestinal enzymes. Different bacterial species are responsible for producing hydrogen and methane. The type of saccharide linkage and the physicochemical nature of the polysaccharide also influence gas production. It is probable that the hydrolysis and fermentation of the different polysaccharides occur at different sites in the colon.[4,5]

Appreciable methane production occurs in only one-third of adults but there are wide variations in different regions of the world. This is a constant trait with a familial tendency. Methanogenesis is probably confined to the transverse and descending colon.[4] Methane is also present in the breath being detected in 54% of healthy subjects, but in fewer with inflammatory bowel disease.[10] Diet, intestinal bacteria, transit time and ethnic origin may all influence methane production. Methane production may be greater in patients with colonic cancer. Floating stools are a feature of patients who produce large volumes of methane, the gas being trapped in the stool thereby increasing its buoyancy. The extent of methanogenesis also determines the pattern of volatile fatty acids produced in the gut with proportionately more propionate and less acetate.[15]

DIFFUSION OF GAS

Hydrogen and methane which are present in very low concentrations in the blood diffuse from bowel lumen into blood. Nitrogen probably diffuses in small quantities from blood to bowel because P_{N_2} (i.e. nitrogen partial pressure) is usually lower in the intestinal tract lumen than blood. The diffusion of oxygen and carbon dioxide is variable.

CLINICAL PRESENTATIONS

Over 2000 years ago, Hippocrates taught that 'passing gas is necessary to well-being' whilst Claudius ruled that 'all Roman citizens shall be allowed to pass gas whenever necessary'. Fienus (Thomas Fyens) in his *'de' Flatibus humanum corpus molestantibus* (1643) gave the symptoms of flatulence as 'rumbling, swelling, and wandering pain coming suddenly and suddenly vanishing; a clear tumour that yields to the touch and that sounds like a drum. Often belching and farting are also signs and ease after breaking of wind doth follow.'

BELCHING

It is normal to eructate (belch or burp) a small volume of air after each meal and this is increased after ingesting carbonated drinks. In some cultures postprandial belching is regarded as an indication that the meal has been enjoyed.

Air that is belched has always been swallowed – aerophagy – but why some patients repeatedly swallow, or more correctly suck in, air is unclear. Normally the superior oesophageal constrictor muscle is closed but it can be relaxed by many individuals who, by a combination of inspiring against a closed glottus and relaxing the superior constrictor muscle, can draw air into the oesophagus. The majority of those who belch are relieving themselves of air in the oesophagus for little air actually enters the stomach. This technique of voluntary air sucking can be learned. It is used in oesophageal speech and is demonstrated as a party trick by those who can burp long and loudly at will.

There have been few studies of factors controlling the oral venting of gas from the stomach. Wyman *et al.*[16] demonstrated that gaseous distension of the stomach will provoke gastro-oesophageal reflux of gas which is cleared mainly by oesophageal peristalsis and not necessarily by belching. It is postulated that gastric distension triggers a neurally mediated response with both sensory and motor components which induces relaxation of the lower oesophageal sphincter. Only a minority of episodes of gastro-oesophageal reflux are associated with abdominal straining. The reflux of gas from the stomach occurs mainly during non-swallowing transient relaxation of the gastro-oesophageal sphincter which is subject to postural control because relaxation occurs more frequently in the upright than in the supine position.

Gastroenterologists will be familiar with the patient who complains of excessive and repeated belching and, while giving the history, burps ostentatiously between each sentence. Such persons are frequently tense, anxious and nervous, and it is thought that belching may relieve a sense of discomfort in the chest or abdomen. Possibly a vicious cycle is established with burping resulting in more air swallowing, further discomfort, and the need to belch for relief.

Talking a great deal may be accompanied by air swallowing and excessive eructation. Hypersalivation or chewing gum may cause flatulence but smoking, sucking sweets, and loss of teeth or dentures are implicated on less certain grounds.[14] Excessive belching is rarely a manifestation of organic disease but occasionally patients with troublesome burping are cured by appropriate treatment for a gastric ulcer, hiatus hernia or gallstones.

TREATMENT

There is always the dilemma of whether to investigate the upper gastrointestinal tract of a patient who complains of belching. The pragmatic approach, which applies to the investigation of dyspepsia, applies to eructation as well: only patients over the age of 45 years presenting for the first time merit investigation, usually by endoscopy.[6]

Therapy is based on an explanation that swallowed air is the cause of gas sitting in the gullet; the author's experience is that this is not always accepted by the patient who is convinced of the presence of gastric or gallbladder disease. Metoclopramide 10 mg three times daily or cisapride 10 mg three times daily for up to 3 weeks is occasionally helpful. Dimethicone, an inert silicone agent which lowers surface tension and causes small bubbles in the stomach to coalesce, is contained in a number of preparations used alone or in combination with an antacid that have been recommended as antiflatulents, but in the author's experience they are unhelpful. In the end the clinician is resigned to the task of repeated explanation and reassurance while resisting requests for repeated investigations, diverse medications or even surgical intervention.

INTESTINAL DISTENSION AND EXCESSIVE FLATUS

It is convenient to consider these two symptoms together because patients usually complain of distension, bloating, borborygmi, discomfort, cramping abdominal pains and the passage of large volumes of flatus. Many are socially embarrassed and some admit to a fear of cancer. The gas may be dispersed throughout the small and large bowel, or collect in certain areas such as the caecum which the examiner can identify as being a soft, squelching, slightly tender swelling in the right iliac fossa. Another site of accumulation is the splenic flexure, giving rise to pain in the left upper quadrant – a condition known as the 'splenic flexure syndrome' and generally held to be a variant of the irritable bowel syndrome. Indeed a disorder of muscle function and motility rather than gas production may be the mechanism for the complaint in some of these patients, because Lasser *et al.* (1975), in a study of 18 subjects who complained of excessive abdominal gas, bloating and discomfort, found no objective evidence of increased bowel gas and suggested a combination of disordered intestinal motility and an abnormal pain response to gut distension as the source of the symptoms.[7]

Malabsorption is an important, if uncommon, cause of excessive intestinal gas which is derived from fermentation of unabsorbed nutrients. Patients with coeliac disease, pancreatic insufficiency or bacterial overgrowth may complain of excessive wind. However, malabsorption of lactose is a significant cause of abdominal discomfort, bloating, excessive flatus and diarrhoea.[1] A reduction in intestinal lactose activity is normal in adults except for those of northern European origin and the Hammitic people of Africa. The ingestion of milk may, therefore, produce unpleasant sensations in many individuals, and lactose intolerance must be considered in those who complain of pain of abdominal distension, particularly if the patients is of African or Asian origin. The diagnostic tests employed for lactose intolerance are discussed on page 389.

Certain types of food are prone to cause flatulence and excessive flatus and these include the storage carbohydrates of vegetable material which are resistant to digestive enzymes and, like lactose, become available as substrates for colonic bacterial enzymes. Most commonly implicated are beans, nuts, raisins, onions, cabbage, Brussels sprouts, prunes and apples. Patients differ greatly in their susceptibility. Fructose and sorbitol are natural constituents of fruit, berries and plants. Fructose is also a commonly used sweetener in soft drinks. Malabsorption may produce flatulence and gastrointestinal distress. Inability to hydrolyse starch, e.g. in rice, potatoes, bananas or beans may also cause increased intestinal gas production. Any suggestion of carbohydrate malabsorption from the history should lead to the performance of a hydrogen breath test to demonstrate that the undigested carbohydrates are reaching the colon in excessive amounts.[9,12,13] Patients on high-fibre diets, e.g. in the treatment of irritable bowel syndrome, often notice an unwelcome increase in intestinal gas.

There is a group of young or middle-aged women who complain bitterly of abdominal distension often prior to the menses or at the time of the menopause. They claim that they cannot fasten belts or skirts and are unable to wear clothing comfortably around the abdomen. They often maintain that they are socially embarrassed and that their lifestyle is adversely affected and yet no abdominal distension is obvious at the time of physical examination.[3]

TREATMENT

It is usually easy to exclude organic disease without recourse to laboratory investigations but occasionally barium studies or a cholecystogram are required. Breath hydrogen tests may be helpful. Patients need to be reassured of the absence of organic pathology and an explanation for their symptoms provided. A low-fibre diet, now so unfashionable, may be of benefit. An attempt should be made to eliminate possible food factors such as lactose, fructose and non-absorbable carbohydrate including various gums, mucilages, pectin, cellulose and hemicellulose. Antibiotics should not be prescribed and there is no evidence for the efficacy of activated charcoal,[11] kaolin or dimethicone preparations. Thus the long-term management of the flatulent patient is often difficult and taxing, requiring a tolerant understanding by the practitioner and a willingness to advise on an experiment with the diet.

REFERENCES

1. Barr, R.G., Levine, M.D. and Watkins, J.B. (1979) Recurrent abdominal pain of childhood due to lactose intolerance. *New England Journal of Medicine*, **300**, 1449–1452.
2. Bond, J.H. and Levitt, M.D. (1977) A rational approach to intestinal gas problems. *Viewpoints on Digestive Diseases*, **9**, 1–4.
3. Bouchier, I.A.D. (1980) Flatulence. *The Practitioner*, **224**, 373–377.
4. Flourie, B., Etachaud, F., Flourent, C., Pellier, P., Bouhnik, Y. and Ramband, J.-C. (1990) Comparative study of hydrogen and methane production in the human colon using caecal and faecal homogenates. *Gut*, **31**, 684–685.
5. Grimble, G. (1989) Fibre, fermentation, flora and flatus. *Gut*, **30**, 6–13.
6. Jones, R. (1989) Dyspeptic symptoms in the community. *Gut*, **30**, 893–898.
7. Lasser, R.B., Bond, J.H. and Levitt, M.D. (1975) The role of intestinal gas in functional abdominal pain. *New England Journal of Medicine*, **293**, 524–526.
8. Levitt, M.D. (1971) Volume and composition of human intestinal gas determined by means of an intestinal washout technique. *New England Journal of Medicine*, **284**, 1394–1398.
9. Levitt, M.D. (1983) Malabsorption of starch: a normal phenomenon. *Gastroenterology*, **85**, 769–770.
10. McKay, L.F., Eastwood, M.A. and Brydon, W.G. (1985) Methane excretion in man – a study of breath, flatus and faeces. *Gut*, **26**, 69–74.
11. Potter, T., Ellis, C. and Levitt, M. (1985) Activated charcoal: in vivo and in vitro studies of effect on gas formation. *Gastroenterology*, **88**, 620–624.
12. Ravich, W.J., Bayless, T.M. and Thomas, M. (1983) Fructose: incomplete intestinal absorption in humans. *Gastroenterology*, **84**, 26–29.
13. Rumessen, J.J. and Gudmand-Hoyer, E. (1988) Functional bowel disease: malabsorption and abdominal distress after ingestion of fructose, sorbitol, and fructose-sorbitol mixtures. *Gastroenterology*, **95**, 694–700.
14. Sircus, W. and Prescott, R.J. (1985) Relation between dentition and dyspeptic disorders. *British Medical Journal*, **290**, 115.
15. Weaver, G.A., Krause, J.A., Miller, T.C. and Wolin, M.J. (1989) Constancy of glucose and starch fermentation by two different human faecal microbial communities. *Gut*, **30**, 19–25.
16. Wyman, J.B., Dent, J., Heddle, R., Dodds, W.J., Toouli, J. and Downton, J. (1990) Control of belching by the lower oesophageal sphincter. *Gut*, **31**, 639–646.

ANOREXIA NERVOSA, AND OTHER PSYCHOLOGICAL DISORDERS OF THE GASTROINTESTINAL TRACT

G. Masterton and C.P.L. Freeman

INTRODUCTION

The justification for this chapter was provided almost 50 years ago by Walter Alvarez[1] in the preface to his book *Nervousness, Indigestion and Pain*, in which he wrote:

> The gastroenterologist just has to be a psychiatrist of sorts and no matter how much he may dislike spending hours each week trying to teach neurotic persons how to live more sensibly, he must do this sort of thing if he is to help them at all. Furthermore if he is to avoid ordering many needless operations and scaring many physically sound patients half to death with diagnoses of serious organic disorder, he must become expert at recognising hysteria, anxiety neurosis, hypochondriasis and mild forms of insanity.

The patients to whom Alvarez was referring present with physical complaints that are invariably attributed to organic disease in the gut. They are not easy to diagnose, often describing puzzling discomforts and dysfunction, sometimes failing to provide crucial information and, rarely, intentionally misleading the doctor. The patients are not easy to manage, often resenting the physician's inability to produce a disease and a cure, or alternatively objecting to being given a psychiatric label and to use of the psychological treatment approach. They also tend to be unrewarding patients – seemingly quick to express dissatisfaction and slow to comply with their treatment.

Yet, in various guises, these patients present in such large numbers to gastroenterology clinics that, as Alvarez puts it, the gastroenterologist must learn to deal as much with sick, unhappy people as with their diseases.

THE PREVALENCE OF FUNCTIONAL PRESENTATIONS IN GASTROENTEROLOGICAL PRACTICE

The description 'functional' is used widely to refer to a diagnosis of a non-organic condition – a disorder as opposed to a disease. This dichotomy is false for several reasons. First, some apparently functional disorders may have an organic basis that has not yet yielded to scientific understanding,[7] or may represent a pre-diagnostic stage in a disease, such as bowel cancer masquerading as functional abdominal pain.[3] Second, patients may present with 'genuine' physical conditions which indisputably have a psychogenic basis, such as laxative abuse, self-induced vomiting and self-inflicted blood loss.[6] Even in truly organic diseases factors such as emotional state, personality traits and life events may play a role in development, relapse or treatment response – more so, for example, in peptic ulcer than in malignancy.

Noting that not a single referral letter had mentioned the presence of psychiatric illness, MacDonald and Bouchier found that 28 of 100 new gastroenterology outpatients had severe psychiatric disorder – 14 of these new patients had functional gastrointestinal disorders and the other 14 had disease.[11] Further, patients who experience prolonged life difficulties may be more likely to have a functional rather than an organic condition,[2] yet one in three functional presentations occur in patients who are neither mentally disordered nor faced with life's adversities.[8]

Gastrointestinal symptoms are very common: roughly 30% of the adult population have dyspepsia to a personally significant extent,[10] whilst about the same proportion report abnormal bowel symptoms or habit.[4,14]

With this prevalence of gastrointestinal dysfunction in the community, it should come as no surprise that around 40–45% of a gastroenterologist's new outpatient referrals can be anticipated to have no identifiable disease[5,8,9,11–13] (*Table 10.7*).

The distribution and frequency of specific presentations are demonstrated in further analysis of the data of Harvey and colleagues[9] (*Table 10.8*). The variety of common functional conditions was as wide as that found in organic presentations; however, among the functional disorders unexplained abdominal pain accounted for half of the total.

Table 10.7 Prevalence of functional gastrointestinal disorders in gastroenterology outpatient practice

Authors	*Source*	*Number of patients*	*Functional disorders (%)*
Ferguson *et al.*[5]	Gastrointestinal clinic (UK)	88	31
Ford *et al.*[8]	Gastrointestinal clinic (UK)	134	40
Harvey *et al.*[9]	Gastrointestinal clinic (UK)	2000	44
MacDonald and Bouchier[11]	Gastrointestinal clinic (UK)	87	48
Switz[13]	Questionnaire to gastroenterologists (USA)	369	19
Mitchell and Drossman[12]	Questionnaire to 704 members of AGA (USA)	–	41

Table 10.8 Distribution and frequency of diagnoses made in 2000 gastroenterology outpatient referrals

Main categories	*n*	*Organic gastrointestinal disease*	*n*	*Functional gastrointestinal disorder*	*n*
Organic gastrointestinal disease	980	Peptic ulceration	197	Abdominal pain with altered bowel habit	449
Functional gastrointestinal disorder	888	Oesophageal reflux/oesophagitis	188	Painless diarrhoea	107
Non-gastrointestinal disease	57	Inflammatory bowel disease	168	Endoscopy negative dyspepsia	77
No diagnosis made	75	Cholelithiasis	48	Depression presenting with abdominal pain	50
		Carcinoma of colon	28	Painless constipation	39
		Coeliac disease	26	Habit disorders (e.g. aerophagy, rumination)	34
		Hepatic cirrhosis	21	Anxiety presenting with gastrointestinal symptoms	24
		Infective diarrhoea	21	'Mad and incurable', including Munchausen's Syndrome	15
		Alcoholism	16	Eating disorders	10
		Post-gastrectomy/vagotomy	14	Others	83
		Carcinoma of stomach	13		
		Hepatitis	11		
		Others (71 diagnoses)	229		

From Harvey *et al.*[9]

REFERENCES

1. Alvarez, W.C. (1944) *Nervousness, Indigestion and Pain.* London: William Heinemann.
2. Craig, T.K. and Brown, G.W. (1984) Goal frustrating aspects of life event stress in the aetiology of gastrointestinal disorder. *Journal of Psychomatic Research*, **28**, 411–421.
3. De Dombal, F.T., Mathan, S.S., Staniland, J.R. *et al.* (1980) Presentation of cancer to hospital as 'acute abdominal pain'. *British Journal of Surgery*, **67**, 413–416.
4. Drossman, D.A, Sandler, R.S., McKee, D.C. and Lovitz, A.J. (1982) Bowel patterns among subjects not seeking health care. *Gastroenterology*, **83**, 529–534.
5. Ferguson, A., Sircus, W. and Eastwood, M.A. (1977) Frequency of 'functional' gastrointestinal disorders. *The Lancet*, **2**, 613–614.
6. Ford, C.V. (1983) Factitious illness. In *The Somatising Disorders*, pp. 135–154. New York: Elsevier Biomedical.
7. Ford, M.J. (1986) The irritable bowel syndrome. *Journal of Psychosomatic Research*, **30**, 399–410.
8. Ford, M.J., Miller, P.M., Eastwood, J. and Eastwood, M.A. (1987) Life events, psychiatric illness and the irritable bowel syndrome. *Gut*, **28**, 160–165.
9. Harvey, R.F., Salih, S.Y. and Read, A.E. (1983) Organic and functional disorders in 2,000 gastroenterology outpatients. *The Lancet*, **1**, 632–634.
10. Jones, R. and Lydeard, S. (1989) Prevalence of symptoms of dyspepsia in the community. *British Medical Journal*, **298**, 30–32.
11. MacDonald, A.J. and Bouchier, I.A.D. (1980) Non-organic gastrointestinal illness: a medical and psychiatric study. *British Journal of Psychiatry*, **136**, 276–283.
12. Mitchell, C.M. and Drossman, D.A. (1987) Survey of the AGA membership relating to patients with functional gastrointestinal disorders. *Gastroenterology*, **92**, 1282–1284.
13. Switz, D.M. (1976) What the gastroenterologist does all day. *Gastroenterology*, **70**, 1048–1050.
14. Thompson, W.G. and Heaton, K.W. (1980) Functional bowel disorders in apparently healthy people. *Gastroenterology*, **79**, 283–288.

PSYCHOLOGICAL FACTORS IN GASTROINTESTINAL DISEASES

PRINCIPLES OF PSYCHOSOMATICS

Psychosomatic research can be defined as any investigation that focuses on the correlation between one or more psychological or social variables, on the one hand, and one or more biological variables, on the other.[5]

Psychosomatic medicine is a subspeciality of neither psychiatry nor medicine; it is a scientific field of interest, an interface among various specialities and allied disciplines. It embraces the pathogenesis and nature of disease: how factors such as conflict, loss, stress and maladaptive coping influence the precipitation, course and outcome of disease and, in turn, how disease affects the psyche (sometimes termed 'somatopsychic medicine').[6]

There are many ways in which psychosocial variables might influence functioning and disorder of the gastrointestinal tract.[2,4] One provisional classification[3,7] divided such aspects into:

1. Primarily psychogenic, such as non-organic abdominal pain and globus hystericus.
2. Primarily behavioural, such as eating disorders and encopresis.
3. Primarily psychophysiological, such as gut motility and regulation of secretions.
4. Primarily symbolic:
   (a) defence or riddance reactions, such as vomiting and altered bowel habit.
   (b) the effects of displaced, incomplete or blocked drives, such as aerophagy.
   (c) the complications of affect (or mood) disturbances, such as the giving-up/given-up complex.[1]

As these concepts indicate, the psychosomatic approach can embrace apparently all disorders and diseases – and devotees may sometimes overstate or investigate inappropriately. When exaggeration and generalization are compounded by lack of scientific rigour, evident, for example, in much individual casework, the clinician's scepticism may turn to discount of the entire subject. Not all psychosomatic research in gastrointestinal disease can be so readily dismissed so the gastroenterologist who over-reacts in this manner risks throwing the baby out with the bathwater.

REFERENCES

1. Engel, G.L. (1976) A psychological setting of somatic disease: The 'giving up–given up' complex. *Proceedings of the Royal Society of Medicine*, **60**, 553–555.
2. Engel, G.L. (1974) The psychosomatic approach to individual susceptibility to disease. *Gastroenterology*, **67**, 1085–1093.
3. Engel, G.L. (1975) In *Comprehensive Textbook of Psychiatry*, Vol. 2, 3rd edn, pp. 1638–1648. (Ed.) Freedman, A.M., Kaplan, H.I. and Saddock, B.I. Baltimore: Williams & Wilkins.
4. Glaser, J.P. and Engel, G.L. (1977) Psychodynamics, psychophysiology and gastrointestinal symptomatology. *Clinics in Gastroenterology*, **6**, 507–531.
5. Lipowski, Z. (1982) Modern meaning of the terms 'psychosomatic' and 'liaison psychiatry'. In *Medicine and Psychiatry: A Practical Approach*, pp. 3–24. (Ed.) Creed, F. and Pfeffer, J.M. London: Pitman.
6. Oken, D. (1989) Current theoretical concepts in psychosomatic medicine. In *Comprehensive Textbook of Psychiatry*, Vol 2, 5th edn, pp. 1160–1169. (Ed.) Kaplan, H.I. and Saddock, B.I. Baltimore: Williams & Williams.
7. Strang, P.J. (1989) Gastrointestinal disorders. In *Psychosomatic Medicine: Theory, Physiology and Practice*, **2** pp. 427–502. (Ed.) Cheren, S. Madison, Connecticut: International Universities Press.

PEPTIC ULCER

Psychophysiology

William Beaumont's classic studies on the stomach of the trapper Alexis St Martin, which he could observe directly through a gastric fistula caused by a shooting accident, advanced physiological understanding into the processes of digestion. Among his careful observations Beaumont noticed changes in secretions and mucosa in response to powerful emotions, and he concluded 'fear, anger, and whatever depresses or disturbs the nervous system check its (gastric) secretions'.[2,27]

The relationship between gastric physiology and psychological factors was investigated in detail during the heyday of psychosomatic research in the first half of this century, often using Beaumont's technique of direct observation upon fistula patients.[27] That stress might induce pathological change was demonstrated in the case of Tom, the New York janitor with a gastrostomy, who appeared to develop gastric ulceration when his life was threatened by a cancer in the exposed gastric mucosa.[27] From this type of 'natural' experiment on single subjects there has followed a series of controlled studies on samples of peptic ulcer patients as well as samples of normals. These have substantially confirmed Beaumont's findings of marked, complex changes in the volume and acidity of gastric secretions and impairment in mucosal function as a direct response to various emotions and stresses.[5,9,25] Accompanying this there have been physiological developments in understanding the role that the central nervous system plays in areas such as the control of acid secretion, although the pathways by which emotional factors are transduced remain unknown.[21]

Psychoanalysis

Perhaps the best known psychosomatic work upon peptic ulceration has been the psychoanalytic contribution, spearheaded by Dunbar and Alexander. From her analytical casework, Dunbar[6] concluded that patients with peptic ulcer disease shared specific personality traits – being distinctively activity-oriented, ambitious and striving – hence launching the concept of ulcer-prone personality. Whilst such traits do indeed appear to be overrepresented among peptic ulcer patients, they are core characteristics of type A behaviour and are also associated with other diseases such as coronary artery disease, asthma, thyroid disorders and rheumatoid arthritis.[16]

However, the psychoanalytic work took the issue of peptic ulcer specificity further, with Alexander espousing that the traits Dunbar had identified were the product of an unconscious conflict focusing upon chronic 'oral' themes, notably the need to be loved, cared for and nourished.[1] He theorized that the patient's struggle to resist dependency needs resulted in inner (psychic) tensions which activated inappropriate physiological processes and consequent ulcer development. Alexander's elegant unification of the disparate threads of chronic oral conflict, psychophysiology and constitutional predisposition proved to be particularly influential.

Much of the theory has been confirmed in women as well as in men, and in all socioeconomic groups, to the satisfaction of most psychoanalytically oriented workers.[20] However, the evidence from most,[19,20] but not all,[18] investigations into psychotherapy as treatment for peptic ulceration is that it has no particular role to play. Supportive psychotherapy is helpful for some ulcer patients and of course patients who happen to have concomitant psychological problems which are amenable to psychotherapy benefit from this treatment – but there has been no specific analytical technique derived from Alexander's theory of unconscious oral conflict.

Further, the generation of hypotheses that could test the validity of Alexander's theory has proved difficult,[25] and the results obtained have been generally inconclusive as a result, although some support has come from the prediction of ulcer disease by independent investigators classifying subjects on the basis of psychoanalytic theory and projective personality tests.[26,28]

However, esoteric theory, uncontrolled research and no effective treatment have essentially marginalized the psychoanalytic contribution.

Life events

There is no evidence of increased numbers of adverse life events among patients with either chronic duodenal[15] or gastric ulcer.[22] Although it has been suggested that life events may precipitate duodenal ulceration more readily than gastric ulceration,[17] a well-controlled study found men with duodenal ulcers had not experienced either more severe or more frequent life events than controls.[7]

The psychophysiologically based idea that ulcer patients may react to such stresses differently[13] was recently re-evaluated in a comparison of men suffering from peptic ulcer against controls who were a mixture of healthy volunteers and gallstone or kidney stone patients.[24] Serum pepsinogen levels correlated with personality traits of hostility, irritability and hypersensitivity, and with impaired coping abilities, but not with cigarette, alcohol or aspirin consumption. The best discriminators between ulcer patients and controls, in rank order, were: (1) depression; (2) a negative perception of life events; (3) the number of relatives with peptic ulcerations; and (4) serum pepsinogen I concentration. The implication is that the key to the relationship between stress and ulceration is not the number or nature of the stresses, but rather how the individual perceives and responds to adversity – and this is mediated directly through physical change, such as hyperpepsinogenaemia, rather than implicated intermediaries such as alcohol and cigarette consumption.[24]

Stressful life events may influence the course of the disease, chronic family and marital difficulties being independent factors associated with delayed healing.[12] Chronic occupational stress also appears to play a role, one example being the greater prevalence of peptic ulceration among air traffic controllers compared with second-class airmen.[4]

An important caveat in this field of research derives from the tendency for patients who have, or have had, physical illness to somatize worries to their target organ, and of course past experience of the disease influences the presenting symptomatology. In ordinary life peptic ulcer is particularly associated with worry, so the belief, and indeed the expectation, that an ulcer will develop or recur when the individual is confronted with stressful circumstances may result in a report of exacerbation of dyspepsia without evidence of actual ulceration. However, this picture is not entirely straightforward, because one study found 54% of ulcer patients had worsening symptoms in association with personal stresses, but one in three actually reported improvement in such circumstances.[10]

Mental illness

An increased prevalence of psychiatric disorder has been reported in both duodenal and gastric ulcer patients,[8,23] the most common conditions being alcoholism, anxiety neurosis, psychopathic personality and less so, depression. There is no evidence of association with psychotic illness,[23] nor does depressive illness appear to predispose to ulcer formation.[14]

The suicide rate is increased in peptic ulcer patients, and indeed mainly explains the excess

Table 10.9 Observed and expected causes of death following Billroth II resection for peptic ulceration

Cause	*Observed*	*Expected*	*Odds ratio*	*Significance*
Infectious disease	5	4.8	1.04	NS
Neoplasm	124	114.7	1.08	NS
Cardiovascular disease	193	198.8	0.99	NS
Respiratory disease	31	27.5	1.12	NS
Gastrointestinal disease	23	19.7	1.16	NS
Peptic ulcer	2	4.9	0.41	NS
Hepatic cirrhosis	13	7.0	1.86	NS
Urogenital disease	17	11.8	1.44	NS
Accident	21	29.6	0.71	NS
Suicide	68	13.4	5.07	$P < 0.01$
Other causes	40	27.5	1.45	–
Total	537	459.7	1.18	$P < 0.05$

NS = not significant.
From Knap and Fischer.[11]

mortality in this disease following surgery (*Table 10.9*). Alcoholism is by far the most common primary psychiatric diagnosis among peptic ulcer suicides,[11] whilst alcoholics who have a peptic ulcer are three times more likely to commit suicide than those who do not have one.[3] This indicates that the explanation for the increased suicide rate in peptic ulceration is not simply attributable to the presence of more high-risk individuals.

REFERENCES

1. Alexander, F. (1950) *Psychosomatic Medicine*. New York: Norton.
2. Beaumont, W. (1833) *Experiments and Observations on the Gastric Juice and the Physiology of Digestion*. Plattsburg: F.P. Allen.
3. Berglund, M. (1986) Suicide in male alcoholics with peptic ulcers. *Alcoholism: Clinical and Experimental Research*, **10**, 631–634.
4. Cobb, S. and Rose, R.M. (1973) Hypertension, peptic ulcer and diabetes in air traffic controllers. *Journal of the American Medical Association*, **224**, 489–492.
5. Dotevall, G. (1985) *Stress and Common Gastrointestinal Disorders*. New York: Praeger.
6. Dunbar, F. (1947) *Emotions and Bodily Change*, 3rd edn. New York: Columbia University Press.
7. Feldman, M., Walker, P., Green, J.L. and Weingarten, K. (1986) Life events stress and psychosocial factors in men with peptic ulcer disease. *Gastroenterology*, **91**, 1370–1379.
8. Gosling, R.H. (1958) Peptic ulcer and mental disorder (I and II). *Journal of Psychosomatic Research*, **2**, 190–198, 258–301.
9. Hojgaard, L. and Bendtsen, F. (1989) Gastric potential difference and pH in ulcer patients and normal volunteers during Stroop's colour word conflict test. *Gut*, **30**, 782–785.
10. Ippoliti, A.F. (1980) The diagnosis and treatment of gastrointestinal ulcer. *Directions in Psychiatry*, **3**, 3–7.
11. Knop, J. and Fischer, A. (1988) Psychiatric morbidity and cause of death following gastrectomy for peptic ulcer. *Acta Chirurgica Scandinavica*, **154** (suppl. 547), 68–70.
12. Mason, J.B., Moshal, M.G., Naidoo, V. and Schlemmer, L. (1981) The effect of stressful life situations on the healing of duodenal ulceration. *South African Medical Journal*, **60**, 734–737.
13. Mittleman, B. and Wolff, H.G. (1942) Emotions and gastroduodenal function: experimental studies on patients with gastritis, duodenitis and peptic ulcer. *Psychosomatic Medicine*, **4**, 5–6.
14. Piper, D.W., Ariotti, D.E., Greig, M. and Brown, R. (1980) Chronic duodenal ulcer and depression. *Scandinavian Journal of Gastroenterology*, **72**, 19–25.
15. Piper, D.W., McIntosh, J.H., Ariotti, D.E., Caloguiri, J.V., Brown, R.W. and Shy, C.M. (1981) Life events and chronic duodenal ulcer: a case control study. *Gut*, **22**, 1011–1017.
16. Rime, B., Ucros, C.G. and Bestgen, Y. (1989) Type A behaviour pattern: Specific coronary risk factor or general disease-prone condition? *British Journal of Medical Psychology*, **62**, 229–240.
17. Sapira, J.D. and Cross, M.R. (1982) Prehospitalisation life change in gastric ulcer versus duodenal ulcer. *Psychosomatic Medicine*, **44**, 121.
18. Sjodin, I., Svedlund, J., Ottoson, J.O. and Dotevall, G. (1986) Controlled study of psychotherapy in chronic peptic ulcer disease. *Psychosomatics*, **27**, 187–200.
19. Stracher, G. (1986) Psychotherapy of peptic ulcer: expectations and reality (German with English

summary). *Fortschritte der Medizin*, **104** (suppl. III), 929–932.
20. Strang, P.J. (1989) Gastrointestinal disorders. In *Psychosomatic Medicine: Theory Physiology and Practice*, Vol. 2, pp. 427–502. (Ed.) Cheren, S. Madison, Connecticut: International Universities Press.
21. Taché, Y. (1987) Central nervous system regulation of gastric acid secretion. In *Physiology of the Gastrointestinal Tract*, Vol. 2, 2nd edn, pp. 911–930. (Ed.) Johnson, L.R. New York: Raven Press.
22. Thomas, J., Greig, M.E. and Piper, D.W. (1980) Chronic gastric ulcer and life events. *Gastroenterology*, **78**, 905–911.
23. Viskum, K. (1975) Mind and ulcer. *Acta Psychiatrica Scandinavica*, **51**, 182–200.
24. Walker, P., Luther, J., Samloff, I.M. and Feldman, M. (1988) Life events stress and psychosocial factors in men with peptic ulcer disease II. Relationships with serum pepsinogen concentrations and behavioural risk factors. *Gastroenterology*, **94**, 323–330.
25. Weiner, H. (1977) *Psychobiology and Human Disease*, pp. 33–101. New York: Elsevier North-Holland.
26. Weiner, H., Thaler, M., Reiser, M.F. and Mirsky, I.A. (1957) Aetiology of duodenal ulcer. I. Relation of specific psychological characteristics to rate of gastric secretion (serum pepsinogen). *Psychosomatic Medicine*, **19**, 1–10.
27. Wolf, S. (1981) The psyche and the stomach. *Gastroenterology*, **80**, 605–614.
28. Yessler, P.G., Reiser, M.F. and Rioch, D.M. (1959) Etiology of duodenal ulcer. II. Serum pepsinogen and peptic ulcer in inductees. *Journal of The American Medical Association*, **169**, 451–456.

INFLAMMATORY BOWEL DISEASE

Psychophysiology

Stress can alter the motility in both the small bowel[3] and colon,[21] and fistula studies have reported superficial changes in the mucosa in response to stress[32] – but there is no evidence that psychological factors can directly, or indirectly, cause lesions of the type and distribution found in inflammatory bowel disease.[32]

Psychoanalysis

Most of the psychoanalytic work has concentrated upon ulcerative colitis, although many of the samples have included cases of Crohn's disease.[19,30] Alexander's theory of specificity of unconscious conflict attributed ulcerative colitis to 'the patient facing a life situation which requires some outstanding accomplishment for which the patient feels unprepared'.[1] Psychodynamically, the patient was seen as regressing to the stage of the first environmental demand for accomplishment which is the period of bowel control development ('anal regression'), and this conflict set in motion psychophysiological processes that led to inflammatory bowel disease in biologically predisposed individuals.

Subsequent analytically oriented work has not supported specificity theory to the same extent as in peptic ulcerations;[36] instead authors have concentrated upon the responses shown to adverse life circumstances.

A range of scenarios has been described, characteristically based upon an intensely dependent relationship with a key figure (most frequently a domineering mother), focusing on themes of threatened insecurity, failure or over-burdening, and with the generation of feelings of hopelessness or helplessness in reaction to bereavement or other loss.[5,8,30,32] Thus, inflammatory bowel disease is envisaged as the outcome of specific biological processes set in motion in predisposed individuals by non-specific, maladaptive, psychological responses to characteristic life events. As in peptic ulcer disease the methodological difficulties arising from trying to validate such findings, which are derived from uncontrolled case studies involving highly selected individuals, has limited the contribution of this approach.[5]

There have been many case reports and studies of psychotherapy in the treatment of ulcerative colitis in particular, although the findings also appear to hold true for Crohn's disease.[30] The best work, having been undertaken over more than 40 years, is the Columbia Ulcerative Colitis Project.[17–19] These controlled studies have confirmed the effectiveness of psychotherapy not only in improving psychological and social adjustment to the disease, but also in assisting a better physiological outcome (as assessed by gastroenterologists). Remissions are not prolonged but there is evidence of diminished severity in subsequent attacks, and possibly fewer complications. The skill and quality of supervision of the therapist had an important bearing upon outcome, as did the duration of psychotherapy, the degree of psychopathology and the severity of the disease.

Finally, relaxation training is an effective (and much briefer) method of ameliorating pain and distress among patients with ulcerative colitis.[27]

Life events

Uncontrolled reports indicate that 80% or more cases of inflammatory bowel disease were initiated or exacerbated by major life events, commonly an important bereavement.[4,5,6,11,12,14,22,23,26,33] However, controlled studies have failed to confirm this.[9,10,24] In general, adverse life events appear to play a greater role in ulcerative colitis than in Crohn's disease and in exacerbations of the disease rather than in the initiation. As the analytical work indicates, how such events are perceived and handled by the individual is probably more important than the event itself.

Mental illness

An increased prevalence of psychiatric illness has been reported in many investigations of this aspect of inflammatory bowel disease.[2,5,7,11,12,13,15,16,19,20,23,28,30,33] There have been a few negative results,[9,10,29,31] and there is no evidence that psychiatric disorder occurs more frequently than in other chronic physical illnesses[13,15] – except perhaps depression in Crohn's disease.[16]

By far the most common psychiatric diagnosis is depressive illness, followed by anxiety and phobic states. Depression appears to be particularly associated with Crohn's disease.[2,5,13,16,20,28] whilst anxiety states occur as often as depression in ulcerative colitis.[2,15] The suicide rate is increased among women with Crohn's disease.[25] Organic mental disorders are not infrequent, being attributable to metabolic disturbances or complications of the disease, or to side effects of treatment.[30] The presence of psychiatric illness appears to be unrelated to disease activity in ulcerative colitis,[2,15] but the findings in respect of Crohn's disease have been conflicting.[2,16] There is an association between emotional disturbance (other than distress) and the amount of diarrhoea,[13] as well as the duration and severity of the disease.[20,33] The presence of a psychiatric disorder adversely affects recovery,[2,19] and perhaps because of this, these patients tend to attend the clinic more frequently.[13] Finally it has not proved possible to tease out emotional illness as an understandable reaction to unpleasant disease from emotional illness as an intrinsic complication of the pathological process.[5,30] However, there is a little evidence that patients with Crohn's disease are more likely to have had psychological problems prior to the presentation of the disease.[28,31]

REFERENCES

1. Alexander, F. (1950) *Psychosomatic Medicine*. New York: Norton.
2. Andrews, H., Barczak, P. and Allan, R. (1987) Psychiatric illness in patients with inflammatory bowel disease. *Gut*, **28**, 1600–1604.
3. Cann, P.A., Read, N.W., Cammack, J. *et al*. (1983) Psychological stress and the passage of a standard meal through the stomach and small intestine in man. *Gut*, **24**, 236–240.
4. Cohn, E.M., Lederman, I.I. and Shore, E. (1970) Regional enteritis and its relation to emotional disorders. *American Journal of Gastroenterology*, **54**, 378–387.
5. Drossman, D.A. (1986) The psychosocial aspects of inflammatory bowel disease. *Stress Medicine*, **12**, 119–128.
6. Engel, G.L. (1954) Studies of ulcerative colitis: I Clinical data bearing on the nature of the somatic process. *Psychosomatic Medicine*, **16**, 496–501.
7. Engel, G.L. (1955) Studies of ulcerative colitis: III The nature of the psychologic process. *American Journal of Medicine*, **9**, 231–256.
8. Engel, G.L. (1958) Studies of ulcerative colitis: V Psychological aspects and their implications for treatment. *American Journal of Digestive Diseases*, **3**, 315–337.
9. Feldman, F., Cantor, D., Soll, S. and Bachrach, W. (1967) Psychiatric study of a consecutive series of 34 patients with ulcerative colitis. *British Medical Journal*, **3**, 14–17.
10. Feldman, F., Cantor, D., Soll, S. and Bachrach, W. (1967) Psychiatric study of a consecutive series of 19 patients with regional ileitis. *British Medical Journal*, **4**, 711–714.
11. Ford, C.V., Glober, G.A. and Castelnuova-Tedesco, P. (1969) A psychiatric study of patients with regional enteritis. *Journal of The American Medical Association*, **208**, 311–315.
12. Fullerton, D.T., Kollar, E.J. and Caldwell, A.B. (1962) A clinical study of ulcerative colitis. *Journal of the American Medical Association*, **181**, 463–471.
13. Goldberg, D. (1970) A psychiatric study of patients with diseases of the small intestine. *Gut*, **11**, 459–465.
14. Grace, W.J. (1953) Life stress and regional enteritis. *Gastroenterology*, **23**, 542–553.
15. Helzer, J.E., Stillings, W.A., Chammas, S., Norland, C.C. and Alpers, D.H. (1982) A controlled study of the association between ulcerative colitis and psychiatric diagnoses. *Digestive Diseases and Sciences*, **27**, 513–518.
16. Helzer, J.E., Chammas, S., Norland, C.C., Stillings, W.A. and Alpers, D.H. (1984) A study of the association between Crohn's disease and psychiatric illness. *Gastroenterology*, **86**, 324–350.
17. Karush, A., Daniels, G., O'Connor, J.F. and Stern, L.O. (1968) The response to psychotherapy in chronic ulcerative colitis. I Pretreatment factors. *Psychosomatic Medicine*, **30**, 255–276.
18. Karush, A., Daniels, G., O'Connor, J.F. and Stern, L.O. (1969) The response to psychotherapy in chronic ulcerative colitis. II Factors arising from the therapeutic situation. *Psychosomatic Medicine*, **31**, 201–226.
19. Karush, A., Daniels, G., Flood, C. and O'Connor, J.F. (1977) *Psychotherapy in Chronic Ulcerative Colitis*. Philadelphia: W.B. Saunders.

20. Latimer, P.R. (1978) Crohn's disease: a review of the psychological and social outcome. *Psychological Medicine*, **8**, 649–656.
21. Latimer, P., Sarna, S., Campbell, D., Latimer, M., Waterfall, W. and Daniel, E.E. (1981) Colonic motor and myoelectrical activity: a comparative study of normal subjects, psychoneurotic patients and patients with irritable bowel syndrome. *Gastroenterology*, **80**, 893–901.
22. Lindemann, E. (1945) Psychiatric problems in conservative treatment of ulcerative colitis. *Archives of Neurology and Psychiatry*, **53**, 322–325.
23. McKegney, F.P., Gordon, R.O. and Levine, S.M. (1970) A psychosomatic comparison of patients with ulcerative colitis and Crohn's disease. *Psychosomatic Medicine*, **32**, 153–166.
24. Mendeloff, A.L., Monk, M., Siegel, C.I. and Lilienfeld, A. (1970) Illness experience and life stresses in patients with irritable colon and with ulcerative colitis. *New England Journal of Medicine*, **282**, 14–17.
25. Prior, P., Gyde, S., Cooke, W.T., Waterhouse, J.A.H. and Allan, R.N. (1981) Mortality in Crohn's disease. *Gastroenterology*, **80**, 307–312.
26. Prugh, D.G. (1951) The influence of emotional factors on the clinical course of ulcerative colitis in children. *Gastroenterology*, **18**, 339–354.
27. Shaw, L. and Ehrlich, A. (1987) Relaxation training as a treatment for chronic pain caused by ulcerative colitis. *Pain*, **29**, 287–293.
28. Sheffield, B.F. and Carney, M.W.P. (1976) Crohn's disease: A psychosomatic illness? *British Journal of Psychiatry*, **128**, 446–450.
29. Sloan, W.P., Bargen, J.A. and Gage, R.P. (1968) Life histories of patients with chronic ulcerative colitis: A review of 2,000 cases. *Gastroenterology*, **54**, 819–822.
30. Strang, P.J. (1989) Gastrointestinal Disorders. In *Psychosomatic Medicine: Theory, Physiology and Practice*, Vol. 2, pp. 427–502. (Ed.) Cheren, S. Madison, Connecticut: International Universities Press.
31. Tarter, R.E., Switala, J., Carra, J. and Edwards, K.L. (1987) Inflammatory bowel disease: Psychiatric status of patients before and after disease onset. *International Journal of Psychiatry and Medicine*, **17**, 173–181.
32. Weiner, H. (1977) *Psychobiology and Human Disease*, pp. 495–574. New York: Elsevier North-Holland.
33. Whybrow, F.C., Kane, F.J. and Lipton, M.A. (1968) Regional ileitis and psychiatric disorder. *Psychosomatic Medicine*, **30**, 209–219.

APPENDICITIS AND APPENDICECTOMY

Appendicectomy, the most common emergency abdominal operation, is recognized as probably unnecessary from the surgical standpoint in the 20–40% of patients (mainly younger females) who have a histologically normal appendix.[4,8,11,13] Whilst a radical surgical approach with operation in over 80% of possible appendicitis presentations may be preferable to a conservative (60%) strategy in terms of less subsequent morbidity and a lower rate of pain recurrence,[9] over half of the patients who have a normal appendix removed continued to suffer clinically significant episodes of unexplained abdominal pain,[6,10] and frequently require readmission.[12] Psychological factors are clearly implicated.

Life events

The role of life events in the precipitation of physical illness is complex and difficult to substantiate,[7] but in the case of appendicectomy for possible acute appendicitis, the frequency of the presentation, the demarcation of the event and the availability of histological confirmation have enabled this contribution to be investigated. Creed reported findings on 119 appendicectomy patients, subdivided into histologically confirmed acute appendicitis and normals (which included lymphoid hyperplasia and chronic inflammatory changes) and compared against a community sample.[6]

Whilst there was no difference among the groups in the frequency of occurrence of any life event, those that were threatening to the individual, i.e. subject focused, were reported much more often in both appendicectomy groups compared with the general population, and severe, lasting threats were particularly associated with the normal appendix subgroup (*Figure 10.3*).

Personality factors and mental disorder

Creed also found 32% of the normal appendix subgroup reported recent psychiatric symptoms, compared to 16% in both the acute appendicitis subgroup and the community sample.[6] An earlier study claimed that 83% of young women who had a normal appendix removed were considered (independently) to have an emotional problem against 17% of those found to have an acute inflammation,[10] whereas Barraclough noted that the subgroup of women who experienced persistent pain were more anxious than those with acute appendicitis or presenting with a single acute attack.[3] Women who have a normal appendix removed have a stronger somatic orientation and greater use of denial when matched against depressed women.[5] They are also more likely to deliberately harm themselves[12,15] and to have subsequent psychiatric contact.[14,15] Men who have a histologically normal appendix removed are also likely to be psychologically abnormal, with high levels of anxiety.[2]

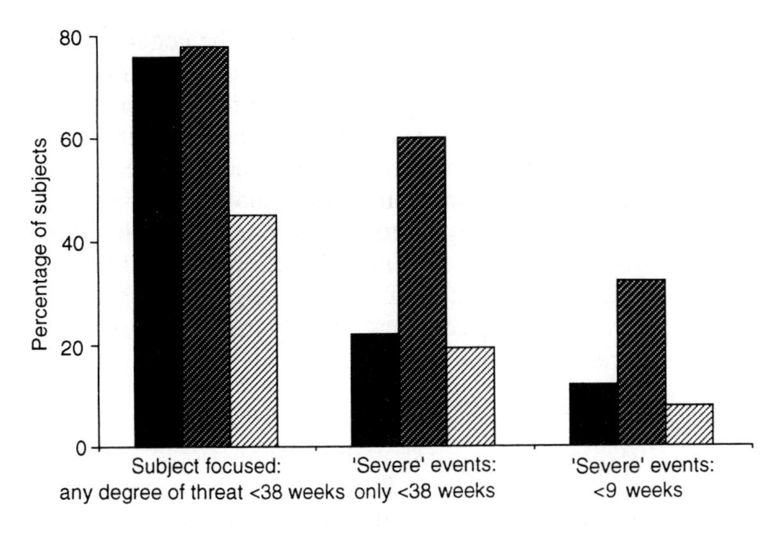

Figure 10.3 Proportion of subjects experiencing a life event: ■ appendix acutely inflamed; ▨ appendix not acutely inflamed; ▨ community comparison group.

Psychoimmunology

Appendicectomy patients confirmed as having acute appendicitis also experienced more adverse life events.[6] Stress and abnormal mental states have diverse effects upon the immune system, including increased susceptibility to acute infection and hypertrophy of lymphoid tissue.[1]

REFERENCES

1. Baker, G.H.B. (1987) Psychological factors and immunity. *Journal of Psychosomatic Research*, **31**, 1–10.
2. Barraclough, B. (1967) Appendicectomy in men. *Journal of Psychosomatic Research*, **11**, 203–206.
3. Barraclough, B. (1968) Appendicectomy in women. *Journal of Psychosomatic Research*, **12**, 231–234.
4. Boerema, W.J., Burnand, K.G. and Fitzpatrick, R.I. (1981) Acute appendicitis. *Australia New Zealand Journal of Surgery*, **51**, 165–168.
5. Canton, G., Santonastosa, P. and Fraccon, I.G. (1984) Life events, abnormal illness behaviour and appendicectomy. *General Hospital Psychiatry*, **6**, 191–195.
6. Creed, F. (1981) Life events and appendicectomy. *The Lancet*, **1**, 1381–1385.
7. Creed, F. (1985) Life events and physical illness. *Journal of Psychosomatic Research*, **29**, 113–123.
8. Harding, H.E. (1962) A notable source of error in the diagnosis of apppendicitis. *British Medical Journal*, **2**, 1028–1029.
9. Howie, J.G.R. (1968) The place of appendicectomy in the treatment of young adult patients with possible appendicitis. *The Lancet*, **1**, 1365–1367.
10. Ingram, P.W. and Evans, G. (1965) Right iliac fossa pain in young women. *British Medical Journal*, **2**, 149–151.
11. Jess, P., Bjerregaard, B., Brynitz, S., Holst-Christensen, J., Kalaja, E. and Lund-Kristensen, J. (1981) Acute appendicitis: prospective trial concerning diagnostic accuracy and complications. *American Journal of Surgery*, **141**, 232–234.
12. Joyce, P.R., Walshe, J.W.B., Bushnell, J.A. and Morton, J.B. (1981) Readmission to hospital after appendicectomy for non-specific abdominal pain. *Australia New Zealand Journal of Surgery*, **51**, 465–476.
13. Lee, J.A.K. (1961) Appendicitis in young women. *The Lancet*, **2**, 815–817.
14. Rang, E.H., Fairburn, A.S. and Acheson, E.D. (1970) An enquiry into the incidence and prognosis of undiagnosed abdominal pain treated in hospital. *British Journal of Preventative and Social Medicine*, **24**, 47–51.
15. Vassilas, C.A. (1988) Parasuicide and appendicectomy. *British Journal of Psychiatry*, **152**, 706–709.

ABDOMINAL PAIN WITH NO EXPLANATORY DISEASE

DEFINITION

This presentation defies classification and understanding in spite of its frequency. The terminology reflects the uncertainty – 'functional', 'non-specific', 'non-organic', 'psychogenic' and 'unexplained' – all apparently referring to the same condition(s), yet each having rather different connotations.

Even the most frequently used term, 'functional', has two distinct meanings. In the gastroenterological sense it applies to disruption of the function rather than the structure of the gut. Yet in its psychodynamic usage functional means how the symptom serves to develop or maintain the individual, and this indeed is a key concept in categorizing psychogenic/idiopathic pain disorders.[24,59]

Nevertheless what is at the core of this confusion is simple – a presentation of abdominal pain, acute or chronic, which fails to yield a physical diagnosis following investigation. Thus it is a retrospective diagnosis made by the exclusion of potentially causative diseases and, no doubt, covering 'a motley collection of conditions'.[15] The description *abdominal pain without explanatory disease* will be preferred for this section. (See also Chronic Functional Abdominal Pain.)

PREVALENCE

Community (*Table 10.10*)

Two major surveys of bowel-related symptoms among the general population reported a high prevelance of functional disorder, with approximately one in three adults significantly affected, and one in four or five experiencing recurrent episodes of abdominal pain.[20,64] Upper abdominal pain is equally common in the adult community with a 38% prevalence of dyspepsia over a 6-month period, of whom three-quarters experienced upper abdominal pain.[38] Interestingly 20% of the sample had either had a barium meal or endoscopy but only 7% claimed to have had peptic ulceration. About one in seven schoolchildren experience recurrent abdominal pain which rarely has an organic cause.[21]

General practice

An audit of 150 consecutive patients with abdominal pain presenting in general practice reported that 89% were managed exclusively by the general practitioner, and over half of these received nothing more than advice or reassurance (i.e. no prescription).[22] Of the remaining 17 patients, 8 were referred to outpatient clinics (2 being psychiatric) and 9 were referred as abdominal emergencies, of whom 3 actually underwent surgery. The diagnosis made by the general practitioner was gastrointestinal in just over half of the cases (56%); unknown, gynaecological, psychiatric and probably viral conditions accounted for most of the remainder.

Hospital practice

Acute/emergency (*Table 10.11*)

As *Table 10.11* illustrates, almost half of all acute or emergency presentations of abdominal pain to hospital are considered to be without explanatory disease.[15,67] This finding is geographically stable.[15]

Chronic/routine outpatients

Most of the surveys of functional presentations in gastroenterological outpatient practice do not delineate types of presentation, but it is probable that pain will frequently be an important feature. The data of Harvey *et al.* (see *Table 10.8*) are sufficiently detailed to enable an estimate of frequency to be reached by combining the three categories that involved pain foremost (abdominal pain with altered bowel habit, endoscopy-negative dyspepsia and predominant depression with abdominal pain); these accounted for 576 (31%) of referrals.[32]

Table 10.10 Prevalence of abdominal pain without explanatory disease: community

Authors	*Source*	*Definition of pain*	*Number of subjects*	*Prevalence (%)*
Thompson and Heaton[64]	UK	>6 attacks/year	301	21
Drossman *et al.*[20]	USA	>6 attacks/year	789	24
Jones and Lydeard[38]	UK	'Indigestion' for more than a few days/6 months	2066	29 (38% including heartburn)

Table 10.11 Prevalence of abdominal pain without explanatory disease: hospital acute/emergency

Authors	*Source*	*Definition of pain*	*Number of subjects*	*Prevalence (%)*
Wilson *et al.*[67]	UK	<1 week's duration	1196	46
De Dombal[15]	Ten countries	<1 week's duration	6097	43

CAUSES

It is certain that abdominal pain without explanatory disease is a common end-point of diverse processes and causes. It is also evident that simplistic, single-element solutions are unusual; recent work has begun to unravel some of the relationships among factors.

Organic conditions

Gray and Collin's review of acute presentations listed a range of physical possibilities – worm infestation, viral and bacterial infections, lactose intolerance, gynaecological disorders, abdominal wall disorders such as hernia, haematoma and shingles, and rarer causes such as 'discitis', abdominal epilepsy and abdominal migraine.[30] Their conclusion was that most adult presentations were attributable to these and other minor self-limiting causes, psychological factors only being significant where recurrent episodes of pain linked to psychological pressures were apparent from childhood.

Serious disease may be subsequently detected. This is rare among children, with only 3 of 161 children with recurrent, severe, abdominal pain developing disease (all inflammatory bowel diseases) during 5 years' follow-up.[58] However, around 10% of presentations in adults over 50 years of age are subsequently found to be linked to malignant disease, most frequently sited in the large bowel.[16,37,53]

Finally putative organic disorders have been inferred from isolated physical findings such as pyrexia, a raised leukocyte count or erythrocyte sedimentation rate, and patients with such non-specific anomalies appear to have less abnormal psychological characteristics when compared with patients who have no potential physical cause for their unexplained abdominal pain.[39]

Psychiatric illness

Medical outpatient surveys of functional gastrointestinal presentations have reported current or previous psychiatric illness in about half the subjects,[25,44] whilst 64% of patients in another sample were rated as depressed.[55] In a prospective study of chronic, non-specific, abdominal pain, 8 of 20 cases were believed to be attributable to psychiatric disorder, and in view of this the authors recommend psychiatric evaluation as a routine component of assessment.[68]

Various psychiatric conditions are associated with abdominal pain without explanatory disease. After excluding obvious diseases detected at initial clinical examination, a series of 96 patients with recurrent or persistent abdominal pain presented to either surgical or gastrointestinal clinics were carefully evaluated by psychiatrists.[29] The diagnoses made were the following: depression (n = 31), chronic tension (21), hysteria (17), gastrointestinal disease (15) and alcoholism (12). Patients with depression or organic disorders were significantly older than the others; patients with alcoholism or organic disorders were predominantly male whilst there was a preponderance of females in the other categories; finally it was notable that early experiences and family patterning of illness were considered aetiologically important in 75% of cases. In patients with unexplained upper abdominal pain, levels of anxiety and tension were greater than those found in peptic ulcer patients, but the groups could not be distinguished in terms of neuroticism, suppression of affect or degree of depression.[43]

Finally psychiatric patients frequently present with, or complain of, pain that is psychogenic in origin. The abdomen is the third most common site following the head and back among acute presentations, and also among chronic pain presentations in which multiple sites are frequent.[46,60]

Life events

The relationship between adverse life events and acute abdominal pain leading to appendicectomy has been delineated (see page 1534), but the technical difficulties associated with this field of research have limited the validity of findings across the spectrum of presentations of abdominal pain without explanatory disease.[4] Concerning recurrences of pain among chronic attenders, Bouchier and Mason reported that half their sample had exacerbations of their complaints in relation to problems in their environment, whilst solution of these problems alleviated their symptoms.[8] However, others have noted that life events did not predict the course of their patients' conditions.[57] Ford and colleagues found that recent adverse life events were reported by 30% of both their functional and organic groups, and concluded that it was not the life event in itself that was crucial, but rather whether the anxiety-provoking situation actually succeeded in generating an anxiety disorder.[25]

However, the most extensive work indicates that both mental disorders and life events are linked to functional abdominal presentations. *Table 10.12* summarizes data combined from three separate investigations.[14] In the community samples and those with organic conditions, subjects found to have

Table 10.12 The relationship between functional/organic abdominal pain or deliberate self-harm, and psychiatric illness and adverse life events

Group	*Number of subjects*	*Chronic difficulties (%)*	*Severe chronic difficulties (%)*	*Psychiatric illness (%)*	*Severe difficulties and psychiatric illness (%)*	*Severe difficulties without psychiatric illness (%)*
Appendicectomy						
Normal appendix	56	38	30	14	78	53
Appendicitis	63	24	13	3	40	25
Normal	62	16	8	3	40	16
Gastrointestinal outpatients with abdominal pain						
Functional	79	47	38	34	70	65
Organic	56	27	11	16	67	17
Normal	135	16	4	8	64	11
Deliberate self-harm	82	32	29	46	68	73

From Creed *et al.*[14]

psychiatric disorders were likely to have experienced adverse life events, as would be anticipated. Notably severe life difficulties occurred frequently in the functional and para-suicide groups in subjects who were not mentally ill, a finding that fits with the concept of somatization of emotional distress.

Studies of children with recurrent abdominal pain confirm that they experience more adverse life events than healthy controls and indeed are similar in this respect to behaviourally disturbed children.[33,54] There is some evidence that these children are more frequently exposed to deaths, illnesses or hospitalization in their family.[33]

Personality traits/illness behaviour

Drossman followed up 24 patients with psychogenic abdominal pain for 6 years and reported abnormal core personality styles in 60% – these were a mixture of histrionic, depressive, hypochondriacal and 'pain-prone' traits.[18] In a larger, controlled study examining what differentiated irritable bowel syndrome sufferers who sought medical treatment from the pool of individuals in the community with the same symptoms, he reported that patient status was primarily associated with pain and diarrhoea; when these symptoms were controlled the patient group was found to suffer more frequently from abnormal personality patterns and accentuated illness behaviours than non-patient irritable bowel syndrome sufferers.[19]

When unexplained upper abdominal pain patients were compared with peptic ulcer patients, the functional group scored higher on personality traits of tension and hostility.[43]

Abnormal illness behaviours, particularly hypochondriasis, somatization and denial, have repeatedly been reported in patients who complain of abnormal pain without explanatory disease.[8,11,18,19,29,39] The conclusion is that many of these patients perceive and act upon symptoms differently from normal, as a consequence of personality traits, previous personal and family illness experiences and predetermined coping responses; hence these are individuals who more often deny, displace or somatize when faced with chronic difficulties or acute stresses in life.

BACKGROUND FACTORS

Age and sex

Investigations into this presentation report an invariable association with female sex and younger age. The peak rates of hospital admission among females were in the three decades between 10 and 40 years of age at 1.6, 1.4 and 1.0 per 1000 population respectively.[53] Among males the pattern differed with peaks of 0.9 per 1000 population at 10–19 and 60–69 years of age.

Physical/sexual abuse

A history of physical abuse by a parent or spouse has been linked to this presentation.[23] The association with previous sexual abuse is intuitively valid, but awaits confirmation.[2,3,26]

Family ill health

Illness in the family may be an important predisposing factor, conditioning how adults cope with life difficulties and precipitating abdominal pain without disease especially in childhood.[29,33]

Appendicectomy (see page 1534)

Patients who have a normal appendix removed for suspected appendicitis often continue to suffer abdominal pain without explanatory disease.[11,13,34,40,53]

Other functional presentations

As might be expected, a past history of somatization involving other sites is not uncommon.[23] Women who suffer pelvic pain without explanatory disease share many of the psychosocial characteristics reported here[56] and gynaecological problems are common in this group.[37,53]

Deliberate self-harm

There is an association between deliberate self-harm and functional abdominal pain, and considerable similarity in the characteristics of the two patient groups.[14,40,65]

Alcohol and drugs

Alcohol or drug abuse may be predisposing factors, although this element may frequently be denied or minimized by the patient.[29]

Psychiatric illness

For details of this factor see page 1537.

PRESENTING FEATURES

General factors that distinguish physical from psychological/behavioural elements in pain presentation[6,47] (*Table 10.13*)

These features apply as much to abdominal pain as to pain in any other site.[28] A further, therapeutic clue is that pain that persists above an opiate dose capable of inducing somnolence is most frequently due to a marked affective component.[45]

Specific issues in abdominal pain without explanatory disease

Character/description

The language of pain is a complex area with conflicting and disputed findings.[35] Three aspects to bear in mind are (1) descriptors; (2) imagery and (3) affect/cognitions.

Table 10.13 The analysis of pain

Factor	*Indicates marked physical elements in a pain state*	*Indicates marked psychological or behavioural elements in a pain state*
Onset	Usually clear cut	Vague Often no precipitant
Nature	Well-recognized characteristics Interferes with sleep	Often poorly described Discrepancy between pain behaviour and severity Sleep often unaffected
Site	Usually recognized by its relation to injury or disease or its site if referred	Ill-defined May occur at site of previous damage More often left than right sided
Increased by	Movement, palpation, etc.	Wide range of stimuli or no stimulus May change markedly with mood
Relieved by	Physical means, e.g. rest, surgery, analgesics	Often unresponsive to any treatment May respond to factors that relieve tension e.g. alcohol
Other features	Psychological factors may be prominent, but are clearly secondary changes, i.e. anxiety/depression develop	Commonly have a premorbid history of mental illness (especially neurotic disorders) or abnormal personality traits evident

From Bond.[6]

DESCRIPTORS

It is most unwise to rely upon the bizarreness of a patient's description of his or her pain as the basis for distinguishing functional from organic complaints. Odd or flamboyant descriptions occur just as frequently in disease, especially when the presentation is acute[17,60] and may be determined by factors such as linguistic ability, previous experience of pain, drugs, the way the questions are phrased by the doctor and the patient's determination that he or she be taken seriously. What is much more characteristic of a non-organic basis is the description of multiple pains, in the same site or different sites, and with distinctly different characteristics.[6,17,28] The use of more than one type of descriptor in chronic pain is associated with greater physical interference, more emotional distress and a poorer treatment response when compared with simply described pains, but this is a correlation rather than a causative relationship.[35]

IMAGERY

The use of imagery to describe abdominal pain was used much more frequently by children and adolescents who had functional pain (78%) than by those suffering from inflammatory bowel disease (23%).[27]

AFFECT/COGNITIONS

The language used to describe pain is powerfully influenced by the degree of emotional distress that is present, and indeed this variable, which of course operates also in organic pain, confounds attempts to relate the type of description to the medical diagnostic category.[42]

Cognitions, essentially the awareness of pain and judgements taken about pain (and its relief), are also powerful factors in determining how pain is experienced and reported. These core attitudes influence not only pain itself, but also mood disturbance and behavioural consequences. It is known that negative cognitions are linked to reported pain severity and concomitant distress: positive cognitions bear no relationship to presenting features.[7] Scales are under development to assess how such attitudes affect the management of pain, and this field holds considerable promise.[7,36]

Severity

Again it is unsafe to rely on exaggerated description of severity to differentiate functional presentations. In general people can rank common pain states in order of intensity with good agreement, but this objective evaluation has to be modified when considering individuals in pain.[9] The perception and reporting of pain severity are influenced by many factors including mood illness (both anxiety and depression), emotional distress and cognitions concerning pain. Most commonly patients who are worried about their condition, or those who perhaps consider that they have not been taken seriously enough, may overstate in this manner; however, individuals whose temperament predisposes to dramatization and overreaction are not immune to gastrointestinal disease. There are two pointers that do aid in distinction – first a marked difference between the reported severity of pain and the level of behavioural impairment,[28] and secondly a tendency for pain in organic conditions to fluctuate in intensity contrasting with the common account of pain of constant severity in functional presentations.[47]

Site

Abdominal pain without explanatory disease can be located anywhere in the abdomen, and may be referred to extra-abdominal sites, most often the back.[49,66] Pain that is diffuse or reported in several sites is characteristic but not invariable, and it should be borne in mind that functional presentations in patients who have had gastrointestinal disease will often be localized to the classic site. Interestingly, colonic distension studies demonstrate that subjects who have functional abdominal pain describe more unusual localization and referral patterns when compared with normal patients.[61] It would appear any part of the gut may be affected and any site on the trunk is possible.[49]

Relieving and exacerbating factors

It is characteristic of functional pain to be relieved or exacerbated either by nothing or by unusual factors. Some examples are the patient who reports pain consistently at work but never during leisure pursuits, who derives no benefit from any drug treatment yet habitually reports plenty of side effects, or who repeatedly indulges in unnecessary behaviour that is reported as exacerbating the pain.

Associated symptoms

Associated symptoms that point towards a disease process include marked anorexia and weight loss, vomiting and blood loss. Scoring systems have been developed for identifying 'high risk' patients who present with dyspepsia and require early investigation, but these have proved too cumbersome and insensitive for routine use.[63] The reverse also holds true in that the presence of many associated symptoms arising in systems other than the gut indicates a functional disorder but is not sufficiently reliable to confirm this. There are two features that are strongly suggestive of a functional basis: first the capacity for sleep to be unaffected by the pain[6,47] and second the denial of emotional experience.[5,24]

Sick role/abnormal illness behaviour

With chronic pain in particular this is an important area where enquiry frequently yields clues as to the origin of the presentation. This fits with the psychological use of the term 'functional', in other words what the patient achieves or gains from his or her pain.

Thus the credits and debits of living in a sick role must be elucidated – and this covers a wide area, e.g. money (including compensation), career, status, social/family/intimate relationships, hobbies/pursuits/interests and life difficulties/crises/events. Of course the patient may either block or mislead such lines of enquiry, for a variety of reasons, ranging from intentional concealment to failing to appreciate the relevance, and if there are doubts or gaps, relatives or other professionals who know the background have to be approached.

The concept and analysis of abnormal illness behaviour have been developed most notably by Pilowsky,[51] who identifies three components, namely the cognitive, behavioural and affective elements of illness.[52] Plainly this sociological–behavioural dimension overlaps considerably with psychological aspects that have already been discussed, and indeed it is not surprising that the level of general illness behaviour correlates with subjective ratings of pain and pain behaviour when other relevant factors including demographic variables and disease status are controlled.[41]

Physical findings

These comprise the following:

1. Either exaggerated or absent pain behaviours and reactions.
2. Either no localizing signs or unusual features such as shifting pain, multiple sites of pain or atypical sites of referral.
3. Changes in the features when the patient is distracted.
4. The closed eyes sign:[12,31] patients who had abdominal pain without explanatory disease more often closed their eyes during abdominal examination, the test having a positive predictive power of 79% and a negative predictive power of 65%.[31] The explanation could be that patients with painful disease keep their eyes open so that they can voluntarily guard as the palpation approaches the tender area: functional patients will have no such fear (*Figure 10.4*).

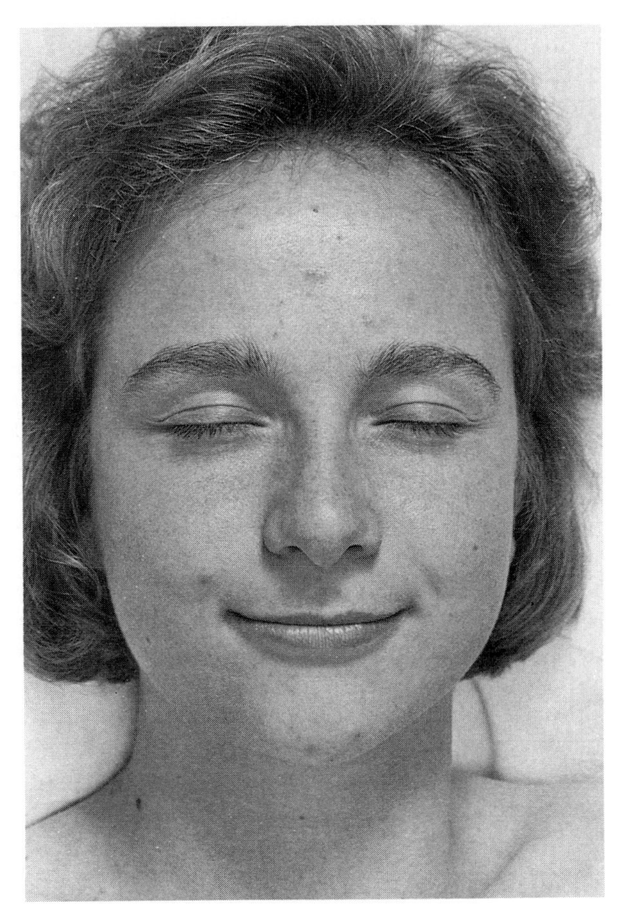

Figure 10.4 The closed eyes sign. The 'patient' shown is actually a medical student simulating the sign.

INVESTIGATIONS

Psychosocial lines of enquiry should not have to wait until an extended series of physical investigations draws a blank. When abdominal pain without explanatory disease is suspected, the physician must embark on obtaining further information about the patient which places the presentation into the life context. This frequently involves enquiries to close relatives and the family practitioner – it takes time but is unavoidable.

There are no hard and fast rules governing the extent or content of physical investigation that is undertaken – this will depend on the clinical features of the case, and the gastroenterologist's personal judgement. In general, the better the psychosocial explanation the less the need to investigate vigorously. Certainly, the frequency with which serious diseases subsequently emerge following presentations among the middle-aged and the elderly[16,37,53] indicates that these patients should not be labelled as having a functional disorder unless there are solid psychosocial grounds – and even then an index of suspicion should remain if this is a first presentation. As older age groups are also more often found to have treatable mental illness, notably depression,[29] a psychiatric assessment or viewpoint may prove particularly valuable in assisting management.

Almost invariably, the gastroenterologist is faced with the dilemma of under-investigating and thereby failing to establish the presence of disease – or over-investigating and thereby reinforcing a maladaptive pattern of behaviour. With non-emergency presentations the solution is to proceed gradually. Four to six weeks of conservative treatment for dyspepsia do not adversely affect the outcome even if there is serious underlying disease,[10] and there is no obvious reason why this policy should not be equally applicable to lower bowel complaints when there are no good grounds for investigation. Of course this may not be welcomed by the patient whose desperation may sway the doctor to investigate against his or her better judgement, but a calm, authoritative approach emphasizing the importance of adequate consideration of the right investigations to establish the correct diagnosis is both truthful and constructive.

TREATMENT

The fundamental point is whether gastroenterologists regard their role as the management of diseases of the gut or disorders of the gut. If they stick to diseases they confine their attention to about half the patients referred to the clinic.[32,48,62] However, if they wish to manage gut disorders, they commit themselves to a hotchpotch of conditions that are frustrating to elucidate and they involve themselves more explicitly with the lives of their patients.[1]

There will be circumstances in which referral to a psychiatrist, clinical psychologist or social worker may not only be the obvious solution, but also proves acceptable to the patient. Although Gomez and Dally reported that 80% of their sample were willing to accept a psychogenic basis for their pain,[29] this seems an unusually high proportion given the well-recognized tendency for patients who somatize, deny or adopt other abnormal illness behaviours, consciously or unconsciously, to reject a psychological explanation and treatment approach.[24] In these circumstances the physician will have to decide how far he or she is competent and able to intervene. The simple function of reassuring the patients, their families and the family practitioners that there is no sinister explanation for the complaint can be a most useful contribution which tends to be overlooked.

Table 10.14 One- to three-year mortality among 427 patients discharged with a diagnosis of unexplained abdominal pain

	Observed	*Expected*	*Odds ratio*
Males	11	0.85	12.9
Females	7	1.92	3.6

From Rang *et al.*[53]

PROGNOSIS

Unexplained abdominal pain affects one in seven children, is best managed along psychological lines and is rarely associated with unidentified disease: over-investigation risks entrenching the condition.[21] A 28-year follow-up of 34 'intractable' childhood cases reported that 18 (53%) continued to have the same complaints in adult life.[50]

In adults with acute presentations requiring hospital admission, 23% of 230 patients had similar presentations during the follow-up period of 5 years.[37] In chronic disorder, a 5- to 7-year follow-up on outpatients with predominantly upper abdominal pain (although 54% were diagnosed as irritable bowel syndrome) reported that a poor outcome was linked to: (1) a low pain threshold, confirmed by an ischaemia test; (2) 'psychic vulnerability'; and (3) poor school and vocational education.[57] Factors that were not predictive included the duration or severity of the pain, bowel habit, associated symptoms, alcohol, smoking, tranquillizer intake, life events and sex, marital state or occupational status.

Among middle-aged and elderly patients the likelihood of underlying disease, especially bowel malignancy, is of the order of 10% in acute presentations of undiagnosed abdominal pain, and about half of these patients remain undiagnosed at discharge.[16,53] As the observed mortality rates indicate, abdominal pain without explanatory disease should be regarded as neither minor nor harmless[53] (*Table 10.14*).

References

1. Alvarez, W.C. (1944) *Nervousness, Indigestion and Pain.* London: William Heinemann.
2. Arnold, R.P., Rogers, D. and Cook, D.A.G. (1990) Medical problems of adults who were sexually abused in childhood. *British Medical Journal*, **300**, 705–708.
3. Bachmann, G.A., Mueller, T.P. and Benett, J. (1986) Childhood sexual abuse and the consequences in adult women. *Obstetrics and Gynaecology*, **7**, 631–642.

4. Bass, C. (1986) Life events and gastrointestinal symptoms. *Gut*, **27**, 123–126.
5. Blumer, D. and Heilbronn, M. (1981) The pain-prone disorder: A clinical and psychological profile. *Psychosomatics*, **22**, 395–402.
6. Bond, M.R. (1984) Pain, emotion and physical symptoms. In *Pain: Its Nature, Analysis and Treatment*, pp. 127–133. Edinburgh: Churchill Livingstone.
7. Boston, K., Pearce, S.A. and Richardson, P.H. (1990) The Pain Cognitions Questionnaire. *Journal of Psychosomatic Research*, **34**, 103–109.
8. Bouchier, I.A.D. and Mason, C.M. (1979) A study of patients with abdominal symptoms of undefined cause. *Scottish Medical Journal*, **24**, 199–205.
9. Brattberg, G., Thorslund, M. and Wikmann, A. (1988) The use of common pain experiences in designing a pain intensity scale for epidemiological purposes. *Journal of Psychosomatic Research*, **32**, 505–512.
10. Brown, C. and Rees, W.D.W. (1990) Dyspepsia in general practice. *British Medical Journal*, **300**, 829–830.
11. Canton, G., Santonastaso, P. and Fraccon, I.G. (1984) Life events, abnormal illness behaviour and appendicectomy. *General Hospital Psychiatry*, **6**, 191–195.
12. Collin, J. and Gray, D.W.R. (1987) The eyes closed sign. *British Medical Journal*, **295**, 1656.
13. Creed, F. (1981) Life events and appendicectomy. *The Lancet*, **1**, 1381–1385.
14. Creed, F., Craig, T. and Farmer, R. (1988) Functional abdominal pain, psychiatric illness and life events. *Gut*, **29**, 235–242.
15. De Dombal, F.T. (1979) Acute abdominal pain – an OMGE survey. *Scandinavian Journal of Gastroenterology*, suppl. 56, 29–43.
16. De Dombal, F.T., Mathan, S.A., Staniland, J.R. *et al.* (1980) Presentation of cancer to hospital as 'acute abdominal pain'. *British Journal of Surgery*, **67**, 413–416.
17. Devine, R. and Merskey, H. (1965) The description of pain in psychiatric and general medical patients. *Journal of Psychosomatic Research*, **9**, 311–316.
18. Drossman, D.A. (1982) Patients with psychogenic abdominal pain: Six years observation in the medical setting. *American Journal of Psychiatry*, **139**, 1549–1557.
19. Drossman, D.A., McKee, D.C., Sandler, R.S. *et al.* (1988) Psychosocial factors in the irritable bowel syndrome. *Gastroenterology*, **95**, 701–708.
20. Drossman, D.A., Sandler, R.S., McKee, D.C. and Lovitz, A.J. (1982) Bowel patterns among subjects not seeking health care. *Gastroenterology*, **83**, 529–534.
21. Editorial (1980) Recurrent abdominal pain in childhood. *British Medical Journal*, **280**, 1096–1097.
22. Edwards, M.W., Forman, W.M. and Walton, J. (1985) Audit of abdominal pain in general practice. *Journal of the Royal College of General Practitioners*, **35**, 235–238.
23. Eisendrath, S.J., Way, L.W., Ostroff, J.W. and Johansen, C.A. (1986) Identification of psychogenic abdominal pain. *Psychosomatics*, **27**, 705–710.
24. Ford, C.V. (1984) Chronic pain syndromes. In *The Somatizing Disorders*, pp. 98–126. New York: Elsevier Biomedical.
25. Ford, M.J., Miller, P.M., Eastwood, J. and Eastwood, M.A. (1987) Life events, psychiatric illness and the irritable bowel syndrome. *Gut*, **28**, 160–165.
26. Fry, R. and Wallis, R. (1990) Medical problems of adults who were sexually abused in childhood (correspondence). *British Medical Journal*, **300**, 941–942.
27. Geist, R. (1989) Use of imagery to describe functional abdominal pain as an aid to diagnosis in a pediatric population. *Canadian Journal of Psychiatry*, **34**, 506–511.
28. Glaser, J.P. and Engel, G.L. (1977) Psychodynamics, psychophysiology and gastrointestinal symptomatology. *Clinics in Gastroenterology*, **6**, 507–531.
29. Gomez, J. and Dally, P. (1977) Psychologically mediated abdominal pain in surgical and medical outpatient clinics. *British Medical Journal*, **1**, 1451–1453.
30. Gray, D.W.R. and Collin, J. (1987) Non-specific abdominal pain as a cause of acute hospital admission. *British Journal of Surgery*, **74**, 239–242.
31. Gray, D.W.R., Dixon, J.M. and Collin, J. (1988) The closed eyes sign: an aid to diagnosing non-specific abdominal pain. *British Medical Journal*, **297**, 837.
32. Harvey, R.F., Salih, S.Y. and Read, A.E. (1983) Organic and functional disorders in 2,000 gastroenterology outpatients. *The Lancet*, **1**, 632–634.
33. Hodges, K., Kline, J.J., Barbero, G. and Flanery, R. (1984) Life events occurring in families of children with recurrent abdominal pain. *Journal of Psychosomatic Research*, **28**, 185–188.
34. Howie, J.G.R. (1968) The place of appendicectomy in the treatment of young adults with possible appendicitis. *The Lancet*, **1**, 1365–1367.
35. Jamison, R.N., Vasterling, J.J. and Parris, W.C.V. (1987) Use of sensory descriptors in assessing chronic pain patients. *Journal of Psychosomatic Research*, **31**, 647–652.
36. Jensen, M.P., Karoly, P. and Huger, R. (1987) The development and preliminary validation of an instrument to assess patients' attitudes towards pain. *Journal of Psychosomatic Research*, **31**, 393–400.
37. Jess, P., Bjerregaard, B., Brynitz, S. *et al.* (1982) Prognosis of acute non-specific abdominal pain. *American Journal of Surgery*, **144**, 338–340.
38. Jones, R. and Lydeard, S. (1989) Prevalence of symptoms of dyspepsia in the community. *British Medical Journal*, **298**, 30–32.
39. Joyce, P.R., Bushnell, J.A., Walshe, J.W.B. and Morton, J.B. (1986) Abnormal illness behaviour

and anxiety in acute non-organic abdominal pain. *British Journal of Psychiatry*, **149**, 57–62.
40. Joyce, P.R., Walshe, J.W.B., Bushnell, J.A. and Morton, J.B. (1981) Readmissions to hospital after appendicectomy for non-specific pain. *Australian and New Zealand Journal of Surgery*, **51**, 465–467.
41. Keefe, F.J., Crisson, J.E., Maltbie, A., Bradley, L. and Gilk, M. (1986) Illness behaviour as a predictor of pain and overt pain behaviour patterns in chronic low back pain patients. *Journal of Psychosomatic Research*, **30**, 543–551.
42. Kremer, E.F. and Atkinson, J.H. (1984) Pain language: affect. *Journal of Psychosomatic Research*, **28**, 125–132.
43. Langeluddecke, P., Goulston, K. and Tennant, C. (1990) Psychological factors in dyspepsia of unknown cause: A comparison with peptic ulcer disease. *Journal of Psychosomatic Research*, **34**, 215–222.
44. MacDonald, A.J. and Bouchier, I.A.D. (1980) Non-organic gastrointestinal illness: a medical and psychiatric study. *British Journal of Psychiatry*, **136**, 276–283.
45. Melzack, R., Ofiesh, G. and Mount, B.M. (1976) The Brompton mixture: effects on pain in cancer patients. *Canadian Medical Association Journal*, **115**, 125–129.
46. Merskey, H. (1965) Psychiatric patients with persistent pain. *Journal of Psychosomatic Research*, **9**, 299–309.
47. Merskey, H. (1968) Psychological aspects of pain. *Postgraduate Medicine*, **44**, 297–306.
48. Mitchell, C.M. and Drossman, D.A. (1987) Survey of the AGA membership relating to patients with functional gastrointestinal disorders. *Gastroenterology*, **92**, 1282–1284.
49. Moriarty, K.J. and Dawson, A.M. (1982) Functional abdominal pain: further evidence that whole gut is affected. *British Medical Journal*, **284**, 1670–1672.
50. Nicol, A.R. (1982) Psychogenic abdominal pain in childhood. *British Journal of Hospital Medicine,* **27**, 351–353.
51. Pilowsky, I. (1978) A general classification of abnormal illness behaviour. *British Journal of Medical Psychology*, **51**, 131–137.
52. Pilowsky, I. (1984) Illness behaviour. In *Textbook of Pain*, pp. 767–775. (Ed.) Wall, P.D. and Melzack, R. Edinburgh: Churchill Livingstone.
53. Rang, E.H., Fairburn, A.S. and Acheson, E.D. (1970) An inquiry into the incidence and prognosis of undiagnosed abdominal pain treated in hospital. *British Journal of Preventative and Social Medicine,* **24**, 47–51.
54. Robinson, J.O., Alvarez, J.H. and Dodge, J.A. (1990) Life events and family history in children with recurrent abdominal pain. *Journal of Psychosomatic Research*, **34**, 171–181.
55. Rose, J.D.R., Troughton, A.H., Harvey, J.S. and Smith, P.M. (1986) Depression and functional bowel disorders in gastrointestinal patients. *Gut*, **27**, 1025–1028.
56. Slocumb, J.C., Kellner, R., Rosenfeld, R.C. and Pathak, D. (1989) Anxiety and depression in patients with abdominal pelvic pain syndrome. *General Hospital Psychiatry*, **11**, 48–53.
57. Sloth, H. and Jorgensen, L.S. (1989) Predictors for the course of chronic non-organic upper abdominal pain. *Scandinavian Journal of Gastroenterology*, **24** 440–444.
58. Stickler, G.B. and Murphy, D.B. (1979) Recurrent abdominal pain. *American Journal of Diseases in Children*, **133**, 486–489.
59. Stoudemire, A. and Sandhu, J. (1987) Psychogenic/idiopathic pain syndromes. *General Hospital Psychiatry*, **9**, 79–86.
60 Spear, F.G. (1967) Pain in psychiatric patients. *Journal of Psychosomatic Research*, **11**, 187–193.
61. Swarbrick, E.T., Hegarty, J.E., Bat, L., Williams, C.B. and Dawson, A.M. (1980) Site of pain from the irritable bowel. *The Lancet*, **2**, 443–446.
62. Switz, D.M. (1976) What the gastroenterologist does all day. *Gastroenterology*, **70**, 1048–1050.
63. Talley, N.J., McNeil, D. and Piper, D.W. (1987) Discriminant value of dyspepsia symptoms: a study of the clinical presentation of 221 patients with dyspepsia of unknown cause, peptic ulceration and cholelithiasis. *Gut*, **28**, 40–46.
64. Thompson, W.G. and Heaton, K.W. (1980) Functional bowel disorders in apparently healthy people. *Gastroenterology*, **79**, 283–288.
65. Vassilas, C.A. (1988) Parasuicide and appendicectomy. *British Journal of Psychiatry*, **152**, 706–709.
66. Waller, S.L. and Misiewicz, J.J. (1969) Prognosis in the irritable-bowel syndrome. *The Lancet*, **2**, 753–756.
67. Wilson, D.H., Wilson, R.G., Walmsley, R.G., Horrocks, J.C. and De Dombal, F.T. (1977) Diagnosis of acute abdominal pain in the accident and emergency department. *British Journal of Surgery*, **64**, 250–254.
68. Woodhouse, C.R.J. and Bochner, S. (1979) Chronic abdominal pain: A surgical or psychiatric symptom? *British Journal of Surgery*, **66**, 348–349.

ENCOPRESIS

DEFINITION

Functional encopresis is the passage of faeces in inappropriate places occurring past the time that bowel control is physiologically possible and after toilet training should have been accomplished, which is taken to be a chronological and mental age of 4 years.[1] Soiling can be involuntary or intentional. If faecal continence has been present for over 1 year the encopresis is categorized as secondary: if not it is primary.[1]

Other types of functional faecal soiling occur, for instance, due to: (1) lack of toilet training; (2) functional constipation with overflow or leakage; (3) emotionally induced diarrhoea; and (4) anal masturbation (digital insertion for pleasure or comfort), and these are sometimes included under the rubric of encopresis.[6,7]

EPIDEMIOLOGY

Encopresis occurs in 1–2% of 5 year olds, the prevalence declining through childhood.[5,6,8,9] It is very rare beyond mid-adolescence. There is a male:female ratio of 3–6:1,[6,8,9] and there may be an association with lower social class[6,9] – but not with family size.[9]

CAUSES

Emotional disorders

The most common basis for encopresis is an emotional problem within the family in which a power struggle develops between the child and parents over issues of autonomy and control, leading to 'the battle of the bowel'.[6,8] The child may have had sluggish bowels and the parents have a preoccupation with regular bowel motions, but the key point appears to be toilet training where a coercive or anxiety-tinged approach establishes bowel control that is precarious and associated with fear, and hence liable to break down under stress. Frequently it is difficult to tease out cause from consequence, because encopresis generates considerable pressure on the child and family – embarrassment, shame, rejection, hostility, 'accusatory cross-fire', all commonly occurring. Where there is a clear-cut precipitant to which the child is reacting, the prognosis is excellent provided it is caught before the family conflicts over the issue become established.[6] Sometimes encopresis can be the expression of what is in effect a phobia of toilets, particularly a social phobia in relation to defaecating in a school toilet.[6,8,9]

Neurophysiological/developmental disorders

Features of developmental delay or difficulties that are associated with encopresis include easy distractibility, short attention span, low frustration tolerance, hyperactivity and poor coordination.[6] In a few patients brain damage or syndromes associated with mental impairment have been reported.[2,3]

Inadequate toilet training

This cause is invariably associated with primary encopresis and is characterized by the child regarding his or her behaviour as normal and therefore displaying no anxiety or shame.

CLINICAL FEATURES

How and where faeces are deposited varies considerably from child to child. Sometimes the behaviour suggests that the child is elaborating or exploiting the situation, e.g. by placing faeces in the parental bed, smearing faeces on the furniture or by making 'special parcels'.[6,7] More complex (and hostile) behaviour points to an emotional basis and sometimes to its nature. Passage of stools of normal consistency also indicates a functional basis, and aids in the exclusion of organic disorders. However, most encopretic individuals have some degree of faecal retention at least occasionally, while 70% of children with functional constipation are encopretic.[5] This considerable overlap means many encopretic individuals present with overflow incontinence, having liquid stools, hard faecal masses on abdominal palpation and local complications such as faecal impaction and anal fissure. Abdominal pain is commonly reported in the early stages but not later because tolerance develops to colonic distension.[9] Loss of appetite and poor weight gain are other features of established encopresis,[5] and 15–25% of patients also have enuresis.[6,8,9]

DIFFERENTIAL DIAGNOSIS

Organic causes of soiling and constipation must be excluded; the list of possibilities is long.[5] These are more likely when the soiling is simple, the stool is not normally formed, toilet training has been straightforward, and emotional problems in the child and family are fairly inapparent.

The important conditions to exclude are the following:

1. A ganglionic megacolon, in which the child has an empty rectum and no desire to defaecate, rarely soils, has marked failure to thrive, constipation from birth (in the congenital form) and commonly experiences abdominal pain.
2. Local causes of constipation such as anal stenosis or fissure.
3. Diarrhoea as a presenting symptom of (most often) infective or inflammatory bowel disease.
4. Endocrine disorders, notably hypothyroidism.
5. Neurological disorders.

6. Psychiatric disorders, notably depression.
7. Drugs, including tricyclic antidepressants that are frequently prescribed in the treatment of enuresis.[4]

TREATMENT

Successful management combines to varying degrees behavioural, medical, counselling and psychotherapeutic elements.[6–9] The behavioural strategy relies upon positive reinforcement of appropriate defaecation in place of punishment of encopresis. The type of reward depends upon the child's age but the goal is always the restoration of normal bowel habit.

The medical strategy is aimed at re-establishing normal bowel tone and function, and may involve enemas, suppositories and/or laxatives with a brief spell of inpatient care for intensive treatment in the more severe and persistent cases. Where enuresis coexists this should not be treated with tricyclic antidepressants. Invariably the parents require counselling to defuse the tensions, recriminations and hostility which otherwise block recovery. Psychotherapy which is frequently family-focused tackles the underlying issues upon the basis that encopresis is not the problem, but rather a symptom of the problem.

PROGNOSIS

The outcome is usually very good when treatment can be properly instituted. Unfortunately this is not always possible, parents' powerful negative emotions engulfing their medical helpers and setting off fresh areas of conflict, or their urgency failing to give treatment sufficient opportunity. An external locus of control in the child (in other words the attitude that what happens is due to fate, luck or other people but not to themselves), the absence of a precipitating stress and the presence of nocturnal encopresis are predictors of a poor response.[6,8,10]

REFERENCES

1. American Psychiatric Association (1987) *Diagnostic and Statistical Manual of Mental Disorders*, 3rd edn – revised, pp. 82–84. Washington DC: American Psychiatric Association.
2. Carpenter, S.P.C. (1989) Development of a young man with Prader–Willi syndrome and secondary functional encopresis. *Canadian Journal of Psychiatry*, **34**, 123–127.
3. Dedman, P. and Numa, S. (1986) A case of parietal lobe atrophy. *British Journal of Psychiatry*, **148**, 725–726.
4. Foxman, B., Valdez, R.B. and Brook, R.H. (1986) Childhood enuresis: Prevalence, perceived impact and prescribed treatments. *Pediatrics*, **77**, 482–487.
5. Hatch, T.F. (1988) Encopresis and constipation in children. *Pediatric Clinics of North America*, **35**, 257–280.
6. Hersov, L. (1985) Faecal soiling. In *Child and Adolescent Psychiatry: Modern Approaches*, 2nd edn, pp. 482–489. (Ed.) Rutter, M. and Hersov, L. Oxford: Blackwell Scientific.
7. Hill, P. (1985) Child psychiatry. In *Essentials of Postgraduate Psychiatry*, 2nd edn, pp. 113–114. (Ed.) Hill, P., Murray, R. and Thorley, A. London: Grune & Stratton.
8. Kaplan, H.I. and Sadock, B.J. (1988) Elimination disorders, In *Synopsis of Psychiatry*, 5th edn, pp. 615–618. London: Williams & Wilkins.
9. Levine, M.D. (1982) Encopresis: Its potentiation, evaluation and alleviation. *Pediatric Clinics of North America*, **29**, 315–330.
10. Rappaport, L., Landman, G., Fenton, T. and Levine, M.D. (1986) Locus of control as predictor of compliance and outcome in treatment of encopresis. *Journal of Pediatrics*, **109**, 1061–1064.

ABNORMAL ILLNESS BEHAVIOURS

ILLNESS AND DISEASE

The difference between a doctor and a patient amounts to more than which side of the desk is occupied: fundamentally the doctor is concerned with disease whilst the patient is concerned with illness.[7] (*Table 10.15*). Disease refers to objective anatomical deformations and pathophysiological conditions which are caused by diverse factors such as heredity, diet and infective organisms. The medical model, which directs the thinking and behaviour of doctors, is a scientific approach to the prevention, diagnosis, treatment and understanding of disease and disease processes. Undoubtedly this has led to major advances in patient care, yet paradoxically the general population has become increasingly dissatisfied with physicians, with problems in communi-

Table 10.15 Illness and disease

Illness	*Disease*
The patient's perspective	The doctor's perspective
Subjective experience	Objective study
Sociological model	Medical model
Major psychosocial element	Major physical element

Table 10.16 Disease–illness relationships

disease – illness		normal adjustment
DISEASE – ILLNESS		
DISEASE – illness		denial/overcompensation
DISEASE – 0		
disease – 0		
disease – ILLNESS		unwarranted illness (sick role) behaviour
0 – ILLNESS		
0 – illness		

cation making an important contribution to this problem.[27]

The source of this paradox is that what concerns the doctor is often not what concerns the patient. In concentrating on disease the doctor may disregard other elements of the patient's illness experience, which embrace a range of psychological and social effects such as the personal nature of suffering and alterations in relationships and activities. The expression of illness, namely illness behaviour, encompasses 'the ways in which individuals react to aspects of their own functioning which they evaluate in terms of "health" and "illness"'.[31] Usually illness and disease accompany one another, and in general the more severe the disease, the greater the illness behaviour. Yet, considerable differences exist among individuals as to how much illness a particular disease generates, and these are linked to diverse factors such as age, culture, social isolation, psychosocial stresses and personality/attitudes,[8] so that the distinction between normal variation and abnormal illness behaviour is often a matter of judgement rather than fact. However, there are indisputably pathological extremes with denial/overcompensation at one pole and unwarranted illness behaviours at the other, and these states are not infrequently encountered in gastroenterological practice (*Table 10.16*).

DENIAL/OVERCOMPENSATION

Denial and overcompensation – which is denial accompanied by behaviours that directly negate the disability – are coping mechanisms that serve to minimize the impact of the disease.[9] Frequently these are healthy, adaptive responses in patients whose courage, resilience and optimism prove an inspiration to others (including their doctors);[5] occasionally they are not.[4]

The advantages and disadvantages are as follows:

1. Advantages:[5,9]
   (a) protection from intolerable or disabling emotional distress;
   (b) enhancing status and self-esteem through public approbation;
   (c) personal development through goal-attaining behaviours;
   (d) better recovery following some diseases;[26]
   (e) better prognosis in some diseases.[16]
2. Disadvantages:[4,9]
   (a) later presentation, sometimes converting a curable into an incurable disease;
   (b) poorer compliance with treatment;
   (c) adverse reactions to successful treatment;
   (d) greater emotional distress in the spouse.[33]

Treatment

The temptation when confronted with an obviously abnormal coping response is to 'treat' it by confronting the patient with reality (as others see it). Denial and over-compensation are potent defence mechanisms adopted consciously, or more often unconsciously, for a purpose: they are challenged at the patient's peril. The exception is when there are clear-cut medical requirements that are being blocked, and in such circumstances psychiatric advice should be sought whenever time permits.

CLASSIFICATION OF UNWARRANTED ILLNESS BEHAVIOURS

Before presenting a classification of unwarranted illness behaviours it is worth while emphasizing what these conditions share – other than the disapproval of most physicians! The core of these disorders is entry to, or maintenance in, a sick role because of advantages accrued:[8] the patient is better off in various ways from being ill rather than well. Obvious advantages from entering or remaining in the sick role include the following:

1. Financial rewards:
   (a) allowances, benefits, grants, pensions;
   (b) compensation, e.g. occupational, criminal.
2. Other privileges, e.g. housing, transport.
3. Removal of responsibilities:
   (a) roles in education, work, parental or other family duties;
   (b) avoidance of difficult situations, e.g. funeral, court, public speaking;
   (c) excuse for failure.
4. Control in relationships:
   (a) avoidance of criticism or rejection;

   (b) avoidance of intimacy;
   (c) obligatory caring.
5. Status, defined role, enhanced self-esteem.
6. Sanctioned self-concern and indulgence.

Unwarranted illness behaviours take four principal forms – malingering, hysteria, factitious disorder and hypochondriasis – and can be differentiated by whether disease is simulated, gain is apparent and the condition is consciously or unconsciously operated (*Table 10.17*).

Such distinctions are not always easy, appreciable gain and the degree of insight sometimes being moot points, and of course different illness behaviours may coexist with disease as well as with each other. A common example of this is epilepsy, where consciously feigned seizures, hysterical psuedo-seizures and self-induced seizures may all occur in different circumstances in an individual who has 'genuine' epilepsy.[6,35] Indeed the considerable extent of overlap between malingering, hysteria and factitious disorder, both in terms of the behaviour and patient characteristics, has cast doubt upon the validity and value of making a distinction.[18]

Table 10.17 Unwarranted illness behaviour: classification and differentiation

	Simulation of disease	*Evident gain*	*Insight/ awareness*
Malingering	Present	Present	Present
Hysteria	Present	Present	Absent
Factitious disorder	Present	Absent	Uncertain
Hypochrondriasis	Absent	Uncertain	Uncertain

MALINGERING

Malingering is the voluntary simulation of disease or disability with the intention of deceit and for an understandable purpose.[12,22]

The behaviour takes three forms:[15]

1. Pure malingering – the symptoms/signs are based upon no disease.
2. Partial malingering – the symptoms/signs are voluntary exaggerations of a real disease.
3. The purposefully false attribution of a disease or disability to an injury or accident that did not cause it.

The most common presentations of malingering involve neurological or sensory disorders, with subjective ill-defined complaints.[12,22] In gastroenterological practice the most probable presentation is abdominal pain, not uncommonly in the setting of established disease. The usual purposes of malingering are financial gain or avoidance of work, but feigning pain to obtain potent analgesics is also common.

Behavioural characteristics[12,22]

1. Incongruous or exaggerated signs/symptoms.
2. Giving up the illness when it suits, e.g. for leisure interests.
3. Querulous, hostile, defensive and/or uncooperative during the medical examination.

Points (2) and (3) help to distinguish malingering from hysteria.

Patient characteristics[12,22]

1. Usually male.
2. Younger patients have immature, inadequate or sociopathic personality disorders; middle-aged patients are less personality disordered but tend to be frustrated or disillusioned with their job.
3. A past history of malingering or litigation/ compensation.
4. The nature of the goal is sensible, e.g. financial gain, avoidance of work, prison or military service.

Treatment[12,22]

First the physician must be sure that the patient is malingering. This involves the demonstration of unwarranted illness behaviour, the exclusion of likely organic causes and the identification of the goal that the patient seeks. Malingering is an accusation as much as a diagnosis;[34] it has ethical and legal implications, and requires skilful management. There is no universally accepted technique, much depending upon the case's circumstances, so it is preferable to discuss the findings with the patient's family practitioner and agree a strategy, rather than proceed independently, precipitately and perhaps intemperately.

Management could involve treating the symptoms as if they were real so that the patient can give them up without losing face, or alternatively ignoring them and treating the patient as if he or she was no longer ill. A third strategy, less frequently employed, is to discourage the continuation of the behaviour by ensuring that the costs outweigh the benefits, although this ploy may sometimes be morally questionable. The obvious solution – to confront the patient directly – may purge the doctor's anger but risks driving the patient's deception to greater levels or provoking him or her into self-destructive behaviour. Sometimes confrontation can be appropriate, although a more subtle and gradual denouement can achieve the same end without demolishing the doctor–patient relationship.

HYSTERIA

Hysteria is the simulation of disease or disability for reasons that are inapparent to the patient, i.e. the hysteric deceives him- or herself as well as other people.[10]

The basic features are the following:[28]

1. The disorder corresponds to an idea in the patient's mind concerning physical, sensory or psychological abnormality.
2. It is definable, if somatic, in terms of positive evidence and, if psychological, by techniques of clinical examination.
3. The disorder is related to emotional conflict.

Other characteristics of hysteria include suggestibility, identification, symbolism of the symptom, belle indifference, secondary gain, hysterical personality. Their presence may support the diagnosis but none of these features is essential.

The behaviour takes three main forms:

1. Conversion disorder, where the psychological conflict is converted into a loss or change in bodily functioning.
2. Dissociative disorder, where the psychological conflict leads to alteration in the normally integrated functions of consciousness.
3. Somatization disorder, or Briquet's syndrome,[10,19] where the emphasis is upon repeated, unexplained, diverse physical complaints not necessarily associated with emotional conflict.

The old maxim that hysteria and syphilis should be included in any differential diagnosis may be valid, but for most practical purposes conversion and dissociative disorders present with neurological, sensory or psychological manifestations. Occasionally a conversion disorder may present as vomiting or altered bowel function. However, somatization disorder frequently presents with gastroenterological complaints and so requires further description: the rest of this section is concerned with this presentation.

Behavioural characteristics[10,19]

1. A history of many physical complaints beginning before the age of 30 and being present for several years, with no or insignificant pathology.
2. Frequent consultations, investigations and treatments with no or limited benefit.
3. The account of the medical history is:
   (a) dramatic, exaggerated, emotional;
   (b) vague, inconsistent, disorganized;
   (c) lengthy.
4. Exhibitionist dress and behaviour; sometimes coy or seductive.
5. Friendly, relaxed demeanour.

Patient characteristics[10,19]

1. Occurs in 1–2% of adult females but extremely rare in men.
2. Any age: behaviour persists through adult life.
3. Lower social class, lower educational attainment and poverty are all associated.
4. Family history of somatization disorder in 10–20% of first-degree female relatives; among first-degree male relatives the prevalences of psychopathy, alcoholism and drug addiction are increased.

Treatment[10,19]

The physician's task is to exclude organic causes for the symptoms. The extent to which a physical diagnosis is pursued will depend upon the findings and the clinician's own opinion: he or she should resist ordering investigations because the patient wants them and it should be borne in mind that this is not a condition that responds to the reassurance of negative physical findings. Thereafter the management is best left to the patient's family practitioner rather than the specialist. Somatization disorder is refractory to change, and even prolonged psychotherapy helps patients in terms of decreasing the rate of hospitalization without improving their sense of well-being or changing their attitudes. Finally, drug treatments should be avoided unless there are strong indications, because compliance is poor despite the vehemence of the complaints.

FACTITIOUS DISORDER

Factitious disorders are characterized by the simulation or induction of disease for no evident reason other than assuming or maintaining the role of a patient.[13]

The behaviour takes four forms:[1,13,21]

1. Simulation of disease by feigning symptoms or signs.
2. Self-induced disease.
3. Aggravation of pre-existing disease.

4. The Munchausen syndrome[2,14] – where the patient travels from hospital to hospital, presenting with acute factitious conditions.

Any of these forms may be encountered in gastroenterological practice, and indeed the gastrointestinal tract appears to be one of the most frequent sites for presentation. The prevalence of factitious disorder is unknown; perhaps most presentations remain unrecognized due to their subtlety and ingenuity. Further, there are no limits to the suffering some patients are prepared to put themselves through. Although well known, The Munchausen syndrome is probably the rarest variant – and the least typical in that cases are often recognized with relative ease.

Characteristics of the behaviour[1,13,21]

These vary considerably owing to the myriad forms of presentation; some features to be aware of include the following:

1. Unusual lesions in terms of site, shape or persistence in spite of treatment.
2. Lesions must be accessible to the patient – but may seem inaccessible, e.g. laceration of the colon with a knitting needle to simulate ulcerative colitis.[3]
3. The development of fresh, unexpected or inexplicable symptoms, signs or complications occurring especially as the condition heals or negative results are obtained upon investigation.
4. Secretive behaviour in the ward, e.g. long spells in the toilet or behind screens.
5. Excessive stoicism.
6. Undue helpfulness with other patients.
7. Unusual interest in disease (their own or other's), asking staff many technical questions or reading medical textbooks.

Patient characteristics[1,2,13,14,21,32]

1. The Munchausen syndrome is more common in males. Other factitious disorders are much more common in females with two major surveys reporting a female : male prevalence of 20:1.[2,32]
2. Young, average age of about 30 years.
3. Around half the identified cases have either training or close relatives in health care professions.
4. Personal or family experiences of serious disease or major disability are common.
5. Typically compliant individuals – employed and socially conforming. Deviant social behaviour much more common in The Munchausen syndrome.
6. Immature, submissive, insecure personality types often with impoverished relationships and impaired psychosexual development. Antisocial/psychopathic personality characteristic only of The Munchausen syndrome.

Treatment[2,13,21,32]

The first and most difficult task is to recognize a factitious disorder. This is partly because of the technical skills of the patient whose presentation rapidly becomes a polished performance, and partly due to the absence of obvious gains that would alert the physician to a functional basis. However, another reason doctors miss the diagnosis is because of conditioning through luridly entertaining case reports in the medical literature about The Munchausen syndrome to associate factitious disorders with wandering, psychopathic, demanding males rather than with socially conforming, immature, helpful females connected with the medical world.

As consideration of a self-inflicted condition is so alien to most doctor's natures, it is generally the case that, when the possibility of a factitious disorder is contemplated, it is warranted. Proof may not always be available and, although this is desirable before confronting the patient, mere suspicion can suffice, especially when the patient's life is threatened. The outraged patient may vehemently resent this line of enquiry or restrictions in opportunities, but recovery in these circumstances corroborates the diagnosis.

The two aims in managing factitious disorders are first to stop the behaviour and second to resolve the underlying issues; whilst there may be no obvious gains, it is widely accepted that these patients have satisfaction of less tangible needs, e.g. the need for punishment or for being cared about without intimacy. Psychotherapy can help those few patients who are willing to examine the deeper issues. For the physician the task is to stop the behaviour. This is achieved by confronting the behaviour, for example by preventing opportunity or not responding to complaints and/or confronting the patient about the nature of the problem. This should never be a hot-headed, accusatory, public attack which is not only unjustified whatever the degree of provocation but frequently proves counterproductive through either exacerbation of the disorder, suicide or rejection of psychological help. The strategy requires careful consideration, preferably in discussions with nursing staff, the family practitioner and the psychiatrist who will be involved if the patient agrees.

Finally, thought must be given to the nursing staff whose relationship with the patient is frequently more intense and who need an opportunity to ventilate their feelings and to learn from their experience in these difficult circumstances.

HYPOCHONDRIASIS

Hypochondriasis differs from other unwarranted illness behaviours in that there is no attempt made by the patient to simulate disease. Consequently the anger generated in the physician is not hostility at deception, but rather exasperation at the persistence and futility of the 'worried well'.

The diagnosis is based upon three characteristics,[11,20] all of which must be present:

1. Preoccupation with the fear of having serious disease in the presence of either no or insignificant pathology.
2. Failure to respond to adequately given medical reassurance based upon appropriate history taking, examination and investigation.
3. Persistence of these beliefs and behaviours for at least 6 months.

The behaviour takes two forms:[30]

1. Primary – which varies in prevalence from 1% to almost 50% of cases, and represents a life-long behaviour pattern.
2. Secondary – in the setting of another psychiatric disorder, most often a depressive illness.

Hypochondriacal features, as opposed to hypochondriasis, occur frequently in the general population,[24] especially in the context of depression or anxiety generated by stresses or setbacks in life, e.g. in bereavement reactions: the distinction depends upon duration.

The gastrointestinal tract is a particularly common focus for hypochondriacal concern,[11,20,25] so gastroenterologists are liable to encounter more than their fair share of these presentations.

Behavioural characteristics[11,20]

1. Features of the diagnosis.
2. Intense self-observation with a detailed history provided, often accompanied by copious notes – 'the organ recital'.
3. Enjoyment of the interview, symptoms with a smile.
4. Arrive early for appointments, talk freely and appear at home in the clinic.

Patient characteristics[11,20,24]

1. Equal sex distribution; primary form slightly more common in males.
2. Older than other illness behaviour patients, peaking at about 40–50 years of age.
3. History of serious illness in the patient or his or her family during childhood is common.
4. Anxiousness and obsessionality more often noted in personality traits.
5. History of mental illness in the patient or family.
6. Features of mental illness evident, especially with more bizarre presentations.

Treatment[11,17,24]

Hypochondriasis is usually easy to recognize; its management, however, is often difficult. The first task is to ascertain whether there is an underlying psychiatric illness. Somatic delusions which might indicate schizophrenia, endogenous depression or organic brain disease may be bizarre or idiosyncratic, but differ fundamentally from hypochondriasis in that the conviction of disease is fixed and unshakeable for even brief periods. Routine enquiry should also be made to establish whether the patient is depressed or has an anxiety state that is generalized beyond health concerns. Psychiatric treatment for the primary mental illness is required, and the physician's role is first to ensure that this is accomplished either by psychiatric referral or, if the patient refuses this (as not infrequently occurs), through the family practitioner, and second to avoid unnecessary reinforcement of the behaviour by injudicious investigation and treatment.

With primary hypochondriasis the prognosis is poorer[24,29] in spite of group psychotherapy and cognitive–behaviour therapy both of which seem to prove effective. The problem is that most hypochondriacs resist psychiatric treatment; they want to interact with physicians and to focus upon their symptoms. Physicians may make progress with these patients but this takes technique, time, patience and motivation. However, whether it is appropriate to continue reassuring the patient by frequent physical examinations or to listen repeatedly and attentively to their complaints[23] on the basis that these actions convey acceptance is debatable,[17] because these very actions could legitimize and even reinforce the presentation.

This arduous task hardly seems an efficient use of a gastroenterologist's time or training. A specific behaviour modification programme perhaps offers the best hope of helping those patients who accept help;[17] for the remainder the physician's main aim should be to avoid reinforcing the behaviour through inappropriate investigations, treatments or referrals.

REFERENCES

1. Bayliss, R.I.S. (1984) The deceivers. *British Medical Journal*, **288**, 583–584.
2. Carney, M.W.P. (1980) Artefactual illness to attract medical attention. *British Journal of Psychiatry,* **136**, 342– 347.
3. Daily, W.J.R., Coles, J.M. and Creger, W.P. (1963) Factitious anaemia. *Annals of Internal Medicine*, **58**, 533–538.
4. Douglas, C.J. and Druss, R.G. (1987) Denial of illness: A reappraisal. *General Hospital Psychiatry,* **9**, 53–57.
5. Druss, R.G. and Douglas, C.J. (1988) Adaptive reponses to illness and disability: Healthy denial. *General Hospital Psychiatry*, **10**, 163–168.
6. Fenton, G. (1986) Epilepsy and hysteria. *British Journal of Psychiatry*, **149**, 28–37.
7. Ford, C.V. (1983) Disease, illness and health. In *The Somatizing Disorders*, pp. 7–23. New York: Elsevier Biomedical.
8. Ford, C.V. (1983) The sick role. In *The Somatizing Disorders*, pp. 24–35. New York: Elsevier Biomedical.
9. Ford, C.V. (1983) Psychological responses to acute and chronic disease. In *The Somatizing Disorders,* pp. 36–48. New York: Elsevier Biomedical.
10. Ford, C.V. (1983) Hysteria. In *The Somatizing Disorders*, pp. 49–75. New York: Elsevier Biomedical.
11. Ford, C.V. (1983) Hypochondriasis. In *The Somatizing Disorders*, pp. 76–97. New York: Elsevier Biomedical.
12. Ford, C.V. (1983) Malingering. In *The Somatizing Disorders*, pp. 127–134. New York: Elsevier Biomedical.
13. Ford, C.V. (1983) Factitious illness. In *The Somatizing Disorders*, pp. 135–154. New York: Elsevier Biomedical.
14. Ford, C.V. (1983) The Munchausen syndrome. In *The Somatizing Disorders*, pp. 155–175. New York: Elsevier Biomedical.
15. Garner, H.H. (1965) Malingering. *Illinois Medical Journal*, **128**, 318–319.
16. Greer, S., Morris, T. and Pettingale, K.W. (1979) Psychological response to breast cancer: Effect on outcome. *The Lancet*, **2**, 785–787.
17. House, A. (1989) Hypochondriasis and related disorders. *General Hospital Psychiatry*, **11**, 156–165.
18. Jonas, J.M. and Pope, H.G. (1985) The dissimulating disorders: a single diagnostic entity. *Comprehensive Psychiatry*, **26**, 58–62.
19. Kaplan, H.I. and Sadock, B.J. (1988) Somatization disorder. In *Synopsis of Psychiatry*, 5th edn, pp. 335–337. (Eds) Kaplan, H.I. and Sadock, B.J., London: Williams & Wilkins.
20. Kaplan, H.I. and Sadock, B.J. (1988) Hypochondriasis. In *Synopsis of Psychiatry*, 5th edn, pp. 340–342. (Eds) Kaplan, H.I. and Sadock, B.J., London: Williams & Wilkins.
21. Kaplan, H.I. and Sadock, B.J. (1988) Factitious disorders. In *Synopsis of Psychiatry*, 5th edn, pp. 396–399. (Eds) Kaplan, H.I. and Sadock, B.J., London: Williams & Wilkins.
22. Kaplan, H.I. and Sadock, B.J. (1988) Malingering. In *Synopsis of Psychiatry*, 5th edn, pp. 448–449. (Eds) Kaplan, H.I. and Sadock, B.J., London: Williams & Wilkins.
23. Kellner, R. (1983) The prognosis of treated hypochondriasis. A clinical study. *Acta Psychiatrica Scandinavica*, **67**, 69–79.
24. Kellner, R. (1985) Functional somatic symptoms and hypochondriasis. *Archives of General Psychiatry*, **42**, 821–833.
25. Kenyon, F.E. (1976) Hypochondriasis. *British Journal of Hospital Medicine*, **14**, 419–428.
26. Levenson, J.L., Kay, R., Monteferrante, J. and Herman, M.V. (1984) Denial predicts favourable outcome in unstable angina pectoris. *Psychosomatic Medicine*, **46**, 25–32.
27. Ley, P. (1988) Patients' satisfaction. In *Communicating with Patients*, pp. 1–3. London: Croom Helm.
28. Merskey, H. (1978) Hysterical phenomena. *British Journal of Hospital Medicine*, **16**, 305–309.
29. Pilowsky, I. (1968) The response to treatment in hypochondriacal disorders. *Australian and New Zealand Journal of Psychiatry*, **2**, 88–94.
30. Pilowsky, I. (1970) Primary and secondary hypochondriasis. *Acta Psychiatrica Scandinavica*, **46**, 273–285.
31. Pilowsky, I. (1978) A general classification of illness behaviours. *British Journal of Medical Psychology*, **51**, 131–137.
32. Reich, P. and Gottfried, L.A. (1983) Factitious disorders in a teaching hospital. *Annals of Internal Medicine*, **99**, 240–247.
33. Stern, M.J. and Pascale, L. (1979) Psychological adaptation post-myocardial infarction: the spouse's dilemma. *Journal of Psychosomatic Research*, **23**, 83–87.
34. Szasz, T.S. (1956) Malingering: 'Diagnosis' or social condemnation? *Archives of Neurology and Psychiatry*, **76**, 432–443.
35. Trimble, M. (1983) Pseudoseizures. *British Journal of Hospital Medicine*, **21**, 326–333.

CHAPTER 11

THE PANCREAS

CLINICAL ANATOMY AND CONGENITAL ABNORMALITIES

R.C.G. Russell

CLINICAL ANATOMY

The pancreas is a soft, lobulated, yellowish gland, 12–15 cm long, extending nearly obliquely across the posterior abdominal wall, behind the stomach, from the duodenum to the spleen. The head fills the curve of the duodenum and, near the ampulla, is embedded within the duodenal wall. From the lower and left part of the head, there is a prolongation, the uncinate process, which measures approximately 1 cm by 1–3 cm in size, extends beyond the left lateral margin of the superior mesenteric vein in all people, and reaches to, but not beyond, the superior mesenteric artery in more than 90% of subjects.[11] The boundary between the head and neck of the pancreas is marked by a groove in which the gastroduodenal artery runs. The left side of the neck is marked posteriorly by the groove in which the portal vein runs. At this point the pancreas is thin and prone to damage, either in acute pancreatitis or trauma. The posterior surface of the head of the pancreas rests on the inferior vena cava; thus to define the head of the pancreas on CT, the vena cava should be identified with the portal vein and superior mesenteric artery. Within these confines, demarcated by contrast medium in the duodenum on the right, lies the head of the pancreas. The normal head is not more than 3 cm in size. The body of the pancreas is an ellipse varying in thickness from 2.5 cm to 1 cm towards the tail. The splenic artery runs along the superior border while the splenic vein is posterior. Just to the left of the portal vein, the pancreas rests on the aorta. To identify the body and tail of the pancreas on CT, the spleen and the aorta are identified; usually the splenic artery or vein can be recognized running across the posterior abdomen, in front of which lies the body of the pancreas. The lienorenal ligament and tail of the pancreas are of importance surgically because of their variability, and the risk of surgical damage. In a quarter of individuals, the pancreas does not enter the ligament, which is about 2.5 cm long. In half, the spleen lies within the ligament to a greater or lesser extent, and in the remaining quarter, the pancreas is intimately involved with the splenic hilum extending into the gastrosplenic ligament.[15]

The main pancreatic duct traverses the pancreas from left to right, lying nearer the posterior than anterior surface. The main duct ascends at an angle of 45° to an identifiable knee, or even a loop, where it joins the body (*Figure 11.1*). The average main

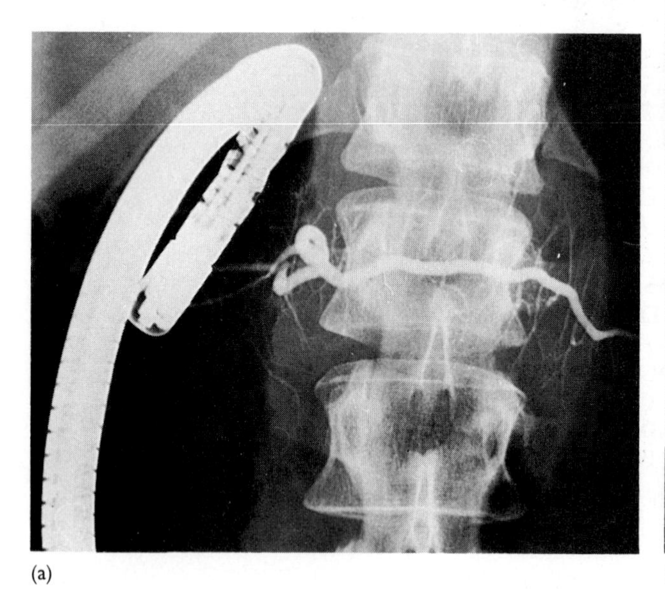
(a)

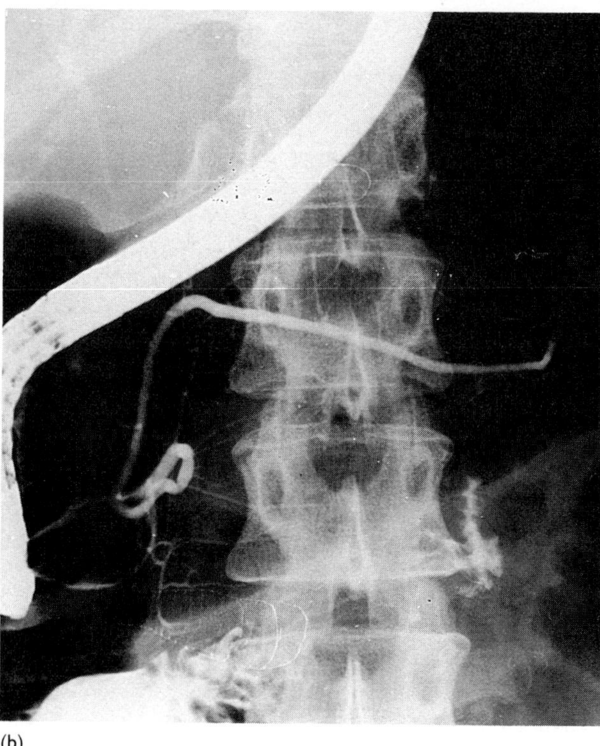
(b)

Figure 11.1 Two normal pancreatograms obtained on endoscopic retrograde cholangiopancreatography.

duct calibre measures 4 mm in the head, 3 mm in the body and 2 mm in the tail with maximum upper limits of 7 mm, 5 mm and 3 mm respectively. There is a slight but significant increase in calibre in patients over 50 years in age. In about 60%, there is an accessory duct derived from the dorsal bud of the pancreatic anlage. This duct drains into the duodenum in 20% by means of the accessory papilla; in approximately 5% of individuals, the dorsal and ventral ducts do not communicate and the condition of *pancreas divisum* is said to exist.

The main pancreatic duct passes obliquely into the wall of the duodenum in conjunction with the bile duct, where the two ducts unite to form a short dilated hepatopancreatic ampulla, which opens on the summit of the major duodenal papilla. This papilla lies in the second part of the duodenum in 75% of the population, at the angle between the second and third parts in 15%, and in 9% in the horizontal third part of the duodenum. There is considerable anatomical variation in relation to the opening of the ducts, with 40% having a completely separate opening in the papilla, 40% having a very short common channel, and the remainder having a longer channel, such that contrast placed in the bile duct will reflux up the pancreatic duct. The normal common channel ranges in length from 1 mm to 12 mm with a mean of 4.4 mm. A channel longer than 15 mm is said to be an anomalous pancreatobiliary junction, and may be associated with a choledochal cyst and gallbladder cancer.[12]

BLOOD SUPPLY

The pancreas has diffuse vascular connections, such that imaging of the entire gland at angiography requires separate cannulation of the coeliac and superior mesenteric trunks. Their branches anastomose in distinct arcades both anterior and posterior to the head of the pancreas. The principle arteries from the coeliac trunk to the head of the gland are the branches of the gastroduodenal artery, anterior superior pancreatoduodenal and posterior pancreatoduodenal artery (*Figure 11.2*). The matching vessels from the superior mesenteric system are the anterior inferior pancreatoduodenal and the posterior inferior pancreatoduodenal arteries. The dorsal pancreatic artery arises from the splenic artery and passes behind the neck of the pancreas to its lower border where it divides into right and left branches which supply the lower part of the body. The left branch is known as the inferior pancreatic artery. There are profuse anastomoses with multiple branches from the splenic artery. Occasionally there is a large vessel to the tail of the pancreas arising from the splenic artery within the hilum of the spleen.

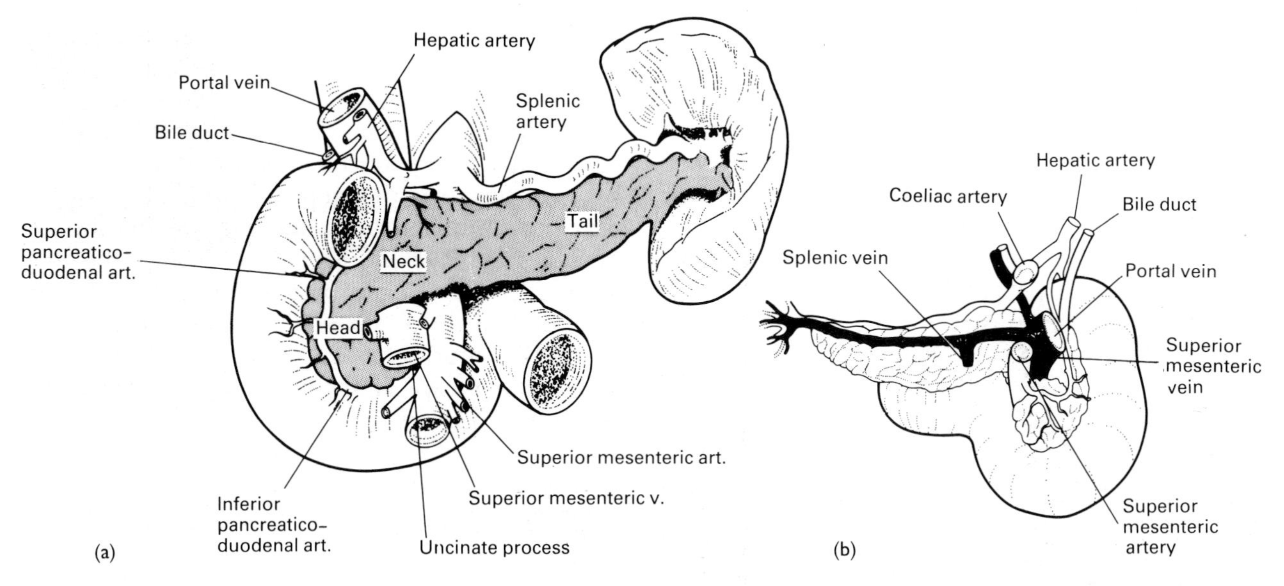

Figure 11.2 The pancreas: (a) anterior view; (b) posterior view.

VENOUS DRAINAGE

The veins correlate with the arteries, and all drain into the portal venous system often as very short tributaries. The intimate relationship of the pancreas to its major draining veins explains the frequent inoperability of quite small pancreatic tumours.

LYMPHATIC DRAINAGE

Just as the venous system is in intimate relationship with the pancreas, so too are the lymphatics. Lymph drains to the splenic nodes, directly to the mass of lymphatics around the coeliac axis, as well as to lymphatics passing beside the bile duct up to the porta hepatis.

INNERVATION

The pancreatic nerve supply is derived from the coeliac plexus, and enters the pancreas with branches of the arteries supplying the pancreas. As well as afferent fibres, there is an efferent supply consisting of sympathetic postganglionic fibres from the coeliac ganglion and parasympathetic preganglionic fibres from the right vagus nerve. The fibres, which are mainly non-myelinated, are vasomotor (sympathetic) and parenchymal (sympathetic and parasympathetic) in their distribution. Fine fibres ramify among the islet cells from the peri-insular plexuses. Fibres frequently make sympathetic contact with the acinar cells before innervating the islets, suggesting a close linkage between the neural control of the exocrine and endocrine components of the pancreas.

Parasympathetic ganglia lie in the inter- and intralobular connective tissue and, in the latter case, are frequently associated with islet cells, together with which they constitute the neuroinsular complexes. The islet cells involved in the complexes include both A and β types. Three types of nerve terminal have been identified in the islets: cholinergic (having 30–50 nm diameter agranular vesicles), adrenergic (having 30–50 nm dense cored vesicles) and peptidergic (having 60–200 nm dense cored vesicles). Pacinian corpuscles are present in the pancreas, and the sensory fibres from them pass through to the paravascular plexuses and sympathetic chains to reach the posterior root ganglion cells from T5–T9.

HISTOLOGY

Exocrine cells

The name 'pancreas' implies that the gland contains relatively little connective tissue and, of 100 g of human pancreas, 98 g are composed of exocrine cells. Interlobular ducts are lined with cuboidal cells and enter the substance of the lobules to join the lumen formed by the acinar cells which are wrapped around the lumen in mulberry fashion. The acinar cells of the exocrine pancreas are typical zymogenic cells, containing a basally situated nucleus, which is surrounded with basophilic cytoplasm seen ultrastructurally as regular arrays of granular endoplasmic reticulum, interspersed mitochondria and dense secretory granules. In the apical, supranuclear compartment of the cell, a prominent Golgi complex is present, surrounded by numerous larger secretory granules; the latter are membrane-bound bodies containing the powerful enzymic constituents of the pancreatic secretion. These enzymes are in an inactive form whilst in the granules, until their discharge into the lumen.

The mechanism of production of non-enzyme bicarbonate with pancreatic juice is discussed on page 1566, but the ultrastructure of the ductal cells is against active secretion by these cells.

Endocrine cells

The endocrine cells of the pancreas are arranged in nests or islets, which are spherical in outline and diffusely distributed in the parenchyma. The islets vary greatly in number (from 170 000 to 2 000 000) and occupy about 1% of the volume of the pancreas. They are surrounded by connective tissue fibres continuous with those of the exocrine interstitial septa, and have a rich vascular supply. The endocrine cells are derived from the ductal system, but no new formation of these cells occurs after birth.

At least four different islet cells exist and are distinguished by their secretory granules. These granules are membrane-bound cytoplasmic particles containing stored hormones: β cells produce insulin: A cells produce glucagon, D cells somatostatin and PP cells pancreatic polypeptide which is confined to the ventral pancreas.[18] Usually the β cells predominate in number. The hormones are synthesized in the endoplasmic reticulum and stored in the cytoplasmic granules from which they are released by the appropriate stimulus.

Islet cells have a significantly higher concentration towards the tail of the gland, and thus this part should not be sacrificed needlessly at surgery.[24]

EMBRYOLOGY

The pancreas is developed in dorsal and ventral parts. The dorsal pancreas arises in the latter half of the fourth week of development as a diverticulum from the dorsal wall of the duodenum, a short distance cranial to the hepatic diverticulum; growing craniodorsally in the mesoduodenum, it enters that part of the dorsal mesogastrium which is forming the dorsal wall of the bursa omentalis. It forms the whole of the neck, body and tail of the pancreas and a part of the head. The ventral part grows out from the primitive bile duct at the point where the duct enters the duodenum. This outgrowth is at first double, but the two soon fuse, and the resulting single mass grows round the gut into the mesoduodenum, where it enlarges to form the remainder of the head of the gland. The duct of the dorsal part (the accessory pancreatic duct) opens directly into the duodenum, whereas that of the ventral part (the main pancreatic duct) opens within the bile duct. Early in the seventh week, the two anlage of the pancreas meet and fuse, and a communication is established between their ducts. After this has occurred, the terminal part of the accessory duct undergoes little or no enlargement, whereas the duct of the ventral part increases in size and forms the terminal part of the main duct of the gland (*Figure 11.3*).

RADIOLOGICAL ANATOMY

The outline of the gland is not definable on plain films, but can be visualized using ultrasound, CT or magnetic resonance imaging. The head of the pancreas usually lies just to the right of the T12/L1 vertebrae, but may be as high as T11 or as low as L5/S1 in the elderly viscerotopic patient. The external contour of the pancreas shows an age-related development. Ninety percent of pancreases display a smooth contour in the third decade but, by the eighth decade, only a quarter have a smooth outline. Pancreatic lobulation increases not only in frequency with age but also in degree. A homogeneous structure is almost exclusively found in the third decade but, by the fourth decade, one third of pancreases show a patchy structure, which is seen in three-quarters of those in the eighth decade. Improved imaging techniques have demonstrated that the ventral pancreas may have a different texture from the dorsal pancreas as a normal variant.[7] With age, an increasing reduction in the anteroposterior diameter of the pancreatic head, body and tail can be seen. For example, in 20–30 year olds, the average diameter is 28 mm, reduced to 21 mm in the 70–80-year-old age group. With increasing age the body and tail shrink, atrophy and fatty infiltration being the cause of these changes.[9]

CONGENITAL ABNORMALITIES

The most important congenital abnormality affecting the pancreas is cystic fibrosis, which is inherited as an autosomal recessive trait. This is described on page 1588.

THE HETEROTOPIC PANCREAS

Pancreatic heterotopia, or aberrant pancreas or accessory pancreas, may be defined as tissue histo-

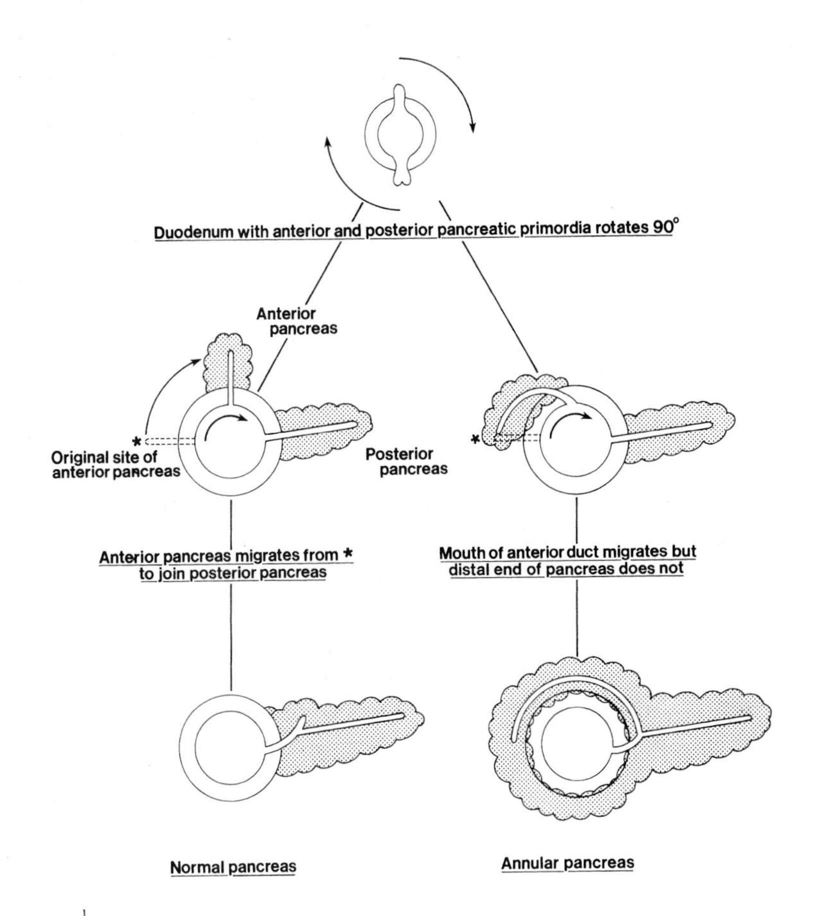

Figure 11.3 Development of normal and annular pancreas. (From Morrell, M.T. and Keynes, W.M. (1981) Annular pancreas. In *The Pancreas* (Eds) Keynes, W.M. and Keith, R.G. pp. 159–168. London: Heinemann Medical, with permission.)

logically similar to normal pancreatic tissue found outside its usual location and having no anatomical or vascular connection with the pancreas itself. Numerous confusing terms including adenomyosis, adenomyoma, and myoepithelial hamartoma have been used but the term heterotopic pancreas is now accepted. The origin of this tissue is controversial: most accept the thesis of separation from the main pancreatic structure during embryonic rotation. The estimated incidence ranges from 0.55% to 13.7% in necropsy analyses. The overall surgical incidence has been estimated as one case in every 500 explorations. By far the most common locations are the stomach, duodenum and jejunum; in childhood, the most common location is within a Meckel's diverticulum. The tissue presents as firm yellow intramural nodules varying in size from 2–4 mm, which are subserosal or submucosal. Histologically the heterotopic pancreas is classified into three main types.

1. Differentiated pancreatic tissue containing acini, ducts or islets.
2. Incompletely differentiated tissue composed predominantly of ducts and a few acini.
3. Adenomyoma, composed of smooth muscle tissue and ducts only.

Clinically, a heterotopic pancreas rarely presents in children; it is encountered most commonly in the fourth, fifth and sixth decades of life. Heterotopic pancreas is subject to all the pathological changes that can occur in the pancreas itself; most symptoms, however, are attributable to obstruction, haemorrhage or peptic ulcer-like disease. For the surgeon it is important to recognize the gross features of this lesion, as frozen section may reveal only duct-like structures obviously infiltrating the muscle layers, which can be mistaken for a carcinoma.

The typical radiological features consist of an intramural nodular prominence with a corresponding indentation and filling defect in barium shadow or central umbilication. A central position of the barium fleck favours heterotopic pancreatic tissue. The lesion may be up to 5 cm in size.

A duodenal diaphragm or a duplication cyst of the ileum may be associated and present with bleeding as a consequence of the heterotopic pancreatic complication.

Pancreatic heterotopia is an uncommon and frequently misdiagnosed condition with variable presentations. Endoscopic biopsy is the preferred diagnostic method, and treatment in the symptomatic patient is local surgical excision.[13]

PANCREAS DIVISUM: DOMINANT DORSAL DUCT SYNDROME

Pancreas divisum, a variant of pancreatic ductal configuration in which the dorsal and ventral analgen do not fuse during organogenesis, has been known since the descriptions by the classical anatomists of the 17th century.[2] The congenital anomaly has been the subject of controversy since its clinical relevance was first postulated.[4] In Western populations, this variant occurs in at least 5% of the population,[6] whereas it is less prevalent in Japan.[23] The condition includes those who have entirely separate dorsal and ventral ducts, those with an absent ventral system, and those with a tiny but functionally inadequate communication between the two systems (*Figure 11.4*). It is for this reason that the term 'dominant dorsal duct syndrome' is preferred.

The presumption has developed that the accessory papilla is too small and inadequate to serve as the daily outflow for up to 2 litres of pancreatic secretions. To support this hypothesis, elevated pressures within the dorsal duct has been described by the technique of inserting endoscopic manometers into the dorsal duct. After placing a stent in the sphincter, the pressures have been shown to fall with improvement in the sphincter pressure gradient.[16,20] It is now accepted that a dominant dorsal duct does not cause pancreatic disease; if associated with accessory papillary stenosis, however, then symptoms may occur.[5] The incidence of accessory papillary stenosis is rare, and hence the dominant dorsal duct syndrome is a rare cause of pancreatitis.

Investigation

The clinical presentation of this condition is controversial, and the diagnosis can only be made when there is unequivocal radiological evidence in the presence of recurrent attacks of acute pancreatitis, which are usually of a mild degree and rarely associated with complications of pancreatitis. It is doubtful if those patients with chronic pancreatic pain should be included in this syndrome.

Clinical features

The diagnosis of dominant dorsal duct syndrome is made by endoscopic cannulation of both the dorsal and ventral ducts to show that the body and tail of the pancreas drain solely or mainly via the accessory sphincter. In 80% of patients, it is possible to cannulate the dorsal duct using metal-tipped guidewire catheters in conjunction with secretin injection.[4] In the remainder, percutaneous puncture of the main duct in the body of the pancreas with contrast injection will elucidate the anatomy. An estimate of the physiologically significant stenosis of the pancreatic duct orifice can be made by ultrasonographical monitoring of duct size before and after administration of intravenous secretin (1 mg/kg). Prolonged dilatation (15–30 minutes) after administration of secretin is considered an index of abnormal resistance of flow through the papillary orifice.

Treatment

Once diagnosed, the preferred treatment is a transduodenal sphincteroplasty. The accessory papilla can usually be identified superior and anterior to the main papilla. The papilla is probed and considered stenotic if it does not accept a 0.75 mm wire. The sphincter is divided for 1 cm and the edges sutured.[22] Alternatively, a stent is placed in the duct endoscopically,[3,20] but attempts at endoscopic sphincterotomy are associated with a high incidence of failure.

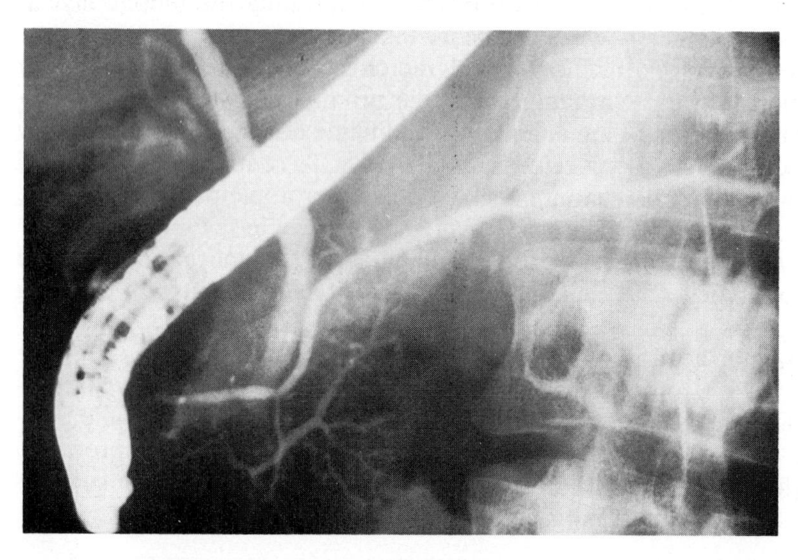

Figure 11.4 Endoscopic retrograde cholangiopancreatogram showing a moderately sized ventral pancreas with the main dorsal duct draining through the accessory papilla. The bile duct is filled with contrast medium which can be traced down to the main papilla.

The results of this procedure suggest that if the patient has a stenosis of the accessory duct there will be a symptomatic benefit in 85%.[22] Once relief of symptoms has been achieved, the benefits appear to be long term.[10]

ANNULAR PANCREAS

Annular pancreas was first described by Tiedman in 1818 and named by Echer in 1862. Its incidence is unclear, but has been calculated at about 1:20 000. The aetiopathogenesis is unknown, but it may be a component of a more generalized disorder of embryogenesis when associated with trisomy 21, tracheo-oesophageal fistula or cardiorenal abnormalities, or may occur alone with local duodenal abnormality only. Neonatal cases are associated with other congenital abnormalities in about 80% of cases and adult cases in about 20%.

Clinical features

Its presentation tends to be bimodal, with peaks neonatally and in the fourth to fifth decades. Neonatal presentation is usually with a congenital duodenal obstruction wherein it contributes to 15% of all cases. The pregnancy may have been associated with polyhydramnios. The obstruction is generally classified as intrinsic, as pancreatic tissue is often intimately related to the wall of the duodenum. The most common adult symptom is upper abdominal pain. The coincident peptic ulcer disease that has been reported in 29–48% of patients may be related to gastric stasis and antral overdistension with secondary hypergastrinaemia. The chronic pancreatitis found in 14–50% of adult cases may be attributed to poor duct drainage from relative outlet obstruction, as well as a possible intrinsic susceptibility of the annular gland to damage. Unless another factor is present, the pancreatitis has always appeared limited to the annulus itself. Biliary obstruction is rare.[8]

Investigation

In the infant, diagnosis is made on a plain radiograph of the abdomen in the erect position; two adjacent fluid levels are present, one in the stomach and one in the dilated proximal duodenum, with absence of air in the rest of the abdomen. In the adult, the diagnosis is made by hypertonic duodenography with narrowing of the duodenum at the level of the papilla, endoscopy and CT (*Figure 11.5*).

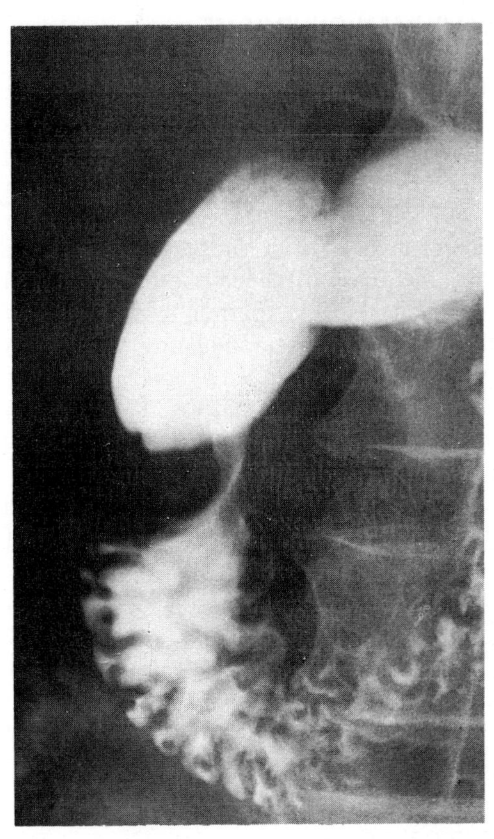

Figure 11.5 Barium filling the duodenum with constriction in the second part produced by an annular pancreas. (From Morrell, M.T. and Keynes, W.M. (1981) Annular pancreas. In *The Pancreas* (Eds) Keynes, W.M. and Keith, R.G. pp. 159–168. London: Heinemann Medical, with permission.)

Treatment

Treatment of the infant is that of a duodenoduodenostomy or duodenojejunostomy. In the adult, the treatment is tailored to the presentation, care being taken to define accurately the cause of the pain. If obstruction is the main problem, then a duodenojejunostomy is preferred, whereas if chronic pancreatitis is the predominant problem, a pancreatoduodenectomy should be undertaken. Lesser procedures are invariably associated with a less favourable outcome.

CONGENITAL SHORT PANCREAS

This is a very rare finding at pancreatography for investigation of upper abdominal symptoms. Its importance lies in the the differential diagnosis of a block in the body of the pancreas. A good CT scan will solve the problem by showing an absence of pancreatic tissue to the left of the presumed block. It is not associated with symptoms.

SCHWACHMAN SYNDROME

In 1964 in separate publications, Bodian, Sheldon and Lightwood,[2] and Schwachman *et al.*[17] drew attention to a rare multiorgan disease characterized by pancreatic insufficiency and bone marrow hypoplasia associated with other abnormalities which included growth retardation, metaphyseal dyschondroplasia, ichthyotic maculopapular rash and immunodeficiencies. The pathogenesis is unknown, but the syndrome is familial and thought to be inherited as an autosomal recessive trait. Patients with this syndrome are predisposed to haematological disorders. The condition is distinguished from cystic fibrosis by a normal sweat test.

The degree of pancreatic insufficiency is variable and the persistence of some residual exocrine function possibly accounts for the delayed presentation of malabsorption. Histologically, exocrine pancreatic tissue is scarce or completely absent, being replaced by a non-infiltrated, non-fibrotic adipose tissue in which intact islets in normal numbers are embedded.[19] As a result of the loss of exocrine tissue the plasma amylase is low. The parotid gland may undergo similar degenerative change.

Clinical features

The affected patient is susceptible to respiratory, cutaneous and systemic infections. The nature and frequency of infection does not correlate with the degree of neutropenia; there is a defective neutrophil mobility[1] and an exaggerated chemoluminescence[14] which may account for the susceptibility to infections. Lymphoproliferative neoplasia has been described in these patients.

Skeletal abnormalities include metaphyseal dyschondroplasia affecting ribs, knees and femoral head. Long bone tabulation with genu and cubitus valgus occur. Malnutrition and metabolic abnormalities retard ossification centres. Growth retardation is a primary feature, as is delayed puberty.

The diffuse abnormality includes hepatic fatty infiltration with raised transaminases and renal tubular dysfunction. Intelligence is inherently below average, with psychomotor retardation.

Investigation

The diagnosis of fatty infiltration can be confirmed by both CT and ultrasound.

Treatment

Treatment is symptomatic, with antibiotics for infections. Pancreatic enzyme replacements are needed, although requirements are variable. The prognosis for this syndrome is probably better than for cystic fibrosis, although it is accompanied by considerable morbidity. Infections and haemorrhagic diatheses can prove fatal.

REFERENCES

1. Agett, P.J., Cavanagh, N.P.C., Matthew, D.J., Pincott, J.R., Sutcliffe, J. and Harries, J.T. (1980) Schwachman's syndrome. A review of 21 cases. *Archives of Diseases in Childhood*, **55**, 331–347.
2. Bodian M., Sheldon, W. and Lightwood, R. (1964) Congenital hypoplasia of the exocrine pancreas. *Acta Paediatrica*, **53**, 282–293.
3. Cooperman, A.M., Siegel, J. and Hammerman, H. (1989) Pancreas divisum—advocates and agnostics. *Journal of Clinical Gastroenterology*, **11**, 489–491.
4. Cotton, P.B. (1980) Congenital anomaly of pancreas divisum can cause obstructive pain and pancreatitis. *Gut*, **21**, 105–114.
5. Cotton, P.B. (1988) Pancreas divisum. *Pancreas*, **3**, 245–247.
6. Delhaye, M., Engelholm, L. and Cremer, M. (1985) Pancreas divisum: Congenital anatomic variant or anomaly? *Gastroenterology*, **89**, 951–958.
7. Donald, J.J., Shorvon, P.J. and Lees, W.R. (1990) A hypoechoic area within the head of the pancreas –a normal variant. *Clinical Radiology*, **41**, 337–338.
8. Dowsett, J.F., Rode, J. and Russell, R.C.G. (1986) Annular pancreas: a clinical, endoscopic, and immunohistochemical study. *Gut*, **30**, 130–135.
9. Heuck, A., Maubach, P.A. and Reiser, M. *et al.* (1987) Age-related morphology of the normal pancreas on computed tomography. *Gastrointestinal Radiology*, **12**, 18–22.
10. Keith, R.G., Shapero, T.F., Saibil, F.G. and Moore, T.L. (1989) Dorsal duct sphincterotomy is effective long-term treatment of acute pancreatitis associated with pancreas divisum. *Surgery*, **106**, 660–667.
11. Martin, D.F. (1988) Computed tomography of the normal pancreatic uncinate process. *Clinical Radiology*, **39**, 195–196.
12. Misra, S.P. and Dwivedi, M. (1990) Pancreatobiliary ductal union. *Gut*, **31**, 1144–1149.
13. Pang, L.-C. (1988) Pancreatic heterotopia: A reappraisal and clinicopathological analysis of 32 cases. *Southern Medical Journal*, **81**, 1264–1275.
14. Repo, H., Savilahti, E. and Leirsalo-Repo, M. (1987) Aberrant phagocyte function in Schwachman syndrome. *Clinical and Experimental Immunology*, **69**, 204–212.
15. Rosen, A., Nathan, H., Luciansky, E. and Sayfan, J. (1988) The lienorenal ligament and the tail of the pancreas: A surgical anatomical study. *Pancreas*, **3**, 104–107.
16. Satterfield, S.T., McCarthy, J.H. and Geenen, J.E. *et al.* (1988) Clinical experience in 82 patients with

pancreas divisum: preliminary results of manometry and endoscopic therapy. *Pancreas*, **3**, 248–253.
17. Schwachman, H., Diamond, L., Oski, F.A. and Khaw, K.-T. (1964) The syndrome of pancreatic insufficiency and bone marrow dysfunction. *Journal of Pediatrics*, **65**, 645–663.
18. Sessa, F., Fiocca, R., Tenti, P., Solcia, E., Tavani, E. and Pliteri, S. (1983) Pancreatic polypeptide rich tissue in the annular pancreas. A distinctive feature of ventral primordium derivatives. *Virchows Archiv. A Pathological Anatomy and Histopathology (Berlin)*, **399**, 227–232.
19. Shmerling, D.H., Prader, A., Hitzig, W.H., Giedion, A., Hadorn, B. and Kuhni, M. (1969) The syndrome of exocrine pancreatic insufficiency, neutropenia, metaphyseal dysostosis and dwarfism. *Helvetica Paediatrica Acta*, **24**, 547–575.
20. Siegel, J.H., Ben-Zvi, J.S., Pullano, W. and Cooperman, A. (1990) Effectiveness of endoscopic drainage for pancreas divisum: endoscopic and surgical results in 31 patients. *Endoscopy*, **22**, 129–133.
21. Stern, C.D. (1986) A histological perspective on the discovery of the accessory duct of the pancreas, the ampulla of Vater and pancreas divisum. *Gut*, **27**, 203–212.
22. Warshaw, A.L., Simeone, J.F., Schapiro, R.H. and Flavin-Warshaw, B. (1990) Evaluation and treatment of the dominant dorsal duct syndrome (Pancreas divisum redefined). *American Journal of Surgery*, **159**, 59–66.
23. Warshaw, A.L. (1990) Dominant dorsal duct syndrome: Pancreas divisum redefined. *Journal of Paediatric Gastroenterology and Nutrition*, **10**, 281–289.
24. Wittingen, J. and Frey, C.F. (1974) Islet concentration in the head, body and tail of the pancreas. *Annals of Surgery*, **179**, 412–414.

PHYSIOLOGY

O.H. Petersen

The pancreas contains exocrine and endocrine components and, although the emphasis in this section is on the exocrine tissue, there are important endocrine–exocrine functional relationships that have to be considered. In terms of volume percentages, the pancreas consists of 82% acinar cells, 4% duct cells, 4% blood vessels, 2% endocrine cells and 8% extracellular matrix.[2] The acinar cell is thus by far the dominant cell type, as well as being the most important for the exocrine function. The acinar cell itself is not, however, the functional unit in this tissue because acinar cells are organized in a network consisting of up to several hundred intercommunicating cells (functional syncytium) surrounding complexly shaped lumina.[14,16] The exocrine pancreas, apart from being an extremely important organ in its own right, has also served as the most useful model system for the study of protein secretion and its control.

PANCREATIC JUICE

COMPOSITION AND SECRETORY RATE

The exocrine pancreas secretes a fluid containing electrolytes as well as a large number of functionally important digestive enzymes. Pancreatic juice collected in a physiological situation (after a meal) will have been produced as a result of a complex mixture of physicochemical processes evoked by a combination of chemical signals. Pancreatic secretion is evoked by both nervous and hormonal mechanisms, and the most important signalling molecules are cholecystokinin, acetylcholine, secretin and vasoactive intestinal polypeptide. Although the precise electrolyte composition will vary with the type of stimulation, some general features are always observed. The juice is isosmolal with plasma and the sodium and potassium concentrations are virtually constant and approximately plasma-like. The sum of the chloride and bicarbonate concentrations is constant, in spite of wide variations in the individual concentrations (*Figure 11.6*). Although it is possible to obtain pure human pancreatic juice,[4] the most detailed studies have been undertaken in the dog, cat, rat and pig. There seem to be species differences, particularly with regard to the ability of cholecystokinin to evoke fluid secretion, but most work has been in vivo where many interactions between nervous and hormonal mechanisms may occur and will complicate the analysis.

In contrast to the view presented in many textbooks, pure cholecystokinin alone evokes marked fluid secretion at least in the isolated perfused rat and pig pancreas.[9,17] In both the intact rat and the isolated perfused rat pancreas, pure cholecystokinin can evoke higher rates of fluid secretion than can be obtained with secretin stimulation.[17,20] Vasoactive

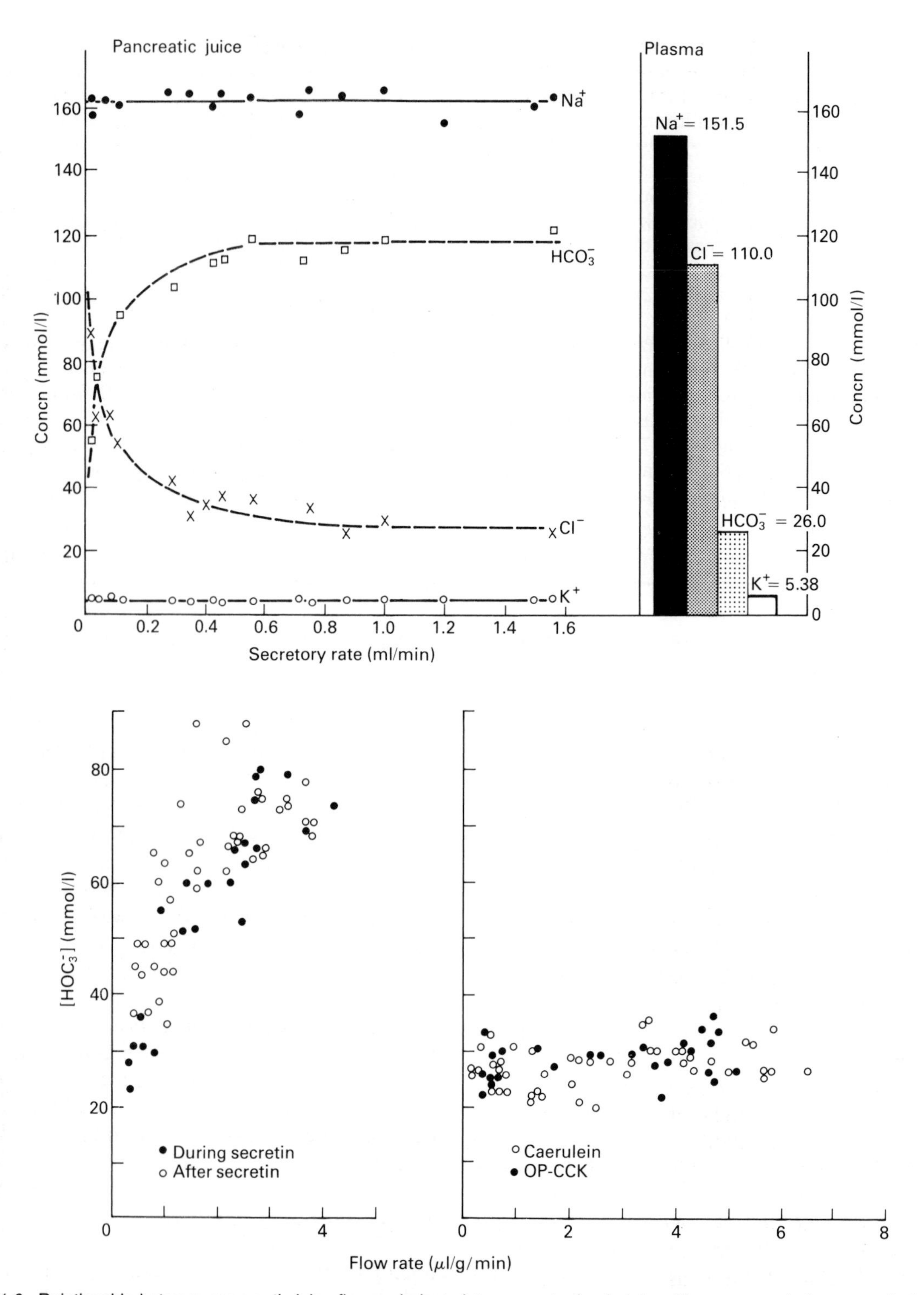

Figure 11.6 Relationship between pancreatic juice flow and electrolyte concentration in juice. The upper part shows results from dog pancreas stimulated with secretin. (From Bro-Rasmussen, Killman and Thaysen,[3] with permission.) The lower part shows results from the rat pancreas stimulated with secretin, the octapeptide cholecystokinin (OP-CCK) or the cholecystokinin analogue caerulein. (From Sewell and Young,[20] with permission.)

intestinal peptide evokes marked fluid secretion at least in the pig.[5] Acetylcholine activates exactly the same type of secretory process as cholecystokinin. Acetylcholine interacts with muscarinic receptors and its effect on fluid secretion is blocked by atropine. This antagonist does not interfere with the action of cholecystokinin and related peptides, gastrin for example. Cholecystokinin interacts with specific receptors and its effects on fluid secretion can be blocked by a specific and competitive antagonist which does not interfere with the action of acetylcholine.[14,16,17] Another peptide, totally unrelated to the cholecystokinin–gastrin family, bombesin (or gastrin-releasing peptide), and other members of the bombesin family can also stimulate the same fluid secretion mechanism as cholecystokinin and acetylcholine. Bombesin also acts in the presence of complete blockage of acetylcholine and cholecystokinin receptors.[14,16] Vasoactive intestinal peptide evokes formation of fluid with the same composition as that evoked by secretin.[16,18]

Figure 11.6 illustrates the relationship between electrolyte concentration and secretory rate in the cat and rat during stimulation with secretin or cholecystokinin. The latter evokes the formation of a juice with a plasma-like composition in both the rat and the pig and there is no tendency for the bicarbonate concentration to rise with increasing flow rate. In the case of secretin stimulation, however, there is a clear pattern of increase in bicarbonate and decrease in chloride concentration as the flow rate goes up.

THE COMPONENTS OF FLUID SECRETION

Cholecystokinin clearly evokes the formation of a fluid with a composition that is quite different from that evoked by secretin. Cholecystokinin receptors have been localized to acinar cells, whereas there is no evidence available to suggest the existence of such receptors on duct cells. On the other hand, duct cells have secretin receptors although they are not the only site for specific secretin binding, as acinar cells have also been shown to possess such receptors.[6,18] There is otherwise substantial, but still indirect, evidence showing that the cholecystokinin-evoked secretion originates from the acinar cells whereas the secretin-evoked juice comes from duct cells.[17,18]

The mechanisms underlying the two types of fluid secretion are also different. In experiments on the isolated perfused rat pancreas, it has been shown that the acinar fluid secretion evoked by activation of cholecystokinin receptors is acutely dependent on the presence of calcium in the extracellular fluid, whereas this is not the case with respect to the secretin-evoked fluid secretion. On the other hand, secretin-evoked fluid secretion is markedly dependent on the presence of carbon dioxide and bicarbonate in the perfusion fluid whereas this is not the case for cholecystokinin-evoked secretion.[17,18]

PROTEIN SECRETION

The pancreatic acinar cells secrete a large number of proteins, electrolytes and water. Amongst the secreted proteins are many important digestive enzymes such as lipase, α-amylase, four (pro)carboxypeptidases, three trypsin(ogen)s, chymotrypsin(ogen), two (pro)elastases, two colipases and (pro)phospholipase A_2. It is generally accepted that these proteins are synthesized at the rough endoplasmic reticulum, processed through the Golgi complex and stored in the zymogen granules. Stimulation of the acinar cells results in the fusion of zymogen granule membrane with luminal plasma membrane, with an opening developing at the point of fusion establishing continuity between the interior of the zymogen granule and the acinar lumen through which the stored proteins can escape. This mode of secretion has been termed exocytosis. The granule membrane inserted into the luminal plasma membrane during exocytosis is subsequently recaptured and can be re-utilized (membrane recycling).[10] In many species, certainly in the rat and the pig, acinar enzyme secretion is accompanied by acinar fluid secretion. The fluid secretion is not merely a passive process secondary to enzyme secretion, as it is possible to reduce cholecystokinin-evoked fluid secretion markedly by the specific sodium-potassium pump inhibitor, ouabain, without reducing amylase output.[17]

HORMONAL AND NERVOUS CONTROL OF EXOCRINE SECRETION

The most important control of acinar enzyme and fluid secretion is exerted by the hormone cholecystokinin and by the parasympathetic nerves with acetylcholine as the transmitter, but several other control mechanisms have also been identified (*Figure 11.7*).

CHOLECYSTOKININ

Cholecystokinin occurs naturally in multiple molecular forms. The most important of these are the classical 33-amino-acid peptide (CCK_{33}), the carboxyl-terminal octapeptide (CCK_8), the intermediate form CCK_{22} and the larger CCK_{39} and CCK_{58}.[23] Good radioimmunoassays and bioassays have shown that the resting cholecystokinin concentration in plasma in humans may be about 1 pM (CCK_8 equivalents) and that a meal may cause an increase of about 5–10 pM (CCK_8 equivalents).[23]

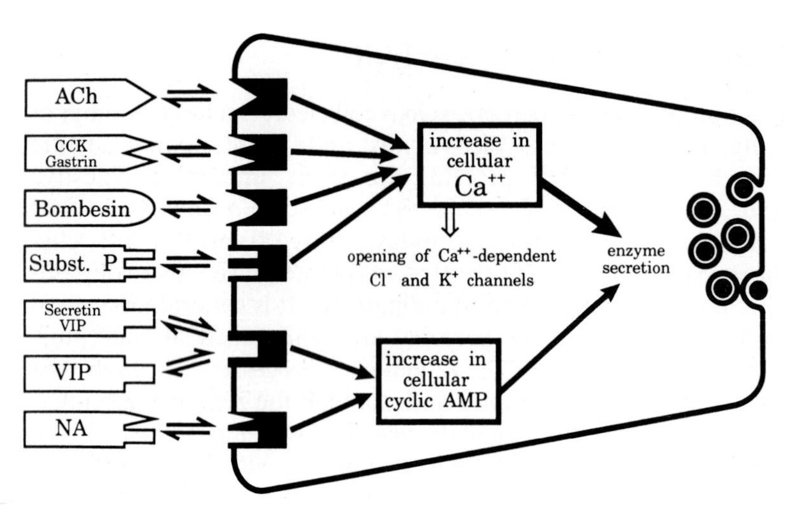

Figure 11.7 Receptors on pancreatic acinar cells. Activation of the first group of receptors, (acetylcholine, ACh; cholecystokinin, CCK; bombesin; substance P) causes elevation of the intracellular free calcium ion concentration (see *Figure 11.9* for more details of the underlying molecular steps) whereas activation of the other receptor group (secretin; vasoactive intestinal polypeptide, VIP; noradrenaline, NA) stimulates the enzyme adenyl cyclase causing increased cyclic AMP production. The receptors linked to the calcium ion signal pathways (and particularly those binding acetylcholine and cholecystokinin) are the most important and are also able to switch on fluid secretion due to opening of ion channels.

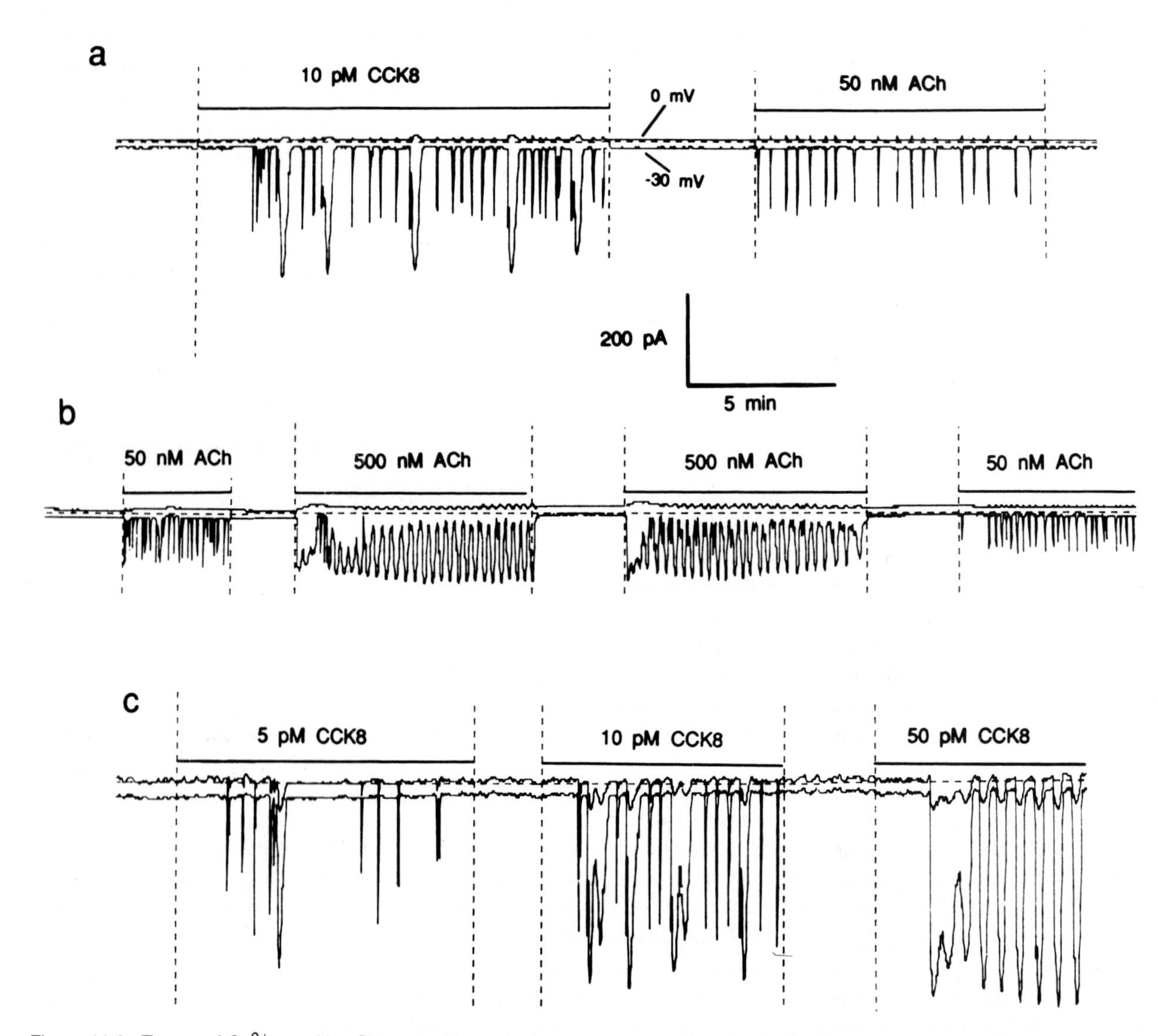

Figure 11.8 Traces of Ca^{2+}-sensitive Cl^- current from single mouse pancreatic acinar cells. The lower of the two traces (at −30 mV) monitors the current in the luminal membrane (downward deflections represent increased current). The different patterns of cytosolic ionized calcium concentration changes seen with different doses of acetylcholine (ACh) and cholecystokinin (CCK) are illustrated in recordings from three different cells (a, b and c). (Adapted from Petersen *et al.*,[12] with permission.)

As seen in *Figure 11.8*, such low CCK_8 concentrations evoke clear increases in the free ionized calcium concentration in the cytosolic compartment close to the luminal membrane where the exocytotic enzyme secretion occurs.

ACETYLCHOLINE

The acinar cells have a good functional innervation, as electrophysiological studies on mouse and rat show that every single acinar unit investigated with an intracellular microelectrode responds with depolarization when the nerves are stimulated.[14,16] In isolated human pancreatic acinar cells it has been shown directly that acetylcholine evokes enzyme secretion, internal ionized calcium release and activation of calcium-dependent ion channels.[15] There is also good evidence from studies in vivo indicating the importance of nervous control. In dogs with a transplanted pancreas the response to intraduodenal stimuli is reduced to about 50% of control indicating a substantial nervous component in the normal response. Furthermore, it has been shown that the pancreatic response to intraduodenal tryptophan or oleate instillation occurs much quicker than can be accounted for by cholecystokinin release. Atropine or vagotomy markedly delays the response, again indicating the functional importance of the vagal cholinergic pathway.[21]

OTHER TRANSMITTERS

A number of putative hormones and transmitters can stimulate the acinar cell, but, in most circumstances, there is still uncertainty about their physiological role in the normal intact organism. The list of substances that can directly activate the acinar cells to secrete includes peptides belonging to the bombesin group, vasoactive intestinal peptide, substance P, noradrenaline and adrenaline. Specific acinar receptor sites for many different agonists seem to coexist in the same acinar units (see *Figure 11.7*). A systematic mapping of the control mechanisms has unfortunately only been undertaken in very few species and not in man.[6,19] The bombesin peptides are perhaps of special interest. Bombesin was originally isolated from amphibian skin but mammalian bombesin has also been isolated. Although bombesin undoubtedly releases gastrin, there is little doubt that it also directly activates acinar cells via the same intracellular mechanism employed by cholecystokinin and acetylcholine.[14,16,19]

CELLULAR SECRETION PROCESSES

Polypeptide hormones, and neurotransmitters in general, activate cellular processes by increasing or decreasing the cytoplasmic level of a messenger. The roles of cyclic nucleotides (cyclic adenosine 3′,5′-monophosphate (cyclic AMP)) and cyclic guanosine 3′,5′-monophosphate) and ionized calcium as intracellular mediators of contraction, secretion and changes in metabolism are widely recognized.[19] The most direct evidence for intracellular messenger effects mediating the action of hormones or neurotransmitters on the acinar cells, comes from two different types of electrophysiological studies. In microelectrode investigations it has been possible to apply substances inside or immediately outside the plasma membrane. It transpires that the peptide secretagogues as well as acetylcholine evoke membrane depolarization when applied to the outside of the plasma membrane, after a minimum delay of about 0.5 s, whereas application inside has no effect. Intracellular injection of the calcium chelator EGTA inhibits the membrane potential changes evoked by extracellular secretagogue application whereas intracellular calcium injection mimics the action normally following extracellular acetylcholine or peptide hormone application.[14,16] In patch-clamp single-channel current recording investigations it has been shown that acetylcholine or cholecystokinin when applied extracellularly, outside a small area of plasma membrane to which there is no access, evokes opening of single ionic channels in that same area. When the isolated membrane patch is excised from the cell, it can be shown that the same channels can be activated by calcium from the internal side.[14,16] Many other less direct approaches confirm that acetylcholine, cholecystokinin and bombesin actions on acinar cells are mediated by a rise in internal ionized calcium concentration. Recent high-resolution single-cell capacitance measurements demonstrate directly that a rise in internal calcium triggers exocytosis,[10] but the precise mechanism by which it activates enzyme secretion by exocytosis is still unknown. The calcium-mediated opening of membrane ion channels allows ion movements important for the formation of the acinar neutral fluid secretion.[14,16]

Three types of calcium-dependent ion channels have been characterized in pancreatic acinar cells, namely ionized chloride, potassium and non-selective cation channels. The Cl^- channels are localized in the luminal membrane, whereas the K^+ and non-selective cation channels are in the basolateral membranes. The Ca^{2+}-activated K^+-selective channels have been characterized in human and pig pancreatic acinar cells whereas the Cl^- channels have only been studied in mouse and rat acinar cells. These localizations correspond to those found in other secretory epithelia (for example the salivary glands) where Cl^- secretion proceeds into the acinar lumen via Ca^{2+}-activated Cl^- channels in the luminal membrane and Cl^- is taken up into the cells via a Na^+–K^+–$2Cl^-$ cotransporter on the basolateral membrane operating together with the Na^+–K^+ pump and the Ca^{2+}-activated K^+ channels. Sodium ions are transported into the lumen via the paracellular route through so-called tight junctions, that are in fact very permeable, attracted by the lumen negativity established by the Cl^- flow across the luminal membrane.[13,14,16] The pancreatic acinar cells secrete very little fluid compared with the salivary gland acinar cells, probably because not all transporters are present in a sufficiently high density.

From an experimental point of view, the Ca^{2+}-activated Cl^- channels are of particular interest as they can be used to monitor changes in internal calcium at the luminal pole of the acinar cells. Recent studies have revealed highly localized internal ionized calcium changes in this region of mouse or rat pancreatic acinar cells[8,11] and electrical recording of Ca^{2+}-dependent Cl^- current under voltage clamp conditions in single cells has shown itself to be a very sensitive system for monitoring the temporal internal calcium changes in this region (*see Figure 11.8*). Although cholecystokinin and acetylcholine qualitatively evoke the same type of effect, the patterns of the responses are clearly different. Acetylcholine predominantly evokes shortlasting repetitive spikes fusing into a quasi-sustained response at higher concentrations, whereas during cholecystokinin stimulation, the apparently same type of short-lasting Ca^{2+} spikes more often trigger larger and longer Ca^{2+} waves. Such waves are not localized but proceed throughout the cell. At higher cholecystokinin concentrations, repetitive wave formation is the predominant response.[12] These single-cell studies reveal that control of internal calcium by acetylcholine or cholecystokinin occurs not by regulation of the amplitudes of the Ca^{2+} spikes or waves, but by regulation of the duration of the periods during which internal calcium is elevated.[12] Internal cell perfusion studies have revealed surprising subtleties in the regulation of internal calcium. *Figure 11.9* shows a model for the mechanism underlying the acetylcholine-evoked Ca^{2+} changes.[22] The effects of cholecystokinin are evoked via different guanosine triphosphatase-binding transducer proteins, but similar components are involved here,

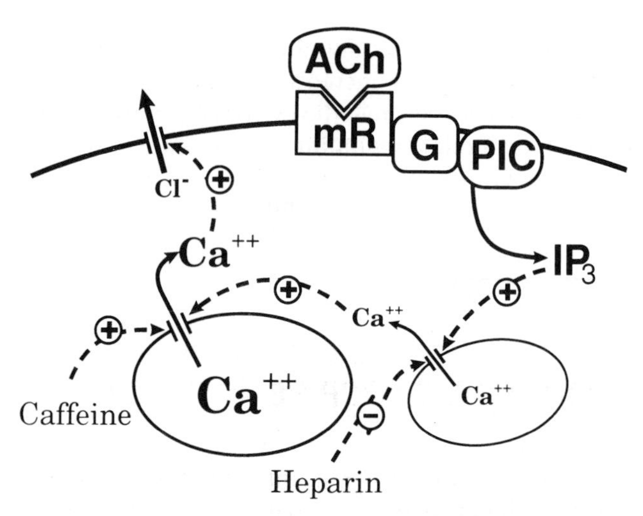

Figure 11.9 Schematic diagram explaining the steps involved in acetylcholine-evoked intracellular ionized calcium release. Acetylcholine (ACh) binds to muscarinic receptors (mR) thereby activating the enzyme phosphoinositidase C (PIC) via a transducing G-protein (G). PIC catalyses the splitting of phosphatidylinositol (4,5) bisphosphate into diacylglycerol (not shown) and inositol (1,4,5) trisphosphate (IP_3). IP_3 binds to and opens a heparin-sensitive Ca^{2+} channel in the endoplasmic reticulum thereby causing a small steady Ca^{2+} release into the cytosol. The IP_3-evoked primary Ca^{2+} release in turn activates a caffeine-sensitive calcium channel in a separate Ca^{2+}-storing compartment (probably also in the endoplasmic reticulum) evoking a larger Ca^{2+} release. This secondary release is pulsatile, either because the Ca^{2+} outflow is so large that the compartment is quickly emptied, and the time taken for reloading of the Ca^{2+} pool would then correspond to the time between Ca^{2+} spikes, or there is negative feedback in this part of the system. The increase in internal calcium stimulates a number of molecular events. This diagram only shows the activation of the Cl^- channel in the cell membrane. (From Wakui *et al.*,[22] with permission).

although there are some indications that there may be additional messengers involved.

The mechanism of action of vasoactive intestinal peptide and secretin on the acinar cells is not so clear. There are strong arguments in favour of cyclic AMP as an intracellular messenger, but the specific transport steps activated by cyclic AMP have not been identified.[19]

In the bicarbonate-secreting duct cells, a cyclic AMP-activated Cl^- channel in the luminal membrane has been identified and studied. This channel can be activated in the intact cell by a secretin-evoked increase in cyclic AMP concentration.[7] Such a Cl^- channel acting in concert with a Cl^-–HCO_3^- exchanger also in the luminal membrane and the Na^+–K^+ pump, K^+ channel and Na^+–H^+ exchanger in the basolateral membrane may explain the secretin-evoked bicarbonate-rich fluid secretion.[7] Recently it has also been shown that bombesin and substance P can evoke fluid secretion in isolated rat pancreatic ducts.[1]

There are marked potentiating interactions between secretagogues acting via changes in internal ionized calcium concentration (cholecystokinin, acetylcholine and bombesin) and those acting via changes in intracellular cyclic AMP concentration (secretin and vasoactive intestinal peptide).[6,19] The mechanism underlying this phenomenon is unknown.

ENDOCRINE–EXOCRINE INTERACTION

It is now clear that a significant proportion of blood draining the islets enters capillaries in the exocrine tissue. Islet hormones can therefore be present in relatively high concentrations in the extracellular fluid surrounding the acinar cells. It has been shown that both exogenous and endogenous insulin markedly augments cholecystokinin-evoked fluid and amylase secretion in the isolated perfused rat pancreas, whilst having no effect on secretion alone.[19]

CONCLUSION

The exocrine pancreas secretes fluid containing a large number of important digestive enzymes. The mechanism of secretion appears to be exocytosis in the acinar cells. Fluid is secreted in both acinar and duct cells in response to a variety of hormonal and nervous stimuli. In both acinar and duct cells, a number of specific transport pathways have been identified and localized.

REFERENCES

1. Ashton, N., Argent, B.E. and Green, R. (1990) Effects of vasoactive intestinal peptide, bombesin and substance P on fluid secretion by isolated rat pancreatic ducts. *Journal of Physiology*, **422**, 471–482.
2. Bolender, R.P. (1974) Stereological analysis of the guinea pig pancreas. *Journal of Cell Biology*, **61**, 269–287.
3. Bro-Rasmussen, F., Killmann, S.A. and Thaysen, J.H. (1956) The composition of pancreatic juice as compared to sweat, parotid saliva and tears. *Acta Physiologica Scandinavica*, **37**, 97–113.
4. Denyer, M.E. and Cotton, P.B. (1979) Pure pancreatic juice studies in normal subjects and patients with chronic pancreatitis. *Gut*, **20**, 89–97.
5. Fahrenkrug, J., Schaffalitzky De Muckadell, O.B., Holst, J.J. and Lindkaer Jensen, S. (1979) Vasoactive intestinal polypeptide in vagally mediated pancreatic secretion of fluid and HCO_3^-. *American Journal of Physiology*, **237**, E535–E540.
6. Gardner, J.D. and Jensen, R.T. (1987) Secretagogue receptors on pancreatic acinar cells. In *Physiology of the Gastrointestinal Tract* (2nd edition) (Ed.) Johnson, L.R. pp. 1109–1127, New York: Raven Press.
7. Gray, M.A., Greenwell, J.R. and Argent, B.E. (1988) Secretin-regulated chloride channel on the apical plasma membrane of pancreatic duct cells. *Journal of Membrane Biology*, **105**, 131–142.
8. Kasai, H. and Augustine, G.J. (1990) Cytosolic Ca^{2+} gradients triggering unidirectional fluid secretion from exocrine pancreas. *Nature*, **348**, 735–738.
9. Lindkaer Jensen, S., Rehfeld, J.F., Holst, J.J. *et al.* (1981) Secretory effects of cholecystokinins on the isolated perfused porcine pancreas. *Acta physiologica Scandinavica*, **111**, 225–231.
10. Maruyama, Y. (1989) Control of exocytosis in single cells. *News in Physiological Sciences*, **4**, 53–56.
11. Osipchuk, Y.V., Wakui, M., Yule, D.I., Gallacher, D.V. and Petersen, O.H. (1990) Cytoplasmic Ca^{2+} oscillations evoked by receptor stimulation, G-protein activation, internal application of inositol trisphosphate or Ca^{2+}: simultaneous microfluorimetry and Ca^{2+}-dependent Cl^- current recording in single pancreatic acinar cells. *EMBO Journal*, **9**, 697–704.
12. Petersen, C.C.H., Toescu, E.C. and Petersen, O.H. (1991) Different patterns of receptor-activated cytoplasmic Ca^{2+} oscillations in single pancreatic acinar cells: dependence on receptor type, agonist concentration and intracellular Ca^{2+} buffering. *EMBO Journal*, **10**, 527–533.
13. Petersen, O.H. (1986) Calcium-activated potassium channels and fluid secretion by exocrine glands. *American Journal of Physiology*, **251**, G1–G13.
14. Petersen, O.H. (1987) Electrophysiology of exocrine gland cells. In *Physiology of the Gastrointestinal Tract* (2nd edition) (Ed.) Johnson, L.R. pp. 745–772. New York: Raven Press.
15. Petersen, O.H., Findlay, I., Iwatsuki, N. *et al.* (1985) Human pancreatic acinar cells: studies of stimulus-secretion coupling. *Gastroenterology*, **89**, 109–117.
16. Petersen, O.H. and Maruyama, Y. (1989) Electrophysiology of salivary and pancreatic acinar cells. In: *Handbook of Physiology, The Gastrointestinal System*, Vol. III (Ed.) Forte, J.G. pp. 25–50. Washington DC: American Physiological Society.
17. Petersen, O.H., Maruyama, Y., Graf, J. *et al.* (1981) Ionic currents across pancreatic acinar cell membranes and their role in fluid secretion. *Philosophical Transactions of the Royal Society of London Series B*, **296**, 151–166.
18. Schulz, I. (1987) Electrolyte and fluid secretion in the exocrine pancreas. In *Physiology of the*

Gastrointestinal Tract (2nd edition) (Ed.) Johnson, L.R. pp. 1147–1171 New York: Raven Press.
19. Schulz, I. (1989) Signaling transduction in hormone- and neurotransmitter-induced enzyme secretion from the exocrine pancreas. In: *Handbook of Physiology, The Gastrointestinal System,* Vol. III (Ed.) Forte, J.G. pp. 443–463. Washington DC: American Physiological Society.
20. Sewell, W.A. and Young, J.A. (1975) Secretion of electrolytes by the pancreas of the anaesthetized rat. *Journal of Physiology*, **252**, 379–396.
21. Solomon, T.E. (1987) Control, of exocrine pancreatic secretion. In: *Physiology of the Gastrointestinal Tract* (2nd edition) (Ed.) Johnson, C.R. pp. 1173–1207. New York: Raven Press.
22. Wakui, M., Osipchuk, Y.V. and Petersen, O.H. (1990) Receptor-activated cytoplasmic Ca^{2+} spiking mediated by inositol trisphosphate is due to Ca^{2+}-induced Ca^{2+} release. *Cell*, **63**, 1025–1032.
23. Walsh, J.H. (1987) Cholecystokinin. In *Physiology of the Gastrointestinal Tract* (2nd edition) (Ed.) Johnson, L.R. pp. 195–205. New York: Raven Press.

EVALUATION OF PANCREATIC DISEASE

A.T.R. Axon and C.J. Mitchell

The evaluation of pancreatic disease remains one of the more difficult problems in gastroenterology. In this section, chronic pancreatitis and pancreatic adenocarcinoma will be the main considerations, because acute pancreatitis, endocrine pancreatic neoplasms, fibrocystic disease and childhood pancreatic disorders are discussed elsewhere.

During the last decade, there has been rigorous assessment of the available investigations so that their limitations and value are more accurately known. Before pancreatic investigation is pursued, the clinician should decide its objective and whether it will affect management. Sometimes the clinical history, examination, and a plain abdominal radiograph are all that is required to make a diagnosis and institute treatment. At other times, a number of tests may be needed before the patient can be properly assessed. This section describes the available investigations and discusses their use in specific situations.

There are several categories of pancreatic investigation. *Morphological* or *imaging* tests detect changes in pancreatic shape, size and duct systems. Other tests aim to detect pancreatic disease by alteration in *function*. A further group of investigations are designed as *markers* of pancreatic disease from abnormalities in blood, urine, faeces or pancreatic juice constituents. Additionally, fine needle aspiration of the pancreas can provide diagnostic information from *cytological* or *histological* samples.

The results of studies of a given investigation should be interpreted with caution, particularly with regard to reported sensitivity and specificity. It is relatively easy to achieve good results when comparing healthy subjects to unrealistic disease controls with patients with advanced pancreatic carcinoma or exocrine insufficiency. Diagnostic problems in clinical practice are mainly encountered in the presence of early chronic pancreatitis or small, and hopefully resectable, pancreatic tumours and this is when good tests are particularly needed. In addition the sensitivity and specificity of a given test is often worse in prospective, as opposed to retrospective, studies. There are also different requirements from a diagnostic test under varying conditions of disease prevalence in the population being studied.

MARKERS OF PANCREATIC DISEASE

SERUM MARKERS

Amylase, trypsin, lipase and gastrointestinal hormones

The use of these tests in the diagnosis of acute pancreatitis is discussed elsewhere (page 1602). Total serum amylase levels are so variable in chronic pancreatitis and carcinoma as to be of little diagnostic value. Measurements of pancreatic isoamylases are now available and recent comparisons suggest that P_3-amylase electrophoresis is the most accurate.[81] Isoamylase determination is frequently normal in chronic pancreatitis until exocrine insufficiency is present and variable levels occur in pancreatic carcinoma.

Similar findings apply to serum immunoreactive trypsin measurement. Some 50% of patients with chronic pancreatitis have a normal serum level, although it is raised during an acute relapse and becomes subnormal in the presence of steatorrhoea.[70,81] In comparative studies, serum lipase performs as well as isoamylase or serum immunoreactive trypsin estimation in the diagnosis of chronic pancreatitis and carcinoma,[65,81] but new methodology makes lipase analysis more easily performed.

The disadvantage of these investigations in the diagnosis of chronic pancreatitis and carcinoma is their variability at different stages of the disease. Elevated levels occur in chronic pancreatitis during early acute relapses whereas levels become subnormal when the disease is well advanced; during the intermediate stage (when a good diagnostic test is most needed) enzyme levels are frequently normal. Similar mechanisms probably apply to pancreatic carcinoma and merely reflect the degree of associated pancreatic damage. Because the finding of a low serum isoamylase, immunoreactive trypsin or lipase is highly specific but not very sensitive, their main use is to provide a simple and reliable confirmation that steatorrhoea is of pancreatic origin.[65] Sufficient numbers of tests must be generated to make them economic to perform.

Measurement of many gastrointestinal hormones is feasible, but some assays are not widely available. High basal levels of motilin and enteroglucagon, but not of pancreatic polypeptide, occur in chronic pancreatitis. When exocrine insufficiency is present, the response of plasma pancreatic polypeptide and cholecystokinin to a test meal is impaired with a less pronounced difference from controls for patients with less severe pancreatitis.[8,46] There are easier ways of deriving the diagnostic information provided by these investigations.

Serum markers of pancreatic carcinoma

The laudable objective of these tests, namely to provide an early diagnosis, has yet to be achieved. Increasing numbers of pancreatic tumour antigens are being described for which space does not allow or merit full description. No single marker has emerged with a marked superiority. The major limitations to this approach are that it is difficult to find a marker which distinguishes benign from malignant pancreatic disease, or which differentiates pancreatic cancer from other tumours, or both. Serum carcinoembryonic antigen fails on both counts; a newer antigen, CA19-9, is more sensitive and specific but levels are unfortunately also raised in jaundiced patients regardless of the cause[24] and may be normal in the presence of small tumours or non-pancreatic malignancies. The carbohydrate antigen CA-50 is more specific, but has a lower positive predictive value. Such markers may, however, be of value in monitoring the progress of disease after treatment. The peanut agglutinin assay is as accurate as CA19-9,[20] but CA125, DU-PAN-2 and tissue polypeptide assays are less sensitive.[35] As more tumour markers are described the choice becomes more bewildering. Comparative studies between the various candidates have provided some help, but results from individual studies vary widely and must reflect selection bias in the studied population. Few studies have demonstrated improved accuracy by combining measurement of more than one tumour marker.

Many of the newer markers remain to be more rigorously tested in prospective studies with realistic controls. At present, sensitivities or specificities of up to 70–80% have been reported, so their accuracy is inadequate for screening an asymptomatic population. These tests are more useful in the investigation of patients with symptoms or signs suggestive of pancreatic carcinoma, particularly as an adjunct to other tests, e.g. ultrasound. It is worth noting that some of the reported sensitivities and specificities compare favourably to those of ultrasound and computed tomography. The practical problem for most clinicians remains that the techniques are often not readily available, and even commercially available kits have drawbacks because of limited shelf-life or requiring batch testing to be economical.

Pancreatic juice markers

Performance of endoscopic retrograde cholangiopancreatography provides an opportunity to collect pancreatic secretions after selective cannulation. Attempts to use this technique for pancreatic function testing have been disappointing. Qualitative assessment of pancreatic juice constitutents has also been studied and immunoglobulin A and G levels are raised in the presence of carcinoma. More detailed analysis of pancreatic juice constitutents, using techniques such as isoelectric focussing, shows abnormal profiles in the presence of pancreatic carcinoma or chronic pancreatitis, but the techniques are not applicable to routine laboratories. Recent studies have not confirmed the discriminatory value of lactoferrin measurement, immunoreactive trypsin levels are more easily obtained from serum samples and carcinoembryonic antigen levels are unhelpful. It should be remembered, however, that the cytology of pancreatic juice obtained at pancreatography consistently enhances the diagnostic accuracy of the technique.[27]

FAECAL ANALYSES

The severity of steatorrhoea that occurs in pancreatic insufficiency, and which may exceed 100 g per day, is rarely encountered in other malabsorptive states. Faecal fat estimation will not identify the cause of steatorrhoea, but it is useful to assess the need and adequacy of enzyme replacement therapy, although oral pancreatic function tests (PFTs) may achieve the latter goal.[43] Accurate and reproducible results require a 7-day constant fat diet with markers and it is an unpopular estimation in the laboratory; recent methodology employing a shorter collection time and easier analysis should be helpful.[7]

The faecal output of pancreatic enzymes can be used to detect exocrine insufficiency. Whereas significant destruction of trypsin occurs during intestinal transit, chymotrypsin is more stable and faecal output has been used as an indication of exocrine insufficiency. A low level is a reliable indication of pancreatic disease in the presence of steatorrhoea, but in comparative studies with oral pancreatic function tests, it is less sensitive (66% versus 88%) and falsely positive results occur in up to 20%.[51] This investigation is useful in screening for cystic fibrosis and in the long-term follow-up of chronic pancreatitis.

FAT ABSORPTION TESTS

In pancreatic disease the failure to assimilate fat is caused by enzymatic triglyceride maldigestion rather than a failure of absorption. Measuring the faecal recovery of orally administered radiolabelled triglycerides and fatty acids has proved unreliable. Several newer studies have measured expired $^{14}CO_2$ released from radiolabelled triglycerides given orally; after initially encouraging results these tests have proved to be both insensitive and non-specific. A recent study of this type using a ^{13}C-octanoate, which requires complex mass spectrometry analysis, discriminated poorly between pancreatic and non-pancreatic steatorrhoea as well as other disease controls.[80]

PANCREATIC FUNCTION TESTING

TESTS INVOLVING DUODENAL INTUBATION

These tests measure exocrine function by analysing duodenal aspirate, either after direct stimulation of pancreatic section using secretin, with or without cholecystokinin,[18,26] or after indirect stimulation by the use of a standard test meal, usually that of Lundh.[57]

For direct stimulation tests, the intubation system must be reliable because incomplete collection or gastric juice contamination of duodenal aspirates invalidates the results. A multi-lumen tube is positioned fluoroscopically to enable duodenal and gastric contents to be collected separately. Basal and sequential 10-minute samples are collected on ice over 30–80 minutes. The methods and dosage of stimulation vary widely, as do the preparations of secretin and cholecystokinin which stimulate bicarbonate and enzyme output respectively. Different protocols have used secretin stimulation alone,[26] secretin followed by cholecystokinin[18] or secretin and cholecystokinin infusion combined.[12] Aspirates are analysed for secretion rates, bicarbonate concentration and output as well as enzyme output if cholecystokinin has been used. Meticulous adherence to technique is required to produce meaningful results. The characteristic finding in advanced chronic pancreatitis or carcinoma is a depression of volume secreted and of bicarbonate and enzyme concentration. Recent large studies have suggested that mean chymotrypsin activity and peak bicarbonate output[39] or secretin stimulated bicarbonate output over 30 minutes[44] provide the best discriminants for detecting pancreatic disease. Impaired bicarbonate secretion, which precedes loss of enzyme output in pancreatitis, will not be detected by indirect tests.

An elaboration of the secretin–cholecystokinin test measures the rate of incorporation of intravenous 75-selenium labelled methionine into the duodenal aspirate as an index of pancreatic enzyme synthesis. This improves the sensitivity at the expense of specificity although the combination of these results with those of the conventional secretin–cholecystokinin test (performed simultaneously) provided a most reliable test.[11]

The indirect test of Lundh[56] is easier to perform and has a more standard protocol. A single lumen tube is positioned fluoroscopically in the duodenum. A test meal of glucose, corn oil and casilan is given orally and four 30-minute aspirates are collected on ice to measure tryptic activity. This test is dependent upon extra-pancreatic factors, such as gastric and vagal function or endogenous secretin and cholecystokinin release; abnormal results should be interpreted with caution especially in the presence of small bowel disease.

The diagnostic accuracy of both types of test is well documented, although largely in retrospective series. Both direct and indirect tests will not distinguish pancreatitis from carcinoma, but do provide an opportunity to collect duodenal aspirates for cytological examination. In the largest series of secretin tests, misleading results occurred in only 5.1% of controls and 5.2% of patients with pancreatic disease.[26] For the secretin–cholecystokinin test, sensitivities of 60–83% and specificities of 89–95% are representative, the lower sensitivities predictably occurring in prospective studies.[11,12,39,44] As indicated above, the specificity of the Lundh test is lower, albeit in defined situations;[66] it is probably also a little less sensitive, although this has been disputed.[13] In clinical practice these differences become less clearly defined and the practical advantages of the Lundh test can offset the higher accuracy of direct stimulation tests.

ORAL (TUBELESS) PANCREATIC FUNCTION TESTS

The practical disadvantages of duodenal intubation tests have led to the development of oral pancreatic function tests which all share a similar basis. An orally administered substrate is hydrolysed by pancreatic enzymes to produce a metabolite that is absorbed and subsequently excreted in the urine. Measurement of urinary recovery of the metabolite provides an indirect index of exocrine function. It should be noted that urinary recovery of the metabolite depends upon its absorption, intermediary metabolism and urinary excretion as much as upon enzyme hydrolysis. These tests must overcome this problem to achieve reasonable specificity, because patients who present with, for example, jaundice or malabsorption (which might lead to a misleadingly abnormal test) may have causes other than pancreatic disease. Furthermore, oral pancreatic function tests depend upon pancreatic digestive capacity, which is not impaired until pancreatic disease is advanced, and which therefore limits the sensitivity of the test.

Synthetic tripeptide test

This test uses N-benzoyl-L-tyrosyl-*p*-aminobenzoic acid (BTP) as a substrate for chymotrypsin hydrolysis to release the metabolite *p*-aminobenzoic acid (PABA) most of which is conjugated before urinary excretion. PABA is measured colometrically or by high-performance liquid chromatography but some foodstuffs and drugs, notably paracetamol and sulphonamides, interfere with estimation so it is important to analyse a pre-test urine sample. The optimal oral dose of BTP is 0.5–1 g[45] is administered with or without a Lundh meal, and urine is collected for 6 hours. The test result is expressed as a percentage urinary recovery of PABA given orally in the BTP.

Considerable experience has accumulated including three reports totalling over 1000 patients.[50,30,41] The overall sensitivity for pancreatic disease was 64–83% and better (86%) for chronic pancreatitis than carcinoma (76%). Specificities of 81–93% were also achieved using controls with other gastrointestinal disease, but this falls to 50% in patients with non-pancreatic steatorrhoea or severe liver disease.[59] The modified BTP test overcomes this problem. The administration of *p*-aminosalicylate (PAS) or a tracer dose of ^{14}C-PABA with the BTP enables a PABA excretion index to be derived from the ratio of urinary recovery of PABA (dependent upon pancreatic function, absorption and conjugation) to PAS or ^{14}C (independent of pancreatic function). Modified BTP tests enable specificities up to 90% to be achieved.[15,40,63]

Misgivings about the reliability of urine collections, which is critical for the unmodified BTP test (but less so for the PABA excretion index), resulted in measurement of the serum rather than urine PABA levels. The practical advantage is that a single blood sample is withdrawn 2–3 hours after BTP administration and clinical results are comparable to those obtained with urine collection.[23] The reservation to this approach is that absorption (and thus peak serum level) varies considerably between individuals. The best of both worlds can be obtained by including a 3-hour serum PABA measurement with estimation of the PABA excretion index, which is the protocol now used routinely by the authors.

Fluorescein dilaurate test

This substance acts as a substrate for pancreatic esterase hydrolysis releasing fluorescein which is absorbed and excreted in the urine. On a second occasion fluorescein alone is given. From the two 10-hour urinary recoveries of fluorescein, a ratio is derived in a similar way to the modified BTP test. The test has achieved high sensitivity (>90%) in the presence of documented exocrine insufficiency[10] although others achieve more representative values of 67% with a poor specificity of 60%[51] which probably relates to the dependence of esterase hydrolysis upon adequate bile salt excretion, as misleadingly abnormal results are frequent with hepatobiliary or extensive small bowel disease. The two-stage test does not seem to overcome this problem in the same way as the modified BTP test. The need for two 10-hour urine collections on days 1 and 3 is a practical disadvantage.

Other tubeless tests

The dual-label Schilling test is based upon the observation that cobalamin can only be transferred to intrinsic factor (by which it is carried for absorption in the terminal ileum) from its complex with R protein after degradation by pancreatic proteases. Coincident administration of cyanocobalamin complexes labelled with ^{59}Co and ^{58}CO to R protein and intrinsic factor respectively allows assessment of exocrine function from a 24-hour urinary recovery of the two isotopes. In the initial study reasonable results were reported except in the presence of steatorrhoea,[16] but a subsequent study showed a poor sensitivity (50%) even among patients with pancreatic steatorrhoea.[53]

A different approach has been to measure changes in plasma amino acid levels after pancreatic stimulation with secretin–cholecystokinin. The normal decrease in plasma amino acid levels was progressively impaired with impressive sensitivities of 67%, 86% and 100% respectively for mild, moderate and severe chronic pancreatitis as judged by the secretin–cholecystokinin test.[25] Amino acid analysis is not widely available and employs quite expensive dedicated equipment. This test requires more rigorous evaluation, particularly with disease controls, to define its specificity.

Which pancreatic function test?

Sufficient information is now available on the accuracy of oral pancreatic function tests to consider the relative merits of the available methods to assess exocrine function. The secretin–cholecystokinin test remains the standard by which to judge other methods. But the technical and practical problems are formidable to most practising clinicians without a specialist unit with its associated manpower and expertise. Duodenal intubation is not popular with patients, fluoroscopy must be available and the tube position must be accurate and maintained throughout the test to prevent gastric contamination. To achieve good results, more tests than most centres can generate must be performed. Even in the best hands up to 10% of tests fail, a factor which is frequently not taken into account in calculation of accuracy. The Lundh test is more 'user-friendly', although not for the patient; it is less demanding of expertise and is claimed to produce as good results[13] in spite of its theoretical disadvantages and it has nearly the same failure rate (7%). In spite of these reservations, the duodenal tests are more sensitive than oral pancreatic function tests by a factor of at least 10%, this being particularly true in patients with moderate rather than severe exocrine dysfunction. The claims for a better specificity, particularly in comparison with the modified pancreatic function tests, are less convincing.

It is now clearer which oral pancreatic function tests are useful. The comparison between the *modified* BTP test and the fluorescein dilaurate test (which is the correct one) shows an equal sensitivity,[51] but worries about the specificity of the fluorescein dilaurate test persist, especially when realistic controls are used in prospective studies. The dual-label Schilling test has proved less accurate than the modified BTP test.[53] Currently the best choice is the modified BTP test using ^{14}C-PABA or PAS. Concerns about the radiation dose from the former test have been overemphasized, as the dose is some 5% of a routine chest radiograph. The simplicity, practical advantages and reproducibility of oral pancreatic function tests allow widespread use in less specialized centres and render them useful for sequential testing[61] or monitoring pancreatic enzyme replacement.[43]

IMAGING

ULTRASOUND

Ultrasound is a sophisticated imaging technique. The newer systems permit real-time imaging with good lateral and axial resolution. Doppler and colour-flow Doppler techniques are becoming more widely available and have had a significant impact on the examination of upper abdominal vascular structures, particularly the portal venous system. Endoscopic ultrasound, employing a higher frequency transducer mounted on a flexible endoscope, is a newer and highly sensitive technique for the examination of the upper gastrointestinal tract and the pancreas.

Most ultrasound imaging of the pancreas is by transabdominal sonography. This relatively quick and cheap technique has the great advantage of flexibility of scan plane which enables the pancreas, with its varying position in the upper abdomen, to be scanned more easily than with some of the static modalities such as CT. It is more subject to technical adversity, however, particularly the presence of bowel gas lying between the transducer and the target organ. High frequency ultrasound is almost totally reflected by such gas resulting in unsatisfactory imaging. Gas poses no such problems for CT or magnetic resonance imaging (MRI).

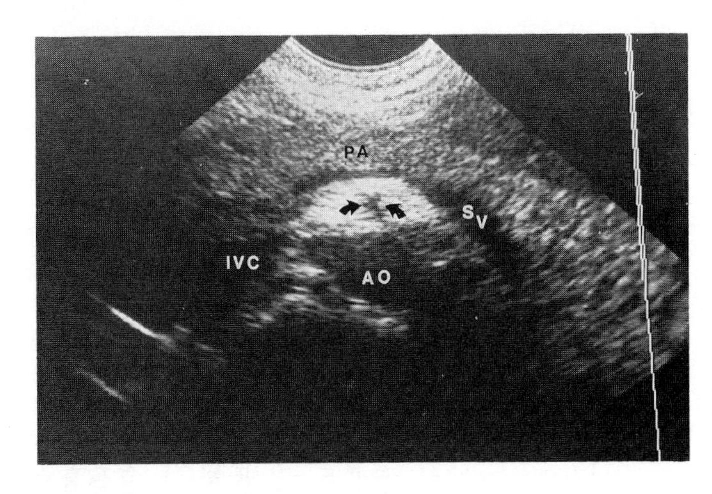

Figure 11.10 Normal anatomy. Transverse scan through the upper abdomen showing pancreas (PA), splenic vein (SV), inferior vena cava (IVC), aorta (AO), and superior mesenteric artery (black arrow heads).

A normal pancreas on ultrasound is a medium amplitude, comma-shaped organ lying obliquely across the upper abdomen (*Figure 11.10*). The uncinate process and dorsal portion may be of reduced echo amplitude compared with the rest of the gland, presumably because of the different embryological origins of the dorsal and ventral pancreas. The posterior border of the pancreas is well demarcated by the splenic vein and portal vein confluence lying under the neck. The right lateral border of the head of the pancreas is demarcated by the gastroduodenal artery and by the duodenum. Water taken by mouth helps to visualize the pancreas by providing an 'acoustic window' and may, when passing into the duodenum, allow better delineation of the head. The normal pancreatic duct can be seen in the main body of the gland using modern equipment. The upper limit of normal on ultrasound examination is 2 mm diameter.

Chronic pancreatitis

The sonographic appearances of chronic pancreatitis include enlargement of the gland with alteration of the normally even echo texture and an increase in echo amplitude in areas of fibrosis. Areas of gland calcification can be more accurately detected by ultrasound (*Figure 11.11*) than by radiography and may also show calculi within the pancreatic duct. Changes assessed at ultrasound compare closely with those of endoscopic retrograde cholangiopancreatography and can be graded similarly.[48]

A normal pancreatic duct can be appreciated on routine examination of the pancreas. Dilatation and irregularity of the duct is seen in chronic disease (*Figure 11.12*), even in mild forms.

Occasionally, duct stenosis may prevent adequate demonstration of the pancreatic duct at pancreatography. On these relatively rare occasions, ultrasound-guided pancreatography may be performed. A fine needle is inserted into the main pancreatic duct via the anterior abdominal wall, often using a transgastric approach, and contrast injected (*Figure 11.13*).

Pancreatic tumours

The demonstration of any mass lesion by ultrasound requires an alteration in the acoustic impedance of tumour tissue compared with the surrounding normal tissue. In pancreatic cancer, the lesions are characteristically hyporeflective compared with the normal pancreatic tissue (*Figure 11.14*). They may be cystic in some cystadenomas and cystadenocarcinomas. The detectability of small lesions depends upon the resolution of the equipment available and upon the quality of the scan obtained. The administration of oral de-gassed water into the stomach aids examination. The diagnostic yield from ultrasound is similar to that of CT, although with thin slice technology and intravenous contrast medium enhancement, CT is probably more accurate and sensitive for smaller lesions.

Colour-flow Doppler studies are a useful adjunct to determine the patency or involvement of the splenic and portal veins. Although occlusion or tumour involvement may be easily appreciated, stenosis and turbulence of flow may be due to compression or invasion, and discrimination between these two (and hence the prediction of resectability) is poor.

Intra-operative ultrasound is a technique that has been available for many years. It is becoming increasingly popular in the field of pancreatic cancer. In particular, endocrine tumours,[69] which may be multiple, are often well shown by ultrasound at operation when they cannot be seen or felt by the surgeon.

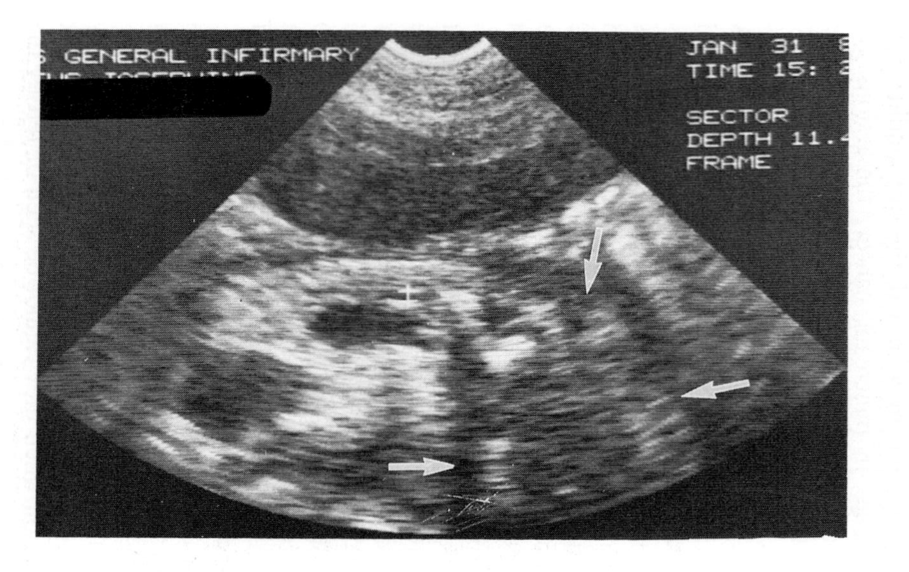

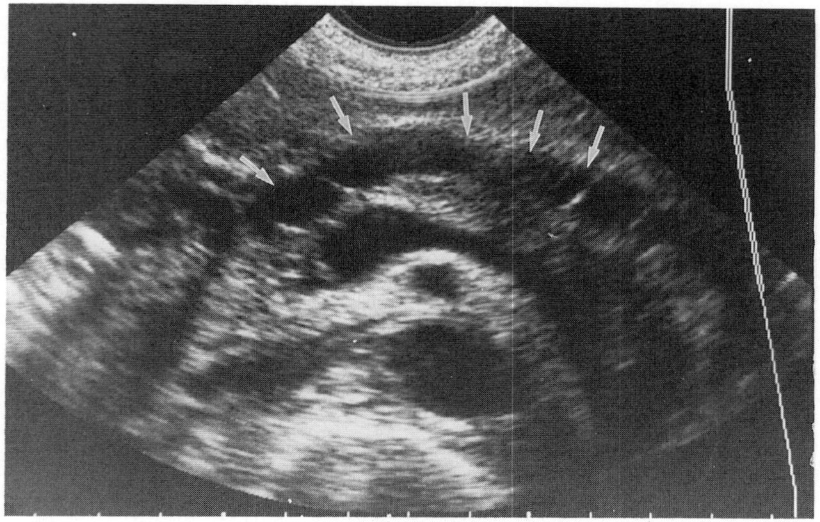

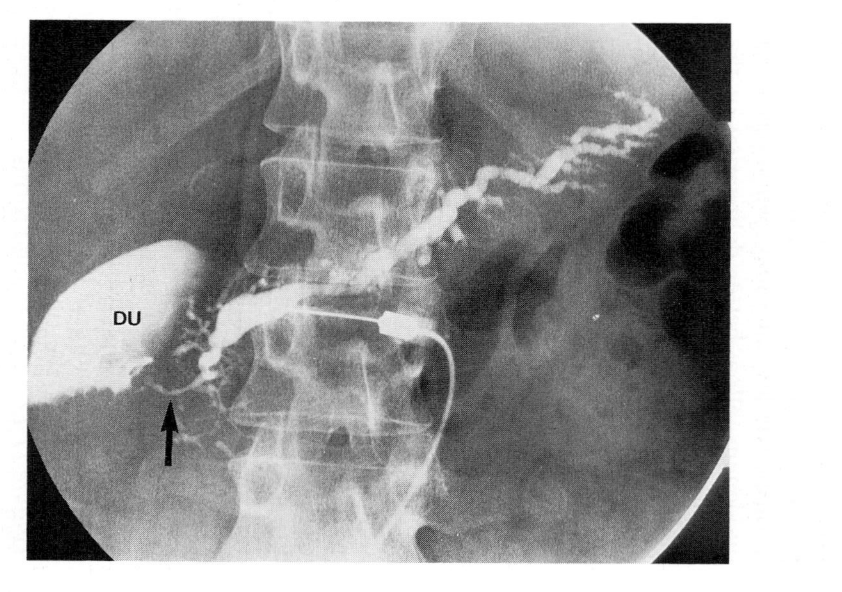

Figure 11.11 (above left) Chronic pancreatitis. Although the head and body of the pancreas are normal and the ducts are of normal calibre, there is an extensive inflammatory mass involving the tail of the pancreas (white arrows). This is swollen and contains an area of calcification.

Figure 11.12 (above right) Gross dilatation of the pancreatic duct. The duct (white arrows) is grossly swollen and tortuous; this degree of distension usually indicates a significant stricture.

Figure 11.13 (left) Percutaneous pancreatogram. A fine needle has been introduced into the pancreatic duct under ultrasound guidance. The duct exhibits the features of chronic pancreatitis and a stricture (black arrow) is shown in the peri-ampullary region. Some contrast has passed into the duodenum (DU).

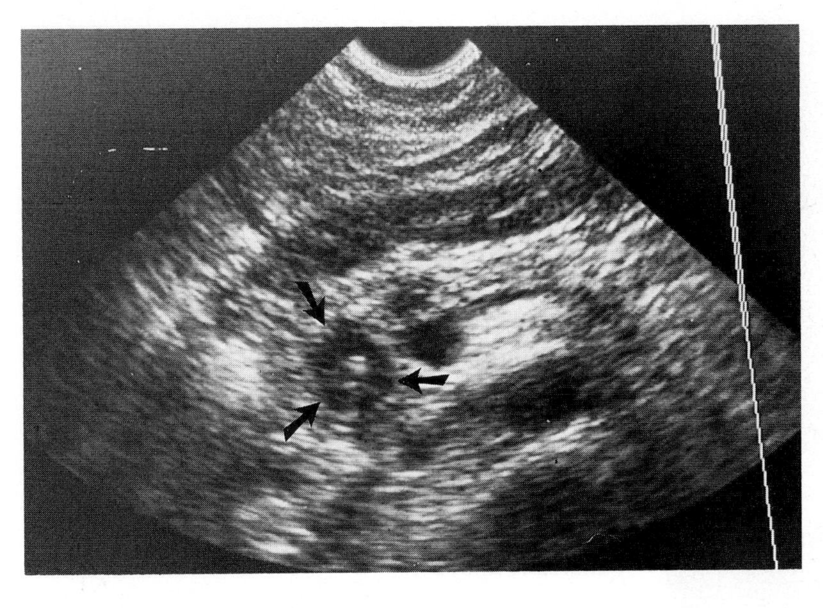

Figure 11.14 Carcinoma of the pancreas. A small hyporeflective lesion (black arrows) is seen in the head of the pancreas. The appearances are typical but non-specific for malignant disease.

ENDOSCOPIC ULTRASOUND

There has been a considerable advance in the technology of endoscopic ultrasound. This equipment, using 7.5 and 10 MHz scanners, enables a detailed assessment of the pancreatic parenchyma. The technique is difficult, however, and requires specialized training both in endoscopy and the interpretation of the ultrasound scan. The precise sensitivity and specificity in distinguishing between benign and malignant disease remains in question, but impressive results have been obtained by Yasuda *et al.*[84] The technique cannot be generally recommended until its merits and limitations have been more precisely defined.[73]

COMPUTED TOMOGRAPHY

With the widespread availability of CT scanners, clinicians now have an imaging technique which will guarantee demonstration of the pancreas. Endoscopic retrograde cholangiopancreatology and ultrasound are valuable in pancreatic imaging but technical failure occurs in up to 10%. CT not only demonstrates the pancreatic morphology (*Figure 11.15*), but provides information about the immediate peripancreatic tissues, the adjacent organs commonly affected by pancreatic pathology, and, when i.v. contrast is given, an assessment of pancreatic parenchymal viability (*Figure 11.16*).

CT technology continues to develop with ever faster scanning times and higher resolution. The availability of shorter scanning times allows more effective examination of ill patients and children, when breath-holding and movement may cause difficulty. The combination of thin slices and intravenous contrast means that smaller lesions can now be imaged.

The disadvantages of CT include exposure to ionizing radiation and its relative high cost compared with ultrasound. Although not as operator dependent as ultrasound, the effectiveness and quality of a CT study largely depend on the degree of supervision of the radiologist and expertise of the radiology staff as well as the quality of the scanner installation.

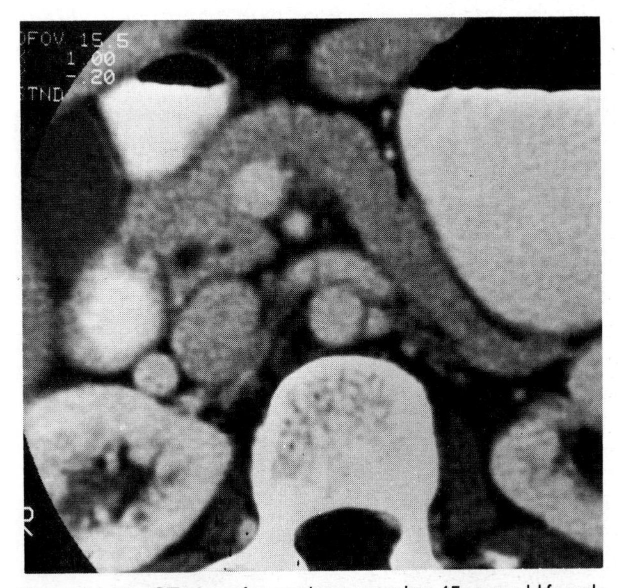

Figure 11.15 CT scan of normal pancreas in a 45-year-old female. Post-contrast section targetted to immediate peripancreatic area showing normal morphology of head, body and tail. The common bile duct and pancreatic duct are seen in the head and the adjacent vasculature is clearly demonstrated.

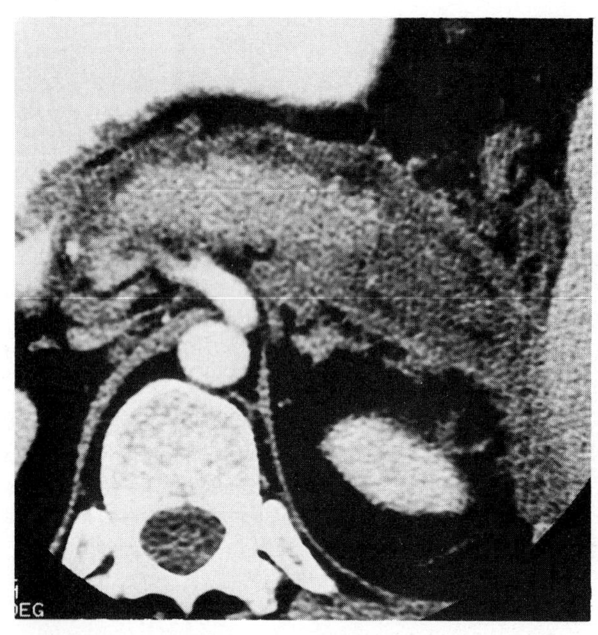

Figure 11.16 Targetted post-contrast CT section from a 40-year-old male showing enhancing viable parenchyma within the body and neck contrasting with absence of parenchymal enhancement in tail. There is also a rind of soft tissue density anterior to the pancreatic body consistent with peripancreatic necrosis or localized phlegmonous change.

Chronic pancreatitis

The impact of CT in chronic pancreatitis has been less marked than in acute pancreatitis.[31] CT features include focal or diffuse gland enlargement, calcification, ductal abnormalities, and pseudocysts which may be intrapancreatic or extrapancreatic (*Figure 11.17*). Endoscopic retrograde cholangiopancreatography remains the imaging 'gold standard' for the diagnosis of chronic pancreatitis, but CT may demonstrate the pancreatic and peripancreatic morphology more readily than ultrasound, particularly when calcification is prominent. Complications of chronic pancreatitis such as portal venous thrombosis may be demonstrated.

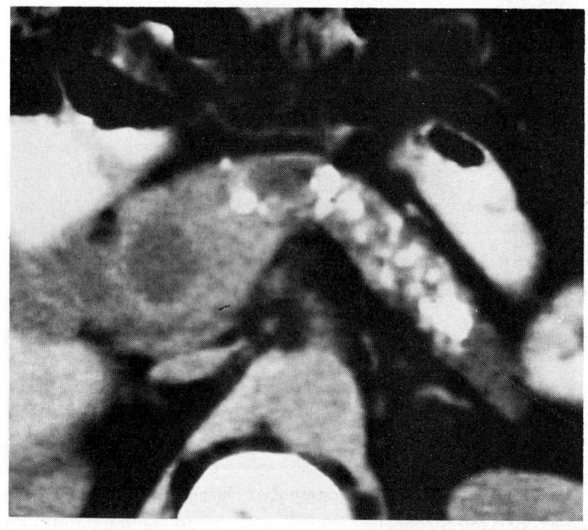

Figure 11.17 Post-contrast CT sections through the pancreatic bed showing calcification throughout the body and tail of pancreas and a short segment of dilated duct around the neck. The common bile duct is also enlarged within the pancreatic head.

Neither ultrasound nor CT can differentiate focal chronic pancreatitis from focal pancreatic malignancy, unless there are secondary signs of the latter. Ultrasound is more accurate than CT in the diagnosis of biliary tract disease.

In those patients to be considered for pancreatic surgery, CT and pancreatography are considered to be the most useful preoperative investigations.

Pancreatic tumours

Although ultrasound and CT are as accurate in the diagnosis of tumours of the pancreatic head and body, CT is superior in the diagnosis and assessment of lesions in the tail. As well as documenting the intrapancreatic abnormality, regional lymphadenopathy, liver metastases and adjacent vasculature can also be shown during the same study (*Figure 11.18*). Although CT is very specific for unresectable tumours, the sensitivity is poor.[32]

Developments in magnetic resonance angiography are encouraging, and may in time replace the need for conventional visceral angiography; at the

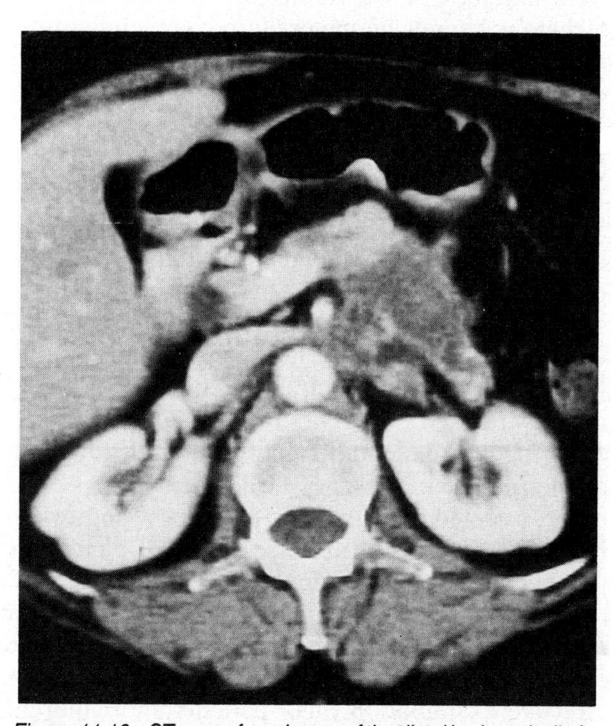

Figure 11.18 CT scan of carcinoma of the distal body and tail of the pancreas. There is a posterior tumour extension adjacent to the superior mesenteric artery and left renal vein.

time of writing it is no better than CT in the assessment of tumour resectability.[75]

CT is useful to detect other pancreatic tumours such as insulinoma and other endocrine lesions, although currently the combination of surgical palpation and intra-operative ultrasound appears to give the best results.[33]

Trauma

The non-invasive diagnosis of pancreatic trauma can be difficult but CT is the best option. A global postcontrast survey examination of the upper abdomen will allow assessment of the liver, spleen, pancreas, and kidneys without restriction by gas, drain sites, dressings etc., all of which may compromise ultrasound.

MAGNETIC RESONANCE IMAGING

The newest of the cross-sectional imaging techniques is MRI which utilizes the behaviour of protons in a magnetic field to create an image. Experience with this technique in pancreatic pathology to date has shown that MRI cannot as yet compete with the resolution of CT (*Figures 11.19* and *11.20*). Bowel contrast agents are still at an experimental stage and until these are more widely

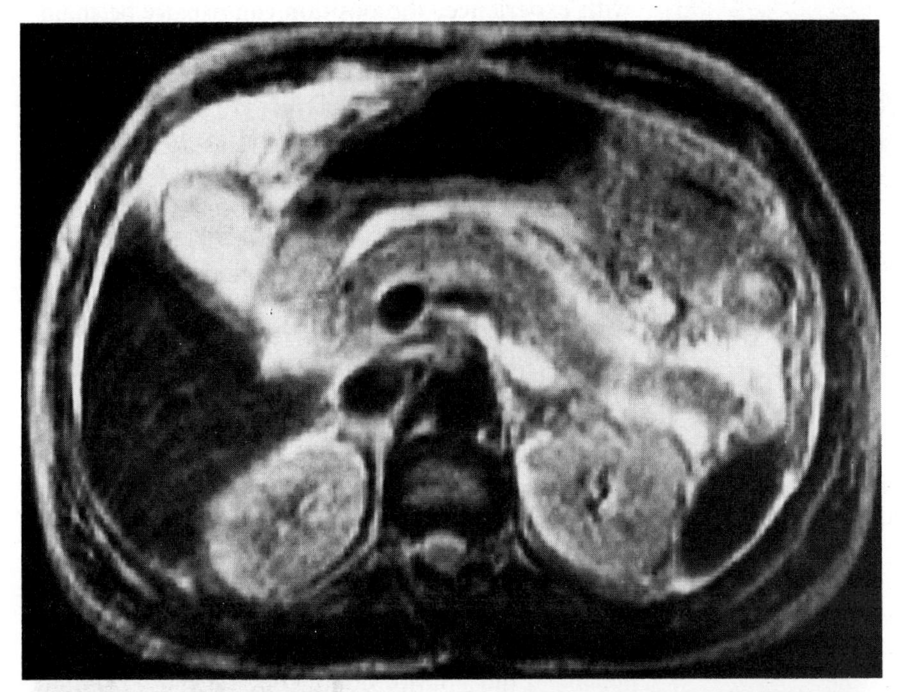

Figure 11.19 Spin echo T2-weighted transverse magnetic resonance image through the pancreas which displays normal parenchymal intensity surrounded by high intensity fluid. Adjacent vascular structures clearly identified without intravenous contrast.

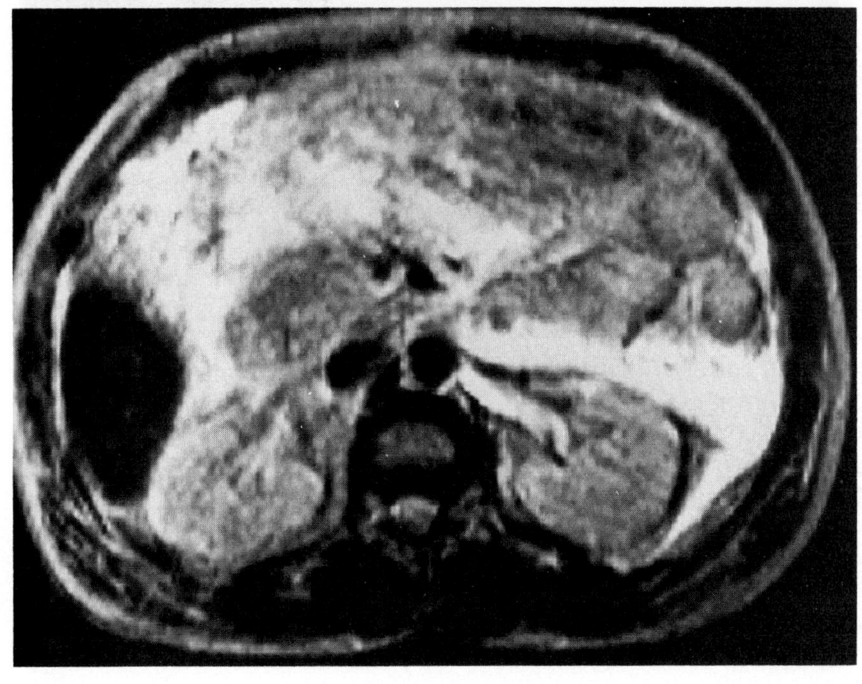

Figure 11.20 Spin echo T2-weighted transverse section through the pancreatic head showing normal parenchymal intensity with adjacent inflammatory fluid. Further fluid is also seen within the left anterior pararenal space in a distribution typical for acute pancreatitis.

available, the differentiation of extrapancreatic pathology from adjacent bowel loops will remain difficult. Magnetic resonance is broadly comparable to state-of-the-art bolus dynamic CT in the detection of liver metastases, but evolving techniques suggest that magnetic resonance may become the best option available in the near future; magnetic resonance is poor in the demonstration of pancreatic calcification.

As pancreatic transplantation becomes more widely available, magnetic resonance shows great promise as the imaging technique of choice for the early detection of pancreatic transplant rejection.[79]

ENDOSCOPIC RETROGRADE CHOLANGIOPANCREATOGRAPHY

Pancreatography is a joint endoscopic and radiological procedure; a team approach is essential for good results. Most patients undergoing this technique are referred for therapeutic procedures so it should be seen as part of an overall gastrointestinal service. The radiologist should be experienced in interventional techniques and there should be a close liaison with specialized pancreaticobiliary surgeons. Radiographs should be reported at joint meetings when clinical aspects of the cases can be discussed in conjunction with the radiology.

TECHNIQUE

Those undergoing pancreatography should receive a full explanation as to the nature of the procedure and why it is being performed, and written consent should be obtained. Venous access is desirable throughout the procedure. Ancillary oxygenation through nasal 'spectacles' or pulse oximetry monitoring, or both, is desirable in selected cases. Patients are usually sedated with intravenous diazepam and pethidine. Duodenal paralysis may be obtained with either hyoscine butylbromide or glucagon; atropine is useful to reduce salivation. The duodenoscope is passed blindly to 40–50 cm and gastric landmarks are sought; full gastroscopy is not usually attempted. The pylorus is identified and, with it virtually filling the field of view, the tip of the instrument is angled up, so that with gentle pressure, the duodenum is entered after a temporary 'red-out'. The cap is examined and the superior duodenal angle identified. The endoscope is rotated approximately 90° clockwise with upward angulation to enter the second part of the duodenum. The papilla is identified at the cephalad end of a longitudinal fold on the medial wall. An accessory papilla may be present anteriorly and proximally. The patient is turned prone. At this point it is desirable to move the endoscope into the 'short' position. Shortening the endoscope enables better positioning and rotational movements and movements of the bridge and of angulation are more direct. In order to achieve this, the tip of the instrument is angled to the right and fixed, and the instrument itself is withdrawn until only 50–60 cm of the endoscope remains in the patient. During this procedure there is a risk of the endoscope falling back into the stomach but, with experience, the position can usually be maintained and once achieved it is relatively stable. An *en-face* view of the papilla must be obtained. This is the most critical phase of the procedure because with poor positioning subsequent cannulation may be impossible.

The cannula, completely filled with full strength contrast medium, is directed at the papilla. An orifice is often visible but, if not, probing of the tip usually results in cannulation. A right-angle approach usually enters the pancreatic duct, whereas upwards angulation towards 11 o'clock favours the bile duct. Deep cannulation selectively opacifies one duct whereas insertion of a few millimetres may result in both ducts filling. Contrast medium is injected under fluoroscopic control; radiographs are taken of the pancreatic duct with the cannula in place. The main pancreatic duct should be filled to the first and second generation of side branches (*Figure 11.21*). High-density (65%) viscous contrast medium gives the best results for the pancreas, but a more dilute contrast (30%) should be used for the biliary system, otherwise small radiolucent stones may be 'whitewashed'. Non-ionic water-soluble contrast has been used by some on the grounds that this may lead to a lower incidence of post-pancreatography pancreatitis. A number of studies suggest that this is not so and the use of these more expensive media cannot be recommended at this stage.

The introduction of air bubbles must be avoided because they prevent side-branch filling and lead to difficulties with interpretation of radiographs. Further films of the pancreaticobiliary system may be obtained after withdrawing the endoscope completely and after the patient has been turned supine. Although the technique has been used to demonstrate pancreatic parenchyma by acinar opacification,[78] this cannot be recommended, as it is associated with an unacceptably high incidence of post-pancreatography pancreatitis, even when nonionic contrast media are used.

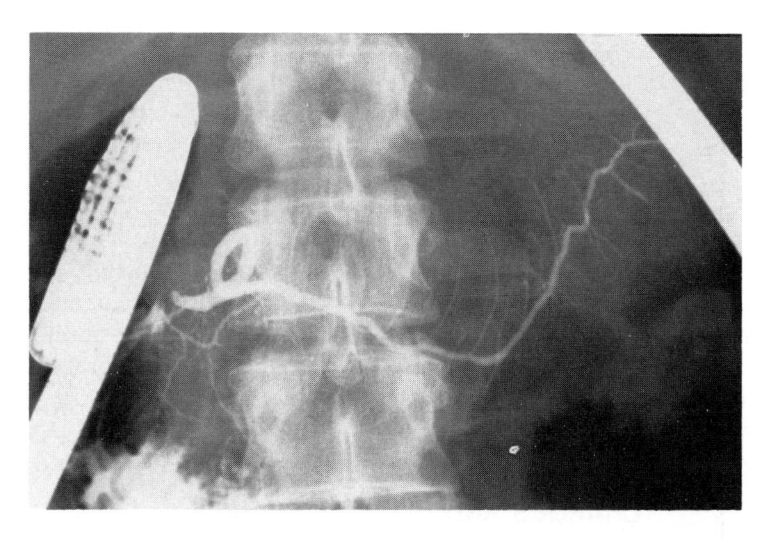

Figure 11.21 Retrograde pancreatogram showing a normal pancreas.

COMPLICATIONS

The complications[9] include those of standard endoscopy such as perforation or inhalation. The risks of over-sedation, however, are greater because patients are usually more heavily sedated and the procedure is performed in a darkened room with the patient lying under radiological apparatus; thus clinical monitoring is more difficult and some authorities recommend the use of pulse oximetry or supplementary oxygen therapy during the procedure. Many patients referred are elderly or infirm. Naloxone and flumazenil must be available in case it is necessary to reverse the sedation. It is for this reason that intravenous access is necessary.

The commonest serious complication is acute pancreatitis. This occurs more commonly when the pancreatic ducts have been either overfilled, leading to parenchymal opacification, or alternatively when the pancreas has been repeatedly filled[38] (usually while attempting to delineate the bile duct). Experienced endoscopists incur fewer complications than those who are still on the upward slope of the learning curve.[9] The commonest cause of death from diagnostic pancreatography is sepsis. This usually occurs in patients who have obstruction to the biliary system leading to acute cholangitis, or where a pancreatic duct is blocked or where it communicates with a cyst or pseudocyst. It is desirable to give a prophylactic antibiotic to patients in these categories, but it is of even greater importance to pay meticulous attention to the cleaning and disinfection of endoscopes and their accessories[5] which should be performed immediately before each individual examination. Most septic complications follow the introduction of organisms which have colonized endoscopic equipment during storage and which then produce serious, sometimes fatal, infection. *Pseudomonas* is the commonest contaminant.

CAMBRIDGE CLASSIFICATION

In 1983, an International group[4] recommended a classification and a terminology to cover the appearances of the normal pancreatogram and changes that arise from chronic inflammation.

Main pancreatic duct

This is the duct that provides the major drainage of the gland. If pancreas divisum is present, the duct is described as dorsal or ventral. The terms proximal and distal should be avoided because they are ambiguous. It is preferable to use upstream (meaning towards the tail), or downstream (towards the head). Stones and other debris within the duct are described as filling defects rather than calculi, as not all filling defects are concretions.

The normal main pancreatic duct tapers smoothly from the head, through the body, to the tail. For the purpose of description, the duct is split into three sections: downstream, middle, and upstream thirds. There is often a physiological narrowing in the head of the gland near the point of embryonic fusion of the ventral and dorsal anlagen. The size of the duct varies, depending upon age, sex, size and racial origin. Collected series give average diameters of 3.6, 2.7, and 1.6 mm for downstream, middle, and upstream thirds respectively. The upper limit of normal is difficult to define because of natural variation, but values of 6.5, 5, and 3 mm respectively have been suggested. When these dimensions are exceeded, the duct is said to be dilated.

It is difficult to define the normal limits for side branches because they are too small to be accurately measured. Similarly it is not possible to give ranges of normal for number or length though subjective assessments can be made.

Chronic pancreatitis

Pancreatograms are classified as normal or showing mild, moderate, or marked changes of chronic pancreatitis. These changes may be diffuse or localized.

Mild changes imply that the abnormality is limited to the side branches, the main duct being normal. At least three side branches must be unequivocally abnormal to make the diagnosis. If only one or two are abnormal, the gland should be classified as equivocal. Side-branch changes include a reduction in the number which may be focal, multi-focal, or diffuse; they may be shortened, and their calibre may be dilated, narrowed, or irregular. 'Nipping' is an appearance where the side branch is narrowed at the origin, this is usually associated with upstream dilatation and shortening as well.

Moderate changes of chronic pancreatitis are present when, in addition to side branch abnormality, the main duct is also affected. It may be dilated, narrowed, or irregular. Narrowing is a subjective assessment, and can be diffuse or focal. A stricture is a narrowing, measuring less than 5 mm in length. Narrowings and strictures may be associated with upstream dilatation, the presence or absence of which should be noted.

Marked changes of chronic pancreatitis are said to be present if, in addition to the changes of moderate pancreatitis, one or more of the following are present: a large cavity, filling defects, or obstruction, severe dilatation (more than 1 cm) or severe irregularity of the main pancreatic duct.

The contour of the main pancreatic duct may be irregular. When multiple strictures or narrowings are present it can be said to be severely irregular.

Cavities are pancreatic or peripancreatic collections that fill with contrast medium. These may be either cysts, pseudocysts, or abscesses and it is for this reason that the term cavity is preferred, as it may be impossible to determine the nature of the cavity at radiology. Cavities are described as large or small (less than 10 mm in diameter).

Occasionally tiny filling defects may be present in patients who have only mild or moderate changes of chronic pancreatitis.

The changes described by the Cambridge classification[4] are descriptive of the pancreatogram only. They are not assessments of the severity of the pathological process, or the clinical condition of the patient.

Common bile duct in pancreatitis

The common bile duct may be obstructed or narrowed either by pressure from a pseudocyst or from oedema or fibrosis in the head of the pancreas.[2,74] With cysts and oedema, the narrowing tends to be longer than with fibrosis. It may be necessary to decompress the bile duct, either endoscopically or surgically. Where the obstruction is due to oedema, biochemical changes will usually resolve spontaneously and a conservative approach is desirable in the first instance.[54]

RELATIONSHIP BETWEEN PANCREATOGRAM CHANGES AND CLINICAL DISEASE

Although pancreatography is very valuable in the diagnosis of chronic pancreatitis, some patients may have abnormalities of their pancreatogram, and yet have few or no symptoms or signs of chronic pancreatitis. Pancreatograms were performed *post mortem* in 69 patients thought not to have chronic pancreatitis; marked changes were shown in 11%, but lesser changes were present in 81%.[72] The abnormalities seem to be associated with perilobular fibrosis, which may accompany ageing. In another study, 49% of 35 patients with alcoholic liver disease had pancreatogram abnormalities, though they had no symptoms to suggest pancreatitis,[76] similar findings have been reported in individuals with sclerosing cholangitis and primary cholangiocarcinoma.[67]

PANCREATOGRAM CHANGES IN DIFFERENT DISORDERS

Alcoholic pancreatitis, hereditary pancreatitis[58] and tropical chronic pancreatitis[6] produce similar pancreatogram abnormalities, and it is impossible to distinguish one from the other. If serial pancreatograms are followed for some years,[64] damage extends in a significant proportion of patients, although improvement may occur after endoscopic removal of protein plugs. Alcoholic patients may worsen more swiftly than those with idiopathic disease. Some patients with chronic pancreatitis have atypical pancreatogram changes, the main duct and side branches taking on a shrunken appearance (*Figure 11.22*). This abnormality may be commoner in individuals with idiopathic pancreatitis.[17]

Chronic pancreatitis and pancreas divisum

In approximately 5% of the population there is malfusion of the ventral and dorsal anlage of the

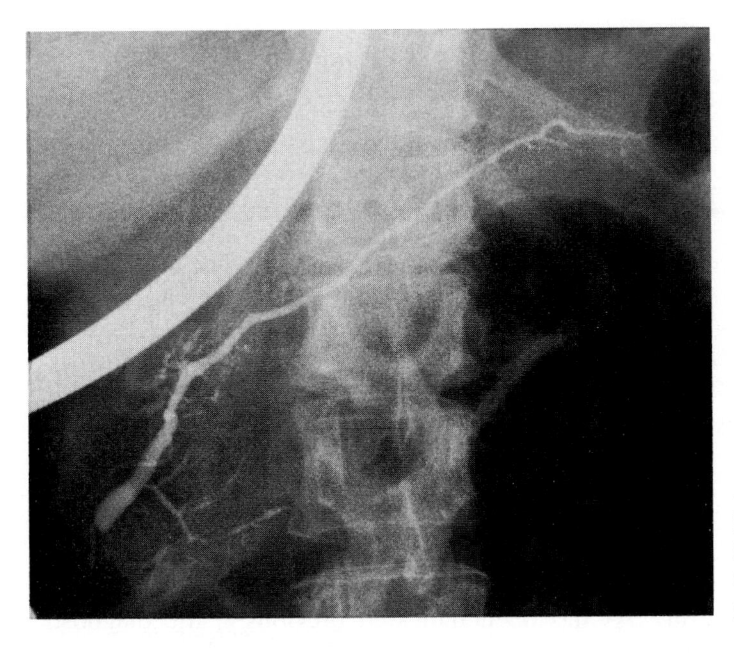

Figure 11.22 Pancreatogram of a patient with chronic pancreatitis secondary to gallstones, showing a normal main pancreatic duct but nipping irregularity, narrowing and dilatation of the side branches typical of mild diffuse chronic pancreatitis.

pancreas during foetal development. This anomaly usually causes the main (dorsal) part of the gland to drain through the minor papilla while the smaller (ventral) duct opens with the bile duct into the ampulla of Vater. Pancreas divisum has been said to be associated with chronic pancreatitis,[21] recurrent acute pancreatitis and episodes of acute abdominal pain that are not associated with a rise in serum amylase. The hypothesis is that, with this anomaly, the small orifice of the accessory ampulla is inadequate and causes relative obstruction during pancreatic secretion leading to symptoms or to obstructive pancreatitis. A number of centres have advocated the use of accessory ampullary sphincterotomy, sphincteroplasty, or stent insertion in some of these patients.[49,71] Although some series have reported good results from these interventions, there has been no satisfactory controlled study and the evidence that pancreas divisum is responsible for pancreatic pathology remains controversial.[60,22]

ERCP and pancreatic cancer

The typical ERCP changes of pancreatic cancer are those of a stenosed or obstructed pancreatic duct (*Figure 11.23*).[68,34] If the lesion is in the head of the pancreas the bile duct is usually obstructed as well (double duct sign). Contrast medium passing upstream from the obstruction will enter a dilated system (*Figure 11.24*). Downstream, the pancreatic ducts should be normal, but parenchymal abnormalities may be found in the region of the obstruction caused by the seepage of contrast medium into necrotic areas of tumour. Occasionally a long stricture of the main pancreatic duct is seen, presumably the result of encasement. Cytology from pure juice or brushings may be diagnostically helpful.[27]

Distinction between cancer and chronic pancreatitis

It may be impossible to distinguish between chronic pancreatitis and pancreatic cancer at pancreatography especially if the patient presents with jaundice.

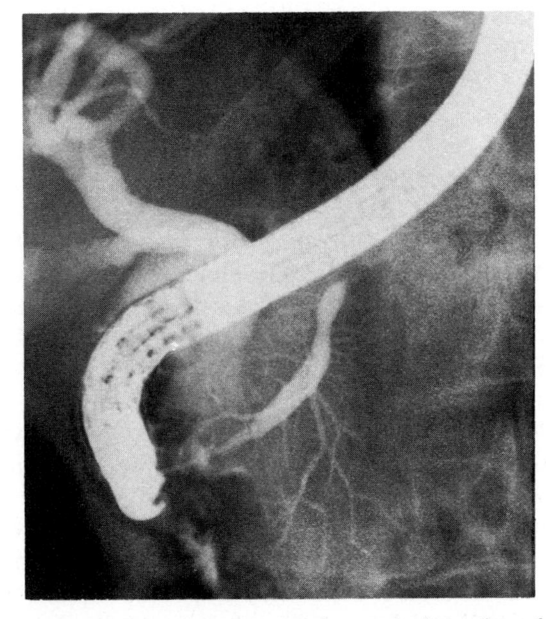

Figure 11.23 Pancreatogram showing total obstruction of the pancreatic duct in the neck of the gland owing to pancreatic cancer.

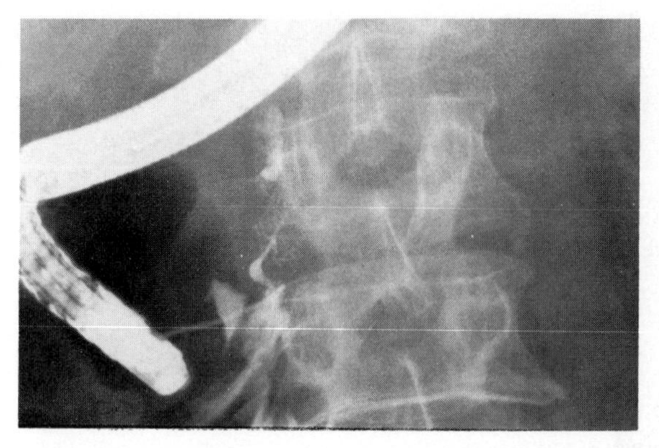

Figure 11.24 Pancreatogram showing stenosis in the neck of the pancreas, with upstream dilatation, caused by carcinoma of the pancreas.

Particular difficulties arise if a definite stricture in the bile duct is shown but ultrasound and CT show no mass lesion. Under these circumstances, a clinical decision must be taken whether to operate in the hope of finding an early cancer or wait and repeat investigations after the lapse of some time. The presence in the pancreas of unequivocal changes of chronic pancreatitis in association with a bile duct stricture is helpful in weighting the decision towards an inflammatory aetiology, although the association of cancer and chronic pancreatitis is not rare. The finding of a bile duct stricture following an episode of abdominal pain or an alcoholic bout may suggest an attack of acute pancreatitis and persuade the clinician towards a conservative approach, but pancreatic cancer may sometimes present as an attack of acute pancreatitis. Cytology may be helpful, but the problem remains where the mass is too small to be biopsied or when cytology is negative.

SPHINCTER OF ODDI MANOMETRY

Considerable interest has developed in the pressure profiles found at the sphincter of Oddi and their relationship to pancreatitis.[77] In a study of 116 patients with idiopathic recurrent pancreatitis,[82] sphincter of Oddi manometry was abnormal in 44 patients. In 17 the basal sphincter pressure was elevated; and 16, treated by sphincterotomy, remained symptom-free for approximately 36 months thereafter. It is perhaps too early to assess the value of sphincter of Oddi manometry and it remains an area of considerable interest to pancreatologists; but pancreatitis may occur following its use.[19]

PANCREATIC ANGIOGRAPHY

Pancreatic angiography[56] is rarely used for evaluation of the pancreas, except in the diagnosis of islet cell tumours where it still has an important part to play. The other circumstance where it may be of use is in the pre-operative assessment of pancreatic cancer when radical surgery is contemplated,[1] providing information about vascular anatomy which sometimes indicates that a lesion is inoperable when other techniques may have underestimated the extent of spread.

ASPIRATION CYTOLOGY AND BIOPSY

As has been indicated previously, the diagnostic accuracy of duodenal intubation tests or pancreatography can be improved by analysis of the specimens obtained for cytology.[26,27]

It is possible to perform direct percutaneous fine needle aspiration of pancreatic mass lesions under ultrasound and CT guidance. The procedure is not difficult. After checking that the patient has a normal coagulation profile, the proposed biopsy track is infiltrated with local anaesthetic. A fine gauge (22 swg) needle mounted on an aspiration syringe is advanced under ultrasound or CT control to the edge of the mass. The needle tip is then advanced and withdrawn through the lesion whilst aspirating the syringe to obtain a specimen for cytological examination. The technique is increasingly referred to as fine-needle aspiration biopsy (FNAB), but this is really a misnomer as only a cytological specimen is obtained. Technical problems relate to the difficulties sometimes experienced in targeting the flexible needle accurately and the need for cytological expertise to prepare and interpret the specimen. Ultrasound, rather than CT, is the preferred modality for guidance because it is both simpler and quicker. The sensitivity of aspiration biopsy is approximately 80% in large series.[42,36] Falsely normal results occur so frequently, however, that a negative result does not exclude malignant disease. The sample is often too small to provide information about cell type or tumour origin.

In attempts to overcome these problems the percutaneous biopsy technique described by Lindgren[54] in 1982 has recently been applied to the pancreas.[47,62] This method employs a 'Tru-cut' needle mounted in a spring-loaded device that operates the cutting biopsy needle automatically ('Biopty™', Radiplast, Uppsala, Sweden). Patients are prepared in the same way as for fine-needle aspiration biopsy. The needle tip is advanced under ultrasound guidance, frequently transgastrically and sometimes transcolonically, to the edge of the lesion to be biopsied and the Biopty gun activated and withdrawn. Biopsy specimens are processed in the normal way for histology. There are several advantages to this technique. The biopsy device can be operated with one hand which leaves the other free to scan continuously throughout the procedure. The speed of activation of the biopsy needle causes no crush artifact in the specimen and also causes microvacuolation in the needle track that can be seen ultrasonically. Thus precise targeting of the biopsy and confirmation of the correct site are provided. Most importantly, an 18 swg needle can be used which provides a histological, rather than cytological sample.

Preliminary results with this technique have been encouraging. Insufficient tissue or equivocal results occur in 4% of patients and false negative results in 6%. The larger series reports a sensitivity for malignancy of 91% and an accuracy of 93%.[47] In the author's experience, the particular benefits have been that a rapid and reliable confirmation of pancreatic carcinoma has been obtained with little distress to the patient. Furthermore, the clinical and imaging diagnosis of malignant or benign pancreatic disease has been correctly refuted by biopsy in 8% of patients and, in a further 7%, tumours other than pancreatic adenocarcinoma have been identified; this includes conditions such as lymphoma, cystadenocarcinoma and ampullary carcinoma which have obvious implications for treatment.[62] If the preliminary results are confirmed, this technique should provide a considerable advance by providing relatively simply histological confirmation of the diagnosis.

A major consideration for either of these techniques is their safety, particularly as complication rates of up to 10% have been reported for open needle biopsy of the pancreas. Potential complications include pancreatitis or fistula formation, haemorrhage, infection and tumour seeding along the needle track. For fine-needle aspiration biopsy, three large surveys of complications, each of which looked at over 10 000 procedures, have been reported. These studies include all intra-abdominal aspiration biopsy procedures and are not restricted to the pancreas. In the most recent survey[28] the mortality was 1 in 5500 which is some two- to threefold higher than in the previous series. The major complication rate was of the order of 1:500 and the risk of tumour seeding has been estimated at 1:21 000.[36] Only preliminary data are available for the newer biopsy technique, but experience in some 200 pancreatic biopsies has no recorded mortality and complications occurring in three patients, with tumour seeding in a further patient. Previous experience with other techniques suggests that the frequency of complications is related to the size of the needle employed. It would therefore be reasonable to assume an eventual complication rate for this procedure intermediate between that of aspiration cytology and open biopsy.

INVESTIGATION OF PANCREATIC DISEASE

In the following section the diagnostic approach to patients who present with known or suspected pancreatic disease is discussed.

ASSESSMENT OF CHRONIC PANCREATITIS

Patients with chronic pancreatitis may be referred for investigation with a view to surgery. Under these circumstances, the aetiology may have a bearing upon management; conditions such as alcohol abuse, cholelithiasis, hypercalaemia or hyperlipidaemia should be sought as they will influence subsequent treatment plans. In general, most surgeons advocate a conservative approach[52] and investigations are designed to elucidate the extent of disease and to identify localized lesions; cysts; strictures of the pancreatic or common bile ducts; and biliary calculi. Ultrasound is useful first, but the most valuable investigation is pancreatography which delineates the pancreatic and biliary ducts and may demonstrate communications with cystic spaces. This assists pre-operative planning and may facilitate a more conservative approach. Exocrine and endocrine function testing may influence the choice between resection or a drainage procedure, particularly if there is residual pancreatic function—for instance, diabetic control in an alcoholic patient may be very difficult.

Although in most patients morphological and functional investigations correlate well,[14] this is not universal and symptoms may bear little relationship to the results of the tests. Some individuals with grossly disorganized pancreatic ductal anatomy may be relatively asymptomatic whereas others with unimpressive findings experience crippling abdominal pain or severe steatorrhoea.

PANCREATIC CANCER

With the exception of ampullary neoplasms, islet cell tumours and some cystic tumours, the prognosis in pancreatic cancer is appalling, but a positive diagnosis must be sought to assist management. Tests are needed to assess extent and to exclude treatable conditions presenting atypically. A diagnosis can be made with varying degrees of confidence by ultrasound, CT, or pancreatography, but an abnormal function test does not distinguish between chronic pancreatitis and cancer, and may be normal in either.

A diagnosis of pancreatic cancer is usually suspected by the finding of a mass lesion either clinically or by imaging. Occasionally the diagnosis is reached from cytology of duodenal aspirate during function testing, pure juice, or brushings taken at pancreatography. More usually, the demonstration of a mass lesion is an indication for fine-needle aspiration or core biopsy.[36] A positive result is reliable and core biopsy in particular, may identify other diseases.[62]

Endoscopic ultrasound may prove to be the most sensitive technique for detecting small mass lesions within the gland and be useful for staging cancer, but at present it is available in only a few centres. Although CT and ultrasound are both helpful for staging, they are not completely reliable but may detect metastatic disease.

RECURRENT ACUTE PANCREATITIS

Modern imaging techniques show that some patients with recurring episodes of acute pancreatitis have anatomical changes in the gland which indicate a diagnosis of chronic pancreatitis.[37] The distinction between acute and chronic pancreatitis is of little consequence in those who have had several episodes of severe abdominal pain associated with an elevated plasma amylase. The main purpose of investigation is to identify a remediable cause for the disease or to exclude cancer-related pancreatitis. Ultrasound and CT will demonstrate mass lesions, cysts and cholelithiasis, whereas pancreatography delineates changes in the duct system and its anatomy (such as pancreas divisum). Ampullary manometry may also have a role.[82] The particular value of pancreatography, however, is to detect common bile duct stones which are difficult to identify by ultrasound. Serum lipids and calcium should also be estimated. Serial oral pancreatic function tests may provide information about the progress of the disease.[61]

PANCREATIC INSUFFICIENCY

Steatorrhoea implies very extensive disease. Plasma isoamylase, immunoreactive trypsin and lipase are likely to be subnormal and function tests confirm pancreatic disease. When these investigations are abnormal, an imaging investigation is required to distinguish pancreatitis from carcinoma. A similar sequence applies in certain patients presenting with diabetes mellitus.

ABDOMINAL MASS

Pancreatic disease may present as a palpable abdominal mass. The investigation of choice is ultrasound or CT, which will reliably demonstrate whether or not the mass is of pancreatic origin and provide other valuable information about the tumour. Both may identify liver metastases. Cystic lesions may be aspirated or, if solid, fine-needle aspiration or core biopsy can be obtained simultaneously. These techniques will provide the diagnosis, so pancreatography and pancreatic function tests are rarely necessary.

CHRONIC ABDOMINAL PAIN

Many patients are referred with suspected pancreatic disease because of undiagnosed abdominal pain and most do not have chronic pancreatitis. It is this presentation that provides the greatest challenge. Before embarking on a pancreatic assessment, it is essential that a plain abdominal radiograph, upper digestive endoscopy, and cholecystogram or ultrasound are performed. Other common causes of abdominal pain should be considered, and only then should the patient be subjected to pancreatic investigations. It is in these cases that a simple, reliable non-invasive test is most needed. Ultrasound can fulfil these criteria,[49] but is dependent on the observer and CT is more objective.[31,75] Serum markers such as isoamylase or immunoreactive trypsin are of only limited usefulness in this context. The modified oral pancreatic function tests may provide a simple non-invasive assessment of exocrine function and identify some patients with pancreatitis, although they are not as sensitive as their duodenal counterparts. Ultrasound or CT, in combination with an oral function test, provides a means of identifying those patients who require further study.[29] Pancreatography and duodenal intubation tests are the most sensitive investigations; of these pancreatography is more widely available and the latter is less specific (in defined situations) and will not distinguish cancer from pancreatitis.

The best diagnostic accuracy will be obtained by a combination of a function and a morphological test. Comparative studies in patients with established pancreatic disease have shown that although both will be abnormal in most cases, the combination will

Table 11.1 Pancreatography (ERCP) and modified oral pancreatic function test (PFT) findings in 50 patients with chronic pancreatitis

ERCP finding	*Normal FPT*	*Abnormal PFT*
	(No. of patients)	
Normal	1	5
Abnormal	9	33
Failed	ND	2
Total	10	40

ND = No data.

increase sensitivity by a factor of some 10–20%. This is hardly surprising because the two investigations detect disease by different methods and it is well established that significant structural abnormality may be associated with normal exocrine function and vice versa.[3,14,83] Duodenal intubation tests and pancreatography are the most accurate combination at present because each test detects some patients missed by the other; function tests diagnose more pancreatitis and pancreatography more carcinoma. Both tests provide an opportunity to take samples for cytology or biochemical analysis. This combination however, is time-consuming, unpleasant for the patient and not widely available. Although it is perhaps surprising in view of the apparent lower sensitivity of oral function tests, even their combination with pancreatography will enhance diagnostic accuracy, as demonstrated in *Table 11.1* of the findings in 50 consecutive patients with chronic pancreatitis.

JAUNDICE

The investigation of choice in patients who present with jaundice is pancreatography which will normally give a diagnosis and in many cases will also provide treatment. If a tumour is suspected and curative resection is under consideration, there are advantages in performing CT and ultrasound with or without biopsy before pancreatography because after stent insertion to palliate jaundice, CT images may be distorted and it may not be possible to assess size or resectability of the lesion.

ACKNOWLEDGEMENTS

We would like to thank our radiological colleagues, Dr D.J. Lintott, Dr R.C. Fowler, and Dr A.G. Chalmers, from the General Infirmary, Leeds for assisting with the preparation of this chapter and for providing the radiographs.

REFERENCES

1. Appleton, G.V.N., Bathurst, N.C.G., Virjee, J., Cooper, M.J. and Williamson, R.C.N. (1989) The value of angiography in the surgical management of pancreatic disease. *Annals of the Royal College of Surgeons of England*, **71**, 92–96.
2. Aranha, G.V., Prinz, R.A., Freeark, R.J. and Greenlee, J.B. (1984) The spectrum of biliary tract obstruction from chronic pancreatitis. *Archives of Surgery*, **119**, 595–600.
3. Ashton, M.G., Axon, A.T.R. and Lintott, D.J. (1978) Lundh test and ERCP in pancreatic disease. *Gut*, **19**, 910–915.
4. Axon, A.T.R., Classen, M., Cotton, P.B., Cremer, M., Freeny, P.C. and Lees, W.R. (1984) Pancreatography in chronic pancreatitis: international definitions. *Gut*, **25**, 1107–1112.
5. Axon, A.T.R., Bond, W.W., Bottrill, P.M., Cowen, A.E., Fleischer, D.E. and Tandon, R.K. (1991) Disinfection and endoscopy. Working Party Report to the World Congress of Gastroenterology, Sydney 1990. *Journal of Gastroenterology and Hepatology*, **6**, 23–48.
6. Balakrishnan, V., Hanriharan, M., Rao, V.R.K. and Anand, B.S. (1985) Endoscopic pancreatography in chronic pancreatitis of the tropics. *Digestion*, **32**, 128–131.
7. Benini, L., Caliary, S., Guidi, C.G. *et al.* (1989) New infra-red spectrometry for faecal fat measurement: comparison with conventional gravimetric and titrimetric method. *Gut*, **30**, 1344–1347.
8. Besterman, H.S., Adrian, T.E., Bloom, S.R. *et al.* (1982) Pancreatic and gastrointestinal hormone in chronic pancreatitis. *Digestion*, **24**, 195–208.
9. Bilbao, M.U., Cotter, C.T., Lee, T.G. *et al.* (1976) Complications of endoscopic retrograde cholangio-pancreatography (ERCP); a study of 10 000 cases. *Gastroenterology*, **70**, 314–320.
10. Boyd, E.J.S., Cumming, J.G.R., Cuschieri, A. *et al.* (1982) Prospective comparison of fluorescein-dilaurate test with the secretin–cholecystokinin test for pancreatic exocrine function. *Journal of Clinical Pathology*, **35**, 1240–1243.
11. Boyd, E.J.S., Wood, H., Clark, G. *et al.* (1985) Pancreatic enzyme synthesis in pancreatic disease. *Scandinavian Journal of Gastroenterology*, **20**, 734–740.
12. Boyd, E.J.S. and Wormsley, K.G. (1987) Laboratory tests in the diagnosis of the chronic pancreatic diseases: Tests of pancreatic secretion. *International Journal of Pancreatology*, **2**, 211–221.
13. Braganza, J.M. and Rao, J.J. (1978) Disproportionate reduction in tryptic response to endogenous compared to exogenous stimulation in chronic pancreatitis. *British Medical Journal*, **ii**, 392–394.
14. Braganza, J.M., Hunt, L.P. and Warwick, F. (1982) Relationship between pancreatic exocrine function

and ductal morphology in chronic pancreatitis. *Gastroenterology*, **82**, 1341–1347.
15. Braganza, J.M., Kay, G.H., Tetlow, V.A. and Herman, K.J. (1983) Observations on the BTP/PABA/^{14}C-PABA tubeless tests of pancreatic function. *Clinica Chimica Acta*, **120**, 339–347.
16. Brugge, W.R., Goffe, J.S., Allen, N.C. *et al.* (1980) Development of a dual label Schilling test for pancreatic exocrine function based on the differential absorption of cobalamin bound to intrinsic factor and R protein. *Gastroenterology*, **78**, 937–949.
17. Bulgim, O., Manning, A., Lintott, D. and Axon, A. (1987) The 'shrunken' pancreas: a morphological variant of idiopathic chronic pancreatitis. *British Journal of Radiology*, **60**, 543–546.
18. Burton, P., Evans, D.G., Harper, A.A. *et al.* (1960) A test of pancreatic function based on the analysis of duodenal contents after administration of secretin and pancreozymin. *Gut*, **1**, 111–124.
19. Cattau, E.L. Jr, Johnson, D.A., Benjamin, S.B., Geenen, J.E. and Hogan, W.J. (1988) Sphincter of Oddi (SO) Manometry: A survey of methodology, complications and clinical application. *Gastrointestinal Endoscopy*, **34**, 185, A60.
20. Ching, C.K. and Rhodes, J.M. (1989) Enzyme-linked PNA lectin binding assay as a diagnostic blood test for pancreatic cancer. *British Journal of Cancer*, **59**, 949–953.
21. Cotton, P.B. (1980) Congenital anomaly of pancreas divisum as cause of obstructive pain and pancreatitis. *Gut*, **21**, 105–114.
22. Delahaye, M., Engelholm, L. and Cremer, M. (1985) Pancreas divisum: Congenital anatomic variant or anomaly? *Gastroenterology*, **89**, 951–958.
23. Delchier, J.-C. and Soule, J.-C. (1983) BT-PABA test with plasma PABA measurements: evaluation of sensitivity and specificity. *Gut*, **24**, 318–325.
24. Del Favero, G., Fabris, C., Plebani, M. *et al.* (1986) CA 19-9 and carcinoembryonic antigen in pancreatic cancer diagnosis. *Cancer*, **57**, 1576–1579.
25. Domschke, S., Heptner, P., Kolb, S. *et al.* (1986) Decrease in plasma amino acid level after secretin and pancreozymin as an indicator of exocrine pancreatic function. *Gastroenterology*, **90**, 1031–1038.
26. Dreiling, D.A. (1975) Pancreatic secretory testing in 1974. *Gut*, **16**, 653–656.
27. Endo, Y., Morii, T., Tamura, H. and Okuda, S. (1974) Cytodiagnosis of pancreatic tumours by aspiration under direct vision using a duodenal fibrescope. *Gastroenterology*, **67**, 944–951.
28. Fornari, F., Civardi, G., Cavanna, I. *et al.* (1989) Complications of ultrasonically guided fine-needle abdominal biopsy. Results of a multicentre Italian study and review of the literature. *Scandinavian Journal of Gastroenterology*, **24**, 949–955.
29. Foster, P.N., Mitchell, C.J., Robertson, D.R.C. *et al.* (1984) Prospective comparison of three non-invasive tests for pancreatic disease. *British Medical Journal*, **289**, 13–16.
30. Friese, J. and Hofmann, R. (1979) Zur Spezifitat des Peptid-PABA-Test. *Zeitschrift für Gastroenterologie*, **17**, 310–317.
31. Freeny, P.C. and Lawson, T.L. (1982) *Radiology of the Pancreas.* New York: Springer-Verlag.
32. Freeny, P.C., Marks, W.M., Ryan, J.A. and Traverso, L.W. (1988) Pancreatic ductal adenocarcinoma: diagnosis and staging with dynamic C.T. *Radiology*, **166**, 125–133.
33. Galiber, A.K., Reading, C.C., Charboneau, J.W. *et al.* (1988) Localisation of pancreatic insulinoma: Comparison of pre- and intraoperative ultrasound with CT and angiography. *Radiology*, **166**, 405–408.
34. Gilinsky, N.H., Bornman, P.C., Girdwood, A.H. and Marks, I.N. (1986) Diagnostic yield of endoscopic retrograde cholangiopancreatography in carcinoma of the pancreas. *British Journal of Surgery*, **73**, 539–543.
35. Haglund, C., Kuusela, P. and Roberts, P.J. (1989) Tumour markers in pancreatic cancer. *Annal Chirurgica Gynaecologica*, **78**, 41–53.
36. Hall-Craggs, M.A. and Lees, W.R. (1987) Fine needle biopsy: cytology, histology or both? (1987) *Gut*, **28**, 233–236.
37. Hamilton, I., Bradley, P., Lintott, D.J. *et al.* (1982) Endoscopic retrograde cholangiopancreatography in the investigation and management of patients after acute pancreatitis. *British Journal of Surgery*, **69**, 504–506.
38. Hamilton, I., Lintott, D.J., Rothwell, J. and Axon, A.T.R. (1983) Acute pancreatitis following endoscopic retrograde cholangiopancreatography. *Clinical Radiology*, **34**, 543–546.
39. Heij, H.A., Obertop, H., Schmitz, P.I.M. *et al.* (1986) Evaluation of the secretin cholecystokinin test for chronic pancreatitis by discriminant analysis. *Scandinavian Journal of Gastroenterology*, **21**, 35–40.
40. Hoek, F.J., Van Den Bergh, F.A.J.T.M., Klein-Elmhurst, J.T., *et al.* (1987) Improved specificity of the PABA test with p-amino salicylic acid (PAS). *Gut*, **28**, 468–473.
41. Hoek, F.J. and Tytgat, G.N.J. (1988) Evaluation of the diagnostic value of the PABA test in the assessment of chronic pancreatic disease. *Netherlands Journal of Medicine*, **32**, 118–129.
42. Holm, H., Als, O. and Gammelgaard, J. (1985) Percutaneous aspiration and biopsy procedures under ultrasound visualisation. In *Diagnostic Ultrasound in Gastrointestinal Disease* (Ed.) Taylor, K.G.M. pp. 137–149. New York: Churchill Livingstone.
43. Hubbard, V.S., Wolf, R.O., Lester, R.A. and Egge, A.C. (1984) Diagnostic and therapeutic applications of bentiromide screening test for exocrine pancreatic insufficiency in patients with cystic fibrosis. *Digestive Diseases and Science*, **29**, 881–889.
44. Hunt, L.P. and Braganza, J.M. (1989) On optimising the diagnostic yield of the secretin-

pancreozymin test. *Clinical Chimica Acta*, **96**, 503–509.

45. Imondi, A.R. (1983) Optimum dose of bentiromide. *Digestive Diseases and Sciences*, **28**, 859–860.
46. Jansen, J.B.M.J., Jebbink, M.C.W., Mulders, J.H.A. and Lamers, C.B.H.W. (1989) Effect of pancreatic enzyme supplementation on post-prandial plasma cholecystokinin secretion in patients with pancreatic insufficiency. *Regulatory Peptides*, **25**, 333–342.
47. Jennings, P.E., Coral, A., Donald, J.J. *et al.* (1989) Ultrasound-guided core biopsy. *Lancet*, **i**, 1369–1371.
48. Jones, S. N., Lees, W.R. and Frost, R.A. (1988) Diagnosis and grading of chronic pancreatitis by morphological criteria derived by ultrasound and pancreatography. *Clinical Radiology*, **39**, 43–48.
49. Keith, R.G., Shapero, T.F., Saibil, G. and Moore, T.L. (1989) Dorsal duct sphincterotomy in effective long term treatment of acute pancreatitis associated with pancreas divisum. *Surgery*, **106**, 660–667.
50. Lang, D., Gyr, K., Stalder, G.A. and Gillessen, D. (1981) Assessment of exocrine pancreatic function by oral administration of N-benzolyl-L-tyrosyl-*p*-aminobenzoic acid; 5 years clinical experience. *British Journal of Surgery*, **68**, 771–775.
51. Lankisch, P.G., Schreiber, A. and Otto, J. (1983) Pancreolauryl test. Evaluation of a tubeless pancreatic function test with other indirect and direct tests for exocrine pancreatic function. *Digestive Diseases and Science*, **28**, 490–493.
52. Leger, I., Lenriot, J.P. and Lemaigre, G. (1974) Five- to twenty-year follow-up after surgery for chronic pancreatitis in 148 patients. *Annals of Surgery (Philadelphia)*, **180**, 185–191.
53. Leung, P.W.C., Frost, R.A., Burgess, R. *et al.* (1988) Modified dual label Schilling test for pancreatic exocrine function. *Clinica Chimica Acta*, **174**, 93–100.
54. Lindgren, P.G. (1982) Percutaneous needle biopsy: a new technique. *Acta Radiol*, **2**, 653–656.
55. Long, D.E., Axon, A.T.R. and Lintott, D.J. (1990) The outcome of patients with an extrahepatic biliary stricture secondary to chronic pancreatitis. *International Journal of Pancreatology*, **4**, 331–341.
56. Lunderquist, A. (1985) Invasive Radiology. The Pancreas. In *Clinics in Gastroenterology*, **14**, pp. 355–369. W.B. Saunders.
57. Lundh, G. (1962) Pancreatic exocrine function in neoplastic and inflammatory disease: a simple and reliable new test. *Gastroenterology*, **42**, 275–280.
58. Makela, P. and Aarimaa M. (1985) Pancreatography in a family with hereditary pancreatitis. *Acta Radiologica: Diagnosis*, **26**, 63–66.
59. Mitchell, C.J., Humphrey, C.S., Bullen, A.W. and Kelleher, J. (1979) The diagnostic value of the oral pancreatic function test. *Scandinavian Journal of Gastroenterology*, **14**, 183–187.
60. Mitchell, C.J., Lintott, D.J., Ruddell, W.S.N. *et al.* (1976) Clinical relevance of an unfused pancreatic duct system. *Gut*, **20**, 1066–1071.
61. Mitchell, C.J., Playforth, M.J., Kelleher, J. and McMahon, M.J. (1983) Functional recovery of the exocrine pancreas after acute pancreatitis. *Scandinavian Journal of Gastroenterology*, **18**, 5–8.
62. Mitchell, C.J., Wai, D., Jackson, A.M. and MacFie, J. (1989) Ultrasound guided percutaneous pancreatic biopsy. *British Journal of Surgery*, **76**, 706–707.
63. Mitchell, C.J., Field, H.P., Simpson, F.G. *et al.* (1981) Preliminary evaluation of a single-day tubeless test of pancreatic function. *British Medical Journal*, **282**, 1751–1753.
64. Miyake, H., Harada, H., Kinichika, K., Ochi, K. and Kimura, I. (1987) Clinical course and prognosis of chronic pancreatitis. *Pancreas*, **2**, 378–385.
65. Moller-Petersen, J., Pedersen, J.O., Pedersen, N.T. and Andersen, B.N. (1988) Serum cathodic trypsin-like immunoreactivity, pancreatic lipase and pancreatic isoamylase as diagnostic tests of chronic pancreatitis or pancreatic steatorrhoea. *Scandinavian Journal of Gastroenterology*, **23**, 287–296.
66. Mottaleb, A., Kapp, F., Noguera, E.C.A. *et al.* (1973) The Lundh test in the diagnosis of pancreatic disease: a review of five years experience. *Gut*, **14**, 835–842.
67. Palmer, K.R., Cotton, P.B. and Chapman, M. (1984) Pancreatogram in cholestasis. *Gut*, **25**, 424–427.
68. Reuben, A. and Cotton, P.B. (1979) Endoscopic retrograde cholangiopancreatography in cancer of the pancreas. *Surgery, Gynecology and Obstetrics*, **148**, 179–184.
69. Rossi, P., Allison, D.J. and Bezzi, M. (1989) Endocrine tumours of the pancreas. *Radiological Clinics of North America*, **27**, 121–125.
70. Ruddell, W.S.J., Mitchell, C.J., Hamilton, I. *et al.* (1981) Clinical value of serum immunoreactive trypsin concentration. *British Medical Journal*, **ii**, 1429–1432.
71. Russell, R.C.G., Wong, N.W. and Cotton, P.B. (1984) Accessory sphincterotomy (endoscopic and surgical) in patients with pancreas divisum. *British Journal of Surgery*, **71**, 954–957.
72. Schmitz-Moormann, P., Himmelman, G.W., Brandes, J.W. *et al.* (1985) Comparative radiological and morphological study of human pancreas. Pancreatitis-like changes in postmortem ductograms and their morphological pattern. Possible implications for ERCP. *Gut*, **26**, 406–414.
73. Sivak, M.V. (1988) Is there an ultrasonographic endoscope in your future? *Gastrointestinal Endoscopy*, **34**, 64–65.
74. Stabile, B.E., Calabria, R., Wilson, S.E. and Passaro, E. (1987) Stricture of the common bile duct from chronic pancreatitis. *Surgery, Gynecology and Obstetrics*, **165**, 121–126.
75. Steiner, E., Stark, D.D., Hahn, P.F. *et al.* (1989) Imaging of pancreatic neoplasms: comparison of

MR and CT. *American Journal of Roentgenology (Baltimore)*, **152**, 487–491.
76. Testoni, P.A., Masci, E., Passaretti, S., Guslandi, M. and Tittobello, A. (1984) Early detection of pancreatic lesions in chronic alcoholism: diagnostic accuracy of ERP. *Journal of Clinical Gastroenterology*, **6**, 519–532.
77. Toouli, J. and Roberts-Thompson, I.C. (1987) Alimentary tract and pancreas: endoscopic manometry of the sphincter of Oddi. *Journal of Gastroenterology and Hepatology*, **2**, 431–442.
78. Twomey, B., Wilkins, R.A. and Levi, A.J. (1982) Pancreatic parenchymography using metrizamide. *Gut*, **5**, A432.
79. Uyuh, W.T.C., Hunsicker, L.G., Ngheim, D.D. *et al.* (1989) Pancreatic transplants: evaluation with MR imaging. *Radiology*, **170**, 171–177.
80. Vantrappen, G.R., Rutgeerts, P.J., Ghoos, Y.F. and Hiele, M.I. (1989) Mixed triglyceride breath test: a noninvasive test of pancreatic lipase activity in the duodenum. *Gastroenterology*, **96**, 1126–1134.
81. Ventrucci, M., Pezzilli, R., Gullo, L. *et al.* (1989) Role of serum pancreatic enzyme assays in diagnosis of pancreatic disease. *Digestive Diseases and Science*, **34**, 39–45.
82. Venu, R.P., Geenen, J.E., Hogan, W., Stone, J., Johnson, G.K. and Soergel, K. (1989) Idiopathic recurrent pancreatitis: an approach to diagnosis and treatment. *Digestive Diseases and Sciences*, **34**, 56–60.
83. Waye, J.D., Adler, M. and Dreiline, D.A. (1978) The pancreas: a correlation of function and structure. *American Journal of Gastroenterology*, **69**, 176–181.
84. Yasuda, K., Mukai, H., Fujimoto, S., Nakajima, M. and Kawai, K. (1988) The diagnosis of pancreatic cancer by endoscopic ultrasonography. *Gastrointestinal Endoscopy*, **34**, 1–8.

CYSTIC FIBROSIS

G.G. Forstner

Cystic fibrosis is an inherited disease which primarily affects the pancreas and lungs but is characterized by abnormal secretion from many exocrine glands. It was first separated from other 'coeliac' syndromes, and the relationship between the pancreatic and lung lesions clarified, by Fanconi, Uehlinger and Knauer[23] in Germany and Dorothy Andersen[1] in the United States. The demonstration of pancreatic insufficiency was the key to the clinical diagnosis until di Sant'Agnese *et al.*[17] showed that patients uniformly secreted sweat containing high concentrations of sodium chloride. The one absolute essential for diagnosis continues to be the finding of sweat with high sodium or chloride levels. Gibbs, Bostick and Smith[30] showed that steatorrhea was not seen in all patients. Since then it has generally become apparent that the clinical expression of the disease may be quite variable.

PATHOGENESIS

The electrolyte abnormalities in sweat reflect a secretory lesion that is probably expressed in all epithelial cells. At maximal flow rates, the concentration of sodium and chloride is much greater in sweat from cystic fibrosis patients than in sweat from normal individuals, and the sweat bicarbonate concentration is lower. Quinton[50] showed that chloride permeation was defective in the sweat duct, preventing reabsorption of chloride and its accompanying cation, sodium. Whereas chloride channels in the sweat duct cells facilitate chloride reabsorption, apical chloride channels in other epithelial cells frequently play an important role in facilitating sodium and chloride secretion, as outlined in *Figure 11.25.* In turn, net secretion of sodium and chloride stimulates fluid secretion, because the accumulation of osmotically active ions exterior to the apical surface encourages water movement from within and between cells toward the lumen. Apical chloride channels in a variety of epithelial cells, including those of the sweat gland,[55] trachea[8] and pancreatic duct,[56] have been shown to be unresponsive to cyclic AMP in cystic fibrosis, although otherwise normal. In cystic fibrosis, therefore, chloride, sodium and fluid secretion might be expected to be defective in those cells and tissues where chloride secretion depends on cyclic AMP for stimulation.

This is the case in the pancreas, where secretin normally stimulates ductal secretion via a cyclic AMP-mediated response,[9] probably involving the activation of an apical chloride channel.[3] In patients with cystic fibrosis, secretin-induced secretion of chloride, bicarbonate, and fluid is deficient even when the pancreatic acini appear to be spared.[27,40] Secretagogues such as cholera toxin and vasoactive intestinal peptide that stimulate secretion via cyclic AMP-responsive chloride channels, induce a pro-

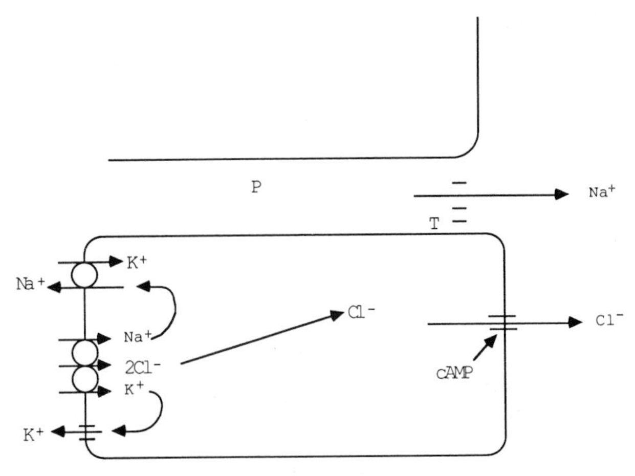

Figure 11.25 The ion channel circuitry in a typical epithelial cell that produces a net secretion of chloride through the apical membrane into the lumen. Sodium follows chloride, but through a paracellular route, in response to the electrical gradient set up by chloride. Note that chloride moves 'downhill', because the three basal channels cause it to accumulate internally. Cyclic AMP encourages the 'open' state of the chloride channel allowing the ion to pass through. Na^+ = sodium; K^+ = potassium; Cl^- = chloride; P = paracellular route; T = tight junction; cAMP = cyclic AMP. The circles in the basolateral membrane denote coupled ion transporters.

nounced secretory response in the intestine. These channels appear to be defective in cystic fibrosis.[6]

Not surprisingly, the secretory abnormalities are associated with increased viscosity of secretions and a tendency to develop highly proteinaceous or mucoid plugging. Protein in meconium[35] and pancreatic secretions[41] is elevated. Mucus glycoproteins appear to be chemically altered as well, with a high ratio of fucose:sialic acid, elongated carbohydrate chains and increased sulfate,[66] perhaps as the result of a related defect in the regulation of exocytosis or assembly. Mucus is particularly thick, tenacious and copious. The result, as shown in *Figure 11.26*, is an obstructive tubulopathy which affects multiple organs, including the pancreas, gut, liver, lungs and testes. Interestingly, the urinary tract is functionally spared, perhaps because high passive flow and low protein concentration prevent the accumulation of organic plugs.

INHERITANCE

Cystic fibrosis is inherited as an autosomal recessive trait, with a very high incidence in white races compared with others. Approximately one individual for every 20 in the population is a heterozygote or gene carrier, and homozygotes occur with a frequency of one in every 2000 live births. The gene is on chromosome 7 and the nucleotide and amino acid sequence of the gene product are known.[51,52] The gene product, known as the cystic fibrosis transmembrane regulator, has the characteristics of a transmembrane protein, with nucleotide binding sites and regulatory segments that could regulate channel activity. A single mutation within the nucleotide-binding region accounts for most cases but other mutations are common, contributing to considerable phenotypic variation.

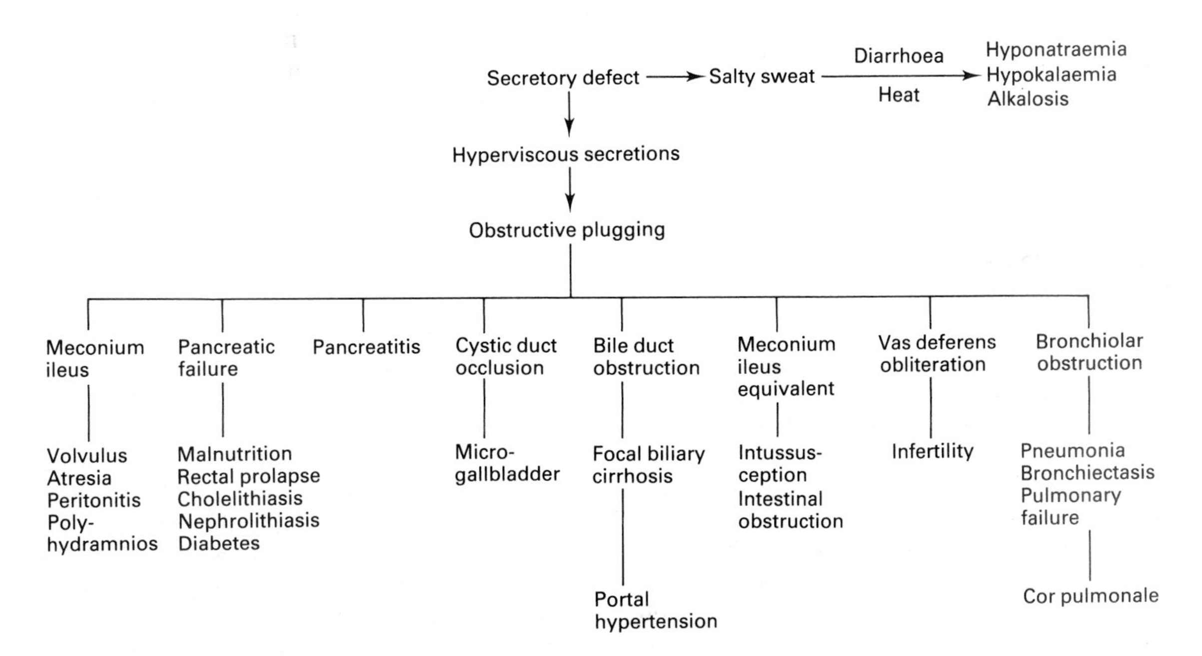

Figure 11.26 Consequences of the secretory defect in cystic fibrosis.

PANCREATIC DISEASE

The classification of pancreatic disease in cystic fibrosis can be quite confusing. Patients who have steatorrhoea are generally considered to have pancreatic insufficiency, whereas those who absorb fat normally are said to have retained pancreatic function. Neither term is satisfactory, as many patients in the latter category lack pancreatic function, and many of the former have some pancreatic function. Nevertheless, a classification based on the presence or absence of fat malabsorption has merit because the clinical course of the disease is quite different in patients from each category. Pancreatic disease will be discussed, therefore, under two headings, pancreatic insufficiency and pancreatic sufficiency, arbitarily defined by the presence or absence of steatorrhoea.

PANCREATIC INSUFFICIENCY (PATIENTS WITH STEATORRHOEA)

Pathology

Pancreatic damage begins in utero and first appears as an arrest of acinar development.[38,49] At birth intralobular ductules are filled with mucus and many are dilated. Acini are still relatively intact, although there is evidence of early atrophy and there are visible degrees of interstitial fibrosis. By the end of the first year of life, advanced acinar destruction is always present and exocrine elements are progressively replaced by fibrous tissue and fat.[42] With time, ductules and acini disappear. Endocrine elements are relatively preserved but, as patients grow older, there is islet cell loss and the gland becomes completely replaced by a fibroadipose stroma.

Clinical features

In the author's clinic approximately 60% of patients are diagnosed before the age of one year, and 85% before the age of 5 years. Although pancreatic acini appear to be relatively preserved in infancy, most patients have steatorrhoea at diagnosis. Stools are bulky, greasy, malodorous, loose and often more frequent than normal, although diarrhoea is rarely reported. In the absence of chest complications the appetite is often well maintained and growth may be unimpaired. If chest problems are severe the appetite falls and there is rapid and profound weight loss. On physical examination infants are often thin with wasted limbs and buttocks and a protuberant abdomen. Rectal prolapse occurs in 20% of patients and should suggest the diagnosis. Finger clubbing is an early and impressive sign. Deficiencies of fat-soluble vitamins are common biochemically but rarely clinically. At birth, bruising and intracranial and gastrointestinal bleeding due to vitamin K deficiency have been reported.[61] In older children it is common to find evidence of vitamin E deficiency but clinical sequelae are unusual. Ophthalmoplegia, absent deep tendon reflexes, hand tremors and positive Rombergism have been described, however,[22] and raise the possibility of vitamin E deficiency (see also page 414). Overt rickets does not occur in cystic fibrosis but, in older children, bony demineralization is not uncommon, and in some patients 25-hydroxy-vitamin D levels may be low. Although vitamin B-12 may be malabsorbed in untreated patients, megaloblastic anaemia has not been reported. Most patients with pancreatic insufficiency have low plasma and tissue levels of linoleic acid, whereas other fatty acids such as palmitoleic, oleic and eicosotrienoic may be elevated, suggesting a mild essential fatty acid deficiency.[36] Urinary oxalate excretion may be increased as with other causes of steatorrhoea.

Investigations

The diagnosis of pancreatic insufficiency can usually be made by looking at the stool smear which is loaded with neutral fat droplets. Deficient secretion of pancreatic enzymes may be suspected from low random or 24-hour stool chymotrypsin activity.[7] Serum levels of pancreatic amylase or trypsinogen may be reduced.[21] Most patients with steatorrhoea will have abnormal excretion or low plasma levels of *p*-aminobenzoic acid (PABA) following the administration of N-benzoyl-L-tyrosyl-PABA.[65] Quantitative determination of 3- or 5-day faecal fat excretion with a known fat intake will establish the presence of steatorrhoea. Faecal fat excretion is surprisingly variable, amounting to as much as 80% of intake in some patients, with a mean of 38% (*Figure 11.27*).

The only truly definitive test for pancreatic insufficiency continues to be the demonstration of very low enzyme output from the pancreas following stimulation by secretin and cholecystokinin. Our studies on patients with steatorrhoea show that all had a lipase output that was less than 1.5% of the average for controls.[28]

Paradoxically, pancreatic damage in cystic fibrosis is associated in very early infancy with elevated levels of serum trypsinogen. High serum trypsinogen values at this age appear to be a very satisfactory screening technique for almost all of the cystic fibrosis population including those with pan-

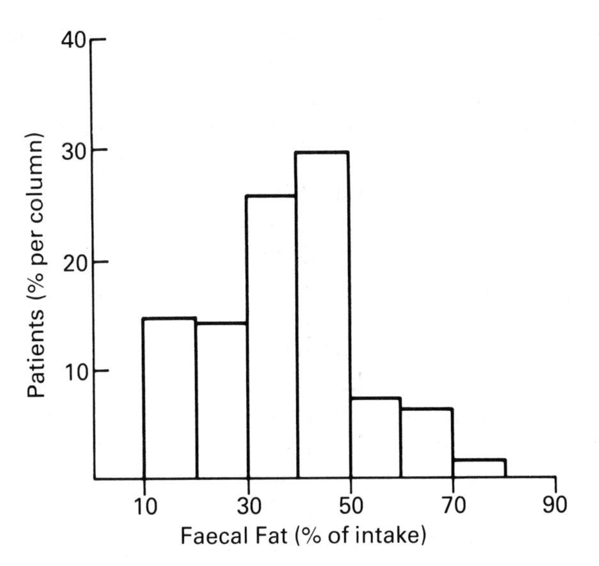

Figure 11.27 Range of steatorrhoea in 190 patients, untreated, with cystic fibrosis, registered with the Cystic Fibrosis Clinic in Toronto, Canada. Note that most of the cases are concentrated in the 10–50% range. (From Forstner *et al.* (1980),[24] with permission.)

creatic sufficiency.[13,63] The high serum trypsinogen levels must be caused by reflux from obstructed acini as most patients have evidence of pancreatic insufficiency at this time. Serum trypsinogen levels fall as patients become older, but low activities do not consistently appear until 6 years of age[21] and, therefore, a normal value in a young patients does not exclude pancreatic insufficiency.

Radiology

Plain radiographs, barium studies, ultrasonography, computed tomography and cholangiopancreatography may all provide useful information with regard to the pancreas. Calcification and macroscopic cyst formation are both relatively rare, but their demonstration may provide the explanation for an extrinsic mass compressing the duodenum.[14] Recurrent episodes of obstructive jaundice have occurred as a result of intrapancreatic compression of the common duct by fibrous tissue, and a similar narrowing and distortion of pancreatic ducts may be seen in patients with pancreatic sufficiency and recurrent pancreatitis.

Treatment

All patients should receive regular supplementation with pancreatic enzymes. Enteric-coated, acid-resistant microspheres that release their pancreatic enzymes at a pH of 5.5–6.0 have largely replaced capsules containing pancreatic extract powders, because in this way the number of capsules required for symptomatic relief is greatly reduced. The recommended dose is 3–4 capsules per meal, and one with each snack, with each capsule containing approximately 30 000 NF (USP) units of protease. It seems reasonable to take the capsules at regular intervals throughout the meal, but this has not been tested systematically. A very few patients appear to be made worse by the acid-resistant preparations and these may have unusually high gastric acid output preventing neutralization of duodenal and upper jejunal secretions to the degree required for pancreatic enzyme release.

It is uncommon to correct the steatorrhoea completely. Our patients with cystic fibrosis excreted 18 times as much fat per gram of fat intake as the normal average when no pancreatic supplement was given, and only improved to 12 times the normal with pancreatic extract powders.[24] When cimetidine and bicarbonate were added to inhibit and neutralize gastric acid secretion, absorption improved significantly but stool fat excretion fell to less than 7% of intake in only 3 of 45 tests. The response to pancreatic supplementation depends on the amount of fat in the diet.[19] Patients taking more than 100 g of fat daily may require one or two additional capsules with meals and snacks. The diet should be adequate in calories. Because fat is the most economical and appetizing energy source, it should not be restricted, but encouraged. When patients are given adequate diets they exhibit normal growth velocity for both height and weight until they develop advanced respiratory failure in their teens.[12]

Vitamins should be given in large daily doses in water-soluble form. Recommended daily amounts are: vitamin A, 8000 iu; vitamin D, 800 iu; and water-soluble vitamin E (DL-α-tocopherol acetate), 300 iu. B vitamins should be administered in twice the daily minimum requirements. Water-soluble vitamin K (menadiol sodium phosphate), 5.0 mg should be given twice weekly.

Amino acid hydrolysate, medium-chain triglycerides and polysaccharide supplements are rarely indicated. In infants under 6 months old with severe pulmonary problems, it is useful to begin feeding with medium-chain triglycerides and hydrolysate formulae because it may be difficult to ensure delivery of pancreatic enzymes with liquid formulae. The triglyceride mixes should be supplemented with essential fatty acids.[31] An attempt should be made to give pancreatic supplements along with the triglyceride formula because the absorption of fat will be improved.[20]

There is no solution for the anorexia and profound malnutrition that overcomes the steatorrhoeic patient as pulmonary function enters the stage of terminal deterioration. These patients are usually adolescents or young adults, and girls fail earlier than boys. Oral supplementation with elemental and high caloric diets are of no value. Nocturnal caloric supplementation by intubation has had little long-term effect, and a tube is poorly tolerated by patients with a chronic cough. Intravenous alimentation or supplements with Intralipid succeed only in younger patients with relatively good pulmonary function who appear to have been underweight on other grounds.

Specific syndromes associated with pancreatic insufficiency

Hypoalbuminaemia, oedema and anaemia

These problems coalesce in infants under the age of 6 months, with a peak incidence at 3–4 months. Affected patients are almost always untreated and often undiagnosed. The cause appears to be profound maldigestion and malnutrition, often aggravated by an inadequate caloric intake due to a poor supply of breast milk or intercurrent illness. Vitamin E levels are low, but the cause of the anaemia is not known. Soy protein has been incriminated because of its low digestibility, but the syndrome occurs on all formulae. Patients improve rapidly with pancreatic supplementation and adequate caloric intake. The diagnosis of cystic fibrosis may be difficult to confirm if the initial presentation is with fluid retention, because oedema may produce spurious low sweat chloride estimations.[44] A negative sweat test should always be repeated in a suspicious case when the oedema subsides.

Rectal prolapse

Rectal prolapse is a useful sign of pancreatic insufficiency because, in almost half of those patients who have cystic fibrosis, the episodes of prolapse precede the diagnosis.[59] Prolapse usually develops between 1 and 2.5 years of age and has a tendency to spontaneous resolution even without treatment. Patients who have not received pancreatic supplements are often improved dramatically when these are given; but if episodes of rectal prolapse develop whilst on pancreatic supplements, dietary and supplement manipulation rarely improve the situation.[59] With time, the children learn to reduce the prolapsed mucosa themselves and the problem seems to fade in significance. Approximately 10% of patients require surgical correction, usually for repeated episodes which are either painful or a nuisance.

Diabetes mellitus

Pancreatic islets are almost the last element to disappear as pancreatic fibrosis develops, but biochemical evidence of insulin deficiency becomes more frequent with increasing age and can be detected in one-third of older patients.[53,67] Clinically significant diabetes mellitus is rare and is easily controlled with small doses of insulin. The immunoreactive insulin response to glucose is delayed and diminished, even before glucose intolerance can be demonstrated. Basal and oral glucose-stimulated gastric inhibitory peptide levels are high once carbohydrate intolerance develops.[29]

Gallstones

Gallstones develop in 11% of patients with cystic fibrosis,[43] the incidence rising with advancing age. Steatorrhoea is associated with an excessive loss of faecal bile acids, a decreased bile acid pool, a shortage of taurine conjugates and increased cholesterol saturation.[31] Excessive leakage of bile acids is the primary problem. It occurs only in patients with steatorrhoea and responds well to pancreatic supplementation.[64] One suspects that cholelithiasis would cease to be a significant complication of cystic fibrosis if it were possible to correct pancreatic insufficiency completely.

Renal stones

Patients with pancreatic insufficiency are at risk to develop both oxalate and uric acid stones but this is a rare complication. The interest in uricolithiasis is in its relationship to pancreatic supplementation. Pancreatic extracts are rich in purine. Patients who take more than 20 capsules of pancreatic powder daily ingest in excess of 150 mg purine, doubling or tripling their normal intake. Both hyperuricosuria and hyperuricosaemia occur. Enteric microspheres virtually eliminate this risk since the total dose of pancreatic extract is reduced by 60–80%.

PANCREATIC SUFFICIENCY (PATIENTS WITHOUT STEATORRHOEA)

Pathology

In perhaps one-fifth of all patients with cystic fibrosis, the relentless progression of pancreatic disease either does not occur or seems to be retarded for one or two decades. Pancreatic morphology has been studied in relatively few instances, but there is ample evidence that there can be considerable pancreatic damage in many of these patients. Large portions of the pancreas are often atrophic and in areas of relative preservation there is irregular plugging of the large and small ducts and variable amounts of fibrous tissue.[16,58] In some patients, however, pancreatic function is within the normal range, presumably a sign that the pancreas is spared pathologically.

Clinical features

The outstanding feature of these patients is their relative freedom from pulmonary disease.[25,26] *Figure 11.28* summarizes the difference in the rates of deterioration of the 1-s forced expiratory volume, in pancreatic sufficient and insufficient patients and shows progressive deterioration in the patients with pancreatic insufficiency, with minimal change in the pancreatic-sufficient group. Similar results were obtained with a variety of other pulmonary function tests. Lung colonization with *pseudomonas* organisms occurs less frequently than in pancreatic-insufficient patients of corresponding age.[11] In the author's series the mean sweat chloride estimation was 105 mmol/l compared with 120 mmol/l in the patients with pancreatic insufficiency. The mean age at presentation was 5 years, considerably later than that of the patients with pancreatic insufficiency.

Approximately one-quarter of our patients presented with respiratory symptoms, 75% exhibited some evidence of clinical chest disease, 39% had clubbing, 30% nasal polyps; and 4% had a rectal prolapse, which suggests that this complication may not be restricted to patients with pancreatic insufficiency.

Eight per cent of the group had had pancreatitis. This is the only complication of cystic fibrosis that appears to be exclusively restricted to patients with pancreatic sufficiency, almost certainly because they are the only patients with sufficient surviving pancreatic tissue after the first few years of life to generate an active inflammatory response.

Diagnosis

Patients with pancreatic sufficiency are diagnosed most commonly as a result of a routine sweat chloride test performed for respiratory symptoms, because of a family history of cystic fibrosis, or through a neonatal screening programme. Occasionally metabolic alkalosis, rectal prolapse, loose stools or an unexplained attack of pancreatitis may prompt investigation.

The range of pancreatic function in these patients stretches from 1–2% to 100% of normal. In contrast to patients with Shwachman's syndrome (see page 1560) in whom the level of pancreatic insufficiency is often in a borderline zone of 1–10%,[33] 64% of 33 patients examined by quantitative pancreatic function testing have had greater than 20% pancreatic function.

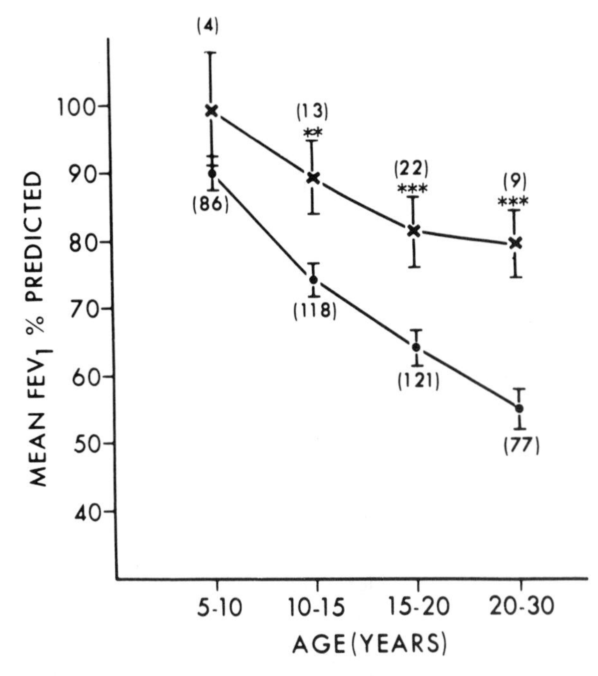

Figure 11.28 Mean FEV_1 (forced expiratory volume in 1 s) as a percentage of the predicted value versus age in cystic fibrosis patients without (×) and with (●) steatorrhoea. The values are mean ± s.e. (mean), $^{**}p < 0.05$, $^{***}p < 0.02$. (From Forstner *et al.* (1980),[25] with permission.)

INTESTINAL TRACT DISEASE

Pathology

The intestinal mucosa is not seriously affected by cystic fibrosis. Villus structure and absorptive cells are normal. Disaccharidase activities may even be increased.[2] Surface and crypt mucus are often increased. Some crypts may be greatly distended and even cyst-like, as if obstructed. At birth and throughout life, the lumen contains masses of rubbery, green-black meconium which adhere very strongly to the intestinal surface. Undegraded proteins, particularly albumin, are the major constituents. The meconium protein content at birth is approximately 6–8 times that of normal meconium.[57]

MECONIUM ILEUS

Approximately 10–15% of patients with cystic fibrosis present at birth or shortly thereafter with signs and symptoms of small bowel obstruction. The cause is a plug of meconium in the terminal ileum

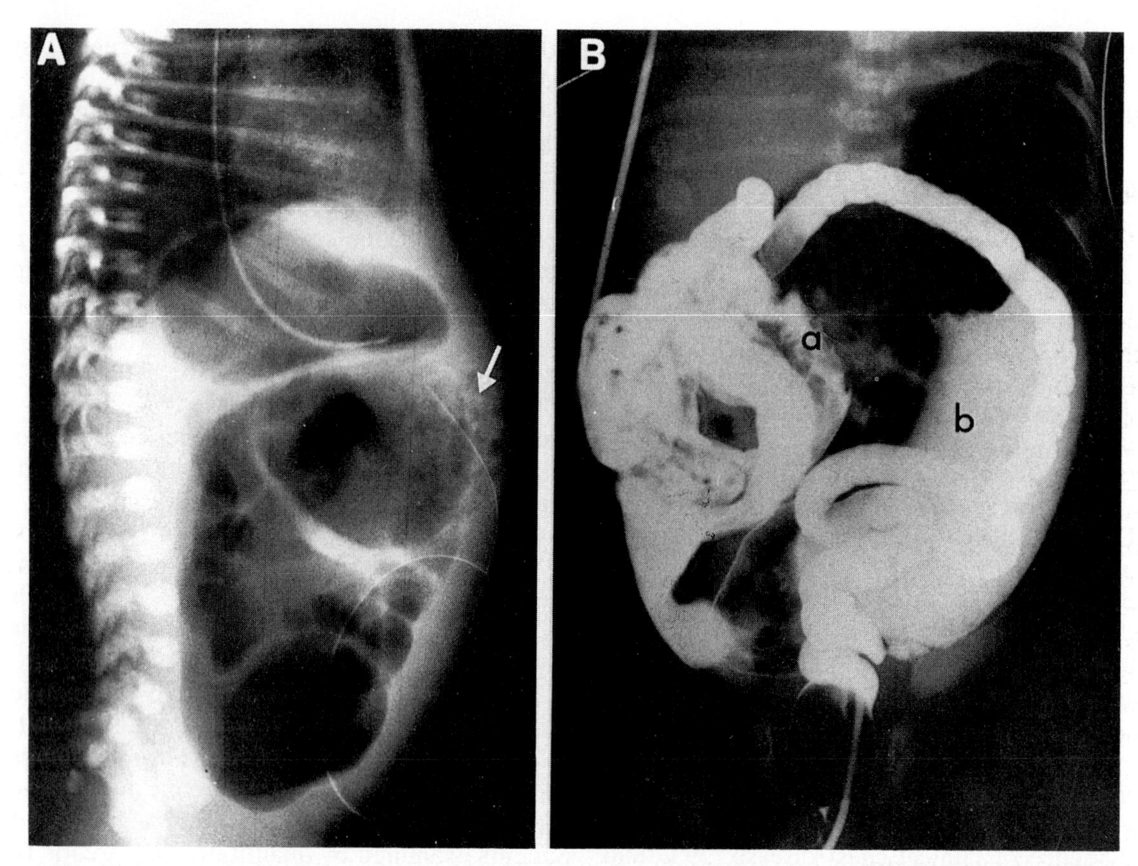

Figure 11.29 Radiological abnormalities in meconium ileus. (a) The plain radiograph shows greatly distended loops of bowel filled with air. The arrow points to a bubbly mass which is typical of meconium. (b) A Gastrografin enema was performed which outlined the small, unexpanded colon. At 'a', the Gastrografin has entered the meconium mass in the distal ileum. At 'b', the Gastrografin has refluxed proximally through an area of incomplete obstruction to fill a huge loop of bowel which proved to be part of a volvulus.

which is acquired in utero as perhaps the first overt manifestation of pancreatic insufficiency. Typically no meconium is passed and there is progressive abdominal distension. Rubbery, firm loops of bowel may be visible or palpable and the rectal examination is unproductive. A history of polyhydramnios may be obtained.

The radiological findings are quite characteristic (*Figure 11.29*). In addition to air fluid levels and distended loops of small bowel, small bubbles of gas can be seen trapped in the meconium of the distal small bowel, giving a ground glass appearance. A barium enema will demonstrate a small collapsed microcolon.

Half of the cases of meconium ileus are complicated by volvulus and atresia or meconium peritonitis or both. Atresia and meconium peritonitis usually result from intrauterine events associated with volvulus or extravasation of meconium through a perforation. Intraperitoneal calcification may be apparent on plain radiographs. Meconium pseudocysts may appear in the inflammatory reaction, ascites may develop and an infective peritonitis may occur if the perforation does not close.

Meconium ileus is almost always associated with cystic fibrosis, but rare reports of the condition have appeared in association with stenosis of the pancreatic duct,[37] with partial pancreatic aplasia,[4] and with normal gastrointestinal tract.[18] Approximately one-third of patients with meconium peritonitis and one-fifth of patients with atresia of the small bowel[47] will have cystic fibrosis.

Treatment

Most patients can be relieved of their intestinal obstruction with diatrizoate (Gastrografin or Hypaque) enemas. The main hazard is that these hypertonic solutions may cause a dangerous loss of fluid and electrolytes into the bowel. Infants ought to be supported with continuous intravenous fluids during the procedure. Colonic perforation has been reported[62] but is rare. Gastrografin enemas are not indicated for complicated meconium ileus. The surgical approach to meconium ileus usually involves removal of the plug with irrigation at the time of surgery and, if there is atresia or peritonitis, a limited resection. Mortality is now less than 10%

acutely and a history of meconium ileus is not a risk factor for long-term survival as previously thought.[46]

DISTAL INTESTINAL OBSTRUCTION SYNDROME (MECONIUM ILEUS EQUIVALENT)

Later in life, about 10% of patients with cystic fibrosis[45] suffer from recurrent complaints attributable to partial or complete bowel obstruction. The failure to digest intraluminal protein is a major cause of constipation and obstruction. Although inspissated masses of meconium play an aetiological role, the resemblance to meconium ileus is somewhat tenuous. Large faecal masses can be palpated in the abdomen, particularly in the caecal area. These masses may persist for many months in spite of the daily passage of several stools. Intermittent abdominal distension and cramping may also occur without further disturbance. Rarely the putty-like obstructive masses in the right colon and terminal ileum precipitate acute obstructive episodes with ileus and vomiting. Holsclaw, Rocmans and Schwachman[34] found that 1% of patients with cystic fibrosis presented with intussusception, presumably using an adherent faecal mass as the lead point. In 22 episodes in 19 patients, only two required intestinal resection. The common site for the intussusception was ileocolic.

Treatment

The syndrome is usually responsive to medical management. The most urgent task is to ensure that the presence of faecal masses and radiological evidence of bubbly faecal material in the distal small bowel and colon are not regarded as a surgical emergency. In chronic cases it is important to ensure adequate pancreatic replacement therapy. A diet that is high in roughage and a mild laxative, such as mineral oil, may be all that is required to relieve the patient. In acute obstructive episodes, characterized by clear evidence of small bowel obstruction, such as vomiting or air fluid levels throughout the small intestine, a nasogastric tube should be introduced and the impaction should be cleared with enemas. Most centres use 10% N-acetylcysteine as a mucus-clearing agent. Even though the masses are not particularly mucoid, this agent seems to be sufficiently irritating to dislodge the faecal plugs.

N-Acetylcysteine may be introduced by mouth, by D-tube or Miller–Abbott tube, depending upon the indication. Gastrografin enemas may be used as a last resort.

In the absence of signs of acute small bowel obstruction, chronic intractable symptoms may be relieved for surprisingly long periods by intestinal lavage with 5–6 litres of a balanced isotonic polyethylene glycol–salt solution (Golytely) delivered orally or through a nasogastric tube.[10] Although this approach may at first sight seem overzealous, it has, in the author's experience, as well as that of others,[15] been greeted with excellent acceptance by patients who have failed to find relief with laxatives and mucolytics. Repeated lavage is well tolerated and can be administered at home by the patient.

Surgery is reserved for those rare patients with intussusception that cannot be relieved by enema, or for the even more unusual patient with clear evidence of an obstructive mass that cannot be removed by the persistent application of conservative measures.

CONSTIPATION

Older patients with cystic fibrosis suffer from a very high incidence of abdominal cramping and decreased stool frequency. Many of these patients also have chronic distal intestinal obstruction syndrome, but constipation appears to be about three times more frequent.[54] The most characteristic radiological finding is copious faecal material throughout the colon. These patients respond to an initial regimen of enemas, followed by long-term oral laxatives. Some may benefit from intermittent gastrointestinal lavage.

GASTRO-OESOPHAGEAL REFLUX

Oesophagitis and oesophageal stricture occur secondary to oesophageal reflux and usually in the absence of any evidence of hiatal hernia (see also Chapter 2, section 5). Chronic pulmonary disease and multiple medications are probable predisposing factors. The incidence is approximately the same as that of overt diabetes mellitus and patients are usually of the same age. Oesophageal reflux should always be considered as a cause of anorexia, weight loss, or unexplained anaemia in an adolescent.

RADIOLOGY OF THE INTESTINAL TRACT

Barium examinations frequently reveal thickened and coarse mucosal folds or nodular indentations which may lead to mistaken diagnoses of duodenal ulcer, neoplasia or inflammatory bowel disease. Adherent faecal masses compound the interpretive difficulties if the primary diagnosis is unclear. Taussig, Saldino and Di Sant'Agnese[60] found radiological abnormalities in one-third of colonic and small intestinal studies, and in 80% of duodenal studies. If an ulcer or a neoplasm is suspected, the diagnosis should be confirmed independently by endoscopy. Pneumatosis intestinales may be seen, particularly in patients with advanced pulmonary disease.[32]

PROGNOSIS

In most patients the outcome of the disease depends almost entirely on the pulmonary complications. These begin, often insidiously, as a chronic pulmonary infection caused by the plugging of small airways by thick, viscid secretions and lead eventually to widespread destruction of terminal bronchioles, bronchiectasis, atelectasis and emphysema with associated respiratory failure, haemoptyses and cor pulmonale. Death results from respiratory failure or overwhelming pulmonary infection. The median survival for patients in Canada is about 30 years for males and 20 years for females. There is no explanation for the great discrepancy between the sexes. Girls appear to do as well as boys until the early teens, but worsen subsequently at a much faster rate.

Gastrointestinal factors may play an important role in deciding overall prognosis, because both male and female patients who lack sufficient pancreatic disease to produce steatorrhoea have been shown to have remarkably well preserved pulmonary function, at least into the third decade.[35] These patients almost invariably lack one or both copies of the common cystic fibrosis mutation.[39]

REFERENCES

1. Andersen, D. (1938) Cystic fibrosis of the pancreas and its relation to celiac disease. *American Journal of Diseases of Children*, **56**, 344–399.
2. Antonowicz, I., Lebenthal, E. and Shwachman, H. (1978) Disaccharidase activities in small intestinal mucosa in patients with cystic fibrosis. *Journal of Pediatrics*, **92**, 214–219.
3. Argent, B.E. Gray, M.A. and Greenwell, J.R. (1987) Secretin regulated anion channel on the apical membrane of rat pancreatic duct cells in vitro. *Journal of Physiology*, **39**, 333.
4. Auburn, R., Feldman, S., Gadacz, T. and Rowe, M. (1969) Meconium ileus secondary to partial aplasia of the pancreas: report of a case. *Surgery*, **65**, 689–693.
5. Bendig, D.W., Seilheimer, D.K., Wagner, M.L. *et al.* (1982) Complications of gastroesophageal reflux in patients with cystic fibrosis. *Journal of Pediatrics*, **100**, 536–540.
6. Berschneider, H.M., Knowles, M.R., Azizkham, R.G. *et al.* (1988) Altered intestinal chloride transport in cystic fibrosis. *FASEB Journal*, **2**, 2625–2629.
7. Bonin, A., Roy, C., LaSalle, R. *et al.* (1973) Fecal chymotrypsin, a reliable index of exocrine pancreatic function in children. *Journal of Pediatrics*, **83**, 594–600.
8. Boucher, R.C., Stutts, M.J., Knowles, M.R., Cantley, L. and Gatzy, J.T. (1986) Na^+ transport in cystic fibrosis respiratory epithelia. *Journal of Clinical Investigations*, **78**, 1245–1252.
9. Case, R.M. and Scratcherd, T. (1972) The actions of dibutyral cyclic adenosine 3′5″-monophosphate and methyl xanthines on pancreatic exocrine secretion. *Journal of Physiology*, **210**, 1–15.
10. Cleghorn, G.J., Forstner, G.G., Stringer, D.A. and Durie, P.R. (1986) Treatment of distal intestinal obstruction syndrome in cystic fibrosis with a balanced intestinal lavage solution. *The Lancet*, **i**: 8–11.
11. Corey, M., Gaskin, K., Durie, P., Levison, H. and Forstner, G. (1984) Improved prognosis in CF patients with normal fat absorption. *Journal of Pediatric Gastroenterology and Nutrition*, **3** (suppl): S99–S105.
12. Corey, M.L. (1980) Longitudinal studies in cystic fibrosis. In *Perspectives in Cystic Fibrosis.* Proceedings of the 8th International Congress on Cystic Fibrosis (Ed.) Sturgess, J. pp. 246–255. Mississauga: Imperial Press.
13. Crossley, J.R., Smith, P.A., Edgar, B.W. *et al.* (1981) Neonatal screening for cystic fibrosis, using immuno-reative trypsin assay in dried blood spots. *Clinica Chimica Acta*, **113**, 111–121.
14. Cunningham, D.G., Henkin, R.E. and Reynes, C.J. (1981) Macroscopic cysts of the pancreas in cystic fibrosis demonstrated by multiple radiological modalities. *Journal of the American Medical Association*, **245**, 72–74.
15. Davidson, A.C., Harrison, K., Steinfort, C.L. and Geddes, D.M. (1987) Distal intestinal obstruction syndrome in cystic fibrosis treated by oral intestinal lavage, and a case of recurrent obstruction despite normal pancreatic function. *Thorax*, **42**, 538–541.
16. di Sant'Agnese, P. (1955) Fibrocystic disease of the pancreas with normal or partial pancreatic function. *Pediatrics*, **15**, 683–695.
17. di Sant'Agnese, P., Darling, R., Perera, G. and Shea, E. (1953) Abnormal electrolyte composition of sweat in cystic fibrosis of the pancreas. *Pediatrics*, **12**, 549–563.
18. Dolan, T. and Touloukian, R. (1974) Familial meconium ileus not associated with cystic fibrosis. *Journal of Pediatric Surgery*, **9**, 821–824.
19. Durie, P.R., Bell, L., Linton, W. *et al.* (1980) Effect of cimetidine and sodium bicarbonate on pancreatic replacement therapy in cystic fibrosis. *Gut*, **21**, 778–786.
20. Durie, P.R., Newth, C.J., Forstner, G.G. and Gall, D.G. (1980) Malabsorption of medium-chain triglycerides in infants with cystic fibrosis:

correction with pancreatic enzyme supplements. *Journal of Pediatrics*, **96**, 862–864.
21. Durie, P.R., Forstner, G.G., Gaskin, K.J. *et al.* (1986) Age related alteration of immunoreactive pancreatic cationic trypsinogen in sera from cystic fibrosis patients with and without pancreatic insufficiency. *Pediatric Research*, **20**, 209–213.
22. Elias, E., Muller, D.P. and Scott, J. (1981) Association of spinocerebellar disorders with cystic fibrosis or chronic childhood cholestasis and very low vitamin E. *Lancet*, **ii**, 1319–1321.
23. Fanconi, G., Uehlinger, E. and Knauer, G. (1936) Das Coelioksyndrom bei angeborener zystisher Pankreas Fibromatose und Branchiektasis. *Weiner Medizinische Wochenschrift*, **86**, 753–756.
24. Forstner, G., Gall, G., Corey, M. *et al.* (1980) Digestion and absorption of nutrients in cystic fibrosis. In *Perspectives in Cystic Fibrosis.* Proceedings of the 8th International Congress on Cystic Fibrosis (Ed.) Sturgess. J. pp. 137–148. Mississauga: Imperial Press.
25. Gaskin, K., Gurwitz, D., Corey, M. *et al.* (1980) Improved pulmonary function in cystic fibrosis patients without pancreatic insufficiency. In *Perspectives in Cystic Fibrosis,* Proceedings of the 8th International Congress on Cystic Fibrosis (Ed.) Sturgess, J. pp. 226–228. Mississauga: Imperial Press.
26. Gaskin, K., Gurwitz, D., Durie, P.R. *et al.* (1982) Improved respiratory prognosis in patients with cystic fibrosis with normal fat absorption. *Journal of Pediatrics*, **100**, 857–862.
27. Gaskin, K.J., Durie, P.R., Corey, M. *et al.* (1982) Evidence for a primary defect of pancreatic HCO_3^- secretion in cystic fibrosis. *Pediatric Research*, **16**, 554–557.
28. Gaskin, K.J., Durie, P.R., Lee, L. *et al.* (1984) Colipase and lipase secretion in childhood onset pancreatic insufficiency. Delineation of patients with steatorrhoea secondary to relative colipase deficiency. *Gastroenterology*, **86**, 1–7.
29. Geffner, M.E., Lippe, B.M., Kaplan, S.A. *et al.* (1984) Carbohydrate tolerance in cystic fibrosis is closely linked to pancreatic exocrine function. *Pediatric Research*, **18**, 1107–1111.
30. Gibbs, G.E., Bostick, W.L. and Smith, P.M. (1950) Incomplete pancreatic deficiency in cystic fibrosis of the pancreas. *Journal of Pediatrics*, **37**, 320–325.
31. Harries, T.J., Muller, D.P.R., McCollum, J.P.K. *et al.* (1979) Intestinal bile salts in CG. Studies in the patient and experimental animal. *Archives of Disease in Childhood*, **54**, 19–24.
32. Hernanz-Schulman, M., Kirkpatrick, J., Shwachman, H., Herman, T., Schulman, G., Vawter, G. (1986) Pneumatosis intestinales in cystic fibrosis. *Radiology*, **160**, 497–499.
33. Hill, R.E., Durie, P.R., Gaskin, K.J. *et al.* (1982) Steatorrhea and pancreatic insufficiency in Shwachman syndrome. *Gastroenterology*, **83**, 22–27.
34. Holsclaw, D., Rocmans, C. and Shwachman, H. (1971) Intussusception in patients with cystic fibrosis. *Pediatrics*, **48**, 51–58.
35. Hopfer, U. (1982) Pathophysiological considerations relevant to intestinal obstruction in cystic fibrosis. In *Fluids and Electrolyte Abnormalities in Exocrine Glands in Cystic Fibrosis.* (Eds) Quinton, P.M., Martinez, J.R., Hopfer, K. p. 241. San Francisco: San Francisco Press.
36. Hubbard, V.S., Dunn, G.D. and diSant'Agnese, P.A. (1977) Abnormal fatty acid composition of plasma lipids in cystic fibrosis. *The Lancet*, **ii**, 1302–1304.
37. Hurwitt, E. and Arnheim, E. (1942) Meconium ileus associated with stenosis of the pancreatic ducts. *American Journal of Diseases in Children*, **64**, 443–454.
38. Imrie, J., Fagan, D. and Sturgess, J. (1979) Quantitative evaluation of the development of the exocrine pancreas in CF and control infants. *American Journal of Pathology*, **95**, 697–707.
39. Kerem, E., Corey, M., Kerem, B. *et al.* (1990) The relationship between genotype and phenotype in cystic fibrosis: analysis of the most common mutation (ΔF 508). *New England Journal of Medicine*, **323**, 1517–1522.
40. Kopelman, H., Corey, M., Gaskin, K., Durie, P., Weizman, Z. and Forstner, G. (1988) Impaired chloride secretion as well as bicarbonate secretion underlies the fluid secretory defect in the cystic fibrosis pancreas. *Gastroenterology*, **95**, 349–355.
41. Kopelman, H., Durie, P., Gaskin, K., Weizman, Z., Forstner, G. (1985) Pancreatic fluid secretion and protein hyperconcentration in cystic fibrosis. *New England Journal of Medicine*, **312**, 329–334.
42. Kopito, L., Shwachman, H., Vawter, G. and Edlow, J. (1976) The pancreas in cystic fibrosis: chemical composition and comparative morphology. *Pediatric Research*, **10**, 742–749.
43. L'Heureux, P., Isenberg, J., Sharp, H. and Warwick, W. (1977) Gallbladder disease in cystic fibrosis. *American Journal of Roentgenology*, **128**, 953–956.
44. Maclean, W. and Tripp, R. (1973) Cystic fibrosis with edema and falsely negative sweat test. *Journal of Pediatrics*, **83**, 85–90.
45. Matseshe, J., Go, V. and DiMagno, E. (1977) Meconium ileus equivalent complicating cystic fibrosis in post neonatal children and young adults. *Gastroenterology*, **72**, 732–736.
46. McPartlin, J., Dickson, J. and Swain, V. (1972) Meconium ileus, immediate and long term survival. *Archives of Disease in Childhood*, **47**, 207–210.
47. Noblett, H. (1979) Meconium ileus. In: *Pediatric Surgery*. (Ed.) Ravitch, M., Welch, K., Benson, C. *et al.* pp. 943–952. Chicago: Year Book Medical Publishers.
48. Nousia-Arvanitakis, S., Stapleton, F., Linshaw, M. and Kennedy, J. (1977) Therapeutic approach to pancreatic extract-induced hyperuricosuria in cystic fibrosis. *Journal of Pediatrics*, **90**, 302–305.
49. Oppenheimer, E. and Esterly, J. (1973) Cystic

fibrosis of the pancreas. *Archives of Pathology*, **96**, 149–154.
50. Quinton, P.M. (1983) Chlorise impermeability in cystic fibrosis. *Nature*, **301**, 421–422.
51. Riordan, J.R., Rommens, J.M. and Kerem, B. (1989) Identification of the cystic fibrosis gene: cloning and characterization of complementary DNA. *Science*, **245**, 1066–1073.
52. Rommens, I.M., Iannuzzi, M.C., Kerem, B. *et al.* (1989) Identification of the cystic fibrosis gene: chromosome walking and jumping. *Science*, **245**, 1059–1065.
53. Rosan, R., Shwachman, H. and Kulczycki, L. (1962) Diabetes mellitus and cystic fibrosis of pancreas. *American Journal of Diseases in Children*, **104**, 625–634.
54. Rubinstein, S., Moss, R., Lewiston, N. (1986) Constipation and meconium ileus equivalent in patients with cystic fibrosis. *Pediatrics*, **78**, 473–479.
55. Sato, K., Sato, F. (1984) Defective beta adrenergic response of cystic fibrosis sweat glands in vivo and in vitro. *Journal of Clinical Investigations*, **73**, 1763–1771.
56. Schoumacher, R.A., Ram, J., Iannuzzi, M.C. *et al.* (1990) A cystic fibrosis pancreatic adenocarcinoma cell line. *Proceedings of the National Academy of Science of the USA*, **87**, 4012–4016.
57. Schutt, W. and Isles, T. (1968) Protein in meconium ileus. *Archives of Disease in Childhood*, **43**, 178–181.
58. Shwachman, H., Lebenthal, E. and Khaw, K. (1975) Recurrent acute pancreatitis in patients with cystic fibrosis with normal pancreatic enzymes. *Pediatrics*, **55**, 86–94.
59. Stern, R., Izant, R.J., Boat, T.F. *et al.* (1982) Treatment and prognosis of rectal prolapse in cystic fibrosis. *Gastroenterology*, **82**, 707–710.
60. Taussig, L.M., Saldino, R.M. and diSant'Agnese, P.A. (1973) Radiographic abnormalities of the duodenum and small bowel in cystic fibrosis of the pancreas. *Radiology*, **106**, 369–376.
61. Torstenson, O., Humphrey, G., Edson, J. and Warwick, W. (1970) Cystic fibrosis presenting with severe hemorrhage due to vitamin K malabsorption. A report of 3 cases. *Pediatrics*, **45**, 857–860.
62. Wagget, H., Bishop, H. & Koop, E. (1970) Experience with Gastrografin enema in the treatment of meconium ileus. *Journal of Pediatric Surgery*, **5**, 649–654.
63. Waters, D.L., Dorney, S.F., Gaskin, K.J. *et al.* (1990) Pancreatic function in infants identified as having cystic fibrosis in a neonatal screening program. *New England Journal of Medicine*, **322**, 303–308.
64. Weber, A., Roy, C., Morin, C. and LaSalle, R. (1973) Malabsorption of bile acids in children with cystic fibrosis. *New England Journal of Medicine*, **289**, 1001–1005.
65. Weizman, Z., Forstner, G.G., Gaskin, K.J., Kopelman, H., Wong, S. and Durie, P.R. (1985) Bentiromide test for assessing pancreatic dysfunction using analysis of para-amino benzoic acid in plasma and urine. Studies in cystic fibrosis and Shwachman's syndrome. *Gastroenterology*, **89**, 596–604.
66. Wesley, A., Forstner, J., Qureshi, R. *et al.* (1983) Human intestinal mucin in cystic fibrosis. *Pediatric Research*, **17**, 65–69.
67. Wilmshurst, E., Soeldner, J., Holsclaw, D. *et al.* (1975) Endogenous and exogenous insulin responses in patients with cystic fibrosis. *Pediatrics*, **55**, 75–82.

ACUTE PANCREATITIS

C.W. Imrie

Acute pancreatitis is a condition resulting from an acute inflammatory process in the pancreas usually characterized by upper abdominal pain and raised concentrations of pancreatic enzymes in blood, urine and peritoneal fluid.

AETIOLOGY

The two most common aetiological factors identified from prospective series of patients are biliary disease and alcohol abuse,[38,56,69] which together account for approximately 80% of patients. Any patient who has suffered an attack of acute pancreatitis may suffer a further attack after recovery from the acute illness when the precipitating factor, for example gallstones, persists. It is therefore mandatory that an immediate search for a possible cause is undertaken and appropriate therapeutic measures instituted. It is customary to describe a patient suffering a series of attacks of acute pancreatitis with full clinical recovery between each attack as having *recurrent acute pancreatitis*. Occasionally subsequent attacks may occur before complete recovery and this may be related to the rapid re-introduction of a normal diet, re-exposure to alcohol or the passage of small stones from the gallbladder down the lower common bile duct in the recovery phase of the disease.

Although sporadic reports of acute pancreatitis and its complications extend back four centuries, it has been well established for about a century[26,61,65] that both gallstones and alcohol abuse are aetiological factors. In the UK it is usual to find that around half the patients have gallstones[38,55,56] which characteristically are smaller than the gallstones in patients presenting with predominantly biliary symptoms. An incidence varying from 9% to almost 40% for alcohol abuse has been reported in the UK[38,76,80] with the highest incidence being found in Scotland. In these patients, there is usually a characteristic time interval of 12–36 hours following a bout of heavy alcohol abuse before the onset of the signs and symptoms of acute pancreatitis. In any individual patient, this period can be remarkably constant where recurrent attacks of acute pancreatitis occur.

There are in addition a considerable number of *minor aetiological factors,* most of which are listed in *Table 11.2.* As with the major factors, the relative incidence of these minor factors varies from area to area within one country and also from country to country. No single factor in this group would be expected to account for more than 5% of all patients with 'de novo' or primary acute pancreatitis.

One prospective study indicated that *viral infections* accounted for approximately 4% of the total patients with primary acute pancreatitis and that the most commonly implicated viruses were the Coxsackie B group and also the mumps virus.[35] These viruses probably attack the pancreatic tissue directly in a preferential fashion and the real incidence of this problem has not yet been studied adequately. It also should be noted that both the hepatitis and Marburg viruses which tend to affect the liver primarily may, coincidentally with the severe hepatitis, cause focal areas of pancreatic necrosis and clinical signs of acute pancreatitis.

Table 11.2 Acute pancreatitis: aetiology

'De novo' acute pancreatitis
Major factors
- Biliary disease (gallstones)
- Alcohol abuse

Minor factors
- Viral infections (Coxsackie B and mumps)
- Tumours (pancreatic and ampullary)
- Ischaemia
- Metastatic tumours
- Hyperparathyroidism
- Hyperlipoproteinaemia
- Drugs
- Previous 'blind loop' surgery

Iatrogenic acute pancreatitis
- Postoperative (especially lower common bile duct exploration and sphincteroplasty)
- After endoscopic retrograde cholangiopancreatography
- After translumbar arteriography

Both *primary*[28] and *secondary*[49,60] *pancreatic tumours* may present initially as an attack of acute pancreatitis, and histologically it is not unusual to find a considerable degree of surrounding inflammation in the tissue immediately adjacent to a carcinoma. Carcinoma of the ampulla of Vater is not infrequently associated with the presence of gallstones and may present clinically with acute pancreatitis. Ischaemic pancreatitis occurs in relation to dissecting aortic aneurysm, mesenteric vascular thrombosis and hypothermia.[27]

The association between *hypercalcaemia, hyperparathyroidism* and acute pancreatitis is ill-understood but this is a much less frequent association than is suggested by many textbooks. Two series, each containing over 500 patients, identified no more than four with hyperparathyroidism[76] and some of these patients had one of the two major aetiological factors present in addition.[10] Suggestions from Australia[71] that the association between recent parathyroidectomy and acute pancreatitis occurred in 9% of patients have been discounted by other authors who found no cases in 334 parathyroidectomies.[79] *Hyperlipaemia* has been claimed to be a causal factor in the pathogenesis of acute pancreatitis[15] but while this metabolic abnormality can induce inflammation in a few patients it is more customary to find hyperlipoproteinaemia as an incidental factor associated with alcohol abuse.[22] In most patients it is type IV or type V hyperlipidaemia,[18] but the occasional patient with the rare type I has been described (see also Chapter 8, Lipid abnormalities).[22]

Many drugs have been implicated in the precipitation of attacks of acute pancreatitis. It is both dangerous and irresponsible to attribute commonly used drugs as possible causative factors in acute pancreatitis without full exploration of the possibilities of the major and minor factors already listed being the cause in an individual patient. Nevertheless, numerous anecdotal reports have appeared over the last 20 or 30 years suggesting that frusemide, cimetidine and oral contraceptives may be involved. Considering the frequency of prescription of these drugs the association with acute pancreatitis may be no more than spurious (*Table 18.2*) but a stronger case can be made for thiazide diuretics. Another group of drugs which have been recorded as precipitants of acute pancreatitis are steroids.[58] The incidence in renal transplant patients varies from 2% to 5.6%. The mortality tends to be high

Table 11.3 Drugs believed to precipitate acute pancreatitis

	Reports	*Patients*
Steroids	Several	50
Oral contraceptives	Several	50
Thiazide diuretics	Several	Few
Azathioprine	Several	Very few
Frusemide (very high dosage)	Several	Very few
Valproic acid	3	Few
L-Asparaginase	3	Few
Phenformin	2	Few
Paracetamol	1	Very few
Warfarin	1	Very few

and many of the patients are on both steroids and azathioprine, another drug which is thought to precipitate acute pancreatitis. All of the many drugs listed in *Table 11.3* have been implicated occasionally as major causative factors of acute pancreatitis. There is no evidence to implicate cimetidine in the pathogenesis of acute pancreatitis. The overall incidence of drug-induced pancreatitis may be much higher than has been appreciated because so few studies have been carried out prospectively with an adequate comparison group, such as that reported from Nottingham in 1978.[11] In that particular study, a diuretic (cyclopenthiazide) together with potassium chloride was found to have been used regularly in 11 of the pancreatitis patients and in only one of the controls. There was no significant difference between the two groups in the use of antihypertensive agents including β-blockers.

Patients who have previously undergone a Billroth II or Polya type gastrectomy creating a blind duodenal loop are significantly more at risk than those who have undergone a Billroth I type gastrectomy.[73,80] The mechanism of acute pancreatitis in these patients may be related to partial obstruction of the blind loop creating a situation similar to the experimental Pfeffer preparation for induction of acute pancreatitis.

IATROGENIC ACUTE PANCREATITIS

This includes pancreatitis that occurs soon after a surgical operation, diagnostic or therapeutic retrograde pancreatography and immediately following translumbar aortography (see *Table 11.2*).[37]

Patients subject to surgical procedures involving instrumentation of the lower end of the common bile duct and sphincteroplasty at the ampulla of Vater are particularly prone to postoperative acute pancreatitis which can be difficult to diagnose.[40] Associated with a delay in diagnosis, is an increased mortality which is at least partly attributable to the delay in recognition of hypovolaemia with consequent increased risk of acute renal failure. Partial gastrectomy may involve direct damage to the pancreas and is known to precipitate immediate postoperative acute pancreatitis[80] but, in addition to those procedures that are performed in the immediate locality of the pancreas, there are a considerable number of isolated reports of pancreatitis occurring after orthopaedic, urological and cardiac[25] operations. In such situations it is believed that pancreatic ischaemia has occurred either during or after surgery.

Although diagnostic pancreatography is believed to be innocuous, there are a number of reports of major attacks of acute pancreatitis following cannulation of the ampulla, some of which have been fatal.[4,72] Therapeutic pancreatography, where stones are removed from the lower common bile duct with sphincteroplasty using a diathermy apparatus, is associated with a higher incidence of post-pancreatitis which can be particularly severe.

Percutaneous translumbar aortography may be associated with direct damage to the pancreas along the course of the needle and a number of patients have been reported with this complication occurring immediately after the investigation.[37] It is necessary to aim the needle at the aorta away from the level of the pancreas to avoid this complication.

Acute pancreatitis may be induced by penetrating injuries to the pancreas but is more frequently associated with blunt abdominal injuries, that inflicted by a seat-belt or steering wheel, for example. In contrast to other forms of acute pancreatitis, where initial conservative management is generally acceptable, direct surgical intervention is warranted as completion of the partial transection of the pancreas following compression against the vertebral column is often the best therapy. Particular difficulty is encountered when the right side of the pancreas is injured by blunt trauma. In such situations, the duodenum and the lower end of the common bile duct, as well as the head of the pancreas, are damaged, and resection with reconstruction is exceedingly difficult. Roux loop drainage and external tube drainage can be fraught with complications but represent possible therapies.

PATHOGENESIS

Material for histology is rarely obtained in vivo in clinical acute pancreatitis. Major changes of autolysis readily occur post mortem and only those specimens obtained for histological purposes within a few hours of death or at operation are entirely satisfactory. In acute pancreatitis from biliary disease and alcohol abuse, *periductal necrosis* is the common post-mortem histological finding, whereas ischaemic forms of pancreatitis are typified by a *perilobular necrosis*.[27] A combination of these elements may be seen in some of the most severe forms of pancreatitis. The details of events in pancreatitis associated with alcohol abuse and gallstones are poorly understood.

In biliary-associated pancreatitis it is typical to find small stones in considerable numbers in the gallbladder and common bile duct. Several studies have shown that it is usually the passage of stones through the common bile duct that is associated with acute pancreatitis.[1,2,41,51] It is believed that a stone or stones are held up at the ampulla of Vater for a varying time only; complete impaction in this area is unusual. The events during the period of hold up are not agreed but the possibilities include duodenal reflux or biliary reflux along the pancreatic duct which acts as the trigger to initiate acute pancreatitis, or both. The eradication of gallstones from the biliary tract invariably prevents further episodes of acute pancreatitis, whilst the presence of even a single stone may allow recurrent attacks to take place.

The traditional explanation for alcohol-induced acute pancreatitis has been that an increase of pancreatic secretion and an associated spasm at the sphincter of Oddi are important factors. Several groups have shown in laboratory studies that both increased vascular levels of ethanol and reflux of ethanol, with or without bile salts being present, increase the permeability of the pancreatic duct epithelium. In addition, in a clinical study from Baltimore of a selected group of patients with previous alcohol-induced acute pancreatitis with induced hyperlipaemia, pain developed.[17] In a proportion of these patients there was elevation of serum amylase, but the small numbers and the lack of a control group of patients causes scepticism that this is the main mechanism in alcohol-induced pancreatitis.[17]

Acute pancreatitis associated with viral infection has been shown in both animals and man to be due to direct attack on the acinar cells by the virus.

CLINICAL FEATURES

The most important feature of acute pancreatitis is abdominal pain which is usually sudden in onset and increases rapidly to reach maximum intensity within a few hours. Such is the rapidity and severity of the pain that it resembles closely that experienced from a perforated viscus. The pain is usually felt in the epigastrium but other common sites are the right and left upper quadrants and, less frequently, peri-umbilical or hypogastric. Characteristically, but only in 50% of patients, the pain radiates centrally through to the back, being felt in the lower thoracic and upper lumbar region.

In the average patient, pain lasts for about 48 hours but occasionally persists for up to a week. Rarely an episode of acute pancreatitis is completely painless. Vomiting may be the most clamant symptom and exceeds the problem of pain.

Physical examination will reveal varying degrees of shock depending upon the severity of the attack. A modest fever is often encountered and there will be tachycardia and hypotension, although a transitory rise in blood pressure is found in 10% of patients. Half the patients show guarding or rigidity but it is a frequent observation that the severity of the pain appears to be out of proportion to the abdominal signs. An epigastric mass is felt in 10–20% of patients. Most patients have a paralytic ileus for 24–96 hours. Other features that occur less commonly and which are discussed below include tachypnoea, hypoxia, ascites and pleural effusions.

Severe hyperglycaemia and diabetic ketoacidosis may be a presenting feature. A fall in serum calcium may be sufficient to cause tetany. Mental confusion may be prominent, particularly in alcoholic patients and where hypoxia is profound. Cardiac failure, pulmonary insufficiency and acute respiratory distress are encountered. Uncommonly, fat necrosis in the subcutaneous tissues manifests as painful areas, particularly in the legs, and there may be associated arthralgia and a mild eosinophilia.

The complications encountered with acute pancreatitis are:

1. Cardiac insufficiency
2. Renal insufficiency
3. Respiratory insufficiency
4. Haematological abnormalities
   (a) Anaemia
   (b) Disseminated intravascular coagulation
   (c) Thrombosis of portal and/or splenic veins
5. Biochemical abnormalities (see text).

The late complications are:

1. Pseudocyst
2. Abscess
3. Fistula
4. Stricture of pancreatic duct
5. Pancreatic ascites
6. Diabetes mellitus.

The biochemical changes in themselves are not specific but, taken together with the clinical setting, they often provide a characteristic diagnostic picture and, furthermore, they can be used to grade the severity of the illness. Mild anaemia, a leucocytosis, hyperglycaemia and glycosuria are found fairly frequently. Other changes include elevated serum bilirubin, alkaline phosphatase and transferase levels and methaemalbuminaemia.

INVESTIGATIONS

Acute pancreatitis should be considered in the differential diagnosis of upper abdominal disease and shock syndromes as follows:

Mild pancreatitis
1. Acute cholecystitis
2. Peptic ulceration
3. Intestinal obstruction with ileus
4. Acute intermittent porphyria
5. Diaphragmatic pleurisy.

Severe pancreatitis
1. Perforated peptic ulcer
2. Gangrenous cholecystitis
3. Intestinal strangulation
4. Mesenteric artery occlusion
5. Ruptured abdominal aneurysm
6. Myocardial infarction.

The most widely used test is serum amylase which may be elevated in acute pancreatitis. Values four times greater than normal favour the diagnosis. Acute inflammation can occasionally occur in the absence of raised amylase values, however, and there are a number of situations in which serum amylase values are increased apart from pancreatitis:

1. Perforated peptic ulcer
2. Ruptured ectopic pregnancy
3. Burns
4. Drugs (including morphine)
5. Intestinal obstruction
6. Mesenteric infarction
7. Renal failure
8. Diabetic ketoacidosis.

They usually follow a different clinical course to acute pancreatitis.

The amylase may be of salivary origin or from macroamylasaemia and the estimation of isoenzymes can be helpful. If there is hypertriglyceridaemia in association with pancreatitis, there is a tendency for the serum, but not the urinary, amylase concentrations to be normal.[22] The rise in amylase level has little prognostic value. Serum amylase levels usually return to normal within one week.

Amylase appears in excess in the urine before the serum, and some authorities believe that the estimation of urinary amylase is of more help than is the serum concentration; but hyperamylasuria has problems of interpretation similar to the serum concentration. Increased amylase levels may also be found in pleural effusions or ascites.

Suggestions that a raised amylase:creatinine clearance ratio is of precise diagnostic value have not been substantiated and this ratio is not regarded as being informative. Serum lipase values are increased in the acute episode and are more specific than amylase as an indication that pancreatitis is present, but not pathognomonic, because serum concentrations may be raised in perforated peptic ulcer, mesenteric vein thrombosis and following the administration of morphine.

Although the plain film of the abdomen may show a localized ileus of small bowel ('sentinel loop') or colon (colon cut-off sign), the information is of limited diagnostic value. Gallstones may be seen. Ultrasonography and computed tomography have had little immediate role in the diagnosis of acute pancreatitis but are of great help in identifying pancreatic pseudocysts and abscesses. CT has an important practical role in confirming the diagnosis and the severity of acute pancreatitis.

Peritoneal aspiration is very helpful where genuine diagnostic doubt is present.[14,53]

ASSESSMENT OF SEVERITY

Attempts before 1974 to grade the severity of acute pancreatitis objectively depended on single or multiple clinical signs, and findings at laparotomy.

CLINICAL ASSESSMENT

A major drawback of most of the many clinical features is that they take a number of hours or days to develop. Only *hypotension* (systolic blood pressure less than 90 mmHg) is a prognostic sign occurring sufficiently early in the course of the disease to be of value.[7,13] It is true that it is usually associated with fairly severe acute pancreatitis but it may simply reflect a delay in hospitalization in the milder case with associated hypovolaemia, rather than intrinsically severe pancreatitis. The use of hypotension as an objective factor in one prospective study from Bristol proved a little disappointing.[19]

Renal failure rarely occurs as a single system failure in hospitals where care is taken in monitoring both urine output and central venous pressure. This regulates the often considerable intravenous volumes required in the initial stages of disease to achieve a minimum 30 ml of urine per hour. At the present time, provided prophylactic steps are taken, renal failure only occurs as a pre-terminal event associated with other major system failures.[8,20,38,54]

The *duration of paralytic ileus* and the presence or absence of abdominal distension are signs that must be monitored for several days and they are therefore of limited value.

Small *pleural effusions,* especially on the left side, occur with great frequency when daily radiological examinations are performed. They do not correlate well with severity but the larger effusions are associated with those patients with the worst prognosis.

Body wall ecchymosis, either at the umbilicus (Cullen's sign) or in the flank, usually on the left side (Grey Turner's sign), occurs in 3% of patients and takes over 24 hours to develop.[23] The signs are undoubtedly associated with a most severe form of acute pancreatitis but cannot be applied universally as an objective grading system. It has been shown that 65% of patients developing these clinical signs survive the pancreatitis, provided active conservative supportive measures are taken.[23]

The development of a later *pancreatic abscess* or *pseudocyst,* although serious for the individual patient, is not necessarily related to an initially severe form of disease. They take a considerable time to develop and cannot be used as markers in a prospective study of any new therapy confined to patients with severe acute pancreatitis where an early separation of severe and mild cases is necessary.

ASSESSMENT AT OPERATION

The presence or absence of fat necrosis, and the volume and colour of free fluid at operation have not been clearly related to outcome. The presence of blood-stained fluid may well be associated with a poorer outcome but less than 10% of patients today undergo laparotomy.[14] Only a few surgeons carefully dissect the anterior surface of the whole pancreas and, of these, only a few remove any possible peripancreatic necrotic tissue to assess the gland directly. This may explain the findings in one French study of over 50 patients where the surgeon considered necrotic pancreatitis to be present and in exactly 50% the pathologist disagreed because the necrotic process was confined to the surrounding tissue rather than the pancreas itself.[47]

MULTIPLE FACTOR OBJECTIVE ASSESSMENT

The drawbacks associated with clinical approaches to grading of severity of pancreatitis prompted Ranson to examine retrospectively a large number of patients admitted to the New York University Hospital with a diagnosis of acute pancreatitis. Of 40 biochemical, haematological and clinical factors which were assessed only 11 were found to be significantly related to the outcome[69] (*Table 11.4*). These 11 factors were then employed prospectively to delineate patients with severe disease from those with a milder form of acute pancreatitis. A minimum of three prognostic factors had to be present for the patient to be considered in the severe category.[69,70] The greater the number of prognostic factors the more severe the disease and the more likely death the outcome. A statistical analysis of this approach validated its use,[67] and in the following year a report from the UK showed that a similar grading system had proved useful in the assessment of 161 patients admitted to one Glasgow hospital.[38] In this modified system only nine factors were employed, but again a minimum of three were taken to indicate severe disease.[40] Comparison of individual factors occurring in the total patients in New York and Glasgow graded as having severe acute pancreatitis indicated that nearly all were more abnormal in the patients with alcohol abuse as the aetiology of the pancreatitis compared with biliary disease.

The main problem of the multiple factor grading scheme was that too many patients with a gallstone aetiology met the criteria for severe disease without running a clinical course of comparable severity to those with the alcohol aetiology. This was because of the higher mean age of patients with biliary disease and the greater frequency of gross elevations in transaminase (transferase) levels. By omitting age as a criterion and increasing the 'cut-off' of the serum aspartate level to 200 units per litre, a more precise system of analysis was produced in which almost half the previously included biliary patients

Table 11.4 The eleven early objective signs used to classify the severity of pancreatitis[69]

At admission
Age > 55 years
White blood cell count > 16 000 per mm^3
Blood glucose > 200 mg/100 ml (11 mmol/l)
Serum lactate dehydrogenase > 350 iu/l
Serum aspartate aminotransferase > 250 Sigma-Frankel units/100 ml
During initial 48 hours
Haematocrit fall > 10 percentage points
Blood urea nitrogen rise > 5 mg/100 ml
Serum calcium level below 8 mg/100 ml (2 mmol/l)
PaO_2 below 60 mmHg
Base deficit > 4 mEq/l
Estimated fluid sequestration > 6000 ml

Table 11.5 Prognostic factors in patients with acute pancreatitis used by Imrie *et al.*[40] (with permission)

White blood cell count (WBC) > 15 × 10^9/l
Glucose > 10 mmol/l (no diabetic history)
Urea > 16 mmol/l (no response to intravenous fluids)
PaO_2 < 60 mmHg (8.0 kPa)
Calcium < 2.0 mmol/l
Albumin < 32 g/l
LDH > 600 units/l
Serum AST > 100 units/l
Age > 55 years

LDH = Lactate dehydrogenase.
AST = Aspartate aminotransferase.

were excluded from the severe category[62] (*Table 11.5*). Although Ranson did not have such a large number of gallstone patients to assess, he reached a similar conclusion[66,68] that is, that a tighter range of criteria is required in gallstone acute pancreatitis.

ANALYSIS OF PERITONEAL ASPIRATE OR LAVAGE FLUID (LEEDS SYSTEM)

An alternative to the assessment of multiple biochemical factors is the analysis of the free peritoneal fluid withdrawn by a catheter introduced below the umbilicus. The presence of a minimum of 20 ml of free fluid, especially if dark in colour, can be considered a good index of the severity of disease.[52] If no free fluid is obtained after the insertion of the peritoneal catheter, 1 litre of isotonic dialysis fluid or saline is run into the peritoneal cavity for 10–15 minutes. The patient is moved from side to side to allow an even distribution of the fluid and aspiration of this lavage fluid is performed. The presence of a dark-coloured fluid with a very high amylase content (with no bacteria present) is indicative of severe acute pancreatitis. The presence of organisms on an immediate Gram film makes the diagnosis of acute pancreatitis very unlikely.[14] Immediate laparotomy is recommended in this situation because bowel ischaemia or perforation is the most likely cause. This is an alternative to the multiple factor grading system and it has the additional advantage of speed and ready availability. The other systems depend on the prompt return of biochemical and haematological assessments which are not necessarily available 24 hours a day.

PRACTICAL ASPECTS OF THE USE OF GRADING SYSTEMS

The large British (Leeds, Glasgow and Bristol) Prospective Study of the place of peritoneal lavage in the management of objectively graded severe acute pancreatitis used both the Glasgow system of multiple prognostic factors and the Leeds system of peritoneal aspirate.[20,55] This determined that 91 (21%) of 428 documented attacks of acute pancreatitis entered the study with an overall mortality of 27.5% for severe acute pancreatitis and 2.9% for milder disease. No benefit in terms of mortality or morbidity was found for the patients with severe disease given additional peritoneal lavage; although the subgroup with an alcohol abuse aetiology was too small to exclude possible benefit from peritoneal lavage.[55,75] Analysis of the accuracy of the Glasgow system showed that 60–70% of those who developed early or late complications of acute pancreatitis with both gallstone and alcohol aetiology were correctly identified early in the disease, whilst the Leeds system had a 90% accuracy for the alcohol abuse group and less than 30% for gallstone patients.[20]

APACHE II

Several recent studies[44,83] have illustrated the advantage of applying the Acute Physiology and Chronic Health Evaluation system of Knaus *et al.*[42] to the grading of severity of pancreatitis. A particular merit is the continuous day-by-day evaluation pointing to the direction of the effect of therapy. This is illustrated in an unusual case where the experimental treatment of plasma exchange (plasmapheresis with fresh frozen plasma replacement) appeared beneficial, the lowering of APACHE score corresponding with clinical improvement and subsequent survival. The cumbersome nature of the 14-factor scheme, which involves different weighting of factors, is a disadvantage.[42]

C-REACTIVE PROTEIN

This well-known acute phase reactant was first suggested to be of possible value in patients with acute pancreatitis by McMahon's group[54] as a predictor of late abscess and pseudocyst formation. Some years later, workers in Germany, Finland and Britain all showed similar findings of good identification of patients with severe forms of the disease from 24–36 hours into the illness (*Figure 11.30*).[16,64,82] It works equally well for the different major aetiologies and, as a single blood test, represents a significant advance in practical assessment of the patients. Other important advantages are the low cost, availability and lack of complexity of laboratory testing. The similar findings of all groups reporting on its use is reassuring, and the only drawback is the delay to significant elevation of C-

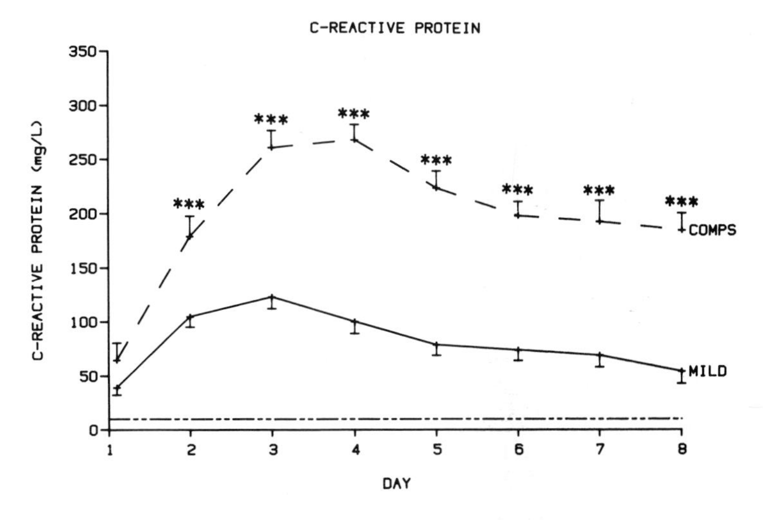

Figure 11.30 Sequential C-reactive protein concentrations in 47 patients with mild pancreatitis (——) and 25 with complicated attacks (– – –). Results are expressed as mean (SE). *$P < 0.05$. **$P < 0.01$. ***$P < 0.001$ (mild versus complicated); (–··–··–) upper limit of normal for C-reactive protein. (From *British Journal of Surgery,*[82] with permission.)

reactive protein. Levels above 150 mg/l indicate the severe form of acute pancreatitis (see *Figure 11.31*).

POLYMORPHONUCLEAR LEUKOCYTE ELASTASE

The elastase released from leukocyte disruption in the course of acute pancreatitis appears on the basis of two pilot studies[24,78] to be potentially an improvement on C-reactive protein measurements. Commercial kits are now available to measure elastase, and the initial studies are encouraging because the speed of response to reach blood levels greater than 120 μg/l in clinically severe acute pancreatitis is more rapid and sensitive than C-reactive protein[24,78] (*Figure 11.31*). The individual tests are not expensive and, should reliability be proved, then future use should be considerable.

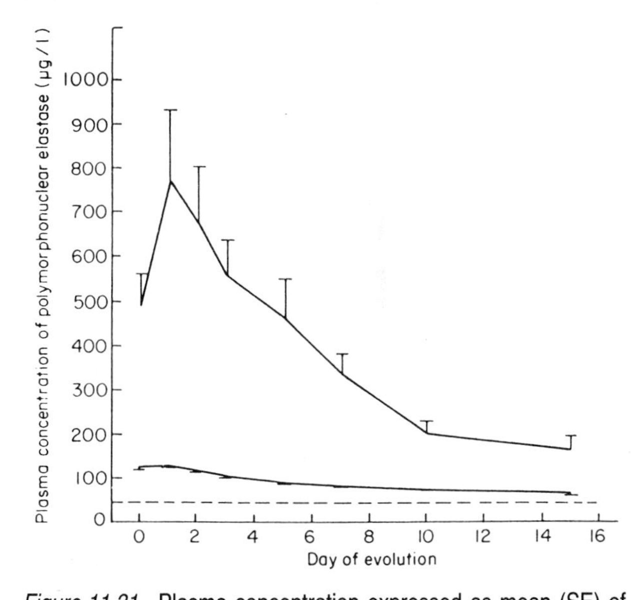

Figure 11.31 Plasma concentration expressed as mean (SE) of polymorphonuclear elastase in patients with severe (upper line) and mild (lower line) acute pancreatitis. (– – –) Upper limit of normal. Days 0–10, $P < 0.001$; day 15, $P < 0.05$. (*British Journal of Surgery,*[24] with permission.)

TRYPSINOGEN ACTIVATION PEPTIDE

When trypsinogen is activated,[5] trypsin is released and a small activation peptide can now be measured accurately in the setting of a research study. Urine levels of the peptide rise rapidly after onset of acute pancreatitis in severe disease and a valuable discrimination with milder disease has been shown.[30] The rate of elevation of trypsinogen activation peptide is similar to elastase, and faster than C-reactive protein. It is hoped that a rapid, reasonably priced method of carrying out this test will be available for regular clinical use. It would be more specific than others, and perhaps the scale of trypsinogen activation might give an accurate indicator of the probability of necrosis.[30] In the context of the initial assessment of patients with upper abdominal pain or vomiting, or both, in the emergency department, this test would be both diagnostic of pancreatitis and enable grading of severity.

OTHER TESTS

The rise in blood interleukin-6 (and pancreatic elastase) levels, as well as the fall in fibronectin have been shown to separate severe from milder acute pancreatitis rather well but, for various reasons (including cost), these markers are unlikely to become established in clinical use.

CT AND SEVERITY ASSESSMENT

Following the introduction of CT in the assessment of acute pancreatitis it is clear that most patients who have an appropriate clinical presentation will show detectable changes on the CT scan. Pancreatic swell-

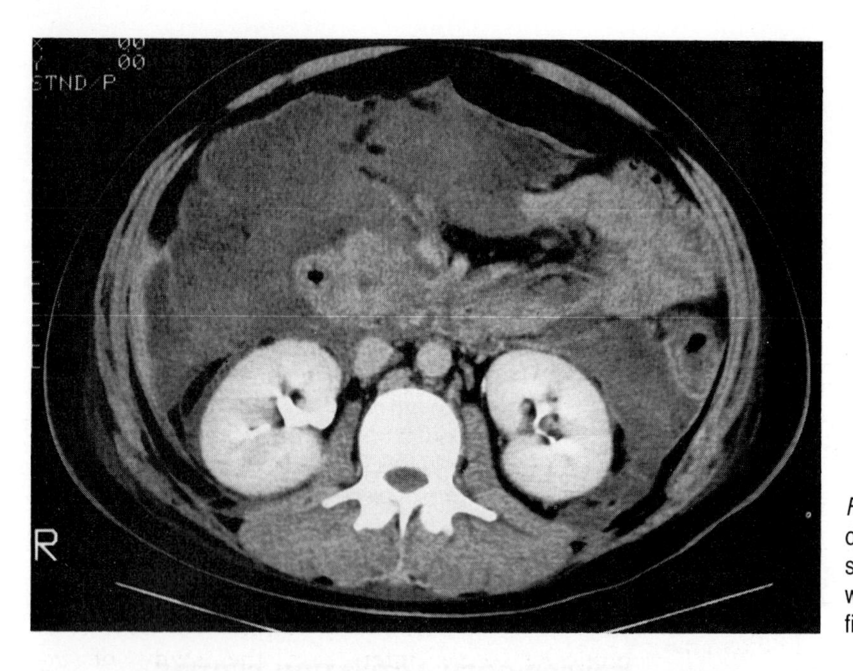

Figure 11.32 Angiogram-enhanced CT scan of severe acute pancreatitis with extensive spread of peripancreatic necrosis and blood, whilst the pancreas remains viable. These findings were confirmed at surgery.

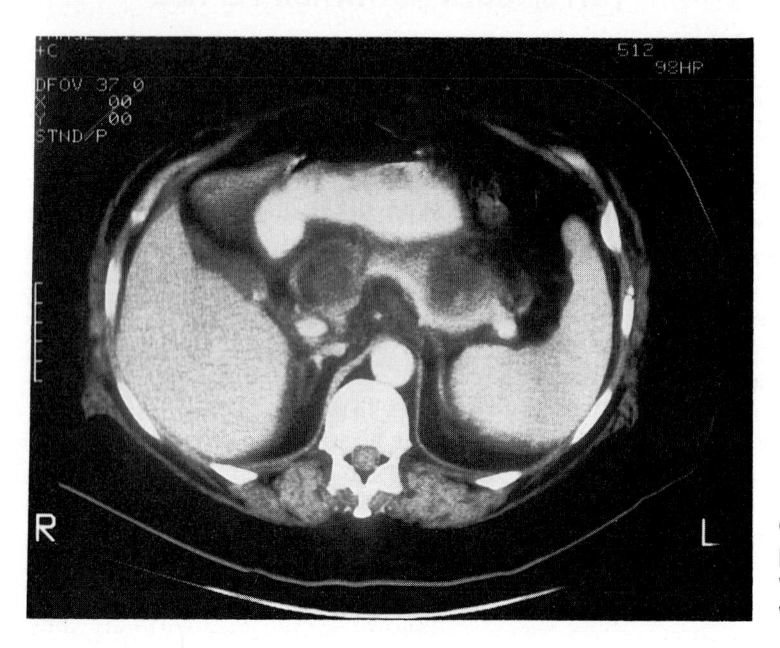

Figure 11.33 Angiogram-enhanced CT scan indicating very poor perfusion of an area of the head of pancreas and another area in the distal body and tail whilst the central part remains viable. These findings were confirmed at surgery.

ing, reduced tissue attenuation, increased peripancreatic and perirenal fluid collections are typical. The greatly increased information yield from angiogram enhancement of the pancreas makes this modification essential in the assessment of such patients.[48] This is especially valuable in the patient with severe acute pancreatitis to demonstrate areas of poor vascular perfusion of the gland (*Figures 11.32* and *11.33*).

The possibility of using CT to grade severity has been evaluated, and the studies of the New York[6] and Leicester[48] groups particularly, have been objective. Unfortunately, the sensitivity and specificity have not compared better than the modified Glasgow criteria used in Leicester in studies of this disease. There is also the drawback of moving a seriously ill patient to the CT scanner and, in practice, these grading systems are not a marked advantage. The patient with a late presentation of acute pancreatitis, on the other hand, may be best diagnosed by CT.

The main advangate of CT scanning is the place of the angiogram-enhanced CT, both in guiding the surgeon to the areas of poorest perfusion and the radiologist to the target area for percutaneous aspiration.

TREATMENT

The two main aims in the initial treatment of acute pancreatitis are:

1. To restore fluid and electrolyte balance.
2. To provide adequate analgesia.

In patients who are moderately or severely ill, central venous pressure monitoring is essential and initial rehydration should be with isotonic saline. The daily administration of an albumin-containing fluid, such as plasma, is necessary and occasionally blood may be required.

It must be appreciated that the hypovolaemia associated with severe acute pancreatitis may approximate that experienced in a severe burn and the total volume replacement may exceed 6 litres in the first 24 hours.[7,13] This replacement of fluid in the intravascular space must be monitored by a combinations of central venous pressure and urinary output. Even in mild pancreatitis intravenous fluids will be required for about 72 hours and for many days in the severely ill. Intravenous nutrition will be essential in a proportion of patients and there is little evidence that the administration of lipids by this route causes a major problem.

Most patients require nasogastric suction for the first 24 to 48 hours and, where paralytic ileus is present, this suction may be necessary for as long as a week. Whereas oral intake can be restarted around the third or fourth day in mild and moderately severe acute pancreatitis, periods greatly in excess of a week are occasionally encountered in the severe disease. Anticholinergic drugs are best avoided because they have no proven value.

Pain control is probably best achieved with pethidine which is usually given in a dose of 50–150 mg 4–6 hourly either intramuscularly or intravenously, depending on the condition of the patient. Good results are also obtained using buprenorphine hydrochloride (Temgesic) 300–600 μg 4–8 hourly by intramuscular or slow intravenous injection. It is unusual for pain relief to be required beyond 72 hours. In patients who have severe pain for a longer period, the addition of a benzodiazepine may be very helpful.

Antibiotics are not recommended for routine use and it is our practice to confine these drugs to clinical situations where infection has been proven. Only in the patient with coincidental early cholangitis would we regularly advocate antibiotic therapy using a third generation cephalosporin, together with metronidazole, or pipericillin, or imipenem.

Many drugs have been considered of specific value in the management of acute pancreatitis but none have proved convincing in the situation of a clinical double-blind controlled trial. Thus glucagon, aprotinin (Trasylol), cimetidine and calcitonin have all been shown to be ineffective. More recently the question of additional intravenous antiprotease support has been re-examined in two ways. Firstly, the provision of purified plasma derivative was examined by the group headed by Leese *et al.* who studied the effects of both low-dose and high-dose plasma derivative in well-controlled clinical trials which showed no benefit from the treatment.[45,46] Likewise, large multicentre controlled studies in Germany using Gabexate mesilate (FOY) have shown no benefit from two different dosages. From this, and previous studies on Trasylol it is now clear that the intravenous antiprotease defence does not require support from any of these substances. A point of some interest is the study of α_2-macroglobulin levels in patients with severe acute pancreatitis by McMahon *et al.*,[50] in which the three patients who died had α_2-macroglobulin levels in the normal range, despite the levels being very low around the fourth or fifth day of illness.

PERITONEAL LAVAGE

This was at one time considered to be an important potential therapy in all patients with severe acute pancreatitis[5,69,75] but the British multicentre study[55] and one from Sweden[31] – which are the only controlled studies performed – did not show any benefit. It remains possible that there may be some efficacy in alcohol-induced severe acute pancreatitis, as the size of this component in these two studies was limited and the statistical evidence of ineffectiveness was not fully established. With regard to the group of patients with gallstones, however, and for those with an unknown aetiology, it certainly confers no benefit.

GALLSTONE ACUTE PANCREATITIS

There is evidence from the pioneering work of Carr Locke and Neoptolemos *et al.*[59] that patients with severe gallstone-induced acute pancreatitis will benefit from an early pancreatography with sphincterotomy if stones are present in the duct. This procedure must be undertaken within the first 72 hours of illness. Their study indicated a distinct trend in favour of this approach in those patients with objectively graded severe disease but, for those with mild disease, there was no benefit from immediate pancreatography.[59] This was a bold piece of work which explored the therapeutic potential of pancreatography at a time when it was still believed that a diagnostic procedure was hazardous in patients with acute pancreatitis. Endoscopic clearance of the duct is undoubtedly preferable to surgical clearance in severe disease.

In all patients who are shown to have gallstones (usually by ultrasound scanning) during their pancreatitis, it is advised that stone clearance be performed before the patient is discharged from hospital. This can be performed during the first week of mild or moderate illness, whereas in those with severe disease, individual timing will depend on recovery from hypoxaemia and a number of other factors.

COMPLICATIONS OF SEVERE ACUTE PANCREATITIS

One of the major purposes in the early grading of a patient in the category of severe pancreatitis is to alert the clinician to the danger and likelihood of certain system failures and to the complications that may develop. A minimum of 50% of patients with severe acute pancreatitis will be candidates for the most intensive conservative, non-surgical therapy, as first-line management.

CARDIAC INSUFFICIENCY OR FAILURE

ECG changes occur in patients with acute pancreatitis but their significance is unknown.[63] This problem is further complicated by the fact that, occasionally, patients present with a clinical condition simulating myocardial infarction; especially when left upper quadrant abdominal pain is the predominant feature. The suggestion that cardiac muscle may be particularly vulnerable in acute pancreatitis is supported by the finding that 6 out of 14 patients who died in one prospective study showed unequivocal evidence of myocardial infarction.[38]

The mechanism of the changes is incompletely understood.[7,13] It may be necessary to digitalize all older patients with acute pancreatitis and many patients do benefit from dopamine, chlobutamine and sometimes noradrenalin. Until there is a more rational understanding of the pathogenesis of this problem, therapy will remain empirical.

RENAL INSUFFICIENCY OR FAILURE

This was formerly a major problem because of the failure to recognize the degree of hypovolaemia but it is now an uncommon complication in those centres where active supportive measures are routine. A minimum urine output of 30 ml per hour can usually be ensured by an appropriate rate of intravenous infusion; many of the severely ill patients require a minimum of 4 litres and sometimes as many as 8 or 9 litres of fluid in the first 24 hours of therapy. It is particularly important to appreciate the need for early reversal of hypovolaemia within the first few hours of hospitalization and for the employment of plasma or albumin-rich fluids as well as electrolyte solutions. In all the severely ill patients, a central venous pressure line is mandatory. Failure to achieve a minimum urine output of 30 ml per hour is an indication for a 20 g bolus of mannitol, once hypovolaemia has been reversed. If this is unsuccessful a repeat of the 20 g bolus is advised. Alternatively, low-dose intravenous dopamine may be very helpful. This drug is preferred to mannitol.

RESPIRATORY INSUFFICIENCY OR FAILURE

This common complication is the most feared.[36,38,57,69] The clinical presentation is insidious with only tachypnoea as an indication of the degree of respiratory insufficiency.[21] Cyanosis is unusual and respiratory distress difficult to detect on clinical grounds alone. It is mandatory that arterial blood gas measurements be performed regularly, especially during the initial period. The levels of arterial gases should be measured at least twice daily and, when the PaO_2 is less than 60 mmHg (8 kPa), supplementary humidified oxygen should be provided. A check of the PaO_2 levels after the provision of oxygen is required to assess whether sufficient reversal of the hypoxaemia has occurred. Restoration of PaO_2 levels to above 70 mmHg is usual, provided a flow rate in the region of 10 litres per minute of 70% oxygen can be achieved.[36] If hypoxaemia cannot be reversed, and particularly when the PaO_2 is less than 52.5 mmHg (7 kPa), assisted ventilation therapy is indicated. Non-invasive measurements of oxygen saturation by the use of pulse oximetry is a most helpful monitoring method. The exact mechanism of the hypoxaemia is ill-understood but there is right-to-left shunting of around 25–30% of cardiac output[57] although this is not the sole factor. The possible causes of the shunting include atelectasis and pulmonary capillary blockage either due to platelet thrombi or leukocyte clumping or combinations of these factors. In addition, hyaline membrane disease has been documented in fatal acute pancreatitis with respiratory failure.[43]

Another factor causing the adult respiratory distress syndrome associated with acute pancreatitis is the varying pressure in the pulmonary artery which has been recorded in severe acute pancreatitis. Airways closure is not an important feature.[43] The presence of pleural effusions, atelectasis and pulmonary oedema may be observed but some patients who are severely hypoxic have remarkably few radiological abnormalities.[35] This respiratory complication is a variant of the adult respiratory distress syndrome with pleural effusions being a particular feature; these require aspiration should they persist. The effusion fluid characteristically has not only a high amylase content but also a high albumin and calcium concentration.[34] In a study involving young patients with no previous history of respiratory disease who suffered from acute pancreatitis, it was shown that a period of 6–12 weeks was required for the hypoxaemia to resolve.[57] This correlates with the length of time a patient may require to remain on assisted ventilator therapy, as patients kept on this type of life support system for periods of around 6–8 weeks may recover sufficiently at this stage to be weaned off the ventilator therapy. Such patients may also develop *peripancreatic sepsis* and require some form of intra-abdominal drainage procedure before withdrawal of the respiratory support. An outline of the steps involved in the management of the respiratory insufficiency of these patients is indicated in *Figure 11.34*.

HAEMATOLOGICAL ABNORMALITIES

The most frequent haematological abnormality is an *apparent drop in haemoglobin* associated with restoration of circulating blood volume. Most patients are admitted initially with a considerable degree of dehydration and have elevated levels of haemoglobin and haematocrit. After restoration of circulating fluid, the haemoglobin may fall markedly and this can be accentuated by any bleeding in or around the pancreas. Only occasionally is blood transfusion required and the need for this requires careful monitoring. Elevated fibrinogen levels have been documented early in the disease[9] and rise progressively to around 300% of normal levels at 5–6 days after admission. Factor V and factor VIII also rise and probably behave as acute phase reactants rather than from any specific coagulopathy. Levels of fibrin degradation products often show a small rise. About one-third of patients with acute pancreatitis have a significant shortening of their clotting time as measured by the kaolin–cephalin clotting time. Although disseminated intravascular coagulation has been described in acute pancreatitis, it is unusual and a consecutive study of 161 patients revealed no evidence of this phenomenon.[38] Deep vein thrombosis and major pulmonary emboli are not common complicating factors.

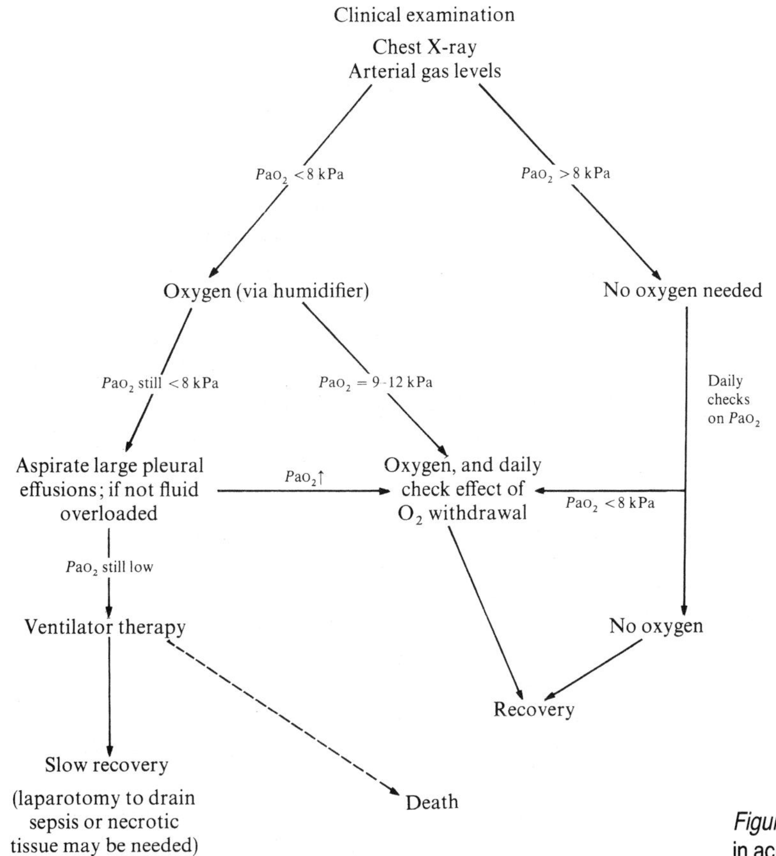

Figure 11.34 Management of respiratory insufficiency in acute pancreatitis.

An activation of the complement system occurs in acute pancreatitis; but it is unclear whether this is simply another manifestation of the response to trauma or whether a more specific explanation must be found.

BIOCHEMICAL ABNORMALITIES

For many years much attention has been focused on the problem of hypocalcaemia, which is mainly due to the loss of circulating albumin from the intravascular space[34] into the retroperitoneum, peritoneal cavity and pleural cavity. This *albumin loss* is an important biochemical phenomenon and requires correction. The restoration of normal serum albumin levels is often impossible in the severely ill patient, however, because of the 'porosity' of the endothelial layer lining capillaries.[3]

There is also a tendency for the ionized fragment of circulating serum calcium to fall[21] and this is associated with elevated parathyroid hormone levels which indicate a satisfactorily functioning calcium homeostatic mechanism.[39] The restoration of circulating ionized calcium by means of infusions of calcium gluconate is rarely necessary but, if it is required, it is essential that sufficient calcium gluconate be given and 50–60 ml of isotonic calcium gluconate is administered slowly, intravenously.[3]

Occasionally, in the most severely ill patients, profound falls in extracellular sodium and elevations of potassium may occur, indicative of the so-called 'sick cell syndrome'. We have documented one such patient who responded well to hourly pulses of 50% dextrose and insulin via a central line.[3] Using this approach, not only did the ionized calcium level rise, but also the sodium and potassium levels returned to normal.

MACROSCOPIC NECROSIS WITH OR WITHOUT SEPSIS

All patients with acute pancreatitis suffer some degree of microscopic necrosis but macroscopic necrosis is the hallmark of the most severe forms of the disease. It is more common to find the necrosis affecting the peripancreatic tissue rather than the pancreatic tissue itself. This is not the bright yellow flecks of fat necrosis that typically appear in the omentum, mesentery and adjacent tissue to the pancreas, but rather a dark grey or black coloured necrosis to which the fatty tissue surrounding the pancreas is particularly vulnerable. The complication may be associated with severe pancreatic necrosis, and poor or zero perfusion of the pancreas can be detected by high quality angiogram-enhanced CT (see *Figures 11.32* and *11.33*). It becomes increasingly clear that clinicians with access to such CT facilities have a major advantage in the managment of these severely ill patients, such that the present prerequisite for satisfactory overall management of these patients includes ready access to such machines, a good quality intensive care unit and expert clinicians. Either ultrasound or CT is essential to guide percutaneous aspiration used to identify the exact location of potential infected foci in and around the pancreas.[17,29]

Once pus is identified, one of the two main criteria for surgical intervention in such patients has been satisfied. Only occasionally can this type of sepsis be successfuly managed by percutaneous aspiration.

The *second major indication* for surgical intervention in such patients is a combination of poor perfusion of the pancreas on angiogram-enhanced CT and a failure for this to improve after 72 hours of intensive care therapy.[8] The results of surgical intervention in such patients for the purpose of digital necrosectomy and the removal of pus is associated with mortality rates (within the severe group of patients) of under 15%. Around 25% of patients will require more than one operative procedure.[8,83] Total hospital stay for such patients is usually in the median of 60–70 days. After digital necrosectomy there is a choice of either continuous focal lavage of between 12 and 24 litres of isotonic warm saline per day and the median duration of lavage is in the region of three-and-a-half weeks.[8] The alternative procedure following digital necrosectomy is to perform intra-abdominal packing with no closure of the main wound. This is also very demanding of both nursing and medical time, but equally good results have been obtained.

This necrosis, with or without sepsis, can be detected as early as 48–72 hours in certain of the most ill patients, although it is typically considered only to develop from 7 days onwards.

LATER COMPLICATIONS OF ACUTE PANCREATITIS

These are listed on page 1601. Pancreatic pseudocyst and abscess are the most common problems.

PANCREATIC PSEUDOCYST

This invariably follows moderate or severe attacks of acute pancreatitis, usually developing within 2–4 weeks. The pseudocyst probably arises from blockage of the foramen of Winslow by fibrinous material with consequent collection of pancreatic juice in the lesser sac. Pancreatography indicates that most major pancreatic pseudocysts are directly linked to the main duct system. Approximately 50% resolve spontaneously and the remainder require some form of drainage procedure. Traditionally this has been a surgical approach, usually by draining the pseudocyst directly into the posterior aspect of the stomach, that is, cystogastrostomy. In this operation it is usual to suture the posterior wall of the stomach to the anterior wall of the pseudocyst, with the size of the incision in the posterior wall of the stomach being 8–10 cm. If the pseudocyst does not lie in direct relationship to the posterior wall of the stomach, drainage by alternative means is necessary; this can be by an anastomosis to a loop of jejunum, or a Roux loop, or less frequently to the duodenum. It is possible to simply aspirate small cysts of the head of the pancreas which can be responsible for considerable symptoms of pain and vomiting,[74] and percutaneous aspiration of pseudocysts guided either by ultrasound or CT is used. This method is particularly attractive in older patients with cardiorespiratory or other complications. A major drawback, however, is the re-accumulation of fluid in the pseudocyst which occurs particularly in larger cysts communicating directly with the main pancreatic duct. Repeated aspirations may be carried out but they increase the risk of introducing sepsis and converting a sterile collection into a pancreatic abscess. A further problem is that many large pseudocysts following attacks of severe acute pancreatitis contain peripancreatic necrotic debris and slough which cannot be aspirated through a percutaneous needle. For these reasons, it is likely that surgical treatment will remain the most important definitive approach to established pseudocysts.

Conservative management beyond 6 weeks for a pseudocyst has been considered at best unpredictable and potentially dangerous[12] but the use of synthetic somatostatin (Octreotide) therapy and percutaneous ultrasound guided drainage catheters are new treatments that may minimize the necessity for surgical external drainage procedures. Such procedures were associated with the need for intervention, sometimes at an early stage in the development of a pseudocyst, when this structure caused severe pain, troublesome vomiting or obstructive jaundice. Percutaneous drainage catheters run the risk of infection occurring in the normally sterile pancreatic juice that fills the pseudocyst associated with acute pancreatitis.

Most deaths associated with pancreatic pseudocyst occur after an episode of acute pancreatitis because the pseudocyst associated with chronic pancreatitis rarely develops major complications. The main complications are sepsis and haemorrhage, both of which are more common in gallstone pancreatitis.[33] Indeed, it is important that the biliary tree is cleared of all stones during the surgical treatment which is required in a patient with pseudocyst following gallstone pancreatitis.[33]

The complication of haemorrhage within a pseudocyst is frequently caused by the incorporation of either the splenic artery or vein into the posterior wall of the lesion but may also be due to leakage from aneurysmal new vessel formation in the wall of the pseudocyst. The exact lesion can be identified by either angiogram-enhanced CT or classic selective catheterization of the feeding vessels. Selective thrombosis of the area of haemorrhage by utilizing a catheter close to the bleeding source is the ideal management, but occasionally surgeons may encounter this difficult problem at operation. Aortic cross-clamping may occasionally be necessary to help control the bleeding in such situations before ligation of the individual offending vessels. *Upper gastrointestinal bleeding* may be a presentation of haemorrhage from a pancreatic pseudocyst and must be differentiated from other sources of upper gastrointestinal bleeding which can occur in patients under stress, such as peptic ulcer or gastric erosions.

PANCREATIC ABSCESS

Considerable confusion occurs with the use of this generic term and it is proposed that a differentiation is made between the well-circumscribed lesion – type 1 abscess, and the diffuse retroperitoneal sepsis – type 2 abscess. This latter type is more difficult to treat and is associated with a higher morbidity and mortality. The use of needle aspiration guided by ultrasound or CT has already been noted.[29]

It was thought that such septic episodes only occurred as a late complication, at least 10 days into the illness, but it is now known that they can occur at a much earlier stage in the disease process.

Sepsis is the most feared complication of severe acute pancreatitis and accounts for much of the morbidity and mortality in patients successfully managed through the initial phase of illness. Prolonged periods of parenteral nutrition are required in many of these patients but a more physiological alternative (with less risk of septicaemia) is to provide a feeding jejunostomy in those patients who come to surgery.

SPLENIC VEIN THROMBOSIS

This usually occurs in severe acute pancreatitis and is associated with splenomegaly and localized portal hypertension. Splenectomy may be indicated at the time of surgical intervention for other complications in the same patient.

PANCREATIC ASCITES (see page 1839)

This is a very unusual complication which can result from spontaneous rupture of a pancreatic pseudocyst into the peritoneal cavity. A breach in the main pancreatic duct is invariably present and can be demonstrated by pancreatography. It is wise to include gentamicin or a cephalosporin antibiotic within the injection fluid at pancreatography in this situation. Synthetic somatostatin (Octreotide) analogue can be helpful in this clinical context.

SUBCUTANEOUS FAT NECROSIS

This author has only witnessed this complication in 2 out of 2000 patients, and on each occasion it was associated with spontaneous rupture of a pancreatic pseudocyst. Painful red nodules develop in the upper and lower limbs and initially can be mistaken for erythema nodosum. Fat necrosis has also been described rarely in the long bones and brain.

DIABETES MELLITUS

The incidence of diabetes mellitus observed in the recovery phase of acute pancreatitis is between 2% and 4%. This is remarkably low and indicates the relative sparing of the endocrine tissue. In the most severe necrotizing forms of acute pancreatitis, however, the islet tissue is also destroyed. The urine is monitored for sugar and ketones and patients will require soluble insulin initially and, subsequently, appropriate long-acting insulin.

RECURRENT ACUTE PANCREATITIS

The diagnosis for recurrent acute pancreatitis is applied to those patients who experience more than one attack of inflammation but who show no morphological or functional evidence of pancreatic disease between episodes of pain. The most frequent cause is the failure to eliminate fine biliary sand or very small stones. Secret alcohol abuse must be excluded and ampullary cancer, hereditary pancreatitis or localized pancreatitis associated with a stricture in the duct system should also be considered. Occasionally malfunction of the sphincter of Oddi with abnormally high pressures being documented at manometry can account for such clinical events which can be cured by endoscopic sphincterotomy. The generic heading for this group of patients is sphincter of Oddi dysfunction.

Non-union of the pancreatic ducts of Wirsung and Santorini, somewhat confusingly known as pancreas divisum (see page 1558) occurs in 1–7% of all patients. Within such anatomical variations, a small number have pancreatitis solely affecting the dorsal duct of Santorini and endoscopic or surgical sphincterotomy can help these patients.

As in all types of acute pancreatitis initial management is conservative. It is important to remember that patients in the recovery phase from pancreatitis are vulnerable to a further attack if re-exposed to the same trigger that precipitated the first attack, and that a heavy meal or alcohol can readily initiate a further episode. When alcohol has induced pancreatitis, total abstinence is the only sensible measure.

REFERENCES

1. Acosta, J.M. and Ledesma, C.L. (1974) Gallstone migration as a cause for acute pancreatitis. *New England Journal of Medicine*, **290**, 484–487.
2. Acosta, J.M., Rossi, R., Galli, O.M.R. *et al.* (1978) Early surgery for acute gallstone pancreatitis: Evaluation of a systemic approach. *Surgery*, **83**, 367–370.
3. Allam, B.F. and Imrie, C.W. (1977) Serum ionized calcium in acute pancreatitis. *British Journal of Surgery*, **64**, 665–668.
4. Ammann, R.W., Deyhle, P. and Butikofer, E. (1973) Fatal necrotizing pancreatitis after peroral cholangiopancreatography. *Gastroenterology*, **64**, 320–323.
5. Balldin, G. and Ohlsson, K. (1979) Demonstration of pancreatic protease-anti-protease complexes in the peritoneal fluid of patients with acute pancreatitis. *Surgery*, **85**, 451–456.
6. Balthazar, E.J., Ranson, J.H., Naidich, D.P. *et al.* (1985). Acute pancreatitis Prognostic value of CT. *Radiology*, **136**, 767–772.
7. Beger, H.G., Bittner, R., Buchler, M. *et al.* (1986) Hemodynamic data patterns in patients with acute pancreatitis. *Gastroenterology*, **90**, 74–79.
8. Beger, H.G., Buchler, M., Bittner, R. *et al.* (1988) Necrosectomy and postoperative local lavage in necrotizing pancreatitis. *British Journal of Surgery*, **75**, 207–212.
9. Berry, A.R., Taylor, T.V. and Davies, G.V. (1982) Diagnostic tests and prognostic indicators in acute pancreatitis. *Journal of the Royal College of Surgeons Edinburgh*, **27**, 345–352.
10. Bess, M.A., Edis, A.J. and Van Heerden, J.A. (1980) Hyperparathyroidism and pancreatitis. *Journal of the American Medical Association*, **234**, 246–247.
11. Bourke, J.B., Mead, G.M., McIllmurray, M.B. and Longman, M.J.S. (1978) Drug associated primary acute pancreatitis. *Lancet*, **i**, 706–708.
12. Bradley, E.L., Clements, J.L. and Gonzales, A.C. (1979) The natural history of pancreatic pseudocysts. A verified concept of management. *American Journal of Surgery*, **137**, 135–141.
13. Bradley, E.L., Hall, J.R., Lutz, J. *et al.* (1983)

Hemodynamic consequences of severe pancreatitis. *Annals of Surgery*, **198**, 130–133.
14. Bradley, J.S., Bradley, P., Cameron, J.L. and McMahon, M.J. (1981) Diagnostic peritoneal lavage in acute pancreatitis, the value of microscopy of the fluid. *British Journal of Surgery*, **68**, 245–246.
15. Buch, A., Buch, J., Carlsen, A. and Schmidt, A. (1980) Hyperlipidemia and pancreatitis. *World Journal of Surgery*, **4**: 307–314.
16. Buchler, M., Malfertheiner, P., Beger, H.G. (1986) Correlation of imaging procedures, biochemical parameters and clinical stage in acute pancreatitis. In: Diagnostic Procedures in Pancreatic Disease. (Eds) Malfertheiner, P. and Ditschuneit, H. pp. 123–129. Berlin: Springer-Verlag.
17. Cameron, J.L., Zuidema, G.D. and Margolis, S. (1975) A pathogenesis for alcoholic pancreatitis. *Surgery*, **77**, 754–763.
18. Cameron, J.L., Capuzzi, D.M., Zinderman, G.D. and Margolis, S. (1975) Acute pancreatitis with hyperlipaemia. *Annals of Surgery*, **177**, 483–499.
19. Cooper, M.J., Williamson, R.C.N. and Pollock, A.V. (1982) The role of peritoneal lavage in the prediction and treatment of severe acute pancreatitis. *Annals of the Royal College of Surgery*, **64**, 422–427.
20. Corfield, A.R., Cooper, M.J., Williamson, R.C.N. *et al.* (1985) Prediction of severity in acute pancreatitis: a prospective comparison of three prognostic indices. *Lancet*, **ii**, 403–406.
21. Croton, R.S., Warren, R.A., Scott, A. and Roberts, N.B. (1981) Ionized calcium in acute pancreatitis. *British Journal of Surgery*, **68**, 241–243.
22. Dickson, A.P. and Imrie, C.W. (1984) Hyperlipidaemia, alcohol abuse and acute pancreatitis, a prospective study. *British Journal of Surgery*, **71**, 685–688.
23. Dickson, A.P. and Imrie, C.W. (1984) Body wall ecchymosis in patients with acute pancreatitis. *Surgery, Gynecology and Obstetrics*, **159**, 343–347.
24. Dominquez-Munoz, J.E., Carballo, F., Garcia, M.J. *et al.* (1991) Clinical usefulness of polymorphonuclear elastase in predicting the severity of acute pancreatitis: results of a multicentre study. *British Journal of Surgery*, **78**, 1230–1234.
25. Feiner, H. (1976) Pancreatitis after cardiac surgery. *American Journal of Surgery*, **131**, 684–688.
26. Fitz, R.H. (1889) Acute pancreatitis. *Boston Medical and Surgical Journal*, **120**, 181, 205, 229.
27. Foulis, A.K. (1982) Morphological study of the relation between accidental hypothermia and acute pancreatitis. *Journal of Clinical Pathology*, **35**, 1244–1248.
28. Gambill, E.E. (1971) Pancreatitis associated with pancreatic carcinoma. *Mayo Clinic Proceedings*, **46**, 174–177.
29. Gerzof, S.G., Banks, P.A., Robbins, A.H. *et al.* (1987) Early diagnosis of pancreatic infection by computed tomography-guided aspiration. *Gastroenterology*, **93**, 1315–1320.
30. Gudgeon, M., Heath, D.I., Hurley, P. *et al.* (1990) Trypsinogen activation peptides assay in the early severity prediction of acute pancreatitis. *Lancet*, **335**, 4–8.
31. Ihse, I., Evander, M.D., Holmberg, M.D. and Gustafson, I. (1986) Influence of peritoneal lavage on objective prognostic signs in acute pancreatitis. *Annals of Surgery*, **202**, 122–127.
32. Imrie, C.W. (1974) Observations on acute pancreatitis. *British Journal of Surgery*, **61**, 539–544.
33. Imrie, C.W., Buist, L.J. and Shearer, M.G. (1988) The importance of etiology in the outcome of pancreatic pseudocyst. *American Journal of Surgery*, **156**, 159–162.
34. Imrie, C.W., Allam, B.F. and Ferguson, J.C. (1976) Hypocalcaemia of acute pancreatitis: the effect of hypo-albuminaemia. *Current Medical Research Opinion*, **4**, 101–116.
35. Imrie, C.W., Ferguson, J.C. and Sommerville, R.G. (1977). Coxsackie and mumps virus infection in a prospective study of acute pancreatitis. *Gut*, **18**, 53–56.
36. Imrie, C.W., Ferguson, J.C., Murphy, D. and Blumgart, L.H. (1977) Arterial hypoxia in acute pancreatitis. *British Journal of Surgery*, **64**, 185–188.
37. Imrie, C.W., Goldring, J., Pollock, J.G. and Watt, J.K. (1977) Acute pancreatitis after translumbar aortography. *British Medical Journal*, **ii**, 681.
38. Imrie, C.W., Benjamin, I.S., Ferguson, J.C. *et al.* (1978). A single centre double blind trial of trasylol therapy in primary acute pancreatitis. *British Journal of Surgery*, **65**, 337–341.
39. Imrie, C.W., Beastall, G.H., Allam, B.F. *et al.* (1978) Parathyroid hormone and calcium homeostasis in acute pancreatitis. *British Journal of Surgery*, **65**, 717–720.
40. Imrie, C.W., McKay, A.J., Benjamin, I.S. and Blumgart, L.H. (1978) Secondary acute pancreatitis: aetiology, prevention, diagnosis and management. *British Journal of Surgery*, **65**, 399–402.
41. Kelly, T.R. (1976) Gallstone pancreatitis: pathophysiology. *Surgery*, **80**, 488–492.
42. Knaus, W.A., Zimmerman, J.E., Wagner, D.P. *et al.* (1981) APACHE-acute physiology and chronic health evaluation: a physiologically based classification system. *Critical Care Med*, **9**, 591–597.
43. Lankisch, P.G., Rahlf, G. and Koop, H. (1983) Pulmonary complications in fatal acute haemorrhagic pancreatitis. *Digestive Diseases and Sciences*, **28**, 111–116.
44. Larvin, M. and McMahon, M.J. (1989) APACHE II score for assessment and monitoring of acute pancreatitis. *Lancet*, **ii**, 201–205.
45. Leese, T., Holliday, M., Heath, D. *et al.* (1987) Multicentre trial of low volume fresh frozen plasma

therapy in acute pancreatitis. *British Journal of Surgery*, **74**, 907–911.
46. Leese, T., Holliday, M., Watkins, M. *et al.* (1991) A multicentre controlled clinical trial of high volume fresh frozen plasma in prognostically severe acute pancreatitis. *Annals of the Royal College of Surgeons*, **73**, 207–214.
47. Leger, L., Lenriot, J.P. and Lemaigre, G. (1974) Five to twenty year follow-up after surgery for chronic pancreatitis in 148 patients. *Annals of Surgery*, **180**, 185–191.
48. London, N.J.M., Neoptolomos, J.P., Lavelle, J. *et al.* (1989) Contrast enhanced abdominal computerised tomography scanning and prediction of severity of acute pancreatitis: a prospective study. *British Journal of Surgery*, **76**, 268–272.
49. McLatchie, G.R. and Imrie, C.W. (1981) Acute pancreatitis associated with tumour metastases in the pancreas. *Digestion*, **21**, 13–17.
50. McMahon, M.J., Bowen, M., Mayer, A.D. and Cooper, E.H. (1984) Relationship of α_2-macroglobulin and other antiproteases to the clinical features of acute pancreatitis. *American Journal of Surgery*, **147**, 164–170.
51. McMahon, M.J., Playforth, M.J. and Booth, E.W. (1981) Identification of risk factors for acute pancreatitis from routine radiological investigation of the biliary tract. *British Journal of Surgery*, **68**, 465–467.
52. McMahon, M.J., Playforth, M.J. and Pickford, I.R. (1980) A comparative study of methods for the prediction of severity of attacks of acute pancreatitis. *British Journal of Surgery*, **67**, 22–25.
53. Mayer, A.D., McMahon, M.J. (1985) The diagnostic and prognostic value of peritoneal lavage in patients with acute pancreatitis. *Surgery, Obstetrics and Gynecology*, **160**, 507–512.
54. Mayer, A.D., McMahon, M.J., Bowen, M. and Cooper, E.H. (1984) C-reactive protein: an aid to assessment and monitoring of acute pancreatitis. *Journal of Clinical Pathology*, **37**, 207–211.
55. Mayer, A.D., McMahon, M.J., Corfield, A.P. *et al.* (1985) Controlled clinical trial of peritoneal lavage for the treatment of severe acute pancreatitis. *New England Journal of Medicine*, **312**, 399–404.
56. MRC Multicentre Trial Study Group (1977) Death from acute pancreatitis. MRC multicentre trial of glucagon and aprotinin. *Lancet*, **ii**, 632–635.
57. Murphy, D., Pack, A.I. and Imrie, C.W. (1980) The mechanism of arterial hypoxia occurring in acute pancreatitis. *Quarterly Journal of Medicine*, **49**, 151–160.
58. Nakashima, Y. and Howard, J.M. (1977) Drug induced acute pancreatitis. *Surgery, Gynecology and Obstetrics*, **145**, 105–109.
59. Neoptolemos, J.P., London, N.J., Slater, N.D. *et al.* (1986) A prospective study of ERCP and endoscopic sphincterotomy in the diagnosis and treatment of gallstone acute pancreatitis. *Archives of Surgery*, **121**, 679–702.
60. Niccolini, D.G., Graham, J.H. and Banks, P.A. (1976) Tumour-induced pancreatitis. *Gastroenterology*, **71**, 141–145.
61. Opie, E.L. (1901) The relation of cholelithiasis to disease of the pancreas and to fat necrosis. *Johns Hopkins Hospital Boston*, **12**, 19.
62. Osborne, D.H., Imrie, C.W. and Carter, D.C. (1981) Biliary surgery at the same admission for gallstone associated pancreatitis. *British Journal of Surgery*, **68**, 758–761.
63. Pollock, A.V. (1959) Acute pancreatitis. *British Medical Journal*, **i**, 6–14.
64. Puolakkainen, P., Valtonen, V., Paananen, A. and Schroder, T. (1987) C-reactive protein (CRP) and serum phospholipase A2 in the assessment of the severity of acute pancreatitis. *Gut*, **28**, 764–771.
65. Prince, M. (1882) Pancreatic apoplexy with a report of two cases. *Boston Medical and Surgical Journal*, **107**, 28, 55.
66. Ranson, J.H.C. (1979) The timing of biliary surgery in acute pancreatitis. *Annals of Surgery*, **189**, 654–663.
67. Ranson, J.H.C. and Pasternack, B.S. (1977) Statistical methods for quantifying the severity of clinical acute pancreatitis. *Journal of Surgical Research*, **22**, 79–91.
68. Ranson, J.H.C. and Spencer, F.C. (1978) The role of peritoneal lavage in severe acute pancreatitis. *Annals of Surgery*, **187**, 565–574.
69. Ranson, J.H.C., Rifkind, K.M. and Turner, J.W. (1976) Prognostic signs and nonoperative peritoneal lavage in acute pancreatitis. *Surgery, Gynecology and Obstetrics*, **143**, 209–219.
70. Ranson, J.H.C., Rifkind, K.M., Roses, D.F. *et al.* (1974) Prognostic signs and the role of operative management in acute pancreatitis. *Surgery, Gynecology and Obstetrics*, **139**, 69–81.
71. Reeve, T.S. and Delbridge, L.W. (1982) Pancreatitis following parathyroid surgery. *Annals of Surgery*, **195**, 158–162.
72. Ruppin, H., Amon, R. and Ettl, W. (1974) Acute pancreatitis after endoscopic radiological pancreatography. *Endoscopy*, **6**, 94–98.
73. Saidi, F. and Donaldson, G.A. (1963) Acute pancreatitis following distal gastrectomy for benign ulcer. *American Journal of Surgery*, **105**, 87–92.
74. Sankaran, S. and Walt, A.J. (1975) The natural and unnatural history of pancreatic pseudocysts. *British Journal of Surgery*, **62**, 37–44.
75. Stone, H.H. and Fabian, T.C. (1980) Peritoneal dialysis in the treatment of acute alcoholic pancreatitis. *Surgery, Gynecology and Obstetrics*, **150**, 878–882.
76. Trapnell, J.E. and Duncan, E.H.L. (1975) Patterns of incidence in acute pancreatitis. *British Medical Journal*, **ii**, 179–183.
77. Trapnell, J.E., Rigby, C.C., Talbot, C.H. and Duncan, E.H.L. (1974) A controlled trial of Trasylol in the treatment of acute pancreatitis. *British Journal of Surgery*, **61**, 177–182.
78. Uhl, W., Buchler, M., Malfertheiner, P. *et al.* (1991) PMN elastase in comparison with CRP,

antiproteases, and LDH as indicators of necrosis in human acute pancreatitis. *Pancreas*, **6**, 253–259.
79. van Lanschott, J.J.B. and Bruining, H.A. (1982) Parathyroidectomy as a cause of pancreatitis. *Langenbecks Archiv für Chirurgie*, **357**, 186–187.
80. Wallensten, S. (1958) Acute pancreatitis and hyperdiasturia after partial gastrectomy. *Acta Chirurgica Scandinavica*, **115**, 182–188.
81. Wilson, C. and Imrie, C.W. (1988) Deaths from acute pancreatitis: why do we miss the diagnosis so frequently . *International Journal of Pancreatology*, **3**, 273–282.
82. Wilson, C., Heads, A., Shenkin, A. and Imrie, C.W. (1989) C-reactive protein, antiproteases and complement factors as objective markers of severity in actue pancreatitis. *British Journal of Surgery*, **76**, 177–181.
83. Wilson, C., Heath, D.I., Imrie, C.W. (1990) Prediction of outcome in acute pancreatitis: a comparative study of APACHE II clinical assessment and multiple factor scoring systems. *British Journal of Surgery*, **77**, 1260–1264.
84. Wilson, C., McArdle, C.S., Carter, D.C. and Imrie, C.W. (1988) Surgical treatment of acute necrotizing pancreatitis. *British Journal of Surgery*, **75**, 1119–1123.

CHRONIC PANCREATITIS

C. Fernández-del Castillo, J.M. Richter and A.L. Warshaw

Chronic pancreatitis is an inflammatory condition of the pancreas characterized by irreversible damage of the acinar and ductular parenchyma and, in its later stages, of the endocrine tissue as well. It is a progressive disease that markedly affects both the quality and life expectancy of most of those affected, and which poses challenges for a better understanding of its natural history and treatment. Although the disease is frequently complicated in its early stages by attacks of acute pancreatitis, with which it shares some clinical similarities, it is generally accepted that these two inflammatory conditions of the pancreas are different processes. This view is supported by the fact that the mean age of presentation of patients with chronic pancreatitis is 13 years *less* than that of acute pancreatitis,[100] as well as by clinical and experimental evidence demonstrating that the acute lesions regress completely, although they may recur if their cause persists.[37,98]

Table 11.6 Aetiology of chronic pancreatitis

Chronic calcifying pancreatitis	*Chronic obstructive pancreatitis*
Alcoholic	Pancreatic tumours
Tropical	Ampullary stenosis
Hyperparathyroidism	Pancreas divisum
Hereditary	Congenital cysts
Idiopathic	Scars (prior pancreatitis, healed pseudocysts, necrosis, trauma)
	Duodenal stenosis
	Ampullary tumours
	Duodenal diverticula
	Mucinous ductal ectasia

AETIOLOGY AND EPIDEMIOLOGY

Chronic pancreatitis can be classified in two broad types:[97] chronic calcifying pancreatitis, which is by far the most commonly encountered, and obstructive chronic pancreatitis (*Table 11.6*). As will be discussed later, the distinction has a pathological basis, but is also very useful clinically.

CHRONIC CALCIFYING PANCREATITIS

Alcoholic

Alcohol abuse accounts for the vast majority of cases of chronic pancreatitis diagnosed in industrialized countries.[2,58,62,74] This is also true for less-developed countries, such as Mexico and Brazil, where alcoholic chronic pancreatitis accounts for 68% and 90%, respectively, of the cases diagnosed.[28,90] The typical patient is an adult male, 35–50 years old, who has been drinking daily an average of 150–200 ml of pure ethanol for more than 10 years.[98] Male predominance is striking, and ranges from 10:1[2] to 77:1,[72] in spite of the observation that women require less ethanol over a shorter time to develop chronic pancreatitis.[98] Sarles *et al.*[100] have shown that the risk of developing chronic pancreatitis increases exponentially with the amount of ethanol consumed, and that for any given amount, the risk increases with duration of consumption. Even small quantities of alcohol are capable of causing the disease in some patients. In contrast, the type of alcoholic beverage (wine, beer or distilled), or the pattern of daily consumption (daily versus intermittent binge drinking), bears no relationship to the development of the disease.

The role of nutrition as a contributory factor in the genesis of alcoholic chronic pancreatitis has also been studied. Although results are conflicting, both clinical and experimental studies seem to indicate that a diet high in fat and proteins potentiates the induction of alcohol-induced chronic pancreatitis.[34] It has also been proposed that deficiency of trace elements, such as zinc and selenium, might play a role in the induction of pancreatic injury by hampering the production of antioxidant enzymes.[86]

Given the high incidence of alcoholism compared with that of chronic pancreatitis (it is estimated that only 5% of alcoholics develop pancreatitis),[33] other factors surely operate in the development of the disease. Individual susceptibility has been explored by means of HLA and blood typing, and the studies show over-representation of some and under-representation of other genetic markers.[136] In spite of the common toxic insult, concomitant chronic pancreatitis and liver cirrhosis is not frequent. In one study, 12.5% of patients with chronic pancreatitis had liver cirrhosis proven by biopsy, and 15% of patients with liver cirrhosis had abnormalities in the pancreatic ducts demonstrated by pancreatography and an abnormal pancreatic function test.[3]

Tropical

Worldwide, this is probably the most common form of chronic pancreatitis, affecting millions of children and young adults in India and other countries of Asia and Africa. Its frequency in the State of Kerala, in southern India, has been estimated at 50 per 1000,[117] as opposed to that of alcoholic chronic pancreatitis in industrialized countries, which has been estimated between 40 and 70 per 100 000 inhabitants. It affects both sexes equally and usually begins during childhood. The aetiology of tropical pancreatitis has not yet been determined. Malnutrition seems to be very closely related to its development, be it in the form of a low-fat or low-protein diet, or both, deficiency of micronutrients such as selenium, copper, and vitamins A and B6, dietary toxins, or maternal undernourishment during gestation.[86,98,117] Ingestion of cassava (*Manihot esculenta*), which has a high content of cyanogenetic glycosides, has been widely implicated, although the results of epidemiological studies are conflicting.[86,98]

Hyperparathyroidism

Both acute and chronic pancreatitis can be part of the spectrum of clinical manifestations that characterize symptomatic primary hyperparathyroidism, and can even lead to its diagnosis.[73,125] Although it has been claimed that such an association is spurious because of bias in patient selection,[9] recent series attest to an incidence of 8–12% of pancreatitis in hyperparathyroidism.[38,108] This discrepancy is probably due to differences in the use of routine serum calcium measurements. Whereas detection of a high calcium level during medical screening can lead to the treatment of hyperparathyroid patients before they develop symptoms or complications, the disease is often diagnosed only in its advanced stages in less-developed countries. Nevertheless, it is important to remember that chronic calcifying pancreatitis can be caused by hyperparathyroidism, because surgical treatment of the latter often leads to improvement in the symptoms of pancreatitis[38] and prevents further renal and osseous damage.

Hereditary

This form of pancreatitis was first described by Comfort and Steinberg in 1952.[23] By 1981, over 195 patients from 40 affected families had been described.[45] The disease is inherited in an autosomal dominant fashion, with a penetrance of 40–80%.[89,105] It affects both sexes equally, and typically has its onset in late childhood (10–13 years), although the range is from 11 months to old age.[45] Hereditary pancreatitis is a distinct entity, with an unknown underlying mechanism, and should not be confused with other forms of chronic pancreatitis which also have familial aggregation. These include certain metabolic defects such as familial hyperlipaemia and hypocalciuric hypercalcaemia, as well as clusters of idiopathic pancreatitis occurring within one generation.[36]

Idiopathic

None of the above-mentioned aetiological factors can be identified in a relatively large number of cases with chronic calcifying pancreatitis. This so-called 'idiopathic' chronic pancreatitis comprised 21%, 29% and 31.5% of patients in three large series from Switzerland, Mexico, and Japan, respectively,[2,72,90] but only 6% in a series of 797 patients from Brazil.[28] Although it has been claimed that many of these patients may have a low threshold for alcohol toxicity to the pancreas, and that others deny actual alcohol abuse[98] (this is certainly true for some cases), epidemiological evidence indicates that, indeed, idiopathic pancreatitis is a distinct form of the disease. This includes an equal male to female ratio, a delayed progression to endocrine and exocrine insufficiency, and a bimodal age at presentation, affecting both younger and older patients as compared with alcoholic pancreatitis.[2,62,64,72,90]

OBSTRUCTIVE CHRONIC PANCREATITIS

This form of chronic pancreatitis is caused by partial or total obstruction of the pancreatic ducts. It can be secondary to tumours, congenital or acquired cysts, ductal anomalies, papillary stenosis, or scars caused by trauma or a previous episode of necrotizing pancreatitis.[122] In most series of chronic pancreatitis, the obstructive variety accounts for less than 2% of total cases.[2,28,62,90] In certain geographical areas, a relatively larger proportion of cases of chronic pancreatitis are ascribed to duct obstruction, although much of the increment is attributed to gallstone disease. A noteworthy example of this are reports from the British Isles where, 25 years ago, biliary disease was considered to be the main aetiologic factor of chronic pancreatitis.[58,69] At present, despite the fact that alcoholic chronic pancreatitis is the most prevalent form of the disease in the UK (probably caused by the increase in per capita alcohol ingestion), gallstone and other forms of obstructive chronic pancreatitis, such as pancreas divisum and trauma, are the cause of over 20% of reported cases.[24,69] A single report from China states that biliary tract disease is responsible for 40–50% of chronic pancreatitis.[47] Both these experiences are in marked contrast to the generally accepted tenet that gallstones can be the cause of acute pancreatitis but rarely, if ever, lead to chronic pancreatitis.[53,64]

Pancreas divisum

Patients with the congenital anomaly pancreas divisum *and* stenosis of the accessory papilla, can develop recurrent episodes of acute pancreatitis. This is also true for variants of this ductal anomaly, which should probably be better termed dominant dorsal duct syndrome.[133] In a few patients, these recurrent attacks lead to the development of chronic pancreatitis,[130] which has been shown to be circumscribed to the inadequately drained area.[10]

PATHOLOGY AND PATHOGENESIS

In the early stages of chronic pancreatitis, the gross appearance of the pancreas may remain normal both to inspection and palpation. During exacerbations the gland is swollen and inflamed, and in later stages it becomes indurated and may be distorted and irregular. Atrophy and extensive scarring develop last, leaving the shrunken pancreas with a firm hard texture and a relatively tubular, rather than flattened, configuration.

On cutting the tissue of advanced chronic pancreatitis, a white uneven surface with very little bleeding is observed. This contrasts sharply with the richly vascularized normal gland. The duct system is characteristically distended, with alternating areas of strictures and dilation (*Figure 11.35*). However, the duct may instead be shrunken and pruned of its branches (*Figure 11.36*). It is not known if the major duct changes are primary, associated directly with the pathogenesis of the disease, or if they are secondary to scarring from chronic parenchymal inflammation or duct disruption during acute pancreatitis. Intraductal calculi (*Figure 11.37*) are present in about half the patients with advanced pancreatitis and may be large enough to occlude the lumen of the duct at the ampulla or at a stricture.

In *chronic calcifying pancreatitis,* microscopical study demonstrates a lobular, patchy distribution of lesions of different intensity from neighbouring lobules.[98] Lesions consist of periductular and perilobular fibrosis, with focal collections or diffuse infiltration of lymphocytes, plasma cells and macrophages in moderate numbers.[61] As the disease progresses, acinar cells disappear and intralobular fibrosis supervens. Ductal epithelium atrophies and occlusion of the small ducts by proteinaceous plugs or stones is observed. Blood vessels are distorted and the intima of small arteries and arterioles becomes thickened. The islets of Langerhans aggre-

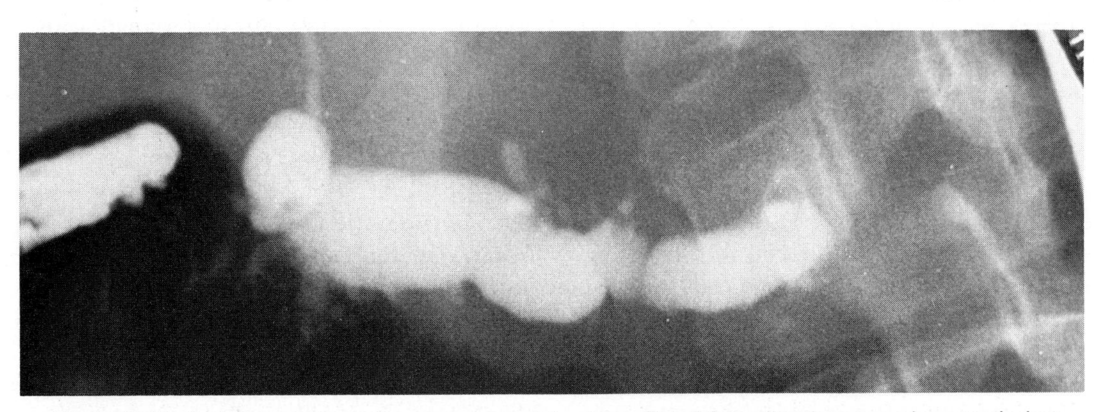

Figure 11.35 Endoscopic retrograde pancreatogram showing a dilated, intermittently narrowed pancreatic duct.

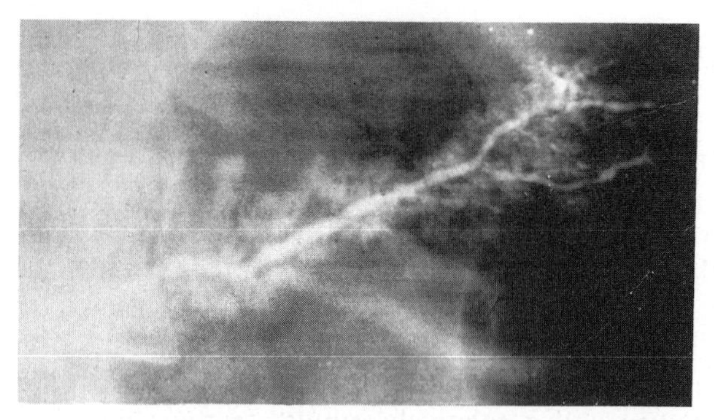

Figure 11.36 Operative pancreatogram demonstrating a diffusely small pancreatic duct.

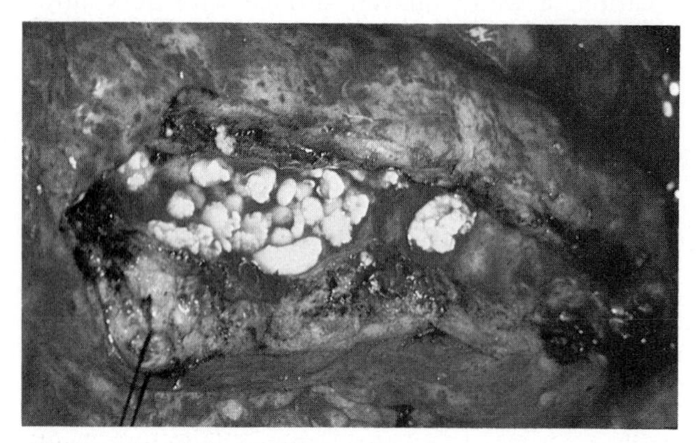

Figure 11.37 Operative photograph showing multiple calculi in a dilated pancreatic duct.

gate and become encased in fibrous tissue but retain adequate function until late in the disease.

By contrast, the lesions in *obstructive chronic pancreatitis* are uniform, being regularly spread in the occluded territory. Ductal epithelium is intact, the duct lumina are empty, and protein plugs and calcifications are rare.[98,107]

Several pathogenetic mechanisms have been proposed to link the previously outlined aetiologic factors to these pathological changes. The most relevant of these are the following.

PANCREATIC STONE PROTEIN AND THE INTRADUCTAL PLUG THEORY

This theory stems from extensive work by Sarles *et al.*[97,98] in Marseille. Pancreatic stone protein is a family of proteins unique to the pancreas. Degraded forms constitute the proteinaceous plugs that are observed histologically, and are the framework on which calcium carbonate is deposited to form pancreatic stones. Stone protein, also known as lithostatine, is synthesized by the pancreatic acinar cell, stored in the zymogen granules, and secreted in parallel with pancreatic enzymes. One of its functions is, paradoxically, to prevent calcium precipitation. Careful distinction should be made between these forms of protein (called PSP-S2-5), and the degraded form found in plugs and stones (called PSP-S1). These investigators have suggested that patients with chronic calcifying pancreatitis have decreased levels of stone protein, and that this deficiency, by facilitating the formation of plugs and stones, is the cause of their disease. Although their results have not been reproduced in other parts of the world, they have found that pancreases from patients with chronic calcifying pancreatitis have decreased levels of messenger RNA responsible for stone protein synthesis, that the zymogen granules of acinar cells contain significantly less stone protein, and that the concentration of stone protein related to secretory protein is also decreased, with almost no overlap between patients with chronic calcifying pancreatitis and normal non-alcoholic controls. Decreased stone protein secretion is observed not only in alcoholic pancreatitis, but also in idiopathic and hereditary cases as well, so it may be congenital or acquired.

DAMAGE DUE TO OXYGEN FREE RADICALS

Free radicals of oxygen have been shown to participate in the tissue injury of both oedematous and necrotizing forms of acute pancreatitis.[96,103] Their role in the pathogenesis of chronic pancreatitis has also been proposed,[20] and increased levels of lipid peroxides (which are formed as a consequence of oxygen radical damage to cell membranes) have been demonstrated in patients with chronic pancreatitis.[6] It is thought that these radicals are generated in excess as a consequence of induction of hepatic and pancreatic drug-metabolizing enzymes (such as cytochrome P450 and xanthine oxidase) by alcohol or other xenobiotics.[95] Damage occurs if the hyperactivity of these enzymatic systems is not balanced by an increase in cellular antioxidant defences. The hepatic load of excess free radicals presumably contributes to pancreatic injury through bile reflux into the pancreatic duct. Successful treatment of four patients with idiopathic recurrent chronic pancreatitis using antioxidants (organic selenium, β-carotene, vitamin C, vitamin E and methionine), was recently reported.[95]

OTHER POSSIBLE MECHANISMS

The only spontaneously occurring animal model of chronic pancreatitis shows ultrastructural changes compatible with ischemia.[80] Interestingly, decreased pancreatic blood flow has also been shown in chronic pancreatitis induced by duct obstruction in the cat.[60] Ischaemia could potentially be linked to the oxygen radicals (see above) through re-perfusion injury.[134]

Another theory suggests that direct injury of alcohol to the acinar parenchyma and duct epithelium is the cause of chronic alcoholic pancreatitis. Although alcohol is not metabolized by the pancreas, it is excreted into pancreatic juice in the same concentration as it is found in the blood and these authors propose that, in patients with functional obstruction of the papilla, alcohol is retained for an extended time and causes cell injury.[114]

The pathogenesis of *obstructive* chronic pancreatitis is presumably different. Stagnation of pancreatic juice eventually leads to acinar atrophy and fibrosis. Experimental studies have shown that, at least for some time, these changes are reversible.[107]

CLINICAL FEATURES

Abdominal pain is the cardinal symptom of chronic pancreatitis. It generally first appears as an attack indistinguishable from acute pancreatitis, although the inflammatory destruction and fibrotic replacement of the gland may have occurred unnoticed for years.[62,99,119] The pain, characteristically severe, constant and penetrating, is occasionally described as a heaviness but rarely as burning. It is almost always localized in the upper half of the abdomen, from which it can radiate directly through to the back or laterally around to the left or right flank. Less frequently, pain is referred to the inferior abdomen or anterior chest. Initially the duration of pain is quite variable, lasting several hours to several days, but as the disease progresses the attacks become more frequent and pain-free intervals shrink and vanish. Painless chronic pancreatitis presenting as pancreatic insufficiency is much less common, at least in alcoholic pancreatitis.

Precipitating factors are difficult to identify. In individuals who drink alcohol sporadically, the pain tends to occur 12–24 hours after episodes of alcohol intake. The influence of meals is not usually significant. Once pain has begun, food frequency exacerbates the discomfort, regardless of the composition of the meal, whereas prolonged fasting may bring relief. Pain is not relieved by antacids, but some patients are improved by vomiting; others feel better when sitting up and leaning slightly forward. The pain seems to grow worse with fatigue.

The mechanism of pain in chronic pancreatitis is not well understood. The inflammatory reaction involving the pancreas and nearby parietal peritoneum, and the recurrent autodigestive necrosis, are probably important in the early episodes but are difficult to implicate in the chronic continuous pain of the later stages of the disease. To explain this, two hypotheses that are not mutually exclusive have been put forward. One relates pancreatic pain to ductal hypertension, a phenomenon that has been documented repeatedly by intraoperative, percutaneous and endoscopic measurements.[35,54] In a recent study, the magnitude of decrease in intraductal pressure after pancreatic duct drainage closely correlated to the length of absence of pain, and in patients with recurrence of pain, a return to increased intraductal pressure was documented.[35] The second hypothesis states that pain in chronic pancreatitis is mainly due to neural changes.[7,11] This is based on histopathological and immunohistochemical studies demonstrating a comparative increase in the number of nerves within the inflammatory pancreatic tissue, disintegration of the perineurium, round cell infiltration, and presence of pain mediators such as substance P and calcitonin gene-related peptide, in increased amounts.[7,11] Probably both of these mechanisms play a role in the genesis of this troublesome symptom of chronic pancreatitis. It should be noted that pain can also be related to the presence of complications of this disease, such as pseudocysts, vascular thrombosis, or duodenal obstruction.

Episodes of anorexia, nausea, and vomiting are associated with abdominal pain when there is acute exacerbation of inflammation. In these instances, loss of weight is caused by decreased caloric intake, even in the absence of pancreatic insufficiency.

Pain is the commonest early feature of chronic pancreatitis, but it is not a *sine qua non.* Some patients will be found to have asymptomatic chronic pancreatitis, perhaps by the incidental finding of pancreatic calcifications seen on radiography or as an unexpected finding at laparotomy for other reasons. Others will present without pain but with advanced disease producing pancreatic insufficiency. When inflammation, atrophy and fibrosis have reduced pancreatic secretion of enzymes and bicarbonate to 10% of normal, significant maldigestion of fat and protein occurs with consequent malabsorption of these nutrients and steatorrhoea.[29] There is also malabsorption of fat-soluble vitamins, especially vitamin D.[21] At this stage, the steatorrhoea causes frequent loose, foul, floating, greasy stools accompanied by bloating, cramping and flatulence. Initially patients may compensate for their malabsorption by hyperphagia but, as the disease advances, weight loss becomes the rule. Some patients will also develop deficiencies of water-soluble vitamins, especially vitamin B12. This defective absorption is reversed by replacement of pancreatic enzymes and seems to be caused by a binding of this vitamin to non-intrinsic factor polypeptides.[118]

Approximately one-third of patients with chronic

pancreatitis will have overt diabetes mellitus and another third will have abnormal glucose tolerance at some time during the course of their disease. The first manifestation will be transient hyperglycaemia associated with an episode of acute pancreatitis or an exacerbation of pain. Diabetes mellitus usually develops about one decade after the onset of symptoms, but can be the first sign of painless chronic pancreatitis. Because the islets of Langerhans tend to resist injury by inflammation and fibrosis longer than the exocrine tissues, most patients who develop diabetes will also have pancreatic exocrine insufficiency and steatorrhoea, as well as pancreatic calcifications.

This form of diabetes is distinct, not only because of its accompanying clinical features, but also hormonally and metabolically.[109] Thus, in the classification of the National Diabetes Data Group, it is referred as 'pancreatic diabetes'.[78] Among the differences that have been pointed out, are low glucagon levels and blunted adrenaline responses to hypoglycaemia. Additionally, because many of these patients have concomitant alcohol abuse and hepatic disease, they have increased levels of circulating gluconeogenic amino acids, decreased insulin requirements, and are more prone to hypoglycaemia while on insulin therapy.[109] It was previously thought that these patients were less likely to develop retinopathy and other microvascular complications of diabetes. Recent, well-controlled studies have shown that this is not the case.[25,48]

Other complications of chronic pancreatitis can occasionally be the presenting feature of the disease. These include obstructive jaundice,[131] gastric outlet obstruction,[18] pancreatic ascites,[22] pleural effusion,[116] and upper gastrointestinal bleeding from oesophageal varices.[67]

Apart from the epidemiological differences (such as age and sex ratio) between alcoholic and idiopathic chronic pancreatitis, there are certain clinical features which are distinct. These include a larger number of patients with idiopathic chronic pancreatitis who have painless disease (more than 50% in the series of Amman *et al.*),[2] a delayed progression to exocrine and endocrine insufficiency[2,90] and, in general, a better prognosis.[74] Patients with tropical pancreatitis characteristically have recurrent episodes of abdominal pain which last for hours or days. Pain usually has its onset during childhood, and is followed a few years later by overt diabetes. The incidence of this form of pancreatitis is so high that, in the State of Kerala in India, pancreatic diabetes accounts for 12–16% of all diabetes.[117] Steatorrhoea almost never occurs in tropical pancreatitis; this has been ascribed to the low-fat content in the diet.[117]

There are few pertinent physical findings, the most common being weight loss, of a degree generally proportional to the severity of anorexia and steatorrhoea. Tenderness in the upper abdomen is common, especially during times of acute inflammation. An enlarged pancreas is occasionally palpable, especially in a thin person, but the finding of a mass usually indicates a pseudocyst. Skin changes caused by a deficiency of fat-soluble vitamins may be present. Other possible findings include: jaundice when there is a stricture of the common bile duct; splenomegaly when there is thrombosis of the splenic vein; ascites when there is a pancreatic–peritoneal fistula; or a succussion splash when there is duodenal obstruction.

INVESTIGATIONS

The diagnosis of chronic pancreatitis relies on two sources of evidence: demonstration of impaired exocrine function or permanent alterations in morphology. Both will be present in most patients with advanced chronic pancreatitis, but in mild and moderate disease, the diagnosis is often established on the basis of only one of these criteria. Current diagnostic methods do not show ductal or parenchymal derangement in all patients with pancreatic insufficiency, nor can the latter be demonstrated in all patients with the radiological or histological changes of chronic pancreatitis.

LABORATORY INVESTIGATIONS

The traditional 'gold standard' of pancreatic function tests is the measurement of pancreatic output of fluid, bicarbonate and enzymes into the duodenum, collected via a duodenal tube, in response to a standard dose of secretin with or without cholecystokinin.[16,44] Low values indicate pancreatic glandular insufficiency or duct obstruction. There is little agreement over which of the components of pancreatic secretion is more able to define pancreatic insufficiency,[16,51] as well as to the cut-off levels for diagnosis. The test is not standardized worldwide, and most institutions have adopted their own criteria based on many years of experience studying different control populations. Pancreatic exocrine function may also be quantified using the Lundh test.[5] In this test a standard meal is given to the patient to stimulate endogenous secretin and cholecystokinin, and the output of trypsin into the duodenum is measured. It is not specific for pancreatic insufficiency, because it involves functional integrity of other digestive processes. A normal test, however, does make chronic pancreatitis unlikely.

Both of the above tests are cumbersome and uncomfortable for the patient because of the requirement of duodenal intubation. Pancreatic secretory capacity can also be assessed by other methods. Measurement of faecal fat excretion over 72 hours on a diet of defined fat intake is one of them. Increased levels (over 10 g) document steatorrhoea. Maldigestion due to pancreatic insufficiency, rather than malabsorption due to intestinal disease, can be demonstrated by normal D-xylose absorption or partial reversal of the steatorrhoea with oral pancreatic enzyme replacement. Severe pancreatic exocrine insufficiency may also be documented by measurement of reduced faecal chymotrypsin.

The *p*-aminobenzoic acid (PABA) and pancreolauryl tests also evaluate pancreatic exocrine function without duodenal intubation.[44] In the former, N-benzoyl-L-tyrosyl-*p*-aminobenzoic acid is given orally as a substrate, and is cleaved by chymotrypsin. Released PABA is absorbed from the small intestine, partially conjugated in the liver, and excreted in the urine where PABA and its metabolites are measured. The test can be repeated on a separate day giving only PABA, thus allowing for other malabsorption causes and individual variability in absorption, conjugation, and excretion. The pancreolauryl test is based on the same principle, using fluorescein dilaurate as substrate (which is hydrolyzed by pancreatic arylesterases), and giving fluorescein alone on a separate day.

Recently, a novel 'tubeless' test based on a different principle has been described. It measures a decrease in total plasma amino acid content following pancreatic stimulation with secretin and cholecystokinin.[30] The degree of amino acid decrease is closely correlated with pancreatic enzyme secretion, and patients with exocrine pancreatic insufficiency have a significantly smaller decrease in amino acid content (presumably because of a diminished protein-synthesizing capacity) compared with controls. The test is attractive because of its simplicity and lack of reliance on other digestive and intestinal factors. Use of cerulein alone (which is a cholecystokinin analogue), and not secretin and cholecystokinin, apparently yields the same results at a fraction of the cost.[49]

Measurement of serum amylase and lipase are helpful in the diagnosis of acute pancreatitis, but are of much less use to evaluate chronic pancreatitis. Serum levels of these enzymes rise with acute exacerbations of inflammation or pancreatic duct obstruction, but are usually normal for much of the time in otherwise uncomplicated chronic pancreatitis. If the amylase isoenzymes in serum or urine are analysed, pancreatic isoamylase can be shown to decrease in chronic pancreatitis. The decline of circulating pancreatic isoamylase is an insensitive index for the disease, however, because it probably occurs only in moderately advance stages when there has been considerable loss of functioning tissue. Abnormal 'aged' pancreatic isoamylases, altered during stagnant incubation, are found in pseudocysts and in the serum of patients with pseudocysts.[127]

Biochemical tests of liver function may demonstrate cholestasis in proportion to the degree of stricture of the common bile duct by surrounding fibrosis. The serum alkaline phosphatase is the most sensitive index and has been reported to be increased in up to one-third of patients.[128,131] The serum bilirubin rises later, as the bile duct obstruction worsens or secondary biliary cirrhosis develops. Fluctuation and transient rises in serum bilirubin also occur with superimposed bouts of pancreatic inflammation or with recurrent cholangitis.[131] It must be emphasized that patients with chronic pancreatitis can also develop intrahepatic cholestasis from concomitant alcoholic liver disease.

The function of the endocrine pancreas can be estimated by determining the fasting and 2-hourly postprandial blood glucose levels, or more formally with a glucose tolerance test.

RADIOGRAPHY

Plain films of the abdomen remain valuable for the detection of patients with suspected chronic pancreatitis.[106] Pancreatic calcifications are found in 50–60% of patients with advanced disease and 30% of patients at earlier stages (*Figure 11.38*). Barium contrast studies of the digestive tract are not helpful

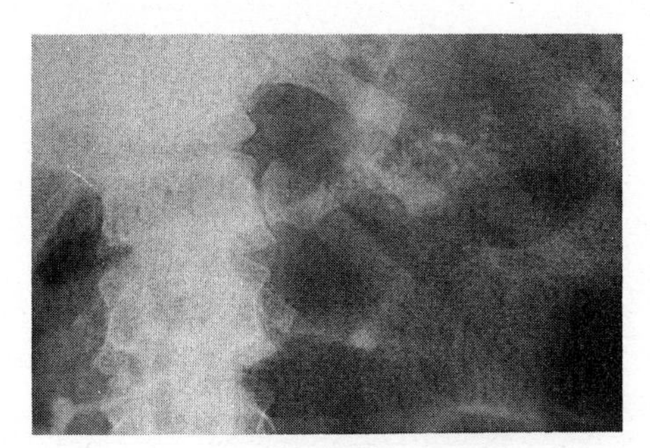

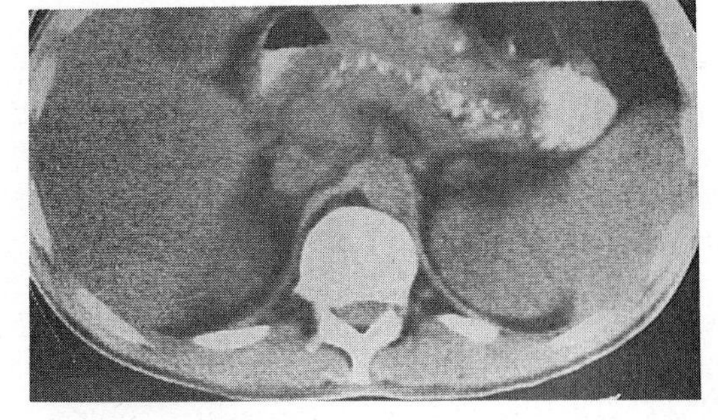

Figure 11.38 A plain radiograph of the abdomen demonstrating calcification of the pancreas (left). A computed tomography scan of the same patient showing enhancement of the calcifications (right).

except when duodenal stenosis is suspected or to define coincident alimentary tract pathology.

Ultrasonography has assumed an increasingly important role in the diagnosis of chronic pancreatitis.[13,120] It can show an increase or decrease in gland size, contour irregularities, changes in echogenicity and calcifications. Real time instruments can readily measure duct diameter and its response to secretin. In normal individuals, pancreatic duct diameter increases over 100% after secretin stimulation; most patients with chronic pancreatitis show minimal or no dilation, and others have persistence of dilation after 15 minutes.[14] This persistence of dilation after secretin stimulation has also been observed by us in patients with pancreas divisum and obstruction of the minor papilla.[132] Additionally, ultrasonography can detect fluid collections, dilation of the biliary tree, and splenic or portal vein obstruction. All this, coupled with its widespread availability and noninvasiveness, makes ultrasonography an ideal first diagnostic step in chronic pancreatitis, although failure to visualize the entire gland because of bowel gas should be anticipated in 20% of patients.

Computed tomography gives better resolution than ultrasonography and does not suffer from obstruction by bowel gas.[40] It is also the most sensitive test in the detection of pancreatic calcifications.[13,120] It does not completely supersede ultrasonography, however, and in most situations should be considered complementary to it.

The most accurate method to detect morphological alterations secondary to chronic pancreatitis is endoscopic retrograde cholangiopancreatography.[120] Although the duct may appear normal in early stages, abnormalities are regularly observed in moderate or advanced disease.[77] The principal earlier changes are irregular dilatation of the main pancreatic duct with occasional narrowing or diffuse constriction and pruning of the ductal system (*Figure 11.39*). Later, the main pancreatic duct either dilates several-fold (see *Figure 11.35*) or may have segmental constrictions ('chain of lakes') or even complete obstruction, sometimes by an intraluminal stone. The presence of pancreatic stones on plain abdominal radiographs tends to correlate with pancreatic duct dilatation. About 30% of patients will have dilated major ducts but well over 60% of those with pancreatic stones have such dilatation. Because the stenotic segments may empty poorly there is a risk of introducing infection during pancreatography; prophylactic antibiotics substantially decrease the incidence of clinical infection.

Extrinsic compression of the common bile duct within the substance of the pancreas occurs in up to one-third of patients with moderate or advanced chronic pancreatitis.[128,131] The typical long, tapered, smooth stricture of the intrapancreatic portion of the bile duct can be shown by pancreatography or by percutaneous transhepatic cholangiography (*Figure 11.40*). Either of these investigations is warranted in any patient with chronic pancreatitis

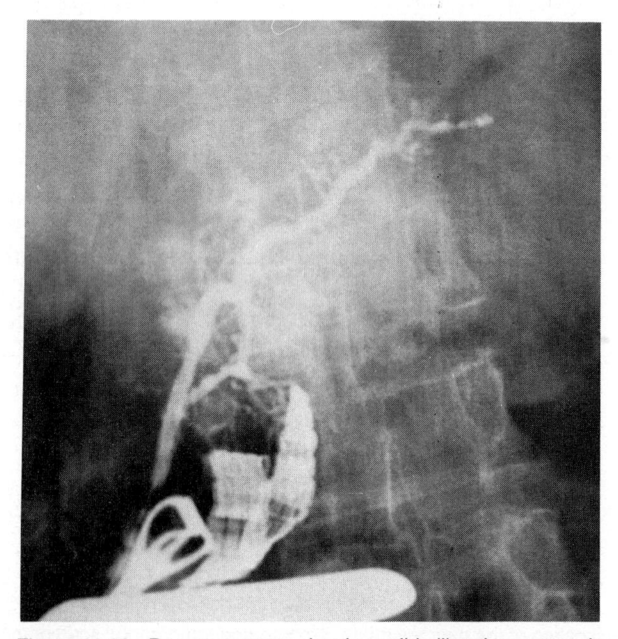

Figure 11.39 Pancreatogram showing mild dilatation, tortuosity and irregularity of the pancreatic duct.

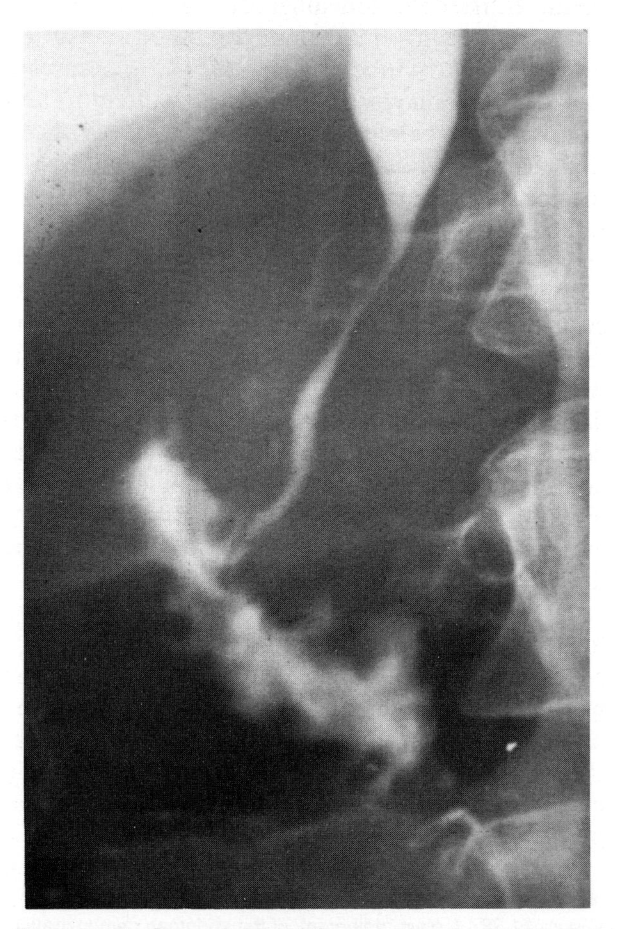

Figure 11.40 Cholangiogram demonstrating a stenotic distal common bile duct caused by chronic pancreatitis.

who is jaundiced or who has a persistently raised serum alkaline phosphatase.

Selective angiography is used mainly when splenic or portal venous occlusion is suspected, or to detect vascular anomalies in advance of major surgical resections.

AN INTEGRATED DIAGNOSTIC APPROACH TO THE PATIENT WITH SUSPECTED CHRONIC PANCREATITIS

The diagnosis of chronic pancreatitis is generally considered in patients who present with chronic epigastric pain, steatorrhoea or weight loss. Diagnostic evaluation of a patient presenting with pain generally begins with radiographical and then endoscopic studies of the upper digestive tracts if there are aspects of the history that suggest gastric or duodenal pathology. A plain film of the abdomen demonstrating characteristic pancreatic calcification virtually establishes the diagnosis. This is not pathognomonic, however, because pancreatic calcifications have been documented in patients without pancreatic insufficiency,[63] and can also be found in pancreatic cancer and cystic tumours of the pancreas. If needed, the diagnostic evaluation then proceeds with an ultrasound examination of the biliary tree and pancreas. When the diagnosis is still in doubt, the evaluation may proceed with computed tomography to visualize the gland more fully. Calcifications undetected on plain film may be observed and solitary solid masses may be identified. Diffuse disease of the pancreas supports the diagnosis of chronic pancreatitis, but localized solid lesions must be distinguished from pancreatic cancer. If this is the case, pancreatography should be the next test. Most of these patients will be jaundiced, and by localizing the site of obstruction and delineating its contour, pancreatography can establish the differential diagnosis. If no jaundice is present, the focal mass will probably be in the body and tail of the organ. An abrupt obstruction of the duct, as opposed to diffuse alterations, would favour the diagnosis of cancer in this setting.

We believe that percutaneous biopsy of these focal lesions should not be attempted if there is a possibility that the patient may harbour carcinoma which is potentially resectable. The biopsy may hasten peritoneal spread of the tumour and a negative result for cancer is never definite. If a suspicion of malignant disease remains after pancreatography, the patient should be staged for pancreatic cancer and treated accordingly.[39] If no such focal mass exists, the diagnosis of chronic pancreatitis can be confirmed by demonstrating decreased pancreatic exocrine function using the secretin stimulation test or the Lundh meal test. When the clinical history is particularly compelling, a clinical diagnosis of chronic pancreatitis may be made without a complete radiological or secretory evaluation.

Patients with painless chronic pancreatitis presenting as steatorrhoea and weight loss require a different diagnostic evaluation. The first step is to document fat malabsorption, usually by collecting stool on a defined diet for 72 hours. A faecal chymotrypsin test may be helpful in identifying pancreatic disease, though a D-xylose test or intestinal biopsy may be needed to exclude intestinal causes in malabsorption. A plain film of the abdomen demonstrating characteristic calcification is once again quite helpful in establishing a diagnosis of chronic pancreatitis. In ambiguous cases, direct measurement of pancreatic exocrine function is helpful. In the absence of the availability of these tests, an empiric trial of therapy with oral pancreatic enzymes may suffice. When the diagnosis of pancreatic cancer is also being entertained, evaluation should proceed with other studies as discussed above.

NATURAL HISTORY

Several studies related to the long-term follow-up of patients with chronic pancreatitis are now available,[2,62,74,90] and show that the natural history of alcoholic chronic pancreatitis varies substantially from that of the idiopathic and other non-alcoholic varieties.

Chronic alcoholic pancreatitis tends to become symptomatic in early adulthood after 10–20 years of heavy alcohol abuse. At least 95% of patients will present with acute abdominal pain and the clinical features of acute pancreatitis. Physiological or histological studies, however, will demonstrate established chronic pancreatitis even at presentation.[99] The first attack of pain generally resolves completely, but if alcohol abuse continues there will be a relapse of pain or acute pancreatitis. With the passage of time, attacks of pain seem to depend less upon alcohol ingestion and resolve more slowly. Initially the serum amylase is significantly elevated with acute attacks, whereas later, the amylase remains at normal concentrations even during symptomatic exacerbations. After a mean of 10 years the discomfort tends to subside in a number of patients. Some authorities believe that this improvement correlates with the development of pancreatic exocrine and endocrine insufficiency, indicative of 'burning out' of the pancreas.[2] Others have found that, after 10 years of follow-up, more than 50% of patients have persistent pain, and no close correlation between the development of pancreatic exocrine or endocrine insufficiency and the abatement of pain.[62] Although it is also claimed that the appearance of calcification on abdominal radiography heralds the abatement of pain, our experience demonstrates many exceptions and we do not find this a clinically useful observation.

Chronic pancreatitis is a relentlessly progressive disease and, although spontaneous improvement and even recovery are occasionally reported, most patients will demonstrate aggravation of exocrine insufficiency and increasing ductal alterations with time.[2,72,77,90] The role of abstinence in arresting the progression of chronic pancreatitis is unproven, but common wisdom emphasizes its importance in limiting the recurrence of acute pancreatitis early in the disease. Continued alcohol abuse significantly increases mortality.[74]

Over 60% of patients survive at least two decades after the diagnosis of chronic pancreatitis has been made. Nevertheless, comparison of survival rates with sex- and age-matched controls demonstrates a significantly higher death rate.[74] The main causes of death include complications of diabetes, infection, and malignant neoplasms (many of which are related to smoking). Very few patients die as a consequence of an acute exacerbation of pancreatitis. In all series, deaths caused by pancreatic cancer can be found. Interestingly, the incidence seems to be higher in patients with idiopathic and hereditary pancreatitis,[2,45] and is definitely increased in patients with tropical pancreatitis.[117]

Patients with idiopathic chronic pancreatitis have a better prognosis. The rate of progression to both exocrine and endocrine insufficiency is slower;[2,90] they have a better survival than their alcoholic counterparts (which becomes even better when compared with age-matched controls because their mean age at diagnosis is 10 years older);[74] and they have the additional advantage of a higher proportion of painless disease.

COMPLICATIONS

CYSTS AND PSEUDOCYSTS

A pancreatic pseudocyst is a fluid collection, usually rich in pancreatic secretions, that has no epithelial lining but is contained by neighbouring viscera and a wall composed of granulation and fibrous tissue. In acute pancreatitis, pseudocysts represent a complication of pancreatic necrosis with resulting rupture of the pancreatic duct or one of its branches and escape of pancreatic juice.[123] In acute pancreatitis, pseudocysts are usually seen in sick, unstable patients and require a waiting period to allow for maturation of their wall, before surgical treatment is attempted. Some will spontaneously regress.[129] In chronic pancreatitis, pseudocysts are most often found in the absence of a recent attack of pain and patients are rarely acutely ill. The pathogenesis is thought to be related to ductal obstruction with continued secretion of pancreatic juice into the obstructed duct.[107] Some authors refer to them as retention cysts and retention pseudocysts, to distinguish them from pseudocysts that follow necrotizing pancreatitis.[15]

Pseudocysts vary in size from 1 to 20 cm in diameter and may be found in any portion of the gland or outside it from the neck of the pelvis. The propensity of pseudocysts to track widely throughout the retroperitoneum and out into the mesenteries, into the thorax, and to develop fistulas into viscera is thought to be by tissue erosion from the activated proteolytic enzymes in the cyst contents. Their most common form of presentation is abdominal pain, usually in the epigastrium, which is frequently aggravated by eating. Some pseudocysts signal their presence by their impingement upon the stomach or duodenum, causing vomiting, or upon the bile duct, causing jaundice. Other pseudocysts do not cause symptoms but are discovered because a mass is palpated, or the serum amylase is found to be elevated or, with increasing frequency, as an unanticipated finding from ultrasound, CT (*Figure 11.41*), or ERCP.

Our understanding of the natural history of pseudocysts is changing now that the new diagnostic techniques, particularly ultrasound and CT, have shown that many pseudocysts remain silent and some resolve spontaneously. In our experience, approximately 15% of pseudocysts following an attack of acute pancreatitis will resolve spontaneously within 6 weeks of the attack.[129] Thereafter the chances of resolution diminish markedly, except for the smallest cysts. The rate of spontaneous resolution of pseudocysts developing in chronic pancreatitis in the absence of an identifiable superimposed acute attack is much less.

The acute life-threatening complications of pancreatic pseudocysts, other than pain, are rupture into the free peritoneal cavity, rupture into a viscus (often with major haemorrhage into the gastrointestinal tract), infection, and erosion of a major blood vessel with massive bleeding into the pseudocyst cavity. It is partly the fear of those consequences that motivates the surgical treatment of symptomatic, persistent pseudocysts, especially those greater than 5 cm in diameter. In one series of 93 patients with pseudocysts, the incidence of complications in medically treated patients was 41%, compared with a 20% incidence in surgically treated patients.[19] Most of the pseudocysts in that series were the product of acute pancreatitis; pseudocysts arising in chronic pancrea-

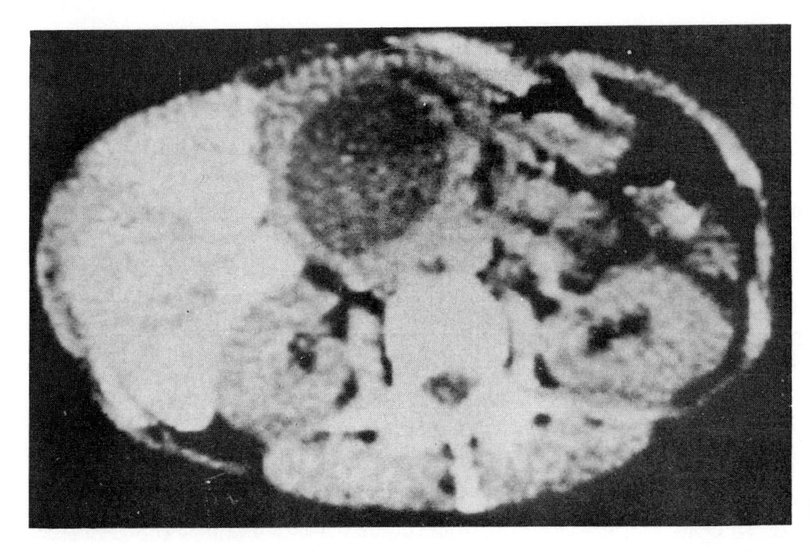

Figure 11.41 CT scan showing a large mature pancreatic pseudocyst.

titis are much less prone to spontaneous complications, and their surgical treatment should be attended by a morbidity rate of less than 5%.

COMMON BILE DUCT STRICTURE

Jaundice is relatively common in chronic pancreatitis and may be caused by common bile duct compression in as many as one-third of patients.[107] In most it will resolve spontaneously within a short time, being secondary to an acute episode of pancreatic inflammation. A fixed stricture of the distal bile duct from surrounding pancreatic fibrosis is less common, affecting between 3 and 8% of patients.[88] The obstruction can also be secondary to compression by an adjacent pseudocyst, although concomitant irreversible fibrosis is usually present.[128] It is usually a long, tapering stricture, with smooth edges, that extends throughout the length of the intrapancreatic common bile duct (see *Figure 11.40*). The earliest functional consequence is cholestasis, first indicated by a persistent increase of serum alkaline phosphatase and later by hyperbilirubinaemia. The frequency with which this obstruction can lead to cholangitis and biliary cirrhosis has not been established. While there is no doubt that a patient with persistent jaundice requires to be drained, the need to treat patients surgically whose only manifestation is increased alkaline phosphatase levels is debatable.[59] We believe that biliary bypass should be performed in all patients with a common bile duct stricture and raised serum alkaline phosphatase who undergo pancreatic drainage, because the added morbidity of the choledochoenteric anastomosis is negligible. Close surveillance and periodic liver biopsies are warranted if the patient's chronic pancreatitis is not amenable to surgery, and an expectant approach is elected for the asymptomatic biliary obstruction. In our experience, secondary biliary cirrhosis and cholangitis are not infrequent in this setting.[131]

DUODENAL OBSTRUCTION

Duodenal obstruction occurs in about 1% of patients with pancreatitis (both acute and chronic).[4,18] In acute pancreatitis it is likely to resolve with conservative treatment in the course of weeks. In chronic pancreatitis, the duodenal wall becomes fibrotic, with destruction of the musuclar wall and inflammation.[107] It is usually present in longstanding disease and in conjunction with a dilated pancreatic or common biliary duct, or both.[88] Upper gastrointestinal barium studies demonstrate narrowing of the second and third portion of the duodenum, with intact mucosa. Endoscopy may be helpful to exclude peptic ulcer disease, and confirm the presence of a concentric narrowing with a normal mucosa. Other cases that must be excluded include pancreatic cancer (which usually causes obstruction in the third and fourth portions of the duodenum), compression by a pseudocyst, and an annular pancreas.[88]

ASCITES

Ascites in an alcoholic patient is usually caused by cirrhosis. It may be present in chronic pancreatitis, however, when a direct communication develops between the pancreatic duct system and the peritoneal cavity, usually the consequence of a ruptured pseudocyst, but sometimes from rupture and necrosis of a duct near the surface of the gland.[22,43] These patients present with ascites, with or without chronic discomfort, but without any acute abdominal catastrophe. The diagnosis of chronic pancreatic ascites is established by paracentesis with the finding of high concentrations of amylase and protein in the ascitic fluid. The pancreatoperitoneal fistula can be demonstrated by pancreatography.[65]

fluid. The pancreatoperitoneal fistula can be demonstrated by pancreatography.[65]

PLEURAL EFFUSION

Chronic pleural effusions may develop in a manner similar to that of pancreatic ascites,[22] and may even lead to its diagnosis.[116] The pancreatic secretions from a ruptured pseudocyst or pancreatic duct leak into the retroperitoneum and dissect cephalad through the oesophageal foramen or behind the attachments of the diaphragm into the chest and rupture into the pleural space. There may also be a fistula into the pericardium. Patients present with dyspnoea and cough from the large effusion which is usually unilateral and most often left-sided. In contrast to the pleural effusions which may follow an attack of acute pancreatitis (and where other pathogenic mechanisms may be at play), there is usually no recent acute episode preceding the development of pancreatic pleural effusions. They do not resolve spontaneously and recur rapidly after thoracentesis. The diagnosis is indicated by the finding of a very high amylase concentration in the effusion and can be established by demonstrating the pancreatopleural fistula with pancreatography (*Figure 11.42*).

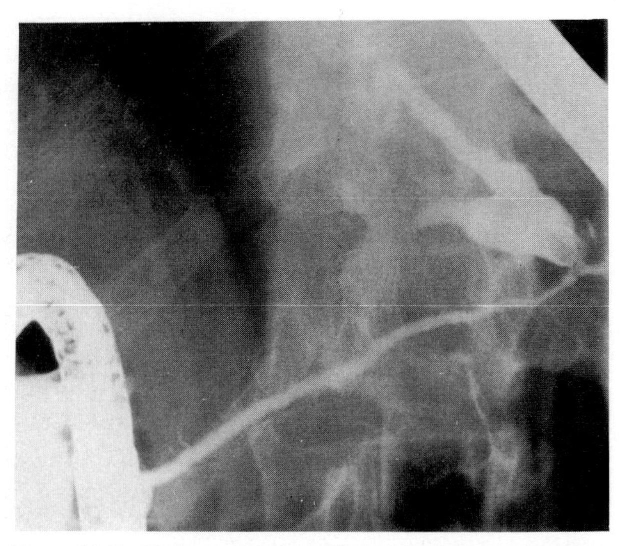

Figure 11.42 Endoscopic retrograde pancreatogram showing a fistula tracking superiorly toward the oesophageal hiatus from a ruptured pseudocyst.

VASCULAR COMPLICATIONS

Both arteries and veins may become involved in chronic pancreatitis. The arterial wall may become weakened by the effect of proteolytic enzymes or inflammation, leading to the formation of false aneurysms and changes in their radiographic appearance.[12] Rarely, the arteries may rupture and lead to spontaneous haemorrhage into the gastrointestinal tract, the peritoneal cavity, the interior of a pseudocyst, or even to the pancreatic duct itself, and from there to the duodenum.[68,111] Venous involvement is more common, with the splenic vein being the most frequently affected. The splenic vein may become occluded by constriction from fibrosis, or thrombosed due to contiguous inflammation. This leads to splenomegaly and left-sided portal hypertension,[88] which in turn may produce upper gastrointestinal bleeding from oesophageal or gastric varices. Involvement of the portal and superior mesenteric veins can also occur (*Figure 11.43*). These are frequently overlooked, and may lead to unanticipated intraoperative blood loss as well as to spontaneous gastrointestinal haemorrhage from duodenal varices.[126]

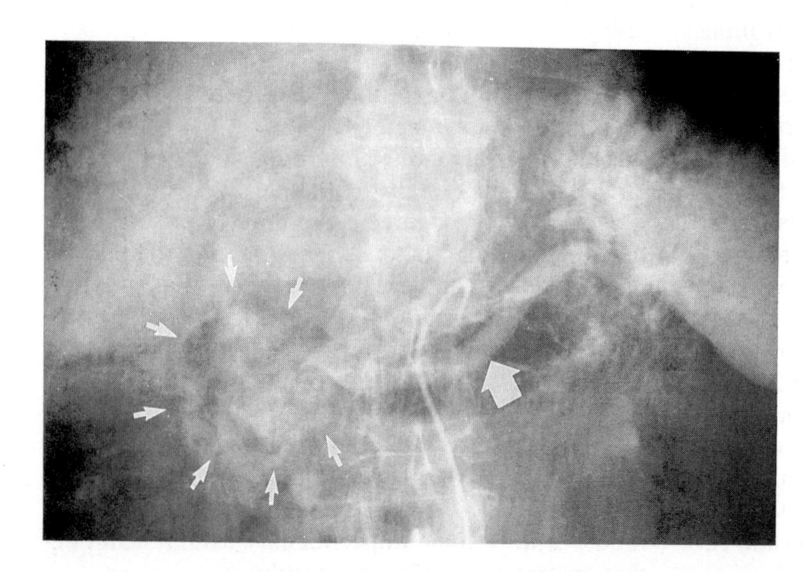

Figure 11.43 Angiogram showing obstruction of the superior mesenteric and portal veins. The splenic vein (large arrow) terminates in a nest of variceal collateral veins (small arrows).

TREATMENT

MEDICAL TREATMENT

The treatment of chronic pancreatitis begins with the identification of aetiological factors and their correction when possible. Alcoholic pancreatitis is often particularly resistant to therapy, both because of the difficulties in ending the alcohol abuse and because cessation of excessive drinking may come too late to be of substantial benefit. If the symptoms are intermittent, abstinence may be rewarded but, as the periods of pain become more frequent and even merge into continuous discomfort, the likelihood of abatement diminishes. At this point, the pain seems to become established and often progresses unremittingly without further exposure to alcohol; none the less, patients with chronic pancreatitis should severely restrict their alcohol consumption.

Beyond the further limitation of toxic factors, the aims of medical treatment in chronic pancreatitis are relief of pain, compensation of exocrine insufficiency and control of diabetes mellitus. There is no present remedy to relieve or even halt the inflammation and scarring of the gland.

Management of pain should be attempted first with non-narcotic analgesics, such as aspirin or other non-steroidal anti-inflammatory drugs, or spasmolytics such as paracetamol.[31] Usually, analgesics should be given before meals to prevent the postprandial exacerbation of pain, and on a fixed schedule. The use of these simpler drugs should be maximised before turning to other alternatives. Tricyclic antidepressants and anxiolytics may have adjuvant value in pain control. If pain control is not otherwise achieved, narcotics may be necessary. Codeine or pethidine (meperidine) are suitable for intermittent use, but methadone or sustained-release morphine are better for long-term maintenance analgesia. Habituation or addiction to narcotics becomes inextricably entwined with the pain of the disease, and it is virtually impossible to differentiate the demands of the two contributing elements. Low-fat diets and anticholinergic medications theoretically decrease stimulation of the pancreas but do not reliably lessen the pain. Large doses of pancreatic enzymes have been reported to decrease pain, presumably by negative feedback on pancreatic secretion.[57,110] Based on the same principle, treatment with cholecystokinin antagonists[56] or a long-acting somatostatin analogue[135] could be used. Some patients with persistent severe abdominal pain have been treated by splanchnic nerve block by percutaneous injection of absolute ethanol or steroids.[50,84] This technique is effective in only 15–20% of patients, and even then the pain tends to return after several months. It is therefore much less helpful in treating chronic pancreatitis than pancreatic cancer where objectives are short-term.

Good nutrition is critical to the management of patients with chronic pancreatitis. Even before pancreatic exocrine insufficiency becomes clinically apparent, many patients with chronic pancreatitis have periods of anorexia, nausea and vomiting which significantly limit their ability to take a satisfactory diet, and the problem is magnified in alcoholic patients with irregular eating habits. Diets that are rich in carbohydrates and somewhat restricted in fat and protein are better tolerated.[115] Care should be taken to anticipate and treat vitamin deficiencies (such as B2, B12 and D).

When pancreatic exocrine capacity falls below 10% of normal, steatorrhoea develops and malnutrition becomes significant.[29] At first, patients may compensate by increasing their total caloric intake, but most patients will benefit from oral replacement of pancreatic enzymes. Treatment of steatorrhoea requires preparations rich in lipase and colipase. It has been estimated that, to substitute for 10% of the maximal pancreatic secretory capacity, 100 000 units of lipase are required.[82] This should be considered when selecting a pharmaceutical preparation. Usually several tablets or capsules are required with each meal, with individual adjustment until the symptoms of diarrhoea and flatulence are controlled. The cost of this treatment is significant.

The availability of the enzymes in the intestine should also be considered. Adequate mixing of food and enzymes is essential (for this reason, breaking tablets before ingestion or use of preparations in the form of pellets or microcapsules is recommended) and lipase needs to be protected from degradation by gastric acid. To avoid the latter, concomitant administration of H_2-receptor antagonists such as cimetidine or ranitidine is recommended, although the acid-secreting status of the patient should probably be determined before starting such treatment.[71]

Diabetes mellitus complicating pancreatitis may be treated initially with a diet and careful attention to overall good nutrition. Later, oral hypoglycaemic agents or insulin therapy are frequently required. Control of the diabetes is often difficult because of the propensity to hypoglycaemic attacks.[109] Diabetic ketoacidosis is rarely seen except after major pancreatic resections.

Recent reports describe the use of extracorporeal shock wave lithotripsy in chronic pancreatitis.[27,102] This modality has been proposed for selected patients with solitary intraductal stones in the vicinity of the ampulla of Vater, when clearance of the duct has been associated with clinical improvement in some patients. The treatment has been combined with endoscopic sphincterotomy to facilitate passage of the stone fragments. It awaits further evaluation.

SURGICAL TREATMENT

The indications for surgical treatment of chronic pancreatitis are:

1. Intractable pain
2. Large pseudocyst (>5 cm)
3. Biliary obstruction
4. Duodenal obstruction
5. Pancreatic ascites
6. Pleural effusion
7. Splenic vein occlusion with variceal bleeding
8. Inability to exclude carcinoma.

Although it has been claimed that drainage of a dilated pancreatic duct can halt the progression of the disease or even lead to improvement in some patients,[79] this is certainly not so in most patients, and the role of surgery in chronic pancreatitis is to alleviate symptoms and treat complications.[124] By far the most common surgical indication is pain uncontrolled by medical therapy. As was described previously, the natural history of the disease shows that pain will subside spontaneously on average 5 years after diagnosis. In about 20% of patients pain relief does not occur, however, or may come after 18 years.[1] As it is not possible to predict which patients will have spontaneous pain relief, and because it is unrealistic to require that a patient bear the pain or continuously take narcotics for years without a determinate end-point, surgical intervention is fully justified.

The two main surgical alternatives for reducing pancreatic pain are operations to improve the drainage of the pancreatic duct or to resect pancreatic tissue.[55,70] In our experience, 40–50% of patients have a dilated pancreatic duct, with or without obstruction in the head of the gland and other partial obstructions along the length of the duct. The remainder have a scarred contracted duct which has been compared to a leafless tree. Only those patients with large, dilated ducts (over 7 mm in diameter) are candidates for drainage procedures; those with the small ducts require resection. Interestingly, patients with the large ducts are more likely to present with concomitant biliary and duodenal obstruction.[121]

Drainage procedures are preferred to pancreatic resection, whenever feasible, because they conserve pancreatic tissue and will not further compromise pancreatic exocrine and endocrine functions. Additionally, they are simpler and probably safer than resection. The prototype of these procedures is the lateral pancreatojejunostomy, also known as the Puestow or modified Puestow operation, the latter having been described by Partington and Rochelle in 1960.[85] It consists of an unroofing of the dilated pancreatic duct throughout its entire length and anastomosis in a side-to-side fashion to a defunctionalized jejunal loop (*Figure 11.44*). Any stones present in the duct or its main branches are removed. The procedure has an operative mortality well below 5%, and renders complete or partial pain remission in about 70% of patients (range 50–100%).[32,46,55,101,121] There are a few reports on pancreatogastrostomy as an alternative drainage procedure,[35,83] however, experience is too limited to allow for adequate comparisons with lateral pancreatojejunostomy. Other drainage procedures, such as caudal pancreatojejunostomy (Duval operation) or transduodenal sphincteroplasty, are associated with poor results and have been largely abandoned.[55]

Patients with the small duct variety of chronic pancreatitis are not candidates for pancreatojejunostomy and are generally managed with resective procedures. Resection of the distal 50–60% of the pancreas (up to the level of the mesenteric vessels) has been used with very little success.[91] The resection level can be extended further to the right, comprising up to 95% of the pancreas.[41] In doing so, the results become somewhat better in terms of pain remission but at the expense of an increased incidence of metabolic complications, particularly diabetes mellitus. Currently, distal pancreatic resection is reserved for the few patients with disease truly lateralized to the tail or with obstructing lesions of the mid-pancreatic duct.

By contrast, resection of the head of the pancreas and uncinate process has good results in terms of pain remittance (60–80%) and metabolic sequelae.[75,92,113] The reported mortality of pancreatoduodenectomy (Whipple's procedure) in this setting is 0–5% in specialized centres, but the operation may be difficult because the anatomical planes are lost due to peripancreatic fibrosis. Gall *et al.*[42] have reported their experience on 289 patients treated with pancreatoduodenectomy combined with occlusion of the remaining distal ductal system with prolamine (Ethibloc). Operative mortality was 1%, and the authors claim that over 88% of patients became either pain free or minimally symptomatic. Prolamine duct occlusion leads to a rapid and complete atrophy of the exocrine tissue, which they believe is the reason for the excellent results. The incidence of overt diabetes increased by about 35%

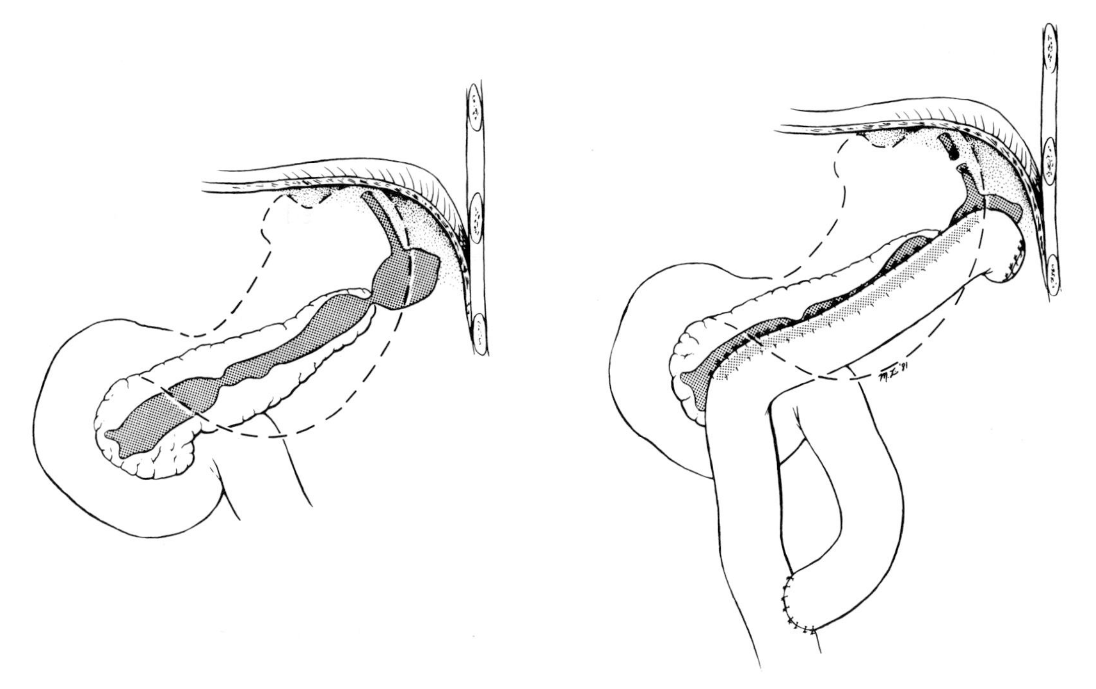

Figure 11.44 Schematic diagram showing (left) a dilated pancreatic duct, with a distal pseudocyst and pancreatopleural fistula. It is treated surgically (right) by lateral pancreatojejunostomy (modified Puestow procedure) and ligation of the fistula tract.

immediately after surgery (as it does after conventional pancreatoduodenectomy), but apparently no further damage was caused by the prolamine injection.

Beger *et al.*[8] have described an extensive experience with a new technique that resects the pancreatic head but spares the duodenum and distal common bile duct. The distal pancreatic duct as well as the rim of pancreatic tissue that is left attached to the duodenum are drained into a Roux-en-Y loop. More than 80% of patients experienced long-lasting relief of pain, and the incidence of postoperative diabetes is claimed to be less than that of the Whipple procedure.

Removal of the entire pancreas is also used in the treatment of chronic pancreatitis.[17,24,66] Even with as radical approach as this, up to 38% of patients may fail to obtain pain relief, which underscores the complexities involved in the pathogenesis of pain in this disease. The procedure is a major undertaking and is associated with a very high late morbidity and mortality closely related to the brittle diabetic state and unreliability of the patient population. We believe total pancreatectomy should be employed only as a last resort in selected patients with unremitting pain. These patients should be closely supervised regarding their diabetic and nutritional status. Successful segmental autotransplantation following extensive pancreatic resection has been described,[93] and would be an attractive option when total or near-total pancreatectomy has to be performed. Islet autotransplantation has also been undertaken in these patients, however the results are not as rewarding.[76]

Aside from drainage and resection, pancreatic denervation offers an alternative approach to the surgical treatment of pain in chronic pancreatitis. Most of the sensory nerves coming from the pancreas pass through the coeliac ganglion and splanchnic nerves, and interruption of these fibres may lessen pain. Stone and Chauvin[12] have recently reported their experience in treating 15 patients with transthoracic left splanchnicectomy with concomitant vagotomy. All patients had prior unsuccessful operative procedures for pain. Denervation gave immediate pain control in the 15 patients; 5 later recurred but were successfully treated with right splanchnicectomy. Hiraoka *et al.*[52] have described a transabdominal pancreatic denervation based on complete mobilization of the organ from the retroperitoneum and report good results. Although similar efforts have been disappointing in other hands, further evaluation of these procedures is warranted.

When biliary obstruction is present, choledochojejunostomy and choledochoduodenostomy are equally effective. Duodenal obstruction is treated by gastrojejunostomy. Addition of these procedures to pancreatic duct drainage does not increase surgical morbidity or mortality.[87,121] This triple drainage operation is very effective and does not require sacrifice of pancreatic tissue.

Symptomatic pancreatic pseudocysts associated with chronic pancreatitis usually require surgical treatment. Internal drainage to the stomach, duodenum, or a Roux-en-Y loop of jejunum (which can be the same one used in the pancreatojejunostomy) is preferred.[104] Recurrence after cyst-enterostomy is about 5% as compared with 25% after external drainage. Endoscopic internal drainage of pancreatic pseudocysts associated with chronic pancreatitis has been described.[94] A study from Belgium reports on endoscopic cystoduodenostomy and cystogastrostomy in 22 and 11 patients respectively, with an overall success of 82%.[26] Endoscopy probably will be used increasingly in the management of this complication of chronic pancreatitis.

Chronic pancreatic ascites and pleural effusions, caused by an internal fistula from the pancreas to the peritoneal cavity or pleural space, occasionally respond to repeated withdrawal of the fluid and pharmacological reduction of pancreatic secretion with somatostatin or its analogues.[81] In most patients, however, surgical treatment is necessary.[22] The leak from the pancreatic duct, usually caused by a ruptured pseudocyst, can be located by pancreatography (see *Figure 11.43*) in more than 80% of patients.[65] The most common surgical procedure used is to bring a Roux-en-Y loop of jejunum to the site of the leak, thereby channelling the pancreatic secretions into the intestinal tract. When the disruption is in the tail of the pancreas, distal pancreatectomy may provide a simple and effective solution. In patients with pancreatic pleural effusions, the retroperitoneal fistula into the chest can be interrupted below the diaphragm (see *Figure 11.44*). Once the origin of the fistula has been dealt with, nothing need be done to the pleural end of the tract other than emptying the fluid from the pleural cavity. The interrupted fistula tract will heal and the pleural effusion will not re-accumulate.

REFERENCES

1. Amman, R.W., Akovbiantz, A., Largiader, F. and Schueler, G. (1984) Course and outcome of chronic pancreatitis. *Gastroenterology*, **86**, 820–828.
2. Amman, R.W., Buehler, H., Muench, R., Freiburghaus, A.W. and Siegenthaler, W. (1987) Differences in the natural history of idiopathic (nonalcoholic) and alcoholic chronic pancreatitis. A comparative long-term study of 287 patients. *Pancreas*, **2**, 368–377.
3. Angelini, G., Merigio, F., Degani, G. *et al.* (1985) Association of chronic alcoholic liver and pancreatic disease: A prospective study. *American Journal of Gastroenterology*, **80**, 998–1003.
4. Aranha, G.V., Prinz, R.A., Greenlee, H.B. and Freeark, R.J. (1984) Gastric outlet and duodenal obstruction from inflammatory pancreatic disease. *Archives of Surgery*, **119**, 833–835.
5. Ashton, M.G., Axon, A.T.R. and Lintott, D.J. (1978) Lundh test and ERCP in pancreatic disease, *Gut*, **19**, 910–915.
6. Basso, D., Panozzo, M.P., Fabris, C. *et al.* (1990) Oxygen derived free radicals in patients with chronic pancreatic and other digestive disorders. *Journal of Clinical Pathology*, **43**, 403–405.
7. Beger, H.G., Buchler, M. and Bittner, R. (1990) The duodenum-preserving resection of the head of the pancreas (DPRHP) in patients with chronic pancreatitis and an inflammatory mass in the head. *Acta Chirurgica Scandinavica*, **156**, 309–315.
8. Beger, H.G., Buchler, M., Bittner, R. and Uhl, W. (1990) Duodenum-preserving resection of the head of the pancreas: an alternative to Whipple's procedure in chronic pancreatitis. *Hepato-Gastroenterology*, **37**, 283–289.
9. Bess, M.A., Edis, A.J. and van Heerden, J.A. (1980) Hyperparathyroidism and pancreatitis: chance or causal association? *Journal of the American Medical Association*, **243**, 246–247.
10. Blair, A.J., Russell, C.G. and Cotton, P.B. (1984) Resection for pancreatitis in patients with pancreas divisum. *Annals of Surgery*, **200**, 590–594.
11. Bockman, D.E., Buchler, M., Balfertheiner, P. and Beger, H.G. (1988) Analysis of nerves in chronic pancreatitis. *Gastroenterology*, **94**, 1459–1469.
12. Boijsen, E. and Tylen, U. (1972) Vascular changes in chronic pancreatitis. *Acta Radiologica Scandinavica*, **12**, 34.
13. Bolondi, L., Bassi, S.L., Gaiani, S. and Barbara, L. (1989) Sonography of chronic pancreatitis. *Radiologic Clinics of North America*, **27**, 815–833.
14. Bolondi, L., Libassi, S., Gaiani, S., Santi, V., Gullo, L. and Barbara, L. (1989) Impaired response of main pancreatic duct to secretin stimulation in early chronic pancreatitis. *Digestive Diseases and Sciences*, **34**, 834–840.
15. Bourliere, M. and Sarles, H. (1989) Pancreatic cysts and pseudocysts associated with acute and chronic pancreatitis. *Digestive Diseases and Sciences*, **34**, 343–348.
16. Boyd, E.J.S. and Wormsley, K.G. (1987) Laboratory tests in the diagnosis of the chronic pancreatic diseases. Part 2. *International Journal of Pancreatology*, **2**, 211–221.
17. Braasch, J.W., Vito, L. and Nugent, F.W. (1978) Total pancreatectomy for end-stage chronic pancreatitis. *Annals of Surgery*, **188**, 317–322.
18. Bradley, E.L. and Clements, J.L. (1981) Idiopathic duodenal obstruction. An unappreciated complication of pancreatitis. *Annals of Surgery*, **193**, 638–648.
19. Bradley, E.L., Clements, J.L. and Gonzales, A.C. (1979) The natural history of pancreatic pseudocysts: a unified concept of management. *American Journal of Surgery*, **137**, 135–141.
20. Braganza, J.M., Wickens, D.G., Cawood, P. and Dormandy, T.L. (1983) Lipid peroxidation (free

radical oxidation) products in bile from patients with pancreatic disease. *The Lancet*, **2**, 375–379.
21. Braunstein, H. (1961) Tocopherol deficiency in adults with chronic pancreatitis. *Gastroenterology*, **40**, 224–231.
22. Cameron, J.L. (1979) Chronic pancreatic ascites and pleural effusions. *Gastroenterology*, **74**, 134–140.
23. Comfort, M.W. and Steinberg, A.G. (1952) Pedigree of family with hereditary chronic relapsing pancreatitis. *Gastroenterology*, **21**, 54–63.
24. Cooper, M.J., Williamson, R.C.N., Benjamin, I.S. *et al.* (1987) Total pancreatectomy for chronic pancreatitis. *British Journal of Surgery*, **74**, 912–915.
25. Couet, C., Genton, P., Pointel, J.P. *et al.* (1985) The prevalence of retinopathy in patients with secondary diabetes following pancretectomy or chronic pancreatitis. *Diabetes Care*, **8**, 323–328.
26. Cremer, M., Deviere, J. and Engelholm, L. (1989) Endoscopic management of cysts and pseudocysts in chronic pancreatitis: long-term follow-up after 7 years of experience. *Gastrointestinal Endoscopy*, **35**, 1–9.
27. Cremer, M., Vandermeeren, A. and Delhaye, M. (1988) Extracorporeal shock wave lithotripsy (ESWL) for pancreatic stones [abstract]. *Gastroenterology*, **94**, A80.
28. Dani, R., Mott, C.B., Guarita, D.R. and Nogueira, C.E.D. (1990) Epidemiology and etiology of chronic pancreatitis in Brazil: a tale of two cities. *Pancreas*, **5**, 474–478.
29. DiMagno, E.P., Go, V.L.W. and Summerskill, W.H.J. (1973) Relations between pancreatic enzyme outputs and malabsorption in severe pancreatic insufficiency. *New England Journal of Medicine*, **288**, 813–815.
30. Domschke, S., Heptner, G., Kolb, S., Sailer, D., Schneider, M.U. and Domschke, W. (1986) Decrease in plasma amino acid level after secretin and panreozymin as an indicator of exocrine pancreatic function. *Gastroenterology*, **90**, 1031–1038.
31. Domschke, W. (1990) The role of analgesic treatment in chronic pancreatitis. In *Chronic Pancreatitis* (Eds) Beger, H.G., Buchler, M., Ditschuneit, H. and Malfertheiner, P. pp. 345–349. Berlin: Springer-Verlag.
32. Drake, D.H. and Fry, W.J. (1989) Ductal drainage for chronic pancreatitis. *Surgery*, **105**, 131–140.
33. Dreiling, D.A. and Koller, M. (1985) The natural history of alcoholic pancreatitis: Update 1985. *Mount Sinai Journal of Medicine*, **52**, 340–342.
34. Durbec, J.P. and Sarles, H. (1978) Multicenter survey of the etiology of pancreatic diseases. Relationship between the relative risk of developing chronic pancreatitis and alcohol protein and lipid consumption. *Digestion*, **18**, 337–350.
35. Ebbehoj, N., Borly, L., Bulow, J., Rasmussen, S.G. and Madsen, P. (1990) Evaluation of pancreatic tissue fluid pressure and pain in chronic pancreatitis. *Scandinavian Journal of Gastroenterology*, **25**, 462–466.
36. Elliot, D.W. (1987) Familial Pancreatitis. In *Surgical Diseases of the Pancreas* (Eds) Howard, J.M., Jordan, G.L. and Reber, H.A. pp. 316–321. Philadelphia: Lea and Febiger.
37. Elsasser, H.P., Adler, G. and Kern, H.F. (1986) Time course and cellular source of pancreatic regeneration following acute pancreatitis in the rat. *Pancreas*, **1**, 421–429.
38. Fernández-del Castillo, C., Cantu-Gonzalez, G., Robles-Diaz, G. and Campuzano, M. (1988) Primary hyperparathyroidism and pancreatitis: further evidence of a true association. *Revista de Gastroenterologia de Mexico*, **53**, 61–65.
39. Fernández-del Castillo, C. and Warshaw, A.L. (1990) Diagnosis and preoperative evaluation of pancreatic cancer, with implications for management. *Gastroenterology Clinics of North America*, **19**, 915–933.
40. Ferruci, J.T., Wittenberg, J. and Black, E.B. (1979) Computed body tomography in chronic pancreatitis. *Radiology*, **130**, 175–182.
41. Frey, C.F., Child, C.G. and Fry, W. (1976) Pancreatectomy for chronic pancreatitis. *Annals of Surgery*, **184**, 403–414.
42. Gall, F.P., Gebhardt, C., Meister, R., Zirngibl, H. and Schneider, M.U. (1989) Severe chronic cephalic pancreatitis: use of partial duodenopancreatectomy with occlusion of the pancreatic duct in 289 patients. *World Journal of Surgery*, **13**, 809–817.
43. Gambill, E.E., Walters, W. and Scanlon, D.W. (1960) Chronic relapsing pancreatitis with extensive subacute peritonitis and chronic, recurrent massive 'chylous' ascites. *American Journal of Medicine*, **28**, 668–670.
44. Gilinsky, N.H. (1989) Pancreatic function testing. Methods to identify exocrine insufficiency. *Postgraduate Medicine*, **86**, 165–172.
45. Girard, R.M., Dube, S. and Archambault, A.P. (1981) Hereditary pancreatitis: report of an affected Canadian kindred and review of the disease. *Canadian Medical Association Journal*, **125**, 576–589.
46. Greenlee, H.B., Prinz, R.A. and Aranha, G.V. (1990) Long-term results of side-to-side pancreaticojejunostomy. *World Journal of Surgery*, **14**, 70–76.
47. Gu, Z.-Y. and Zhang, K.-H. (1990) Chronic pancreatitis in China: Etiology and management. *World Journal of Surgery*, **14**, 28–31.
48. Gullo, L., Parenti, M., Monti, L., Pezzilli, R. and Barbara, L. (1990) Diabetic retinopathy in chronic pancreatitis. *Gastroenterology*, **98**, 1577–1581.
49. Gullo, L., Pezzilli, R., Ventrucci, M. and Barbara, L. (1990) Cerulein induced plasma amino acid decrease: a simple, sensitive, and specific test of pancreatic function. *Gut*, **31**, 926–929.

50. Hegedus, V. (1990) Relief of pancreatic pain by radiology-guided block. *American Journal of Roentgenology*, **133**, 1101–1103.
51. Heij, H.A., Obertop, H. and Van Blankenstein, M. (1986) Relationship between functional and histological changes in chronic pancreatitis. *Digestive Diseases and Sciences*, **31**, 1009–1013.
52. Hiraoka, T., Watanabe, E., Katoh, T. *et al.* (1986) A new surgical approach for control of pain in chronic pancreatitis: complete denervation of the pancreas. *American Journal of Surgery*, **152**, 549–551.
53. Howard, J.M. (1987) Gallstone pancreatitis. In *Surgical Diseases of the Pancreas* (Eds) Howard, J.M., Jordan, G.L. and Reber, H.A. pp. 265–283. Philadelphia: Lea and Febiger.
54. Ihse, I. (1990) Pancreatic pain. *British Journal of Surgery*, **77**, 121–122.
55. Ihse, I., Borch, K. and Larsson, J. (1990) Chronic pancreatitis: Results of operations for relief of pain. *World Journal of Surgery*, **14**, 53–58.
56. Ihse, I. and Permerth, J. (1990) Enzyme supplementation for pain in chronic pancreatitis. In *Chronic Pancreatitis* (Eds) Beger, H.G., Buchler, M., Ditschuneit, H. and Malfertheiner, P. pp. 354–357. Berlin: Springer-Verlag.
57. Isaksson, G. and Ihse, I. (1983) Pain reduction by an oral pancreatic enzyme preparation in chronic pancreatitis. *Digestive Diseases and Sciences*, **28**, 97–102.
58. James, O., Agnew, J.E. and Bouchier, I.A.D. (1974) Chronic pancreatitis in England: a changing picture? *British Medical Journal*, **2**, 34–38.
59. Kalvaria, I., Bornman, P.C., Marks, I.N., Girdwood, A.H., Bank, L. and Kottler, R.E. (1989) The spectrum and natural history of common bile duct stenosis in chronic alcohol-induced pancreatitis. *Annals of Surgery*, **210**, 608–613.
60. Karanjia, N.D. and Reber, H.A. (1990) The cause and management of the pain of chronic pancreatitis. *Gastroenterology Clinics of North America*, **19**, 895–904.
61. Kloppel, G. (1990) Pathology of chronic pancreatitis and pancreatic pain. *Acta Chirurgica Scandinavica*, **156**, 261–265.
62. Lankisch, P.G., Lohr, A., Otto, J. and Creutzfeldt, W. (1993) Natural course of chronic pancreatitis. I. Pain in relation to the duration of the disease, functional/morphological parameters, and prognosis of the disease. *Gastroenterology* (in press).
63. Lankisch, P.G., Otto, J., Lohr, A., Schirren, C.A. and Schuster, R. (1989) Pancreatic calcifications in patients with normal pancreatic function. *International Journal of Pancreatology*, **5**, 281–293.
64. Layer, P. and Singer, M.V. (1990) Non-alcohol-related etiologies in chronic pancreatitis. In *Chronic Pancreatitis* (Eds) Beger, H.G., Buchler, M., Ditschuneit, H. and Malfertheiner, P. pp. 35–40. Berlin: Springer-Verlag.
65. Levine, J.B., Warshaw, A.L., Falchuck, K.R. and Schapiro, R.H. (1977) The value of endoscopic retrograde pancreatography in the management of pancreatic ascites. *Surgery*, **81**, 300–302.
66. Linehan, I.P., Lambert, M.A., Brown, D.C., Kurtz, A.B., Cotton, P.B. and Russell, R.C.G. (1988) Total pancreatectomy for chronic pancreatitis. *Gut*, **358**, 365.
67. Little, A.G. and Moosa, A.R. (1981) Gastrointestinal hemorrhage from left-sided portal hypertension, an unappreciated complication of pancreatitis. *American Journal of Surgery*, **141**, 153–158.
68. Longmire, W.P. and Rose, A.S. (1973) Hemoductal pancreatitis. *Surgery, Gynecology and Obstetrics*, **136**, 246–250.
69. MacLaren, I.F. (1990) Observations and surgical management of chronic pancreatitis in the British Isles: a review of the twentieth century. *World Journal of Surgery*, **14**, 19–27.
70. Mannell, A., Adson, M.A., McIlrath, D.C. and Ilstrup, D.M. (1988) Surgical management of chronic pancreatitis: long-term results in 141 patients. *British Journal of Surgery*, **75**, 467–472.
71. Marotta, F., O'Keefe, S.J.D., Marks, I.N., Girdwood, A. and Young, G. (1989) Pancreatic enzyme replacement therapy. Importance of gastric acid secretion, H2 antagonists, and enteric coating. *Digestive Diseases and Sciences*, **34**, 456–461.
72. Miuake, H., Harada, H., Kunichika, K., Ochi, K. and Kimura, I. (1987) Clinical course and prognosis of chronic pancreatitis. *Pancreas*, **2**, 378–385.
73. Mixter, C.G., Keynes, M. and Cope, O. (1962) Further experience with pancreatitis as a diagnostic clue to hyperparathyroidism. *New England Journal of Medicine*, **266**, 265–272.
74. Miyake, H., Harada, H., Ochi, K., Kunichika, K., Tanake, J. and Kimura, I. (1989) Prognosis and prognostic factors in chronic pancreatitis. *Digestive Diseases and Sciences*, **34**, 449–455.
75. Moreaux, J. (1984) Long-term follow-up study of 50 patients and pancreatoduodenectomy for chronic pancreatitis. *World Journal of Surgery*, **8**, 346–353.
76. Morrow, C.E., Cohen, J.I., Sutherland, D.E.R. and Najarian, J.S. (1984) Chronic pancreatitis: Long-term surgical results of pancreatic duct drainage, pancreatic resection, and near-total pancreatectomy and islet autotransplantation. *Surgery*, **96**, 608–614.
77. Nagata, A., Homma, T., Tamai, K. *et al.* (1981) A study of chronic pancreatitis by serial endoscopic pancreatography. *Gastroenterology*, **81**, 884–891.
78. National Diabetes Data Group (1979) Classification and diagnosis of diabetes mellitus and other categories of glucose intolerance. *Diabetes*, **28**, 1039–1057.
79. Nealon, W.H., Townsend, C.M. and Thompson, J.C. (1988) Operative drainage of the pancreatic

duct delays functional impairment in patients with chronic pancreatitis. *Annals of Surgery*, **208**, 321–329.
80. Ohashi, K., Kim, J.-H., Hara, H., Aso, R., Akimoto, T. and Nakama, K. (1990) WBN/KOB rats. A new spontaneously occurring model of chronic pancreatitis. *International Journal of Pancreatology*, **6**, 231–247.
81. Oktedalen, O., Nygaard, K. and Osnes, M. (1990) Somatostatin in the treatment of pancreatic ascites. *Gastroenterology*, **99**, 520–521.
82. Otte, M. and Heufelder, A. (1990) Modern treatment of exocrine pancreatic insufficiency. In *Chronic Pancreatitis* (Eds) Beger, H.G., Buchler, M., Ditschuneit, H. and Malfertheiner, P. pp. 351–353. Berlin: Springer-Verlag.
83. Pain, J.A. and Knight, M.J. (1988) Pancreato-gastrostomy: The preferred operation for pain relief in chronic pancreatitis. *British Journal of Surgery*, **75**, 220.
84. Pap, A., Nauss, L.A. and DiMagno, E.P. (1990) Is percutaneous celiac plexus block associated with pain relief in chronic pancreatitis? A comparison among analgesic, alcohol and steroid blocks (abstract). *Pancreas*, **5**, 725.
85. Partington, P.F. and Rochelle, R.E. (1960) Modified Puestow procedure for retrograde drainage of the pancreatic duct. *Annals of Surgery*, **152**, 1037–1043.
86. Pitchumoni, C.S. (1990) Role of nutrition in chronic pancreatitis. In *Chronic Pancreatitis* (Eds) Beger, H.G., Buchler, M., Ditschuneit, H. and Malfertheiner, P. pp. 15–25. Berlin: Springer-Verlag.
87. Prinz, R.A., Aranha, G.V. and Greenlee, H.B. (1985) Combined pancreatic duct and upper gastrointestinal and biliary tract drainage in chronic pancreatitis. *Archives of Surgery*, **120**, 361–366.
88. Rattner, D.W. and Warshaw, A.L. (1990) Venous, biliary, and duodenal obstruction in chronic pancreatitis. *Hepato-Gastroenterology*, **37**, 301–306.
89. Riccardi, V.M., Shih, V.E., Holmes, L.B. and Nardi, G.L. (1975) Hereditary pancreatitis. Nonspecificity of aminoaciduria and diagnosis of occult disease. *Archives of Internal Medicine*, **135**, 822–825.
90. Robes-Diaz, G., Vargas, F., Uscanga, L. and Fernández-del Castillo, C. (1990) Chronic pancreatitis in Mexico City. *Pancreas*, **5**, 479–483.
91. Rossi, R.L. (1990) Pancreatic resections for chronic pancreatitis. *Hepato-Gastroenterology*, **37**, 277–282.
92. Rossi, R.L., Rotschild, K., Braasch, J.W., Munson, J.L. and ReMine, S.G. (1987) Pancreatoduodenectomy in the management of chronic pancreatitis. *Archives of Surgery*, **122**, 416–420.
93. Rossi, R.L., Soeldner, J.S., Braasch, J.W. *et al.* (1990) Long-term results of pancreatic resection and segmental pancreatic autotransplantation for chronic pancreatitis. *American Journal of Surgery*, **159**, 51–58.
94. Sahel, J., Bastid, C., Pellat, B., Schurgers, P. and Sarles, H. (1987) Endoscopic cystoduodenostomy of cysts of chronic calcifying pancreatitis: a report of 20 cases. *Pancreas*, **2**, 447–453.
95. Sandilands, D., Jeffrey, I.J.M., Haboubi, N.Y., MacLennan, I.A.M. and Braganza, J.M. (1990) Abnormal drug metabolism in chronic pancreatitis. Treatment with antioxidants. *Gastroenterology*, **98**, 766–772.
96. Sanfey, H., Buckley, G.B. and Cameron, J.L. (1985) The pathogenesis of acute pancreatitis. The source and role of oxygen-derived free radicals in three different experimental models. *Annals of Surgery*, **201**, 633–639.
97. Sarles, H., Bernard, J.P. and Gullo, L. (1990) Pathogenesis of chronic pancreatitis. *Gut*, **31**, 629–632.
98. Sarles, H., Bernard, J.P. and Johnson, C. (1989) Pathogenesis and epidemiology of chronic pancreatitis. *Annual Review of Medicine*, **40**, 453–468.
99. Sarles, H. and Laugier, R. (1981) Alcoholic pancreatitis. *Clinics in Gastroenterology*, **10**, 401–415.
100. Sarles, H., Sarles, J.C., Camatte, R. *et al.* (1965) Observations on 205 confirmed cases of acute pancreatitis, recurring pancreatitis and chronic pancreatitis. *Gut*, **6**, 545–559.
101. Sato, T., Nono, N., Matsuno, S. and Miyakawa, K. (1981) Follow-up results of surgical treatment for chronic pancreatitis. *American Journal of Surgery*, **142**, 317–323.
102. Sauerbruch, T., Holl, J., Sackmann, M. and Paumgartner, G. (1989) Extracorporeal shock wave lithotripsy of pancreatic stones. *Gut*, **30**, 1406–1411.
103. Schoenberg, M.H., Buchler, M., Gaspar, M. *et al.* (1990) Oxygen free radicals in acute pancreatitis of the rat. *Gut*, **31**, 1138–1143.
104. Shatney, C.H. and Lillehei, R.C. (1979) Surgical treatment of pancreatic pseudocysts. Analysis of 119 cases. *Annals of Surgery*, **189**, 386–901.
105. Sibert, J.R. (1978) Hereditary pancreatitis in England and Wales. *Journal of Medical Genetics*, **15**, 189–201.
106. Simeone, J.F., Wittenberg, J. and Ferruci, J.T. (1980) Modern concepts of imaging the pancreas. *Investigative Radiology*, **1**, 6–18.
107. Singh, S.M. and Reber, H.A. (1990) The pathology of chronic pancreatitis. *World Journal of Surgery*, **14**, 2–10.
108. Sitges-Serra, A., Alonso, M., de Lecea, C., Gores, P.F. and Sutherland, D.E.R. (1988) Pancreatitis and hyperparathyroidism. *British Journal of Surgery*, **75**, 158–160.
109. Sjoberg, R.J. and Kidd, G.S. (1989) Pancreatic diabetes mellitus. *Diabetes Care*, **12**, 715–724.
110. Slaff, J., Jacobson, D., Tillman, C.R., Curlington,

C. and Toskes, P. (1984) Protease-specific supression of pancreatic exocrine secretion. *Gastroenterology*, **87**, 44–52.
111. Stanley, J.L., Frey, C.F., Miller, A., Lindenbauer, S.M. and Child, C.G. (1976) Major arterial hemorrhage: as a complication of pancreatic pseudocysts and chronic pancreatitis. *Archives of Surgery*, **111**, 435.
112. Stone, H.H. and Chauvin, E.J. (1990) Pancreatic denervation for pain relief in chronic alcohol associated pancreatitis. *British Journal of Surgery*, **77**, 303–305.
113. Stone, W.M., Sarr, M.G., Nagorney, D.M. and McIlrath, D.C. (1988) Chronic pancreatitis. Results of Whipple's resection and total pancreatectomy. *Archives of Surgery*, **123**, 815–819.
114. Tanaka, T., Ichiba, Y., Miura, Y., Itoh, H. and Dohid, K. (1990) Pathogenesis of chronic alcoholic pancreatitis. *American Journal of Gastroenterology*, **85**, 1536–1537.
115. Taubin, H.C. and Spiro, H.M. (1973) Nutritional aspects of chronic pancreatitis. *American Journal of Clinical Nutrition*, **26**, 367–373.
116. Tewari, S.C., Jayaswal, R., Chauhan, M.S., Kaul, S.K. and Narayanan, V.A. (1989) Bilateral recurrent hemorrhagic pleural effusion in asymptomatic chronic pancreatitis. *Thorax*, **44**, 824–825.
117. Thomas, P.G., Augustine, P., Ramesh, H. and Rangabashyam, N. (1990) Observations and surgical management of tropical pancreatitis in Kerala and southern India. *World Journal of Surgery*, **14**, 32–42.
118. Toskes, P.P., Hansell, J., Cerda, J. and Deren, J.J. (1971) Vitamin B12 malabsorption in chronic pancreatic insufficiency: studies suggesting the presence of a pancreatic 'intrinsic factor'. *New England Journal of Medicine*, **284**, 627–631.
119. Trapnell, J.E. (1979) Chronic relapsing pancreatitis: a review of 64 cases. *British Journal of Surgery*, **66**, 471–475.
120. Van Dyke, J.A., Stanley, R.J. and Berland, L.L. (1985) Pancreatic imaging. *Annals of Internal Medicine*, **102**, 212–217.
121. Warshaw, A.L. (1985) Conservation of pancreatic tissue by combined gastric, biliary, and pancreatic duct drainage for pain from chronic pancreatitis. *American Journal of Surgery*, **149**, 563–569.
122. Warshaw, A.L. (1989) Obstructive pancreatitis: acute and chronic pancreatitis due to ductal obstruction by causes other than gallstones. In *Pancreatitis* (Eds) Carter, D.C. and Warshaw, A.L. pp. 71–89. Edinburgh: Churchill Livingstone.
123. Warshaw, A.L. (1989) Pancreatic cysts and pseudocysts: new rules for a new game. *British Journal of Surgery*, **76**, 533–534.
124. Warshaw, A.L. (1990) Indications for surgical treatment in chronic pancreatitis. In *Chronic Pancreatitis* (Eds) Beger, H.G., Buchler, M., Ditschuneit, H. and Malfertheiner, P. pp. 395–399. Berlin: Springer-Verlag.
125. Warshaw, A.L., Heizer, W.D. and Laster, L. (1968) Pancreatic insufficiency as the presenting feature of hyperparathyroidism. *Annals of Internal Medicine*, **68**, 161–167.
126. Warshaw, A.L., Jin, G. and Ottinger, L.W. (1987) Recognition and clinical implications of mesenteric and portal vein obstruction in chronic pancreatitis. *Archives of Surgery*, **122**, 410–415.
127. Warshaw, A.L. and Lee, K.-H. (1980) Aging changes of pancretic isoamylases and the appearance of 'old amylase' in the serum of patients with pancreatic pseudocysts. *Gastroenterology*, **79**, 1246–1251.
128. Warshaw, A.L. and Rattner, D.W. (1980) Facts and fallacies of common bile duct obstruction by pancreatic pseudocysts. *Annals of Surgery*, **192**, 33–37.
129. Warshaw, A.L. and Rattner, D.W. (1985) Timing of surgical drainage for pancreatic pseudocyst. *Annals of Surgery*, **202**, 720–724.
130. Warshaw, A.L., Richter, J.M. and Schapiro, R.H. (1983) The cause and treatment of pancreatitis associated with pancreas divisum. *Annals of Surgery*, **198**, 443–452.
131. Warshaw, A.L., Schapiro, R.H., Ferrucci, J.T. and Galdabini, J.J. (1976) Persistent obstructive jaundice, cholangitis, and biliary cirrhosis due to common bile duct stenosis in chronic pancreatitis. *Gastroenterology*, **70**, 562–567.
132. Warshaw, A.L., Simeone, J., Schapiro, R.H., Hedberg, S.E., Mueller, P.E. and Ferrucci, J.T. (1985) Objective evaluation of ampullary stenosis with ultrasonography and pancreatic stimulation. *American Journal of Surgery*, **149**, 65–72.
133. Warshaw, A.L., Simeone, J.F., Schapiro, R.H. and Flavin-Warshaw, B. (1990) Evaluation and treatment of the dominant dorsal duct syndrome (Pancreas divisum redefined). *American Journal of Surgery*, **159**, 59–66.
134. Weisiger, R.A. (1986) Oxygen radicals and ischemic tissue injury. *Gastroenterology*, **90**, 494–496.
135. Williams, S.T., Woltering, E.A., O'Dorisio, T.M. and Fletcher, W.S. (1989) Effect of octreotide acetate on pancreatic exocrine function. *American Journal of Surgery*, **57**, 459–462.
136. Wilson, J.S., Gossaat, D., Tait, A., Rouse, S., Jeng Juan, X. and Pirola, R.C. (1984) Evidence for an inherited predisposition to alcoholic pancreatitis. A controlled HLA typing study. *Digestive Diseases and Sciences*, **29**, 727–730.

CANCER OF THE EXOCRINE PANCREAS

P. Watanapa and R.C.N. Williamson

Carcinoma of the exocrine pancreas accounts for at least 95% of the malignant tumours arising in the pancreas. Increasing incidence, obscure aetiology and virtual incurability make this cancer the greatest oncological challenge in developed countries today.[108] Its incidence is rising in many areas of the world.[28,44,73] In Britain, pancreatic cancer is now the third most frequent cause of death from gastrointestinal cancer (after large bowel and stomach carcinomas) and the sixth leading cause of cancer death overall (*Figure 11.45*).[82] Over 6000 Britons die of this disease each year. In the USA 27 000 new cases and 24 500 deaths were attributed to this cancer in 1988; the mortality rate has risen steadily since 1930.[28] It is estimated that the incidence of pancreatic cancer has doubled in western Europe, trebled in the USA and more than quadrupled in Japan over the last 40 years.[37,44,82]

At present, the overall prognosis of this cancer is extremely poor. Regardless of therapy, median survival time is a paltry 2–3 months from diagnosis. The survival rate after 1 year is about 10% and, after 5 years, less than 3%. When first seen, 90% of patients have metastases. Success in early diagnosis of pancreatic cancer still seems remote. The first symptoms are often vague and non-specific, leading to an average delay of 6 months before diagnosis. By this time the disease has usually progressed beyond any current ability to effect a cure. Although under active scrutiny, effective screening tests for high-risk groups remain elusive, hence the current interest in the aetiology and epidemiology of the disease.

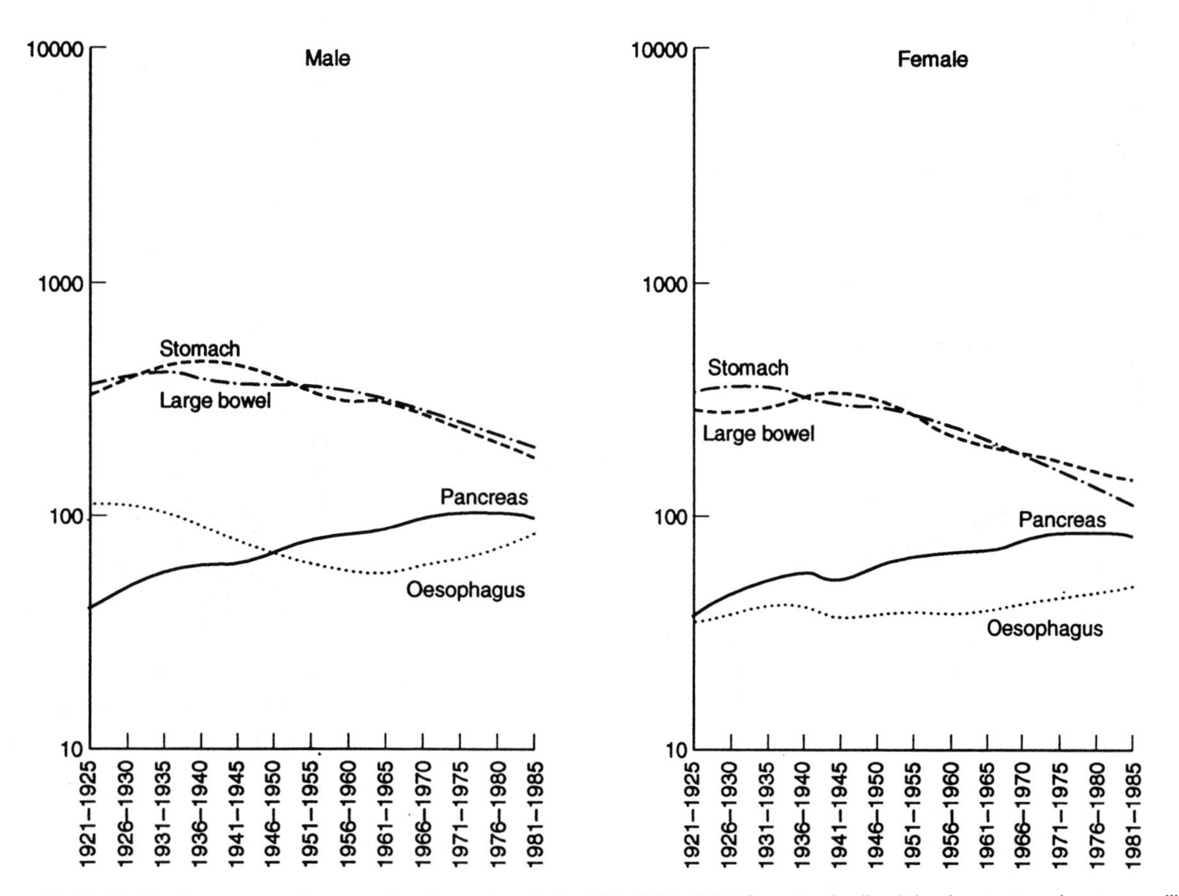

Figure 11.45 Deaths from pancreatic cancer by site and sex in the UK, 1921–1985. Age-standardized death rates are shown per million population (log scale).

EPIDEMIOLOGY

DEMOGRAPHIC CHARACTERISTICS

Age and sex

Age-specific incidence rates indicate that pancreatic cancer is rare before the age of 40 years. Incidence and mortality rates increase with age in both men and women, and this pattern is consistent throughout the world.[5,73] In Britain and the USA, the overall incidence is 110–120 per million population, increasing to 800–1000 per million for those aged 75 or older.[71]

Pancreatic cancer is more common in men. The male to female ratio (1.5–2.0:1) has remained constant over the years and is seen worldwide.[28,37,44,73] The relevance of this fact is not clear, because men on the whole are more exposed to the risk factors for the disease. Biological differences in susceptibility might account for the lower rates in women, who predominate among the elderly population.

Socioeconomic status

Variable over the years, the effect of social class on the risk of pancreatic cancer is small or non-existent (unlike for other gastrointestinal cancers). Most studies have shown that neither income or education have any effect.[80,111]

Racial and geographical differences

The lowest incidence of pancreatic cancer has been reported from Senegal and India, especially Madras, Bangalore, Poona, Nagpur and Bombay. The highest incidences of pancreatic cancer are to be found in affluent countries including Japan, Israel, Canada, Sweden, the UK and USA (*Figure 11.46*). In areas of low incidence, the rates are roughly similar for each sex, whereas in areas of high incidence, males predominate.[73]

Throughout the USA, black Americans have incidence rates that are 1.5–2.0 times higher than those of the white population, except in Connecticut where the incidence rate for males of each colour is only 80 per million.[73] Because this high rate in black Americans is not paralleled in African populations, environmental factors must play an important part in the distribution of the disease.

As one means of evaluating the relative contribution of genetic and environmental factors, several studies have compared the risk of pancreatic cancer between migrant populations and their countries of origin. In the USA, Issei (migrants from Japan) have a higher risk than either Nisei (children born in the USA of migrants from Japan) or American whites.[39] A similar pattern of increased risk has been noted among first-generation migrants to Australia from seven European countries.[65] Perhaps the exocrine activity of the pancreas is stimulated by marked dietary changes in the immediate aftermath of migration.

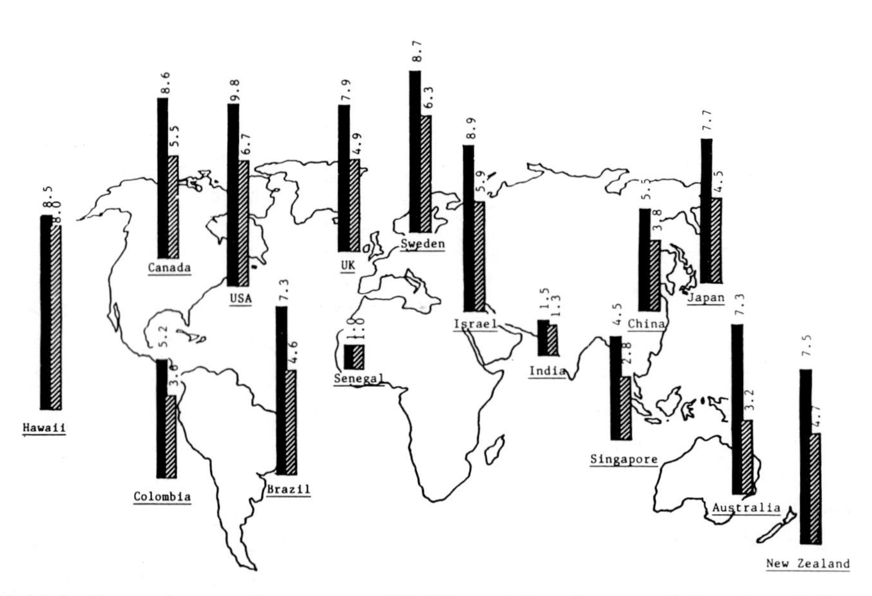

Figure 11.46 Worldwide incidence of pancreatic cancer per 100 000 population. Cancer registries shown in the graph are from Hawaii (whites), Canada, USA (New York City), Colombia (Cali), Brazil (Sao Paulo), Senegal, UK (England and Wales), Sweden, Israel (all Jews), India (Poona), Singapore (Chinese), China (Shanghai), Japan (Osaka), Australia (Queensland), New Zealand (non-Maori). (From Muir *et al.*[2] with permission.)

OCCUPATIONAL FACTORS

Several occupations have been implicated in pancreatic carcinogenesis. A fivefold increase in mortality rate was observed among a cohort of white men employed in a chemical plant manufacturing naphthylamine and benzidine who were followed for more than 25 years.[61] Evidence from either case-control or cohort studies, or both, shows an excess risk with a history of employment in the petrochemical industry or exposure to welding materials, paint thinners, detergents and floor-cleansing agents.[74] There is some biological credibility underlying the 'high risk' of pancreatic cancer previously reported among radiologists[17] and atomic energy workers,[47] but the case remains unproven. Two recent British surveys on the death of nearly 40 000 employees of the Atomic Energy Authority and about 15 000 workers at the Sellafield plant of British Nuclear Fuels showed no significant association between radiation exposure and cancer of the pancreas.[11,94]

DIETARY FACTORS

Fats, meats, vegetables and fruits

There is a positive correlation between per capita consumption of fats and incidence of pancreatic cancer.[26] In support of this statement, high-fat diets enhance pancreatic carcinogenesis in rats exposed to azaserine.[83] It may be that cholecystokinin secreted in response to dietary fat stimulates cell proliferation in the exocrine pancreas.

Increased consumption of meat leads to a higher incidence of pancreatic cancer.[27,44] In contrast, consumption of vegetable proteins (notably soy products), fruits and vegetables (especially carrots and citrus fruits) is associated with decreased risk.[37,58,66] Many of these foods have a high protease inhibitor content. Although foods rich in trypsin inhibitors (such as raw soy flour) have been shown to act as promoters of pancreatic carcinogenesis in some animal models,[64] these deleterious effects of protease inhibitors are species-specific: they occur in rats, chicks, mice and young guinea pigs but not in dogs, growing swine, calves, adult guinea pigs and primates such as man.[7] There is evidence that protease inhibitors in the diet contribute to the prevention of at least three human cancers: breast, colon and prostate. Their possible protective effect against human pancreatic cancer remains to be determined.[102]

Coffee and tea

Considerable attention has focused on the relationship between coffee and cancer of the pancreas. Some investigators have found a positive association[44,58] whilst others have not.[21,43,111] A recent large case-control study conducted in a area of high risk showed that the risk of pancreatic cancer was unrelated to coffee consumption after adjustment for smoking habits, alcohol intake, diet and demographic factors.[27] As heavy coffee drinkers were found to eat little fruit, any link with pancreatic cancer could merely reflect the dietary correlates of coffee drinking. It also seems unlikely that tea drinking is causally related to cancer of the pancreas.[43,58]

Alcohol

No clear relationship between alcohol consumption and pancreatic cancer emerged from an extensive review of the subject in 1986.[101] Subsequent case-control and cohort studies have supported this negative finding.[27,43,44]

Smoking

The most established risk factor for pancreatic cancer is cigarette smoking. Several studies also show a dose-response relationship.[21,27,37,43,44,58] The increased risk associated with current smoking in each sex is estimated at two- to threefold. The use of tobacco products other than cigarettes has not been clearly shown to increase risk.[27,111]

Many mechanisms of action have been postulated. Nitrosamines, which are potent pancreatic carcinogens in the hamster, may be absorbed from tobacco smoke and reach the pancreas through the blood stream. Alternatively, the procarcinogen might be activated by the liver, excreted into the bile and then refluxed into the pancreatic duct. In addition, pancreatic cancer could be potentiated indirectly by hyperlipidaemia induced by cigarette smoking.

MEDICAL HISTORY

Family history

Familial occurrence of pancreatic cancer is rare but has been reported. Several anecdotal reports have shown familial clustering of the disease. A population-based, case-control study in Quebec, Canada, has shown that 6.7% of cases and 0.7% of controls had a positive family history,[33] findings that are supported by a recent American report.[57]

Several genetic (autosomal dominant) disorders predispose to pancreatic cancer, including hereditary pancreatitis, multiple endocrine neoplasia type

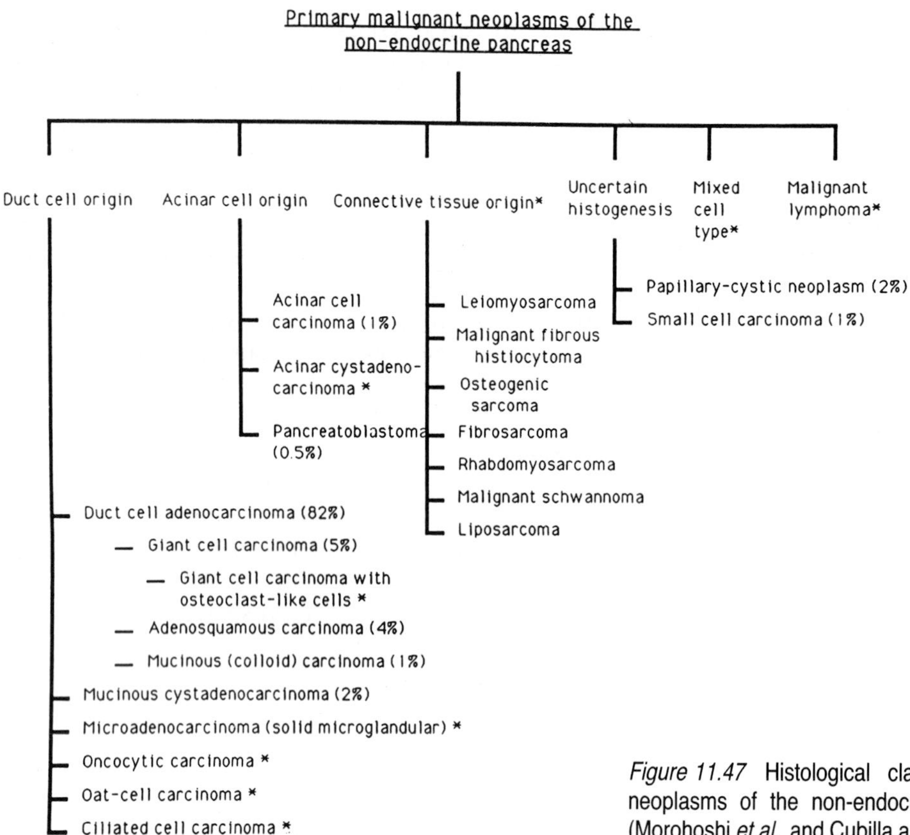

Figure 11.47 Histological classification of primary malignant neoplasms of the non-endocrine pancreas. * = Rare tumour (Morohoshi *et al.* and Cubilla and Fitzgerald, with permission.)

I, glucagonoma syndrome, Gardner's syndrome and Lynch syndrome type II, which comprises proximal colonic carcinoma, often multiple, occurring at an early age, with an increased risk for certain other cancers such as breast and pancreas.

Diabetes mellitus

Several case-control and cohort studies have shown an increased risk of pancreatic cancer among diabetics.[21,43,66] A strong association has emerged between islet cell dysfunction and clinically manifest cancer of the exocrine pancreas. This association often appears even when the location of size of the tumour makes simple destruction of endocrine tissue an unlikely explanation. The interval between onset of diabetes and appearance of the tumour varies in an exponentially declining manner, suggesting that diabetes is an early symptom of pancreatic cancer rather than an actual risk factor.

Pancreatitis

Chronic pancreatitis has been alleged to predispose to pancreatic carcinoma,[9] but this may hold true only for patients with the hereditary form of pancreatitis. In acquired chronic pancreatitis, usually of alcoholic aetiology, there are several case reports of associated pancreatic cancer, but a definite predisposition has not yet been confirmed.[9,36] The inflammatory changes often seen in patients with pancreatic carcinoma result from duct occlusion by the tumour, that is distal obstructive pancreatopathy.

Allergic diseases and tonsillectomy

Relative protection against pancreatic cancer has been reported in patients with asthma, allergic skin reactions, allergy to natural antigens or indeed any allergic disease.[58,66] Previous tonsillectomy may also reduce the risk,[36] conceivably because the tonsils provide a source of antigenic stimulus that plays a role in carcinogenesis.

Gastrectomy

Between three- to sevenfold increments in the incidence of pancreatic cancer have been described in patients undergoing gastric resection 20 years previously.[15,58,66] The following hypotheses might explain this link:

1. Altered gastric regulation of pancreatic function following gastrectomy affects the homeostatic

responses of the gland to 'toxic' substances in the bile, blood or gastric juice.

2. Detoxification of substances metabolized in the small intestine may be impaired after gastrectomy, thereby increasing pancreatic exposure to ingested carcinogens.
3. Decreased gastric acidity permits endogenous nitrosation in gastric juice with formation of N-nitroso carcinogens.[58]

Gallstone disease

Two studies show a positive association between gallstones and pancreatic carcinoma,[21,75] possibly because they have aetiological factors in common.

PATHOLOGY

Although pancreatic ductal tissue accounts for a small proportion of the gland, it gives rise to nearly all the non-endocrine tumours. Less than 5% of tumours originate from either acinar cells or connective tissue elements (leaving aside those that are of uncertain histogenesis).

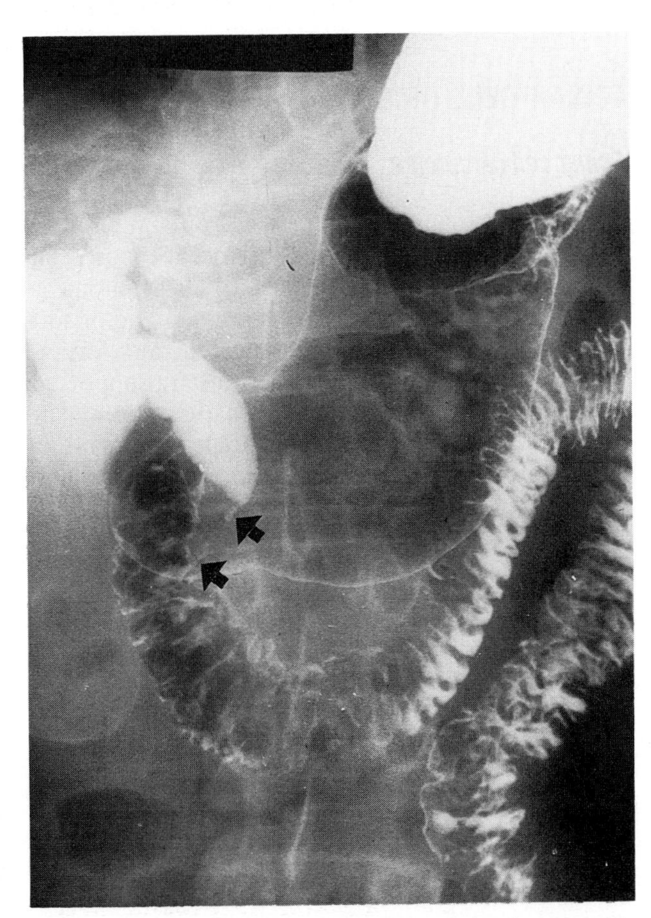

Figure 11.48 Percutaneous transhepatic cholangiogram with concomitant hypotonic duodenography in a 65-year-old man with carcinoma of the pancreatic head. There is a tight stricture (arrowed) in the terminal segment of the common bile duct.

Table 11.7 UICC classification of exocrine pancreatic cancer (1987)

T: Primary tumour

TX	Primary tumour cannot be assessed
T0	No evidence of primary tumour
T1	Tumour limited to the pancreas
	T1a Tumour 2 cm or less in greatest dimension
	T1b Tumour more than 2 cm in greatest dimension
T2	Tumour extends directly to any of the following: duodenum, bile duct, peripancreatic tissues
T3	Tumour extends directly to any of the following: stomach, spleen, colon, adjacent large vessels

N: Regional lymph nodes

NX	Regional lymph nodes cannot be assessed
N0	No regional lymph node metastasis
N1	Regional lymph node metastasis

M: Distant metastasis

MX	Presence of distant metastasis cannot be assessed
M0	No distant metastasis
M1	Distant metastasis

Stage grouping

Stage I	T1	N0	M0
	T2	N0	M0
Stage II	T3	N0	M0
Stage III	Any T	N1	M0
Stage IV	Any T	Any N	M1

Several classifications of exocrine pancreatic tumours have been published but none is accepted worldwide. *Figure 11.48* shows a classification that correlates well with prognosis. The important types are described below. The TNM staging system for exocrine pancreatic cancer recently recommended by International Union Against Cancer (UICC) is given in *Table 11.7*. Survival is clearly affected by stage.

DUCT CELL ORIGIN

Duct cell adenocarcinoma (ductal adenocarcinoma, adenocarcinoma of the pancreas)

Duct cell carcinoma and its variants (giant cell carcinoma, adenosquamous carcinoma and mucinous carcinoma) comprise over 90% of pancreatic exocrine tumours. This cancer is characterized by its expression of carcinoembryonic antigen, carbohydrate antigen 19-9 and the keratins 7, 8, 18 and 19.

Histologically, most differentiated ductal adenocarcinomas display an intensive desmoplasia. Immunocytochemical and biochemical tests demonstrate type I and V collagen, as well as fibronectin within the dense fibrous stroma, but rarely type III collagen.[54] As this is the dominant pancreatic malignancy, all demographic and epidemiological data concerning pancreatic cancer relate to the biological behaviour of duct cell adenocarcinoma.

Giant cell carcinoma (pleomorphic large cell carcinoma)

Giant cell carcinoma is characterized by bizarre giant cells and sarcomatous elements. The tumour is usually large (average diameter 11 cm), moderately firm and grey in colour with many areas of necrosis. Massive retroperitoneal adenopathy and haematogenous metastases are frequent findings. It has a similar age and sex distribution to 'ordinary' duct carcinoma but carries a worse prognosis; median survival time is a bare 2 months.[70] A variant of giant cell carcinoma with osteoclast-like cells seems to have a less aggressive course.

Adenosquamous carcinoma

Adenosquamous carcinoma contains a mixture of both epithelial types, but its clinical behaviour is similar to that of duct adenocarcinoma.

Mucinous (colloid) adenocarcinoma

This carcinoma is characterized by a marked excess of mucin production. These tumours are usually larger and softer than duct cell adenocarcinomas. The cut surface is glistening and yellowish-white, containing tiny cystic spaces filled with mucoid or creamy material. Histologically, clusters of neoplastic cells sometimes have a signet ring appearance. The prognosis is a little better.

Mucinous cystadenocarcinoma

This accounts for about 2% of pancreatic exocrine tumours. The peak age of presentation is 40–60 years with a 6:1 female to male ratio. The tumour contains unilocular or multilocular cysts filled with sticky mucin; its fibrous capsule may be calcified. The clinical presentation sometimes resembles that of chronic pancreatitis. High-grade lesions have often metastasized before they are diagnosed, yet the survival rate after 5 years is 18%.[48] The 'benign' variant, *mucinous cystadenoma,* is now usually categorized in the same group as cystoadenocarcinoma (under the heading of mucinous cystic tumour), as it is potentially malignant.[54,112] Both mucinous cystadenoma and cystadenocarcinoma stain positive for carcinoembryonic antigen, carbohydrate antigen 19-9, epithelial membrane antigen and keratin.[112] By contrast, *microcystic* (*serous*) *adenoma* is a benign and slow-growing tumour of elderly women. This tumour has a typical honeycomb appearance on cross-section. Histologically, there are multiple cysts lined with glycogen-rich epithelium, a vascular stroma, dystrophic calcification and cholesterol clefts. Microcystic adenoma may be derived from the centroacinar cells of the pancreas, whereas mucinous cystadenoma is derived from ductular cells.[2]

Microadenocarcinoma

This is a rare but aggressive tumour, which affects a slightly younger age group (30–70 years). It contains small rosette-like glands with solid cellular areas separated by fine fibrous septa. The absence of both zymogen and neurosecretory granules on electron microscopy is consistent with a duct cell origin.

ACINAR CELL ORIGIN

Acinar cell carcinoma

Acinar cell carcinoma comprises about 1% of non-endocrine pancreatic cancers. It occurs mostly in elderly patients of both sexes.[72] The tumour is lobulated, large, fairly well demarcated and of soft consistency. Histologically, typical acinar formations and partly trabecular structures are supported by a scanty stroma; solid and anaplastic patterns may also be found. Acinar cell carcinoma is characterized by the presence of pancreatic enzymes and zymogen granules demonstrated by immunocytochemistry and in the ultrastructure.[72] Non-suppurative panniculitis of the extremities (and sometimes of the bone marrow) probably reflects release of lipase from the tumour. As with most pancreatic cancers, the prognosis is poor.

Pancreatoblastoma

Pancreatoblastoma is a rare tumour confined to young children aged between 3 and 7 years. The term pancreatoblastoma was proposed because of the mixed histological pattern containing either epithelial structures with acinar cell differentiation and squamoid nests or more primitive epithelial and mesenchymal components.[72] Most children present with abdominal pain or a palpable mass, or both;

one-third have jaundice.[14] α-Fetoprotein is occasionally produced by the tumour.[45] Most pancreatoblastomas are encapsulated, and complete surgical removal is associated with a good prognosis.

CONNECTIVE TISSUE ORIGIN

Primary sarcoma of the pancreas comprises less than 1% of all pancreatic malignancies. Types include leiomyosarcoma, malignant fibrous histiocytoma, malignant haemangiopericytoma, fibrosarcoma and malignant schwannoma.

PAPILLARY CYSTIC NEOPLASM (SOLID AND CYSTIC TUMOUR)

This is a rare tumour that affects adolescent girls and young women almost exclusively, with a mean age of 23 years (range 2–47 years).[109] This tumour usually presents with a mass that is either palpable or seen on CT undertaken for vague upper abdominal symptoms. The tumour contains solid tissue with areas of haemorrhage and cystic degeneration. Its histogenesis is uncertain: the solid components resemble an endocrine neoplasm but without the typical immunocytochemical and ultrastructural features. Papillary cystic neoplasm is of low-grade malignancy and can generally be cured by wide resection, which usually entails pancreatoduodenectomy if the lesion is located in the pancreatic head. The prognosis is excellent following radical surgery.

MALIGNANT LYMPHOMA

This tumour can arise within the pancreas but this is very rare. Most pancreatic lymphomas are secondary to generalized disease. They are often of the malignant histiocytic type. Chemotherapy can sometimes provide effective control.[92]

CLINICAL FEATURES

CARCINOMA OF THE HEAD OF PANCREAS

Cancer of the exocrine pancreas arises from the head of the gland in 68–87% of patients.[77,98] Clinical presentations are shown in *Table 11.8*. Typically, patients present with weight loss, obstructive jaundice, variable abdominal pain, malaise and anorexia. Average weight loss is about 12 kg:[46,77] anorexia, nausea, vomiting, maldigestion owing to exocrine pancreatic insufficiency and diabetes may all be contributory factors.

Table 11.8 Clinical features of cancer of the exocrine pancreas (From Howard and Jordan, with permission)

Head of pancreas (% patients)		*Body/tail of pancreas (% patients)*	
Symptoms		*Symptoms*	
Weight loss	92	Weight loss	100
Jaundice	82	Pain	87
Pain	72	Weakness	43
Anorexia	64	Nausea/vomiting	40
Nausea/vomiting	41	Anorexia	33
Signs		*Signs*	
Jaundice	87	Palpable liver	33
Palpable liver	83	Tenderness	27
Palpable gallbladder	29	Abdominal mass	23
Tenderness	26	Ascites	20
Ascites	14	Jaundice	13

Jaundice occurs in 80–90% of patients and follows either invasion or compression of the common bile duct. The jaundice is relatively painless but it tends to be unrelenting and rapidly progressive. If the tumour arises from the uncinate process or neck of pancreas, jaundice is a relatively late feature and is commonly accompanied by marked weight loss.

Pain is a presenting symptom in 70% of patients. It may be vague, diffuse and limited to the epigastrium and hypochondrium. Pain radiates to the back in 25% and is confined to the back in 5% or less. Back pain usually means irresectability and is associated with short survival.[62]

Physical examination at the time of presentation reveals jaundice and hepatomegaly in more than 80% of cases. Courvoisier's sign of a palpable gallbladder is a useful indication that is present in most patients with obstructive jaundice caused by carcinoma of the pancreas (unlike those with gallstones or hilar cholangiocarcinoma). Benign obstruction of the common bile duct is seldom as complete as the obstruction of pancreatic cancer. It is probably this fact that explains Courvoisier's law rather than the indistensibility of the gallbladder in chronic cholecystitis because, in our experience, the gallbladder has been palpable in a number of patients with concomitant gallstones and pancreatic cancer.

CARCINOMA OF THE BODY AND TAIL OF PANCREAS

The tumours are 'silent' in their early stages and are generally more advanced than lesions in the head by the time of presentation. Their clinical features (see *Table 11.8*) are dominated by weight loss, which is often profound (mean 15 kg),[77] and back pain which occurs in up to 60% of patients. Jaundice is less common and usually reflects an advanced cancer with involvement of the porta hepatis. Vomiting can arise at a late stage from malignant invasion of the duodenojejunal flexure. An abdominal mass is palpated more frequently than in patients with cancer of the pancreatic head (20–25% versus 10%). Commonly, diagnosis is preceded by several months of vague ill health.

Trousseau's sign of migratory thrombophlebitis has been reported in 7% of patients with pancreatic cancer, mostly lesions in the body and tail.[79] Perhaps the partial anticoagulation of obstructive jaundice prevents its occurrence with lesions in the head. Standard coagulation tests are unhelpful in predicting the development of Trousseau's sign, though the platelet count may be reduced. The phenomenon is quite often seen with other occult or overt visceral malignancies, notably carcinoma of the bronchus. Superficial thrombophlebitis, deep vein thrombosis and pulmonary embolism are difficult to control with standard methods of anticoagulation.

Between 20 and 70% of pancreatic cancer patients show glucose intolerance on testing and some are frankly diabetic.[51,90] An increase in insulin requirement in an established and stable diabetic patient should always raise suspicion of pancreatic carcinoma.

INVESTIGATIONS

FULL BLOOD COUNT

Most pancreatic cancer patients are anaemic, partly from nutritional deficiency but more importantly, from chronic blood loss. Stool examination usually reveals occult blood in patients with cancer of the pancreatic head.

BIOCHEMISTRY

Serum levels of lipase, amylase and glucose may be elevated in patients with pancreatic cancer, but these changes are non-specific.[35] Serial measurement of liver function tests is much more valuable than a single set of values. Pancreatic cancer is suggested by a rapid elevation of serum bilirubin and alkaline phosphatase but relatively modest increments in transaminases (as the hepatocytes are injured by unrelieved bile duct obstruction).

PANCREATIC FUNCTION TESTS AND SECRETORY PROTEIN PROFILES

Pancreatic exocrine function is impaired in 90–95% of patients with pancreatic cancer. Malnutrition and damage to the pancreatic parenchyma compound the effects of an obstructed pancreatic duct. Fat malabsorption is aggravated by the absence of bile salts from the intestinal lumen in jaundiced patients. As already mentioned, glucose intolerance is common. These abnormalities of exocrine (and endocrine) function are non-specific and do not help to differentiate pancreatic cancer from chronic pancreatitis. If a microcomputer is used to analyse isoelectric focusing patterns, however, a characteristic profile of exocrine secretion may be found in cancer patients.[106] Similarly, lactoferrin content is elevated in pure pancreatic juice obtained from patients with chronic pancreatitis but not in those with pancreatic cancer.[16]

IMAGING STUDIES

Radiology

Plain abdominal films are of limited value. Although diffuse calcification indicates chronic pancreatitis, some endocrine and cystic tumours may be calcified. Barium meal and especially hypotonic duodenography may show widening of the duodenal loop and distortion or invasion of the descending duodenum, but appearances are normal in many cancers of the head and all but the most extensive cancers of the body and tail (*Figure 11.49*).

Ultrasound

Satisfactory visualization of the pancreas can be obtained in 70–90% of patients, and similar sensitivity rates are reported for the diagnosis of pancre-

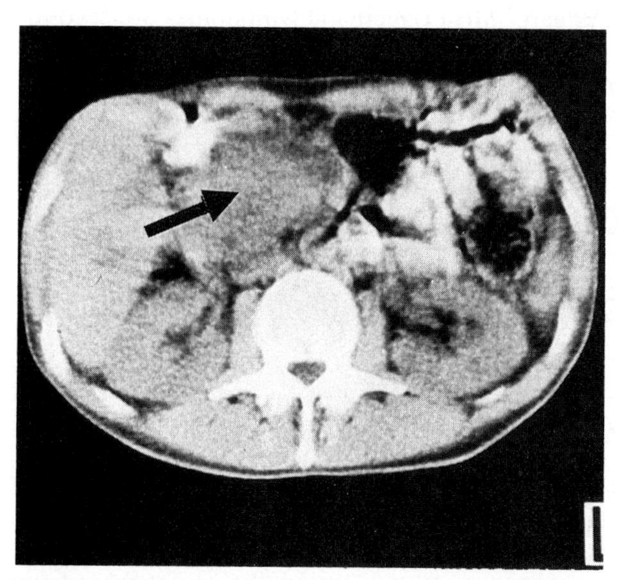

Figure 11.49 CT scan shows a large mass (arrowed) in the pancreatic head/neck in a 51-year-old man without obstructive jaundice.

Table 11.9 Detection rates (%) for pancreatic cancer with different imaging techniques. (From Yasuda *et al.*, with permission.)

Tumour diameter	*Endoscopic ultrasound*	*Conventional ultrasound*	*ERCP*	*CT*	*Angiography*
≤20 mm	100	29	57	29	14
20–30 mm	100	70	80	60	66
≥30 mm	100	82	97	94	96
Total	100	72	88	78	75

atic tumours. Parenchymal defects as small as 2 cm in diameter can sometimes be detected before overall changes in the size and contour of the gland. Several recent studies indicate that ultrasound scanning has achieved a sensitivity approaching that of CT in detecting pancreatic carcinoma.[78] As ultrasound costs less than a third of CT or endoscopic retrograde cholangiopancreatography, it should be the initial investigation in patients with a suspected pancreatic cancer.

Ultrasonographic diagnosis of early cancer is hampered by overlying bowel gas, obesity and the relative inaccessibility of the organ. To overcome these problems a new approach has been developed, namely *endoscopic ultrasound*. By means of balloon contact and a water-filled stomach, the whole organ can be visualized without any blind spots on the ultrasonographic images. This technique discloses the presence or absence of pancreatic cancer with an accuracy rate of 75–100%.[52,97,113] It is also valuable for determining resectability based on the evidence of vascular invasion and involvement of lymph nodes or other organs.[97,113] Current experience in detecting small cancers under 2 cm diameter is promising. (*Table 11.9*), but endoscopic ultrasound still has certain drawbacks that limit its value:

1. The echoendoscope is not as easy to manipulate as a conventional endoscope because of the rigidity of the long tip, and this causes difficulty in placing the transducer in the descending duodenum.
2. The water-filled balloon method of contact with the gut wall is unreliable.
3. The echoendoscope does not have biopsy capability.

Computed tomography

CT has become an invaluable diagnostic modality in the evaluation of pancreatic cancer in both icteric and anicteric patients. CT scanners with rapid sequence acquisition allow good visualization of the pancreas in well over 90% of patients. The most frequent finding in pancreatic cancer is the presence of a localized mass (*Figure 11.49*). Because recognition of a pancreatic mass by CT depends upon distortion of gland contour, tumours must usually attain a size of 2–3 cm to be detected. CT will accurately demonstrate 60–90% of such lesions.[78,85] In addition, it can determine the extent of local (nodal) and distant (hepatic) spread of the disease, providing useful information about staging. When intravenous contrast material is injected during scanning, the crucial relationship of the tumour to the portal vein and its tributaries can be delineated, thus providing further information about the resectability of the cancer. CT is 92% accurate when it predicts irresectability but only 56–72% sensitive. Conversely, it is only 38–45% accurate in predicting resectability.[85,104]

Dynamic CT is superior to conventional high-dose contrast enhancement in displaying the relatively low density of the hypovascular pancreatic carcinoma. At present, CT is best utilized in conjunction with other available investigations when assessing patients with early and potentially resectable tumours. The combined performance of CT, angiography and laparoscopy allows 89% of irresectable tumours and 90% of resectable tumours to be identified correctly.[104]

Endoscopic retrograde cholangiopancreatography

Pancreatography has become one of the most reliable investigations for the detection of pancreatic carcinoma, with a sensitivity and specificity of nearly 90%. Delineation of ductal anatomy enables early diagnosis of resectable tumours. Cannulation of the ampulla can also produce specimens for a reliable cytological diagnosis of malignancy. The sensitivity of cytology of pure pancreatic juice varies between 54–84%, whilst specificity is always high (97–98%).[22] Combining ductography with cytology increases diagnostic accuracy to over 90%.

Although not infallible, it is one of the best techniques for discriminating between chronic pancreatitis and pancreatic cancer[25,34] and even to detect pancreatic carcinoma coexisting with chronic

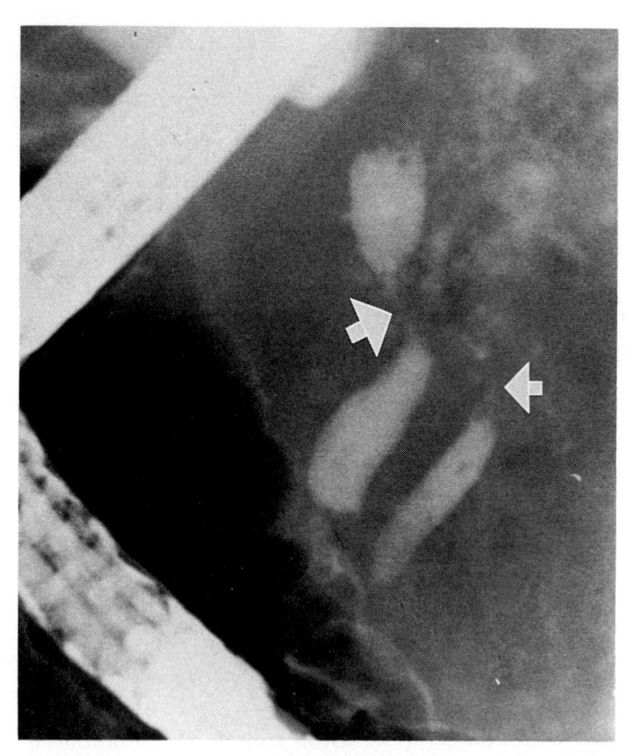

Figure 11.50 Pancreatogram showing the 'double duct' sign. Both the pancreatic duct and the common bile duct are narrowed close to their terminations by a carcinoma of the pancreatic head (arrows).

pancreatitis.[91] The usual pancreatographic abnormalities in cancer are obstruction and encasement of the pancreatic duct. With a tumour in the head, simultaneous involvement of the pancreatic duct and common bile duct produces the classical 'double duct' sign (*Figure 11.50*). In malignant disease the pancreatic duct obstruction is usually abrupt, but in chronic pancreatitis the narrowing is tapered. Limitations of pancreatography include a cannulation failure rate of 15–20% in experienced hands and complications of sepsis or acute pancreatitis following injection of contrast into the obstructed ductal systems.

Angiography

Pancreatic angiography is an important step in the preoperative determination of resectability once the tumour has been identified by ultrasound, CT or pancreatography.[6] Encasement of the splenic, hepatic or superior mesenteric arteries indicates irresectability, likewise the demonstration of hepatic metastases (*Figure 11.51a*). In addition, mapping of the branches of the coeliac and superior mesenteric arteries will demonstrate congenital anomalies in 25% of patients in whom a pancreatic resection is considered.[6] The most common deviant (14%) is an accessory or replaced right hepatic artery arising from the superior mesenteric artery, and the entire hepatic artery may spring from this vessel.[6] The anomalous right (or common) hepatic artery generally passes behind the pancreatic head and portal vein. During pancreatoduodenectomy it may be mistaken for the gastroduodenal artery and accidentally ligated, a manoeuvre that is hazardous in deeply jaundiced patients.

It is important to obtain late films during both the coeliac and superior mesenteric 'runs' so as to demonstrate the confluence of the splenic and superior mesenteric veins to form the portal vein. The most reliable sign of an irresectable pancreatic cancer is clear-cut invasion or obstruction of the portal or superior mesenteric vein, especially when collaterals show that this finding is not an artefact (*Figure 11.51b*). Arterial encasement is a less reliable criterion, although if a major extrapancreatic artery is encased, resection is usually fruitless.[6] The accuracy of angiography in predicting irresectability varies between 58–95%,[6,104] but its accuracy for predicting resectability is lower.[104]

FINE NEEDLE ASPIRATION CYTOLOGY

Preoperative cytological diagnosis of pancreatic cancer is possible using either a percutaneous fine needle aspiration technique or at pancreatography (see above). At present, percutaneous aspiration is a well-established procedure for the accurate diagnosis of neoplasms in the pancreas and is usually performed under CT or ultrasound guidance. It may also be used preoperatively. True-positive diagnosis of pancreatic cancer by cytological evaluation of percutaneous aspiration samples correlates with the definitive histological diagnosis in 60–90% of cases.[55,87] The sensitivity rate for detecting malignant disease is 67–86% and the specificity is 95–100%.[55,87] The false negative rate varies between 10–24%, but there is no false-positive result reported from most series.[55,87] Preoperative aspiration yields the same sensitivity rates as the percutaneous technique.[87] As percutaneous aspiration can only be employed when the mass can be imaged on ultrasound scan, it has no role in the early detection of pancreatic cancer.

A positive result from preoperative cytology is always useful. In patients without biliary or duodenal obstruction, in whom resection is inappropriate, it may obviate laparotomy. The main limitations of percutaneous aspiration are:

1. The relatively high false-negative results, which may reflect inadequacies in sampling, technical preparation or interpretation.
2. The need for an experienced cytologist.

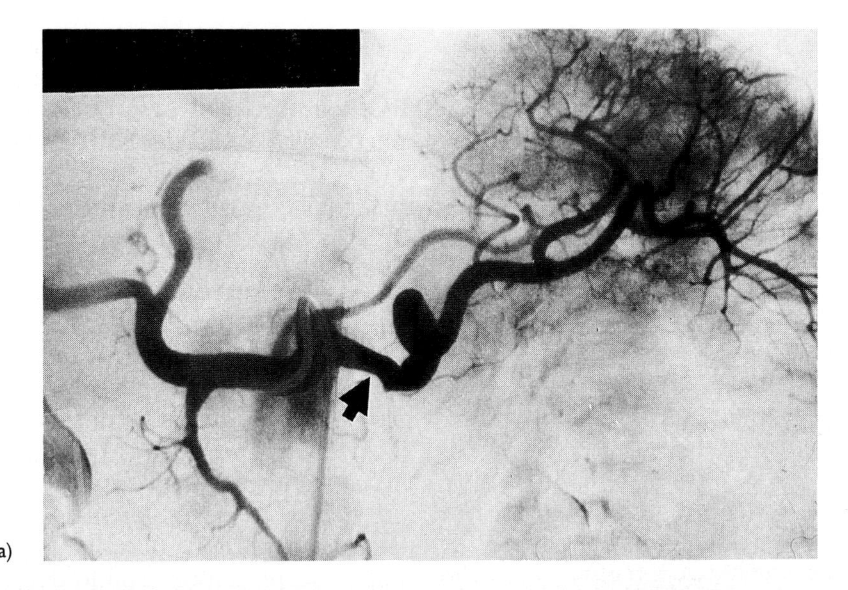
(a)

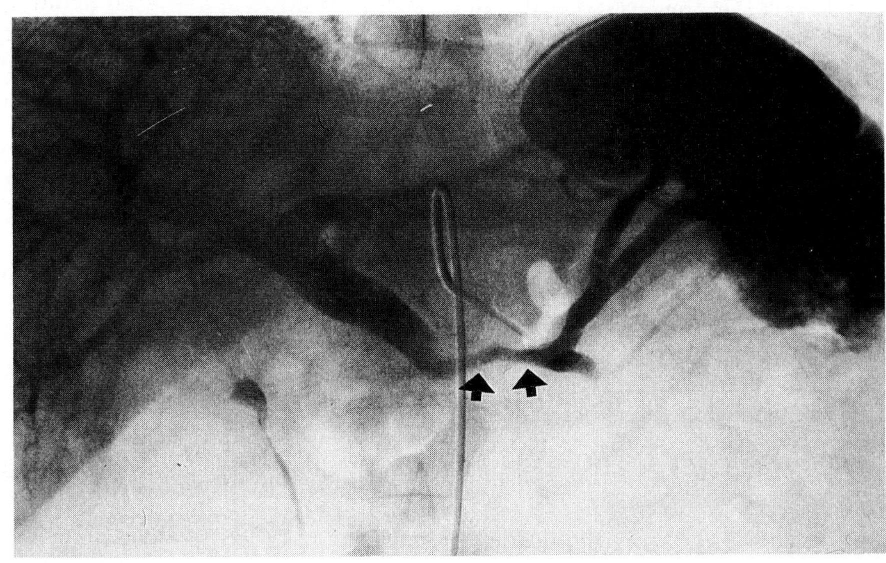
(b)

Figure 11.51 Angiography in a 45-year-old man with an irresectable carcinoma of the body of pancreas. (a) Arteriogram shows encasement of the origin of the splenic artery; the short rigid segment of vessel (arrowed) failed to relax with an injection of adrenalin and was therefore not due to spasm. (b) Venous phase films show stenosis of the distal segment of splenic vein (arrowed) up to its point of junction with the superior mesenteric vein (not visualized) to form the portal vein.

3. The very small risk of acute pancreatitis or needle tract seeding of malignant cells. Nevertheless, percutaneous aspiration is now accepted as a quick, safe, inexpensive and comparatively reliable method for diagnosing pancreatic carcinoma.

TUMOUR MARKERS

Because pancreatic cancer is notoriously difficult to diagnose in its early stages, particularly in the non-jaundiced patient, several serum markers have been extensively studied. Tumour markers include carcinoembryonic antigen, pancreatic oncofetal antigen, pancreatic cancer-associated antigen, α-fetoprotein, ribonuclease, ferritin, lactoferrin and various gastrointestinal hormones. None of these markers has so far proved to be specific or gained widespread clinical use.[4] A new generation of tumour markers is now available, based on monoclonal antibodies to tumour-associated antigens, notably CA 19-9, CA 50, CA 125, Span-1 and DU-PAN 2. Sensitivity and specificity rates of these tumour markers are summarized in *Table 11.10*.

CA 19-9 has been identified as a sialylated sugar moiety. This antigen occurs mainly as a monosialoganglioside in the tissue and can be detected in the serum of patients with adenocarcinoma. Because

Table 11.10 Sensitivity and specificity rates obtained with single and combined assays of tumour markers in pancreatic exocrine cancer. (From references [10,38,41,53,59,76,88])

Tumour markers	*Sensitivity (%)*	*Specificity (%)*
CA 19-9[a]	80	90
CA 50[b]	81	80
CA 125[c]	49	72
Span-1[d]	81	76
DU-PAN 2[e]	66	92
CA 19-9[a] + CA 50[b]	96	82
CA 50[b] + CEA	96	79
CA 19-9[a] + CEA	92	77
CA 125[c] + CA 50[b]	96	79
CA 125[c] + CEA	76	75
CA 19-9[a] + CA 125[c]	96	76

[a]Cut-off value = 37u/ml; [b]cut-off value = 17 u/ml; [c]cut-off value = 26 u/ml; [d]cut-off value = 30 u/ml; [e]cut-off value = 400 u/ml.
CA = Carbohydrate antigen.
CEA = Carcinoembryonic antigen.

the production of CA 19-9 requires the expression of the Lewis blood group gene, the antigen cannot be used as a biomarker in patients with Le^{a-b-} phenotype (4–7% of the population).[96] CA 19-9 radioimmunoassay is currently the most successful serological test for pancreatic cancer. Patients with irresectable or metastatic disease tend to have much higher levels of this antigen than those with resectable disease.[41,88] Assay of CA 19-9 in pancreatic juice is even more sensitive than serum assay in detecting resectable pancreatic cancer.[59]

CA 50 is found in serum as a high-molecular-weight glycoprotein fraction and on cell surfaces in gangliosides. The CA 50 assay is based on an IgM monoclonal antibody (C 50) which, like CA 19-9, has been obtained by immunization of mice with cells from a human colorectal adenocarcinoma.

CA 125 is an established marker for epithelial ovarian tumours and has recently been investigated in pancreatic cancer.

Span-1 is a high molecular weight glycoprotein recognized by a murine monoclonal antibody produced against a human pancreatic cancer cell line. Unlike CA 19-9, Span-1 is not affected by the patient's Lewis phenotypes, but chronic liver disease gives a high false positive rate.

DU-PAN 2 is an antigen defined by a monoclonal antibody raised to a human pancreatic adenocarcinoma cell line. It is exposed more frequently in pancreatic tumour tissue than in serum.

Several combinations of tumour antigen assays have been investigated to improve the diagnostic rate of pancreatic cancer. The best combination at present is CA 19-9 plus CA 50.[10] These serum markers (especially CA 19-9 and CA 50) may also be useful in the follow-up of patients treated radically for pancreatic cancer. Postoperative normalization of CA 19-9 levels indicate a radical resection, and a subsequent increase in levels suggest recurrence.[4,88]

LAPAROSCOPY

Although modern imaging techniques such as ultrasound, CT, pancreatography and visceral angiography are reported to be reliable in the detection of advanced disease, 35% of patients in whom spread of the pancreatic cancer is excluded by these tests are still found to have small metastatic lesions in the liver, omentum or peritoneum at laparotomy.[105] Laparoscopy can be used to detect such metastatic lesions and perhaps avoid laparotomy in selected patients.[20,105] In one series, laparoscopy was 82% sensitive when macroscopic nodules were present, 88% specific in excluding metastases and 93% accurate overall.[105] Although morbidity and mortality rates are very low, the examination has limitations in patients with obesity or adhesions from previous operation. In most centres it is not performed routinely at present, perhaps because a high proportion of patients receive laparotomy for palliation if not attempted cure.

LAPAROTOMY

Nowadays there is a very limited role for diagnostic laparotomy in the management of pancreatic cancer. Preoperative investigation can usually permit a strong presumptive diagnosis with or without cytological confirmation of malignancy (see above). In patients with resectable tumours, histological confirmation of malignancy and staging of the tumour can be achieved by examination of the resection specimen. In those with irresectable tumours it is essential to confirm the existence (and type) of cancer by obtaining appropriate biopsies at operation, both to provide a rational basis for planning adjuvant therapy and to obtain an accurate prognosis.

The techniques for histological confirmation during operation include core needle biopsy, incision (wedge) biopsy, shave biopsy of the edge of the lesion plus fine needle aspiration for cytology. The positive biopsy rate is approximately equal with either the Tru-cut core needle (86%) or wedge biopsy (80%).[13] A higher complication rate (especially pancreatic fistula) has been noted with core needle biopsy than wedge biopsy,[81] perhaps because removal of a wedge of tissue allows close inspection of the biopsy site or because needle biopsy is preferred in more deeply placed and difficult lesions. If there is much leakage of pancreatic fluid following biopsy and if no further procedure is anticipated, it is wise to cover the biopsy site with a Roux-en-Y jejunostomy. Transduodenal needle biopsy may reduce the risk of pancreatic fistula but is only appropriate for lesions close to the duodenal loop. Indirect biopsy by taking the tissue from suspected metastases in lymph nodes or elsewhere is safe but results in a lower positive yield (18%).[13] As percutaneous aspiration has lower morbidity but similar accuracy rates to core or wedge biopsy, it has become the procedure of choice in many centres.[87]

TREATMENT

RESECTIONAL SURGERY

Herein lies the only chance for cure in pancreatic cancer. Unfortunately only 11–28% of patients with carcinoma of the head have lesions suitable for resection and many fewer of those with carcinoma of the body or tail.[23,30,98,99] Resectability rates have improved recently in some leading centres either because the diagnosis is established more quickly or because of selected referral patterns. Although sophisticated modern imaging has improved the preoperative assessment of resectability, laparotomy remains the final arbiter.

Appropriate preoperative preparation in jaundiced patients includes correction of coagulopathy (by parenteral vitamin K administration), rehydration and correction of electrolyte imbalance (to prevent postoperative renal failure), improvement of nutritional status (sometimes by parenteral nutrition) and prophylactic antibiotic therapy. Preoperative biliary decompression can be achieved either radiologically by percutaneous transhepatic insertion of a pigtail catheter or endoscopically by papillotomy and insertion of a suitable stent. These techniques are used in many centres nowadays with low complication rates,[23] but they do contaminate the biliary tree and introduce an element of delay. Some surgeons prefer to proceed direct to pancreatectomy in most patients, reserving biliary decompression for those with cholangitis or incipient hepatorenal failure.

Intraoperative assessment of resectability

After excluding distant metastatic lesions, determination of technical resectability requires thorough examination of the pancreas and surrounding structures. Lymph node involvement may be confirmed by frozen-section examination but does not necessarily preclude resectability provided the nodes can be excised *en bloc*. It is seldom justifiable to proceed to pancreatoduodenectomy unless it seems likely that resection of tumour will be macroscopically complete. The crucial step is to separate the superior mesenteric and portal veins from the overlying neck of pancreas. This manoeuvre requires quite an extensive trial dissection, and sometimes it can be safely achieved in patients with doubtfully resectable tumours on preoperative imaging. Patients with carcinoma of the head or uncinate may be found to have tethering or invasion of the right border of the vein at a late stage of resection, in which case the surgeon has the option of leaving a small sliver of affected tissue (and marking it for subsequent radiotherapy) or, in a few selected patients, of excising and reconstructing a short segment of vein.

Types of pancreatic resection

There are four main types of pancreatic resection: proximal pancreatoduodenectomy (Whipple's operation), distal pancreatectomy, total pancreatoduodenectomy and regional pancreatectomy.

Proximal pancreatoduodenectomy

This resection has undergone numerous modifications and technical refinements since introduced by Whipple and colleagues in 1935. It is indicated when the carcinoma is confined to the head or uncinate process of the pancreas; it is wise to confirm the absence of tumour at the line of pancreatic transection through the neck by sending tissue for frozen-section examination. Conventional proximal pancreatoduodenectomy comprises resection of the distal stomach, duodenum and head of pancreas *en bloc*. The reason for including a gastrectomy is to reduce gastric acidity and prevent the potentially lethal complication of stress ulceration and bleeding in the early postoperative period; some surgeons remove half the stomach, others combine a lesser resection (antrectomy) with truncal vagotomy.

The past decade has seen a sharp decline in operative morbidity and mortality rates for Whipple's operation. The mortality rate has fallen from 20–40% during the 1960s and early 1970s to less than 10% nowadays.[30,98] Serious complications such as bleeding, sepsis, acute pancreatitis and anastomotic leakage similarly have diminished. Proximal pancreatoduodenectomy remains a major undertaking. It generally requires 5–6 hours of operating time divided roughly equally into mobilization and resection of the specimen and reconstruction, which

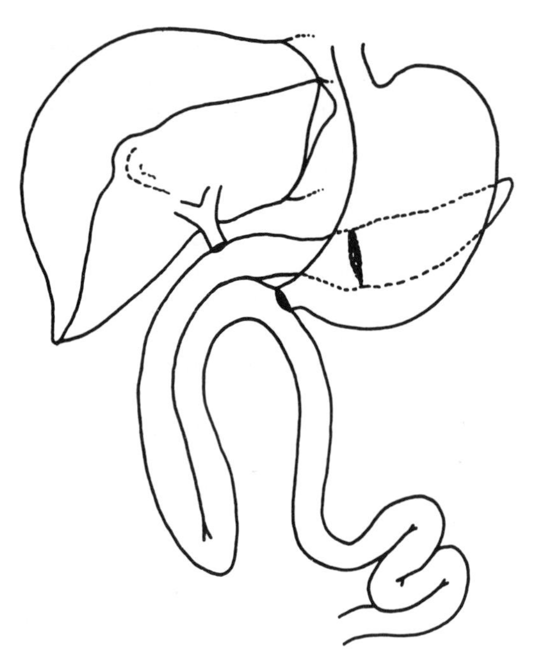

Figure 11.52 Pylorus-preserving proximal pancreatoduodenectomy.

necessitates anastomosing the neck of pancreas, bile duct and stomach to the upper jejunum. The technical details are beyond the scope of this chapter, but it should be noted that particular care is needed in constructing the pancreatojejunostomy because of the serious sepsis and haemorrhage that can follow disruption of this anastomosis. At present, the actuarial survival rate after 5 years among patients with pancreatic head cancer undergoing pancreatoduodenectomy ranges from 3–24%.[12,30,49,99]

Since 1978, the modification of proximal pancreatoduodenectomy preserving the pylorus (*Figure 11.52*) has gained in popularity in several centres. Preservation of an intact pylorus and duodenal cap should prevent enterogastric reflux, erosive gastritis and postoperative bleeding, although the prophylactic use of H_2-receptor antagonists has probably played a part in the reduction of these complications. The survival rate of pancreatic cancer patients undergoing this procedure is similar to that of patients undergoing a standard Whipple's procedure, despite the retention of nodes along the greater and lesser curvatures of the gastric antrum.[12] We favour this operation provided that the tumour is not abutting onto the pyloroduodenal segment. We aim to preserve 4–5 cm of healthy well-vascularized proximal duodenum, and the end-to-side duodenojejunostomy is easy to construct. Postoperative gastric stasis has seldom proved troublesome in our experience, and it seems likely that subsequent weight gain and nutritional status will be better than in those with conventional pancreatoduodenectomy.

Distal pancreatectomy

This operation is indicated for lesions in the body or tail of the gland and includes splenectomy. It is seldom feasible for typical ductal carcinoma because nearly all of these tumours have encased the superior mesenteric vessels by the time of presentation and many will have disseminated. Distal pancreatectomy may be appropriate for slow-growing cancers such as cystadenocarcinoma, papillary cystic neoplasm and islet cell carcinoma.

Total pancreatoduodenectomy

This technique offers the theoretical advantages of avoiding the hazardous pancreatojejunal anastomosis and removing multicentric disease (reported in up to a third of resection specimen) at the expense of obligate diabetes and the need for exocrine supplements; combined insulin and glucagon deficiency results in rather a brittle diabetes. Unfortunately most series have shown higher mortality and morbidity rates than for partial pancreatectomy and no clear gain in long-term survival.[30,49,100] Therefore, total pancreatoduodenectomy should be reserved for the following indications:

1. Pancreatic cancer in an insulin-dependent diabetic.
2. Extensive involvement of the whole pancreas by tumour without evidence of spread, especially in a young patient.
3. Cancer at the site of pancreatic transection demonstrated on frozen section during a radical pancreatoduodenectomy.
4. Inability to perform a safe pancreatojejunostomy because of friability of the residual pancreas. The pylorus can be preserved but the spleen should be removed.

Regional (super-radical) pancreatectomy

This refers to removal of a tumour in (or adjacent to) the pancreas with an adequate soft tissue margin and with its regional lymphatic drainage *en bloc*. This procedure usually includes resection of any or all of the three major vessels near the neck of the pancreas: portal vein, superior mesenteric artery and coeliac axis. The portal vein is usually reconstructed by end-to-end anastomosis (type 1 operation). The superior mesenteric artery is directly reimplanted into the aorta, and the hepatic artery is revascularized via a communicating graft from the aorta (type 2 operation). The advantage of this heroic procedure is to extend resection to a group of patients whose tumour could otherwise only be palliated, hence the high resectability rate of 40%.[29] The disadvantage – and it is a serious one – is the risk of complications from such a complex and extensive procedure. Since the introduction of regional pancreatectomy, most of the data on the operation have been published from a single centre. Although the mortality rate may now be as low as 8%, the morbidity rate remains very high (55%).[29,69] Moreover, there is little to suggest that survival is improved over conventional pancreatectomy. There seems little justification for regional pancreatectomy in routine practice, but local resection of the portal vein followed by reconstruction is one expedient for venous invasion that is discovered late in the operation.

PALLIATIVE SURGERY

Once laparotomy has confirmed the irresectability of a pancreatic cancer, tissue diagnosis must be obtained and staging assessed by means of frozen-section examination of the primary tumour or metastases, or both (see above). The mass may then be marked with metal clips to facilitate postoperative irradiation.

There are three objectives for surgical palliation in patients with irresectable pancreatic cancer:

1. To relieve jaundice and pruritus.
2. To maintain gastric emptying.
3. To control pain.

Obstructive jaundice is the dominant clinical feature in at least two-thirds of patients with pancreatic cancer. Besides causing intolerable itching and suppressing appetite, it has a deleterious effect on most organ systems. Relief of biliary obstruction can normalize hepatic function, correct metabolic derangements, restore nutritional health, eliminate coagulopathy and improve overall well-being. It should therefore be attempted in patients with all but the most advanced disease. The advantage of operation in a reasonably fit patient is that long-term biliary drainage can be achieved without the necessity for tubes and their potential for blockage. Cholecystojejunostomy is simple to perform but unsatisfactory in those destined to live more than a very few weeks because of the risk of subsequent tumour encroachment on the cystic duct; the incidence of recurrent jaundice is at least 10%.[86] It takes longer to remove the gallbladder, transect the common hepatic duct well above the 'leading edge' of tumour and bring up a Roux loop of jejunum for end-to-side anastomosis, but the mortality rate is no higher and the subsequent benefits are greater.[84,86] In one series, survival after choledochojejunostomy (10.4 months) was longer than after cholecystojejunostomy (7.5 months), and the incidence of recurrent jaundice was lower.[84]

Gastric outflow obstruction is present in only 5% of pancreatic cancer patients at the time of diagnosis, although nausea and vomiting are common presenting symptoms. Cancer of the pancreatic head usually obstructs the second part of the duodenum, whereas cancer of the body invades and obstructs the fourth part. In such patients, the need for a gastrojejunostomy is clear. On average another 21% of patients (range 8–50%) develop duodenal obstruction at a later stage of the disease if only bypass (or stenting) or the biliary tract is performed.[93] The question arises whether this incidence justifies routine gastrojejunostomy, bearing in mind the possibility that bile gastritis may increase the risk of postoperative bleeding. Moreover, some patients with advanced disease continue to vomit despite a patent stoma or pylorus, or both, possibly because extensive nodal disease denervates the stomach. In our view prophylactic gastroenterostomy should ordinarily be performed, and we use the same Roux loop for biliary and gastric bypass (*Figure 11.53*).

Pain of some degree is very common at first but will often subside after biliary decompression. Some patients present with constant and more intense pain, which radiates to the back and reflects malignant retroperitoneal extension involving visceral afferent fibres around the coeliac plexus. The simplest and most effective treatment in such patients is

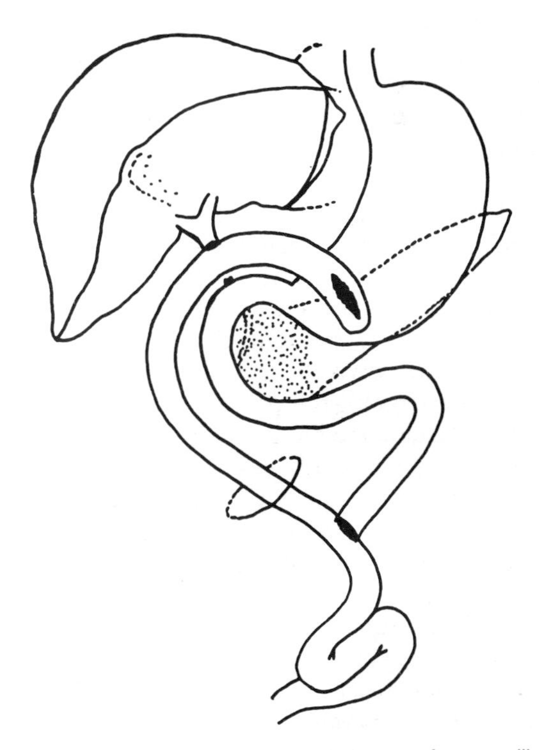

Figure 11.53 The authors' technique for palliative choledochojejunostomy and gastrojejunostomy in patients with irresectable pancreatic cancer.

a chemical splanchnicectomy carried out at the time of laparotomy. The coeliac ganglia are destroyed by injecting 20 ml of 6% phenol or 50% alcohol on each side. More than 80% of patients experience relief of pain, and this relief persists until death in 70% of cases.[32] Severe preoperative pain and evidence of marked pancreatitis distal to the cancer are indications to consider decompression of the obstructed pancreatic duct into the stomach or jejunum.[107]

NONOPERATIVE PALLIATION

During the past decade, several alternatives for palliative treatment of pancreatic cancer patients have been introduced especially for elderly or frail patients unsuitable for operation. External biliary decompression by means of percutaneous transhepatic biliary drainage can be carried out with a high rate of technical success (85–97%), that is, adequate decompression of the obstructed biliary system, but at the risk of serious complications.[50,63] Early complications in 33–43% of patients include cholangitis, haemorrhage, bile duct perforation, haemopneumothorax, electrolyte disorders and catheter malfunction.[24,63] Long-term complications in up to 86% of those surviving their initial hospitalization include catheter dislodgement, tube obstruction, cholangitis and sepsis.[63]

Although permanent external drainage alone is inappropriate, therefore, percutaneous placement of an endoprosthesis overcomes many of its drawbacks. Such prostheses can be applied either percutaneously, endoscopically or by a combined percutaneous–endoscopic technique with success rates of 90% (percutaneous), 81% (endoscopic) and 89% (combined).[1,40,95] The wider the prosthetic stent, the less likely it is to become occluded. Various percutaneous stents are available, but we have increasing experience with an expandable metal stent that can be inserted through a 7 Fr catheter but springs open to produce a 10 mm channel through the stricture (*Figure 11.54*). Similarly, wide-channel endoscopes are now available for placement of stents up to 10 Fr in size (external diameter).

(a)

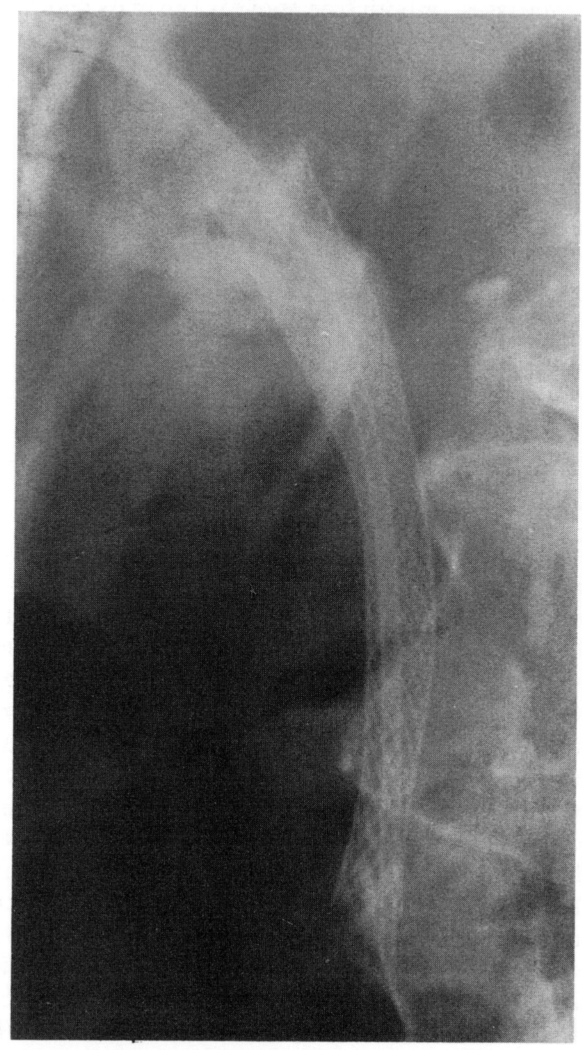

(b)

Figure 11.54 Palliative stenting (by the percutaneous transhepatic route) of an irresectable carcinoma of the pancreatic head in an 89-year-old patient with obstructive jaundice. (a) A 7 Fr catheter has been passed over a guidewire which was threaded through the malignant bile-duct stricture under radiological control. (b) A few days later the catheter is replaced by an expandable metal stent (Wallstent^{R}), which can be seen to lie across the stricture. A temporary external catheter is seen within the stent. (Courtesy of Dr A. Adam.)

For both percutaneous and endoscopic stenting of pancreatic cancers, the complication rate and hospital stay of the initial procedure are less than those of surgical bypass. These benefits are counterbalanced by the complications of stent failure, notably cholangitis and recurrent jaundice, which usually necessitate readmission to hospital and replacement of the stent. Long-term problems of percutaneous and endoscopic stents are similar as there are now no significant differences in size or stent materials. Stents placed endoscopically can simply be extracted and replaced if they block. Stents placed percutaneously are more difficult to replace, but sometimes the radiologist can displace them into the duodenum or insert another stent alongside the original.[40]

Troublesome pain also can be managed non-operatively by means of percutaneous coeliac plexus block under radiographic or CT control or by irradiation (see below). Good results can be anticipated from coeliac plexus block in up to 95% of patients with a very low complication rate.[56] Although obstructive jaundice and pain can be managed by non-operative means, surgical bypass is the only effective palliation in patients with duodenal obstruction.

In our opinion, younger and fitter patients should still receive operative palliation for irresectable pancreatic cancer, non-surgical treatment being reserved for the elderly or frail. Laparotomy provides the opportunity to obtain definitive histology, confirm irresectability beyond any doubt, provide permanent biliary and duodenal bypass and address the problem of intractable pain all in one session.

ADJUVANT THERAPIES

Radiotherapy

Approximately 40% of patients with pancreatic cancer present with locally advanced disease, that is, involvement of regional nodes or major blood vessels, or both, precluding resection but without evidence of distant metastases. Clinical improvement can be achieved in 60% or less of such patients using single modality treatment such as external beam radiation, intraoperative radiation therapy with electrons or brachytherapy. Unfortunately none of these treatments has a major impact on median or long-term survival.[42,103]

There are five major radiotherapeutic approaches to cope with pain in irresectable pancreatic cancer patients. These include conventional external beam, high linear energy transfer external beam, intraoperative radiation therapy with electrons or brachytherapy, and a combination of conventional external beam and intraoperative techniques. Although conventional external beam radiation treatment is the most common method used, pain relief occurs in only half the patients.[56] Less favourable results have been reported following local irradiation with high-energy neutrons (30% pain relief). By contrast, intraoperative radiation therapy with electrons or brachytherapy (radium-222 or iodine-125 implants) can alleviate pain in 70–90% of pancreatic cancer patients, but combining intraoperative with external beam treatment does not improve the results.[67]

Chemotherapy

Despite several studies undertaken during the past 10 years, the results of chemotherapy for pancreatic cancer remain very disappointing. 5-fluorouracil is the single agent most extensively evaluated; it has a median response rate of 28% (range 0–67%). Broadly similar response rates are reported for single-agent treatment with mitomycin-C (27%), streptozotocin (36%) and ifosfamide (22%); all other drugs tested, including epirubicin, have response rates below 20%.[110] The combination regimens most frequently employed are firstly, 5-fluorouracil, adriamycin and mitomycin, and secondly, streptozotocin, mitomycin and 5-fluorouracil, but they have not been shown to be superior to single agents. With currently available drugs, it is doubtful whether the potential toxicity of chemotherapy is justified by the likely benefits in this particular cancer.

Radiotherapy plus chemotherapy

In a co-operative American study, the combination of low dose radiotherapy (40 Gy) and 5-fluorouracil produced a better median survival time (42 weeks) in pancreatic cancer than radiotherapy alone (23 weeks). Survival was no better (40 weeks) after high dose radiotherapy (60 Gy) plus 5-fluorouracil, but leucopaenia occurred more often (60 versus 46%).[68] The combination of 40 Gy (split course) and 5-fluorouracil has become the standard treatment for locally advanced pancreatic cancer in several centres.[68,103] The addition of external beam radiotherapy and 5-fluorouracil chemotherapy to pancreatoduodenectomy showed a clear survival advantage over operation alone in an American study of patients with carcinoma of the pancreatic head.[31]

Hormonal therapy

Investigation of the role of sex hormones in pancreatic carcinogenesis stemmed from several discoveries:

1. The presence of high oestrogen receptor activity and specific oestrogen-binding proteins in pancreatic carcinoma as well as in normal pancreatic tissue.
2. The increased incidence of pancreatic cancer among women with previous oophorectomy, spontaneous abortion or uterine fibroids.
3. Low plasma testosterone levels in pancreatic cancer patients.
4. A twofold increase in 5α-reductase content in malignant pancreatic tissue (this enzyme converts testosterone into the more potent androgen 5α-dihydrotestosterone). Agents that interfere with male sex-steroid metabolism might therefore be of value in the management of pancreatic cancer.[3] The elderly age of onset in many patients with pancreatic cancer, however, would not suggest a major aetiological role for sex hormones in this disease.

The anti-oestrogenic drug, tamoxifen, accumulates to a greater extent in the pancreas than in established oestrogen target organs such as the mammary gland and uterus. Tamoxifen prolonged the survival of patients with irresectable pancreatic carcinoma in two small uncontrolled studies, but subsequent investigations have failed to confirm any benefit.[8,18]

Both cholecystokinin and epidermal growth factor promote experimental pancreatic carcinogenesis. Cholecystokinin antagonists, somatostatin and luteinizing hormone releasing hormone are now under active scrutiny as potential inhibitors of pancreatic carcinogenesis.

Immunotherapy

Exciting development in the fields of cellular immunology and recombinant DNA technology are providing new monoclonal antibodies and cytokines/lymphokines that could be of benefit in the control of pancreatic cancer. To date, clinical experience with interferon has been disappointing.[89]

SUMMARY OF TREATMENT

One algorithm for the treatment of patients with carcinoma of the exocrine pancreas is given in *Figure 11.55*.

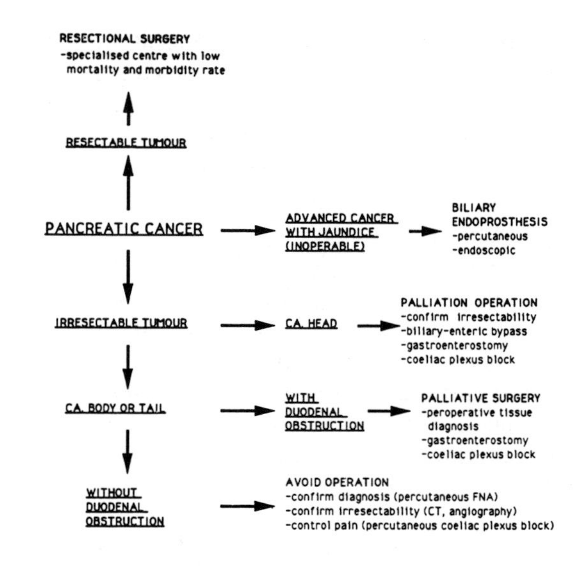

Figure 11.55 Algorithm for treatment of patients with cancer of the exocrine pancreas.

OUTCOME OF TREATMENT AND THE WAY AHEAD

Although survival rates after five years for pancreatic cancer have improved over the past few years, the prognosis remains dismal. Survival following resection rarely exceeds 10% at 5 years (7% reported from Mayo Clinic)[100] and is usually much lower. The best results have been reported from Japan, where 17 patients with very small pancreatic cancers (less than 2 cm in diameter) have undergone 'curative' resection with a survival rate after five years of 33%. These patients comprised only 5% of the total number treated for pancreatic cancer.[60] There remains a serious problem in detecting tumours at such an early stage, although better tumour markers and (perhaps) the development of endoscopic ultrasonography may improve the situation and lead to real gains in curability. Meantime it seems unlikely that further refinements in surgical technique can improve survival, and the search continues for more effective adjuvant therapies.

REFERENCES

1. Adam, A., Chetty, N., Roddie, M. *et al.* (1991) Self-expandable stainless steel endoprostheses for treatment of malignant bile duct obstruction. *American Journal of Roentgenology*.
2. Alpert, L.C., Truong, L.D., Bossart, M.I. and Spjut, H.J. (1988) Microcystic adenoma (serous adenoma) of the pancreas: a study of 14 cases with immunohistochemical and electron-microscopic correlation. *American Journal of Surgical Pathology*, **12**, 251–263.
3. Andren-Sandberg, A. (1989) Androgen influence on exocrine pancreatic cancer. *International Journal of Pancreatology*, **4**, 363–369.

4. Andren-Sandberg, A. (1989) CA 50 and CA 19-9 in serum as tumour markers for pancreatic cancer: a review of the literature. *Acta Chirurgica Scandinavica*, **549** (suppl), 75–81.
5. Aoki, K. and Ogawa, H. (1978) Cancer of the pancreas: international mortality trends. *World Heath Statistics Quarterly*, **31**, 2–27.
6. Appleton, G.V.N., Bathurst, N.C.G., Virjee, J. *et al.* (1989) The value of angiography in the surgical management of pancreatic disease. *Annals of the Royal College of Surgeons of England*, **71**, 92–96.
7. Armstrong, B. and Doll, R. (1976) Environmental factors and cancer incidence and mortality in different countries, with special reference to dietary factors. *International Journal of Cancer*, **15**, 617–631.
8. Bakkevold, K.E., Petterson, A., Arnesjo, B. and Espehaug, B. (1990) Tamoxifen therapy in unresectable adenocarcinoma of the pancreas and the papilla of Vater. *British Journal of Surgery*, **77**, 725–730.
9. Becker, V. (1978) Carcinoma of the pancreas and chronic pancreatitis-a possible relationship. *Acta Hepato-gastroenterology*, **25**, 257–259.
10. Benini, L., Cavallini, G., Zordan, D. *et al.* (1988) A clinical evaluation of monoclonal (CA 19-9, CA 50, CA 12-5) and polyclonal (CEA, TPA) antibody-defined antigens for the diagnosis of pancreatic cancer. *Pancreas*, **3**, 61–66.
11. Beral, V., Inskip, H., Fraser, P. *et al.* (1985) Mortality of employees of the United Kingdom Atomic Energy Authority 1946–1979. *British Medical Journal*, **291**, 440–447.
12. Braasch, J.W., Rossi, R.L., Watkins, E. Jr. *et al.* (1986) Pyloric and gastric preserving pancreatic resection: experience with 87 patients. *Annals of Surgery*, **204**, 411–418.
13. Buice, W.S. and Walker, L.G. Jr. (1989) The role of intraoperative biopsy in the treatment of resectable neoplasms of the pancreas and periampullary region. *American Surgeon*, **55**, 307–310.
14. Camprodon, R. and Quintanilla, E. (1984) Successful long-term results with resection of pancreatic carcinoma in children: favorable prognosis for an uncommon neoplasm. *Surgery*, **95**, 420–426.
15. Caygill, C.P.J., Hill, M.J., Hall, C.N. *et al.* (1987) Increased risk of cancer at multiple sites after gastric surgery for peptic ulcer. *Gut*, **28**, 924–928.
16. Colomb, E., Estevenon, J.P., Figarella, C. *et al.* (1974) Characterization of an additional protein in pancreatic juice of men with chronic calcifying pancreatitis. Identification of lactoferrin. *Biochimica et Biophysica Acta*, **342**, 306–312.
17. Court-Brown, W.M. and Doll, R. (1958) Expectation of life and mortality from cancer among British radiologists. *British Medical Journal*, **2**, 181–187.
18. Crowson, M.C., Dorrell, A., Rolfe, E.B. and Fielding, J.W.L. (1986) A phase II study of evaluate tamoxifen in pancreatic adenocarcinoma. *European Journal of Surgical Oncology*, **12**, 335–336.
19. Cubilla, A.L. and Fitzgerald, P.J. (1984) Tumours of the exocrine pancreas. In: *Atlas of Tumour Pathology,* Second series, fasc. 19. Armed Forces Institute of Pathology, Washington.
20. Cuschieri, A. (1988) Laparoscopy for pancreatic cancer: does it benefit the patient? *European Journal of Surgical Oncology*, **14**, 41–44.
21. Cuzick, J. and Babiker, A.G. (1989) Pancreatic cancer, alcohol, diabetes mellitus and gall-bladder disease. *International Journal of Cancer*, **43**, 415–421.
22. Del-Favero, G., Fabris, C., Angonese, C. *et al.* (1988) Cytology in the diagnosis of pancreatic cancer. International Journal of Pancreatology, **3**, S137–S141.
23. Deschamps, G. and Bourbeau, D. (1984) Pancreatic carcinoma: surgical treatment. *Canadian Journal of Surgery*, **27**, 559–560.
24. Devereux, D.F. and Greco, R.S. (1986) Biliary enteric bypass for malignant obstruction. *Cancer*, **58**, 981–984.
25. Dimagno, E.P. (1988) Early diagnosis of chronic pancreatitis and pancreatic cancer. *Medical Clinics of North America*, **72**, 979–992.
26. Durbec, J.P., Chevillotte, G., Bidart, J.M. *et al.* (1983) Diet, alcohol, tobacco and risk of cancer of the pancreas: a case-control study. *British Journal of Cancer*, **47**, 463–470.
27. Falk, R.T., Pickle, L.W., Fontham, E.T. *et al.* (1988) Lifestyle factors for pancreatic cancer in Lousiana: a case-control study. *American Journal of Epidemiology*, **128**, 324–336.
28. Fontham, E.T.H. and Correa, P. (1989) Epidemiology of pancreatic cancer. *Surgical Clinics of North America*, **69**, 551–567.
29. Fortner, J.G. (1984) Regional pancreatectomy for cancer of the pancreas, ampulla and other related sites. Tumor staging and results. *Annals of Surgery*, **199**, 418–425.
30. Funovics, J.M., Karner, J., Pratschner, T. and Fritsch, A. (1989) Current trends in the management of carcinoma of the pancreatic head. *Hepatogastroenterology*, **36**, 450–455.
31. Gastrointestinal Tumour Study Group. (1987) Further evidence of effective adjuvant combined radiation and chemotherapy following curative resection of pancreatic cancer. *Cancer*, **59**, 2006–2010.
32. Gardner, A.M.N. and Solomou, G. (1984) Relief of the pain of unresectable carcinoma of pancreas by chemical splanchnicectomy during laparotomy. *Annals of the Royal College of Surgeons of England*, **66**, 409–411.
33. Ghadirian, P., Simard, A. and Baillargeon, J. (1988) Family aggregation of pancreatic cancer: a population-based case-control study. *Proceedings of the American Association of Cancer Research*, **29**, 257.

34. Gilinsky, N.H., Bornman, P.C., Girdwood, A.H. and Marks, I.N. (1986) Diagnostic yield of endoscopic retrograde cholangiopancreatography in carcinoma of the pancreas. *British Journal of Surgery*, **73**, 539–543.
35. Go, V.L.W., Taylor, W.F. and Dimagno, E.P. (1981) Efforts at early diagnosis of pancreatic cancer: the Mayo Clinic experience. *Cancer*, **47**, 1698–1705.
36. Gold, E.B., Gordis, L., Diener, M.D. *et al.* (1985) Diet and other risk factors for cancer of the pancreas. *Cancer*, **55**, 460–467.
37. Gordis, L. and Gold, E. B. (1984) Epidemiology of pancreatic cancer. *World Journal of Surgery*, **8**, 808–821.
38. Habib, N.A., Hershman, M.J., Haberland, F. *et al.* (1986) The use of CA 50 radioimmunoassay in differentiating benign and malignant pancreatic disease. *British Journal of Cancer*, **53**, 697–699.
39. Haenszel, W. and Kurihara, M. (1968) Studies of Japanese migrants I: mortality from cancer and other diseases among Japanese in the United States. *Journal of the National Cancer Institute*, **40**, 43–68.
40. Hall, R.I., Denyer, M.E. and Chapman, A.H. (1989) Palliation of obstructive jaundice with a biliary endoprosthesis. Comparison of insertion by the percutaneous-transhepatic and the combined percutaneous-endoscopic routes. *Clinical Radiology*, **40**, 186–189.
41. Hayakawa, T., Kondo, T., Shibata, T. *et al.* (1988) Sensitive screen markers for detecting pancreatic cancer. *Cancer*, **61**, 1827–1831.
42. Heijimans, H.J., Hoekotra, H.J. and Melita, D.M. (1989) Is adjuvant intraoperative radiotherapy (IORT) for resectable and unresectable pancreatic carcinoma worthwhile? *Hepatogastroenterology*, **36**, 474–477.
43. Hiatt, R.A., Klatsky, A.L. and Armstrong, M.A. (1988) Pancreatic cancer, blood glucose and beverage consumption. *International Journal of Cancer*, **41**, 794–797.
44. Hirayama, T. (1989) Epidemiology of pancreatic cancer in Japan. *Japanese Journal of Clinical Oncology*, **19**, 208–215.
45. Horie, A., Haratake, J., Jimi, A. *et al.* (1987) Pancreatoblastoma in Japan, with differential diagnosis from papillary cystic tumours (ductuloacinar adenoma) of the pancreas. *Acta Pathologica Japonica*, **37**, 47–63.
46. Howard, J.M. and Jordan, G.L. Jr. (1977) Cancer of the pancreas. *Current Problems in Cancer*, **2**, 6–22.
47. Hutchinson, G.B. and MacMahon, B. (1979) Review of report by Mancusco, Stewart and Kneale of radiation exposure of Hanford workers. *Health Physics*, **37**, 207–220.
48. Itai, Y., Ohhashi, K., Nagai, H. *et al.* (1986) "Ductectatic" mucinous cystadenoma and cystadenocarcinoma of the pancreas. *Radiology*, **161**, 697–700.
49. Jordan, G.L. Jr. (1989) Pancreatic resection for pancreatic cancer. *Surgical Clinics of North America*, **69**, 569–597.
50. Joseph, P.K., Bizer, L.S., Sprayregen, S.S. and Gliedman, M.L. (1986) Percutaneous transhepatic biliary drainage: results and complications in 81 patients. *Journal of American Medical Association*, **225**, 2763–2767.
51. Karmody, A.J. and Kyle, J. (1969) The association between carcinoma of the pancreas and diabetes mellitus. *British Journal of Surgery*, **56**, 362–364.
52. Kaufman, A.R. and Sivak, M.V. Jr. (1989) Endoscopic ultrasonography in the differential diagnosis of pancreatic disease. *Gastrointestinal Endoscopy*, **35**, 214–219.
53. Kiriyama, S., Hayakawa, T., Kondo, T. *et al.* (1990) Usefulness of a new tumour markers, Span-1, for the diagnosis of pancreatic cancer. Cancer, **65**, 1577–1561.
54. Kloppel, G. (1989) Cancer of the pancreas. In: *Cancer of the Bile Ducts and Pancreas,* (Eds) Preece, P.E., Cuschieri, A. and Rosin, R.D. pp. 113–138. Philadelphia: W.B. Saunders Company.
55. Kocjan, G., Rode, J. and Lees, W.R. (1989) Percutaneous fine needle aspiration cytology of the pancreas: advantage and pitfalls. *Journal of Clinical Pathology*, **42**, 341–347.
56. Lebovits, A.H. and Lefkowitz, M. (1989) Pain management of pancreatic carcinoma: a review. *Pain*, **36**, 1–11.
57. Lynch, H.T., Fitzsimmons, M.L., Smyrk, T.C. *et al.* (1990) Familial pancreatic cancer: clinicopathologic study of 18 nuclear families. *American Journal of Gastroenterology*, **85**, 54–60.
58. Mack, T.M., Yu, M.C., Hanisch, R. and Henderson, B.E. (1986) Pancreas cancer and smoking, beverage consumption, and past medical history. *Journal of the National Cancer Institute*, **76**, 49–60.
59. Malesci, A., Evangelista, A., Mariani, A. *et al.* (1988) CA 19-9 in serum and pancreatic juice: its role in the differential diagnosis of resectable pancreatic cancer from chronic pancreatitis. *International Journal of Pancreatology*, **3**, S119–S124.
60. Manabe, T. and Tobe, T. (1989) Progress in the diagnosis and treatment of pancreatic cancer- the Kyoto University experience. *Hepatogastro-enterology*, **36**, 431–436.
61. Mancuso, T.F. and el-Attar, A.A. (1967) Cohort study of workers exposed to betanaphthylamine and benzidine. *Journal of Occupational Medicine*, **9**, 277–285.
62. Mannell, A., Weiland, L.H., van Heerden, J.A. and Ilstrup, D.M. (1986) Factors influencing survival after resection for ductal adenocarcinoma of the pancreas. *Annals of Surgery*, **203**, 403–407.
63. McGrath, P.C., McNeil, P.M., Neilfield, J.P. *et al.* (1989) Management of biliary obstruction in patients with unresectable carconima of the pancreas. *Annals of Surgery*, **209**, 284–288.

64. McGuinness, E.E., Morgan, R.G.H., Levison, D.A. *et al.* (1981) Interaction of azaserine and raw soya flour on the rat pancreas. *Scandinavian Journal of Gastroenterology*, **16**, 49–56.
65. McMichael, A.J., McCall, M.J., Hartshorne, J.M. *et al.* (1980) Patterns of gastrointestinal cancer in European migrants to Australia: the role of dietary change. *International Journal of Cancer*, **25**, 431–437.
66. Mills, P.K., Beeson, W.L., Abbey, D.E. *et al.* (1988) Dietary habits and past medical history as related to fatal pancreas cancer risk among Adventists. *Cancer*, **61**, 2578–2585.
67. Minsky, B.D., Hilaris, B. and Fuks, Z. (1988) The role of radiation therapy in the control of pain from pancreatic carcinoma. *Journal of Pain and Symptom Management*, **3**, 199–205.
68. Moertel, C.G., Frytak, S., Hahn, R.G. *et al.* (1981) Therapy of locally unresectable pancreatic carcinoma: a randomized comparison of high dose (6000 rads) radiation alone, moderate dose radiation (4000 rads + 5 fluorouracil), and high dose radiation + 5 fluorouracil. *Cancer*, **48**, 1705–1710.
69. Moossa, A.R., Scott, M.H. and Lavelle-Jones, M. (1984) The place of total and extended total pancreatectomy in pancreatic cancer. *World Journal of Surgery*, **8**, 895–899.
70. Morohoshi, T., Held, G. and Kloppel, G. (1983) Exocrine pancreatic tumours and their histological classification. A study based on 167 autopsy and 97 surgical cases. *Histopathology*, **7**, 645–661.
71. Mortality statistics. Office of population censuses and surveys (1985–1988), series DH2, No. 12–15.
72. Morohoshi, T., Kanda, M., Horie, A. *et al.* (1987) Immunocytochemical markers of uncommon pancreatic tumours: acinar cell carcinoma, pancreatoblastoma and solid-cystic (papillary-cystic) tumours. *Cancer*, **59**, 739–747.
73. Muir, C., Waterhouse, J., Mack, T., Powell, J. and Whelan, S. (1987) "Cancer incidence in five continents" Vol V, IARC Scientific Publications, No. 88. Lyon. International Agency for Research on Cancer.
74. Norell, S., Ahlbom, A., Olin, R. *et al.* (1986) Occupational factors and pancreatic cancer. *British Journal of Industrial Medicine*, **43**, 775–778.
75. Norell, S., Ahlbom, A., Erward, R. *et al.* (1986) Diabetes, gall stone disease, and pancreatic cancer. *British Journal of Cancer*, **54**, 377–378.
76. Paganuzzi, M., Onetto, M., Marroni, P. *et al.* (1988) CA 19-9 and CA 50 in benign and malignant pancreatic and biliary diseases. *Cancer*, **61**, 2100–2108.
77. Parker, G.A. and Postlethwait, R.W. (1985) The continuing problem of carcinoma of the pancreas. *Journal of Surgical Oncology*, **28**, 36–38.
78. Piavansalo, M. and Lahde, S. (1988) Ultrasonography and computed tomography in pancreatic malignancy. *Acta Radiologica*, **29**, 343–344.
79. Pinzon, R., Drewinko, B., Trujillo, J.M. *et al.* (1986) Pancreatic carcinoma and Trousseau's syndrome: experience at a large cancer center. *Journal of Clinical Oncology*, **4**, 509–514.
80. Pukkala, E. and Teppo, L. (1986) Socioeconomic status and education as risk determinants of gastrointestinal cancer. *Preventive Medicine*, **15**, 127–138.
81. Reuben, A. and Cotton, B.B. (1978) Operative pancreatic biopsy: a survey of current practice. *Annals of the Royal College of Surgeons of England*, **60**, 53–57.
82. Review of the national cancer registration system. Office of population censuses and surveys (1990), series MB 1, No. 17.
83. Roebuck, B.D. (1986) Effects of high levels of dietary fats on the growth of azaserine-induced foci in the rat pancreas. *Lipids*, **21**, 281–284.
84. Rosemurgy, A.S., Burnett, C.M. and Wasselle, J.A. (1989) A comparison of choledochoenteric bypass and cholecystoenteric bypass in patients with biliary obstruction due to pancreatic cancer. *American Surgeon*, **55**, 55–60.
85. Ross, C.B., Sharp, K.W., Kaufman, A.J. *et al.* (1988) Efficacy of computerized tomography in the preoperative staging of pancreatic carcinoma. *American Surgeon*, **54**, 221–226.
86. Sarr, M.G. and Cameron, J.L. (1984) Surgical palliation of unresectable carcinoma of the pancreas. *World Journal of Surgery*, **8**, 906–918.
87. Savarino, V., Ceppa, V., Biggi, E. *et al.* (1986) Comparative study of percutaneous and peroperative fine-needle aspirations in the diagnosis of pancreatic cancer. *Hepato-Gastroenterology*, **33**, 75–78.
88. Schmiegel, W. (1989) Tumour markers in pancreatic cancer-current concepts. *Hepato-Gastroenterology*, **36**, 446–449.
89. Schmiegel, W. (1989) Biological response modifier-immunotherapeutic approaches in pancreatic cancer. *Hepatogastroenterology*, **36**, 456–458.
90. Schwartz, S.S., Zeidler, A., Moossa, A.R. *et al.* (1978) A prospective study of glucose tolerance, insulin, C-peptide, and glucagon responses in patients with pancreatic carcinoma. *Digestive Diseases*, **23**, 1107–1114.
91. Shemesh, E., Czerniak, A., Nass, S. and Klein, E. (1990) Role of endoscopic retrograde cholangio-pancreatography in differentiating pancreatic cancer coexisting with chronic pancreatitis. *Cancer*, **65**, 893–896.
92. Shtamler, B., Bickel, A., Manor, E. *et al.* (1988) Primary lymphoma of the head of the pancreas. *Journal of Surgical Oncology*, **38**, 48–51.
93. Singh, S.M. and Reber, H.A. (1989) Surgical palliation for pancreatic cancer. *Surgical Clinics of North America*, **69**, 599–611.
94. Smith, P.G. and Douglas, A.J. (1986) Mortality of workers at the Sellafield plant of British Nuclear Fuels. *British Medical Journal*, **293**, 845–854.

95. Speer, A.G., Cotton, P.B., Russell, R.C.G. *et al.* (1987) Randomised trial of endoscopic versus percutaneous stent insertion in malignant obstructive jaundice. *Lancet*, **ii**(8550), 57–62.
96. Tempero, M.A., Uchida, E., Takasaki, H. *et al.* (1987) Relationship of carbohydrate antigen 19-9 and Lewis antigens in pancreatic cancer. *Cancer Research*, **47**, 5501–5503.
97. Tio, T.L. and Tytgat, G.N.J. (1986) Endoscopic ultrasonography in staging local resectability of pancreatic and periampullary malignancy. *Scandinavian Journal of Gastroenterology*, **21** (suppl 123), 135–142.
98. Trede, M. (1985) The surgical treatment of pancreatic carcinoma. *Surgery*, **97**, 28–35.
99. Trede, M., Schwall, G. and Saeger, H. (1990) Survival after pancreatoduodenectomy. 118 consecutive resections without an operative mortality. *Annals of Surgery*, **211**, 447–458.
100. Van Heerden, J.A., McIlrath, D.C., Ilstrup, D.M. and Weiland, L.H. (1988) Total pancreatectomy for ductal adenocarcinoma of the pancreas: an update. *World Journal of Surgery*, **12**, 658–662.
101. Velema, J.P., Walker, A.M. and Gold, E.B. (1986) Alcohol and pancreatic cancer: insufficient epidemiologic evidence for a causal relationship. *Epidemiologic reviews*, **8**, 28–41.
102. Troll, W., Frenkel, K. and Wiesner, R. (1986) Protease inhibitors: their role as modifiers of carcinogenic processes. *Advances in Experimental Medicine and Biology*, **199**, 153–165.
103. Wagener, D.J. and deMulder, P.H.M. (1989) The treatment of locally advanced pancreatic cancer. *Anticancer Research*, **9**, 1009–1012.
104. Warshaw, A.L., Gu, Z., Wittenberg, J. and Waltman, A.C. (1990) Preoperative staging and assessment of resectability of pancreatic cancer. *Archives of Surgery*, **125**, 230–233.
105. Warshaw, A.L., Tepper, J.E. and Shipley, W.U. (1986) Laparoscopy in the staging and planning of therapy for pancreatic cancer. *American Journal of Surgery*, **151**, 76–80.
106. White, T.T., Allan, B.J., Schilling, J.J. and Miyashita, H. (1985) Human pancreatic secretory protein profiles in pancreatic cancer and chronic pancreatitis. *Digestive Diseases and Sciences*, **30**, 200–203.
107. Williamson, R.C.N. (1987) The pancreas. In: Operative Surgery & Management, (Ed.) Keen, B.Y.G. pp. 155–178. Bristol: Wright.
108. Williamson, R.C.N. (1988) Pancreatic cancer: the greatest oncological challenge. *British Medical Journal*, **296**, 445–446.
109. Williamson, R.C.N. (1989) Endocrine and other unusual pancreatic tumours. *Current Opinion in Gastroenterology*, **5**, 728–732.
110. Wils, J.A. (1989) Current status of chemotherapy in metastatic pancreatic cancer. *Anticancer Research*, **9**, 1027–1032.
111. Wynder, E.L., Dieck, G.S. and Hall, N.E. (1986) Case-control study of decaffeinated coffee consumption and pancreatic cancer. *Cancer Research*, **46**, 5360–5363.
112. Yamaguchi, K. and Enjoji, M. (1987) Cystic neoplasms of the pancreas. *Gastroenterology*, **92**, 1934–1943.
113. Yasuda, K., Mukai, H., Fujimoto, S. *et al.* (1988) The diagnosis of pancreatic cancer by endoscopic ultrasonography. *Gastrointestinal Endoscope*, **34**, 1–8.

TUMOURS OF THE ENDOCRINE PANCREAS

P.J. Hammond, D. Wynick and S.R. Bloom

THE GASTRINOMA SYNDROME (ZOLLINGER–ELLISON SYNDROME)

The gastrinoma syndrome was first described in 1955 by Zollinger and Ellison as a triad of fulminating ulcer diathesis, recurrent ulceration and failure of response to standard medical and surgical approaches in the presence of non-β-cell islet tumours of the pancreas.[59] Gregory *et al.*[18] extracted gastrin from these tumours in 1960, and they are now the second most commonly diagnosed pancreatic islet cell tumours with an incidence in the population of about one per million, similar to that of insulinoma. At least 60% are malignant, but the impact of a precise diagnostic tool in gastrin radioimmunoassay and the use of, firstly, H_2-receptor antagonists and, more recently, the proton pump (H^+-K^+-ATPase) inhibitor omeprazole, has changed the natural history and therapy of the disorder. Approximately one-third of patients have the autosomal dominant syndrome, multiple endocrine neoplasia type 1, in which gastroenteropancreatic neuroendocrine tumours are associated with hyperparathyroidism and pituitary tumours (*Figure 11.56*). The gastrinoma is more likely to be malignant in these patients. Most gastrinomas are sited in the pancreas but tumours can also be found in the duodenum, stomach, structures adjacent to the pancreas and,

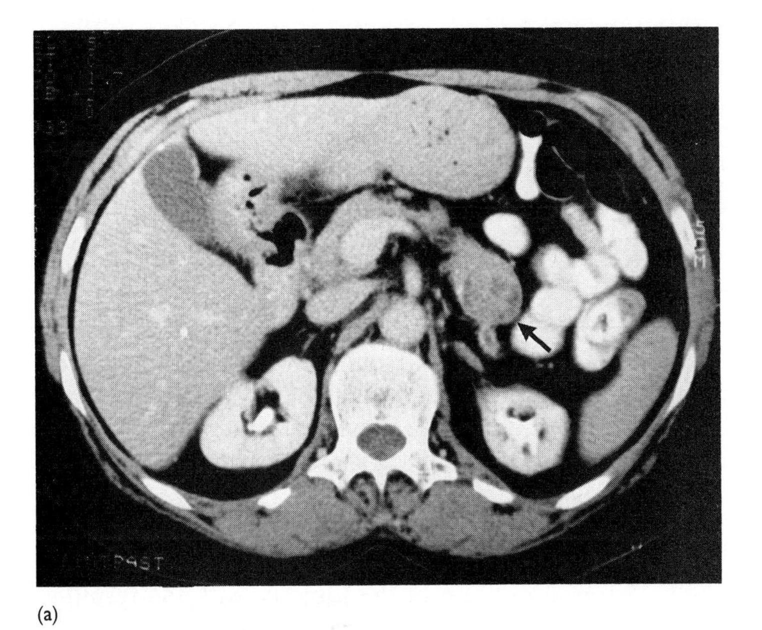

(a)

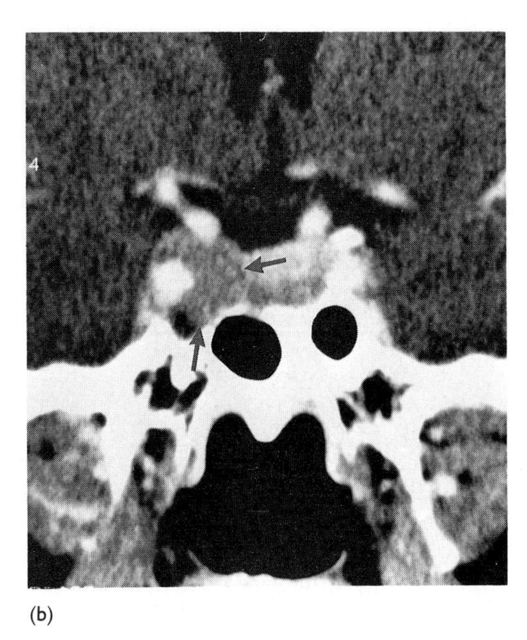

(b)

Figure 11.56 Tumours in multiple endocrine neoplasia type 1. (a) CT scan of the pancreas showing a large tumour in the tail of the pancreas (arrowed). (b) CT scan of the pituitary gland in the same patient, showing a tumour of low attenuation in the right lobe (arrowed).

rarely, in the ovaries and parathyroids. Other peptides may also be secreted from the tumour and thus the clinical syndrome may be mixed, or one syndrome may predominate.[54]

CLINICAL FEATURES

The history is often less than 2 years and the usual clinical presentation is of peptic ulceration, which is often multiple and atypical in site, including the oesophagus, distal duodenum and upper jejunum. Complications are frequent including perforation, pyloric stenosis, haemorrhage and gastrojejunocolic fistulas. The syndrome inevitably recurs after standard surgical procedures. It has become apparent, however, that diarrhoea and malabsorption caused by acid-related inactivation of enzymes and mucosal damage in the upper small bowel often predates ulceration by up to twelve months and may be the presenting feature. The advent of H_2 receptor antagonists and the routine availability of gastrin radioimmunoassay have changed the nature of the gastrinoma syndrome such that the classical presentation and catastrophic complications are less common than a decade ago, and the diagnosis is often made at an earlier stage in the disease.

INVESTIGATIONS

The clinician is confronted with the problem of attempting to differentiate the patient with the uncommon gastrinoma from the mass of peptic ulcer sufferers who do not have a gastrinoma. Clinical features alone are not helpful but suspicion should be heightened by the finding of multiple ulcers in unusual sites, diarrhoea, complications of peptic ulcer, recurrence after gastric surgery, a family history of peptic ulcer, hepatomegaly and other endocrine disorders, particularly hyperparathyroidism. The absence of such features, however, does not exclude the diagnosis.

The combinations of an elevated fasting gastrin and an elevated basal gastric acid output is essential to the diagnosis of a gastrinoma. The highest gastrin levels, 50–100 times the upper limit of normal, are associated with hypo- or achlorhydria, or chronic renal failure, rather than gastrinoma. Raised gastrin levels may also be found after vagotomy, in association with hypercalcaemia, in patients on H_2-antagonists and rarely in the short-gut syndrome. The gastrin assay used identifies the G8 species and a fasting level of greater than 40 pmol/l is abnormal. Other pancreatic and gut hormones should also be assayed to exclude multiple peptide secretion and, at the Hammersmith Hospital in London, glucagon, somatostatin, vasoactive intestinal polypeptide, pancreatic polypeptide and neurotensin are routinely assayed. Provocative tests for gastrin release, particularly with intravenous secretin, have been advocated but these are generally unhelpful with a significant rate of false-positive and false-negative results.

Gastric hypersecretion in association with the gastrinoma syndrome is usually greater than 1 litre, containing more than 100 mmol of acid, on a 12-hour overnight collection. In practice, a 1-hour basal acid output is sufficient and should exceed 10 mmol/h. If the patient has had a previous gastric surgical procedure, the diagnosis should be considered when the basal acid output exceeds 5 mmol/h. In addition, patients with the gastrinoma syndrome have a blunted response to maximal stimulation with pentagastrin (maximum acid output), and therefore have a reduced ratio of maximum to basal acid output.

TUMOUR LOCALIZATION

Ultrasound and high resolution computed tomography are the initial investigations for localization of tumour. Ultrasound will only detect about 20% of tumours and, although CT will detect up to 80% of gastrinomas, they can be difficult to localize, being frequently extra-pancreatic and 38% being less than 1 cm in diameter at presentation. Tumours association with type 1 multiple endocrine neoplasia can be particularly difficult to localize, because they are often multiple, and frequently occur in the duodenum (*Figure 11.57*).[36] The combination of CT and highly selective visceral angiography gives the highest detection rate, approximately 90%. More recently indium-111 labelled somatostatin analogues have been used, which visualize 60%–80% of gastrinomas, but the reported experience is limited.[24] Newer techniques of intraoperative and endoscopic ultrasound and nuclear magnetic resonance have yet to be fully evaluated. Patients with

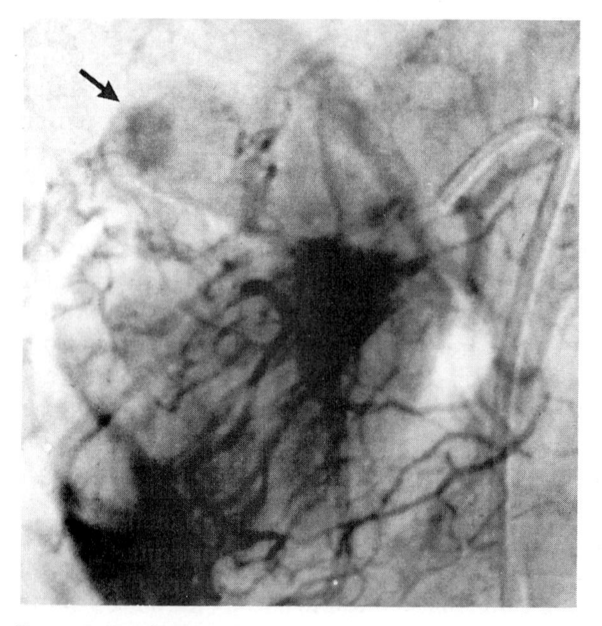

Figure 11.57 Oblique views of the venous phase of a selective hepatic arteriogram, showing the blush of a gastrinoma in the duodenum (arrowed).

an elevated gastrin and basal acid output, but a source which is not found, should be treated with omeprazole and attempts at tumour localization repeated at 2–3-year intervals.

TREATMENT

Morbidity reflects gastrin hypersecretion, so management is directed primarily at the control of the hormone and its action. Control of the tumour, if effectively dealt with, will also eradicate the effects of gastrin hypersecretion. The ultimate aim should be eradication of the tumour, but this is possible in less than 20% of patients.

Surgery

Surgical excision of the tumour, with the resultant cure of the syndrome, is indicated in the rare circumstance when a single simple tumour is clearly identified and is amenable to surgical resection. Cure is indicated by return of circulating gastrin and acid secretion to normal levels. Where there are multiple tumours, as in the multiple endocrine neoplasia type 1 syndrome, or local metastases, a cure is very unlikely. Palliative surgery may be indicated, which will reduce peptide production, and this should always be combined with omeprazole therapy.[32]

Medical therapy

Acid hypersecretion from the stomach could only be controlled by total gastrectomy until H_2-receptor antagonists became available. More recently, omeprazole, a substituted benzimidazole, which competitively inhibits gastric hydrogen potassium adenosine triphosphatase, has become the treatment of choice preoperatively, and for maintenance. Omeprazole 80–120 mg daily effectively produces a medical gastrectomy, reducing basal acid output to less than 5 mmol/h after 2 days of treatment, and healing 98% of ulcers within 2 weeks of commencing therapy, and 100% within 1 month. These ulcers do not recur if treatment is maintained.[31]

Metastatic disease

Many patients with metastatic disease can lead a normal life, and further therapeutic intervention should only be considered if clinical improvement is likely; for example, if metastatic tumour bulk is causing symptoms through compression or infiltration. Two options are then available: cytotoxic chemotherapy or tumour embolization.

The cytotoxic regimen used at Hammersmith Hospital is an intravenous infusion of streptozotocin 500 mg/m^2 and of 5-fluorouracil 400 mg/m^2, on alternate days for 10 days. The course can be repeated every 2–3 months with close monitoring of renal, hepatic and bone marrow function. The commonest side-effects of this therapy are anorexia, nausea and vomiting. Only 20% of gastrinomas respond to chemotherapy, compared with 80% of VIPomas.

Hepatic artery embolization may provide good palliation in those patients with hepatic metastases, but requires a patent portal vein and considerable expertise.

PROGNOSIS

When the syndrome is controlled and the tumour excised, the prognosis is excellent, even with small metastatic deposits in regional lymph nodes. The prognosis is more guarded when there are metastases to the liver or extra-abdominal sites with a 20% survival rate at 5 years, compared with a greater than 80% survival rate for a single resectable lesion. In many cases, however several years of good quality life can be enjoyed despite a large tumour bulk.

CONCLUSION

The advent of H_2-receptor antagonists with routine availability of gastrin radioimmunoassay has changed the presentation of the gastrinoma syndrome and made earlier diagnosis possible. Whether this and the introduction of omeprazole will affect the overall morbidity and mortality remains to be seen.

INSULINOMAS, INCLUDING NESIDIOBLASTOSIS

Insulinoma is the most common pancreatic islet cell tumour, with an incidence of about one per million of the population. It was first described by W.J. Mayor in 1927 in a physician with recurrent hypoglycaemia which was later discovered to result from the inappropriate secretion of insulin into the circulation by tumours of pancreatic β-cells.[53] About 70% are single small benign tumours, 10% are multiple (usually microadenomas), 10% are part of the multiple endocrine neoplasia type I syndrome and 10% are malignant, with metastases.[14,19,30] Occasional cases of generalized islet hyperplasia and nesidioblastosis are recorded. Identification is made by histological methods, immunocytochemistry and the presence of insulin in tumour extracts.

CLINICAL FEATURES

Symptoms result from neuroglycopenia and the effect of hypoglycaemia on the nervous system; there also may be psychiatric and neurological disturbances. The excess of insulin secretion is offset by eating. The symptoms are therefore most common in the early morning and late afternoon and are increased by alcohol and attempts to diet and exercise. Sympathetic stimulation is rare as the blood glucose falls slowly, so that the characteristic features of iatrogenic insulin overdose are not seen. Weight gain is uncommon, except in those who treat their symptoms by overeating.

Psychological disturbances are often subtle and noticed either because they become more severe or are cumulatively striking. Episodes occur during fasting and are stopped by eating. Alterations in mood, attitude, behaviour and personality may all be seen. The subtlety of these changes commonly leads to delays in diagnosis, the mean interval between the onset of symptoms and diagnosis being 4 years, and periods of 10–20 years are not uncommon. The differential diagnosis is usually of psychiatric disorder, temporal lobe epilepsy or drug abuse.

The most common neurological disturbances are circumoral paraesthesiae and numbness, headaches, which may be severe, and mental dysfunction, which may progress to coma. Many organic neurological syndromes have been described. The differential diagnosis is of cerebrovascular disease, cerebal tumour, or infiltrative or metabolic syndromes.

INVESTIGATIONS

When symptoms occur the diagnosis is established by demonstrating hypoglycaemia and inappropriately raised plasma insulin levels. Initially blood should be taken after a 12-hour overnight fast, and if the blood glucose is less than 2.2 mmol/l, insulin and C-peptide are measured as well. If hypoglycaemia is not detected, the patient should be admitted for a 48–72 hour fast, in which free fluids are given and exercise is encouraged. If no symptoms occur during the fast, it should be terminated with 15–30 minutes of exercise, after which a final blood sample should be taken for glucose estimation, again saving plasma for insulin and C-peptide measurement. Normal subjects should not become hypoglycaemic and, if the blood glucose is less than 2.2 mmol/l, endogenous insulin production estimated by C-peptide should be undetectable. An insulin concentration greater than 50 pmol/l and C-peptide of greater than 300 pmol/l is diagnostic of insulinoma, unless there is evidence of ingestion of oral hypoglycaemic agents. If the insulin is raised, but there is a low C-peptide, this suggests factitious hypoglycaemia as a result of self-administration of insulin.

TUMOUR LOCALIZATION

Most insulinomas are 4 cm or less in diameter, highly vascular and found in all parts of the pancreas and occasionally in the duodenal wall or spleen hilum. The radiological investigation of choice is selective coeliac and superior mesenteric angiography, which has an accuracy of 55–75%, compared with 25–60% for ultrasonography.[17] If doubt remains, portal and splenic venous blood sampling for insulin assay may be helpful.[50]

TREATMENT

Ninety per cent of patients will have a single benign tumour which can be cured by resection if the tumour can be accurately localized. Perioperatively, blood sugar levels fall but subsequently hyperglycaemia is seen, and should be monitored for at least 24 hours. When the tumour cannot be resected, the patient is treated with appropriately spaced carbohydrate meals and diazoxide, 5–15 mg/kg of body weight, which directly inhibits insulin release and enhances glycogenolysis. It is usually given with a diuretic to prevent fluid retention. Hirsutism is common, but nausea and hypertension are rare at these doses. Verapamil, to a daily dose of 240 mg, may increase blood glucose, although it appears to have no effect on insulin release.[43] The long-acting somatostatin analogue octreotide (SMS 201-995) is effective in suppressing circulating insulin levels by more than 50%, and intermittent injections or continuous subcutaneous infusion, via a pump, may prevent hypoglycaemic episodes. Octreotide may suppress levels of counter-regulatory hormones to a greater extent however, particularly when the insulinoma is malignant, thus exacerbating the hypoglycaemia. It should thus be introduced with caution, in hospital.[25,55]

In the rare patients in whom the insulinoma is malignant, tumour bulk may be reduced by surgery, and the residual tumour treated by cytotoxic chemotherapy, or embolization of the arterial supply to hepatic metastases, to reduce its secretory capacity. Chemotherapy is with streptozotocin and 5-fluorouracil using the same regimen as for gastrinomas (see above), and the response rate is in the order of 50–60% for insulinomas.[34]

PROGNOSIS

Benign tumours run a prolonged course, and 20 or 30 years may lapse before the diagnosis is made. Mean survival of malignant tumours is approximately 14 months, but extreme variation is encountered.

NESIDIOBLASTOSIS

In this rare condition, nesidioblasts differentiate from pancreatic duct epithelium and from A, B, D, and PP cells, which are separate from the true islets, and increase the endocrine content of the pancreas fivefold.[6] The clinical picture is of a somnolent baby with ataxia and fits, who may become comatose, frequently suffering permanent brain damage. This is the result of hypoglycaemia and hyperinsulinism, which does not improve with time, in contrast to other forms of neonatal hypoglycaemia. The diagnosis is made by finding fasting hypolycaemia and hyperinsulinism, true insulinomas being very rare in infancy. Treatment used to be frequent feeds and diazoxide, usually in an attempt to gain time and weight before partial or total pancreatectomy. The long-acting somatostatin analogue octreotide (SMS 201-995) has proved very effective at preventing hypoglycaemia, and is now in widespread use for this condition.[56]

VIPOMAS AND OTHER TUMOURS

Over the last two decades a considerable number of regulatory peptides have been isolated. These are known to be important neurotransmitters in the central and peripheral nervous system, and a number of them also have role as circulating hormones. They can be identified by immunocytochemistry and radioimmunoassay. Islet cell tumours of the pancreas may produce both those peptides found in the normal adult pancreas (orthotopic secretions, for example, insulin, glucagon and somatostatin) and those usually found in other glands and tissues (ectopic secretion such as gastrin and vasoactive intestinal peptide). The tumours often secrete more than one peptide (*Table 11.11*). Neuroendocrine pancreatic tumours may be non-functioning and these have accounted for up to 50% of patients in some series.[13,46] Non-functioning tumours have

Table 11.11 Peptides secreted by gut neuroendocrine tumours, their functions and associated clinical syndromes

Peptides	*Action*	*Syndrome*
Gastrin	Gastric acid secretion Mucosal growth	Peptic ulceration Diarrhoea
Glucagon	Catabolism fat, protein, carbohydrate Inhibition of intestinal secretion	Rash Impaired glucose tolerance Venous thrombosis
Enteroglucagon	? Trophic to gut mucosa	Small intestinal growth
Insulin	Anabolism of fat, protein, carbohydrate	Recurrent hypoglycaemia Neuroglycopenia
Somatostatin	Inhibition of release and action of gut hormones Inhibition of GH release	Diabetes mellitus Gallstones Steatorrhoea
VIP	Stimulation of intestinal secretion Smooth muscle relaxation	Profuse watery diarrhoea Cardiovascular collapse
GRF	Stimulation of GH release	Acromegaly
CRF	Stimulation of ACTH release	Cushing's syndrome
PTHrP	? Foetal calcium regulation	Hypercalcaemia
Neurotensin	Inhibition of gastric acid and pancreatic secretions Stimulation of gut motility	
PP	? Inhibition of pancreatic and biliary secretion	

VIP = Vasoactive intestinal peptide; GRF = growth hormone releasing factor; PTHrP = parathyroid hormone related peptide; PP = pancreatic polypeptide; GH = growth hormone; ACTH = corticotrophin.

often been mistakenly diagnosed as pancreatic adenocarcinomas, but they are correctly recognized with increasing frequency. Islet cell tumours tend to be slow growing, and early mortality is usually due to systemic effects of peptide hypersecretion rather that the result of increasing tumour mass. Among the different types of pancreatic endocrine tumour, insulinomas stand out as usually being benign and thus curable by resection. The other tumour types are usually malignant, and late recurrence is frequent after apparently successful resection of a single tumour.[16] Metastases occur most frequently in the liver, but may be found in bone and lung (*Figure 11.58*), the latter carrying a very poor prognosis. Metastatic tumours are treated by surgical debulking, cytotoxic chemotherapy and hepatic artery embolisation. Peptide secretion may be reduced by using the long acting somatostatin analogue octreotide.

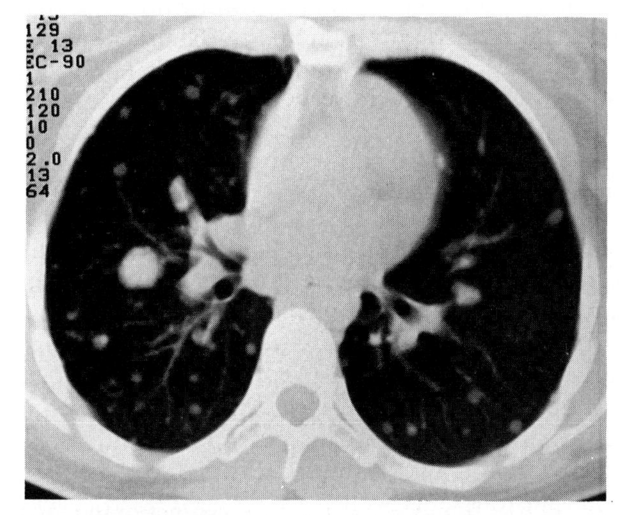

Figure 11.58 CT scan of the thorax showing multiple metastatic nodules to the lung from a non-functioning pancreatic neuroendocrine tumour.

CLINICAL FEATURES

VIPoma

Vasoactive intestinal peptide is a 28-amino acid peptide and its structure puts it in the glucagon–secretin family of peptides. It relaxes smooth muscle, lowers blood pressure and stimulates watery secretion from the intestine and pancreas.[40] It is widely distributed throughout the body in both the central and peripheral nervous system, and is thought to act physiologically as a neurotransmitter or neuromodulator rather than as a circulating hormone. Infusion of the peptide can cause watery diarrhoea in animals and has a dramatic affect on water and ion transport in the human small and large bowel.[22] Two other peptides, peptide histidine valine and peptide histidine methionine are derived from the same precursor, prepro-vasoactive intestinal peptide, and also stimulate intestinal secretion. It is now thought that both vasoactive intestinal peptide and peptide histidine methionine contribute to the aetiology of the VIPoma syndrome.[58]

In 1958 Verner and Morrison[51] described two cases of severe watery diarrhoea associated with non-insulin secreting islet cell adenomas of the pancreas. The syndrome became known by various synonyms: Verner–Morrison syndrome, the watery diarrhoea syndrome, watery diarrhoea hypokalaemia and achlorhydria syndrome or pancreatic cholera syndrome. Bloom, Polak and Pearse[11] were able to show that these tumours were associated with vasoactive intestinal peptide production. In a series of 62 patients, Long *et al.*[27] found that all pancreatic tumours associated with watery diarrhoea produced the peptide. Ten patients were shown to have ganglioneuroblastomas, which are the main extra-pancreatic vasoactive intestinal peptide producing tumours. Phaeochromocytomas producing the peptide have also been described.

The most important clinical feature of the VIPoma syndrome is the very severe watery diarrhoea without steatorrhoea. Stool volumes may be up to 20 litres a day. There is a specific potassium losing enteropathy, resulting in hypokalaemic acidosis, which may end in cardiac standstill. Initially the diarrhoea may be intermittent but, when severe, the hypotensive action of vasoactive intestinal peptide may precipitate vascular collapse and even death. Weight loss is not an early feature but can become extreme in advanced cases. Mild diabetes mellitus and hypercalcaemia occur in a sizeable minority of cases. Vasoactive intestinal peptide has been shown to have a direct glucagon-like effect, causing increased hepatic gluconeogenesis, and the hypercalcaemia may be due to secretion of parathyroid hormone related peptide, or rarely to primary hyperparathyroidism in association with the multiple endocrine neoplasia type I syndrome. Hypochlorhydria may distinguish the VIPoma syndrome from the gastrinoma syndrome, which may also be associated with diarrhoea, but 50% of patients with VIPoma have normal gastric acid secretion. The diagnosis of a VIPoma can only be made by demonstrating both elevated vasoactive intestinal peptide and peptide histidine methionine in the same plasma sample.

Neurotensinoma

Neurotensin is a peptide of 30 amino acids which inhibits gastric acid and stimulates small-intestinal juice production and small-intestinal motor activity. Neurotensin is particularly potent in stimulating contractions of the large bowel. Ten per cent of VIPomas also secrete neurotensin, and, occasionally, neurotensin is produced by other types of tumour or by a pure neurotensinoma.[9] No particular clinical syndrome has been associated with neurotensin production by pancreatic tumours and patients present at a late stage with a high tumour bulk and multiple liver metastases.[17]

Pancreatic polypeptide

Pancreatic peptide consists of 36 amino acids, and was accidentally discovered contaminating insulin preparations. It has been demonstrated to have a weak action in man, inhibiting gallbladder contraction and pancreatic enzyme secretion. Cells producing pancreatic polypeptide comprise approximately 10% of the population of the islet of Langerhans. It is therefore not surprising that pancreatic endocrine tumours frequently secrete pancreatic polypeptide. Approximately a third of gastrinomas, three-quarter of VIPomas, half of glucagonomas and one quarter of insulinomas also release large amounts into the circulation, and nearly 100% of pancreatic endocrine tumours contain significant extractable amounts.[37] Although measurement of the hormone in the blood is a good indicator of the presence of a pancreatic endocrine tumour, no clinical features have yet been recognized in association with elevation of plasma levels.[49]

SOMATOSTATINOMA

Somatostatin is a peptide produced by D-cells which, like the pancreatic polypeptide cell, form about 10% of the cells of the islet of Langerhans. Somatostatin is remarkable for its widespread inhibitory actions on the release of gastrointestinal hormones, and it directly inhibits the action of the same hormones on target tissues. Somatostatinomas are associated with steatorrhoea, diabetes mellitus and gallstones, as well as a reduced gastric acid secretion, although 50% are asymptomatic.[41] These tumours are often extremely slow growing, with a natural history possibly in excess of 25 years. It seems likely that escape occurs from the powerful effects of somatostatin when hypersecretion is prolonged.[41] At presentation tumour bulk may be considerable, so that resection is difficult.[21] There have been a number of reports of the co-existence of somatostatinoma with phaeochromocytoma and neurofibromatosis.[45]

ENTEROGLUCAGONOMA

One patient has been reported with an enteroglucagonoma,[10] a renal tumour associated with gross slowing of gastrointestinal transit and a striking elongation of small intestinal mucosal villi.

OTHER PEPTIDES

Recently, pancreatic endocrine tumours have been described that secrete growth hormone releasing factor with secondary acromegaly,[47] corticotrophin-releasing factor or corticotrophin with associated Cushing's syndrome,[26] and parathyroid hormone related peptide with associated hypercalcaemia and hypophosphataemia.[57]

DIAGNOSIS

Diagnosis of VIPomas and other endocrine tumours is based mainly on clinical awareness of the particular syndrome. Confirmation of the clinical suspicion is provided by the finding of elevated plasma levels of the appropriate gut hormones. A fresh fasting plasma sample containing the enzyme inhibitor aprotinin (Trasylol) is taken and is sent to the nearest major radioimmunoassay laboratory (in the UK via the Supra Regional Assay Service). Plasma levels of the respective peptide are usually extremely elevated and provide no diagnostic problem. In the case of the VIPoma syndrome, for example, levels above 60 pmol/l are compatible with a tumour. If the level is above 30 pmol/l, further samples are required for repeated estimations and the clinical situation should be re-examined. Healthy subjects normally have vasoactive intestinal peptide concentrations of approximately 2 pmol/l. Gastrin, glucagon, vasoactive intestinal peptide, somatostatin, neurotensin and pancreatic polypeptide are routinely assayed together and elevation of more than one peptide helps confirm the diagnosis. Of those patients with islet cell tumours, 7% develop elevation of other hormone levels with associated syndromes and in 50% of cases this would be a gastrinoma. Thus gut hormone assays should be performed at 6-monthly intervals for the rest of the patient's life, irrespective of the tumour syndrome at presentation.[55]

LOCALIZATION

Non-invasive procedures such as CT and ultrasound are followed by highly selective angiography with background subtraction. Rapid dynamic CT following bolus injection of contrast gives detection rates of 80%–90%.[48] Meticulous angiography can localize 92% of cases (*Figure 11.59*), and this detection rate may be improved by the use of selective venous sampling, although this is a procedure to be undertaken only in centres with highly experienced personnel.[39] The use of indium-111 labelled somatostatin analogues is still under evaluation.[23]

Tissue obtained by hepatic biopsy or at surgery may be examined histologically. The appearance of the tissue gives little indication of a tumour's metastatic potential and cannot usually be used to indicate prognosis. Immunocytochemical staining with antibodies and, more recently, techniques of in situ hybridization and northern blotting, allow localization and quantification of peptides within neoplastic cells.[57] Radioimmunoassay of tumour extracts provides further confirmation of hormone production.

TREATMENT

Surgery

Surgical removal of a lone tumour is optimal, but, even when achieved, later recurrences are common to all pancreatic endocrine tumours other than insulinomas, although occasionally cure may be affected in VIPoma and glucagonoma. Excellent palliation can be achieved by tumour bulk reduction if total excision is impossible,[46] because the tumours are slow growing and produce their clinical symptoms by elevated circulating hormone concentrations.

Hepatic artery embolization

Embolization of the hepatic artery supply to liver metastases requires considerable expertise and a patent portal vein, but can result in good palliation.[2,3,4] The procedure should be covered by broad spectrum antibiotics such as imipenem but, despite this, all patients become pyrexial and have striking increases in liver function tests during the first week following embolization. Duration of response ranges from 3–10 months, with a median of 5 months, and the procedure can be repeated when symptoms recur, providing the portal vein remains patent.

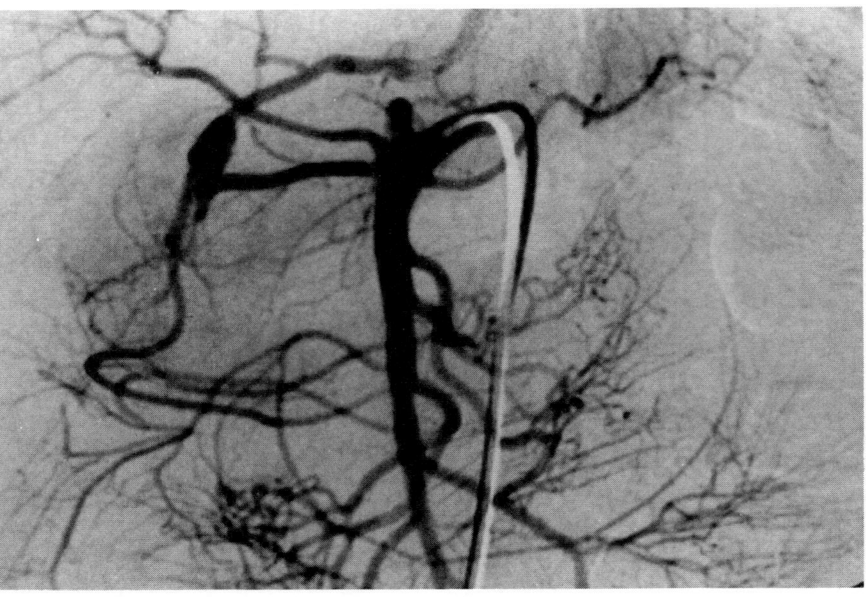

(a)

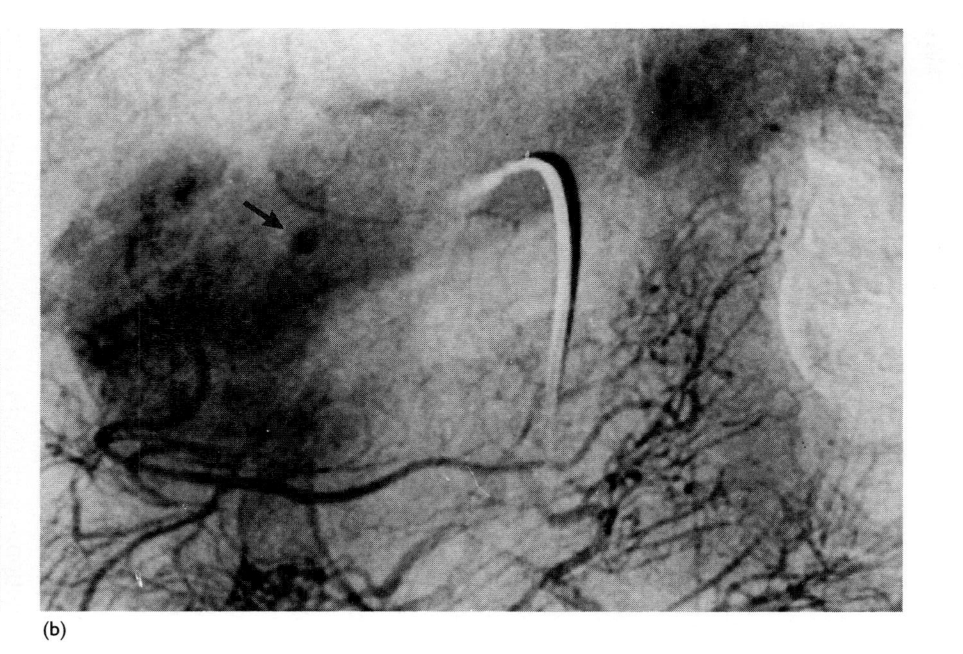

(b)

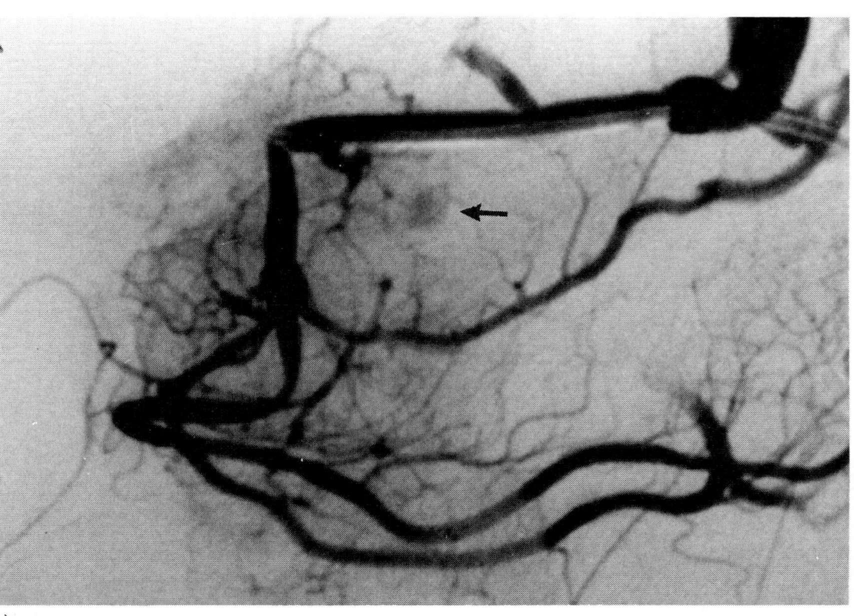

(c)

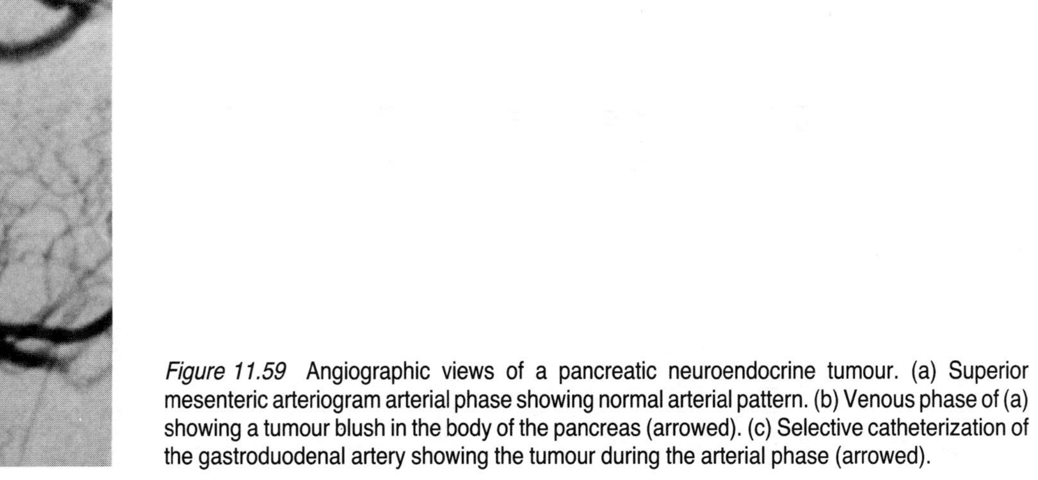

Figure 11.59 Angiographic views of a pancreatic neuroendocrine tumour. (a) Superior mesenteric arteriogram arterial phase showing normal arterial pattern. (b) Venous phase of (a) showing a tumour blush in the body of the pancreas (arrowed). (c) Selective catheterization of the gastroduodenal artery showing the tumour during the arterial phase (arrowed).

Cytotoxic chemotherapy

The cytotoxic regimen of 5-fluorouracil and streptozotocin was reported by Moertel,[34] with a response rate for islet cell tumours of 63%. Further studies of this combination using different dosages, and in combination with vincristine and adriamycin, have shown little improvement in this response rate.[7,15,20] The regimen used at the Hammersmith Hospital is streptozotocin 500 mg/m^2 and 5-fluorouracil 400 mg/m^2 given as an intravenous bolus on alternate days for 10 days. Renal, hepatic and bone marrow function are closely monitored. The course is repeated every 2–3 months, and normally three to four courses would be given, followed by a 6-month wait to assess reduction in tumour bulk, before concluding whether there is a response. Oberg and Eriksson[35] have used α-recombinant interferon, with 25% of patients showing a reduction in hormone secretion, but less than 10% showing a decrease in tumour bulk. Other groups have shown poor response rates with many side-effects, including autoimmune haemolytic anaemia, leucopenia with associated flu-like symptoms and liver fibrosis, and we do not advocate the use of interferon as a routine.

Long-acting somatostatin analogue

The long-acting somatostatin analogue octreotide (SMS 201-995)[8] significantly lowers basal plasma levels of pancreatic polypeptide, glucagon, insulin, vasoactive intestinal peptide and gastrin, and suppresses postprandial release of vasoactive intestinal peptide and gastrin in patients with pancreatic endocrine tumours. The clinical symptoms associated with peptide hypersecretion are diminished or abolished in most patients with pancreatic endocrine tumours treated with octreotide.[5] It may be life saving in patients with VIPoma crisis, with reduction of diarrhoea almost to normal in 24 hours, and resolution of electrolyte imbalance within 48 hours. In 10 patients with pancreatic endocrine tumours treated over a 5-year period with a mean treatment period of 29 months (range 13–54 months), treatment was initially very effective, but symptoms worsened about 5 months after the start of therapy (100 μg twice daily). This was initially reversed by increasing the dose of octreotide over the next 6–12 months to a twice daily maximum of 500 μg. After a further 24 months at this maximum dosage, symptoms recurred and were unresponsive to even higher doses or other therapeutic intervention, and all patients died within a 5-month period once this resistant phase has been reached.[53]

Other treatments

In the VIPoma syndrome acute crisis should be managed with fluid and electrolyte support and, if other measures fail, prednisolone 40–60 mg daily, may control symptoms for up to 6 months.

Prognosis

The overall survival after 5 years is between 40% and 70%, with a worse prognosis in those with non-functioning tumours or those who have hepatic metastases at the time of presentation.[3,46]

CONCLUSION

Widespread availability of radioimmunoassay and immunocytochemistry for a variety of peptides has allowed the diagnosis of an increasing number of different tumour types and clinical syndromes. Although many islet cell tumours are malignant, and metastases at the time of diagnosis make surgical cure rare, effective treatment with cytotoxic agents, hepatic artery embolization and, more recently, the long-acting somatostatin analogue octreotide, produce useful palliation, allowing the patient to return home with a much improved quality of life.

GLUCAGONOMA

Glucagonomas are pancreatic islet cell tumours containing or secreting pancreatic glucagon, and are invariably malignant. They produce a characteristic, largely unexplained clinical syndrome, and have an incidence of about one per 20 million.[29]

CLINICAL FEATURES

The cardinal feature is a necrolytic migratory erythematous rash, which occurs in nearly 75% of patients. The rash usually starts in the groins but often affects the thighs, buttocks and perineal area and can spread to involve any parts of the body. It is often associated with angular stomatitis and glossitis. Histologically and clinically it is similar to the rash of acrodermatitis enteropathica, which occurs in zinc deficiency. Other proposed aetiological factors are the hypercatabolic state and the depression of plasma amino acid levels caused by glucagon hypersecretion.[44]

The other clinical features are impaired glucose tolerance, but only usually mild diabetes mellitus, a marked tendency to severe, life-threatening venous thrombosis resistant to conventional treatment, moderate normochromic normocytic anaemia and, less commonly, weight loss, intermittent diarrhoea and severe depression.

The clinical features develop in random order and may have been present for many years before diagnosis, even when associated with malignant tumours.[33]

Diagnosis

Plasma glucagon levels are usually elevated 10–20-fold, much higher than in stress, burns or ketoacidosis. In 50% of cases, pancreatic polypeptide levels are also elevated and, when estimation is available, the depression of plasma amino acids is also diagnostic. Tumour localization is by ultrasonography and CT followed by visceral angiography.

TREATMENT

Surgery is curative in less than 5% of patients. Debulking of the tumour may be helpful. Recently, excision of the primary tumour coupled with liver transplantation for metastatic disease confined to the liver has been reported, with disease-free survival of at least 36 months.[28] This technique may ultimately offer potential cure, and its use could be extended to other metastatic neuroendocrine tumours. Cytotoxic chemotherapy with streptozotocin and 5-fluorouracil can occasionally have dramatic results and hepatic artery embolization may provide useful palliation. Chronic therapy with the long-acting somatostatin analogue octreotide reduces the length and severity of the glucagonoma rash exacerbation. Other therapeutic measures for the rash include oral and topical zinc with a high protein diet, and acute exacerbations may be managed by amino acid and blood transfusions.

PROGNOSIS

This is highly variable and depends entirely on the response to treatment. Many glucagonomas present relatively late despite the presence of widespread metastases.

ACKNOWLEDGEMENTS

With thanks to Dr J. Jackson, Consultant Radiologist at Hammersmith Hospital, London for help with the illustrations.

REFERENCES

1. Adrian, T.E., Uttenhal, L.O., Williams, S.J. and Bloom, S.R. (1986) Secretion of pancreatic polypeptide in patients with pancreatic and endocrine tumours. *New England Journal of Medicine*, **315**, 287–291.
2. Ajani, J.A., Carrasco, C., Charnsangavej, C. *et al.* (1988) Islet cell tumours metastatic to the liver: effective palliation by sequential hepatic artery embolisation. *Annals of Internal Medicine*, **1083**, 340–344.
3. Alison, D.M., Modlin, I.M. and Jenkins, W.J., (1977) Treatment of carcinoid liver metastases by hepatic artery embolisation. *Lancet*, **ii**, 1323–1325.
4. Alison, D.M. (1978) Therapeutic embolisation. *British Journal of Hospital Medicine*, **20**, 707–715.
5. Anderson, J.V. and Bloom, S.R. (1986) Neuroendocrine tumours of the gut: long-term therapy with the somatostatin analogue SMS 201-995. *Scandinavian Journal of Gastroenterology*, **21**(Suppl.119), 115–128.
6. Aynsley-Green, A., Polak, J.M., Keeling, J. *et al.* (1978) Averted sudden neonatal death due to pancreatic nesidioblastosis. *Lancet*, **i**, 550.
7. Bauer, W., Brimer, U., Doepfner, W. *et al.* (1982) SMS 201-995: a very potent and selective octapeptide analogue of somatostatin with prolonged action. *Life Sciences*, **31**, 1133–1141.
8. Blackburn, A.M., Bryant, M.G., Adrian, T.E. and Bloom, S.R. (1981) Pancreatic tumours produce neurotensin. *Journal of Clinical Endocrinology and Metabolism*, **52**, 820–822.
9. Bloom, S.R. (1972) An enteroglucagon tumour. *Gut*, **13**, 520–523.
10. Bloom, S.R., Polak, J.M. and Pearse, A.G.E. (1973) Vasoactive intestinal polypeptide and watery diarrhoea syndrome. *Lancet*, **ii**, 14–16.
11. Broder, L.E. and Carter, S.K. (1973) Pancreatic islet cell carcinoma. II. Results of therapy with streptozotocin in 52 patients. *Annals of Internal Medicine*, **79**, 108–118.
12. Case Records of the Massachusetts General Hospital (1983) *New England Journal of Medicine*, **308**, 30–37.
13. Eriksson, B., Oberg, K. and Skogseid, B. (1989) Neuroendocrine pancreatic tumors. *Acta Oncologica*, **28**, 373–377.
14. Fajans, S.S. (1979) Diagnosis and treatment of insulinomas. *Annual Review of Medicine*, **30**, 313–329.
15. Frame, J., Kelsen, D., Kemeny, J. *et al.* (1988) A phase II trial of streptozotocin and adriamycin in advanced APUD tumours. *American Journal of Clinical Oncology*, **11**, 490–495.
16. Friessen, S.R. (1982) Tumours of the endocrine pancreas. *New England Journal of Medicine*, **306**, 580–590.
17. Galiber, A.K., Reading, C.C., Charboneau, J.W. *et al.* (1988) Localisation of pancreatic insulinoma:

comparison of pre- and intraoperative US with CT and angiography. *Radiology*, **166**, 405–408.
18. Gregory, R.A., Tracy, H.J., French, J. and Sircus, M. (1960) Extraction of a gastrin-like substance from a pancreatic tumour in a case of Zollinger-Ellison syndrome. *Lancet*, **i**, 1045–1048.
19. Hall, R., Anderson, J., Smart, G.A. and Breese, M. (1978) Hypoglycaemia. *Fundamentals of Clinical Endocrinology* 3rd ed, pp. 583–599. Tunbridge Wells: Atman.
20. Hansen, R., Helm, J., Wilson, J.F. and Wilson, S. (1988) Nonfunctioning islet cell carcinoma of the pancreas. Complete response to continuous 5-Fluorouracil infusion. *Cancer*, **62**, 15–17.
21. Krejs, G.J., Orci, L., Conlon, J.M. *et al.* (1979) Somatostatinoma syndrome: biochemical, morphologic and clinical features. *New England Journal of Medicine*, **301**, 285–292.
22. Krejs, G.J. (1990) Effect of VIP infusion on water and ion transport in the human large intestine. *Gastroenterology*, **78**, 1200–1204.
23. Krenning, E.P., Bakker, W.H., Breeman, W.A. *et al.* (1989) Localisation of endocrine-related tumours with radioiodinated analogue of somatostatin. *Lancet*, **i**, 242–244.
24. Krenning, E.P., Bakker, W.H., Kooij, P.P., Breeman, W.A., Oei, H.Y., De Jong, M. *et al.* (1992) Somatostatin receptor scintigraphy with indium-111-DTPA-D-Phe-I-octreotide in man: metabolism, dosimetry and comparison with iodine-123-Tyr-3 octreotide. *Journal of Nuclear Medicine*, **33**, 652–658.
25. Laron, Z. (1990) Somatostatin analogues in the management of benign insulinomas. *Israeli Journal of Medical Science*, **26**, 1–2.
26. Lokich, J., Botha, A., O'Hara, C. and Fedamen, D. (1987) Metastatic islet cell tumour with ACTH, gastrin and glucagon secretion: clinical and pathological studies with multiple therapies. *Cancer*, **59**, 2053–2058.
27. Long, R.G., Bryant, M.G., Mitchell, S.J. *et al.* (1981) Clinicopathological study of pancreatic and ganglioneuroblastoma tumours secreting vasoactive intestinal polypeptide (VIPomas). *British Medical Journal*, **282**, 1767–1771.
28. Makowka, L., Tzakis, A.G., Mazzaferro, V. *et al.* (1989) Transplantation of the liver for metastatic endocrine tumors of the intestine and pancreas. *Surgery, Gynecology and Obstetrics*, **168**, 107–111.
29. Mallinson, C.N., Bloom, S.R., Warin, A.P. *et al.* (1974) A glucagonoma syndrome. *Lancet*, **ii**, 1–3.
30. Marks, V. and Samols, E. (1974) Insulinoma: Natural history and diagnosis. *Clinics in Gastroenterology*, **3**, 559–573.
31. McArthur, K.E., Collen, M.J., Maton, P.N., Cherner, J.A., Howard, J.M. *et al.* (1985) Omeprazole: Effective, convenient therapy for Zollinger–Ellison syndrome. *Gastroenterology*, **88**, 939–944.
32. McCarthy, D.E. (1980) The place of surgery in the Zollinger–Ellison syndrome. *New England Journal of Medicine*, **302**, 1344–1347.
33. McGavran, M., Unger, R.H. and Recant, L. *et al.* (1966) A glucagon secreting alpha-cell carcinoma of the pancreas. *New England Journal of Medicine*, **274**, 1408.
34. Moertel, C.G., Hanley, J.A. and Johnson, L.A. (1980) Streptozotocin alone compared with streptozotocin plus fluorouracil in the treatment of advanced islet-cell carcinoma. *New England Journal of Medicine*, **303**, 1189–1194.
35. Oberg, K. and Eriksson, B. (1989) Medical treatment of neuroendocrine tumours. *Acta Oncologica*, **28**, 425–431.
36. Pipeleers-Marichal, M., Somers, G., Willems, G. *et al.* (1990) Gastrinomas in the duodenums of patients with multiple endocrine neoplasia type 1 and the Zollinger-Ellison syndrome. *New England Journal of Medicine*, **322**, 723–727.
37. Polak, J.M., Bloom, S.R., Adrian, T.E. *et al.* (1976) Pancreatic polypeptide in insulinomas, gastrinomas, VIPomas and glucagonomas. *Lancet*, **i**, 328–330.
38. Rosell, S., Rokaeus, A. and Theodorsson-Norheim, E. (1983) The role of neurotensin in disease. *Scandinavian Journal of Gastroenterology*, **18**, 59–67.
39. Rossi, P., Allison, D.J., Bezzi, M. *et al.* (1989) Endocrine tumours of the pancreas. *Radiology Clinics of North America*, **27**, 129–161.
40. Said, S.J. (Ed.) (1982) *Vasoactive Intestinal Peptide.* New York: Raven Press.
41. Schuszdiarra, V. (1983) Somatostatin – physiological and pathophysiological aspects. *Scandinavian Journal of Gastroenterology*, **18**, 69–84.
42. Stacpoole, P.W., Kassleberg, A.G., Berelewitz, M. and Chey, W.Y. (1983) Somatostatinoma syndrome: does a clinical entity exist? *Acta Endocrinologica*, **102**, 80–87.
43. Stehouwer, C.D., Lems, W.F., Fischer, H.R. and Hackeng, W.H. (1989) Malignant insulinoma: is combined treatment with verapamil and the long-acting somatostatin analogue octreotide more effective than single therapy with either drug. *Netherlands Journal of Medicine*, **55**, 86–94.
44. Sweet, D. (1984) A dermatosis specifically associated with a tumour of pancreatic alpha cells. *British Journal of Dermatology*, **90**, 301–308.
45. Swinburn, B.A., Yeong, M.L., Lane, M.R. *et al.* (1988) Neurofibromatosis associated with somatostatinoma. *Clinical Endocrinology Oxford*, **28**, 353–359.
46. Thompson, G.B., van Heerden, J.A., Grant, C.S. *et al.* (1989) Islet cell carcinomas of the pancreas: a twenty-year experience. *Surgery*, **104**, 1011–1017.
47. Thorner, M.O., Perriman, R.L., Cronin, M.J. *et al.* (1982) Somatotroph hyperplasia. Successful treatment of acromegaly by removal of a pancreatic islet tumour secreting a growth hormone-releasing

factor. *Journal of Clinical Investigation*, **79**, 965–977.
48. Tjon, A., Tham, R.T., Jansen, J.B. *et al.* (1989) MR, CT, and ultrasound findings of metastatic VIPoma in the pancreas. *Journal of Computer Assisted Tomography*, **13**, 142–144.
49. Tomita, T., Friessen, S., Kimmel, J.R. *et al.* (1983) Pancreatic polypeptide secreting islet cell tumours: a study of three cases. *American Journal of Pathology*, **113**, 134–142.
50. Turner, R.C., Morris, P.J., Lee, E.C.G. and Harris, E.A. (1978) Localisation of insulinomas. *Lancet*, **i**, 515–518.
51. Verner, J.V. and Morrison, A.B. (1958) Islet cell tumour and a syndrome of refractory, watery diarrhoea and hypokalaemia. *American Journal of Medicine*, **25**, 374–380.
52. Wynick, D., Anderson, J.V., Williams, S.J. and Bloom, S.R. (1988) Resistance of metastatic pancreatic endocrine tumours after long term treatment with the somatostatin analogue octreotide (SMS 201-995). *Clinical Endocrinology*, **30**, 385–388.
53. Wilder, R.A., Allan, F.A., Power, A.H. and Roberston, H.E. (1927) Carcinoma of the islands of the pancreas: hyperinsulinism and hypoglycaemia.
54. Wynick, D., Williams, S.J. and Bloom, S.R. (1988) Symptomatic secondary hormone syndromes in patients with established malignant pancreatic endocrine tumours. *New England Journal of Medicine*, **319**, 599–604.
55. Wynick, D., Polak, J.M. and Bloom, S. R. (1989) Somatostatin and its analogues in the therapy of gastrointestinal disease. *Pharmacology and Therapeutics*, **41**, 353–370.
56. Wynick, D. (1990) Gastrinoma syndrome in multiple endocrine neoplasia: new approaches to localisation and management. *British Medical Journal*, **301**, 489–490.
57. Wynick, D., Ratcliffe, W.A., Heath, D.A. *et al.* (1990) Treatment of a malignant pancreatic endocrine tumour secreting parathyroid hormone related protein. *British Medical Journal*, **300**, 1314–1315.
58. Yiangou, Y., Williams, S.J., Bishop, A.E. *et al.* (1987). Peptide-Histidine-Methionine-Immunoreactivity in plasma and tissue from patients with VIP secreting tumours and watery diarrhoea. *Journal of Clinical Endocrinology and Metabolism,* **64**, 131–139.
59. Zollinger, R.M. and Ellison, E.H. (1955) Primary peptic ulceration of the jejunum associated with islet cell tumours of the pancreas. *Annals of Surgery*, **142**, 709–773.

Chapter 12

Gallbladder and Biliary Tract

ANATOMY AND EMBRYOLOGY

I.S. Benjamin

The liver primordium appears in the third week of the conceptus as an outgrowth from the foregut which penetrates the septum transversum to form both the liver and bile ducts. A small ventral outgrowth is formed from the developing bile duct and gives rise to the gallbladder and cystic duct (*Figure 12.1*). The gallbladder can be recognized on fetal ultrasound at 20 weeks in 38% of cases.[19] Bile is formed by hepatocytes by the 12th week, and is able to enter the duodenum at this stage. The entry point of the bile duct to the duodenum gradually shifts from anterior to posterior, so that the duct comes to lie behind the duodenum.

Grossly, the gallbladder is pear shaped, some 6–8 cm long and 2–3 cm in diameter, with a capacity of some 50 ml. It is partly embedded in the underside of the right liver at the junction of segments IV and V,[7] and is covered by peritoneum continuous with Glisson's capsule which invests the liver. The body gives rise to the neck from which a small pouch (Hartmann's) may project. From here the cystic duct (3–4 cm) runs to join the common hepatic duct which together then form the common bile duct (*Figure 12.2*). The cystic duct lumen contains a series of crescentic mucosal folds which form the spiral valves of Heister which may help to hold the lumen open. There is considerable variation from this general description: in particular, several common anomalies of the cystic duct/hepatic duct junction exist (see Congenital abnormalities, p. 1676),

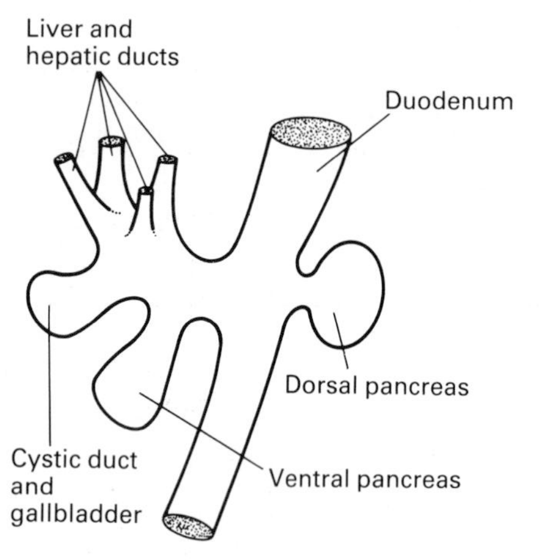

Figure 12.1 Embryology of the biliary system: the four primordia of the hepaticopancreatic complex in the fifth week. (Reproduced, with permission, from Gray, S.E. and Skandalakis, J.E. (1972) *Embryology for Surgeons*, p. 252. Philadelphia: W.B. Saunders.)

and the cystic duct may run in a common sheath with the common hepatic duct for a variable distance. Some of these anomalies are important in that they may give rise to operative difficulties and lead to biliary injury at cholecystectomy. The blood supply of the extrahepatic bile ducts is derived from the hepatic artery and the pancreatoduodenal arterial arcade, and is carried mainly by two narrow vessels running along the axial direction of the bile duct on its medial and lateral border – the '3 o'clock and 9 o'clock arteries';[38] the importance of these vessels has been noted in the causation of ischaemic biliary strictures following biliary anastomosis for injury or in liver transplantation. The gallbladder receives its blood supply from the cystic artery, an end-artery arising usually from the right hepatic artery: its origin and course are also somewhat variable.[33]

Anatomical anomalies of the gallbladder and ducts include agenesis of the gallbladder,[2,24] left-

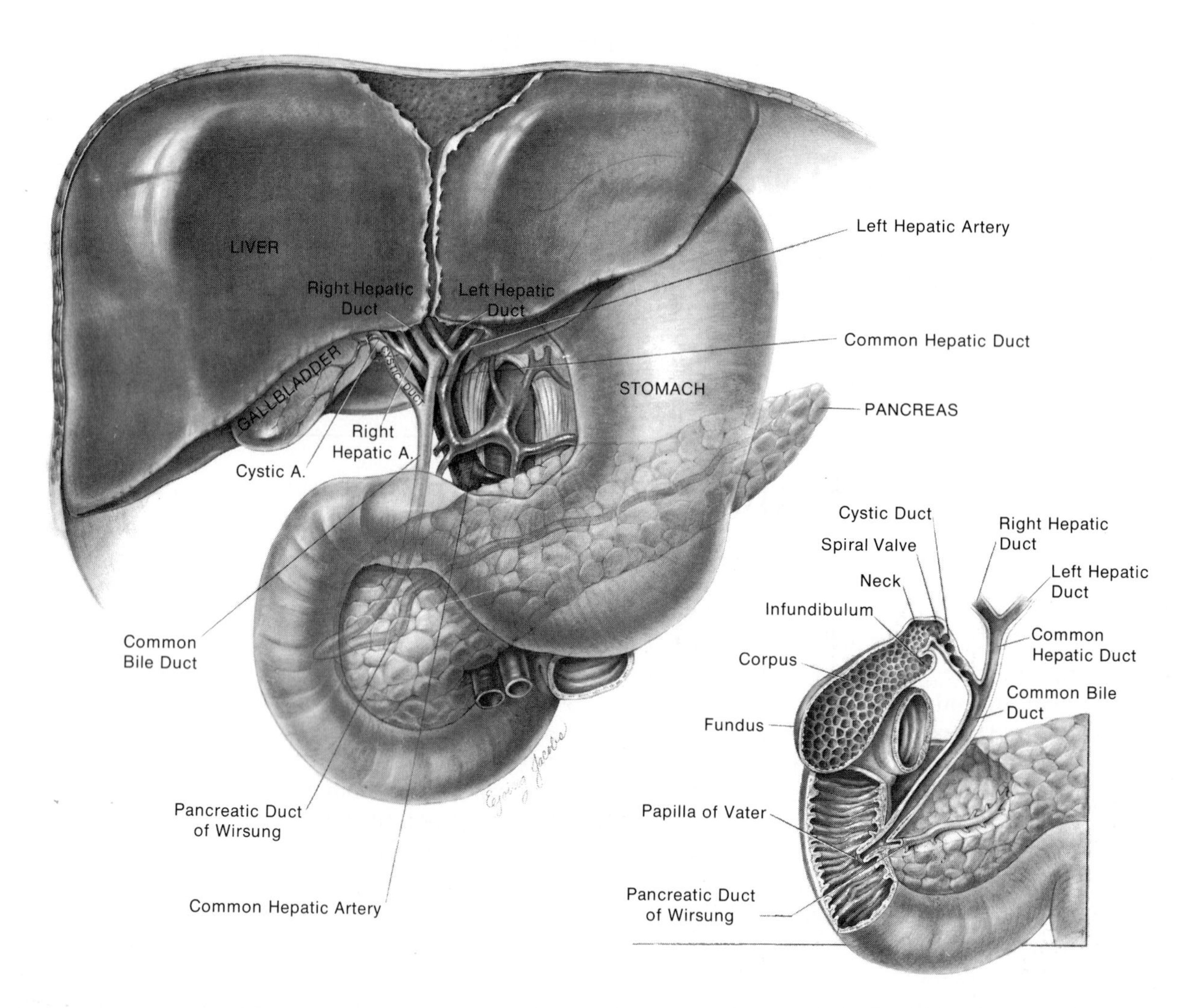

Figure 12.2 Anatomy of the biliary system. (Reproduced, with permission, from Orloff, M.J. (1981) The biliary system. In: *Davis-Christopher Textbook of Surgery* (Ed.) Sabiston, D.C. p. 1230. Philadelphia: W.B. Saunders.)

sided gallbladder,[40] double gallbladder, triple gallbladder (including a case of stone in the 'middle gallbladder'[5]), absent common hepatic duct and cystic ducts,[45] and absent common hepatic duct with drainage of the right and left hepatic ducts into the duodenum via the gallbladder and cystic duct.[12,39] Biliary atresia and congenital cystic disease are considered elsewhere (see Chapter 11).

The biliary tract receives both sympathetic (from the coeliac plexus) and parasympathetic (vagal) innervation, and gives rise to afferent fibres. The sympathetic fibres supply the muscle coat, which also receives a small cholinergic innervation. A myenteric plexus is present in the submucosa and subserosa. Receptors for vasoactive intestinal polypeptide have been described on gallbladder nerve fibres and pharmacological techniques have revealed a variety of receptors on the smooth muscle.

HISTOCHEMISTRY

ENZYMES

Acid phosphatase activity has been demonstrated in human *gallbladder* epithelium at the ultrastructural level[28] chiefly in the lysosomes, although some is seen in the Golgi apparatus. Thiamine pyrophosphatase is present in the Golgi apparatus too, and small amounts are also seen in mucus droplets. This may represent a route for various lysosomal enzymes to be secreted into the bile along with mucus.[41] Mucosal β-glucuronidase activity measured biochemically is higher in acalculous patients despite the fact that this enzyme has been thought to play a role in the formation of the nidus for lithogenesis.

Alkaline phosphatase has been demonstrated in gallbladder capillary endothelium[49] and in the brush border of the epithelium[27] (*Figure 12.3*). Three patterns are found – complete, patchy and absent – which can be related to the biliary lipid composition, suggesting that the biliary epithelium may be able to modify biliary lipids. Alkaline phosphatase is found in the embryologically related small intestinal brush border, a known site of lipid absorption. Human gallbladder epithelial esterase activity is chiefly lysosomal (*Figure 12.4*). Using inhibitors and activators, it appears that at least two enzyme complexes are involved, one of which has cholesterol esterase activity. Bile acids are able to modulate the mucosal enzyme activity.

MUCOSUBSTANCES

Wallraff and Dietrich[49] provided one of the earliest comprehensive surveys of gallbladder histochemistry, documenting the presence of glycoproteins, neutral and acidic mucosubstances, in the apical epithelium. This was confirmed by Esterly and Spicer,[13] who showed that the amount of mucus present increased with inflammation; this has also been described in experimental lithogenesis in animals.[20,31] The neck cells secrete both neutral and carboxymucins. In carcinoma of the gallbladder,

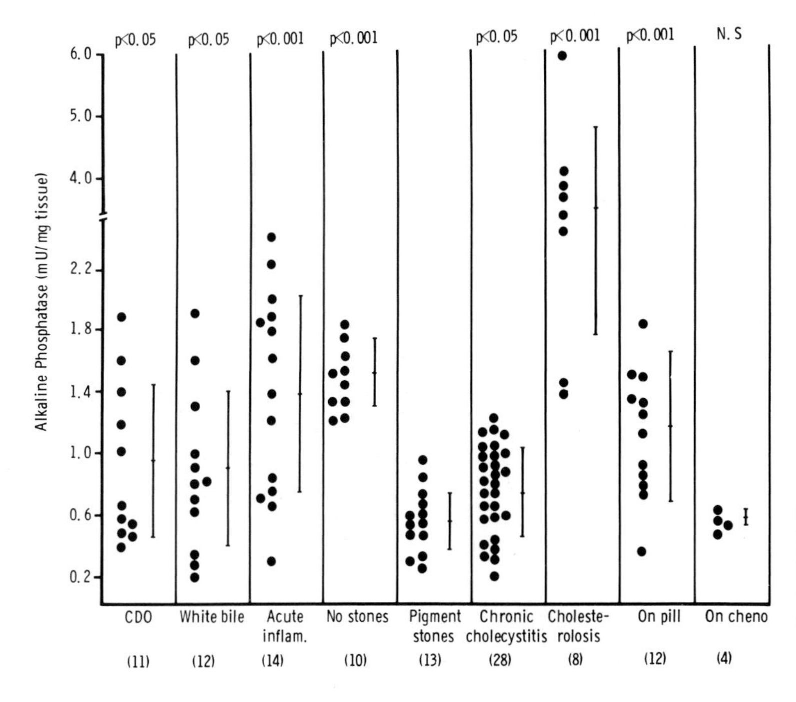

Figure 12.3 Alkaline phosphatase (mU/mg tissue) activity in gallbladder mucosa of various groups of patients (numbers are given in parentheses). The pigment stone group is taken as an arbitrary control for comparison and statistical differences between the groups are shown at the tops of the columns. CDO, common duct obstruction.

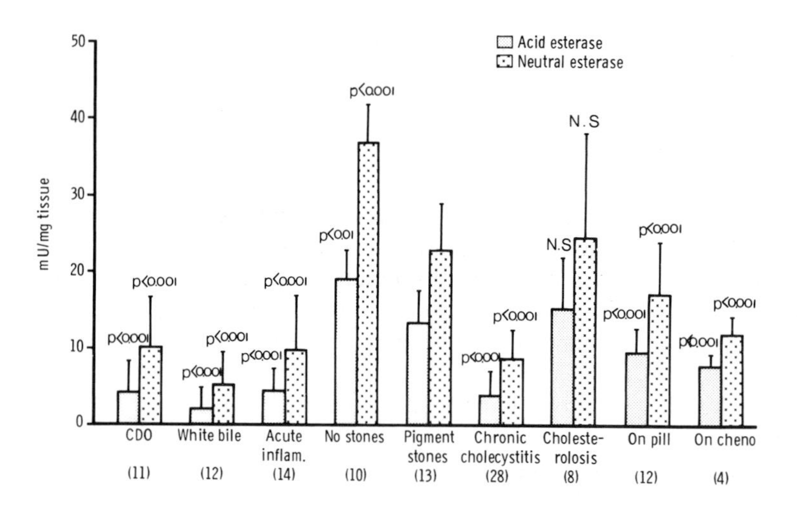

Figure 12.4 Acid and neutral esterase activity (mU/mg tissue) in gallbladder mucosa from various groups of patients (numbers are shown in parentheses). The pigment stone group is taken as an arbitrary control for comparison and statistical differences between the groups are shown at the tops of the columns. DCO, common duct obstruction.

carboxymucins predominate. Immunological techniques[18] have demonstrated a sulphoglycoprotein specific for the human gallbladder, and three others which are common to the stomach and intestine. There is considerable variation in lectin binding both between and within cases.[25] There are a few reports of the localization of mucosubstances at the ultrastructural level.[26,32]

The glycoprotein content of the intrahepatic *bile ducts* has been shown to change in patients with intrahepatic cholangiocarcinoma.[50] In the intrahepatic ducts two populations of mucus-secreting glands have been described. Those within the ductal wall communicate with the duct lumina directly, and may originate from the bile duct epithelium. Those outside the wall communicate via their own conduits, and may arise from peribiliary glands. Both are rich in neutral, carboxylated and sulphated mucoglycoproteins.

LIPIDS

Lipid droplets were first described in the gallbladder epithelium by Virchow in 1857.[47] More recently, cholesterol and its esters, fatty acids and some unsaturated lipids have been documented.[4] There is evidence in the guinea-pig of lipid uptake from the lumen by the epithelial cells, using labelled oleic acid, cholesterol lecithin and lysolecithin.[36] Extremes of this phenomenon may lead to cholesterolosis and it is possible that one of the lipid components may act as an irritating agent to initiate and maintain cholecystitis.

HISTOLOGY

LIGHT AND ELECTRON MICROSCOPY

There are numerous accounts of transmission electron microscopy on normal animal tissues, but most studies of the human *gallbladder* have been performed on diseased tissue.[21] Three epithelial cell types have been described in the fundus. The principal ordinary cells have regular microvilli on their apical cell membrane with some intervening pits. Anions may play a role in the stability of the apical cell membrane.[43] The lateral cell border has irregular microvilli and the space between the cells varies with their functional state in the rabbit.[3] The cells are joined at their apices by tight junctions but these are not the site for net fluid transport.[16] Coated and non-coated pits may be found on the basolateral membrane. The epithelium rests on a basement membrane. There is a normal complement of organelles. At the apex, there are secretory droplets derived from a well-developed Golgi apparatus. The residual bodies have many forms, including some with lipid inclusions. Lipid droplets may be found especially in the basal part of the cells. A fibrillary system is well developed by the lateral cell membrane and as a terminal web.

Pencil cells may be seen in over 60% of gallbladders with compact cytosol but their exact state is uncertain. Basal cells represent intraepithelial lymphocytes, probably T cells, and mast cells. Macrophages, some containing lipid, are also found between the epithelial cells and in the lamina propria.

Various cell types have been described in the neck glands.[29] The glands have tall antral cells with numerous pale secretory droplets and tall microvilli, whereas the cells in the neck are cuboid with short, irregular microvilli and few or no secretory granules. Endocrine-like cells are also present.

There are several scanning electron microscopy reports on normal and pathological material.[34] Mucosal folds are seen, and at high magnifications the hexagonal boundaries of the cells and the apical microvilli are identified. Cholesterolosis produces broadened folds, and chronic cholecystitis effaces the folds to give irregular undulating areas.

The surface of the *bile duct* is lined by tall epithelium which extends into diverticula. Apically they contain neutral and sialated mucosubstances; the membrane is lined with microvilli and the cells have a well-developed rough endoplasmic reticulum and Golgi apparatus. In biliary tract obstruction and choledocholithiasis, many lipid-laden macrophages can be seen basally.[23] Adaptive changes have been described in the common bile duct epithelium following choledochoduodenostomy, with hyperplasia of the epithelium, metaplastic goblet cells containing predominantly acid sialomucins, and pyloric-like gland formations containing neutral mucins.[10]

CELL PROLIFERATION

The labelling index is very low in 'normal' human gallbladder, some 10 times lower than the 1–1.5% reported for laboratory animals.[42] There is a significantly higher labelling index in distended gallbladders, for example when pancreatic cancer causes distal biliary tract obstruction. There is no preferential site for cell labelling on the crests or valleys of the mucosal folds.

TISSUE CULTURE

It is possible to culture guinea-pig gallbladder epithelium in a number of media.[11] Growth of epithelial cells is established by 1–2 days into culture extending over the explant and into colonies. The fine structure and biochemical activity is maintained for at least 7 days, as is the ability to take up cationized ferritin in vitro, as an index of integrated behaviour.

IMMUNOCYTES

Lymphocytes and *plasma cells* (predominantly IgA) are found in the lamina propria of the gallbladder and their numbers are increased in cholecystitis. IgA and IgM cells also increase in severe acute cholecystitis,[17] and IgM cells are the most numerous in the muscle layers. These cells also increase in chronic inflammation. Using electron immunoperoxidase techniques, Nagura *et al.*[35] have shown a basolateral distribution of IgA over bile duct epithelium, which suggests a secretory component-mediated transfer of IgA. There are coated pits on the basolateral surface of gallbladder epithelium.

Eosinophils may be noted in increased numbers infiltrating the gallbladder in 2.5% of specimens, often simply a prominent component of a mixed inflammatory cell infiltrate. Rarely, there may be a purely eosinophilic cholecystitis.[15]

Mast cells are found in relatively small numbers in the gallbladder.[37] Their ratios are 40:20:10 in serosa, muscle and mucosa per high-power field. Mast cells are also present between the epithelial cells, where they stain relatively little, possible due to low quantities of heparin in the granules and the presence of lower sulphated glycosaminoglycans.[46]

METAPLASIA/ECTOPIA

Chronic inflammation and the presence of stones may induce metaplasia, usually in the form of cells resembling pyloric antrum or goblet cells but occasionally as squamous cells. Argentaffin cells occur chiefly in relation to neck glands.[9] Enterochromaffin cells are common in the gallbladders of some species, e.g. the ox, pig and guinea-pig. Endocrine cell types and Paneth cells are seen on electron microscopy of metaplastic gallbladders removed for stones.[30] Inappropriate mucin secretion with the production of carcinoembryonic antigen and intestinal mucin has been noted in metaplasia.[8] Ectopic gastric mucosa occurs rarely and contains gastric mucous cells and parietal cells. Such patients may present with cholecystitis.[44] Heterotopic gastric mucosa has also been described in the common bile duct.[14]

STRUCTURE/FUNCTION CORRELATIONS

CONCENTRATION OF BILE

The principal function of the gallbladder is to concentrate bile 4- to 10-fold by the absorption of water and electrolytes. Horseradish peroxidase (molecular weight 40 000) and cationized ferritin (molecular weight 480 000) are absorbed in vivo.[6,22] Horseradish peroxidase, following fluid phase endocytosis, appears in the lateral intercellular space within 5 minutes of an intraluminal injection. Cationized ferritin is internalized by adsorption endocytosis, stripped from the membrane and after 2 hours, exocytosed in clumps into the lateral intercellular space (*Figures 12.5* and *12.6*). These observations represent both rapid and somewhat slower pathways for the transport of large molecules from the bile to the lamina propria.

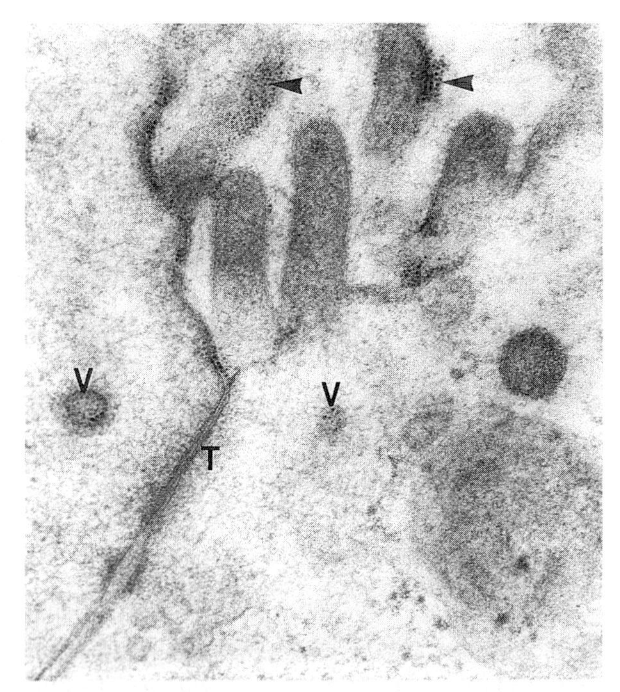

Figure 12.5 Apex of guinea-pig gallbladder epithelial cell showing binding within 5 minutes' exposure of cationized ferritin by microvilli (arrowheads) and internalization in vesicles (V). There is no marker in the tight junction (T). Uncounterstained electron micrograph, × 70 000.

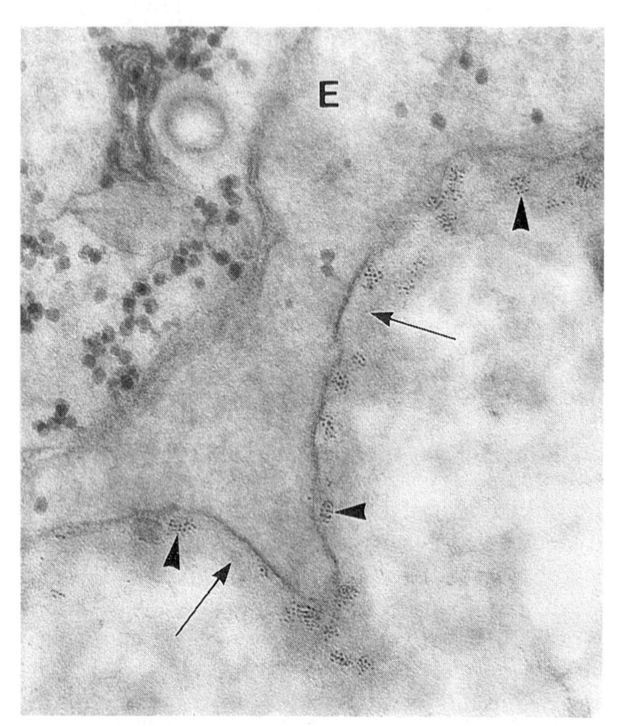

Figure 12.6 Base of guinea-pig gallbladder epithelial cell (E) showing clumps of cationized ferritin against the basement membrane (arrow). At this stage (2 hours after labelling) no marker has passed into the underlying connective tissue. Uncounterstained electron micrograph, × 60 000.

SECRETION OF MUCUS

The secretion of mucus is a further important function of gallbladder epithelium. This occurs spontaneously but discharge of mucus droplets may also be induced by intragastric olive oil,[48] systemic cholecystokinin, vagal stimulation or pilocarpine.[1] The secretion of mucus by exocytosis will place more packages of membrane into the apical cell membrane and this will induce membrane retrieval.

REFERENCES

1. Axelsson, H., Danielsson, A., Henriksson, R. and Wahlin, R. (1979) Secretory behaviour and ultrastructural changes in mouse gallbladder principal cells after stimulation with cholinergic and adrenergic nerves. *Gastroenterology*, **76**, 334–340.
2. Bennion, R.S., Thompson, J.E. Jr and Tompkins, R.K. (1988) Agenesis of the gallbladder with extrahepatic biliary atresia. *Archives of Surgery*, **123**, 1257–1260.
3. Blom, H. and Helander, H.F. (1977) Quantitative electron microscopical studies on in vitro incubated rabbit gallbladder epithelium. *Journal of Membrane Biology*, **37**, 45–61.
4. Boyd, W. (1922) Studies in gallbladder pathology, *British Journal of Surgery*, **10**, 337–356.
5. Carter, R. and Imrie, C.W. (1992) Stone in the middle gallbladder. *Journal of the Royal College of Surgeons of Edinburgh* (in press).
6. Coghill, S.B., Hopwood, D. and Milne, G. (1983) The uptake of horseradish peroxidase and its subsequent redistribution by guinea pig gallbladder in vivo. *Journal of Pathology*, **139**, 89–95.
7. Couinaud, C. (1957) Le foie. Les hepatectomies e'largies. In *Etudes Anatomiques et Chirurgicales*, pp. 400–409. Paris: Masson et Cie.
8. De Boer, W.G.R.M., Ma, J., Rees, J.W. and Nayman, J. (1981) Inappropriate mucin production in gallbladder metaplasia and neoplasia: an immunological study. *Histopathology*, **5**, 295–303.
9. Delaquerrier, L., Tremblay, G. and Riopelle, J.L. (1962) Argentaffine cell in chronic cholecystitis. *Archives of Pathology*, **74**, 142–151.
10. Eleftheriadis, E., Tzioufa, V., Kotzampassi, K. and Aletras, H. (1988) Common bile-duct mucosa in choledochoduodenostomy patients – histological and histochemical study. *HPB Surgery*, **1**, 15–20.
11. Elhamady, M.S., Hopwood, D., Milne, G. *et al.* (1983) Tissue culture of guinea pig gallbladder. *Journal of Pathology*, **140**, 221–235.
12. Elhamel, A. (1989) A rare extrahepatic biliary anomaly. *HPB Surgery*, **1**, 353–358.
13. Esterly, J.R. and Spicer, S.S. (1968) Mucin histochemistry of human gallbladder and changes in adenocarcinoma, gastric fibrosis and cholecystitis. *Journal of the National Cancer Institute*, **40**, 1–11.
14. Evans, M.M., Nagorney, D.M., Pernicone, P.J.

and Perrault, J. (1990) Heterotopic gastric mucosa in the common bile duct. *Surgery*, **108**, 96–100.
15. Fox, H. and Mainwaring, A.R. (1972) Eosinophilic infiltration of the gallbladder. *Gastroenterology*, **63**, 1049–1052.
16. Frederickson, D., Mollgaard, K. and Rostgaard, J. (1979) Lack of correlation between transepithelial transport capacity and paracellular pathway ultrastructure in Alcian blue treated rabbit gallbladder. *Journal of Cell Biology*, **83**, 383–393.
17. Green, F.H.Y. and Fox, H. (1972) An immunofluorescent study of the distribution of immunoglobulin containing cells in the normal and inflamed human gallbladder. *Gut*, **13**, 379–384.
18. Hakkinen, I. and Laito, M. (1970) Epithelial glycoproteins of human gallbladder. *Archives of Pathology*, **90**, 137–142.
19. Hata, K., Aoki, S., Hata, T., Murao, F. and Kitao, M. (1987) Ultrasonographic identification of the human fetal gall bladder in utero. *Gynecologic and Obstetric Investigation*, **23**, 79–83.
20. Hayward, A.F., Freston, J.W. and Bouchier, I.A.D. (1968) Changes in the ultrastructure of gall bladder epithelium in rabbits with experimental gall stones. *Gut*, **9**, 550–556.
21. Hopwood, D., Kouroumalis, E., Milne, G. and Bouchier, A.I.D. (1980) Cholecystitis: a fine structural analysis. *Journal of Pathology*, **130**, 1–4.
22. Hopwood, D., Milne, G. and Wood, R.A.B. (1982) The uptake of cationized ferritin and its subsequent redistribution by gallbladder epithelium in vivo. *Journal of Pathology*, **136**, 95–109.
23. Hopwood, D., Wood, R. and Milne, G. (1988) The fine structure of histochemistry of human bile duct in obstruction and choledocholithiasis. *Journal of Pathology*, **155**, 49–59.
24. Jackson, R.J. and McClellan, D. (1989) Agenesis of the gallbladder. A cause of false-positive ultrasonography. *American Surgeon*, **55**, 36–40.
25. Karayannopoulou, G. and Damjanov, I. (1988) Lectin histochemistry of goblet cells in metaplastic epithelium and human gallbladder. *Modern Pathology*, **1**, 132–134.
26. Koga, A. (1973) Electron microscopic observations on the mucous secretory activity of the human gallbladder epithelium. *Zeitschrift für Zellforschung*, **139**, 463–471.
27. Kouroumalis, E., Hopwood, D., Ross, P.E. *et al.* (1983) Gallbladder epithelium acid hydrolases in human cholecystitis. *Journal of Pathology*, **139**, 179–191.
28. Kouroumalis, E., Hopwood, D., Ross, P.E. and Bouchier, I.A.D. (1983) Mucosal alkaline phosphatase and bile lipids in gallbladder in cholecystitis. *Journal of Pathology*, **141**, 169–179.
29. Laitio, M. and Nevalainen, T. (1975) Gland ultrastructure in human gallbladder. *Journal of Anatomy*, **120**, 105–112.
30. Laitio, M. and Nevalainen, T. (1975) Ultrastructure of endocrine cells in metaplastic epithelium of human gallbladder. *Journal of Anatomy*, **120**, 219–225.
31. Lee, S. (1981) Hypersecretion of mucous glycoprotein by the gallbladder epithelium in experimental cholecystitis. *Journal of Pathology*, **134**, 199–207.
32. Luciano, K., Reale, E. and Wolpers, C. (1974) Die Fein struktur der Gallenblase und Gallengange V. Histochemische Lokalisierung von Mukosubstanzen in menschlichen Gallenblasenepithel. *Histochemistry*, **38**, 57–70.
33. Michels, N.A. (1960) Newer anatomy of the liver: variant blood supply and collateral circulation. *Journal of American Medical Association*, **172**, 125.
34. Myllarneimi, H. and Nickels, J.I. (1972) Observations by scanning electron microscopy of normal and pathological human gallbladder epithelium. *Act Pathologica et Microbiologica Scandinavica*, **A85**, 42–48.
35. Nagura, H., Smith, P.D., Nakane, P.K. and Brown, W.R. (1981) IgA in human bile and liver. *Journal of Immunology*, **126**, 587–595.
36. Niederheiser, D.H., Harmon, C.K. and Roth, H.P. (1976) Absorption of cholesterol by the gallbladder. *Journal of Lipid Research*, **17**, 117–124.
37. Norris, H.T., Zamcheck, N. and Gottlieb, L.S. (1963) The presence and distribution of mast cells in the human gastrointestinal tract at autopsy. *Gastroenterology*, **44**, 448–455.
38. Northover, J.M.A. and Terblanche, J. (1979) A new look at the arterial supply of the bile duct in man and its surgical implications. *British Journal of Surgery*, **66**, 379–384.
39. Olsha, O., Steiner, A., Rivkin, L.A. and Sheinfeld, A. (1987) Congenital absence of the anatomic common bile duct. Case report. *Acta Chirurgica Scandinavica*, **153**, 387–390.
40. Ozeki, Y., Onitsuka, A., Hayashi, M. and Sasaki, E. (1987) Left-sided gallbladder: report of a case and study of 26 cases in Japan. *Nippon Geka Gakkai Zasshi*, **88**, 1644–1650.
41. Palade, G. (1975) Ultracellular aspects of the process of protein secretion. *Science*, **189**, 347–358.
42. Putz, P. and Willems, G. (1979) Cell proliferation in the human gallbladder epithelium: effect of distension. *Gut*, **20**, 246–248.
43. Quinton, P.M. and Philpott, C.W. (1973) A role for anionic sites in epithelial architecture. *Journal of Cell Biology*, **56**, 787–796.
44. Runge, P.M., Schwartz, J.N, Seigler, H.F. *et al.* (1978) Gallbladder with ectopic gastric mucosa. *Archives of Pathology*, **102**, 209–211.
45. Stringer, D.A., Dobranowski, J., Ein, S.H., Roberts, E.A., Daneman, A. and Filler, R.M. (1987) Interposition of the gallbladder – or the absent common hepatic duct and cystic duct. *Pediatric Radiology*, **17**, 151–153.
46. Tas, J. and Berndsen, R.G. (1977) Does heparin occur in mucosal mast cells of the rat small intestine. *Journal of Histochemistry and Cytochemistry*, **35**, 1058–1062.

47. Virchow, R. (1857) Uber das Epithel der Gallenblase und uber einen intermediaren Stoffwechsel das Fettes. *Virchows Archiv*, **11**, 574–578.
48. Wahlin, T., Bloom, G.D. and Danielsson, A. (1976) Effect of cholecystokinin–pancreozymin (CCK-PZ) on glycoprotein secretion from mouse gallbladder epithelium. *Cell Tissue Research*, **171**, 425–435.
49. Wallraff, J. and Dietrich, K.F. (1957) Die Morphologie und Histochemie der Steingallenblase des Menschen. *Zeitschrift für Zellforschung*, **46**, 155–231.
50. Zhang, S.M., Wu, M.C., Chen, H. and Zhang, X.Z. (1989) Expression of glycoconjugates in intrahepatic cholangiocellular carcinoma. *Virchows Archiv A*, **415**, 395–401.

CONGENITAL ABNORMALITIES

S. Cywes, A. Millar and J. Terblanche

Most apparent congenital anomalies of the gallbladder and biliary tract are really variants of the normal anatomy. The rare anomalies that do occur are related to alterations and variations in embryological budding from the foregut.[11] These abnormalities are usually asymptomatic and of no clinical significance but may occasionally predispose to stasis, inflammation and stone formation. They are, however, important to the radiologist in interpreting radiological investigations and to the surgeon when operating on the biliary system.

ANOMALIES OF THE BILE DUCTS

HEPATIC DUCTS (*Figure 12.7*)

The intrahepatic ducts are remarkably constant and drain named segments of the liver. The confluence of the right and left hepatic ducts is always extrahepatic. In 75% of individuals there is a single right hepatic duct but in 25% the right anterior and posterior segmental ducts enter the left hepatic duct

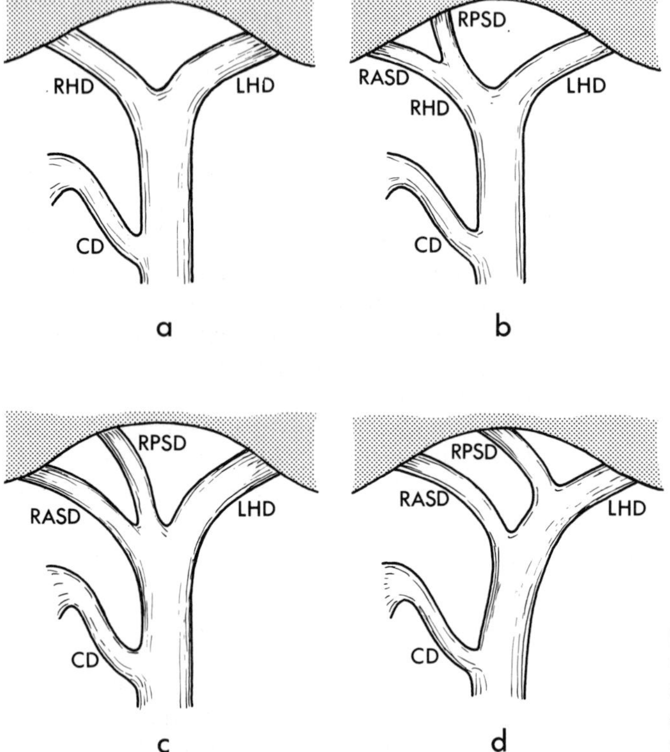

Figure 12.7 Variations of the hepatic ducts. (a) A single right hepatic duct (RHD) is usually formed within the liver and is present in 75% of individuals; (b) sometimes it is formed outside the liver; (c) in 25% the segmental ducts form a triple confluence with the left hepatic duct (LHD); or (d) join it separately. RASD, right anterior segmental duct; RPSD, right posterior segmental duct; CD, cystic duct.

separately, which has led to the erroneous concept of an 'accessory' hepatic duct. This is a variant of normal and not a congenital anomaly.[25] Occasionally the hepatic ducts enter the duodenum separately, with the cystic duct joining the right hepatic duct. This has been termed duplication of the common bile duct. Bile ducts passing directly from the liver to the gallbladder are rare, and probably secondary to disease rather than congenital.[26]

COMMON HEPATIC AND COMMON BILE DUCT

Most anomalies are variants of normal anatomy. Variations of the intrapancreatic portion depend on the extent to which the common duct is covered by the pancreas. Although of no functional significance they are important to the surgeon. Very rarely the retroduodenal portion may be atretic and bypassed by an accessory duct.

The relationship of the bile duct to the pancreatic duct at the ampulla and the site of opening of the bile duct into the duodenum are also variants of normal anatomy. With duplications of the bile duct, two separate openings may be present. Duplications may be associated with duodenal atresia with separate openings proximal and distal to the atresia.

CONGENITAL CYSTIC DILATATION OF THE COMMON BILE DUCT – CHOLEDOCHAL CYSTS

The currently accepted classification (*Figure 12.8*) is a modification of the original of Alonso-Lej *et al.*[2] by the addition of intrahepatic cystic or fusiform dilatation:[34,51] (I) concentric dilatation – this is the classical choledochal cyst and is usually (a) cystic but may be (b) fusiform; (II) diverticulum or eccentric dilatation of the common duct; (III) choledochocoele – this may be extra- or intramural; (IV) multiple cystic dilatations[31,51] – this may be (a) intra- and extrahepatic or (b) extrahepatic only; (V) intrahepatic cystic dilatation – Caroli's disease.[6]

All forms are uncommon in Western countries, where choledochal cyst is usually unassociated with intrahepatic cystic dilatation. Choledochal cysts are commoner in Oriental countries and are four times more common in the Japanese than in other races. About half of the patients have associated intrahepatic cystic dilatation.[41,53] Increasing use of endoscopic retrograde cholangiopancreatography (ERCP) has indicated that choledochocoeles may be more common than previously suspected.[18,42] The relationship between Caroli's disease and congenital hepatic fibrosis, of which it may be a variant, is recognized.

One-quarter of choledochal cysts present during the first year of life, some 60% between 1 and 10 years of age and the remaining 10–20% during the second decade. Presentation later in life may occur, but is rare. Although many patients are diagnosed after the age of 1 year, very few are symptom-free during the first year of life. Choledochal cysts are commoner in females (3:1).

Pathology

Choledochal cysts vary greatly in size and may contain from a few millilitres to several litres of fluid. The content is usually inspissated bile but rarely frankly purulent. Associated gallstones are rarely found in children (2 out of 34 patients in Cape Town), but may be more frequent in adults. The gallbladder is usually normal. The cyst wall varies in thickness from 1 mm to about 1 cm and microscopically it consists of fibrous tissue. Muscle is conspicuously absent although smooth muscle fibres may occasionally be identified. There is no epithelial lining although islets of cuboidal or columnar mucosa may remain. The incidence of carcinoma is approximately 20 times greater than in the normal population.[35,50,52]

Types associated with biliary atresia are either (1) bile lakes in the porta hepatis or (2) cystic structures protruding from the porta hepatis, usually associated with a dilated gallbladder containing clear mucoid fluid, 'white bile'. With both there is significant hepatic pathology (inflammation with fibrosis to frank cirrhosis).[31]

Aetiology

The aetiology is unknown but suggested aetiological mechanisms range from distal common bile duct obstruction to congenital weakness of the wall. Distal obstruction alone is an insufficient mechanism and requires concomitant damage to epithelium and duct wall to produce a choledochal cyst.[7,22] Reflux of pancreatic juice in situations where a common channel of pancreatic and bile duct above the ampulla have been shown, could cause the damage, and this theory is supported by the finding of elevated amylase concentrations in the cyst.[3,23] Intraoperative manometry of the biliary tract has shown a high pressure zone in the area of the sphincter of Oddi but not in the area of abnormal choledochopancreatic ductal junction which further supports the reflux of pancreatic juice theory.[16] Although not previously suggested, the authors consider that an intrauterine vascular accident affecting the tenuous blood supply to the supraduodenal bile duct could

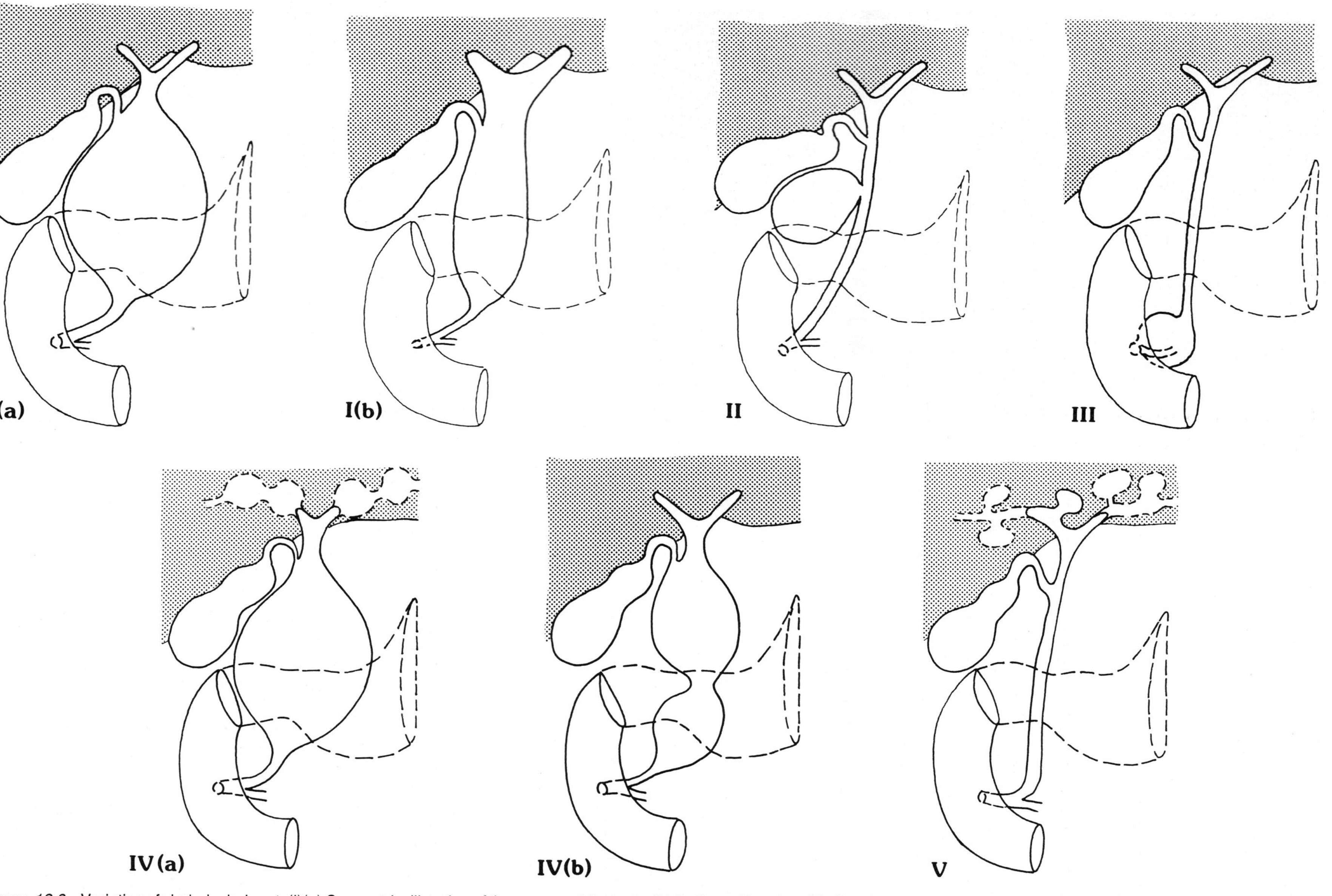

Figure 12.8 Varieties of choledochal cyst. (I)(a) Concentric dilatation of the common bile duct – (b) fusiform dilatation; (II) diverticulum or excentric dilatation; (III) choledochocoele; (IV) multiple cystic dilatations – (a) intra- and extrahepatic or (b) extrahepatic alone; (V) intrahepatic cystic dilatation – Caroli's disease.

be an alternative mechanism.[38] Oligoganglionosis in the narrow portion of the bile duct has also been incriminated.[27] Infantile choledochal cysts are usually associated with complete bile flow obstruction and significant liver pathology and may be a forme fruste of biliary atresia.[20]

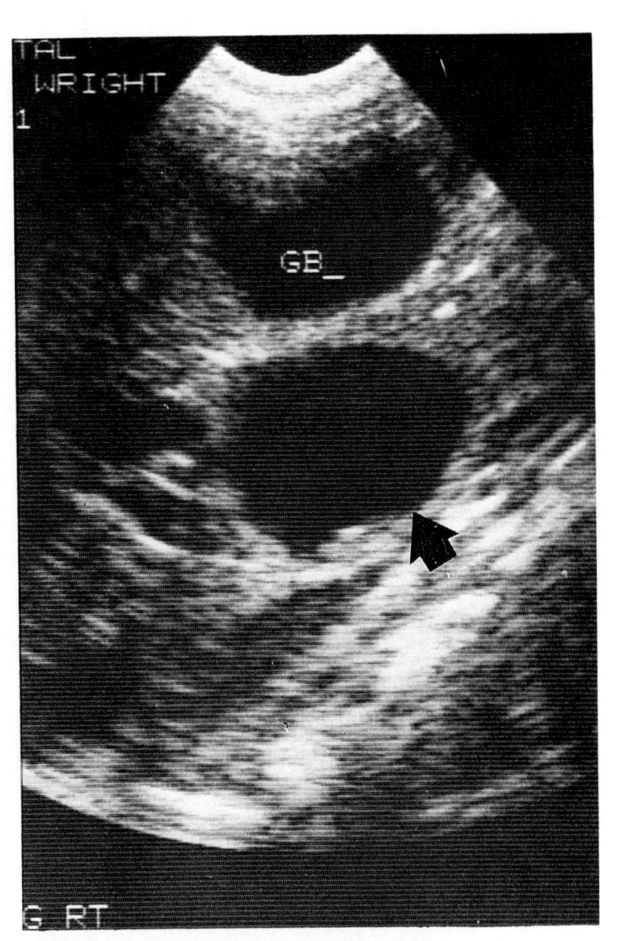

Figure 12.9 Ultrasonogram of a choledochal cyst. The echolucent choledochal cyst is indicated by the arrow.

Clinical features

The classical triad is intermittent obstructive jaundice, abdominal pain and an abdominal mass. Jaundice is the most constant feature, occurring in about 75% of reported cases. Pain is usually a feature in about two-thirds of patients but occurred in only half of those seen by the authors. A smooth mass continuous with the liver is palpable in the right upper quadrant in about half the patients. The full triad was only present in 20% of Cape Town patients.[36] Occasionally there may be associated pancreatitis (one of the Cape Town children had evidence of chronic pancreatitis at surgery). In infancy the most common symptom is persistent jaundice often associated with abdominal distension, fever and vomiting while in older children there is frequently a history of recurrent mild episodes of jaundice with pale stools and dark urine. Important late complications include cholangitis and cirrhosis. Portal vein thrombosis has been rarely observed.

INVESTIGATIONS

Liver function tests will merely confirm obstructive jaundice, when present. The most important definitive diagnostic tests today are ultrasound (*Figure 12.9*) or computed tomography (CT) scanning to demonstrate the cyst and the status of the intrahepatic ducts (*Figure 12.10*). In older children and adults, ERCP will confirm the diagnosis (*Figure 12.11*). This technique has replaced operative cholangiography, except in the case of small children (*Figure 12.12*). ^{99m}Tc-labelled iminodiacetic acid derivative radionuclide scanning can be helpful in confirming the biliary origin of the cyst, if doubt exists and ERCP is not successful. These methods have superseded previously used radiological investigations.

Treatment

The only acceptable treatment today for the classic choledochal cyst is surgical excision of the cyst with reconstruction of the bile duct by hepaticojejunostomy using a Roux-en-Y loop. An alternative, which is seldom used, is interposition of an isolated segment of jejunum between the proximal bile duct and the duodenum. The cyst may be removed in its entirety or, if the adjacent vascular structures are adherent to the cyst, the anterior wall is first excised. Posteriorly the cyst lining is then stripped, leaving the outer wall intact where it abuts on the portal vein and hepatic artery.[30] The upper anastomosis should be performed to normal duct above the cyst, preferably to the confluence and left duct in the porta hepatis to prevent subsequent stricture.[47] An anastomosis to normal duct may not always be possible because of intrahepatic extension. Intrahepatic choledochal cystenterostomy at the porta hepatis with further incision and laying open of the major hepatic ducts may be required for a type IVa anomaly.[31,49] Following surgery, dilatation of the intrahepatic ducts can be expected to decrease with improvement of biliary excretory function.[39] Anastomotic stenosis may develop; thus, long-term follow-up is essential. Distally, the opening of the bile duct is oversewn, taking care not to damage the pancreatic duct.

External drainage is unjustified except as first stage treatment of an infected choledochal cyst that does not respond to antibiotic therapy. Internal

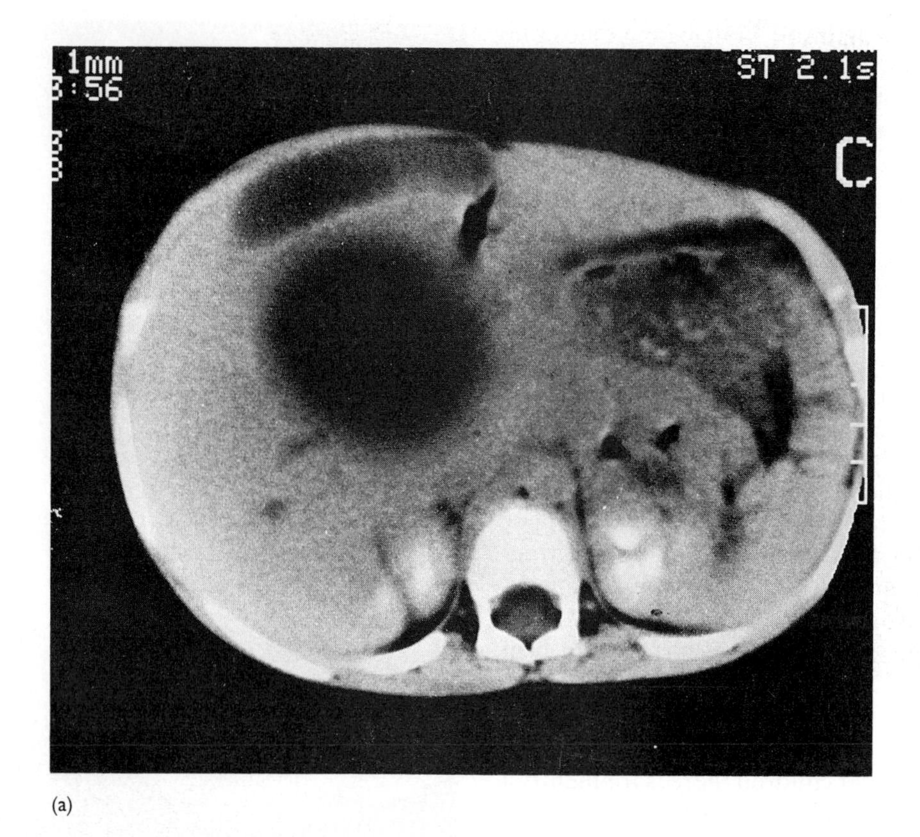

(a)

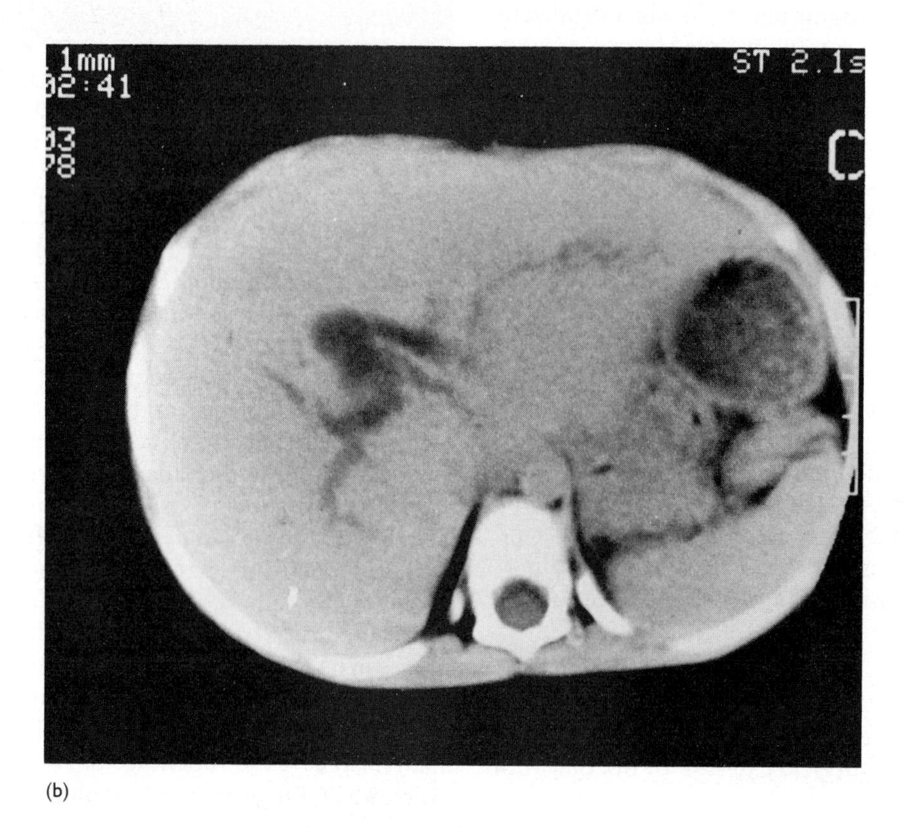

(b)

Figure 12.10 CT scan showing (a) the choledochal cyst with a dilated gallbladder lying anteriorly and (b) intrahepatic biliary dilatation.

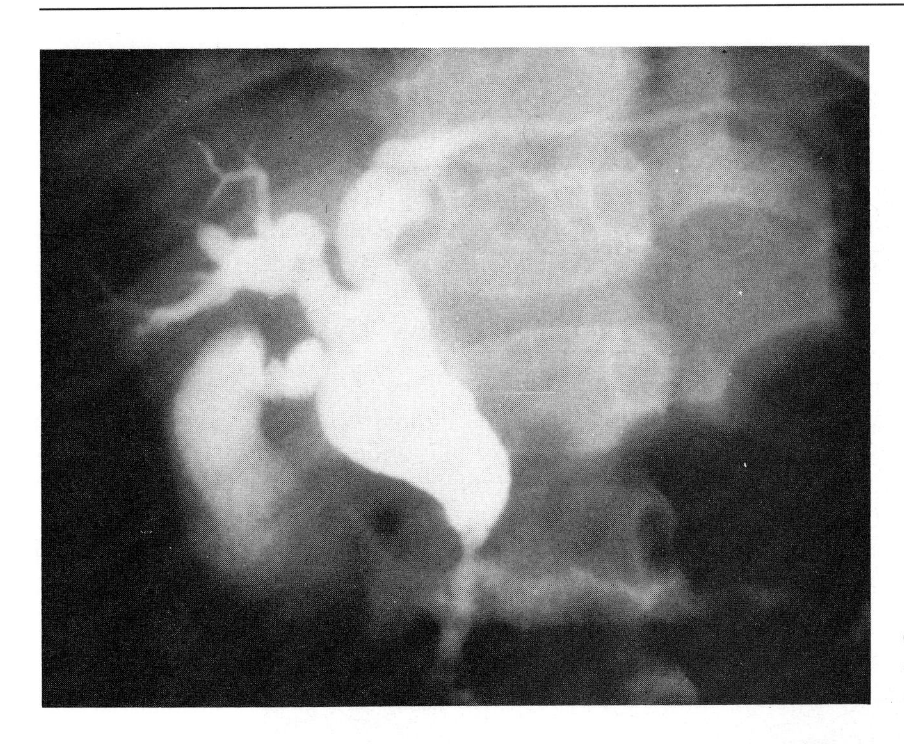

Figure 12.11 ERCP showing a fusiform cyst and intra- and extrahepatic bile duct dilatation with tapering of the distal common bile duct.

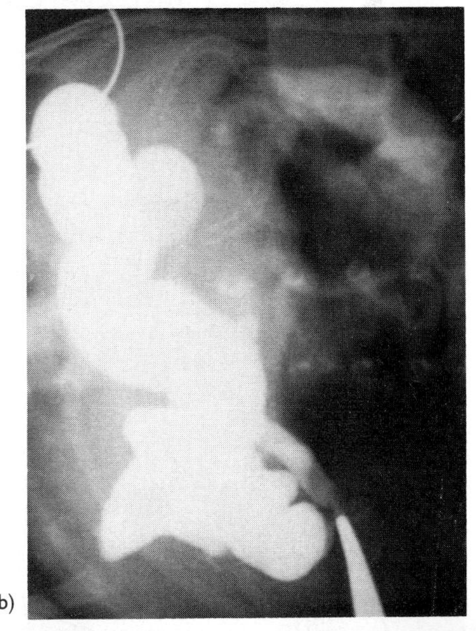

(b)

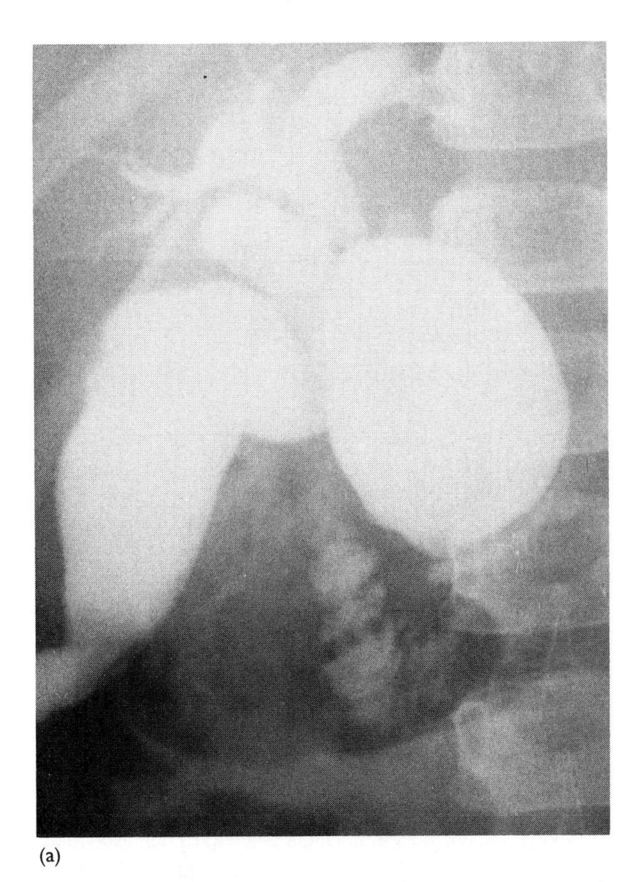

(a)

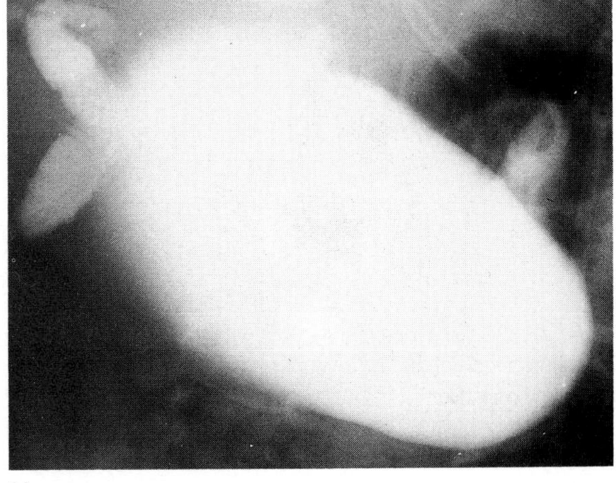

(c)

Figure 12.12 Operative cholangiograms. (a) The concentric dilatation of the common bile duct is outlined on cholangiography; (b,c) a large choledochal cyst with gross dilatation of the intrahepatic ducts in a 3-week-old baby.

drainage to the duodenum or a Roux loop of jejunum was practised in the past, but is unacceptable because drainage is inadequate, anastomotic strictures form and recurrent cholangitis leads to secondary biliary cirrhosis and portal hypertension. Biliary sludge or stones may form within the cyst. In addition, the increased hazard of carcinoma persists unless the cyst is excised.[24,50]

The treatment of other varieties of choledochal cyst depends upon the symptoms and the type of anomaly. Eccentric diverticula should be excised. Treatment for Caroli's disease remains unsatisfactory. Choledochocoeles should only be treated if symptomatic, as the pancreatic duct is in danger at operation. Vaterian cysts can be treated by sphincteroplasty or endoscopic sphincterotomy.[18] Symptomatic peri-Vaterian cysts pose a very difficult management problem but partial excision was successful in one of the authors' patients.

ANOMALIES OF THE GALLBLADDER AND CYSTIC DUCT

GALLBLADDER ANOMALIES

This is the least variable part of the biliary tree. The only common anomaly (18%) is the Phrygian cap deformity in which the distal fundus of the gallbladder is folded upon itself. Very rarely the gallbladder may be absent, vestigial, duplicated, bilobed, or may be misplaced. The anomaly is found usually by chance at radiology or at laparotomy;

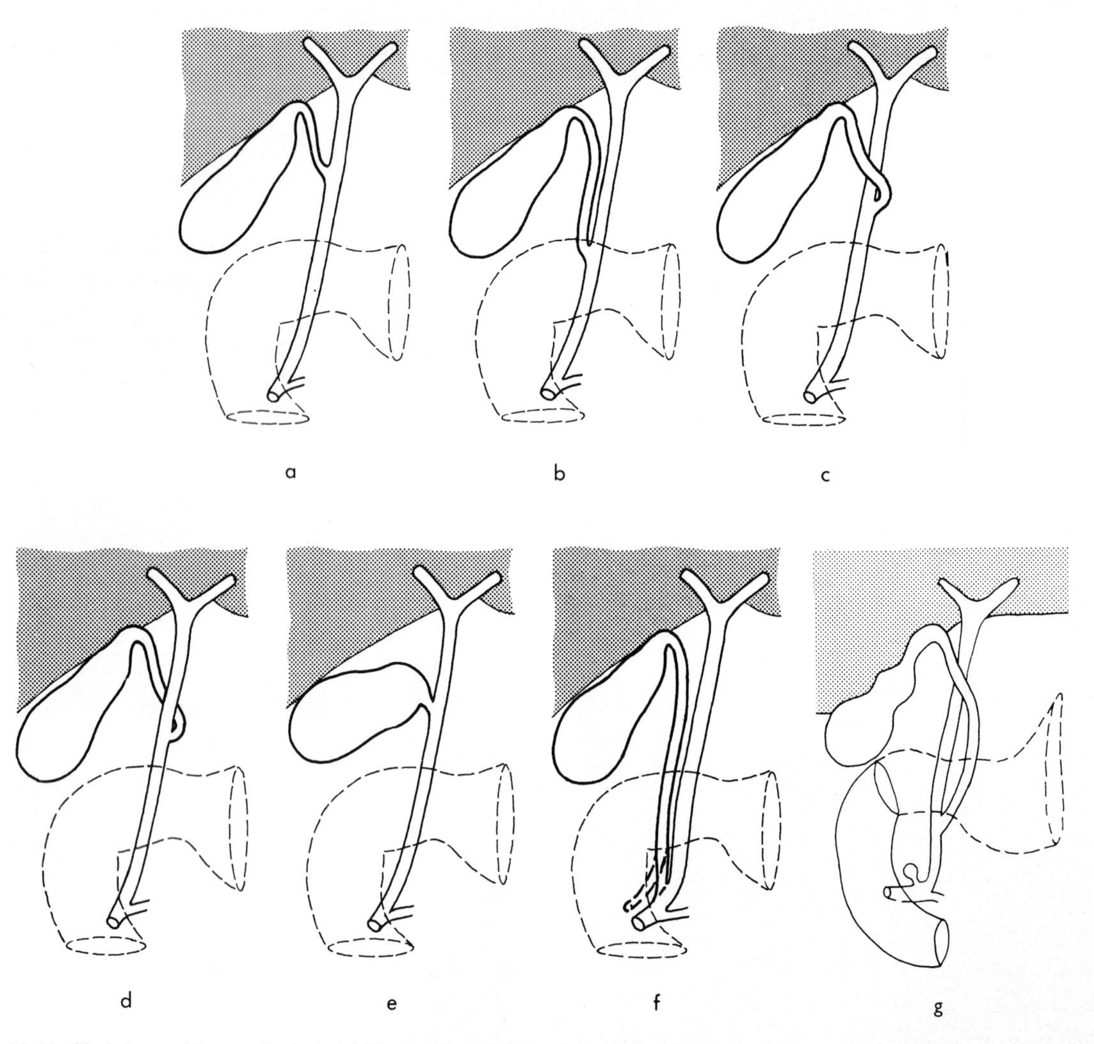

Figure 12.13 Variations of the cystic duct. (a) The cystic duct joins the common hepatic duct at an angle entering its right side in about two-thirds of individuals. In the remaining one-third it either (b) runs parallel with the duct, often incorporated in its wall, or (c,d) spirals around it, entering on the left side. The cystic duct may be (e) short or (f) long, entering separately into the duodenum or joining the common hepatic duct low down, giving a short common duct. In these situations, the common duct or its blood supply may be damaged when removing the whole cystic duct. (g) A low left-sided entry is commonly associated with an ampullary diverticulum and predisposes to stones in the common bile duct.

occasionally, gallstones develop in the common bile duct. A mobile gallbladder attached by a mesentery, may undergo torsion and strangulation. If the gallbladder is absent, then so is the cystic duct. Duplications are rare. Only two abnormalities of position are of importance to the surgeon: very rarely the gallbladder may lie on the left side of the liver without situs inversus, but more important is an intrahepatic gallbladder which is completely submerged in the liver substance. It may be missed and mistaken for absence of the gallbladder. When associated with symptomatic gallstones, treatment is difficult. The alternatives are cholecystostomy and removal of the gallstones, or, preferably, a partial cholecystectomy and ligation of the cystic duct if possible.

CYSTIC DUCT ANOMALIES

The cystic duct may be absent, with the gallbladder draining directly into the common duct. This is almost certainly not a congenital defect, but due to erosion of a large gallstone, which is invariably present, into the duct.[25] Most cystic duct anomalies are variants of the normal anatomy, in which the duct runs a longer course parallel with or spiralling around the common hepatic duct (*Figure 12.13*). The Cape Town group have shown that a low left entry of the cystic duct into the common bile duct is associated with an increased incidence of common bile duct stones.[4] Double cystic ducts may drain a single normal gallbladder and enter the bile duct or right hepatic duct.

BILIARY ATRESIA

Although considered here, biliary atresia should be regarded as an acquired and not a congenital or developmental anomaly. In the past it was regarded as congenital and classified into 'correctable' and 'non-correctable' types. In the correctable type (5%) the proximal bile ducts are patent and dilated but end blindly before the duodenum (*Figure 12.14*). In non-correctable types the proximal extrahepatic bile ducts are obliterated, and this may extend throughout the entire liver. The modern concept is based on the work of Kasai *et al.*,[21] who demonstrated convincingly that biliary atresia was a treatable, and in some instances a curable, condition. The common anatomical types encountered at operation are depicted in *Figure 12.15*.

AETIOLOGY AND PATHOLOGY

Biliary atresia arises as a result of an inflammatory process, best described as a progressive, obliterative sclerosing cholangitis, which usually affects both the extrahepatic and intrahepatic biliary tree but may occasionally be segmental and localized. Some have suggested that this is a result of an abnormal blood

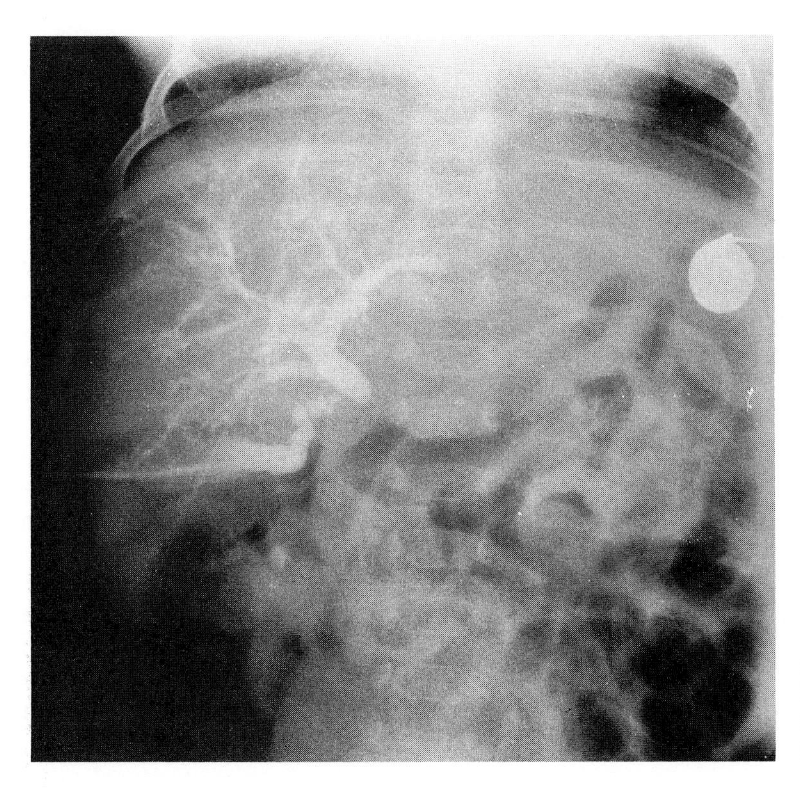

Figure 12.14 'Correctable' type of biliary atresia (5%). The proximal bile ducts are patent and dilated but end blindly before the duodenum – type (e) depicted in *Figure 12.15*.

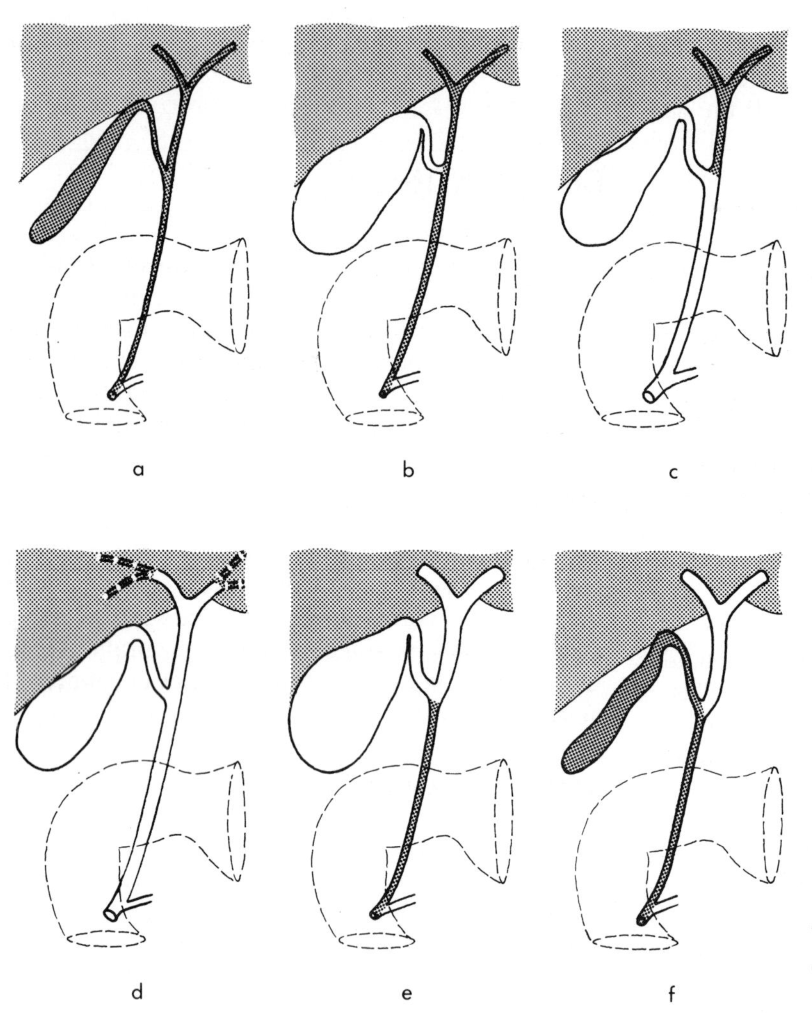

Figure 12.15 Common anatomical types of biliary atresia. Obliteration of (a) gallbladder and extrahepatic bile duct; (b) the extrahepatic bile duct; (c) the common hepatic bile duct; (d) the intrahepatic bile ducts; (e) the common bile duct and (f) the gallbladder and common bile duct. Types (a)–(d) were formerly considered 'non-correctable' and (e) and (f) 'correctable' biliary atresia.

supply plus a circulatory disturbance.[46] Although no specific agents have been identified consistently, an infective virus seems most likely. Rubella cytomegalovirus, hepatitis A and B viruses and, more recently, REOvirus have been implicated, with conflicting evidence being reported.[5,10] There appears to be a progression from hepatitis to ductal hypoplasia or obliteration. Liver damage is present in all patients but the extent of the damage varies. The rarity of the disease in the immediate neonatal period or in stillborn infants, suggests that complete obliteration of the bile ducts occurs some time after birth. It is thought to occur in about 1 in 10 000 infants.[43]

CLINICAL FEATURES

The clinical features are persistent jaundice, clay-coloured faeces and hepatomegaly. The jaundice is usually noticed within the first few weeks after birth. An infant with persistent jaundice requires urgent investigation to determine the cause.

INVESTIGATIONS

Full investigations must be undertaken to exclude other causes of jaundice and to determine ductal patency. There are no absolutely reliable tests available to confirm a diagnosis of biliary atresia, and ultrasound scanning, radioactive isotope scintigraphy and percutaneous liver biopsy can all be misleading. Furthermore, extensive tests are time-consuming and time is crucial for successful surgical management. Once biliary atresia is strongly suspected or cannot be ruled out, surgical exploration for definitive diagnosis is essential. The diagnosis depends on surgical biopsy of the liver, which is submitted to an expert pathologist for frozen section, and operative cholangiography. Surgical treatment depends on the findings. The earlier laparotomy policy improves the results of treatment for biliary atresia at the expense of a more accurate preoperative diagnosis.

TREATMENT

In approximately 5% of patients a large enough extrahepatic bile duct is found to permit an anastomosis to a Roux loop of jejunum. In the remainder, a hepatic portoenterostomy (Kasai operation) is performed.[13,14,18,21] The basis of hepatic portoenterostomy is that the intrahepatic bile ducts are patent in early infancy and extend 1–2 mm from the porta hepatis into the fibrous tissue which replaces the extrahepatic biliary ducts. When this portal fibrous tissue is transected deep in the porta hepatis behind the bifurcation of the portal vein, minute bile ducts communicating with intrahepatic ducts are opened and bile drainage can be established in many patients younger than 3 months of age. With time the intrahepatic ductules are progressively destroyed and by the age of 2 months there is a rapid decrease in the rate of cure by surgery. Thus, an operation should be performed within 60 days of birth.

The Kasai operation (hepatic portoenterostomy) has been fully described in standard texts,[13,14,21] and various modifications devised to prevent postoperative cholangitis are demonstrated in *Figure 12.16*. Currently, a long (30–45 cm) Roux loop of jejunum without a stoma is favoured with an acceptable low incidence of cholangitis.[8,15] Some have advocated various forms of valves, e.g. the intussusception valve, to avoid cholangitis.[33,40]

A variety of choleretic agents have been recommended for use in the postoperative period and, with antibiotic prophylaxis, are used in an attempt to promote bile flow and prevent cholangitis.[21,33]

RESULTS

The results largely depend upon: (1) the age at the time of operation; (2) the degree of cirrhosis and liver damage; (3) the presence (or absence) and size of microscopically demonstrable ducts in the fibrous mass at the porta hepatis – ducts over 150 μm in size appear to have a better prognosis; (4) the technique of the surgical procedure; and (5) the incidence and severity of postoperative cholangitis.

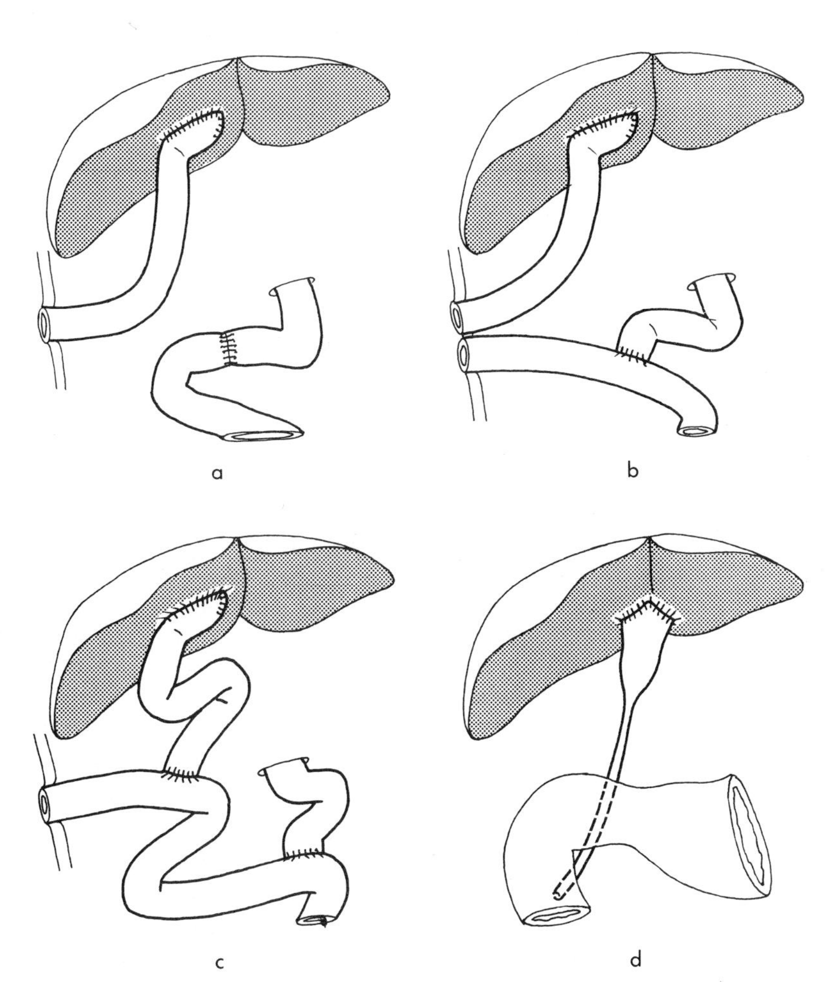

Figure 12.16 Various modifications of portoenterostomy to prevent ascending cholangitis. (a) The Sawaguchi procedure completely diverts biliary flow to an abdominal wall stoma. (b) In the Suruga procedure a double-barrelled stoma is devised. (c) The Kasai II procedure provides a biliary conduit system that is not completely diverting but allows decompression of the conduit via a stoma. (d) The Kasai gallbladder operation or hepatic portocholecystostomy is performed where the gallbladder, cystic duct and common bile duct are patent.

A 'cure rate' of 40–50% in infants operated on at less than 90 days of age has been quoted from various centres. However, this 'cure' means bile drainage and loss of jaundice with survival for more than 1 year. Even when good bile drainage has been achieved and the serum bilirubin level returns to normal, progression of fibrosis may occur after portoenterostomy. This fibrosis is often aggravated by recurrent attacks of cholangitis. Persisting long-term problems are those of cirrhosis and portal hypertension.

Where bile drainage stops and jaundice returns some time after an early successful result, re-exploration and removal of the fibrous plaque in the porta hepatis with a revision of the portoenterostomy may re-establish bile flow.[33]

LIVER TRANSPLANTATION

Liver transplantation is an accepted treatment in children in whom the Kasai operation has failed,[44,45] and biliary atresia is the most common indication for transplantation in children. Current long-term good-quality survival following liver transplantation for biliary atresia is projected at 65% at 5 years. Advances in surgical management and immunotherapy are likely to improve these results. Because of this, the role of portoenterostomy in the management of biliary atresia has been questioned. However, there is consensus that a single appropriately timed portoenterostomy is indicated as there is always the potential for cure.[12,32] More than 50% of these patients will grow and develop normally for some years despite the presence of liver disease, which later enables them to compete for a much larger donor pool.[9] Re-exploration for a failed portoenterostomy should not be undertaken lightly as it rarely results in sustained bile drainage and significantly increases the morbidity of a subsequent liver transplantation.[37,45]

BILIARY HYPOPLASIA

Biliary hypoplasia is a descriptive term which has been used both to denote paucity of intrahepatic, specifically interlobular bile ducts, as well as small but visible and radiographically patent extrahepatic bile ducts. Intrahepatic biliary hypoplasia may be non-syndromic and is associated with various metabolic (α_1-antitrypsin), viral and genetic abnormalities. The syndromic hypoplasia (Alagille's syndrome, arteriohepatic dysplasia) is a rare disorder (1 in 100 000 live births) of chronic cholestasis and is associated with a specific facial appearance, cardiovascular anomalies (mainly pulmonary stenosis or tetralogy of Fallot), vertebral arch defects and the ocular anomaly of posterior embryotoxon.[1] The pathogenesis of biliary hypoplasia is unclear, with a destructive inflammatory process being observed in some. In others it is thought to result simply from reduced bile flow with subsequent atrophy.

TREATMENT

Progression from biliary hypoplasia to biliary atresia in the non-syndromic group has been observed and in these cases portoenterostomy is advised. However, spontaneous resolution of jaundice may occur. Thus, timing of surgical intervention in a patient with unremitting jaundice is difficult and an arbitrary time limit of 6 weeks' observation has been suggested.[28] In the syndromic variety, treatment is conservative and is directed at the nutritional consequences of chronic cholestasis and management of other associated anomalies. Thus, early recognition is important to avoid needless surgery. Although on long-term follow-up the mortality is high (25%), liver complications are a surprisingly uncommon cause of death. In both types where cholestasis is progressive, liver transplantation must be considered.

REFERENCES

1. Alagille, D., Estrata, A., Hadchouel, M. *et al.* (1987) Syndromic paucity of interlobular bile ducts (Alagille syndrome or arteriohepatic dysplasia): review of 80 cases. *Journal of Pediatrics*, **110**, 195–200.
2. Alonso-Lej, F., Rever, W.G. Jr and Pessagno, D.J. (1959) Congenital choledochal cyst, with report of 2, and an analysis of 94 cases. *International Abstracts of Surgery*, **108**, 1–30.
3. Babbitt, D.P. (1969) Congenital choledochal cysts; new etiological concept based on anomalous relationships of common bile duct and pancreatic bulb. *Annals of Radiology*, **12**, 231–240.
4. Bornman, P.C., Kottler, R.E., Terblanche, J. *et al.* (1988) Does low entry of cystic duct predispose to stones in the common bile duct? *British Medical Journal*, **297**, 31–32.
5. Brown, W.R., Sokol, R.J., Levin, M.J. *et al.* (1988) Lack of correlation between infection with reo virus and extrahepatic biliary atresia or neonatal hepatitis. *Journal of Pediatrics*, **113**, 670–676.
6. Caroli, J., Soupalt, R., Kossakowski, J. *et al.* (1958) La dilatation polycystique congénitale des voies biliares intrahépatiques. Essai de classification. *Semaine des Hôpitaux de Paris*, **34**, 488–495.
7. Donahue, P.K. and Hendren, W.H. (1976) Bile duct perforation in a newborn with stenosis of the

ampulla of Vater. *Journal of Pediatric Surgery*, **11**, 823–825.
8. Dorney, S.F.A., Middleton, A.W., Martin, H.C.O. *et al.* (1989) Outcome of surgery for biliary atresia. *Australian and New Zealand Journal of Surgery*, **59**, 855–858.
9. Esquivel, C.O., Koneru, B., Karrer, F.M. *et al.* (1987) Liver transplantation before 1 year of age. *Journal of Pediatrics*, **110**, 545–548.
10. Glaser, J.H., Balistreri, W.F. and Morecki, R. (1984) Role of reovirus 3 in persistent cholestasis. *Journal of Pediatrics*, **103**, 912–915.
11. Gray, S.W. and Skandalakis, J.E. (1972) *Embryology for Surgeons*, Philadelphia: W.B. Saunders.
12. Hall, R.J. and Karrer, F.M. (1990) Biliary atresia: perspective on transplantation. *Pediatric Surgery International*, **5**, 94–99.
13. Hays, D.M. and Kimura, K. (1980) *Biliary atresia: The Japanese Experience*. Cambridge MA: Harvard University Press.
14. Hays, D.M. and Kimura, K. (1981) Biliary atresia: new concepts of management. *Current Problems in Surgery*, **18**, 541–608.
15. Howard, E.R., Driver, M., McClement, J. and Mowat, A.P. (1982) Results of surgery in 88 consecutive cases of extrahepatic biliary atresia. *Journal of the Royal Society of Medicine*, **75**, 408–413.
16. Iwai, N., Tokiwa, K., Tsuto, T. *et al.* (1986) Biliary manometry in choledochal cyst with abnormal choledochopancreatico ductal junction. *Journal of Pediatric Surgery*, **21**, 873–876.
17. Jones, P.G., Smith, E.D., Clarke, M. *et al.* (1971) Choledochal cysts: experience with radical excision. *Journal of Pediatric Surgery*, **16**, 112–120.
18. Kagiyama, S., Okazaki, K., Yamamoto, Y. *et al.* (1987) Anatomic variants of choledococele and manometric measurements of pressure in the cele and the orifice zone. *American Journal of Gastroenterology*, **82**(7), 641–649.
19. Kasai, M. (1974) Treatment of biliary atresia with special reference to hepatic porto-enterostomy and its modifications. *Progress in Pediatric Surgery*, **6**, 5–52.
20. Kasai, M., Asakura, Y. and Taira, Y. (1970) Surgical treatment of choledochal cyst. *Annals of Surgery*, **172**, 844–850.
21. Kasai, M., Kimura, S., Asakura, Y. *et al.* (1968) Surgical treatment of biliary atresia. *Journal of Pediatric Surgery*, **3**, 665–675.
22. Kato, T., Asakura, Y. and Kasai, M. (1974) An attempt to produce choledochal cyst in puppies. *Journal of Pediatric Surgery*, **4**, 509–513.
23. Kimura, K., Tsugawa, C., Ogawa, K. *et al.* (1978) Choledochal cyst. *Archives of Surgery*, **113**, 159–163.
24. Komi, N., Tamura, T., Miyoski, Y. *et al.* (1985) Histochemical and immunocytological studies in forty-seven patients with choledochal cysts – special reference to intestinal metaplasia in the biliary duct. *Japanese Journal of Surgery*, **15**, 273–278.
25. Kune, G.A. (1970) The influence of structure and function in the surgery of the biliary tract. *Annals of the Royal College of Surgeons of England*, **47**, 78–91.
26. Kune, G.A. and Sali, A. (1980) *The Practice of Biliary Surgery*, 2nd edn. Oxford: Blackwell.
27. Kusonoki, M., Saitoh, N., Yamamura, T. *et al.* (1988) Choledochal cysts. Oligoganglionosis in the narrow portion of the choledochus. *Archives of Surgery*, **123**, 984–986.
28. Lilly, J.R. (1976) The surgery of biliary hypoplasia. *Journal of Pediatric Surgery*, **11**, 815–821.
29. Lilly, J.R. (1977) Surgical jaundice in infancy. *Annals of Surgery*, **186**, 549–558.
30. Lilly, J.R. (1978) Total excision of choledochal cyst. *Surgery, Gynecology and Obstetrics*, **146**, 254–256.
31. Lilly, J.R. (1979) Surgery of co-existing biliary malformations in choledochal cysts. *Journal of Pediatric Surgery*, **14**, 643–647.
32. Lilly, J.R., Hall, R.J. and Altman, P.O. (1987) Editors column. Liver transplantation and the Kasai operation for biliary atresia in the first year of life: therapeutic dilemma in biliary atresia. *Journal of Pediatrics*, **110**, 561–562.
33. Lilly, J.R., Karrer, F.M., Hall, R.J. *et al.* (1989) The surgery of biliary atresia. *Annals of Surgery*, **210**, 289–296.
34. Longmire, W.P., Mandiola, S.A. and Gordon, H.E. (1971) Congenital cystic disease of the liver and biliary system. *Annals of Surgery*, **174**, 711–726.
35. Lorenzo, G.A., Seeds, R.W. and Beal, J.M. (1971) Congenital dilatation of the biliary tract. *American Journal of Surgery*, **121**, 510–517.
36. Louw, J.H. (1975) Choledochal cysts. *South African Journal of Surgery*, **13**, 199–205.
37. Millis, M.J., Brems, J.J., Hiatt, J.R. *et al.* (1988) Orthotopic liver transplantation for biliary atresia – evolution of management. *Archives of Surgery*, **123**, 1237–12239.
38. Northover, J.M.A. and Terblanche, J. (1979) A new look at the arterial supply of the bile duct in man and its surgical implications. *British Journal of Surgery*, **6**, 379–384.
39. Ohi, R., Koike, N., Matsumoto, Y. *et al.* (1985) Changes of intrahepatic bile duct dilatation after surgery for congenital dilatation of the bile duct. *Journal of Pediatric Surgery*, **20**, 138–142.
40. Reynolds, M., Luck, S.R. and Raffensperger, J.G. (1985) The valved conduit prevents ascending cholangitis: a follow-up. *Journal of Pediatric Surgery*, **20**, 695–672.
41. Saito, S. and Ishida, M. (1974) Congenital choledochal cyst (cystic dilatation of the common bile duct). *Progress in Pediatric Surgery*, **6**, 63–90.
42. Scholz, F.J., Carrera, G.F. and Larse, C.R. (1976) The choledochocele – correlation of radiological, clinical and pathological findings. *Radiology*, **118**, 25–28.
43. Shim, W.K.T., Kasai, M. and Spence, M.A. (1974)

Racial influence on the incidence of biliary atresia. *Progress in Pediatric Surgery*, **6**, 53–62.
44. Starzl, T.E., Koep, L.J., Schröter. G.P.J. *et al.* (1979) Liver replacement for pediatric patients. *Pediatrics*, **63**, 825–829.
45. Stewart, B.A., Hall, R.J. and Lilly, J.R. (1988) Liver transplantation and the Kasai operation in biliary atresia. *Journal of Pediatric Surgery*, **23**, 623–626.
46. Schweizer, P. and Kerremans, J. (1988) Discordant findings in extrahepatic bile duct atresia in 6 sets of twins. *Zeitschrift für Kinderchirurgie*, **43**, 72–75.
47. Terblanche, J., Allison, H.F. and Northover, J.M.A. (1982) An ischaemic basis for biliary strictures. *Surgery*, **94**, 52–57.
48. Terblanche, J., Koep, L.J. and Starzl, T.E. (1979) Liver transplantation. *Medical Clinics of North America*, **63**, 507–521.
49. Todani, T., Narusue, M., Watanabe, Y. *et al.* (1978) Management of choledochal cyst with intrahepatic involvement. *Annals of Surgery*, **187**, 272–280.
50. Todani, T., Tabachi, K. and Watanabe, Y. (1979) Carcinoma arising in the wall of congenital bile duct cysts. *Cancer*, **44**, 1134–1141.
51. Todani, T., Watanabe, Y., Narusue, M. *et al.* (1977) Congenital bile duct cysts. Classification, operative procedures and review of thirty-seven cases including cancer arising from choledochal cyst. *American Journal of Surgery*, **134**, 263–269.
52. Todani, T., Watanabe, Y., Toki, A. *et al.* (1987) Carcinoma related to choledochal cysts with internal drainage operations. *Surgery, Gynecology and Obstetrics*, **164**, 61–64.
53. Tsuchida, Y. and Ishida, M. (1971) Dilatation of the intrahepatic bile ducts in congenital cystic dilatation of the common bile duct. *Surgery*, **69**, 776–781.

PHYSIOLOGY OF EXTRAHEPATIC BILE TRANSPORT

J.S. Davison

The flow of bile is determined by the pressure difference between the hepatocytes and the intestinal lumen. The origin of this gradient is the 'secretory pressure' of the hepatocytes themselves, which in humans is about 29–39 mmHg. However, control of the gradient, and thus of bile flow, is achieved mainly by regulating the resistance of the gallbladder and biliary duct system.

GALLBLADDER FILLING

During the interdigestive period, bile flows into the gallbladder because for much of the time the sphincter of Oddi remains closed. Closure of the common bile duct, however, depends not only on the activity of the sphincter muscle but also on the state of tone of surrounding duodenal muscle. The gallbladder tone at this stage is low, as is the resistance of the cystic duct, thus favouring flow in the gallbladder. This is generally regarded as being due simply to the intrinsic properties of the gallbladder and cystic duct muscle in the absence of the excitatory hormonal and neural stimuli which operate during feeding. However, recent evidence suggests that there may be active inhibition of muscle tone by vagal, non-adrenergic non-cholinergic inhibitory nerves during this period.[2] Evidence has accumulated suggesting that vasoactive intestinal polypeptide is the inhibitory transmitter. Thus, the gallbladder may demonstrate receptive relaxation analogous to that of other storage organs such as the gastric corpus.[1] Gallbladder filling in humans can be observed by HIDA scanning[9] and typically has a time-course as shown in *Figure 12.17*.

GALLBLADDER EPITHELIAL TRANSPORT

During this phase of filling and storage there is rapid absorption of fluid by the gallbladder epithelium. This is significant, not so much as a device for water conservation by the body, but as a means of preventing the build-up of an excessive volume because the capacity of the gallbladder in humans is limited to approximately 20 ml. As a consequence of the absorption of water and electrolytes there is a five- to 10-fold increase in concentration in the gallbladder bile of organic constituents such as bile salts, bile pigments, cholesterol and other biliary lipids (*Table 12.1*).

Fluxes of water occur in both directions across gallbladder epithelium but the net flux is from gallbladder to blood. The absorptive capacity of the gallbladder epithelium is greater than that of the ileum or the urinary bladder and for that reason the

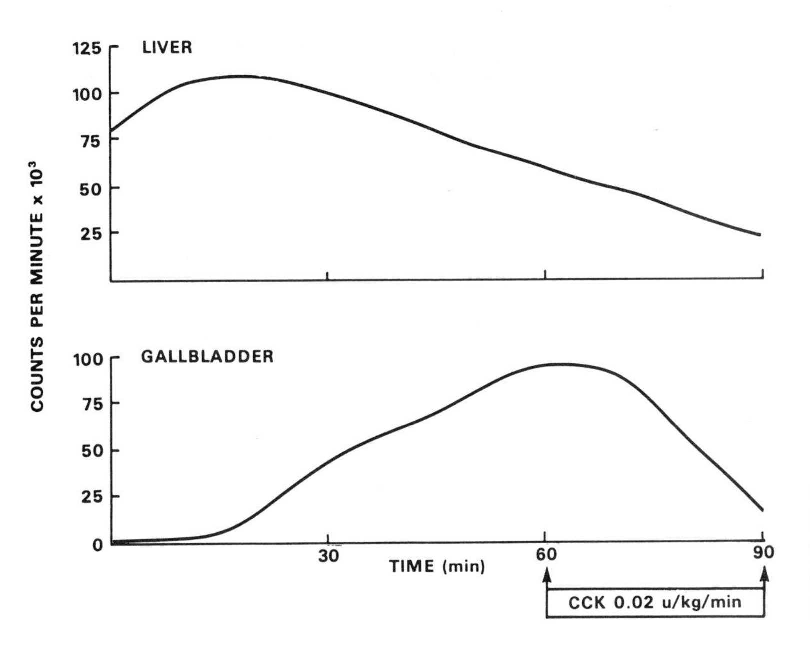

Figure 12.17 Dynamic curves from a ^{99m}Tc HIDA scan in a normal subject showing the time course of gallbladder filling in relation to hepatic secretion and gallbladder emptying in response to intravenous cholecystokinin infusion.[9]

Table 12.1 Composition of normal bile

	Hepatic bile (mmol/l)	*Gallbladder bile (mmol/l)*
Blue salts[a]	0.8–38.1	47.9–275.4
Bilirubin	6.8	51.0
Cholesterol[a]	0.3–3.0	0.1–87.1
Fatty acids[a]	0.1–2.9	0.1–55.4
Lecithin[a]	4.1–6.6	11.2–39.0
Na^+	145	130
K^+	5	12
Ca^{2+}	10	46
Cl^-	100	25
HCO_3^-	28	10

[a]Data provided by P.E. Ross.

gallbladder has become a widely used model for electrolyte and water transport across epithelia.

As in other transport systems, the movement of water is passive and secondary to the active uptake of other substances, principally sodium. The fluid absorbed from the gallbladder is iso-osmotic with respect to plasma but the passive permeability of the epithelium to water is too low to permit simple iso-osmotic fluid absorption. Hence, a mechanism exists which restricts the diffusion into the blood of the actively transported solutes until sufficient water has followed. The lateral intercellular spaces play an important part in this process.[3]

Until recently, the most widely accepted explanation was the standing gradient hypothesis (*Figure 12.18a*). Solute, actively pumped into the long lateral intercellular space, diffuses along its concentration gradient to emerge at the serosal end of the space. Water can then diffuse from the epithelial cells along their entire length. Hence, in the steady stage of fluid absorption there will be an osmotic gradient along the length of the intercellular space. However, evidence has shown that the so-called 'tight' junctions between gallbladder epithelial cells are leaky to water and small solute molecules and that most of the fluid transported by the gallbladder epithelium follows a paracellular route (i.e. via the junctions and spaces) rather than a transcellular route through the epithelial cells. The paracellular or 'shunt' pathway is thought to comprise two paral-

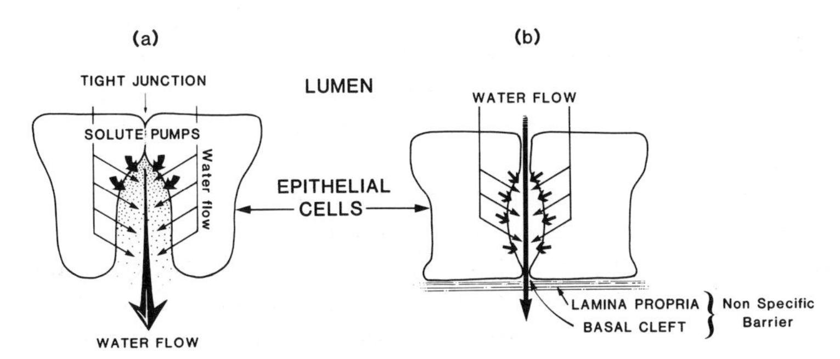

Figure 12.18 Two hypotheses for iso-osmotic fluid absorption by the gallbladder epithelium. (a) The standing gradient hypothesis and (b) the serial membrane hypothesis. In (a) the osmotic gradient is indicated by the density of stippling (for explanation see text). In (b) the paracellular route for water and ion movement is shown in addition to the originally proposed transcellular route.

lel components: (1) a solution 'leak', permeable to all ions and small molecules in free solution, and (2) selective cation channels. As much as 95% of transepithelial ionic diffusion has been estimated to occur via these paracellular routes.

Micropuncture studies of intercellular space fluid have not confirmed the existence of an osmotic gradient. Hence, the older, and until recently less accepted, serial membrane model (*Figure 12.18b*) with modification might provide a better explanation. In this model, the solute is pumped into the intercellular space or passes through cation-selective channels in the junctional complex but does not readily diffuse out of this region because of a non-specific barrier provided by the basal clefts and lamina propria. Water can then diffuse into the intercellular space, taking with it other ions in free solution (bulk flow), producing an osmotic equilibrium and, of course, increasing the hydrostatic pressure. This predicted rise in pressure would account for the observed swelling on the intercellular spaces during fluid absorption and is consistent with micropuncture studies showing an iso-osmotic intercellular fluid. Moreover, although the original hypothesis envisaged a transcellular route for water movements, a predominantly paracellular route would still be consistent with the model.

Transcellular transport of ions involves entry into the cell across the apical membrane and exit via the basolateral membrane.[4] Sodium and chloride entry across the apical membrane is electroneutral but the mechanism is still controversial.[6] Two models have been proposed (see *Figure 12.19*). In one there is a simple symport of sodium and chloride. In the

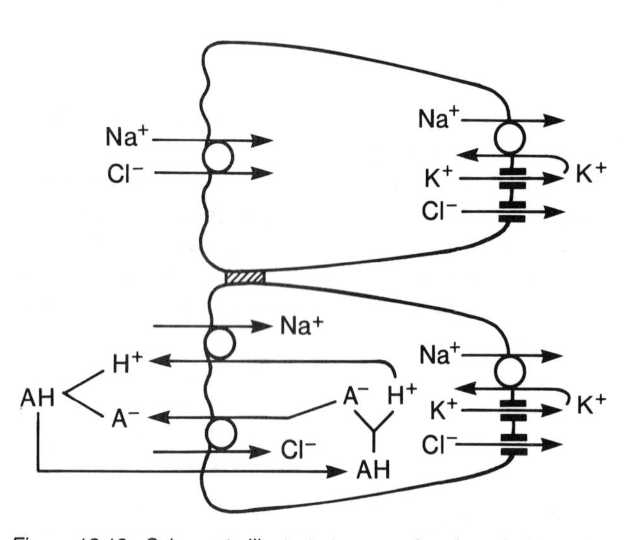

Figure 12.19 Scheme to illustrate two postulated mechanisms for the uptake of sodium chloride by the apical (luminal) membrane of gallbladder epithelium. In this scheme A^- could be HCO_3^- or a fatty acid anion such as butyrate. Also shown is a proposed exit mechanism on the basolateral membrane.

second, there are two parallel but linked exchange (antiport) processes (Na^+/H^+ and Cl^-/HCO_3^-). Transport across the basolateral membrane is more complex. Sodium exit is via the sodium pump (NA^+/K^+ exchange). Potassium and chloride exit is electroneutral and downhill driven, possibly by the combined electrochemical gradient for potassium and chloride. In addition, there may also be a chloride/bicarbonate exchanger that would account for the excess of chloride over sodium absorption.

The gallbladder epithelium of several species, including humans, also absorbs certain amino acids and sugars using specific carriers. Although the gallbladder maintains a high concentration gradient of bile salts and bile pigments across the epithelium, certain salts and pigments can be absorbed. In general, weakly ionized compounds such as chenodeoxycholic acid and unconjugated bilirubin are absorbed more readily than highly ionized compounds such as taurocholic acid.

While the gallbladder epithelium is considered to be the main site for modification of bile, it is now recognized that the bile ductules and ducts are also sites of secretion and reabsorption. Secretin-induced choleresis is now considered to be mainly through its effect on the duct system rather than the hepatocyte.[4]

GALLBLADDER EMPTYING

Throughout the interdigestive period there is periodic emptying of the gallbladder.[8] These bouts of emptying are associated with phase 2 of the migrating myoelectrical complexes, recurring bursts of electrical activity, and associated mechanical activity, which sweep down the gut during periods of fasting. While some of the mechanisms controlling the migrating myoelectrical complexes have been identified, nothing is known about what links gallbladder and biliary tract motility to this intestinal activity.

The physiological significance of this periodic emptying, however, is readily evident. It prevents stasis of bile in the gallbladder and, hence, reduces the risk of gallstone formation. Stasis is now recognized as an important contributing factor in the genesis of cholesterol gallstones. In part, this is simply because of an increased probability of crystal formation during prolonged storage of lithogenic bile. However, stasis may itself contribute to the production of lithogenic bile – not because of the concentrating effect of epithelial absorption of water which also increases bile salt concentration in proportion to the increase in biliary lipid concentration – but because of the effect of stasis on the enterohepatic circulation of bile salts. It is established that a reduction in the enterohepatic circulation of bile salts results in the production of a more lithogenic bile. So by maintaining the enterohepatic circulation, the periodic emptying of the gallbladder, linked to the propulsive activity of the ileum during the final phase (3) of the migrating myoelectrical complexes, should reduce the likelihood of lithogenic bile being formed and, hence, of cholesterol stone formation. The 'housekeeper' role of the migrating myoelectrical complexes may apply also to the biliary tract in that periodic emptying may prevent the build-up of bacterial flora and cell debris in the biliary tree.

In normal subjects the gallbladder empties rapidly after ingestion of a meal. The gallbladder contracts, increasing the intravesicular pressure. Since, at the same time, the resistance to bile flow through the sphincter decreases, bile enters the duodenum. The cystic duct resistance increases in response to the same mechanisms which elevate gallbladder pressure. This probably has less effect in restricting the expulsion of bile from the gallbladder than in preventing the diversion of hepatic bile into the gallbladder. Hepatic secretion increases as a result of the increase in the rate of the enterohepatic circulation of the bile salt pool, and perhaps as a consequence of neural and hormonal signals.

The mechanisms controlling gallbladder emptying are summarized in *Figure 12.20*. The principal mechanism for the stimulation of gallbladder emptying has long been considered to be the release of the hormone cholecystokinin from the duodenal mucosa, stimulated by the presence of food. The establishment of this hormonal mechanism by classical physiological methods involving transplanted intestinal loops or cross-circulation experiments was eventually followed by the isolation and purification of cholecystokinin. It is a linear polypeptide containing 33 amino acids of which the *C*-terminal octapeptide is considered to be the biologically active fragment although the *C*-terminal tetrapeptide retains much of the activity.

Cholecystokinin is released from the endocrine cells of the small intestine in response to stimulation by a variety of digestion products including amino acids such as phenylalanine and tryptophan, fatty acids and hydrogen ions.

Cholecystokinin acts directly on gallbladder smooth muscle.[7] Contraction of the gallbladder induced by cholecystokinin is preceded by an increase in phosphodiesterase activity, leading to a fall in intracellular cAMP levels. It is not clear what role this plays in initiating gallbladder contraction because a rise in the free cytosolic calcium concentration is generally regarded as the significant intracellular mediator of the contractile process. There is dispute, however, over the relative contribution of intracellular (bound) and extracellular sources of calcium to the rise in free calcium levels. In contrast, cholecystokinin causes relaxation of the sphincter of Oddi.

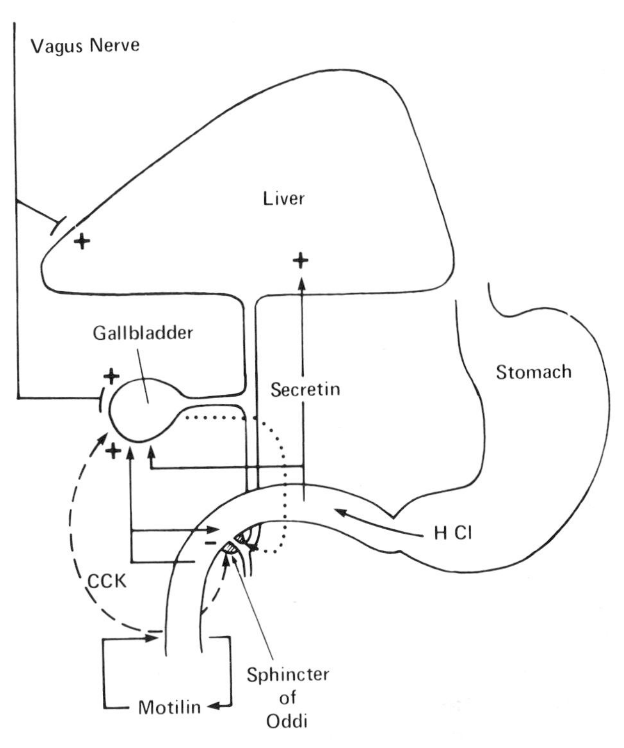

Figure 12.20 Control of gallbladder emptying. During a meal cholecystokinin released from the duodenal mucosa contracts the gallbladder and relaxes the sphincter of Oddi. Secretin, released by gastric acid passing into the duodenum, can enhance the cholecystokinin action on the gallbladder contraction. Secretin also stimulates bile secretion by its action on the liver ductules. The vagus nerve also stimulates gallbladder contraction. Bile flow into the duodenum is also enhanced by the actions of the vagus and secretin on hepatic bile secretion. A pathway between the gallbladder and sphincter of Oddi has been postulated (dotted line). Pathways also exist which link gallbladder emptying to fasting duodenal motility (dashed lines) and these probably account for the action of motilin.

Other hormones and peptides will also stimulate or inhibit gallbladder contraction.[7] Gastrin and the amphibian peptide caerulein are structurally similar to cholecystokinin and can both activate the cholecystokinin receptors, leading to gallbladder contraction. Gastrin, although less potent than cholecystokinin, may play a physiological role in the regulation of gallbladder contraction during the gastric phase of digestion. Secretin is without effect on the gallbladder when administered alone but augments responses to cholecystokinin. Vasoactive intestinal polypeptide inhibits responses to cholecystokinin and the existence of vasoactive intestinal polypeptide immunoreactive nerves has been demonstrated in feline and human gallbladder.

Motilin and pancreatic polypeptide also appear to influence gallbladder contractility, the former causing gallbladder contraction and the latter relaxation. In both cases, isolated gallbladder strips from several species, including man, fail to respond to these peptides indicating that their site of action is probably remote from the gallbladder muscle. In the case of motilin, activation of gallbladder contraction may be secondary to initiation of migrating myoelectrical complexes by this peptide. The mode of action of pancreatic polypeptide on the gallbladder muscle is obscure.

Neural control of gallbladder emptying generally has been relegated to a fairly unimportant role. Although the vagus appears to have little importance in regulating the sphincter of Oddi, it is well established that stimulation of cholinergic, parasympathetic nerves, or exogenous administration of acetylcholine or cholinomimetic drugs will stimulate vigorous gallbladder contractions, though less powerfully than cholecystokinin. Perhaps more significantly, concomitant cholinergic nerve and cholecystokinin (or gastrin) stimulation will produce synergistic responses (i.e. greater than the sum of the responses to each individual stimulus)[5] and this is largely ignored in most textbook accounts of the control of gallbladder emptying.

The time-course of gallbladder emptying also suggests that the control mechanism involves much more than merely the release of cholecystokinin consequent upon entry of chyme into the duodenum. The gallbladder emptying response to a liquid meal in humans is very rapid and cannot be accounted for by release of cholecystokinin alone. The gallbladder can empty by over 50% in the first 15 minutes before any appreciable gastric emptying has occurred and long before there is any real elevation of serum cholecystokinin levels. It seems probably that there are significant interdigestive, cephalic and gastric phases of gallbladder emptying involving vagal cholinergic nerves and perhaps gastrin and an early intestinal phase which may involve complex neurohormonal and hormonal–hormonal interactions. While individual mechanisms have been identified (see *Figure 12.20*), we need much more information about the integration of these processes before their physiological importance in the regulation of the motility of the gallbladder and biliary tree can be evaluated.

REFERENCES

1. Davison, J.S. and Al-Hassani, M. (1980) The role of non-cholinergic, nonadrenergic nerves in regulating distensibility of the guinea-pig gallbladder. In *Gastrointestinal Motility* (Ed.) Christensen, J. pp. 89–95. New York: Raven Press.
2. Davison, J.S., Al-Hassani, M., Crowe, R. and Burnstock, G. (1978) The non-adrenergic inhibitory innervation of the guinea-pig gallbladder. *Pflugers Archivs*, **337**, 43–49.
3. Diamond, J.M. (1979) Osmotic water flow in leaky epithelia. *Journal of Membrane Biology*, **51**, 195–216.
4. Erlinger, S. (1987) Physiology of bile secretion and enterohepatic circulation. In *Physiology of the Gastrointestinal Tract*, 2nd edn (Ed.) Johnson, L.R. pp. 1557–1580. New York: Raven Press.
5. Pallin, B. and Skoglund, S. (1964) Neural and humoral control of the gallbladder-emptying mechanism in the cat. *Acta Physiologica Scandinavica*, **60**, 358–362.
6. Rose, R.C. (1987) Absorptive functions of the gallbladder. In *Physiology of the Gastrointestinal Tract*, 2nd edn (Ed.) Johnson, L.R. pp. 1455–1468. New York: Raven Press.
7. Ryan, J.P. (1987) Motility of the gallbladder and biliary tree. In *Physiology of the Gastrointestinal Tract,* 2nd edn (Ed.) Johnson, L.R. pp. 695–721. New York: Raven Press.
8. Scott, R.B., Eidt, P.B. and Shaffer, E.A. (1985) Regulation of fasting canine duodenal bile acid delivery by sphincter of Oddi and gallbladder. *American Journal of Physiology*, **249**, G622–G633.
9. Shaffer, E.A., McOrmond, P. and Duggan, H. (1980) Quantitative cholescintigraphy: assessment of gallbladder filling and emptying and duodenogastric reflux. *Gastroenterology*, **79**, 899–906.

PHYSIOLOGY OF BILE SECRETION

S. Erlinger

Bile secretion is one of the major functions of the liver. Bile is an aqueous solution of organic and inorganic compounds. Bile acids, bile pigments, cholesterol and phospholipids are the chief organic compounds. Bile also contains small amounts of proteins. Because of the peculiar aggregation properties of the bile acids, which readily form micelles at physiological concentrations, bile is more complex than most other secretions, especially in regard to the osmotic properties of its constituents. Bile formed by the hepatocytes is secreted into the bile canaliculi. It is then modified during its passage in the bile ductules and ducts, and in the gallbladder, where water and inorganic electrolytes are reabsorbed, with, as a result, concentration of the organic constituents. Most conclusions regarding canalicular bile formation are derived from indirect evidence and are hypothetical. Here, the available experimental data are summarized and the current theories of hepatic bile formation discussed. More detailed references may be found in other reviews.[3,8]

BILE COMPOSITION

In general, *inorganic electrolytes* are present in common duct bile at concentrations closely reflecting those in plasma (*Table 12.2*). Bile concentrations of sodium, potassium, calcium and bicarbonate may, however, be appreciably higher than in plasma, while the chloride level may be lower.

In spite of these variations, bile *osmolality*, as measured by freezing point depression, is usually approximately 300 mosmol/kg and it varies in parallel with plasma osmolality. The total osmotic activity is accounted for only by the inorganic electrolytes because it is generally assumed that bile acids, which are in micellar form, have little or no osmotic activity.

The concentration of bicarbonate in bile is often higher than that in plasma. This may be due to bicarbonate transport mechanisms which have been postulated in the hepatocytes and in the bile ductules and ducts, in response to secretin (see below).

The major *organic constituents* of bile are the conjugated bile acids, the bile pigments, cholesterol and phospholipids. The concentration and physicochemical properties of these compounds, which are important for the understanding of cholesterol and pigment gallstone formation, are discussed on p. 1704.

STRUCTURE–FUNCTION RELATIONSHIPS IN THE BILIARY SYSTEM

Bile is secreted primarily by the hepatocytes into bile canaliculi, which are formed by a groove of the lateral plasma membrane between two hepatocytes[20] and are about 1 μm in diameter (*Figure 12.21*). The bile canalicular membrane forms numerous microvilli which increase the surface area, and it represents about 13% of the hepatocyte plasma membrane. The bile canaliculi connect to bile ducts, lined by biliary epithelial cells. The smallest bile duct, the ductule, connects the canaliculus with the portal (interlobular) bile ducts. The interlobular bile ducts drain into larger bile ducts which form the intra- and extrahepatic biliary tree (*Figure 12.22*). With respect to bile secretion, the liver may be regarded as an epithelium transporting a variety of substrates from blood to bile. This vectorial transport is made possible by the high degree of polarization of the hepatocyte plasma membrane. As in other transporting epithelia, the canalicular lumen is sealed by intercellular junctions.

THE POLARIZATION OF THE HEPATOCYTE PLASMA MEMBRANE

Three domains of the hepatocyte plasma membrane may be recognized: sinusoidal (facing the blood sinusoids), lateral (or intercellular) and canalicular. They demonstrate important morphological, biochemical and enzymic differences. Especially im-

Table 12.2 Flow and electrolyte concentrations of hepatic bile

Species	*Flow* (μ*l/(min kg)*)	*Concentration (mmol/l)* Na^+	K^+	Ca^{2+}	Mg^{2+}	Cl^-	HCO_3^-	*Bile acids*
Human	1.5–15.4	132–165	4.2–5.6	0.6–2.4	0.7–1.5	96–126	17–55	3–45
Dog	10	141–230	4.5–11.9	1.5–6.9	1.1–2.7	31–107	14–61	16–187
Sheep	9.4	159.6	5.3	—	—	95	21.2	42.5
Rabbit	90	148–156	3.6–6.7	1.3–3.3	0.15–0.35	77–99	40–63	6–24
Rat	30–150	157–166	5.8–6.4	—	—	94–98	22–26	8–25
Guinea-pig	115.9	175	6.3	—	—	69	49–65	—

Numbers indicate range or means of published values.

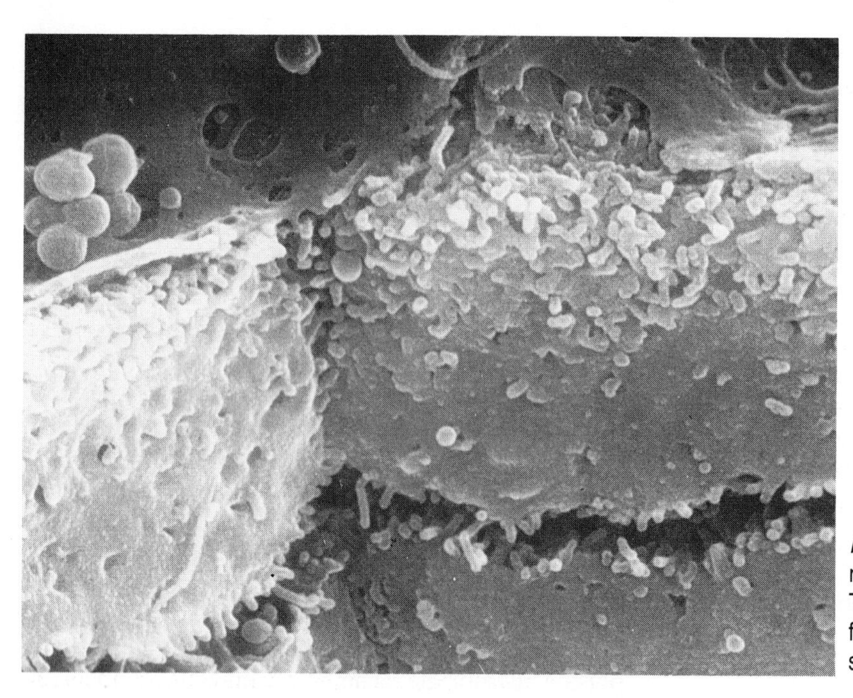

Figure 12.21 Scanning electron micrograph of a hemi-bile canaliculus. The bile canaliculus runs on the lateral face of the hepatocyte. At the top the sinusoid with red cells can be seen.

portant for transepithelial transport is the localization of Na^+/K^+-activated adenosine triphosphatase (Na^+/K^+-ATPase), which is mainly in the sinusoidal and intercellular membrane, with little or no activity in the canalicular membrane.[2,17,30] A wide range of epithelia, including iso-osmotic and hyperosmotic absorbers and secretors, have (with the exception of the choroid plexus) the Na^+ pump (Na^+/K^+-ATPase) preferentially on the basolateral surface of the epithelial cells. In the hepatocyte, the sinusoidal and intercellular membrane is the equivalent of the basolateral membrane of other epithelial cells: the liver is therefore no exception among transporting epithelia regarding the localization of the enzyme.

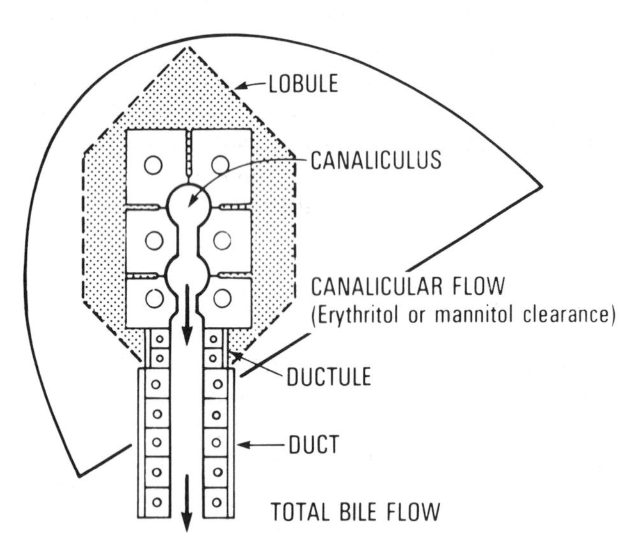

Figure 12.22 Schematic diagram of the biliary system. (Reproduced, with permission, from Erlinger.[8])

Alkaline phosphatase, whose role in transport and in bile secretion is unknown, is, in contrast, preferentially located on the canalicular membrane.[2]

THE TIGHT JUNCTION AND THE PARACELLULAR PATHWAY

A substrate in plasma can enter canalicular bile in one of two ways (*Figure 12.23*): either by the transcellular pathway, that is, entering the hepatocyte through the sinusoidal membrane, crossing the

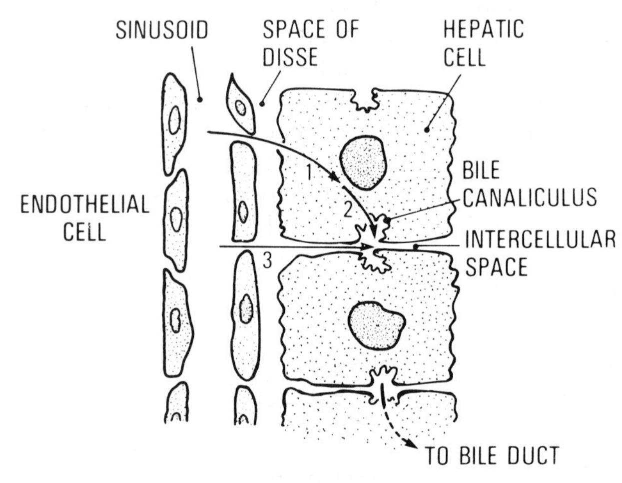

Figure 12.23 Possible anatomical pathways of bile formation. A substrate can enter bile either after being taken up by the sinusoidal membrane (1) and transported into the cell (2) (transcellular pathway) or directly from the intercellular space through the tight junction (3) (paracellular pathway). (Reproduced, with permission, from Erlinger.[8])

hepatocyte and entering the canaliculus through the canalicular membrane; or by the paracellular pathway. In the latter, the solute crosses the intercellular junction. The junction includes the tight junction, which is a sealing structure between the lumen of the bile canaliculus and the intercellular space and, hence, the sinusoidal blood. Tight junctions differ among epithelia. In impermeable epithelia (such as the toad bladder), the tight junction provides a high transepithelial resistance to the movement of water and ions (and, hence, to electrical current) whereas in relatively permeable epithelia (such as the gallbladder, intestine or proximal kidney tubule) the tight junction is 'leaky', permitting some passage of water and ions (with, as a result, a low electrical resistance). The liver is of an intermediate type and there is evidence for a paracellular ion and fluid flux into bile which could play an important role in choleresis and possibly cholestasis. The existence of a negative charge barrier in the tight junction has also been postulated.

THE HEPATOCYTE CYTOSKELETON

The canaliculus is surrounded by a narrow zone or organelle-poor cytoplasm, known as pericanalicular ectoplasm, where actin microfilaments (7 nm in diameter) are especially prevalent. They form a pericanalicular network, insert in the intercellular junction and extend into the microvilli, where they appear to insert on the inner part of the membrane. They may have a key role in maintaining the shape of the cell, particularly its microvilli. Agents that interfere with the structure and function of microfilaments affect bile flow, which suggests a role for these organelles in secretion.[20,21]

Microtubules, which are 24 nm in diameter, are more randomly distributed within the liver cell cytoplasm than are microfilaments. They play a role in the intracellular transport and secretion by the liver cell of proteins and lipoproteins, and possibly in the transport of bile acids and other anions into bile. Antimicrotubular agents may affect bile formation (see below).

CANALICULAR BILE FLOW

The maximum bile secretory pressure (about 25–30 cmH_2O) exceeds the sinusoidal perfusion pressure (about 5–10 cmH_2O), which excludes hydrostatic filtration as an important mechanism of canalicular bile secretion. Canalicular bile flow is regarded mainly as an osmotic water flow in response to active solute transport. *Bile acids*, which are potent choleretics, are most probably one of these solutes but the transport of *other organic compounds* and *inorganic ions* also plays a role.

ESTIMATION OF CANALICULAR BILE FLOW

Canalicular bile flow may be estimated by measuring the biliary clearance of non-metabolized solutes that enter canalicular bile by passive processes and are neither secreted nor reabsorbed by the biliary epithelium.[9,33] The most widely used of such solutes are erythritol and mannitol (labelled with ^{14}C). Briefly, when injected into the systemic circulation, the biliary secretion rate of such a solute during a steady state should depend on the permeability of the canaliculus and on canalicular bile flow. The biliary clearance (C) is calculated as $C=F[B]/[P]$, where F is the bile flow, and [B] and [P] the biliary and plasma concentrations, respectively. The technique implies that the selected solute is unable to cross the biliary epithelium and has a permeability in the canaliculi high enough to achieve diffusion equilibrium at the highest rates of canalicular flow. Neither of these assumptions is presently accessible to direct experimental testing. However, an operational test of adequate canalicular permeability is the finding that increments in bile flow induced by bile acids are accompanied by parallel increases in solute clearance. Depending on the species, erythritol (molecular weight 122) and mannitol (molecular weight 182) meet these requirements.

The original assumption that erythritol and mannitol do not cross the biliary epithelium was based on the observation that their clearance was not modified by secretin,[9,33] which acts presumably on the ductules or ducts. However, small increases in erythritol and mannitol biliary clearance in response to secretin have been observed in dogs because either canalicular bile flow is stimulated by this hormone, or there is some permeability of the bile ductules or ducts to erythritol and mannitol.[31]

BILE ACID-DEPENDENT FLOW

Canalicular bile flow includes two major components, designated as bile acid-dependent and bile acid-independent flow. Bile acid-dependent flow is related to bile acid transport and secretion into the canalicular lumen. Bile acid transport by the hepatocyte involves three steps: uptake by the sinusoidal membrane, intracellular transport and canalicular secretion.

Uptake of bile acids

The uptake of conjugated bile acids by the hepatocyte is an active process utilizing the transmembrane sodium gradient as its source of energy (it is called secondary active transport because it does not use the energy source ATP directly, but through a secondary ion gradient). The transmembrane sodium gradient is continuously maintained by the Na^+/K^+-ATPase located on the sinusoidal and lateral domains of the plasma membrane (see above). The enzyme uses ATP as its energy source and exchanges three sodium ions for two potassium ions. Sodium is pumped out of the cell and the intracellular sodium concentration is maintained at a low level. The sodium concentration difference (high outside, low inside) can be used to drive substrates into the cell. This is the case for conjugated bile acids.

The protein responsible for the transport has been identified by photoaffinity labelling techniques[15] as a 48 kDa protein. The system is called symport, or cotransport. It has been reconstituted in artificial liposomes[19,32] and in xenopus oocytes.[14] These types of experiments clearly establish that the putative protein is responsible for transport.

Intracellular transport

Cytosolic protein binding

After uptake by the sinusoidal membrane, bile acids are, in part, bound to cytosolic proteins. Several proteins with a high binding affinity for bile acids have been identified. Glutathione *S*-transferases of the Ya family have high-affinity binding sites for monohydroxylated and dihydroxylated bile acids.[28] Binders I and II, also designated as Y′, which are proteins of approximately 33 kDa, have high-affinity binding sites for several bile acids with overlapping but distinct specificities.[28] They exhibit 3α-hydroxysteroid dehydrogenase activity and may reduce 3-oxo-bile acids into 3α-hydroxy-bile acids. Other cytosolic proteins may bind bile acids. After injection of a labelled bile acid, 30–60% of the intracellular bile acid is found in the cytosolic fraction. The exact role of protein binding in the transport of bile acids is not known. It is assumed that protein binding plays a role in facilitating bile acid entry into the cell and/or in reducing bile acid efflux out of the cell after entry.

Evidence for vesicular transport

Existing evidence supports the view that intracellular organelles play a role in the vectorial transport of bile acids by the hepatocyte towards the canalicular membrane. High-affinity binding sites have been identified in the Golgi apparatus:[25] the binding affinity was similar to that of the plasma membrane. The existence of a vesicular transport for bile acids is supported by studies with microtubule inhibitors, morphological observations, and experiments using autoradiography and immunoperoxidase techniques.

Pretreatment of rats with microtubule inhibitors, such as colchicine and vinblastine, inhibits bile acid secretion. Studies from the author's laboratory and by others have indicated that these agents do not inhibit basal bile acid secretion or bile acid secretion after a tracer dose of a labelled bile salt, but strongly inhibit secretion after injection of a substantial load of bile acid.[6]

It is known that a variety of vesicular transport processes in cells require the integrity of microtubules. Inhibition of transport when microtubules are disrupted by colchicine and vinblastine is consistent with a vesicular transport. The above-mentioned observations are best explained by the existence of two transport pathways: a colchicine-insensitive (possibly diffusional) pathway at low concentrations or tracer doses; and a colchicine-sensitive (possibly vesicular) pathway at higher concentrations.

More direct evidence for such vesicular transport is derived from morphological observations. After a 48-hour taurocholate loading, significant increases in the amounts of Golgi-rich area, Golgi membranes and pericanalicular vesicles have been observed. Autoradiographic studies using two labelled bile acid analogues (cholylglycylhistamine and cholylglycyltyrosine) have shown preferential distribution of grains over the Golgi complex and the endoplasmic reticulum.[12,29]

Immunoperoxidase experiments with specific anti-bile acid polyclonal antibodies have shown preferential staining of the Golgi apparatus, and, to a lesser extent, of the endoplasmic reticulum.[16] These experiments also suggest that, at some stage of their intracellular transport, bile acids interact with these organelles.

It is noteworthy that a taurocholate transport system has been identified in isolated purified Golgi fractions from rat liver.[18,26] This system appears to be sodium-independent and, therefore, distinct from the sinusoidal transporter.

Collectively, these observations support the view that, after uptake by the sinusoidal membrane and cytosolic protein binding, bile acids may be transported by the hepatocyte by two distinct pathways (*Figure 12.24*). One is a non-vesicular pathway by simple diffusion to the canalicular carrier and secretion into bile by carrier-mediated transport, facilitated by the membrane potential. The other is a

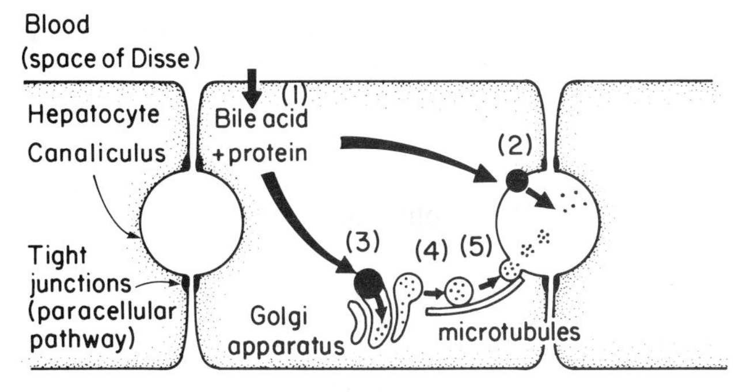

Figure 12.24 Proposed pathways for transport of bile acids by the hepatocytes. After uptake by the sinusoidal membrane (1), bile acids are bound to proteins. They can be transported to the canalicular membrane by diffusion and secreted into bile by a carrier (2). Alternatively, they can enter the Golgi apparatus through a carrier (3), transfer into Golgi-derived vesicles (4), which move to the canaliculus by a microtubule-dependent process, and be secreted by exocytosis (5).

vesicular pathway involving the Golgi apparatus: bile acids are transported by a specific carrier of the Golgi membrane into the Golgi lumen, and then into Golgi-derived vesicles. These vesicles move towards the canaliculus by a microtubule-dependent process and could be secreted into bile by exocytosis. The latter pathway becomes increasingly important when the transcellular flux of bile acid increases. It is important to recognize that such vesicular transport systems are energy-dependent: they are mediated, in part, by the microtubule-associated ATPase kinesin, which is abundant in hepatocytes. They may be extremely rapid: their speed can be of the order of 1–5 μm/s, and allow the transport of a molecule across the hepatocyte in less than 1 minute. This is consistent with the known kinetics of taurocholate biliary secretion. At present, however, no direct morphological data supporting exocytosis has been obtained.

Canalicular secretion

From the preceding discussion, two mechanisms can be proposed for canalicular secretion. One is via the canalicular carrier protein, which has been identified by photoaffinity labelling and reconstituted in artificial liposomes;[19,24] it is a 100 kDa transmembrane protein. This protein does not use energy but utilizes the membrane potential (−35 mV inside the cell, −5 mV in the canalicular lumen) to drive bile acids out of the cell into the canalicular lumen; a typical example of facilitated diffusion. Recently, an ATP-dependent taurocholate transport system has been identified on canalicular membrane vesicles from rat liver. The second mechanism could be exocytosis of Golgi-derived vesicles after membrane fusion. Direct proof of such a mechanism, as indicated above, is currently lacking.

Direct information on canalicular secretory processes should be obtained in the near future by an elegant technique of isolated hepatocyte couplets in culture,[11] developed first by Phillips and associates[22] and, more recently, by Boyer and colleagues.[13] These hepatocytes reform well-constituted canaliculi which can be micropunctured and used to estimate canalicular flow. This preparation has already provided precise information on electrical potential and on the rate of canalicular bile production under various circumstances. It should help to clarify the mechanisms of canalicular bile formation which cannot be studied directly in vivo, and perhaps to elucidate canalicular cholestasis.

Effect of bile acid secretion on canalicular flow

An apparently linear relationship between the bile acid secretion rate and bile flow has been demonstrated in many animal species, including humans[8] (*Figure 12.25*). Bile acid-induced choleresis is presumably of canalicular origin, because bile acids are secreted into the canaliculi, and as there is a linear relationship between erythritol clearance and bile acid secretion (*Figure 12.25*).

The hypothesis that bile acids increase bile flow by providing an osmotic driving force for water and electrolytes was proposed by Sperber.[27] However, because bile acids are in micellar form in bile, most osmotic activity must be accounted for by their counter-ions (or cations accompanying the bile acid anions to maintain electroneutrality).

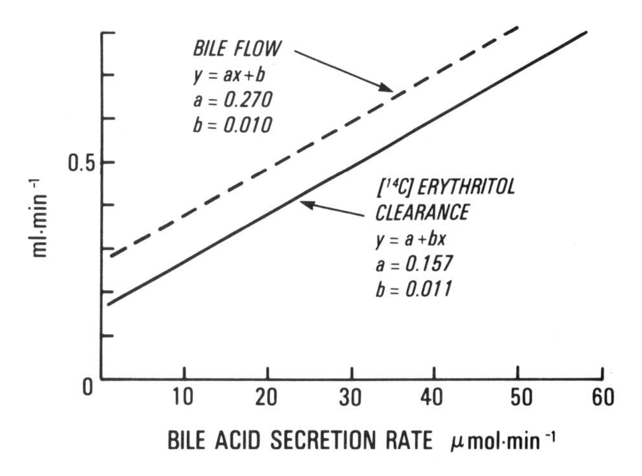

Figure 12.25 Relationship between the bile flow (dashed line), [^{14}C]erythritol clearance (full line) and bile acid secretion in cholecystectomized patients with T tubes in the common bile duct. (After Erlinger.[8])

Hypercholeretic bile acids and the cholehepatic shunt hypothesis

In 1980, it was demonstrated that ursodeoxycholic acid ($3\alpha,7\beta$-dihydroxycholanoic acid, the 7β epimer of chenodeoxycholic acid), a bile acid which is widely used in the medical dissolution of cholesterol gallstones, had a much more pronounced choleretic effect than taurocholate[7] or even than its own conjugate, tauroursodeoxycholate (*Figure 12.26*). Subsequently, several other bile acids were shown to have a similar 'hypercholeretic effect'; for example, 23-norursodeoxycholate or 23-norchenodeoxycholate. In all cases, hypercholeresis is associated with a marked stimulation of bicarbonate concentration and secretion into bile.

The mechanism of this curious phenomenon is not yet established. At present, the best explanation is probably the so-called cholehepatic shunt hypothesis, proposed by Hofmann and his colleagues.[34] According to this hypothesis, ursodeoxycholate is transported into bile in part in the unconjugated form. It becomes protonated in the canalicular lumen to form ursodeoxycholic acid. The proton comes from carbonic acid (H_2CO_3) and the process generates one bicarbonate ion which is secreted into bile. The protonated ursodeoxycholic acid is lipid-soluble and readily absorbed by the biliary epithelial cells into the peribiliary vascular plexus and returns to the hepatocyte, which resecretes it into bile. The bile acid does not appear in final bile, but, at each cycle, one bicarbonate ion is secreted and stimulates bile flow (*Figure 12.27*). Other explanations have been proposed, involving hepatocytic mechanisms, including stimulation of Na^+/H^+ exchange in the plasma membrane. This hypothesis rests on the observation that amiloride, an inhibitor of the Na^+/H^+ exchanger, inhibits ursodeoxycholate-induced choleresis.[14] Direct proof, however, is not available.

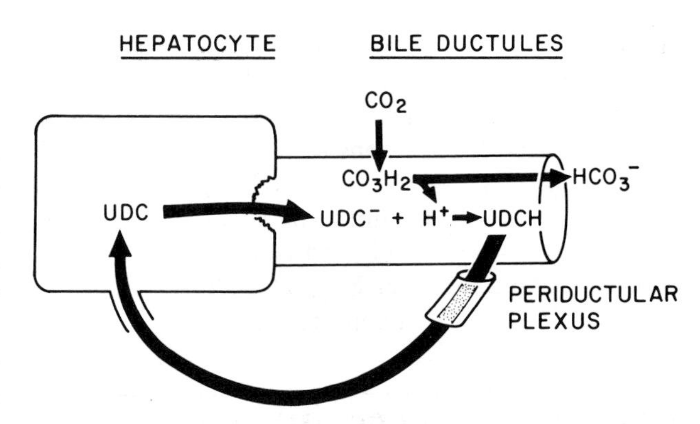

Figure 12.27 The cholehepatic shunt hypothesis. See text for explanation.

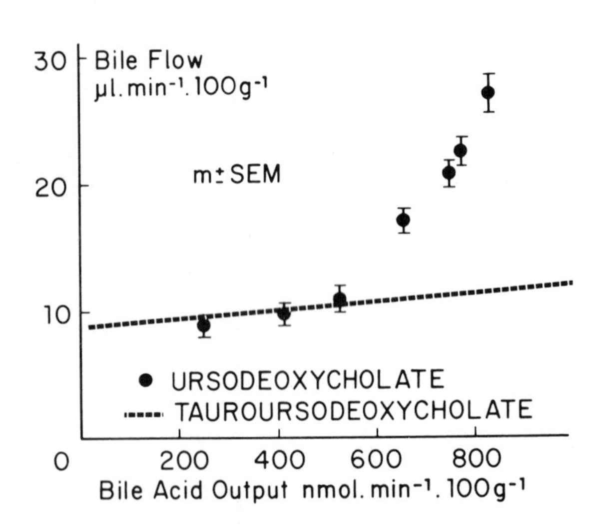

Figure 12.26 Hypercholeretic effect of ursodeoxycholate. Bile flow induced by ursodeoxycholate, at bile acid outputs in bile higher than 500 nmol/min per 100 g, far exceeds that induced by tauroursodeoxycholate.

BILE ACID-INDEPENDENT FLOW

When the linear relationship between bile flow and bile acid secretion is extrapolated for a zero bile acid secretion, a positive intercept (bile flow) is obtained (*Figure 12.28*). This bile flow is generally designated as canalicular bile acid-independent flow. Although this procedure of estimation is subject to criticism, the value obtained is similar to that measured directly in the isolated perfused liver in the absence of bile acids in the system. Bile acid-independent flow differs markedly between animal species (*Figure 12.28*). It is increased by phenobarbitone, other

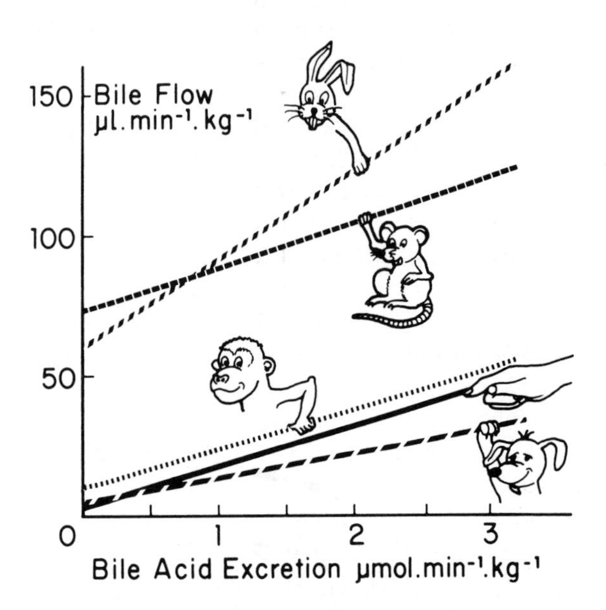

Figure 12.28 Relationship between bile flow and bile acid excretion in several animal species. Note that the positive intercept for a zero bile acid excretion is markedly higher in rats and rabbits than in the three other species.

inducers of the microsomal drug-metabolizing system, and thyroid hormones. It is inhibited by chronic oestrogen administration.

The mechanism responsible for this secretion is not clearly established. An active secretion of inorganic ions (such as sodium or bicarbonate) has been postulated but not established. Secretion into bile of organic compounds, such as glutathione or other amino acids, has also been proposed.

ROLE OF DUCTULES AND DUCTS

SECRETION (DUCTULAR/DUCTAL BILE ACID-INDEPENDENT FLOW)

Secretion occurs in the ductules and ducts in many species including humans, mostly in response to secretin administration.[23] Secretin choleresis is generally accompanied by changes in bile composition, chiefly a rise in bicarbonate and pH, and a fall in bile acids. The intraduodenal infusion of hydrochloric acid in dogs induces the same response as endogenous secretin.

The evidence for a ductular/ductal site of action of secretin is three-fold: secretin choleresis does not enhance the maximal biliary secretory capacity of sulphobromophthalein (BSP) whereas bile acids, which act on the bile canaliculi do; the biliary 'washout' volume during constant-rate BSP infusions is less with secretin choleresis than bile acid choleresis, suggesting that secretin acts distal to the canaliculi; biliary clearances of erythritol and mannitol are increased during bile acid choleresis and not (or minimally) during secretin choleresis. Secretion in the bile ductules or ducts is inhibited by somatostatin.

The secretory activity of the bile ductules and ducts explains the choleresis that occurs in certain diseases. Elevated bile flow has been recorded in patients with cirrhosis, other chronic liver diseases associated with ductular proliferation, and in congenital dilatation of the intrahepatic biliary tree (Caroli's syndrome). An augmentated surface of the biliary epithelium is common to these conditions.

REABSORPTION

The bile ductules or ducts may also have a reabsorptive function. Thus, in cholecystectomized dogs, the composition of bile stored in the common bile duct is similar to typical gallbladder bile. Bile-to-plasma concentration ratios above unity in the steady state have been found for mannitol and erythritol in various species, which suggests that there is water reabsorption distal to the canaliculi because neither solute is thought to be transported by concentrative processes. No studies in humans are available.

MECHANISMS OF CHOLESTASIS

Cholestasis is defined as a diminution (or cessation) of bile flow and may be due to extrahepatic and intrahepatic causes (*Figure 12.29*). *Extrahepatic cholestasis* is the result of mechanical obstruction of the extrahepatic bile ducts usually by a gallstone, a tumour or a stricture. *Intrahepatic cholestasis* may be the result of two different mechanisms: (1) mechanical obstruction of intrahepatic bile ducts, for example by a primary or secondary liver tumour, granulomata, infiltration by lymphoma or any other space-occupying lesion; (2) disturbance of canalicular bile flow, for example during viral or drug-induced hepatitis, or drug-induced cholestasis. Cholestasis must be distinguished from necrosis during liver parenchymal disease: both can occur separately or together. For instance, during viral hepatitis, necrosis can occur alone (anicteric hepatitis), or in association with cholestasis (common acute hepatitis with jaundice), while cholestasis can occur alone or predominantly (cholestatic hepatitis).

The cellular mechanisms of intrahepatic cholestasis due to disturbance of canalicular bile flow are not well understood and it is possible that there are several. Experimentally, four main mechanisms have been implicated:

1. *A decrease in Na^+/K^+-ATPase*. Cholestasis could result from decreased bile acid secretion

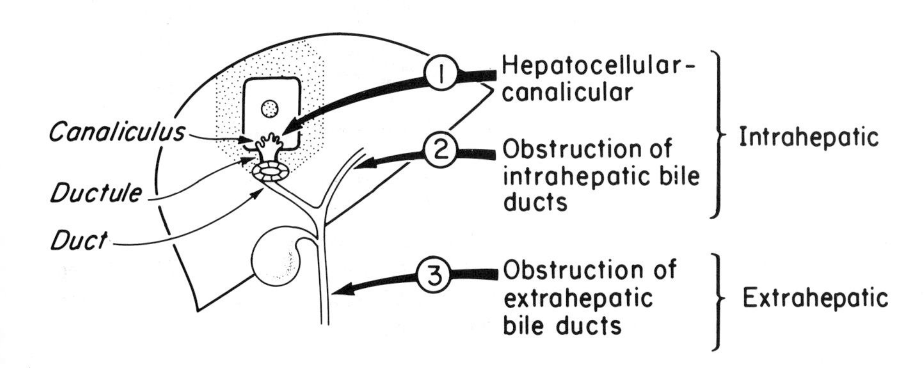

Figure 12.29 Types of cholestasis.

due to a decreased Na^+ gradient, or from decreased Na^+/K^+-ATPase-mediated transport. Drugs which affect the Na^+/K^+-ATPase activity to produce cholestasis include oestrogens, chlorpromazine, and 17α-alkylated steroids. Interference with hepatocyte membrane transport processes may be a common mechanism of cholestasis.

2. *An alteration of the cytoskeleton.* Interference with *microfilament* structure and function by cytochalasin B or phalloidin[22] causes a decrease in or even a complete cessation of bile flow. This provides circumstantial evidence that microfilament dysfunction leads to cholestasis and that microfilaments may have a role in secretion. This could be by: altering the structural organization necessary for normal secretion, particularly microvilli; interfering with a *contractile* function;[22] or modifying the *permeability* of the *paracellular* pathway that may be regulated by microfilaments. The role of *microtubules* has been studied with colchicine and vinblastine. No effect on basal (spontaneous) bile flow is observed but colchicine markedly decreases bile flow and bile acid secretion induced by a bile acid load.[6]
3. *An increase in the permeability of the paracellular pathway.* This was first postulated to explain oestrogen-induced cholestasis.[10] Any increased permeability may allow regurgitation of bile constituents (such as bile acids or bilirubin, and water) from the canalicular lumen into the circulation. Structural evidence that absorption (regurgitation) can take place in human bile ductules has been obtained in cholestasis from various causes.
4. *Intracellular calcium alterations.* Several monohydroxylated bile acids, such as lithocholate and its conjugates, induce cholestasis. One possible mechanism by which they might stop bile secretion is by precipitation into the bile canaliculi because of their poor water solubility. However, some are water-soluble, in particular lithocholate sulphate or lithocholate glucuronide, and these are even more potent cholestatic agents than the parent compounds. Lithocholate and taurolithocholate induce an increase in cytosolic ionized calcium concentration.[1,4] This increase appears to be due mostly to a permeabilization of the endoplasmic reticulum membrane to calcium.[5] The author has proposed that this permeabilization and depletion of this essential intracellular calcium pool may result in alteration of intracellular transport processes (in particular of bile acids) and lead to cholestasis. Direct proof of this hypothesis is lacking and it is not known whether such a mechanism could be involved in cholestasis induced by other agents.

CHOLERETICS: MECHANISMS OF ACTION

A choleretic drug might act by one of several possible mechanisms:

1. Concentrative (usually active) secretion into bile canaliculi followed by osmotic filtration of water and electrolytes. This process may be conveniently called 'bile acid-like choleresis' and operate for most commercial choleretics. However, this type of choleresis is not accompanied by an increase in biliary lipid secretion, in contrast to the choleresis induced by physiological bile acids.
2. Stimulation of canalicular bile acid-independent mechanisms by, for example, phenobarbitone and other drugs (spironolactone or clofibrate in the rat) that are microsomal enzyme inducers.
3. Stimulation of secretion by the ductules or ducts, for example with secretin.

There is no evidence that any of these choleretics is of therapeutic value in patients with cholestasis, with the possible exception of phenobarbitone in children with intrahepatic cholestasis.

BILIARY SECRETION IN HUMANS

Although the existence of most of the processes described previously has been inferred from animal studies, similar processes may well operate in humans (*Figure 12.30*). Patients with T tubes in the common bile duct show a linear relationship between bile flow (and erythritol or mannitol clearance) and bile acid secretion rate, with a mean of

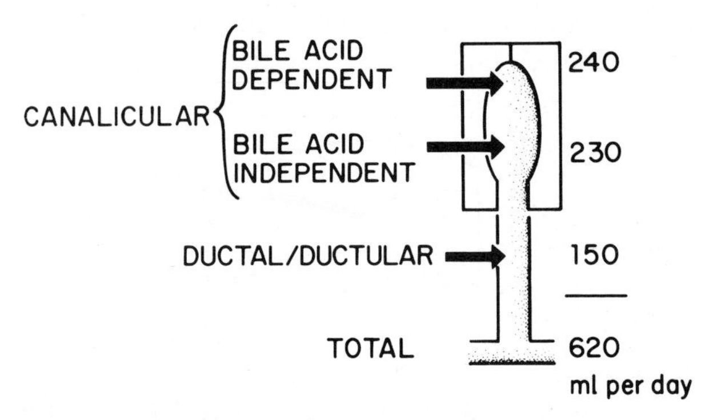

Figure 12.30 Bile secretion in humans. The data was collected in cholecystectomized patients with T tubes in the common bile duct.

11 μl of canalicular bile secreted per micromole of bile acids. When the enterohepatic circulation is intact, a mean of approximately 15 μmol of bile acids is secreted per minute, which gives a mean flow associated with bile acids of 0.15–0.16 ml/min. The estimated canalicular bile acid-independent flow is 0.16–0.17 ml/min, and the estimated ductular/ductal secretion is about 0.11 ml/min. The daily hepatic bile production under these circumstances (i.e. after cholecystectomy) is therefore approximately 600 ml.

REFERENCES

1. Anwer, M.S., Engelking, L.R., Nolan, K., Sullivan, D., Zimniak, P. and Lester, R. (1988) Hepatotoxic bile acids increase cytosolic Ca^{++} activity of isolated rat hepatocytes. *Hepatology*, **8**, 887–891.
2. Blitzer, B.L. and Boyer, J.L. (1978) Cytochemical localization of Na^{+}/K^{+}-ATPase in the rat hepatocyte. *Journal of Clinical Investigation*, **62**, 1104–1108.
3. Blitzer, B.L. and Boyer, J.L. (1982) Cellular mechanisms of bile formation. *Gastroenterology*, **82**, 346–357.
4. Combettes, L., Dumont, M., Berthon, B., Erlinger, S. and Claret, M. (1988) Release of calcium from the endoplasmic reticulum by bile acids in rat liver cells. *Journal of Biological Chemistry*, **263**, 2299–2303.
5. Combettes, L., Berthon, B., Doucet, E., Erlinger, S. and Claret, M. (1989) Characteristics of bile acid-mediated Ca^{2+} release from permeabilised liver cells and liver microsomes. *Journal of Biological Chemistry*, **264**, 157–167.
6. Crawford, J.M., Berken, C.A. and Gollan, J.L. (1988) Role of the hepatocyte microtubular system in the excretion of bile salts and biliary lipid: implications for intracellular vesicular transport. *Journal of Lipid Research*, **29**, 144–156.
7. Dumont, M., Uchman, S. and Erlinger, S. (1980) Hypercholeresis induced by ursodeoxycholic acid and 7-ketolithocholic acid in the rat. Possible role of bicarbonate transport. *Gastroenterology*, **79**, 82–89.
8. Erlinger, S. (1988) Bile flow. In *The Liver, Biology and Pathobiology*, 2nd edn. (Ed.) Arias, I.M., Jakoby, W.B., Popper, H., Schachter, D. and Shafritz, D. A. pp. 643–661. New York: Raven Press.
9. Forker, E.L. (1967) Two sites of bile formation as determined by mannitol and erythritol clearance in the guinea pig. *Journal of Clinical Investigation*, **46**, 1189–1195.
10. Forker, E.L. (1969) The effect of estrogen on bile formation in the rat. *Journal of Clinical Investigation*, **48**, 654–663.
11. Gautam, A., Ng, O.C., Strazzabosco, M. and Boyer, J.L. (1989) Quantitative assessment of canalicular bile formation in isolated hepatocyte couplets using microscopic optical planimetry. *Journal of Clinical Investigation*, **83**, 565–573.
12. Goldsmith, M.A., Huling, S. and Jones, A.L. (1983) Hepatic handling of bile salts and protein in the rat during intrahepatic cholestasis. *Gastroenterology*, **84**, 978–986.
13. Graf, J. and Boyer, J.L. (1990) The use of isolated rat hepatocyte couplets in hepatobiliary physiology. *Journal of Hepatology*, **10**, 387–394.
14. Hagenbuch, B., Lübbert, H., Stieger, B. and Meier, P.J. (1990) Expression of the hepatocyte Na^{+}/bile acid cotransporter in *Xenopus laevis* oocytes. *The Journal of Biological Chemistry*, **265**, 5357–5360.
15. Kramer, W., Bickel, U., Buscher, H.P., Gerok, W. and Kurz, G. (1982) Bile-salt-binding polypeptides in plasma membranes of hepatocytes revealed by photoaffinity labelling. *European Journal of Biochemistry*, **129**, 13–24.
16. Lamri, Y., Roda, A., Dumont, M., Feldmann, G. and Erlinger, S. (1988) Immunoperoxidase localization of bile salts in rat liver cells. Evidence for a role of the Golgi apparatus in bile salt transport. *Journal of Clinical Investigation*, **82**, 1173–1182.
17. Latham, P.S. and Kashgarian, M. (1979) The ultrastructural localization of transport ATPase in the rat liver at non-bile canalicular plasma membranes. *Gastroenterology*, **76**, 988–996.
18. Levy, D., Alves, C. and von Dippe, P. (1990) Functional expression of the 49 kDa organic anion transport protein in endoplasmic reticulum and Golgi vesicles (abstract). *Hepatology*, **12**, 872.
19. Meier, P.J. (1989) The bile salt secretory polarity of hepatocytes. *Journal of Hepatology*, **9**, 124–129.
20. Phillips, M.J., Latham, P.S. and Poucell, S. (1982) Electron microscopy of human liver diseases. In *Diseases of the Liver*, 6th edn. (Ed.) Schiff, L. and Schiff, E. R. pp. 47–76. Philadelphia: Lippincott.
21. Phillips, M.J. and Satir, P. (1988) The cytoskeleton of the hepatocyte: organization, relationships, and pathology. In *The Liver, Biology and Pathobiology*, 2nd edn. (Ed.) Arias, I.M., Jakoby, W.B., Popper, H., Schachter, D. and Shafritz, D.A. pp. 11–27. New York: Raven Press.
22. Phillips, M.J., Poucell, S. and Oda, M. (1986) Biology of disease. Mechanisms of cholestasis. *Laboratory Investigation*, **54**, 593–608.
23. Preisig, R., Cooper, H.L. and Wheeler, H.O. (1962) The relationship between taurocholate secretion rate and bile production in the unanesthetized dog during cholinergic blockade and during secretin administration. *Journal of Clinical Investigation*, **41**, 1152–1162.
24. Ruetz, S., Hugentobler, G. and Meier, P.J. (1988) Functional reconstitution of the canalicular bile salt transport system of rat liver. *Proceedings of the National Academy of Sciences of the USA*, **85**, 6147–6151.
25. Simion, F.A., Fleischer, B. and Fleischer, S. (1984)

Subcellular distribution of bile acids, bile salts and taurocholate binding sites in rat liver. *Biochemistry* **22**, 6459–6466.
26. Simion, F., Fleischer, B. and Fleischer, S. (1984) Two distinct mechanisms for taurocholate uptake in subcellular fractions from rat liver. *Journal of Biological Chemistry*, **259**, 10814–10822.
27. Sperber, I. (1959) Secretion of organic anions in the formation of urine and bile. *Pharmacological Reviews*, **11**, 109–134.
28. Stolz, A., Takikawa, H., Ookhtens, M. and Kaplowitz, N. (1989) The role of cytoplasmic proteins in hepatic bile acid transport. *Annual Review of Physiology*, **51**, 161–176.
29. Suchy, F.J., Balistreri, W.F., Hung, J., Miller, P. and Garfield, S.A. (1983) Intracellular bile acid transport as visualized by electron microscopic autoradiography using a bile acid analogue. *American Journal of Physiology*, **245**, G681–G689.
30. Sztul, E.S., Biemesderfer, D., Caplan, M.J., Kashgarian, M- and Boyer, J.L. (1987) Localization of Na^+/K^+-ATPase a-subunit to the sinusoidal and lateral but not canalicular membrane of hepatocytes. *Journal of Cellular Biology*, **104**, 1239–1248.
31. Tavoloni, N. (1988) Biliary clearance of inert carbohydrates. Expectations and reality. *Gastroenterology*, **94**, 217–228.
32. Von Dippe, P., Ananthanarayanan, M., Drain, P. and Levy, D. (1986) Purification and reconstitution of the bile acid transport system from hepatocyte sinusoidal membrane. *Biochimica et Biophysica Acta*, **862**, 352–360.
33. Wheeler, H.O., Ross, E.D. and Bradley, S.E. (1968) Canalicular bile production in dogs. *American Journal of Physiology*, **214**, 866–874.
34. Yoon, Y.B., Hagey, L.R., Hofmann, A.F., Gurantz, D., Michelotti, E.L. and Steinbach, J.H. (1986) Effect of side-chain shortening on the physiologic properties of bile acids: hepatic transport and effect on biliary secretion of 23-norursodeoxycholate in rodents. *Gastroenterology*, **90**, 837–852.

FORMATION OF CHOLESTEROL GALLSTONES

J.M. Donovan and M.C. Carey

Cholesterol gallstones are composed principally of cholesterol monohydrate crystals. Crystals and gallstones form only in the gallbladder and are a result of alterations in both hepatocellular and gallbladder functions. The principal pathophysiological abnormality in cholesterol gallstone disease is a relative excess of biliary cholesterol, produced by hepatic hypersecretion of cholesterol, and/or hyposecretion of bile salts and lecithin, the solubilizers of biliary cholesterol. Potentially, gallstones can form whenever biliary lipids fail to solubilize cholesterol completely in a thermodynamically stable system. However, the kinetics of stone formation depends upon other factors, including rapid nucleation and crystal growth that result, in part, from an imbalance in anti- and pro-nucleating factors, and gallbladder dysfunction characterized by decreased contractility and mucin hypersecretion. These steps are followed by retention of cholesterol monohydrate crystals within a mucin glycoprotein gel in the gallbladder ('biliary sludge') where macroscopic gallstones grow by the continuous formation and agglomeration of discrete crystals cemented together by mucin glycoproteins and admixed with variable proportions of inorganic and organic calcium salts. This section will describe the physiochemical basis of cholesterol solubilization in normal bile, outline the pathophysiological defects responsible for each of the steps leading to cholesterol gallstone formation, correlate clinical risk factors for gallstones with specific pathophysiological defects, and conclude with recent pharmacological interventions that promise to prevent cholesterol gallstones in selected high-risk individuals.

BILIARY BILE SALTS, PHOSPHOLIPIDS AND CHOLESTEROL

Bile salts (*Figure 12.31*) are the major solutes in human bile.[12] Primary bile salts (cholates and chenodeoxycholates) are synthesized in the liver from cholesterol and represent the major catabolic products of the sterol. Secondary bile salts (deoxycholates, ursodeoxycholates and lithocholates) are colonic bacterial products of primary bile salts. They are formed by selective removal (deoxycholate, lithocholate) or epimerization (ursodeoxycholate) of the 7α-hydroxyl function of primary bile salts. The steroid nucleus of lithocholate undergoes further hepatic metabolism to form lithocholate sulphate.

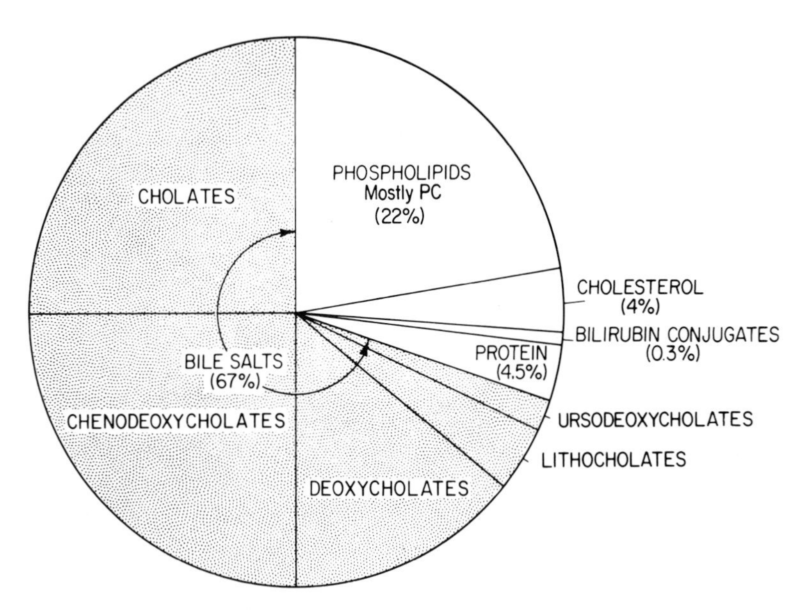

Figure 12.31 Typical solute composition (wt%) of gallbladder and hepatic bile in healthy humans. PC represents phosphatidylcholine.

Bile salts are secreted as conjugates, that is, their isopentyl side-chains are linked via amide bonds with amino acids, either glycine or taurine, in a 3:1 ratio. Together, the family of bile salts molecules acts as detergents and solubilizes otherwise insoluble endogenous lipids in bile and exogenous as well as endogenous lipids in the upper small intestine.

Biliary phospholipids are mostly (>95%) a mixture of lecithins, i.e. phosphatidylcholines. Their fatty acid compositions are distinct in that more than 80% of bile lecithins has palmitic acid (C_{16}) esterified at the *sn*-1 position and an unsaturated fatty acid, principally oleic ($C_{18:1}$), linoleic ($C_{18:2}$) or arachidonic acid ($C_{20:4}$) esterified at the *sn*-2 position of the molecules. Biliary lecithins with di- and tetraenoic fatty acids may have pathophysiological importance since these fatty acids are potential precursors of prostaglandin synthesis by the gallbladder mucosa. The predominant sterol of bile (>95%) is free (unesterified) cholesterol; in addition, small amounts of cholesterol precursors and derivatives (but not cholesteryl esters), as well as dietary phytosterols, are present in varying proportions. Bilirubin conjugates, inorganic and organic salts, and a large variety of proteins constitute minor components of bile (*Figure 12.31*).

All biliary lipids are amphiphiles, that is, each molecule is partly hydrophobic (literally, water fearing) and partly hydrophilic (literally, water loving). Conventional and space-filling structures of the major biliary lipids as well as their physicochemical behaviour in bulk water are depicted in *Figure 12.32*.[3] The molecules align at an oil–water interface with their hydrophobic portions directed towards the oil and their hydrophilic portions directed towards the water. In bulk aqueous solution, these physicochemical properties force biliary lipid molecules to aggregate so that exposure of their hydrophobic portions to water is minimized. The hydrophobic portion of cholesterol (A) is the steroid nucleus (cross-hatched) and branched hydrocarbon side-chain; the hydrophilic portion is a single hydroxyl function (oval). By itself, cholesterol is virtually insoluble in bulk water (monomeric solubility approximately 10^{-8} mol/l), and above this concentration forms a precipitate of cholesterol monohydrate crystals. The hydrophobic portions of lecithin (B) consist of two long (and dissimilar) fatty acid chains (R,R′) with glycerol (oval) and a zwitterionic (positive and negative charged) phosphorylcholine group constituting the hydrophilic portions. Lecithin is also insoluble (monomeric solubility approximately 10^{-10} mol/l) in bulk aqueous solution, but by itself or with cholesterol forms membrane bilayers (liquid crystals) wherein the hydrophobic fatty acid chains of lecithin are in the interiors and the hydrophilic head groups protrude into water. Bile salts (C) have a hydrophobic steroid nucleus (cross-hatched), to which are attached one to three hydrophilic hydroxyl groups, or a sulphate group in the case of the lithocholates (closed circles), and an ionic side-chain (enclosed negative sign) with its hydrophilic amide bond (closed circle). In contrast to cholesterol and lecithin molecules, bile salts are very soluble in bulk water. Bile salt molecules exist as monomers in dilute solution, but in excess of their critical micellar concentrations (approximately 0.5–5 mmol/l) all additional monomers self-associate to form small polymolecular aggregates called simple micelles.[3]

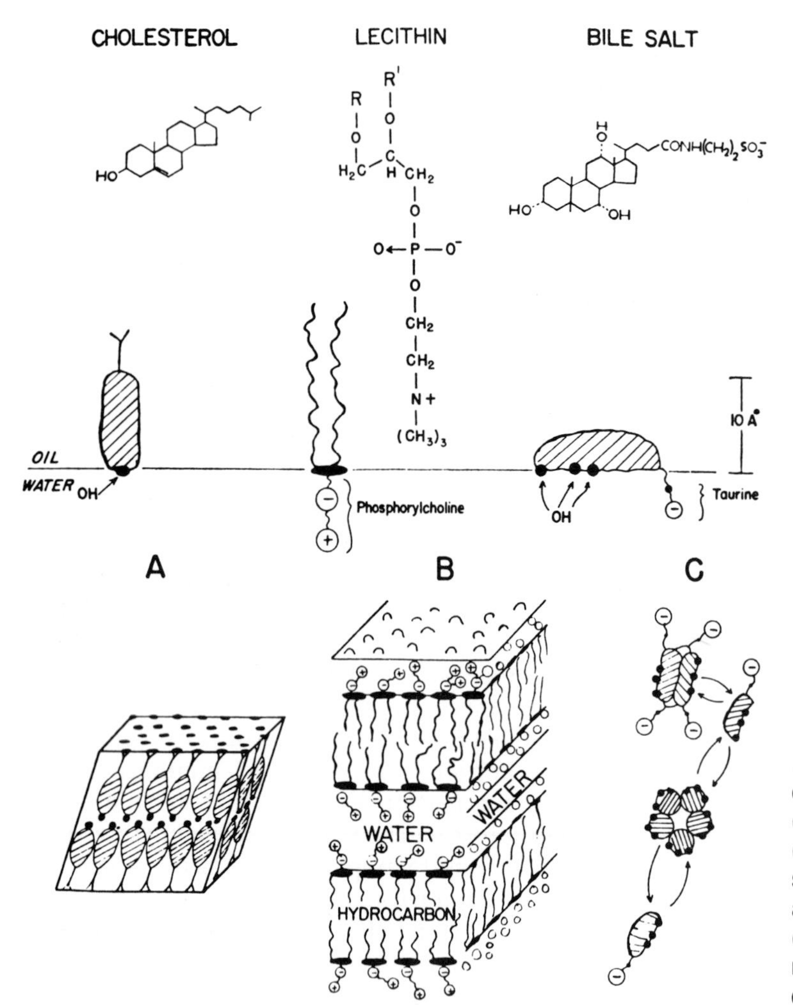

Figure 12.32 The major biliary lipids, free (unesterified) cholesterol, the phospholipid lecithin (phosphatidylcholine) and a typical common bile salt (taurocholate). The figure displays conventional structures (top) space-filling structures, with their amphiphilic orientation at an oil–water interface (middle) and physicochemical characteristics of the molecules in bulk water (bottom) (see text for details).

PHYSICOCHEMICAL STATE OF UNSATURATED AND SUPERSATURATED BILE

Bile salts interact with themselves and with cholesterol and lecithin to form three distinct multimolecular aggregates (*Figure 12.33*) that are often called the cholesterol solubilizers (or 'carriers') of bile.[7] These are: (1) simple micelles, aggregates 2–4 nm in diameter, that contain bile salt molecules interacting with one another via their hydrophobic portions, and in turn solubilizing a small fraction of biliary cholesterol molecules but not lecithin; (2) mixed micelles, aggregates 4–6 nm in diameter which contain a core of lecithin, cholesterol and even bile salt molecules, enveloped by a perimeter of bile salt molecules acting as a water-solubilizing surface; and (3) unilamellar vesicles, which are closed bilayers composed predominantly of lecithin and cholesterol molecules with minor amounts of bile salts. These liquid crystalline fragments (see B in *Figure 12.32*) have diameters of 40–100 nm, and are distinct from micelles in size and structure (*Figure 12.33*). Using symbols for each of these particles (*Figure 12.33*), we will now define the physicochemical states of both normal and supersaturated biles in the context of these cholesterol 'carriers'.

The limits of cholesterol solubility in simple and mixed micelles have been well established from in vitro studies on model biles.[5] In the case of a physiological bile salt mixture, solubility limits depend upon both the bile salt:lecithin ratio and total lipid concentration. When these two conditions are fixed, the ratio of the cholesterol content to the maximum equilibrium solubility of cholesterol is defined as the cholesterol saturation index. As shown in *Figure 12.34*, below the limit of cholesterol solubility in the micellar phase of model bile, that is, at CSI values less than 1.0, cholesterol is solubilized completely as micelles, principally by mixed micelles and to a minor extent by simple micelles. In biles with CSI values greater than 1.0, simple and mixed micelles also cooperate in solubilizing cholesterol, but excess cholesterol is dispersed as unilamel-

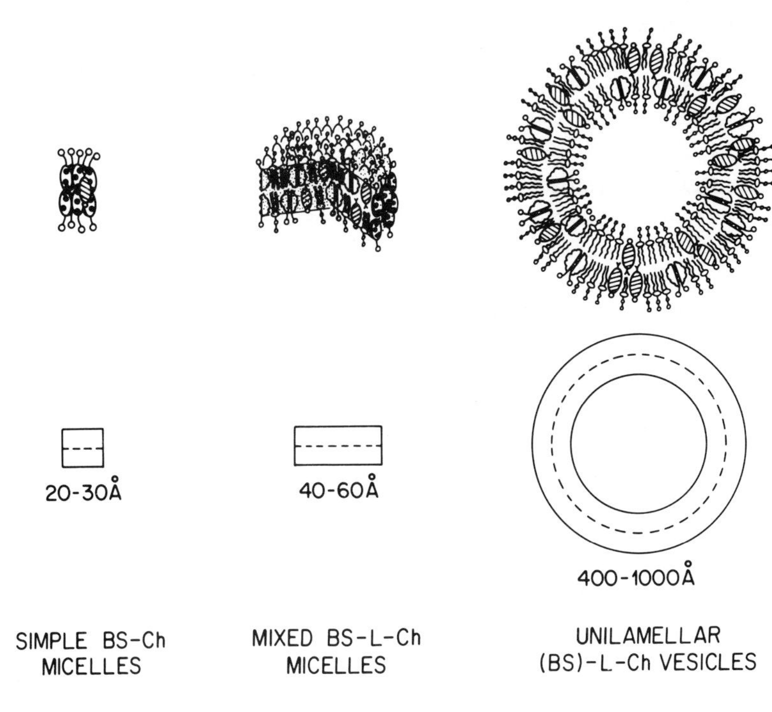

Figure 12.33 Cholesterol solubilizers (also termed 'carriers') of human bile: they are simple micelles, mixed micelles and unilamellar vesicles. Suggested molecular packing of bile salt (BS), lecithin (L) and cholesterol (Ch) in each structure is shown in the upper part of the figure. Schematic block diagrams of each particle with typical diameters given in angstroms (10^{-10} m) are used in subsequent illustrations (lower part of figure).

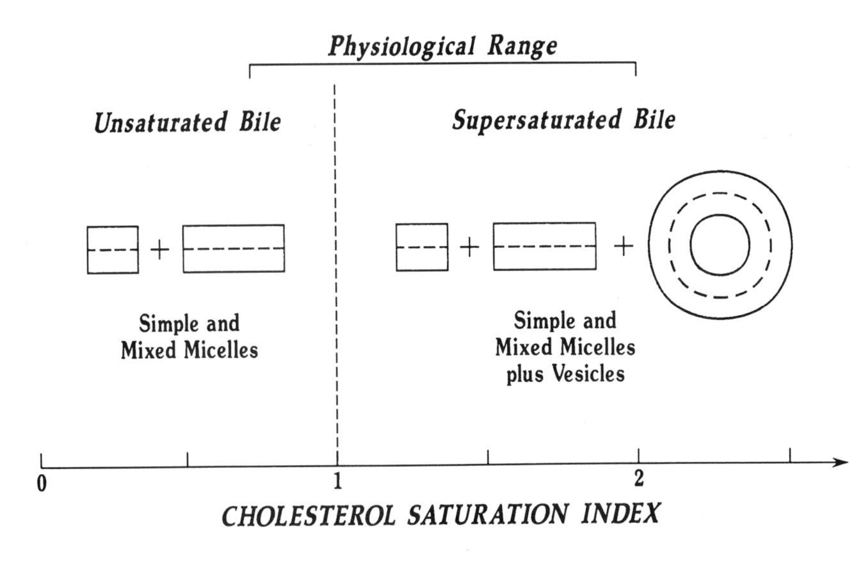

Figure 12.34 Lipid aggregates present in unsaturated and supersaturated biles over the physiological range of cholesterol saturation index (CSI) values. Note that CSI values of most human biles lie above 1, where vesicles and both simple and mixed miscelles are present.

lar cholesterol/lecithin vesicles. For thermodynamic reasons, the cholesterol:lecithin ratio of the vesicles has an important influence on the cholesterol distribution in the whole system. Supersaturation of vesicles, i.e. a cholesterol:lecithin ratio greater than unity, necessitates simultaneous supersaturation of both simple and mixed micelles as well as supersaturation of the aqueous cholesterol monomeric concentration (i.e. $\gg 10^{-8}$ mol/l), which is a prerequisite for formation of cholesterol monohydrate crystals.

PHYSICAL CHEMISTRY AND PATHOBIOLOGY OF BILIARY LIPID SECRETION

Approximately 98% of all bile salts secreted into bile return to the hepatocytes from the small and large intestines in a continuous but fluctuating flow called the enterohepatic circulation.[4] Bile salt concentrations in the enterohepatic circulation vary considerably, approximating 0.1 and 0.3 mmol/l in hepatocytes, 20–50 mmol/l in hepatic ducts, 100–400 mmol/l in the gallbladder and 20–40 mmol/l in the postprandial duodenum and, because of continuous absorption as the small intestine is traversed, decrease from 2–8 mmol/l in the jejunum to 0.1–2 mmol/l in the distal ileum. Intrahepatic bile salt movement stimulates lecithin and cholesterol co-secretion from hepatocyte membranes into bile in the form of small unilamellar vesicles by a process that is not understood fully. Bile salts are secreted as monomers via an 100 kDa membrane transport protein that is driven by the strong (approximately −40 mV) inside negative potential of hepatocytes.[4]

As bile water is progressively reabsorbed in the biliary tree, bile salt concentrations exceed their critical micellar concentrations (0.5–5.0 mmol/l) and simple micelles form, which dissolve cholesterol/lecithin vesicles to form mixed micelles.[6] In dilute bile the process is incomplete, because as much as 90% of cholesterol in hepatic duct bile is carried in vesicles (*Figure 12.34*). At higher total lipid concentrations, bile salts and lecithin solubilize proportionally more cholesterol; hence, the CSI falls as bile becomes more concentrated. As bile resides in the gallbladder, the dramatic increase in bile salt concentration induces further information of mixed micelles from vesicles. In cholesterol-unsaturated bile, all cholesterol and lecithin molecules that were present in vesicles have been transferred to mixed micelles, forming a thermodynamically stable solution incapable of precipitating cholesterol.

When the capacity of mixed micelles to solubilize cholesterol is exceeded, unilamellar vesicles disperse the excess cholesterol and bile is supersaturated with cholesterol and potentially unstable. Since the capacity of mixed micelles to solubilize lecithin is greater than the capacity to solubilize cholesterol,[5] selective extraction of vesicular lecithin results in vesicle enrichment with cholesterol. In cholesterol-supersaturated model hepatic biles (total lipids approximately 3 g/dl), these cholesterol-rich vesicles remain stable, without precipitating or fusing, for intervals of several days to weeks. However, within the gallbladder both higher total lipid concentrations and higher vesicle cholesterol/lecithin ratios, produce favourable thermodynamic conditions for cholesterol nucleation. In gallstone-prone individuals, cholesterol-rich vesicles aggregate and fuse to form large cholesterol-rich multilamellar vesicles (liposomes or liquid crystals), which are visible by light microscopy (>500 nm) (*Figure 12.35*).[11] Cholesterol-rich multilamellar vesicles are metastable and, when retained within gallbladder bile, they are progressively transformed into cholesterol monohydrate crystals, a process that may take several days. Cholesterol monohydrate crystals grow by diffusion of cholesterol monomers from supersaturated micelles and unilamellar vesicles to the crystal surfaces. Nevertheless the cholesterol: lecithin ratio of vesicles is maintained above unity because vesicular lecithin molecules are preferentially depleted by transfer from vesicles to micelles. Eventually, all vesicular cholesterol precipitates, as crystals and all vesicular lecithin are dissolved by bile salts, forming mixed micelles (*Figure 12.35*).

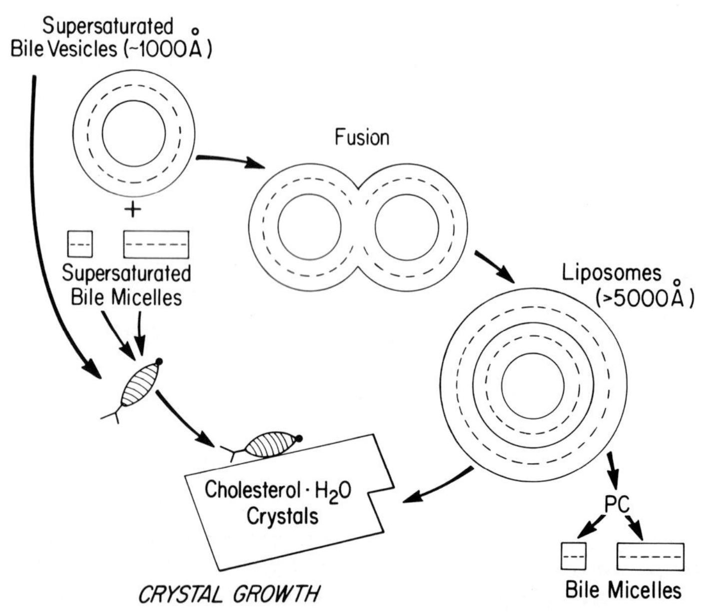

Figure 12.35 Proposed pathways for cholesterol nucleation and crystal growth in bile (further described in text).

HEPATIC DEFECTS: CHOLESTEROL HYPERSECRETION AND BILE SALT HYPOSECRETION

Cholesterol supersaturation of bile is the *sine qua non* of cholesterol gallstone formation. In normal subjects, the cholesterol content of bile fluctuates diurnally since the mass ratio of cholesterol/lecithin vesicles to bile salts in bile varies inversely with the bile salt secretion rate. During fasting, when the rate of bile salt return to the hepatocytes and thereby biliary secretion rates are diminished, cholesterol-supersaturated bile is produced (*Figure 12.34*). Although cholesterol crystals and even gallstones could form theoretically under these conditions, they do not do so in the majority of humans. Following a meal, the enterohepatic circulation is driven by gallbladder emptying and small intestinal motility and bile salt secretion rates increase. Although lecithin/cholesterol vesicular secretion rates also increase, bile salt secretion rates increase disproportionately, and cholesterol-unsaturated bile is produced.

Cholesterol balance in human beings is controlled principally by the parenchymal cells of the liver.[8] Despite alterations in the rates of cholesterol uptake, synthesis and export, the free cholesterol pool in hepatocytes, largely in the form of membrane cholesterol, remains constant. The major sources of cholesterol for hepatocyte metabolism (*Figure 12.36*) are from uptake of plasma lipoproteins principally low-density lipoproteins and chylomicron remnants, mediated by specific apolipoprotein receptors. These emulsion-like particles transport endogenous and dietary cholesterol, respectively, to the liver for further processing. Like all cells in the organism, hepatocytes synthesize cholesterol from acetate, with the rate-limiting step being controlled by 3-hydroxymethylglutaryl-coenzyme-A (HMG-CoA) reductase. Cholesterol is exported from hepatocytes in the form of newly synthesized lipoproteins – principally very low-density lipoproteins and high-density lipoproteins. A small fraction of total cholesterol resides on the surface coats of lipoproteins as free cholesterol molecules; quantitatively more important are cholesterol ester molecules in the cores of lipoproteins synthesized in the liver from free cholesterol by the enzyme acyl:cholesterol:lecithin transferase (ACAT). Cholesteryl esters can be stored in hepatocytes as oil droplets and are recruitable for formation of lipoprotein cores. When hydrolysed by neutral cholesterol-ester hydrolase, free cholesterol molecules are released from these stores and returned to the free cholesterol pool of the hepatocyte as membrane cholesterol. Net elimination of cholesterol from the body utilizes the free cholesterol pool and is accomplished principally by secretion into bile via two major pathways: directly as free (unesterified) cholesterol, or after metabolic conversion via the rate-limiting enzyme 7α-hydroxylase as primary bile salts (*Figure 12.36*).

Alterations in the relative activity of hepatocyte apolipoprotein receptors and the key enzymes in cholesterol flux can produce biliary cholesterol supersaturation (*Table 12.3* and *Figure 12.36*). During hyperoestrogenaemic states, as in the case of females compared with males, and especially during pregnancy, increased cholesterol uptake occurs via

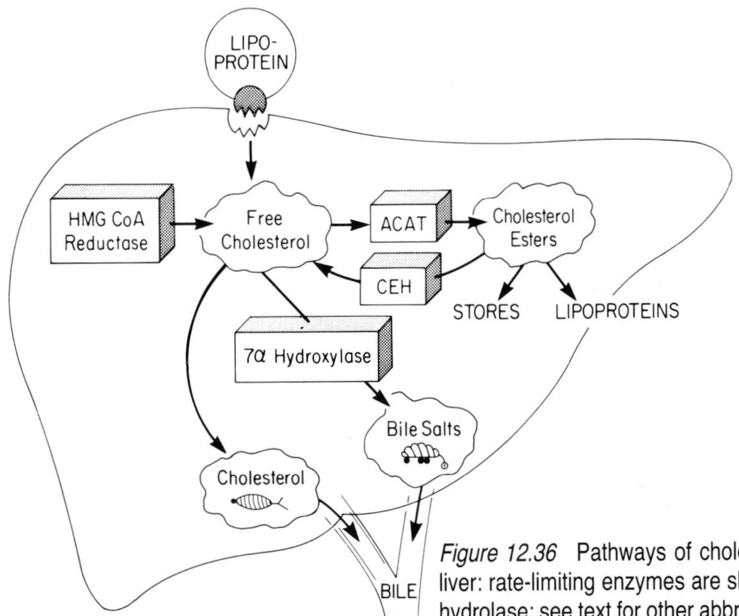

Figure 12.36 Pathways of cholesterol uptake, synthesis and disposition in the human liver: rate-limiting enzymes are shown by abbreviations in boxes (CEH, cholesterol-ester hydrolase; see text for other abbreviations).

Table 12.3 Risk factors for cholesterol gallstones

	Increased cholesterol secretion	*Decreased bile salt secretion*	*Impaired gallbladder motility*
Ethnicity	+	±	–
Age	+	+	–
Female gender	+	–	–
Pregnancy	+	+	+
Heredity	+	–	–
Hyperestrogenemic states	+	–	–
Medications			
Fibrates	+	–	–
Obesity	+	–	–
Rapid weight loss	+	–	+
Hypertriglyceridaemia	+	–	–
Gallbladder stasis	–	±	+
Spinal cord injury	±	–	+

up-regulation of the hepatocytes low-density lipoprotein receptors. When HMG-CoA reductase activity is increased, such as in obesity and hypertriglyceridaemia, cholesterol synthesis increases, as does biliary cholesterol secretion. When cholesterol conversion to cholesterol esters by the enzyme ACAT is inhibited by progestogens or by the 'fibric' acids (e.g. clofibrate), biliary cholesterol secretion increases. In humans, 7α-hydroxylase (*Figure 12.36*) is not appreciably stimulated by its cholesterol substrate, and its activity is far less than that of other animal species, and falls continuously with ageing. Therefore, human biles have much higher cholesterol:lecithin and cholesterol:bile salt ratios than biles of other animal species, and both ratios are further elevated in gallstone-prone subjects. For example, the average cholesterol:lecithin ratios in two large human studies were 0.37 in control subjects and 0.47 in gallstone subjects, and for the cholesterol:bile salt ratio, respective values were 0.11 compared with 0.14 (Hofmann *et al.*[9] and G. Salvioli and M.C. Carey, unpublished observations). Assuming that there is no appreciable secretion or absorption of cholesterol or lecithin molecules distal to the canaliculi and since biliary lecithin:bile salt ratios do not differ between control and gallstone subjects (approximately 0.30), this implies that the hepatic vesicles exocytosed into bile are cholesterol enriched by about 27% in gallstone patients compared with controls. Hence, humans, with their hepatic resistance to catabolize cholesterol to bile salts, have the dubious distinction of forming the only naturally occurring cholesterol gallstones in the animal kingdom.

Hepatic hyposecretion of bile salts was considered until recently to play the most important role in inducing cholesterol supersaturation of bile. It was postulated that there was an inborn or acquired defect in the enterohepatic circulation of bile salts with associated depletion of the bile salt pool. By employing better techniques for assessing biliary secretion rates, it has now become apparent that biliary cholesterol supersaturation is more often due to hepatic hypersecretion of cholesterol. As shown in *Table 12.3*, it appears that hyposecretion of bile salts alone is associated with few risk factors for acquiring cholesterol gallstones, whereas cholesterol hypersecretion is common among those epidemiologically most likely to suffer from gallstones, e.g. females, obese subjects, subjects undergoing rapid weight loss etc. Lecithin hyposecretion could theoretically produce cholesterol supersaturation of bile but, apart from an experimentally induced decrease in biliary lecithin secretion in response to dietary legumes in human volunteers,[19] this has not been documented in gallstone subjects.

NUCLEATION DEFECTS

All cholesterol-supersaturated biles are not lithogenic, i.e. they do not form crystals or gallstones. Since CSI values alone do not rigorously differentiate biles in patients with and without gallstones, investigators recently turned their attention to cholesterol crystal detection ('nucleation') times in bile. Holan and colleagues[14] were the first to remove cholesterol crystals from control and cholesterol gallstone biles and, by observing 'isotropic' biles microscopically, they timed the appearance of the first plate-like cholesterol crystals. As shown in *Figure 12.37*, 'nu-

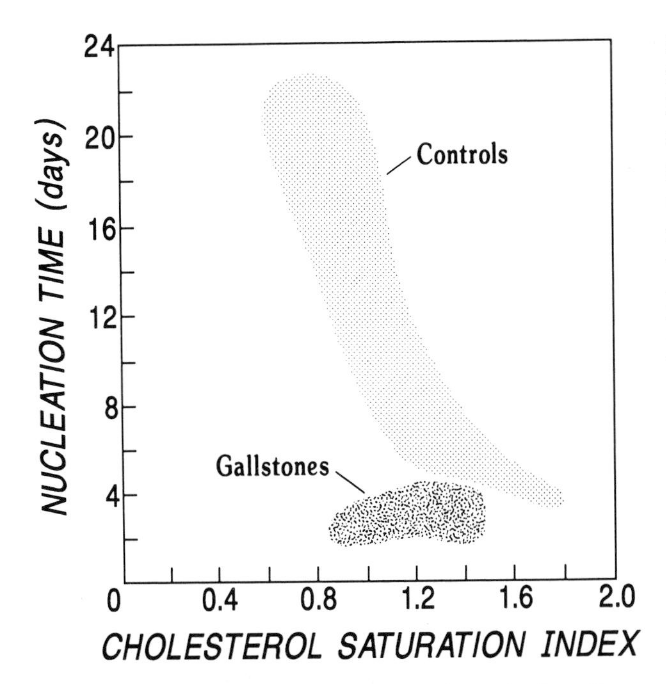

Figure 12.37 Dependence of cholesterol nucleation times (actually, cholesterol crystal detection times) upon CSI values for control gallbladder biles and biles from patients with cholesterol gallstones. Note that there is complete discrimination between normal and abnormal biles. (Redrawn, with permission, from Holan *et al.*[14]).

cleation' times in biles were measured in days to weeks. Clear-cut differences in 'nucleation' times were observed in biles with similar (supersaturated) CSI values obtained from cholesterol gallstone patients (2–4 days), compared with biles from control subjects without gallstones (>5 days). Although these widely confirmed experiments clearly distinguish cholesterol gallstone-containing biles from controls, they do not, by their nature, distinguish rates of nucleation, i.e. initial cholesterol crystal formation, from crystal growth. A more quantitative assay for the development of cholesterol crystals has been developed recently.[2] This promises to allow insights into the relative importance of inhibitors and promoters of cholesterol crystal nucleation as opposed to crystal growth.

Several components of bile have been identified as pro- and anti-nucleating agents. Changes in the molecular species of bile salts, lecithin and bilirubin conjugates, as well as in inorganic constituents of bile, particularly calcium ions, may influence the rate of cholesterol crystal formation in biles with high CSI values. Mucin glycoproteins, which are secreted in increased quantities in animal models of cholesterol lithogenesis as well as in humans prior to the development of cholesterol crystals, promote cholesterol nucleation in in vitro experiments. Systematic studies have demonstrated that nucleation is mediated in part via the high binding affinity of mucin glycoproteins for biliary lipids. Biliary apolipoproteins A-I and A-II, which occur in bile in concentrations less than 1% of their serum levels, and at least one non-mucin glycoprotein, inhibit cholesterol crystallisation in vitro, whereas several non-mucin glycoproteins promote cholesterol crystal formation. With the exception of a 150 kDa non-mucin glycoprotein found in considerably higher levels in gallbladder and hepatic biles from patients with multiple but not single gallstones,[10] the clinical relevance of these pro- and anti-nucleating factors has yet to be determined. Unfortunately most human biles have not been studied during active lithogenesis, but rather months to many years following gallstone formation; therefore, the roles of these factors in the pathogenesis of gallstones are difficult to assess.

GALLBLADDER 'DEFECTS'

The healthy human gallbladder has multiple functions:[9] (1) absorption of electrolytes and water, thus elevating solute concentrations in bile; (2) absorption of some biliary cholesterol and perhaps lecithin, which together with lipid concentration produces a gallbladder bile with lower CSI values than hepatic bile; (3) secretion of H^+ ions in exchange for absorbed Na^+ ions, thus neutralizing alkaline hepatic bile; (4) continuous production of mucin glycoproteins that constitute a mechanical and electrical barrier protecting mucosal cells from the destructive effects of concentrated bile salts; and (5) regular emptying in response to cholecystokinin released from the upper small intestine during a meal. Concentrated cholesterol-supersaturated gallbladder biles form cholesterol crystals far more rapidly than do dilute hepatic biles, despite the higher CSI values of hepatic biles. When the gallbladder fails to acidify bile, precipitation of inorganic and organic calcium salts is enhanced, a crucial factor in formation of pigment gallstones (see next section), but also precipitation of calcium carbonate and phosphate on the surface of cholesterol gallstones that can hinder pharmacological dissolution. As discussed above, mucin glycoproteins accelerate cholesterol crystal formation and, moreover, hinder their clearance from the gallbladder. Clearly, if the gallbladder evacuated newly formed cholesterol crystals efficiently, their coalescence to form gallstones would never occur.

In experimental animals, cholesterol-supersaturated bile depresses gallbladder contractility and stimulates mucin hypersecretion with the result-

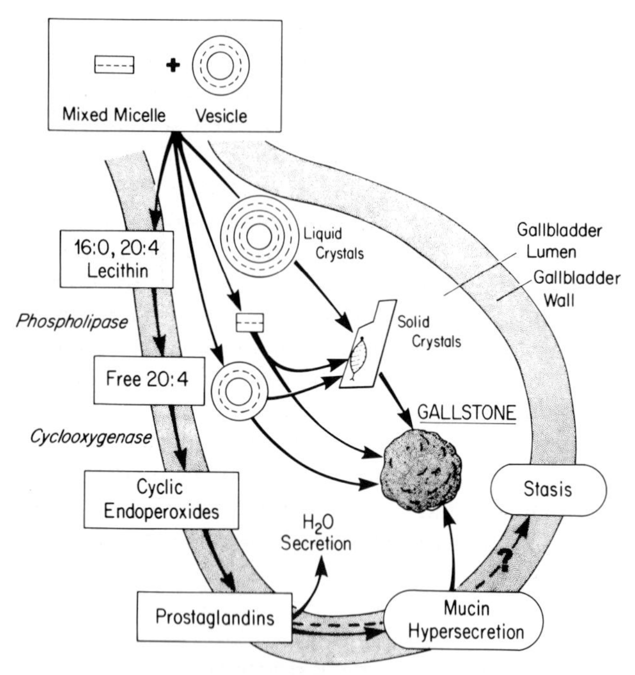

Figure 12.38 Postulated gallbladder mucosal and luminal events during cholesterol lithogenesis in human beings. Many of these concepts are currently in a state of maturation (see text for details).

ant formation of a mucin gel adherent to the gallbladder mucosa. A current hypothesis is that both phenomena are mediated via increased prostaglandin production by the gallbladder mucosa (*Figure 12.38*). Aspirin and, possibly, non-steroidal anti-inflammatory drugs (NSAIDs) that inhibit cyclo-oxygenase are capable of inhibiting mucin hypersecretion, mucin gel formation and gallstone formation without altering cholesterol-supersaturated bile.

The majority of cholesterol gallstone patients have clear-cut defects in gallbladder motility, particularly gallbladder emptying. Although, on average, gallstone patients have increased fasting and residual gallbladder volumes that are believed to be a consequence of biliary cholesterol supersaturation, primary gallbladder dysmotility amounting to 'paralysis' is rare. Risk factors that mainfest the most severe depression of gallbladder muscle function induce 'biliary sludge' and cholesterol gallstones with extraordinary frequency. These include the last trimester of pregnancy (thought to be secondary to progesterone effects), rapid weight loss, especially with diets containing less than 5 g of triglyceride per day that provide a suboptimal stimulus for cholecystokinin release, and other stasis syndromes (*Table 12.3*) such as spinal cord injury, somatostatinoma and therapy with its biologically active peptide (octreotide).

SEQUENCE OF EVENTS: SUPERSATURATION, CRYSTALLIZATION AND STONE GROWTH

Cholesterol hypersecretion, mucin hypersecretion, formation of cholesterol crystals and impairment of gallbladder motility are not isolated processes but interact synergystically to produce gallstones (*Figure 12.38*). Cholesterol supersaturation not only promotes more rapid crystal formation, but may also play a part in increased mucin production and gallbladder hypomotility. In experimental animal models and in humans, cholesterol-supersaturated bile is associated with impaired gallbladder motility *before* the development of cholesterol crystals and gallstones. Gallbladder mucin forms a gel matrix that enhances formation of cholesterol crystals, and impairs crystal clearance from the gallbladder. Cholesterol crystals (>50 μm in size) in a mucin matrix, together with pigment granules of calcium bilirubinate, constitute 'biliary sludge', a key intermediate in gallstone formation. Although only a minority of individuals with 'biliary sludge' will eventually form macroscopic gallstones,[17] 'biliary sludge' is now believed to be a transient but often clinical silent phenomenon in all patients forming gallstones.

In addition to its nucleating role, mucin acts as a scaffold to cement crystals together and transform discrete crystals into mature gallstones (*Figure 12.38*). Once macroscopic cholesterol gallstones form, further growth occurs from cholesterol molecules transferred to the stones' surface from supersaturated vesicles or micelles. The anatomy of gallstones gives us further clues to this sequence of events. Human gallstones are either single, or if numerous are usually equal in size, an indication that multiple nucleation occurred at one point in time. Once gallstones are present in cholesterol-supersaturated bile, further growth occurs in preference to the development of new gallstones. The centres of human gallstones invariably contain an amorphous substrate containing calcium bilirubinates, and mucin glycoproteins together with crystalline calcium carbonate and phosphate salts, suggesting a possible role for these substances in the earliest stages of nucleation and gallstone growth. Moreover, human gallstones tend to have cholesterol crystals layered in different topologies often with concentric calcium bilirubinate and carbonate/phosphate-containing rings. These may represent periodic changes in the degree of saturation with cholesterol and with other solute concentrations in bile (see Formation of pigment gallstones, p. 1713), with interruption of gallstone growth, or even temporary dissolution.

Conjugates of the hydrophobic secondary bile salt deoxycholate are relatively enriched in the bile salt pool of cholesterol gallstone patients. Because there is a documented evidence for a lower proportion of deoxycholate conjugates in the centre of gallstones compared with the outer portions and the surrounding bile[20] this enrichment is most likely secondary to defects in gallbladder motility with consequent increased exposure to the bile salt pool to intestinal bacteria. Deoxycholates conjugates are known to have multiple effects on biliary pathophysiology: they (1) increase biliary cholesterol secretion rates compared with more hydrophilic bile salts, (2) induce rapid cholesterol crystal formation in supersaturated model bile systems, and (3) increase secretion rates of gallbladder mucin glycoproteins. Several of the groups at highest risk for development of cholesterol gallstones (*Table 12.3*), including advanced age and severe hypertriglyceridaemia, have the highest levels of deoxycholate conjugates in bile.[18]

PREVENTION OF GALLSTONES

An understanding of cholesterol gallstone pathophysiology has allowed investigators to explore ways of preventing gallstone formation in high-risk groups. The triple set of defects that must be present simultaneously for gallstones to form are shown by the Venn diagram in *Figure 12.39*. Ablation of any one defect is sufficient to prevent formation of gallstones. Cholesterol supersaturation can be reversed by chronic administration of the bile acid ursodeoxycholic acid, which also inhibits nucleation of cholesterol crystals even in cholesterol-supersaturated biles.[16] Primary prevention studies in the obese who are undergoing rapid weight loss have shown that the administration of adequate doses of ursodeoxycholic acid significantly decreases the incidence of new gallstones.[1] Secondary prevention studies with low-dose ursodeoxycholic acid in gallstone patients, who had previously undergone successful bile acid dissolution therapy, also suggest a decreased incidence of new gallstones. In patients receiving total parenteral nutrition who form predominantly pigment gallstones, the intravenous administration of cholecystokinin octapeptide stimulates gallbladder contractility, abolishes the development of 'biliary sludge', and prevents gallstone formation.[21] Furthermore, in experimental animals that form cholesterol gallstones such as the cholesterol-fed prairie dog, strategies that inhibit the gallbladder from concentrating hepatic biles (high doses of amiloride, caffeine and ethyl alcohol) all prevent gallstone formation despite the persistence of bile with CSI values greater than 1. Since NSAID administration inhibits gallbladder mucin production in experimental animals, which in turn prevents nucleation of cholesterol crystals, it is not surprising that in an obese population undergoing weight loss there was a decreased trend to form new gallstones in those taking 1 g/day of aspirin.[1] Moreover, in a retrospective study, patients who had previously undergone successful bile acid dissolution therapy and chronically took NSAIDs for unassociated reasons displayed a significantly decreased rate of gallstone recurrence.[15]

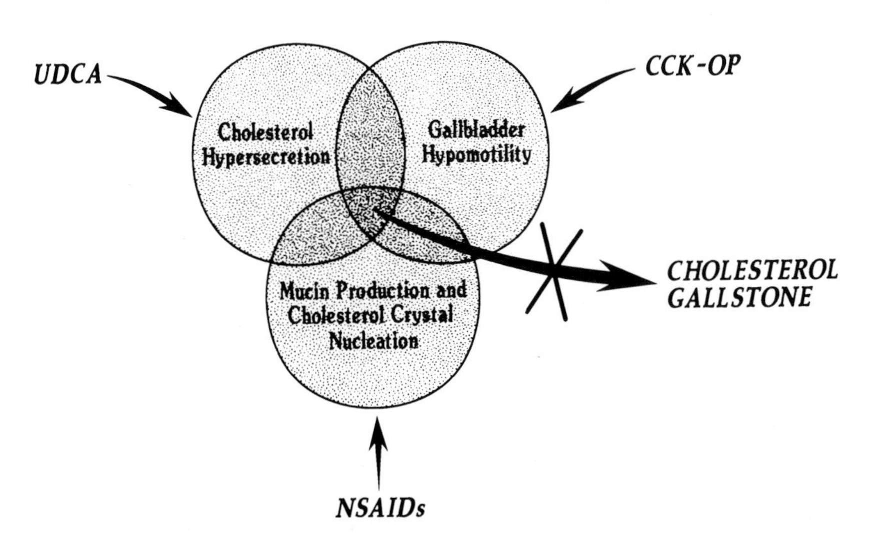

Figure 12.39 Venn diagram of the triple defect necessary for cholesterol gallstone formation and showing possibilities for primary pharmacological prevention of gallstones by elimination of at least one defect. Administration of ursodeoxycholic acid (UDCA) primarily blocks cholesterol hypersecretion. Administration of NSAIDs blocks mucin production, which in turn slows or suppresses formation of cholesterol crystals. Intravenous cholecystokinin octapeptide (CCK-OP) stimulates gallbladder motility, resulting in more rapid and complete gallbladder evacuation, preventing mucin accumulation and cholesterol crystallization and removing crystals already formed.

This overview has pointed out how biliary cholesterol hypersecretion bile targets the gallbladder, and how the organ responds, often to its own detriment, by forming gallstones. Three defects that are simultaneously required for cholesterol crystal formation in gallbladder bile have been outlined, and how pharmacological interruption of any one of these steps can prevent gallstones from forming has been discussed. This a posteriori reasoning further attests to the combined importance of thermodynamic (cholesterol supersaturation) as well as kinetic (nucleating and impaired emptying) events in the formation of cholesterol gallstones. This section began with the statement that cholesterol gallstones form only in the gallbladder and not in the ductal system of the biliary tree. It is known that strategies that mechanically prevent gallbladder filling such as defunctioning of the sphincter of Oddi can prevent cholesterol gallstone formation in lithogenic experimental animals. It will be of interest to see if this salutary effect might be achieved by pharmacological interventions in humans at high risk of developing cholesterol gallstones.

REFERENCES

1. Broomfield, P.H., Chopra, R., Sheinbaum, R.C. *et al.* (1988) Effects of ursodeoxycholic acid and aspirin on the formation of lithogenic bile and gallstones during loss of weight. *New England Journal of Medicine*, **319**, 1567–1572.
2. Busch, N., Tokumo, H. and Holzbach, R.T. (1990) A sensitive method for determination of cholesterol growth using model solutions of supersaturated bile. *Journal of Lipid Research*, **31**, 1903–1990.
3. Cabral, D.J. and Small, D.M. (1989) Physical chemistry of bile. In *Handbook of Physiology – The Gastrointestinal System III,* Section 6 (Ed.) Schultz, S.G., Forte, J.G. and Rauner, B.B. pp. 621–662. Baltimore: American Physiological Society, Waverly Press.
4. Carey, M.C. and Cahalane, M.J. (1988) Enterohepatic circulation. In *The Liver: Biology and Pathobiology* (Ed.) Arias, I.M., Jakoby, W.B., Popper, H., Schachter, D. and Shafritz, D.A. pp. 573–616. New York: Raven Press.
5. Carey, M.C. and Small, D.M. (1978) The physical chemistry of cholesterol solubility in bile: Relationship to gallstone formation and dissolution in man. *Journal of Clinical Investigation*, **61**, 998–1026.
6. Cohen, D.E. and Carey, M.C. (1990) Physical chemistry of biliary lipids during bile formation. *Hepatology*, **12**, 143S–148S.
7. Donovan, J.M. and Carey, M.C. (1990) Separation and quantitation of cholesterol "carriers" in bile. *Hepatology*, **12**, 94S–105S.
8. Einarsson, K. and Angelin, B. (1988) Pathogenesis of cholesterol gallstone disease: the secretory defect. In *Bile Acids in Health and Disease* (Ed.) Northfield, T., Jazrawi, R. and Zentler-Munro, P. pp. 117–133. Dordrecht: Kluwer.
9. Forgacs, I.C. (1988) Pathogenesis of cholesterol gallstone disease: the motility defect. In *Bile Acids in Health and Disease* (Ed.) Northfield, T., Jazrawi, R. and Zentler-Munro, P. pp. 135–153. Dordrecht: Kluwer.
10. Groen, A.K., Noordam, C., Drapers, J.A., Egbers, P., Jansen, P.L. and Tytgat, G.N. (1990) Isolation of a potent cholesterol nucleation-promoting activity from human gallbladder bile: role in the pathogenesis of gallstone disease. *Hepatology*, **11**, 525–533.
11. Halpern, Z., Dudley, M.A., Lynn, M.P., Nader, J.M., Breuer, A.C. and Holzbach, R.T. (1986) Vesicle aggregation in model systems of supersaturated bile: relation to crystal nucleation and lipid composition of the vesicular phase. *Journal of Lipid Research*, **27**, 295–306.
12. Hay, D.W. and Carey, M.C. (1990) Chemical species of lipids in bile. *Hepatology*, **12**, 6S–16S.
13. Hofmann, A.F., Grundy, S.M., Lachin, J.M. *et al.* (1982) Pretreatment biliary lipid composition in white patients with radiolucent gallstones in the National Cooperative Gallstone Study. *Gastroenterology*, **83**, 738–752.
14. Holan, K.R., Holzbach, R.T., Hermann, R.E., Cooperman, A.M. and Claffey, W.J. (1979) Nucleation time: a key factor in the pathogenesis of cholesterol gallstone disease. *Gastroenterology*, **77**, 611–617.
15. Hood, K., Gleeson, D., Ruppin, D.C. and Dowling, R.H. (1988) Prevention of gallstone recurrence by non-steroidal anti-inflammatory drugs. *The Lancet*, **ii**, 1223–1225.
16. Jüngst, D., Brenner, F., Pratschke, E. and Paumgartner, G. (1989) Low-dose ursodeoxycholic acid prolongs cholesterol nucleation time in gallbladder bile of patients with cholesterol gallstones. *Journal of Hepatology*, **8**, 1–6.
17. Lee, S.P., Maher, K. and Nicholls, J.F. (1988) Origin and fate of biliary sludge. *Gastroenterology*, **94**, 170–176.
18. Marcus, S.N. and Heaton, K.W. (1988) Deoxycholic acid and the pathogenesis of gallstones. *Gut*, **29**, 522–533.
19. Nervi, F., Covarrubias, C., Bravo, P. *et al.* (1989) Influence of legume intake on biliary lipids and cholesterol saturation in young Chilean men: identification of a dietary task factor for cholesterol gallstone formation in a highly prevalent area. *Gastroenterology*, **96**, 825–830.
20. Schoenfield, L.J., Sjövall, J. and Sjövall, K. (1966) Bile acid composition of gallstones from man. *Journal of Laboratory and Clinical Medicine*, **68**, 186–194.
21. Sitzmann, J.V., Pitt, H.A., Steinborn, P.A., Pasha, Z.R. and Saunders, R.C. (1990) Cholecystokinin prevents parenteral nutrition induced biliary sludge in humans. *Surgery, Gynecology and Obstetrics*, **170**, 25–31.

FORMATION OF PIGMENT GALLSTONES

J.M. Donovan and M.C. Carey

There are two types of pigment gallstones, known trivially as 'black' and 'brown' gallstones. They differ in chemical composition, pathophysiology and pathogenesis, as well as in clinical risk factors. Like cholesterol gallstones, black pigment gallstones precipitate in *sterile* gallbladder bile when concentrations of normal biliary constituents exceed their maximum solubilities. Black pigment gallstones are composed predominantly of oxidized and polymerized calcium salts of unconjugated bilirubin (UCB), together with calcium phosphate and carbonate. Brown pigment gallstones form in the bile ducts or rarely in the gallbladder as a result of supersaturation of bile with calcium salts of UCB and two long-chain fatty acids, palmitate or stearate, neither of which is present in bile normally. Brown pigment gallstones are *always* associated with biliary stasis and bacterial infection with subsequent hydrolysis and precipitation of biliary lipids. First, the chemical compositions of both types of gallstones will be reviewed, then current insights into biliary solubilization and precipitation of their constituents will be discussed, and known pathophysiological abnormalities correlated with clinical risk factors for pigment gallstone disease.

COMPOSITION OF BLACK AND BROWN PIGMENT GALLSTONES

Typical compositions of black and brown pigment gallstones are shown in *Figure 12.40*.[14,20] Both types of gallstones are composed principally of calcium salts of UCB, deposited in a mucin glycoprotein matrix. Depending on solution pH (see below), UCB exists either as the dianion (UCB^{2-}), monoanion ($HUCB^{-}$) or diacid (H_2UCB) species and, consequently at least two calcium salts can form – the neutral salt Ca(UCB), and the acid salt $Ca(HUCB)_2$. Since at physiological pH the monoanion predominates in solution,[15] the acid salt $Ca(HUCB)_2$ is most likely the principal species in both black and brown pigment gallstones. It is believed that, in black pigment gallstones, free radical-induced polymerization of calcium bilirubinates takes place to form this insoluble polymer, the solid state structure of which has not been determined. The insolubility of this black pigment polymer in both aqueous and organic solvents has posed a major obstacle not only to chemical analysis of black pigment gallstones, but also to pharmacological and contact dissolution in vivo. In contrast, calcium salts of UCB in brown pigment gallstones are not polymerized unless a migrating black pigment gallstone from the gallbladder acts as a nidus for brown pigment gallstone formation in the ducts. Consequently, most brown pigment gallstones can be dissolved by complex mixtures of chemicals that split the salt bond, chelate calcium and solubilize UCB.[11] The physical properties of gallstones are determined by the degree of polymerization of bilirubinate and the presence of crystalline inorganic calcium salts or calcium soaps ('grease'): brown pigment gallstones are laminated and soft, whereas black pigment gallstones are amorphous and hard.

Several different crystalline (polymorphic) forms of calcium carbonate (vaterite, aragonite and calcite) and calcium phosphate (hydroxyapatite and whitlockite) have been demonstrated by radiological diffraction and infrared spectroscopy in black pigment gallstones. Only one polymorph is usually

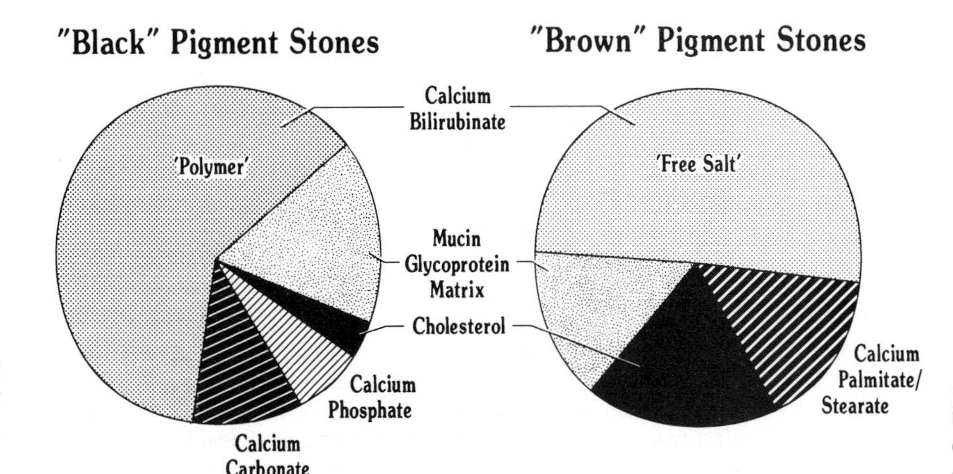

Figure 12.40 Pie charts illustrating chemical compositions (wt%) of black and brown pigment gallstones.

found in a gallstone, but the pathophysiological significance of a particular polymorph is uncertain.[3] The calcium palmitate and stearate salts that typify brown pigment gallstones may be crystalline or amorphous. Stones that are rich in inorganic calcium salts, i.e. most black (gallbladder) pigment gallstones, are radiopaque, whereas most brown (ductal) pigment gallstones are radiolucent.

Only a minor amount of cholesterol (less than 20%), if any, is found in black pigment gallstones, as biles from which they precipitate are generally unsaturated with cholesterol (cholesterol saturation index, CSI <1). Hence, black pigment lithogenesis may be related pathophysiologically to the absence of cholesterol/lecithin vesicles in such biles (see below). In contrast, a variable amount of cholesterol (20–80%) is present in most brown pigment gallstones as a consequence of their formation in ductal biles where CSI values invariably exceed 1; furthermore, cholesterol 'carriers' are depleted during their formation. Gallstones with cholesterol contents between 20 and 50% do not form in sterile bile.

Mucin glycoproteins are a major component (10–30%) of the total weight of both black and brown pigment gallstones[10] (*Figure 12.40*). In black pigment gallstones, histochemical stains show a glycoprotein matrix throughout, which is derived from mucin secreted by the gallbladder epithelium. Brown pigment gallstones contain mucin glycoproteins of ductal origin, as well as bacterial glycoproteins shown by the presence of sugars (e.g. rhamnose) unique to Gram-negative bacteria. Frequently, the cytoskeletal remains of bacteria can be visualized by scanning electron microscopy in the interiors of brown pigment gallstones.

The major biliary lipids, bile salts and lecithin (see *Figure 12.31*, p. 1703), are found in minute quantities in black pigment gallstones. Because sterile bile is never supersaturated with lecithin, its presence in trace quantities (1–2%) in black pigment gallstones and the fact that lecithin accelerates $Ca(HUCB)_2$ precipitation in vitro suggests that it lowers the free energy of nucleation.

PHYSICAL CHEMISTRY OF BILIRUBIN CONJUGATES AND UCB IN BILE

UCB, the end-product of haem degradation, is a bislactam open-chain tetrapyrrole with six hydrocarbon as well as two hydrophilic ('water-loving') propionic acid side-chains (*Figure 12.41*).[4] Because the molecule is composed of both hydrophilic regions (the carboxylic acids) and hydrophobic ('water-fearing') regions (the hydrocarbon skeleton and side-chains), UCB may be considered amphiphilic. However, its amphiphilicity depends critically on the ionization state of the two carboxylic acid groups. The pK_a values of the carboxylic acids of UCB differ from one another, and are in dispute, but are certain to be much higher than 4.8, the pK_a of short-chain carboxylic acids such as acetate. At pH values both below pK_a values, the carboxylic acids are protonated and uncharged; at pH values above both pK_a values the carboxylic acids are ionized; at intermediate pH values (typical of bile) only one carboxylic acid is ionized ($HUCB^-$).[15] Internal hydrogen bonding between the protonated

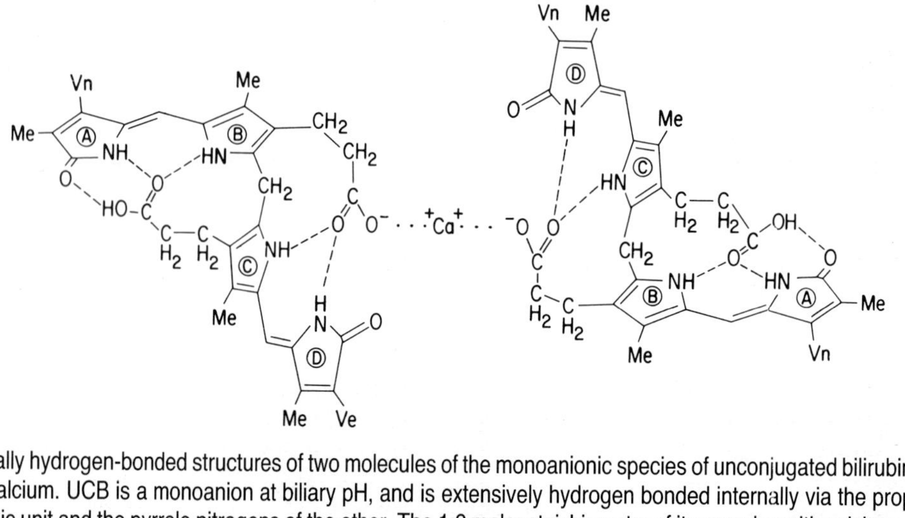

Figure 12.41 Internally hydrogen-bonded structures of two molecules of the monoanionic species of unconjugated bilirubin ($HUCB^-$) in a salt bond with ionic calcium. UCB is a monoanion at biliary pH, and is extensively hydrogen bonded internally via the propionic carboxyl groups of one dipyrrolic unit and the pyrrole nitrogens of the other. The 1:2 molar stoichiometry of its complex with calcium, $Ca(HUCB)_2$, is believed to be the principal calcium salt of UCB in both black and brown pigment gallstones. Because of its high binding affinity, the salt is not dissociated to any appreciable extent in bile.

carboxylic acids and the nitrogens of the opposite pyrrole rings renders the protonated form far more hydrophobic than the fully ionized molecule. Thus, the aqueous solubility of the dianion (UCB^{2-}), which is approximately 10 mmol/l at pH 10, exceeds by several orders of magnitude that for the uncharged, protonated form (H_2UCB), which approaches 1 nmol/l at pH 5.

Because of the extreme insolubility of UCB at physiological pH, it is excreted by the liver as soluble bilirubin conjugates, predominantly as bilirubin diglucuronide and two bilirubin monoglucuronide isomers. In normal biles, less than 1% of total bilirubin is present as UCB. Only minor amounts of bilirubin, diglucuronide and bilirubin monoglucuronide occur in human pigment gallstones.[21] However, the calcium salt of bilirubin monoglucuronide precipitates as the insoluble pigment in gallstones of a haemolytic mouse model,[22] and bilirubin monoglucuronide and traces of bilirubin diglucuronide are components of human biliary sludge.[1] Nonenzymic[22] and enzymatic hydrolysis[3] produces UCB from bilirubin diglucuronide and bilirubin monoglucuronide, the latter being more readily hydrolysed because of its single conjugated bond. The enzyme β-glucuronidase is believed to originate from hepatocytes and bile ductular epithelium (black pigment gallstones), as well as from bacteria during biliary infection (brown pigment gallstones). Activity of β-glucuronidase has been reported to be increased slightly in black pigment gallstone biles, and is very high during anaerobic bacterial infections that result in brown pigment gallstone formation.[9]

In sterile bile at approximately pH 7.5, UCB concentrations can be as high as 100 μmol/l (M.J. Cahalane and M.C. Carey, unpublished observations), a concentration that greatly exceeds aqueous solubility. Therefore, virtually all UCB must be solubilized by aggregates of the three major biliary lipids, which form simple bile salt micelles, bile salt/lecithin/cholesterol mixed micelles and lecithin/cholesterol vesicles, the latter present only in biles with CSI values greater than 1 (see *Figure 12.33*, p. 1705).[7] Model bile studies have shown that bile salts alone solubilize physiological concentrations of UCB in simple bile salt micelles.[17] The addition of physiological concentrations of lecithin decreases UCB solubility appreciably, implying that mixed bile salt/lecithin micelles are less efficient in solubilizing UCB. Although the relative quantities of UCB solubilized by each of the biliary lipid aggregates are unknown, the absence of lecithin/cholesterol vesicles in biles containing black pigment gallstones suggests that lecithin/cholesterol vesicles may be important in UCB solubilization.[18] However, low concentrations of the monoanionic form of UCB ($HUCB^-$) are very sensitive to the presence of quite small concentrations of calcium, and the insoluble salt $Ca(HUCB)_2$ forms and readily precipitates (*Figure 12.41*).

ROLE OF IONIZED (UNBOUND) CALCIUM

Since the major components of both types of pigment gallstone are inorganic and organic calcium salts, divalent ionized calcium plays a pivotal role in their formation. Calcium is passively transported into bile, and is in equilibrium with serum ionized calcium. Most biliary calcium is bound in soluble anion–cation complexes, primarily with bile salts[13] and to a lesser extent with bilirubin conjugates, bicarbonate, and mucin glycoproteins via their sialic acids. The crucial calcium concentration that determines insoluble salt formation with UCB, carbonate or phosphate is the free ionized fraction, $[Ca^{2+}]$, which only constitutes a small (about 20%) proportion of total biliary calcium. The maximum solubility of each of these calcium salts in bile is expressed as a solubility product (K_{sp}), that is, the product of the concentrations of each of their respective *unbound* ions. For example, the solubility product of the acid salt of UCB is equal to $[Ca^{2+}]$ $[HUCB^-)^2$. When the product of the actual measured quantities (the ion product) exceeds the solubility product, bile becomes supersaturated with respect to that salt, which can then form and precipitate when kinetic factors are favourable.

Bile can become supersaturated with $Ca(HUCB)_2$ by increases in either $[Ca^{2+}]$ or $[HUCB^-]$ or both. As indicated earlier, each ion is in rapid equilibrium with a large excess of calcium and $HUCB^-$, both of which are bound to biliary lipid aggregates. Since it is believed that only a tiny fraction (<1%) of $HUCB^-$ is free, K_{sp} values cannot be determined accurately. Apparent solubility products, utilizing total biliary UCB concentrations rather than free $HUCB^-$ concentrations and ionized calcium (which can be measured accurately), have been estimated to be approximately 10^{-13} (mol/l)^3.[16] Thus, in contrast to the well defined millimolar limits of cholesterol solubility in bile, the limits of calcium bilirubinate solubility in bile are extradordinarily low. Hence, the degree of unsaturation or supersaturation of normal and pigment gallstone biles remains elusive. The appearance of pigment precipitates after incubation of cholesterol gallstone biles[18] suggests that UCB calcium salt supersaturation is frequent. As in the case for cholesterol gallstones, it is difficult to draw conclusions from analysis of biles containing pigment gallstones since lithogenesis occurred months or years before collection of bile.

PATHOPHYSIOLOGICAL EVENTS IN BLACK PIGMENT GALLSTONE FORMATION

Figure 12.42 shows a Venn diagram where biliary supersaturation with $Ca(HUCB)_2$, accelerated nucleation of $Ca(HUCB)_2$ and gallbladder dysfunction with increased mucin production and impaired motility are postulated as critical elements in black pigment gallstone formation. Biliary supersaturation with $Ca(HUCB)_2$ can occur in several ways: via increases in concentrations of either UCB (and consequently $HUCB^-$) or calcium, or by decreases in the binding capacity of biliary lipid aggregates for each. Elevations in UCB concentrations in pigment gallstone biles have been demonstrated in some human studies and in animal models. Theoretically, elevations may be due to (1) increased secretion of UCB precursors such as bilirubin diglucuronide or bilirubin monoglucuronide, (2) increased levels of non-bacterially derived β-glucuronidase, or (3) decreased levels of the naturally occurring β-glucuronidase inhibitor, β-1,4-glucurolactone. Increased bilirubin diglucuronide and bilirubin monoglucuronide secretion rates occur in chronic haemolytic states and hepatic cirrhosis (*Table 12.4*), both of which are associated with the development of black pigment gallstones. The respective roles of β-glucuronidase activity and its inhibitors in human biles are unknown. Since both calcium and $HUCB^-$ are bound by monomeric and micellar bile salts, decreased bile salt secretion may result in $Ca(HUCB)_2$ supersaturation. As demonstrated in animal models and in chronic hypercalcaemic states in humans, isolated elevations in biliary ionized calcium also produce $Ca(HUCB)_2$ supersaturation.[12]

Virtually nothing is known concerning factors that promote or inhibit calcium bilirubinate precipitation. Pigment gallstone biles have lower CSI values compared with cholesterol gallstone biles, and consequently have few or no biliary vesicles.[18]

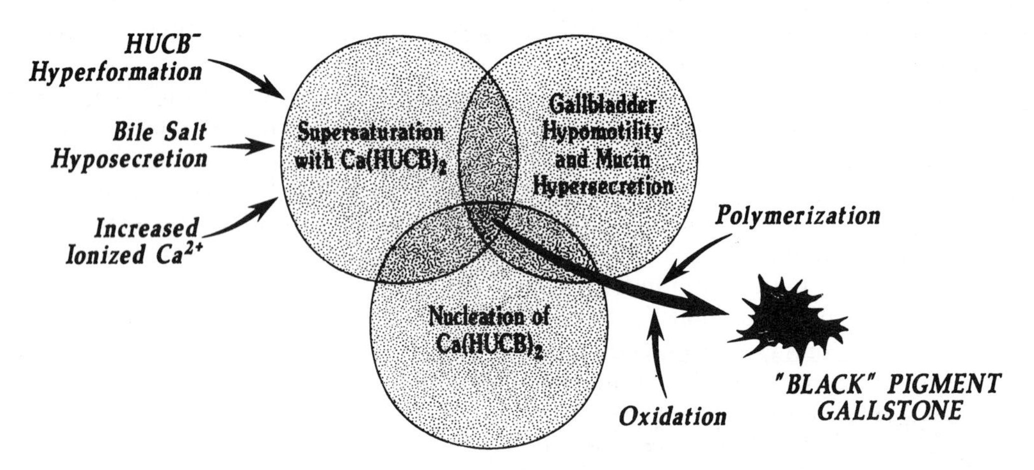

Figure 12.42 Venn diagram demonstrating the key factors contributing to the formation of black pigment gallstones.

Table 12.4 Risk factors for black pigment gallstones[a]

	Increased UCB formation	*Decreased bile salt secretion*	*Altered calcium metabolism*	*Impaired gallbladder motility*
Haemolytic disorders	+	–	–	–
Age	+	+	–	–
Hepatic cirrhosis	+	+	–	–
Ileal disease/resection	+	–	+	–
Total parenteral nutrition	–	+	+	+

[a]Risk factors are, as yet, undefined for most patients with this disease.

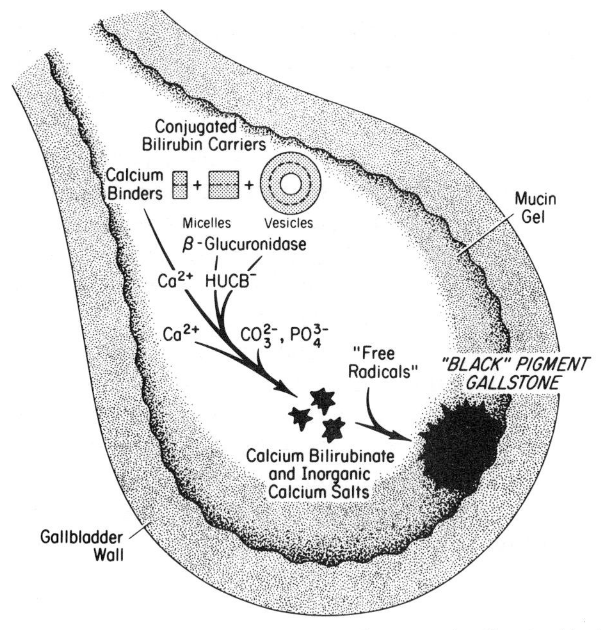

Figure 12.43 Postulated sequence of events leading to black pigment gallstone formation (see text for details).

As suggested earlier, biliary vesicles may be important either in solubilizing $HUCB^-$ or in binding early $Ca(HUCB)_2$ precipitates. Inhibitors of calcium phosphate and carbonate precipitation are also present in bile, but have not been well characterized, nor is their role in the pathogenesis of black pigment gallstones understood. Hyperproduction of a mucin gel by the gallbladder mucosa occurs in animal models of black pigment gallstones, and provides a matrix that binds $Ca(HUCB)_2$, induces adherence of precipitates to the gallbladder wall, and impairs their clearance.

Figure 12.43 shows the progression of this sequence of events in the formation of 'biliary sludge', an earlier stage in the formation of both cholesterol and black pigment gallstones (see previous section). Sludge is a viscous gel containing mucin and microscopic precipitates of multilamellar vesicles, cholesterol monohydrate and calcium bilirubinate.[1] Free radical polymerization of precipitated $Ca(HUCB)_2$ probably occurs over a time-scale of months, as shown by the variable polymer content of black pigment gallstones, as well as the reversibility of black pigment gallstone formation in a subacute canine model.[16] Increased alkalinity increases concentrations of the calcium-sensitive anions, carbonate (from bicarbonate) and phosphate (from hydrogen phosphate), and promotes precipitation of their calcium salts in bile. Hence, the demonstrated impairment of gallbladder acidification in human gallstone biles may be important in accelerating inorganic calcium salt precipitation.

PATHOPHYSIOLOGY OF BROWN PIGMENT GALLSTONE FORMATION

Bile stasis and bacterial infection invariably precede the development of brown pigment gallstones.[5] Cholesterol and black pigment gallstones that migrate from the gallbladder, as well as parasites and surgical suture material, may serve as the nidus for initial bacterial colonization. As shown in *Figure 12.44*, bacterial enzymes hydrolyse biliary lipids, forming insoluble products as well as depleting bile

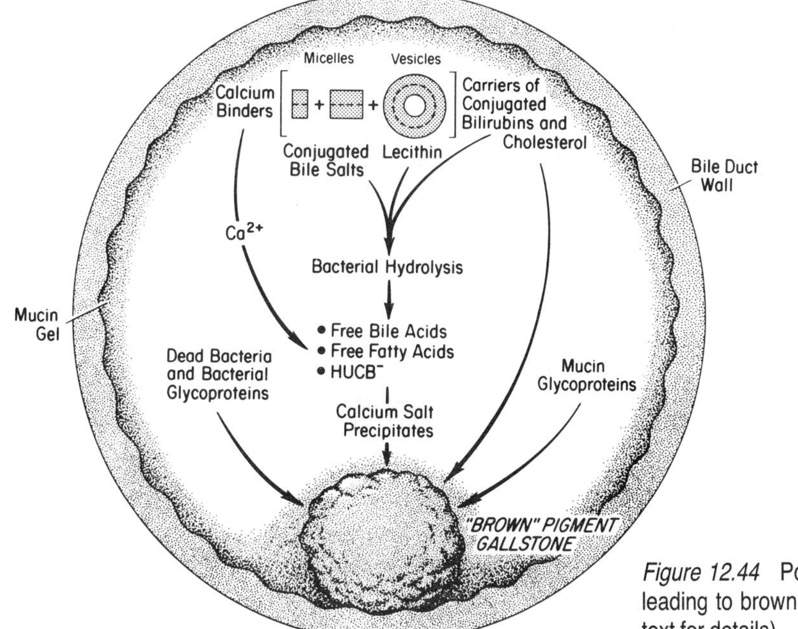

Figure 12.44 Postulated sequence of events leading to brown pigment gallstone formation (see text for details).

of the carriers for cholesterol and UCB. Bacterial phospholipase A_1 hydrolyses lecithin to form free fatty acids, palmitic and stearic acids, and lysolecithin, which is soluble in aqueous solution. In the presence of ionized calcium, insoluble calcium soaps of the free fatty acids form and precipitate. Bacterial deconjugases hydrolyse conjugated bile salts to produce free bile acids, which may also precipitate as their calcium salts or as the protonated bile acids. Bacterial β-glucuronidase hydrolyses bilirubin diglucuronide and bilirubin monoglucuronide, producing UCB in far higher concentrations than in biles containing black pigment gallstones. Once brown pigment gallstone formation is initiated, a vicious cycle may ensue, with brown pigment gallstones themselves obstructing and ulcerating the biliary ductal system, thus further promoting biliary stasis and chronic infection. Thus, during bacterial infection of bile, soluble biliary lipids are hydrolyzed to insoluble products and the degraded biliary lipids are unavailable to solubilize cholesterol, which then precipitates as part of brown pigment gallstones. The pathophysiology of brown pigment gallstones differs distinctly from that of black pigment and cholesterol gallstones, both of which result from an excess of normal biliary constitutents, and form because of metabolic and physicochemical defects in biliary homeostasis.

CLINICAL RISK FACTORS FOR PIGMENT GALLSTONES

Table 12.4 correlates the pathophysiology, where known, of black pigment gallstone formation with major clinical risk factors for developing these gallstones. In chronic haemolytic disorders there is an isolated defect: greatly increased production of bilirubin from haem, resulting in elevated biliary levels of both bilirubin monoglucuronide and bilirubin diglucuronide. Normal levels of β-glucuronidase and non-enzymic hydrolysis produce increased biliary UCB concentrations. Consequently, the majority of children with severe, chronic haemolytic syndromes, such as sickle cell anaemia, develop black pigment gallstones by puberty. With advancing age in otherwise normal individuals, biliary UCB concentrations increase while absolute quantities of secreted bile salts decrease, leading to higher biliary supersaturation with $Ca(HUCB)_2$. Patients with chronic liver disease not only have increased bilirubin diglucuronide and bilirubin monoglucuronide production secondary to haemolysis of hypersplenism, but also secrete less bile salts,[22] and therefore solubilize less $HUCB^-$ and bind less calcium in their biles. Patients with impaired ileal absorption of bile salts develop black pigment gallstones, *not* cholesterol gallstones as was previously believed. Following ileal resection in animal models, increased biliary concentrations of both calcium and UCB have been demonstrated. Patients undergoing total parenteral nutrition have greatly impaired gallbladder motility and, at least in animal models, both biliary calcium and UCB levels are elevated for reasons that remain unclear. After several weeks of total parenteral nutrition, this combination of defects results in the almost universal development of biliary sludge, and the subsequent development of black pigment gallstones in 30–40% of patients.

In summary, although important advances have been made in our understanding of the multiple factors that affect the solubilities of organic and inorganic calcium salts in bile, advances in pharmacological therapies that could reverse the earliest stages of black pigment gallstone formation and prevent their progression are still awaited. Prevention of brown pigment gallstones relies on prevention of cholesterol and black pigment gallstones that commonly serve as a ductal nidus, and the avoidance of other causes of bile stasis that result in chronic anaerobic bacterial infection.

REFERENCES

1. Allen, B., Bernhoff, N. and Blankaert, N. (1981) Sludge is calcium bilirubinate associated with bile stasis. *American Journal of Surgery*, **141**, 51–56.
2. Alvaro, D., Angelico, M., Gandin, C., Corradini, S.G. and Capocaccia, L. (1990) Physico-chemical factors predisposing to pigment gallstone formation in liver cirrhosis. *Journal of Hepatology*, **10**, 228–234.
3. Cahalane, M.J., Neubrand, M.W. and Carey, M.C. (1988) Physical–chemical pathogenesis of pigment gallstones. *Seminars in Liver Disease*, **8**, 317–328.
4. Carey, M.C. and Spivak, W. (1986) Physical chemistry of bile pigments and porphyrins with particular reference to bile. In *Bile Pigments and Jaundice, Molecular, Metabolic, and Medical Aspects* (Ed.) Ostrow, J.D. pp. 81–132. New York: Marcel Dekker.
5. Cetta, F. (1991) The role of bacteria in pigment gallstone disease. *Annals of Surgery*, **213**, 315–326.
6. Dawes, L.G., Nahrwold, D.L., Roth, S.I. and Rege, R.V. (1989) Reversal of pigment gallstone disease in a canine model. *Archives of Science*, **124**, 463–466.
7. Donovan, J.M. and Carey, M.C. (1990) Separation and quantitation of cholesterol "carriers" in bile. *Hepatology*, **12**, 94S–105S.
8. Gallinger, S., Harvey, P.R.C., Petrunka, C.N. and Strasberg, S.M. (1986) Effect of binding of ionised

calcium on the in vitro nucleation of cholesterol and calcium bilirubinate in human gall bladder bile. *Gut*, **27**, 1382–1386.
9. Ho, K.-J., Hsu, S.-C., Chen, J.-S. and Ho. L.-H.C. (1986) Human biliary β-glucuronidase: correlation of its activity with deconjugation of bilirubin in the bile. *European Journal of Clinical Investigation*, **16**, 361–367.
10. LaMont, J.T., Ventola, A.S., Trotman, B.W. and Soloway, R.D. (1983) Mucin glycoprotein content of human pigment gallstones. *Hepatology*, **3**, 377–382.
11. Leuschner, U. (1990) Topical treatment of calcified and pigment stones. *Seminars in Liver Disease*, **10**, 191–196.
12. Magnuson, T.H., Lillemoe, K.D., Peoples, G.E. and Pitt, H.A. (1989) Oral calcium promotes pigment gallstone formation. *Journal of Surgical Research*, **46**, 286–291.
13. Moore, E.W. (1984) The role of calcium in the pathogenesis of gallstones: Ca^{++} electrode studies of model bile salt solutions and other biologic systems: With a hypothesis on structural requirements for Ca^{++} binding to proteins and bile acids. *Hepatology*, **4**, 228S–243S.
14. Ostrow, J.D. (1984) The etiology of pigment gallstones. *Hepatology*, **4**, 215S–222S.
15. Ostrow, J.D. and Celic, L. (1984) Bilirubin chemistry, ionization and solubilization by bile salts. *Hepatology*, **4**, 38S–45S.
16. Ostrow, J.D. and Celic, L. (1987) Apparent solubility products (K''_{sp}) of the calcium salts of unconjugated bilirubin (B) indicate supersaturation of human gallbladder bile with $Ca(HB)_2$ but not CaB (abstract). *Hepatology*, **7**, 1111.
17. Ostrow, J.D., Celic, L. and Mukerjee, P. (1988) Molecular and micellar associations in the pH-dependent stable and metastable dissolution of unconjugated bilirubin by bile salts. *Journal of Lipid Research*, **29**, 335–348.
18. Schriever, C.E. and Jüngst, D. (1989) Association between cholesterol–phospholipid vesicles and cholesterol crystals in human gallbladder bile. *Hepatology*, **9**, 541–546.
19. Spivak, W., DiVenuto, D. and Yuey, W. (1987) Non-enzymic hydrolysis of bilirubin mono- and diglucuronide to unconjugated bilirubin in model and native bile systems. Potential role in the formation of gallstones. *Biochemical Journal*, **242**, 323–329.
20. Trotman, B.W. (1983) Pigment gallstone disease. *Seminars in Liver Disease*, **3**, 112–119.
21. Trotman, B.W., Ostrow, J.D. and Soloway, R.D. (1974) Pigment vs cholesterol cholelithiasis: comparison of stone and bile composition. *American Journal of Digestive Diseases*, **199**, 585–590.
22. Trotman, B.W., Nair, C.R. and Bernstein, S.E. (1988) Monoconjugated bilirubin is a major component of hemolysis-induced gallstones in mice. *Hepatology*, **8**, 919–924.

CLINICAL FEATURES AND NON-SURGICAL TREATMENT OF GALLSTONES

I.A.D. Bouchier and J. Neoptolemos

EPIDEMIOLOGY

Although it is difficult to obtain firm data, the evidence suggests that gallstones are becoming more frequent, and this is supported by autopsy data from Scotland.[6] It has been suggested that about 5 million persons in the UK and 15 million in the USA may have gallstones, with an overall prevalence of 10–20%; but single figures are misleading because of the large variation with age.[10]

There have been many studies on the prevalence of gallstones in different racial groups and these are summarized in *Table 12.5*, in which the prevalence is expressed as an overall percentage for a population. Factors responsible for these racial differences are not known but genetic and dietary factors, and obesity, may all play a role. The genetics of this disease have not been elucidated but cholelithiasis may well have a polygenetic inheritance, as indicated by the following:

- Gallstones are five times commoner in gallstone families.

Table 12.5 Racial prevalence of gallstones

	Prevalence (%)
Pima Indians	80
Chilean Indians	65
Germany	45
UK	27
India	20
Italy	20
Denmark	19
Africa	14
Japan	10
China	5

- Gallstones are twice as common in first-degree relations.
- There is no increase in spouses.

Environmental factors probably override a genetic influence, as shown by the increased prevalence of gallstones in those who come from low-prevalence areas to countries with a high frequency of gallstones; for example, Japanese who move to the USA or Europe, or African blacks who live in the USA.

Until recently, prevalence studies in communities were derived from post-mortem data or the records of cholecystectomies. The advent of ultrasonography has permitted studies on asymptomatic populations of all ages, thereby providing more realistic information on prevalence. Some of the best data come from Italy.[3] The Sirmione data, based on ultrasonography and a history of previous cholecystectomy, indicate that the disease affects 6.7% of males and 14.6% of females aged 18–65 years with an overall prevalence of 11%. The prevalence in females ranged from 2.9 (18–29 years) to 27% (50–65 years). Males were 1.1 and 11% respectively, for the same time period.[5] Studies from Rome give a prevalence in females of 5.9 (30–39 years), 10.9 (40–49 years) and 17.8% (50–59 years). Comparable figures for males were 3.8, 5.2 and 6.2, and 11.1% for the 60–69-year age group. The male:female ratios were 1:2.9, 1:1.6 and 1:1.2, respectively, indicating that gallstone formation occurs at a younger age in women.[4]

CHOLESTEROL GALLSTONES

All studies are consistent in finding a higher prevalence of gallstones in females than males, the difference becoming less obvious with age. In high-prevalence populations such as Mexian–American females the prevalence of gallstones is 44.1%.[47] The reason for the increased frequency of gallstones in premenopausal females has still to be clarified but may be related particularly to alterations in biliary lipids and gallbladder motility. There is an increased risk of gallstone disease in women using supplemental oestrogens,[50,64] the effect of which is most marked in younger women. Scragg *et al.* also observed that endogenous oestrogen concentrations appeared to be of more importance in postmenopausal women.[64] Gallstone disease is more frequent in males taking oestrogens for prostatic cancer,[29] because of a raised hepatic secretion of cholesterol, possibly due to increased hepatic low-density lipoprotein receptor capacity with a reduction in the serum low-density lipoprotein levels. High plasma insulin concentrations are found in gallstone subjects, which may relate to the activation of low-density lipoprotein receptors, thereby enhancing low-density lipoprotein cholesterol transport from blood to liver.[36,62] Thus, factors determining the flux of cholesterol through the liver determine the development of gallstones and there is a reduced prevalence in individuals using 3-hydroxymethylglutaryl-coenzyme-A (HMG-CoA) reductase inhibitors such as Lovastatin (*Table 12.6*).[2]

Table 12.6 Relative risks of gallstone formation

Factor	*Relative risk*
Hypertriglyceridaemia	1.6
Clofibrate	1.6
Nicotinic acid	1.2
Hypercholesterolaemia	1.0
Lovostatin	1.0

Gallstones are commoner in women who have had children and increased parity is associated with an increased frequency of gallstones, although not all studies support this observation.[43] The explanation is probably the development of gallbladder stasis during pregnancy. With each trimester there is an increased amount of gallbladder sludge and stones, and by the time of delivery 50% of women have sludge and 15% have gallstones. One year postpartum, sludge will have disappeared but 4% of women still retain their gallstones.

There is considerable evidence for the association of obesity and gallstones and this is seen in children as well as adults.[49] Weight gain need only be modest (relative weight 24–29.9 kg/m^2) for the risk to be increased. There is a linear relationship between relative weight and risk, and the risk remains when the weight gain has occurred in late adolescence.[43,51,63] The most consistent dietary factor associated with gallstones is an increased energy intake. This acts independently of obesity.[43,63] It has not been possible to establish with certainty whether any specific dietary component has a positive association with gallstones. Perhaps the best evidence is for polyunsaturated fatty acids, particularly the ω-6 fatty acid linoleic acid, although Diehl *et al.*[20] found the association of high fat intake and linoleic acid to be a risk in males only. In Chile, where gallstones are relatively more common, diets rich in legumes have been implicated, possibly by inducing a relative deficiency in biliary phospholipid. Data from Australia support the association with an increased intake of simple sugars in the form of soft drinks and sweets.[20,63] A consistent observation in all studies have been the negative association with moderate alcohol intake.[43,63] The difficulties of identifying dietary factors are highlighted by the study of Pixley and Mann,[51] which was unable to identify differences in nutrient intake between vegetarian and non-vegetarian women with gallstones. Age and sex appear to be the overriding factors determining prevalence and may well dominate over dietary influence.

Other factors associated with an increased frequency of gallstones include clofibrate therapy, where there is an increased cholesterol saturation of bile, and diabetes mellitus, somatostatinoma, and the treatment of acromegaly with somatostatin analogues.[10,74] Cholelithiasis follows total gastrectomy for the Zollinger–Ellison syndrome.[16] The Sirmione study failed to demonstrate an association with diabetes mellitus[5] but recent data from Edinburgh support the association of diabetes with gallstones.[27]

PIGMENT STONES

There are two types of pigment stone, 'black' and 'brown', both formed of calcium bilirubinates. The stones tend to be multiple, 2–5 mm in diameter, and smooth or irregular in shape. In contrast to cholesterol stones, there is no male/female difference in prevalence and the stones tend to occur in an older age group than cholesterol stones.

Black stones

These are the type of pigment stone found in Western communities and they account for 25% of all gallstones. About 5% of these stones are radiolucent. The stones are hard and shiny and the pigment is cross-linked and oxidized to form a black polymer which is insoluble in all solvents. The stones contain substantial amounts of calcium carbonate and calcium phosphate.[14] Black pigment stones occur in association with haemolytic disease. However, most patients with pigment stones do not have haemolytic disease. Other associations are hepatic cirrhosis,[9] sclerosing cholangitis, ileal disease and resection, vagotomy, and prolonged parenteral nutrition[15,46] and prolonged fasting.[8] The frequency of gallstones is 23–37% in sickle cell anaemia, 43–66% in hereditary spherocytosis and 23% in thalassaemia major. The more severe the anaemia, the greater the prevalence of gallstones. The probable explanation is the excess load of unconjugated bilirubin in the bile, and this also accounts for the greater frequency of gallstones in liver cirrhosis.[10,42] Ultrasonographic studies suggest a frequency of 30% in patients with chronic liver disease.[1,42] Mechanical destruction of erythrocytes by prosthetic heart valves is the reason for the increased prevalence of gallstones in such patients.

Brown stones

These are soft, easily crushed and formed by calcium bilirubinates, which can be completely hydrolysed, solubilized and extracted. Typically they contain coprecipitates of calcium palmitate and stearate which are the consequence of bacterial phospholipase A_1 hydrolysis of biliary lecithin.[14] Indeed, it is a characteristic of brown stones that they occur when there is infection in the intra- or extrahepatic biliary systems. Brown pigment stones occur most frequently in the Orient. β-Glucuronidase-producing bacteria hydrolyse bilirubin diglucuronide to free bilirubin either as a primary phenomenon or in association with biliary obstruction or secondary to parasitic infection of the biliary tree. Brown stones typically occur in the bile ducts. Stewart *et al.*[68] have emphasized the role of an ionic glycoprotein secreted by bacteria which promotes crystal formation and stone growth. These authors claim that bacteria actually form a substantial part of a gallstone. Their observation that bacteria are responsible for the formation of most black pigment stones has not been confirmed.[35]

Gallstones are not associated with gastrointestinal malignancies other than gallbladder cancer, where the prevalence is high in Chile and Pima Indians and increases with age and the size of the gallstone. There is a 10% risk of gallbladder cancer with gallstones greater than 3 mm in diameter. Gallstone acute pancreatitis is associated particularly with small black pigment stones.

Gallstones in children

While it is true that cholelithiasis is a disease of adults, gallstones have been recorded in neonates[32] and adolescents.[17,26,65] Haemolysis is a cause in less than 10% of all children. Extrabiliary infections in various organs are often implicated and it is possible that dehydration, gallbladder stasis, and biliary sludge are important. Congenital abnormalities of the biliary tree are a rare association and heredity plays no clear role. There is surprisingly little information on the nature of the gallstones.

NATURAL HISTORY

Little is known about the rate at which gallstones grow, which is surprising because it could be postulated that the growth rate might be relevant to the development of symptoms. Using the excess ^{14}C in the atmosphere as a biological marker for the age of gallstones, Mok *et al.*[46] concluded that the growth rate was 1–4 mm annually. It took at least 2 years, with a mean of 8.0 ± 5.2 years, for symptoms to develop after stone formation. There was no difference in the growth rate of symptomatic as opposed to asymptomatic stones.

Nothing is known about factors which determine why gallstones cause symptoms. Size, number or composition of stones do not appear to be relevant.[13] It is possible that gallstones are less frequently symptomatic in males than females.[22,45,65]

Until recently it was believed that the presence of gallstones in either the gallbladder or bile ducts inevitably led to major medical problems and carried a significant morbidity and mortality. A paper by Gracie and Ransohoff in 1982[25] demonstrated that, in a healthy white population, gallstones were usually asymptomatic. The cumulative probability of biliary pain developing in their study was 10% at 5 years and 18% at 15 and 20 years. Thus, the yearly risk of biliary pain decreased with time. Medical problems, when they developed, were not severe. Their observations confirm the findings of the authors' group and others that untreated gallstones rarely cause death.[7,44] The conclusion of Gracie and Ransohoff have been confirmed in the main by a number of studies over the ensuing decade.

Asymptomatic stones are defined as gallstones that have not caused biliary colic or other biliary symptoms.[61] This is important because there is general agreement that once gallstones cause symptoms they will continue to do so with the development of significant complications.[75] Patients experiencing one episode of biliary pain over a 12-month period are much more likely to have further episodes during the subsequent 24 months.[73] A large study of patients with 'mild' or no symptoms followed for 25 years found the annual probability of developing a severe complication to be 1% with little change over time. The risk of surgery or continuing symptoms was greater (6%) during the first 5 years after diagnosis and decreased to 1–0.5% after 15 years.[22] The excellent Italian studies on truly asymptomatic stones indicate that between 66 and 87% of adults with gallstones are free of complaints.[74] A study from Duke University Medical Center found only 11% of patients in whom gallstones were diagnosed coincidentally at ultrasonography developed abdominal pain over a period of 5 years.[18]

Although gallstones are more frequent in cirrhotics, they are seldom symptomatic and the development of jaundice in a cirrhotic patient is more likely to be due to liver decompensation than choledocholithiasis. None-the-less, it is wise to proceed to endoscopic retrograde cholangiography if ultrasonography in the jaundiced patient indicates either gallstones or duct dilatation.[21] Patients with diabetes and gallstones fare less well and are more prone to acute cholecystitis and perforation than the non-diabetic patient with gallstones.[59] Cholecystectomy in both cirrhotic and diabetic patients has a higher morbidity than in the general population.

CLINICAL FEATURES

It is important to appreciate that the majority of patients with gallstones never have symptoms and never present with the clinical syndromes of cholelithiasis – 'silent gallstones'. Their stones are usually discovered as an incidental finding at post-mortem examination. No pain will be experienced and complications will not occur provided the stones remain free in the lumen of the gallbladder and do not migrate into the cystic duct or bile duct.

A further 5% of gallstones are discovered incidentally as a result of laparotomy or radiological investigation performed for some other reason. Until recently, only those gallstones which contained enough calcium to render them radio-opaque tended to be identified, for instance at the time of a barium meal or intravenous pyelogram. With the increasing use of abdominal ultrasound and whole body computed tomography and magnetic resonance imaging, many more radiolucent gallstones are likely to be discovered.

Biliary colic, obstructive jaundice and acute cholecystitis are all specific symptoms or complications that can be ascribed to gallstones. In contrast, symptoms such as fatty food intolerance, 'dyspepsia', eructation, flatulence, pyrosis, bad breath and vague epigastric discomfort occur with equal frequency in patients with and without gallstones. Such non-specific symptomatology should not be taken as an indication that gallstones are causing symptoms. It is probable that about 15% of all patients with cholelithiasis are identified not because they have specific symptoms but rather because they have complained to their medical practitioner of a variety of these non-specific symptoms that have served as an indication for an oral cholecystogram which subsequently demonstrates gallstones. If the 50% of all patients whose stones are discovered at autopsy are excluded together with the 5% discovered incidentally and the 15% whose stones are not giving rise to true symptoms, a hard core of 35% of patients remains who have genuine signs and symptoms or complications which develop as a result of cholelithiasis.

PAIN

If a gallstone becomes acutely impacted in the cystic duct or common bile duct the patient will experience pain as the gallbladder responds by contracting down in an attempt to expel the stone. The term gallbladder or biliary 'colic' is a misnomer, because the pain does not increase and decrease in intensity (as occurs in intestinal colic). Instead, the pain is of sudden onset, is severe and constant for up to three hours and does not have the characteristic waxing and waning element of colic. The characteristics of the pain cannot distinguish between stones occluding the cystic duct, and those in the common bile duct. The pain lasts less than an hour in 40% of patients. Should the pain continue for more than 6 hours it is probable that some other complication such as cholecystitis or pancreatitis has developed.

The pain of biliary origin is usually located in the epigastrium or upper right quadrant and classically radiates to the infrascapular region or tip of the right scapula. The patient frequently describes the pain as band-like, extending round the upper abdomen, and through into the back. Less commonly, discomfort is experienced in the lower chest, when it may be confused with intrathoracic diseases such as oesophagitis, myocardial infarction or a dissecting aneurysm. Conversely, the pain associated with myocardial infarction or ischaemia may be upper abdominal and band-like and may mimic gallbladder disease. It is less well recognized that biliary colic pain may occasionally be felt predominantly or exclusively in the left upper quadrant, which may suggest a high posterior gastric ulcer, pancreatitis or even renal disease especially when the pain radiates into the back.

One of the commonest conditions to be confused with biliary disease is a variant of the irritable bowel syndrome, which is sometimes referred to as the 'hepatic flexure syndrome'. In this disorder the symptoms of fatty intolerance and right hypochondrial pain radiating into the back appears indistinguishable from those of gallbladder disease but the association with other symptoms such as abdominal bloating, alternating diarrhoea and constipation, and the fact that the pain is relieved by defecation should suggest a diagnosis of functional colonic disorder rather than gallstones. Typical biliary pain associated with an elevation of serum conjugated bilirubin, alkaline phosphatase or transaminase is virtually diagnostic of biliary tract disease; bilirubin and alkaline phosphatase levels are higher in common duct obstruction than in cystic duct obstruction.

The consequences of gallstones in the gallbladder include acute cholecystitis, chronic cholecystitis, empyema of the gallbladder, fistulas and choledocholithiasis, all of which are described below.

NON-SURGICAL TREATMENT

Following the demonstration by Langenbuch in 1881 that cholecystectomy could be undertaken safely, the treatment of gallstone disease has been primarily by surgical techniques. The recent introduction of agents that can safely dissolve gallstones and the advent of lithotripsy have added new dimensions to managing this common and economically important disorder. There is a danger that we will become overwhelmed by a prodigality of treatments and techniques (*Table 12.7*) but it is important to appreciate that the different forms of therapy, whether they be surgical or non-surgical, should not be seen in competition because gastroenterologists are now in the happy position of being able to select from a variety of procedures the one that will be most suitable for the individual patient.[1]

The main methods of treating gallstones by non-surgical techniques include the use of oral bile salts, Rowachol, inhibitors of cholesterol metabolism, extracorporeal shock wave lithotripsy and agents which work by contact dissolution. There have been a number of recent reviews of non-surgical management of gallstones and these contain an extensive bibliography to which the reader is referred.[8,13,27] Medical treatment will first be discussed, followed by extracorporeal shock wave lithotripsy.

Table 12.7 Treatment of gallstones

Treatment	Applicable to
No treatment Open abdominal surgery Minimal scar surgery (percutaneous cholecystolithotomy) Laparoscopic cholecystectomy	All gallstones
Oral dissolution Lithotripsy and oral dissolution Contact dissolution	Cholesterol gallstones
Endoscopic retrograde cholangiopancreatography plus contact dissolution Percutaneous rotary lithotripsy Chemical cholecystectomy – gallbladder ablation	New techniques

MEDICAL TREATMENT OF GALLBLADDER STONES

Oral dissolution therapy

There are no chemical methods known for effectively dissolving pigment gallstones and the various forms of treatment listed below apply solely to cholesterol stones.

Three bile acid preparations are in general use to dissolve cholesterol gallstones: chenodeoxycholic acid, ursodexycholic acid and a combination of the two.

Chenodeoxycholic acid

The pioneer studies by Danziger and his colleagues in 1972 demonstrating that chenodeoxycholic acid could dissolve cholesterol gallstones initiated the modern era of oral dissolution of gallstones. Chenodeoxycholic acid is a naturally occurring dihydroxy bile acid with hydroxyl groups in the 3α and 7α positions. Absorption occurs to some extent in the jejunum by passive non-ionic diffusion but is mainly via an active transport system situated in the distal ileum. Chenodeoxycholic acid enters the enterohepatic circulation and is excreted in the bile after being conjugated to glycine or taurine. The majority of the conjugated chenodeoxycholic acid is reabsorbed in the distal ileum but some is deconjugated by intestinal bacteria, part is reabsorbed to mix with the pool of endogenous chenodeoxycholic acid while the remainder is dehydroxylated in the 7α position by colonic bacteria to form the monohydroxy lithocholic acid. This is a toxic bile acid but, fortunately, most of it is lost in the stool, one-fifth being reabsorbed, conjugated and sulphated in the liver and thereafter secreted into bile to be lost from the body in the stool. Chenodeoxycholic acid is a potent suppressor of cholesterol biosynthesis and causes a significant decrease in the hepatic HMG-CoA reductase level. Chenodeoxycholic acid also decreases to some extent intestinal absorption of cholesterol. The drug reduces cholesterol saturation of bile mainly by suppressing endogenous bile acid synthesis and hepatic cholesterogenesis. Chenodeoxycholic acid is effective in a dose of 12–15 mg/kg per day but larger doses may be required in the obese patient.

Ursodeoxycholic acid

Like chenodeoxycholic acid, ursodeoxycholic acid is a naturally occurring bile acid which is found to a small extent in human bile. It is the 7β epimer of chenodeoxycholic acid and undergoes a similar enterohepatic circulation. Absorption is less complete and, on full therapeutic doses, ursodeoxycholic acid comprises only 50% of the total bile acid pool. Ursodeoxycholic acid suppresses neither cholesterol nor bile acid biosynthesis and its main mechanism of action is to diminish intestinal absorption of cholesterol. The usual therapeutic dose is 8–10 mg/kg per day.

Because of the potential toxic side-effects of chenodeoxycholic acid (see below), ursodeoxycholic acid has more or less replaced chenodeoxycholic acid when single bile salt therapy is given.

Chenodeoxycholic acid and ursodeoxycholic acid differ in the way in which they remove cholesterol from gallstones. Chenodeoxycholic acid solubilizes cholesterol into a micellar phase. Ursodeoxycholic acid enhances the transport of cholesterol in the liquid crystalline phase as well as into mixed micelles. Ursodeoxycholic acid has the additional benefit of prolonging cholesterol crystal nucleation and retarding the growth of crystals.[34,70]

Combination therapy

Because of the potential side-effects of chenodeoxycholic acid, and the differing modes of action to solubilize cholesterol between chenodeoxycholic acid and ursodeoxycholic acid, it is common practice to prescribe these two drugs in combination.[52,56] The dose of each bile acid used in combination therapy is 5–7 mg/kg per day. The combination treatment reduces the daily cost by 25% because ursodeoxycholic acid is about twice as expensive as chenodeoxycholic acid. Two other factors improve the efficacy of therapy: a low-cholesterol diet may enhance the effect of oral bile acid therapy, and the bile acids should be given as a single dose at night-time. Overnight there is an interruption of the enterohepatic circulation of bile salts and an increase in the secretion of supersaturated bile. The bed-time administration of bile acids prevents this and improves the potential for gallstone dissolution.[38]

Unwanted effects

Chenodeoxycholic acid does have a few side-effects, most of which are of little consequence but have led to the drug being less favoured than ursodeoxycholic acid. The most important is a dose-dependent diarrhoea which occurs in 30–60% of patients, and is easily correctible by withdrawing the drug and reintroducing it at a lower dose. The other major side-effect is mild hypertransaminasaemia, which occurs in 30% of patients. There is, in addition, a modest increase in low-density lipoprotein cholesterol. Ursodeoxycholic acid, on the other hand, is completely free of side-effects, with no significant changes taking place in fasting serum lipids or liver biochemical tests.[24] Mixed ursodeoxycholic and chenodeoxycholic acid therapy is free from toxic side-effects. There is no evidence that, used in the dose and duration which is commonly prescribed for treating gallstones, oral bile acid has any risk of carcinogenesis in the gastrointestinal tract.

Patient selection

Patients suitable for bile acid therapy should have a functioning gallbladder as demonstrated by oral cholecystography. The gallstones must be radiolucent for this suggests that they are formed mainly of cholesterol. Unfortunately, about 25% of radiolucent stones are pigment stones and there is, as yet, no accurate method for detecting these stones, which are not amenable to oral bile salt therapy. Rambow *et al.*[53] have suggested that computed tomography may be a way of differentiating between cholesterol and pigment stones and confirmation of this important observation is eagerly awaited.[53] Gallstones that are calcified will also fail to solubilize on bile salt therapy. Calcification may be detected on plain radiography of the abdomen but this is not sufficiently accurate for clinical purposes and many stones are identified as being non-responsive to therapy because of their high calcium content which has not been identified on a plain radiograph. Recent observations suggest that computed tomography may serve a very useful role and that stones which have attenuation values greater than 100 Hounsfield units contain sufficient calcium to prevent complete dissolution with bile salts.

Stone size is important and stones should be less than 15 mm in diameter. The patient should not be suffering from acute symptoms. Women who are fertile should be taking adequate contraceptive precautions.

Efficacy

The overall efficacy of oral dissolution is difficult to determine because of different points of entry into the various studies and the differing ways of expressing outcome, such as partial dissolution or complete dissolution or intention to treat. Most studies do not indicate whether ideal conditions for dissolution such as bile unsaturation have been achieved. The likelihood of successful dissolution in compliant patients is around 60%; but a more realistic figure is between 30–40% of patients using chenodeoxycholic acid and 20–30% on ursodeoxycholic acid.[24] Dissolution may be faster initially with combined therapy but there is no evidence that this is more effective than using a single bile acid.

Response to treatment

Stones of 5–10 mm diameter usually dissolve within 1–2 years and smaller stones may do so within 6–12 months. Obese patients are more resistant to therapy and may require doses of up to 20 mg/kg per day of chenodeoxycholic acid or 13 mg/kg per day of ursodeoxycholic acid. Regular 6-month ultrasound or cholecystography follow-up is necessary. It usually takes 6 months before there is any change in the size of gallstones and treatment is unlikely to be effective if no reduction in size is observed after 1 year of continuous therapy. The risk of gallstone complications is not increased during stone dissolution.

Disadvantages

Despite their inherent attraction, cholelitholytic drugs have not proved popular in clinical use. Fewer than 30% of all patients with gallstones fulfil the criteria for oral dissolution therapy, and factors such as obesity and failure to comply may cause the figure to be as low as 10%. The duration of treatment is a problem too because gallstones may take up to 24 months to dissolve. Furthermore, the gallbladder may become non-functioning on oral cholecystography, possibly because of impaction of a stone in the cystic duct, or the stone may become calcified. In both these events, oral therapy becomes ineffective. Another problem is the inevitable and inappropriate treatment of radiolucent stones which are formed by bilirubin and which will not respond to bile acid therapy. Recurrence is a problem, and this is discussed below.

However, the advent of extracorporeal shockwave lithotripsy has been a new stimulus to the use of bile acid therapy and all patients undergoing lithotripsy are given bile acids shortly before lithotripsy. The therapy is continued until all stone fragments have disappeared.

Rowachol

This is an inexpensive preparation of six cyclic monoturpines (menthol, menthone, pinene, borneol, camphene and cineol) in olive oil. It has choleretic and spasmolytic properties and has been used to treat cholesterol stones in the gallbladder and bile ducts at a dose of one capsule per 10 kg body weight per day. The duration of treatment is similar to that for the bile acids. Rowachol has been combined with bile acids in a dose of one capsule twice daily. The preparation has been recommended for use on its own or in combination with bile acids to treat gallstones or for use in patients who have undergone extracorporeal shockwave therapy and thereafter require cholelitholytic drugs. Rowachol works by altering the saturation of bile[40] and also preventing the formation of cholesterol crystals. To date, Rowachol has not been used widely in the management of gallstones.

HMG-CoA reductase inhibitors

The recent introduction of agents which competitively inhibit HMG-CoA reductase such as Lovastatin and Simvastatin have added a new dimension to oral dissolution therapy.[41,55] Limited experience with these drugs suggests that these inhibitors do not affect other enzymes involving cholesterol metabolism such as cholesterol 7-α-hydroxylase, and acyl-Coenzyme A-cholesterol acyltransferase (ACAT). These agents may be used alone or in combination with ursodeoxycholic acid to produce a more powerful combination to dissolve gallstones. Further studies are necessary to determine whether these agents are effective, safe and will have a role in gallstone therapy.

Direct contact dissolution

Two agents have been used particularly to dissolve gallstones, methyl tert-butyl ether, which has been used to dissolve cholesterol gallbladder stones, and monooctanoin, which has been used in the dissolution of cholesterol stones lodged in the common bile duct.

Methyl tert-butyl ether

This is an alkyl ether differing from deithyl ether in that it remains liquid at body temperature (boiling point 55°C in contrast to 35°C for diethyl ether). It is a highly effective solvent for cholesterol but has no effect on pigment stones. Experimental studies demonstrate that the agent does not cause significant damage to the gallbladder mucosa. It is delivered by percutaneous transhepatic catheterization and will dissolve virtually all cholesterol stones that are radiolucent on computed tomography, leaving only a small residue of non-cholesterol debris such as calcium bilirubinate. However, the problem is that the remaining debris can form the nidus for new stone formation. In contrast to oral dissolution therapy and extracorporeal shock wave lithotripsy, stone number or size is not a contraindication to direct contact dissolution with methyl tert-butyl ether. The technique of percutaneous transhepatic catheterization is familiar to most experienced interventional radiologists and, using small volumes of around 5 ml of methyl tert-butyl ether, the gallbladder is continually infused and aspirated using glass syringes. Automatic pump systems are being developed to induce vigorous stirring of the gallbladder contents which will achieve more rapid fragmentation of stones. Most cholesterol gallstones can be removed in one session.[72]

Methyl tert-butyl ether is inflammatory and potentially explosive and a general anaesthetic and therefore must be used in small volumes and all spillage avoided. Overflow from the gallbladder into the duodenum can cause anaesthesia and duodenitis. Other complications include bleeding from the gallbladder, intravascular haemolysis, and a painful bile leakage from the transhepatic catheter site. This latter complication can be avoided by using a Gelfoam plug in the transhepatic tract.[28] Poor results are obtained if gallstones contain significant amounts of calcium or pigment. Methyl tert-butyl ether is not used to dissolve retained cholesterol bile duct stones because of the danger that it will cause duodenitis or that systemic absorption will lead to anaesthesia.

Monooctanoin

This agent is used to dissolve retained cholesterol gallstones in the bile duct and is discussed below.

Stone recurrence

Experience with all forms of non-surgical gallstone treatment such as bile acid therapy, methyl tert-butyl ether and extracorporeal shock wave lithotripsy indicates clearly that, as long as the gallbladder remains in situ after gallstones have been eradicated, the stones may recur. It appears that the recurrence rate is similar regardless of how the stones have been treated. Bile will return to the supersaturated state within 4 weeks of discontinuing bile acid therapy. The recurrence rate is then about 10% per year for the first 3–5 years, after which further stones do not develop. The overall recurrence rate is 50%; but the other way of interpreting the results is that 50% of patients have been cured. Gallstones recur three times more frequently in patients who have had multiple stones prior to stone dissolution compared to those with single stones. The stones that recur are usually asymptomatic.[48,58,76]

There is no accepted method of preventing gallstone recurrence, which remains a problem to be resolved. Recurrence must be considered when comparing different methods of treating gallstones, some of which leave the gallbladder in situ. Low-dose bile acid therapy, low-cholesterol diets or high-fibre diets have all proved ineffective in preventing recurrence. There has been no widespread acceptance of long-term full-dose bile acid therapy except in those patients who have serious medical problems where life expectancy is reduced.

The management of patients in whom stones have been completely dissolved has yet to be established but currently it is suggested that they be followed 6-monthly with an ultrasonogram so that small stones can be identified and bile acid treatment instituted immediately. Most stones which recur are asymptomatic, and also of the same composition as the stones originally present in the gallbladder. Prompt treatment of small recurrent stones enables short courses of therapy to be given which are highly effective. Patients receiving bile acid therapy or any other form of treatment which does not remove the gallbladder thus require long-term surveillance even after the stones have dissolved, and this is one of the drawbacks of all of these treatments compared with cholecystectomy.

MANAGEMENT OF ASYMPTOMATIC GALLSTONES

While there is no doubt that symptomatic gallstones require treatment, there is no consensus regarding the management of asymptomatic gallstones. Epidemiological evidence indicates that only a minority of patients with gallstones will become symptomatic and that the onset of symptoms is seldom urgent or severe (see above). Thus, many gastroenterologists believe that asymptomatic stones should not be treated.[23] There are exceptions, however, and this applies particularly to those populations in which there is a greater risk of gallbladder cancer developing in association with gallstones such as the Chilean and Pima Indian populations, and patients who have very large but asymptomatic gallstones. In addition, it has been suggested that patients with diabetes mellitus, who, it is claimed, have a higher prevalence of postoperative complications following cholecystectomy, should undergo elective cholecystectomy for silent stones rather than waiting for symptoms to develop. This view is controversial.

There is, however, another school of thought which believes that most silent stones should be treated. This applies particularly to those patients who have been told of the presence of gallstones and become anxious as a consequence. The ease with which non-invasive or minimally invasive techniques can be used to remove the gallstones has encouraged some gastroenterologists to recommend that all gallstones should be treated whether symptomatic or not. This view is not held by the author.

At one time it could be argued that the risks of cholecystectomy meant that a prophylactic cholecystectomy could not be recommended for treating asymptomatic gallstones. Cholecystectomy has now become a very safe operation in most major medical centres. Using decision analysis to study whether or not patients with asymptomatic stones would benefit from a cholecystectomy, Friedman *et al.* concluded that there was little reason either to accept or reject early elective cholecystectomy for asymptomatic stones purely on the basis of average survival.[22] Two factors could determine whether or not patients with asymptomatic stones should be treated: (1) the preference of the patient and (2) the high cost to society of treating all patients with gallstones with a routine elective cholecystectomy.

MEDICAL TREATMENT OF COMMON BILE DUCT STONES

The introduction of endoscopic sphincterotomy has revolutionized the treatment of stones in the common bile duct, and has largely replaced gallstone dissolution using cholelitholytic agents or extraction via a T-tube tract.[33] Extracorporeal shock wave lithotripsy is a newly introduced and highly effective method of dealing with common bile duct stones.

Monooctanoin (Capmul and Moctanin)

This viscous agent comprises about 70% glyceryl monooctanoate and 30% glyceryl dioctanoate with traces of glyceryl trioctanoate and caprilic acid. Before use, monooctanoin is diluted with water in a ratio of 10:90 parts of oil and infused into the common bile duct at a rate of 3–5 ml/h using a drip or infusion pump. It is important that the pressure does not exceed 12 cm of monooctanoin. The agent can be administered either via a T-tube drain or a nasobiliary catheter or a catheter positioned in the bile duct via the percutaneous transhepatic route. Infusion should be upstream from the stones. The time for dissolution is between 1 and 3 weeks. Monooctanoin is irritating to the biliary and gastrointestinal mucosa and can induce pulmonary oedema. The duration of therapy, the potential for side-effects, and the introduction of more convenient forms of treating bile duct stones has meant that monooctanoin is used to a limited extent only in current gastroenterological practice.[69]

TREATMENT OF CALCIUM AND PIGMENT STONES

No effective method other than cholecystectomy exists for treating calcium-containing gallstones or those composed primarily of brown or black pigment. Although there is much work under way to develop agents which will dissolve these stones, none is as yet effective. Glyceryl monooctanoate, Palmidrol, Pluronic F-68, bile salts, methyl hexyl ether and urea EDTA (ethylenediaminetetraacetic acid) have all been used singly or in combination in an attempt to dissolve these stones. No effective combination or dose is available. The regimens are complicated and experience is limited presently to only one or two centres.

EXTRACORPOREAL SHOCK WAVE LITHOTRIPSY

Successful gallstone fragmentation by extracorporeal shock wave lithotripsy was first reported in patients in 1986.[60] Since then it has been shown to be a relatively safe and effective method of treatment in the short term in selected cases,[31,39,54,57] and the vast majority of patients can now be treated on an outpatient basis. Oral bile salt therapy is additionally necessary for complete elimination of fragments.

Principles

The fragmentation of a gallstone is dependent on the amount of energy generated when focused shock waves converge on it. Shock waves behave in a similar manner to ultrasound waves and obey the laws of acoustics. The important and unique features of different types of shock wave are:

1. Energy density (or pressure).
2. Focal zone (area volume with over 50% of the peak pressure).
3. Energy of each pulse (integration of the energy density over the duration of the shock wave).

The shock wave is in the shape of a sharp spike with a prolonged tail. The positive pressure front is generated in nanoseconds and lasts for about 1 ms. This is followed by a negative pressure front of lower amplitude, but longer duration, which may give rise to cavitation. Shock waves are normally generated in degassed water to avoid dissipation of energy. Water is also used as the coupling agent with the skin; the impedence of soft tissues is similar so that little energy is lost (less than 3%/cm).

It is important to avoid solid tissues such as the ribs, vertebral column and the liver and also tissues with a large air content such as the gastrointestinal tract and the lungs. Pain is dependent upon the energy density and the area of the skin through which the shock waves are focused. Thus, shock waves of a lower energy density delivered over a wide area are relatively pain-free.

Types of shock wave generators (*Figure 12.45*)

Spark gap[57,60]

An electric current is passed between two electrodes, which produces an explosion. An elliptical reflector is used to focus the shock waves. The first-generation machines required powerful analgesia for use (general anaesthetic or epidural analgesia, or parenteral opiate analgesia) and the patient had to be partially immersed in water. Modifications including the use of a water bag have largely overcome these limitations. Gating of the electrocardiograph is required as the forward (unreflected) wave is non-focused and may therefore cause arrhythmias. The focal zone is about 6–12 mm in diameter.

Piezoelectric[31]

With this system about 4000 piezoceramic crystals are used to produce ultrasonic waves. These may be directed in a converging manner or, alternatively, focused by an acoustic lens. As these ultrasound waves converge they become more intense and transform into shock waves over the focal zone. This zone is only 3–6 mm in diameter. The final energy density is greater than for the spark gap system. Neither analgesia nor electrocardiograph gating is required.

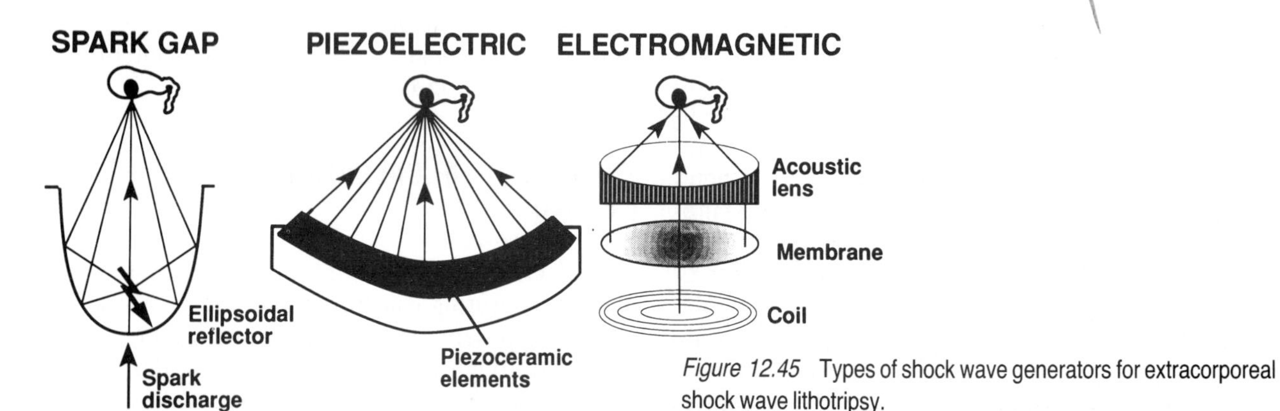

Figure 12.45 Types of shock wave generators for extracorporeal shock wave lithotripsy.

Electromagnetic[39]

The focal zone and the energy density produced by this system are intermediate to those produced by the spark gap and piezoelectric systems.

In comparing the different systems it is important to consider the total energy delivered rather than the number of pulses (shocks) given. Efficacy of treatment is dependent as much on the accuracy of focusing (fluoroscopic and/or ultrasonic) as the type of shock waves used. The shock waves are delivered anteriorly for gallbladder stones and posteriorly for bile duct stones.

Patient selection (*Table 12.8*)

The selection criteria for patients with gallbladder stones for extracorporeal shock wave lithotripsy have been devised to maximize the efficiency of treatment and minimize serious complications (extracorporeal shock wave lithotripsy for bile duct stones is discussed on p. 1728). A functioning gallbladder is necessary for the efficacy of bile acid therapy. Non-calcified stones of the cholesterol variety fragment much better than calcified stones. Thus, significant calcification seen on a plain radiograph or by computed tomography is a contra-indication to treatment. Shock wave treatment in most patients produces maximum stone fragments of 2–6 mm, so that patients with stones of this size can be treated by oral dissolution therapy without recourse to extracorporeal shock wave lithotripsy. Early reports that pre-existing gallbladder motility shows no correlation with stone clearance[67] have been contradicted. The patient's habitus and position of the gallbladder also have important bearings on outcome. Obesity and a gallbladder high up above the costal margin will interfere with treatment in up to 18% of patients.

Because petechiae are a complication of extracorporeal shock wave lithotripsy, patients with a bleeding tendency are excluded. The effect of shock waves on the diseased liver is not known. Because repeat oral and cholecystographic studies are required, allergy to contrast agents is an exclusion criterion. Complicated gallstone disease should be avoided.

Using the above criteria, probably no more than 30%, possibly only 15–20%, of patients referred for extracorporeal shock wave lithotripsy are suitable for treatment. Reasons for exclusion include more than three stones (44%), failure to visualize the gallbladder (17%), calcified stones (15%), stone diameter over 30 mm (10%) and inability to focus the shock waves (2%).[5] More liberal criteria of stone number and size are being tried, but this may be at the expense of reduced efficacy.[19]

Efficacy

Oral dissolution should be started in the week before shock wave delivery and continued for at least 3 months afterwards, and certainly until all stone fragments are clear. Several treatment sessions may be required. Assessment of stone clearance is most accurate with a combination of ultrasonography and oral cholecystography. Successful clearance of stones depends both upon the dissolution of fragments as well as ejection from the gallbladder and bile duct. In the experience of the Munich group, complete clearance was achieved in 63% of patients at 4–8 months and in 91% at 12–18 months. Ninety-six per cent of patients with a single stone achieved clearance at this time compared to only 67% of patients with two or three stones.[57]

Complications include biliary colic (35%), which can occur up to 18 months after extracorporeal shock wave lithotripsy, and acute pancreatitis (1%) necessitating endoscopic sphincterotomy for extraction of fragments from the bile duct.[57]

With the spark gap lithotriptor, cutaneous petechiae occur in 14% and transient haematuria in 3% of patients. A slight fever and a leukocytosis may

Table 12.8 Selection and exclusion criteria of patients with extracorporeal shock wave lithotripsy of gallbladder stones

Inclusion criteria	*Exclusion criteria*
1. A history of biliary colic	1. Coagulopathy or anticoagulation therapy, aspirin, non-steroidal anti-inflammatory drugs
2. A functioning gallbladder on oral cholecystography	2. Allergy to contrast media
3. One, two or three stones with a total diameter of >30 mm	3. Liver disease
4. No calcification except for a fine rim or small nidus (<3 mm)	4. Pregnancy
5. No cysts or aneurysms in the shock wave path	5. Pacemaker or significant arrhythmia
6. Positioning of the patient avoiding bone and lungs in the shock wave path	6. Gastric or peptic ulcer
	7. Presence of acute pancreatitis, acute cholecystitis, cholangitis and choledocholithiasis

occur immediately after treatment, but acute cholecystitis is rare. There may be fewer side-effects with piezoceramic lithotripsy, but 66% of patients require more than two treatments compared to 5% for spark gap lithotripsy.[31,57,60] Examination of the gallbladders in patients who have subsequently undergone cholecystectomy shows that there is bruising and partial loss of the mucosa early on, but little abnormality later on (other than the expected changes of chronic cholecystitis).[71]

REFERENCES

1. Acalovschi, M., Baden, R., Dumitrascu, D. and Varga, C. (1988) Prevalence of gallstones in liver cirrhosis: a sonographic survey. *American Journal of Gastroenterology*, **83**, 954–956.
2. Angelico, M. and The Rome Group for Epidemiology and Prevention of Cholelithiasis (GREPCO) (1988) The epidemiology of gallstone disease in Rome, Italy. Part II. Factors associated with disease. *Hepatology*, **8**, 907–913.
3. Attili, A.F. and The Rome Group for the Epidemiology and Prevention of Cholelithiasis (GREPCO) (1987) *Digestive Diseases and Sciences*, **32**, 349–353.
4. Attili, A.F. and The Rome Group for the Epidemiology and Prevention of Cholelithiasis (GREPCO) (1988) The epidemiology of gallstone disease in Rome, Italy. Part I. Prevalence data in men. *Hepatology*, **8**, 904–909.
5. Barbara, L., Samo, C., Labate, A.M.M. *et al.* (1987) A population study on the prevalence of gallstone disease: the Sirmione study. *Hepatology*, **7**, 913–917.
6. Bateson, M.C. (1984) Gallbladder disease and the cholecystectomy rate are independently variable. *The Lancet*, **ii**, 621–624.
7. Bateson, M.C. and Bouchier, I.A.D. (1992) Unpublished data.
8. Bolondi, L., Gaiani, S., Testa, S. and Labo, G. (1985) Gallbladder sludge formation during prolonged fasting after gastrointestinal surgery. *Gut*, **26**, 734–738.
9. Bouchier, I.A.D. (1969) Postmortem study of the frequency of gall stones in patients with cirrhosis of the liver. *Gut*, **10**, 705–710.
10. Bouchier, I.A.D. (1988) Gallstones: formation and epidemiology. In *Surgery of the Liver and Biliary Tree* (Ed.) Blumgart, L. pp. 503–516. Edinburgh: Churchill Livingstone.
11. Bouchier, I.A.D. (1988) Non-surgical treatment of gallstones: many contenders but who will win the crown? *Gut*, **29**, 137–142.
12. Bouchier, I.A.D. (1990) Gall stones. *British Medical Journal*, **300**, 592–597.
13. Bouchier, I.A.D., Rhodes, K. and Brien, M. (1968) A study of symptomatic and “silent” gallstones. *Scandinavian Journal of Gastroenterology*, **3**, 299–304.
14. Cahalane, M.J., Neubrand, M.W. and Carey, M.C. (1988) Physical–chemical pathogenesis of pigment gallstones. *Seminars in Liver Disease*, **8**, 317–328.
15. Cano, F., Cicero, F., Ranieri, R., Martin, J. and Di Costanzo, J. (1986) Ultrasonographic study of gallbladder motility during total parenteral nutrition. *Gastroenterology*, **91**, 313–317.
16. Cattey, R.P. and Wilson, S.D. (1989) Cholelithiasis follows total gastrectomy in Zollinger–Ellison syndrome. *Surgery*, **106**, 1070–1073.
17. Crichlow, R.W., Seltzer, M.H. and Jannetta, P.T. (1972) Cholecystitis in adolescents. *American Journal of Digestive Diseases*, **17**, 68–72.
18. Cucchiaro, G., Rossitch, J.C., Bowie, J. *et al.* (1990) Clinical significance of ultrasonographically detected coincidental gallstones. *Digestive Diseases and Science*, **35**, 417–421.
19. Darzi, A., Monson, J.R.T., O’Morain, C., Tanner, W.A. and Keane, F.B.V. (1989) Extension of selection criteria for extracorporeal shock wave lithotripsy for gall stones. *British Medical Journal*, **299**, 302–303.
20. Diehl, A.K., Haffner, S.M., Knapp, J.A. Hazuda, H.P. and Stern, M.P. (1989). Dietary intake and the prevalence of gallbladder disease in Mexican Americans. *Gastroenterology*, **97**, 1527–1533.
21. Dunnington, G., Alfrey, E., Sampliner, R., Kogan, F. and Putman, C. (1987) Natural history of cholelithiasis in patients with alcoholic cirrhosis (Cholelithiasis in cirrhotic patients). *Annals of Surgery*, **205**, 226–229.
22. Friedman, G.D., Raviola, C.A. and Fireman, B. (1989) Prognosis of gallstones with mild or no symptoms: 25 years of follow-up in a health maintenance organisation. *Journal of Clinical Epidemiology*, **42**, 127–136.
23. Gibney, E.J. (1990) Asymptomatic gallstones. *British Journal of Surgery*, **77**, 368–372.
24. Gleeson, D., Ruppin, D.C., Saunders, A., Murphy, G.M. and Dowling, R.H. (1990). Final outcome of ursodeoxycholic acid treatment in 126 patients with radiolucent gallstones. *Quarterly Journal of Medicine*, **76**, 711–729.
25. Gracie, W.A. and Ransohoff, D.F. (1982) The natural history of silent gallstones. *New England Journal of Medicine*, **307**, 798–800.
26. Hawkins, P.E., Graham, F.B. and Holliday, P. (1966) Gallbladder disease in children. *American Journal of Surgery*, **111**, 741–744.
27. Hayes, P.C., Patrick, A., Roulston, J.E. *et al.* (1992) Gall stones in diabetes mellitus: prevalence and risk factors. *European Journal of Gastroenterology and Hepatology*, **4**, 55–59.
28. Hellstern, A., Leuschner, M., Frenk, H., Dillinger, H.W. *et al.* (1990) Gallstone dissolution with methyl tert-butyl ether: how to avoid complications. *Gut*, **31**, 922–925.
29. Henriksson, P., Einharsson, K., Eriksson, A., Kelter, U. and Angelin, B. (1989) Estrogen-induced gallstone formation in males. *Journal of Clinical Investigation*, **84**, 811–816.

30. Hofmann, A.F. (1989) Medical dissolution of gallstones by oral bile acid therapy. *American Journal of Surgery*, **158**, 198–294.
31. Hood, K.A., Keightley, A., Dowling, R.H., Dick, J.A. and Mallinson, C.N. (1988) Piezo-ceramic lithotripsy of gallbladder stones: initial experience in 38 patients. *The Lancet*, **ii**, 1322–1324.
32. Hughes, R.G. and Mayell, M.J. (1975) Cholelithiasis in a neonate. *Archives of Disease in Childhood*, **50**, 815–816.
33. Johnson, A.G. and Hosking, S.W. (1987) Appraisal of the management of bile duct stones. *British Journal of Surgery*, **74**, 555–560.
34. Jungst, D., Brenner, G., Pratschke, E. and Paumgartner, G. (1989) Low-dose ursodeoxycholic acid prolongs cholesterol nucleation time in gallbladder bile of patients with cholesterol gallstones. *Journal of Hepatology*, **8**, 1–6.
35. Kaufman, H.S., Magnuson, T.H., Lillemoe, K.D., Frasca, P. and Pitt, H.A. (1989) The role of bacteria in gallbladder and common duct stone formation. *Annals of Surgery*, **209**, 584–592.
36. Laakso, M., Suhonen, M., Julkunen, R. and Pyorala, K. (1990) Plasma insulin, serum lipids and lipoproteins in gall stone disease in non-insulin dependent diabetic subjects: a case control study. *Gut*, **31**, 344–347.
37. Lanzini, A. and Northfield, T.C. (1990) Bile acid therapy. *Alimentary Pharmacology and Therapy*, **4**, 1–24.
38. Lanzini, A., Facchinetti, D. and Northfield, T.C. (1988) Maintenance of hepatic bile acid secretion rate during overnight fasting by bedtime bile acid administration. *Gastroenterology*, **95**, 1029–1035.
39. Lee, S.H. and Burhenne, H.J. (1990) Symptoms after gallbladder clearance with biliary lithotripsy. *The Lancet*, **335**, 1108.
40. Leiss, O. and von Bergmann, K. (1985) Effects of Rowachol on biliary lipid secretion and serum lipids in normal volunteers. *Gut*, **26**, 32–37.
41. Logan, G.M. and Duane, W.C. (1990) Lovastatin added to ursodeoxycholic acid further reduces biliary cholesterol saturation. *Gastroenterology*, **98**, 1572–1576.
42. Lucariello, A., Francica, G., Morante, R. *et al.* (1989) Cholelithiasis and chronic liver disease. *Italian Journal of Gastroenterology*, **21**, 59–63.
43. Maclure, K.M., Hayes, K.C., Colditz, G.A. *et al.* (1989) Weight, diet and the risk of symptomatic gallstones in middle-aged women. *New England Journal of Medicine*, **321**, 563–569.
44. McSherry, C.K., Ferstenberg, H., Calhoun, W.F., Lahman, E. and Virshup, M. (1985) The natural history of diagnosed gallstone disease in symptomatic and asymptomatic patients. *Annals of Surgery*, **202**, 59–63.
45. Messing, B., Bories, C., Kunstlinger, F. and Bernier, J.J. (1983) Does total parenteral nutrition induce gallbladder sludge formation and lithiasis? *Gastroenterology*, **84**, 1012–1019.
46. Mok, H.Y.I., Druffel, E.R.M. and Rampone, W.M. (1986) Chronology of cholelithiasis. *New England Journal of Medicine*, **314**, 1075–1077.
47. Maurer, K.R., Everhart, J.E., Ezzati, T.M., Johannes, R.S. *et al.* (1989) Prevalence of gallstone disease in Hispanic populations in the United States. *Gastroenterology*, **96**, 487–492.
48. O'Donnell, L.D.J. and Heaton, K.W. (1988) Recurrence and re-recurrence of gall stones after medical dissolution: a long term follow up. *Gut*, **29**, 655–658.
49. Palasciano, G., Portincasa, P., Vinciguerra, V. *et al.* (1989) Gallstone prevalence and gallbladder volume in children and adolescents. *American Journal of Gastroenterology*, **84**, 1378–1382.
50. Petitti, D.B., Sidney, S. and Perlman, J.A. (1988) Increased risk of cholecystectomy in users of supplemental estrogen. *Gastroenterology*, **94**, 91–95.
51. Pixley, F. and Mann, J. (1988) Dietary factors in the aetiology of gall stones: a case control study. *Gut*, **29**, 1511–1515.
52. Podda, M., Zuin, M., Battezzati, P.M. *et al.* (1989) Efficacy and safety of a combination of chenodeoxycholic acid and ursodeoxycholic acid for gallstone dissolution: a comparison with ursodeoxycholic acid alone. *Gastroenterology*, **96**, 222–229.
53. Rambow, A., Staritz, A., Wosiewitz, U. *et al.* (1990) Analysis of radiolucent gallstones by computed tomography for in vivo estimation of stone components. *European Journal of Clinical Investigation*, **20**, 475–478.
54. Rege, R.V., Nemcek, A.A. and Nahrwold, D.L. (1989) Selection of patients for gallstone lithotripsy. *American Journal of Surgery*, **158**, 184–187.
55. Reihner, E., Rudling, M., Stahlberg, D. *et al.* (1990) Influence of provastatin, a specific inhibitor of HMG-CoA reductase, on hepatic metabolism of cholesterol. *New England Journal of Medicine*, **323**, 224–228.
56. Roehrkasse, R., Fromm, H., Malavolti, M., Tunuguntla, A.K. and Ceryak, S. (1986) Gallstone dissolution treatment with a combination of chenodeoxycholic and ursodeoxycholic acids. *Digestive Diseases and Sciences*, **31**, 1032–1040.
57. Sackmann, M., Delius, M., Sauerbruch, T. *et al.* (1988) Shock wave lithotripsy of gallbladder stones. The first 175 patients. *New England Journal of Medicine*, **318**, 393–397.
58. Sackmann, M., Ippisch, E., Sauerbruch, T. *et al.* (1990) Early gallstone recurrence rate after successful shock-wave therapy. *Gastroenterology*, **98**, 392–396.
59. Sandler, R.S., Maule, W.F. and Baltus, M.E. (1986) Factors associated with postoperative complications in diabetes after biliary tract surgery. *Gastroenterology*, **91**, 157–162.
60. Sauerbruch, T., Delius, M., Paumgartner, G. *et al.* (1986) Fragmentation of gallstones by extracorporeal shock waves. *New England Journal of Medicine*, **314**, 818–822.

61. Schoenfield, L.J., Carulli, N., Dowling, R.H., Sama, C. and Wolpers, C. (1987) Asymptomatic gallstones: definition and treatment. *Gastroenterology International*, **1**, 25–29.
62. Scragg, R.K.R., Calvert, G.D. and Oliver, J.R. (1984) Plasma lipids and insulin in gallstone disease: a case–control study. *British Medical Journal*, **289**, 521–524.
63. Scragg, R.K.R., McMichael, A.J. and Baghurst, P.A. (1984) Diet, alcohol and relative weight in gall stone disease: a case–control study. *British Medical Journal*, **288**, 1113–1119.
64. Scragg, R.K.R., McMichael, A.J. and Seamark, R.F. (1984) Oral contraceptives, pregnancy and endogenous oestrogen in gall stone disease: a case–control study. *British Medical Journal*, **288**, 1795–19799.
65. Sears, H.F., Golden, G.T. and Horsley, S. III (1973) Cholecystitis in childhood and adolescence. *Archives of Surgery*, **106**, 651–653.
66. Soloway, R.D., Trotman, B.W. and Ostrow, J.D. (1977) Pigment stones. *Gastroenterology*, **72**, 167–182.
67. Spengler, U., Sackmann, M., Sauerbruch, T., Holl, J. and Paumgartner, G. (1989) Gallbladder motility before and after extracorporeal shock wave lithotripsy. *Gastroenterology*, **96**, 860–863.
68. Stewart, L., Smith, A.L., Pellegrini, C.A., Motson, R.W. and Way, L.W. (1987). Pigment gallstones form as a composite of bacterial microcolonies and pigment solids. *Annals of Surgery*, **206**, 242–250.
69. Summerfield, J.A. (1989) Dissolution of gallstones in the biliary tree. *Alimentary Pharmacology and Therapeutics*, **3**, 211–221.
70. Tazuma, S., Sasaki, H., Mizuno, S. *et al.* (1989) Effect of ursodeoxycholic acid administration on nucleation time in human gallbladder bile. *Gastroenterology*, **97**, 173–178.
71. Teichmann, R.K., Sauerbruch, T., Sackmann, K., Holl, J., Paumgartner, G. and Heberer, G. (1989). Surgical intervention following fragmentation of gallstones by extracorporeal shock waves. *World Journal of Surgery*, **13**, 317–320.
72. Thistle, J.L. and Petersen, B.T. (1990) Nonsurgical treatment of gallstones. *Viewpoints on Digestive Diseases*. **22**, 1–4.
73. Thistle, J.L., Cleary, P.A., Lachin, J.M. *et al.* (1984) The natural history of cholelithiasis: the National Cooperative Gallstone Study. *Annals of Internal Medicine*, **101**, 171–175.
74. Van Liessum, P.A., Hopman, W.P.M., Pieters, G.F.F.M. *et al.* (1989) Postprandial gallbladder motility during long term treatment with the long-acting somatostatin analog SMS 201-995 in acromegaly. *Journal of Clinical Endocrinology and Metabolism*, **69**, 557–562.
75. Wenckert, A. and Robertson, B. (1966) The natural course of gallstone disease. *Gastroenterology*, **50**, 376–381.
76. Villanova, N., Bazzoli, F., Taronia, F. *et al.* (1989) Gallstone recurrence after successful oral bile acid therapy. *Gastroenterology*, **97**, 726–731.

CHOLECYSTITIS AND CHOLEDOCHOLITHIASIS

J. Neoptolemos and I.A.D. Bouchier

Approximately 12% of all individuals with gallstones develop symptoms of biliary colic each year.[100] The complications of gallstones confined to the gallbladder include chronic and acute cholecystitis, empyema of the gallbladder, Mirizzi's syndrome, perforation of the gallbladder with generalized peritonitis and cholecystoenteric fistulas. Secondary complications that can ensue include pyogenic liver abscess, empyema of the thorax, subhepatic abscess and septicaemia. Spontaneous formation of a cholecystocutaneous fistula with discharge of pus and gallstones may lead to symptomatic resolution.

Perhaps 50% of patients with symptoms eventually undergo cholecystectomy;[100] of these, approximately 20% have acute cholecystitis; altogether some 8% present with jaundice. The incidence of empyema of the gallbladder may be as high as 11%[55] but is more likely to be 2.4%.[175] Mirizzi's syndrome, gallbladder perforation with free peritonitis and cholecystoenteric fistula will each contribute about 1% to complicated gallbladder stone disease.

About 10% of patients with symptomatic gallbladder stones pass small bile duct stones into the duodenum.[1] On the other hand, 15–20% of patients undergoing cholecystectomy have bile duct stones as determined by operative cholangiography.[112] The true incidence of bile duct stones is uncertain, as is the proportion of these patients that have jaundice. In one autopsy study, the incidence of choledocholithiasis was 3.8% of those patients with gallbladder stones.[84] Nearly all patients with gallstone-associated acute pancreatitis pass bile duct stones into the duodenum although few become jaundiced.[1,112] Up to 45% of patients with bile duct stones may remain asymptomatic.[106]

About 10% of patients with symptomatic bile duct stones present with acute cholangitis or 2% of all symptomatic patients with gallstones.[112] Acute pancreatitis develops in about 8% of patients with gallstones although this is 22% of those with small stones.[71] Acute pancreatitis may be present in 12–23% of patients with acute cholangitis. Conversely, acute cholangitis may occur in up to 14.4% of patients with acute pancreatitis.[118]

BENIGN DISEASES OF THE GALLBLADDER

CHRONIC CHOLECYSTITIS

Symptoms of biliary colic might develop in patients with gallstones but a group of patients with acalculous chronic cholecystitis of various aetiologies is also being increasingly recognised (see p. 1742).

Chronic gallstone cholecystitis

Aetiology

In Western patients 70% of gallbladder stones are of the cholesterol variety, the remainder being of the black pigment variety.[116] It is uncertain whether the presence of gallstones is responsible for the development of chronic cholecystitis or whether it is due to supersaturated bile and/or associated bacterial infection. There is a poor correlation between any of these factors, the degree of chronic inflammation and the level of symptoms.

Pathology

The mucosa loses its normal honeycomb appearance and becomes flattened and, initially, there is increased secretory activity by the epithelial cells. Intramural mucosal diverticula develop which extend between the muscle bundles of the gallbladder wall; these are called Rokitansky–Aschoff sinuses. The gallbladder wall becomes thickened and is associated with fibrosis and hypertrophy of the muscle coat, mucosal ulceration may be present both macroscopically and microscopically and there is a variable chronic inflammatory infiltrate. Follicular cholecystitis refers to an intense infiltration by lymphocytes arranged in aggregate patterns.

The cystic duct may become occluded by fibrosis or, more commonly, a stone impacted in Hartmann's pouch. Continued mucus secretion and resorption of bile will lead to a mucocoele (hydrops of the gallbladder). A blocked gallbladder with secondary infection may result in more serious complications (*Table 12.9*).

Table 12.9 Complications of chronic cholecystitis

Mucocoele
Empyema of the gallbladder
Acute cholecystitis
Acute on chronic cholecystitis
Gangrenous cholecystitis
Liver abscess
Subhepatitis abscess
Mirizzi's syndrome
Cholecystoduodenal fistula
Cholecystocolic fistula
Cholecystocutaneous fistula
Gallstone ileus
Porcelain gallbladder
Gallbladder carcinoma

Clinical features

The cardinal symptom is biliary colic. The pain is sudden in onset, originating in the right upper quadrant or epigastrium and usually radiating around to the back to the right scapular region; it may radiate to the left subcostal region. The pain is constant and not colicky, although the patient is restless, and lasts for at least 20 minutes and up to several hours if not treated. The patient often has nausea; vomiting if it occurs happens rather late and may terminate the attack. Attacks are brought on after a heavy meal or after a fatty snack. A night-time attack may be related to the tendency of a stone to block the cystic duct in the prone sleeping position.

Retrosternal pain of sudden onset may occur and can be misinterpreted as a myocardial infarction. Conversely, a myocardial infarction may present with the typical history and findings of a severe attack of biliary colic. An electrocardiogram is therefore important in the investigation of such patients.

On clinical examination, there is usually no pyrexia but the patient may perspire. The pulse is fast and there is no hypotension. On abdominal palpation there is usually tenderness in the epigastrium or right upper quadrant. Murphy's sign (see below) may not be clearly present. In the absence of a mucocoele, the gallbladder is not usually palpable.

So called 'biliary dyspepsia' should not be confidently ascribed to gallstones. These non-specific symptoms comprising flatulence, fullness and dyspepsia after a heavy meal are as common in patients without gallstones as those with gallstones.

Young women with the *Curtis–Fitz–Hughes syndrome* may present with the typical features of biliary colic. Occasionally there may be a rub to hear over the liver. The syndrome is caused by transcoelomic spread from the vagina (rarely the rectum) of

Neisseria gonorrhoeae and, less commonly, *Chlamydia trachomatis*.[193]

Investigations

ORAL CHOLECYSTOGRAPHY

The technique relies on the absorption of an orally administered contrast agent, its uptake by the liver and excretion into the biliary tract, its entry into the gallbladder via the cystic duct, and its concentration as normally occurs with gallbladder bile.[17] Thus, a failure of uptake will occur if: (1) the patient does not take the contrast agent; (2) there is inadequate absorption due to achalasia, pyloric stenosis, vomiting, diarrhoea, malabsorption or concomitant use of cholestyramine; (3) there is inadequate hepatic clearance due to liver disease; (4) the sphincter of Oddi has been divided, allowing permanent egress of bile into the duodenum; (5) the cystic duct is blocked from whatever cause, including carcinoma; (6) there is an absent gallbladder either because of agenesis (0.03%) or cholecystectomy.[109]

If the contrast agent enters the gallbladder, poor or non-visualization of the gallbladder may occur due to: (1) severe fibrosis leading to loss of gallbladder mucosal function; (2) ejection of contrast material either because of spontaneous gallbladder contraction or, more commonly, because the patient has not remained fasted.[109]

Thus, it is important that clear instructions are given to the patient regarding oral cholecystography. Ideally, a control roentgenogram should be taken the day before the final radiographs because radiopaque stones (10–30%) may not be seen once contrast is in the gallbladder, but this is not always performed. A fractionated dose of 4.5–6 g of either Telepaque (iopanoic acid), Biloptin (sodium iopodate) or Solubiloptin (calcium iopodate), all of which are equally effective, should be given over the next 12 hours. A minimum of 2 litres of fluids, avoiding milk, should be taken. Avoidance of a fatty meal and overnight fasting will usually give excellent results. It is preferable that liver function should be normal but the test is effective up to a serum bilirubin level of 35 μmol/l.

Radiographs should be taken in the supine–oblique and prone–oblique positions to avoid duodenal or colonic gas shadows and faeces. An erect film should be taken to demonstrate layering by small cholesterol stones which might otherwise be missed (*Figure 12.46*). A fatty meal to induce gallbladder contraction can then be used because this may help to identify abnormalities. Often, some visualization of the common bile duct can be obtained.

Faint opacification of the gallbladder may only be revealed by computed tomography (CT) scans. A radiograph of the whole abdomen may indicate non-absorption of the contrast agent.

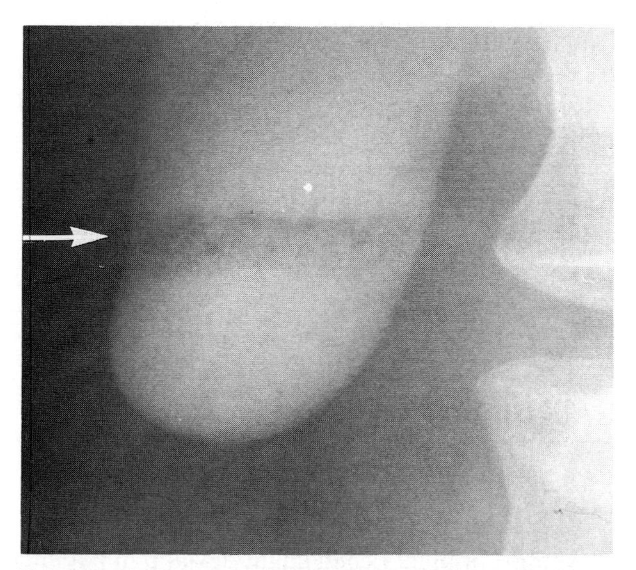

Figure 12.46 Oral cholecystogram taken with the patient in the erect position demonstrating multiple small stones floating in the gallbladder (arrow). This appearance is typical of cholesterol calculi.

Minor side-effects with oral contrast agents, which include nausea, vomiting, diarrhoea, dysuria and urticaria, occur in 30% of patients. Serious side-effects are exceptional, with death occurring in less than 1 in 3 million cases. The most frequently reported severe side-effect is renal failure (usually in patients with pre-existing renal damage), but hypotension, anaphylaxis and myocardial ischaemia have also occurred. Toxicity seems to be least frequent with sodium iopodate.[149]

Contraindications to oral cholecystography include: (1) repeated investigation over short intervals, because toxicity reactions increase; (2) a history of severe skin reactions or anaphylaxis; (3) renal failure, in the presence of which oral cholecystography is in any case often unsuccessful; (4) liver disease, especially if the bilirubin concentration is greater than 35 μmol/l.

The accuracy of oral cholecystography for detecting gallbladder stones is 92–95%.[44] Its main current indications are for assessing patients for oral dissolution therapy, extracorporeal shock wave lithotripsy and following the course of disolution therapy for gallstones. It still has an important place in routine diagnosis where ultrasonography is not available or in situations where stones are suspected but ultrasound proves to be unhelpful.[22]

ULTRASONOGRAPHY

The accuracy of gallbladder stone detection by ultrasonography is high, being in the region of 98%.[97] This is largely replacing oral cholecystography, as

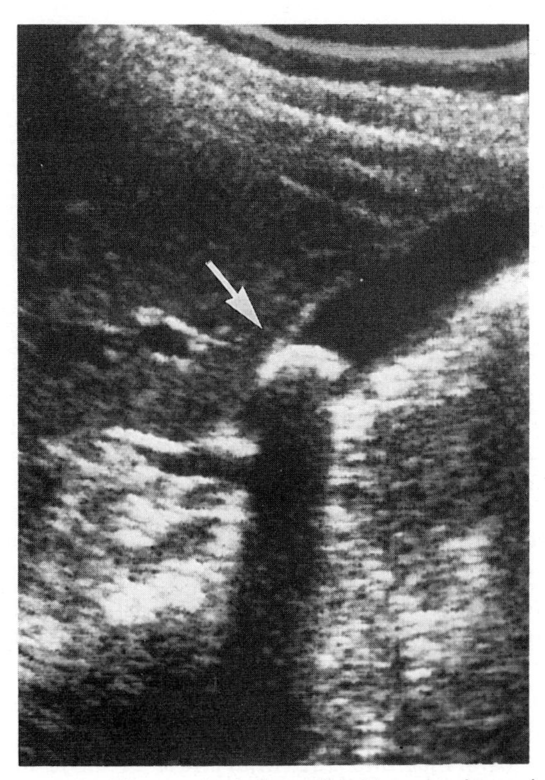

Figure 12.47 Ultrasound of the gallbladder, showing a large calculus (arrow) in the fundus of the gallbladder casting a prominent acoustic shadow.

adverse reactions are avoided and additional diagnostic information of the liver and biliary tree may be obtained.[22]

It is preferable for the patient to be fasted because a morning examination minimizes the presence of intestinal gas and results in a full gallbladder, both of which enhance diagnostic accuracy. The long axis of the gallbladder is identified by making multiple, longitudinal and transverse scans in the right upper quadrant. The patient normally lies in the supine or left oblique supine position; sitting or standing positions may also be required. A gallstone appears as a strong bright echogenic area (due to the stone–bile interface) with an acoustic (black) shadow behind (*Figure 12.47*). The echogenicity of a stone is unrelated to its composition. Stones must be shown to move as the patient is moved because a structure which is fixed relative to the gallbladder is indicative of a polyp or carcinoma. Sludge, secondary to prolonged gallbladder non-contraction such as during intravenous nutrition, does not cast a shadow. Bright echoes without a shadow may be caused by bleeding into the gallbladder (as in haemophiliacs) or by air due to previous biliary–enteric anastomosis or gas-forming organisms.

Multiple transverse scans of the gallbladder are required to detect the smallest stones, the limit being 2 mm. Non-visualization of the gallbladder lumen and inability to detect stones may be due to a fibrotic gallbladder packed with stones with little if any space for bile; thus, the bile–gallstone interface is lost. In such a situation alternative investigations are warranted and, in particular, oral cholecystography.[67] Radionuclide biliary scanning (vide infra) is diagnostic in over 80% of patients with biliary colic.[114] Endoscopic retrograde cholangiopancreatography may be indicated if small stones in a contracted gallbladder are suspected.[164] CT and intravenous cholangiography (vide infra) are alternatives but are rarely indicated.[23,107]

Treatment

Supportive therapy

Pain relief is the most important immediate objective. The use of pethidine (100–150 mg intramuscularly) is well established; morphine (15–20 mg intramuscularly) may be required with the severest of pains. The addition of an antiemetic such as prochlorperazine is usually required. Newer approaches to pain relief such as the use of glucagon, indomethacin and cholecystokinin receptor antagonists have yet to find acceptance. Intravenous fluids may be required for a short period but the patient can usually be adequately managed with oral clear fluids for the first 24 hours.

Definitive treatment

The definitive treatment of gallbladder stones is no longer restricted to surgical cholecystectomy. The decision as to which treatment should be applied to an individual will be dependent upon the presence or absence of concomitant medical disease, the availability and applicability of various forms of new techniques, the skill and preference of those giving the treatment and, increasingly of importance, the choice of the patient (*Table 12.10*).

Surgical approaches

Conventional cholecystectomy has often been quoted as the 'gold standard' of treatment. It has a low procedural mortality (0.5%) and morbidity (5%) and, unlike forms of treatment aimed at the gallstones per se, has a high long-term success rate.[98] In a large series, patients aged 50 years or less undergoing cholecystectomy for chronic cholecystitis had a mortality of 0.1%; in older patients the mortality was 1%.[99] Deaths were attributable to cardiovascular disease and respiratory disease in 37% of patients.

The mortality risk from cholecystectomy in patients with cirrhosis is around 5%; this is 1.1% in patients with normal clotting studies rising to 83% in those with a prothrombin time 2.5-fold normal.[6]

Table 12.10 Different approaches to the treatment of gallbladder stones

Non-invasive	*Invasive surgical*	*Invasive non-surgical*
Conservative	Incisional	Percutaneous
	Conventional cholecystectomy	Cholecystostomy (transhepatic)
	'Mini' cholecystectomy	Cholecystostomy (transperitoneal)
	Cholecystostomy	Dissolution therapy
Oral dissolution	'Mini' cholecystostomy	Lithotripsy
	Cystic duct obliteration	Cholecystoscopy
Extracorporeal shock wave		Chemical cholecystectomy
lithotripsy	Laparoscopic	Cystic duct obliteration
	Cholecystectomy	Cystic duct obliteration
	Cholecystolithotomy	Endoscopic retrograde cholangiopancreatography
	Chemical cholecystectomy	Dissolution therapy (NBC)

Whereas diabetes mellitus has little effect on the results of elective cholecystectomy,[110] the complications are greatly increased in diabetics requiring emergency cholecystectomy for acute cholecystitis (mortality 4.2–31.4%).[69] Thus, there should be little hesitation in offering elective cholecystectomy to the young healthy adult with symptomatic gallstones, the cirrhotic patient with minimal hepatic disease and patients with diabetes mellitus.

Cholecystostomy is a lesser procedure, but it is invariably associated with a higher morbidity and mortality (*Table 12.11*). Although it tends to be chosen for the patient who is 'unfit' for major surgery, it is usually the result of an inexperienced surgeon finding a rather difficult situation for cholecystectomy at laparotomy. This operation is rarely indicated, although it still has its advocates for acute cholecystitis.[189]

Rapid developments in laparoscopic cholecystectomy has meant that this has become the treatment of choice for the majority of patients currently undergoing cholecystectomy. The main advantages of the laparoscopic approach are a dramatic reduction in hospital stay (1–3 days versus 4–12 days) and an even more striking reduction in time to return to work (1–2 weeks versus 6–12 weeks). Avoidance of a long abdominal incision with associated risks of wound infection and incisional hernia is another important consideration. Although there are few published reports at present,[49,147] presentations to surgical societies in 1990 collectively involving over 3500 patients showed a complication rate of 4.1%, bile duct injury rate of 0.3% and a mortality of 0.07%. These figures are entirely comparable to conventional cholecystectomy.

A number of other minimally invasive surgical procedures have been developed. The aim of these procedures is to reduce the length of the surgical incision or, alternatively, to avoid it with the result that hospital stay and the time to return to work is much reduced. Cholecystostomy done through a mini-incision[59] or by laparoscopy[31] has the disadvantage that stone recurrence is likely in 50% or more patients by 5 years.[130] Moreover retained gallbladder stones may result in continuing gallbladder symptoms and will necessitate cholecystectomy in 30–60% of patients.[129,162] Stone recurrence might be reduced by obliterating the cystic duct by diathermy or chemical destruction of the gallbladder mucosa.[7,13]

Table 12.11 Results of surgical treatment in chronic acute cholecystitis

Operation	*Number of patients*	*Deaths*	*Mortality (%)*
Chronic cholecystitis			
Cholecystectomy	8910	38	0.4
Cholecystostomy	161	12	7.5
Cholecystectomy and choledocholithotomy	1798	55	3.1
Acute cholecystitis			
Cholecystectomy	1839	22	1.2
Cholecystostomy	438	44	10.9
Cholecystectomy and choledocholithotomy	428	34	7.9

After McSherry.[98]

Cholecystectomy performed through a mini-incision does achieve early hospital discharge and an earlier return to work compared to conventional cholecystectomy. In a prospective study comparing this technique with laparoscopic cholecystectomy, however, the laparoscopic technique was shown to be significantly superior both in terms of hospital stay (2 versus 3 days) and return to work (6.5 versus 34 days).[147]

Perioperative cholangiography

The two main arguments in favour of routine perioperative cholangiography are (1) detection of incidental bile duct stones and (2) assessment of biliary anatomy and, by implication, reduction in the number of bile duct injuries. Both of these reasons have been increasingly questioned; moreover, the arguments will be coloured by the emerging use of laparoscopic cholecystectomy.

Accepted indicators for undertaking perioperative cholangiography are shown in *Table 12.12*. More sophisticated approaches based on logistic regression analysis have been derived but the practicalities remain much the same. Such an approach would result in only 20% of cholangiograms being performed with less than an estimated 1% of bile duct stones being overlooked.[171] With the widespread availability of endoscopic retrograde cholangiopancreatography for dealing with retained stones, this is a powerful argument. The main saving is in cost rather than time, which in most institutions adds no more than 5–10 minutes of operating time.

The incidence of iatrogenic bile duct stricture following cholecystectomy varies between 0.09 and 0.31%. The evidence that routine use of perioperative cholangiography reduces this in any way is unconvincing; what matters most is the experience of the surgeon undertaking the procedure.[4]

Should these particular arguments be altered by laparoscopic cholecystectomy? The answer is no: the principles of surgery (good exposure and delineation of structures and good training) apply equally to whatever method of cholecystectomy is used.

Table 12.12 Factors associated with an increased chance of finding bile duct stones at routine cholecystectomy

History of jaundice
History of acute pancreatitis
Multiple small gallbladder stones
A wide cystic duct
Common bile duct >10 mm
Raised bilirubin level
Raised alkaline phosphatase level
Raised liver transaminase level

An alternative question is whether routine preoperative endoscopic retrograde cholangiopancreatography should be used with a view to undertaking endoscopic sphincterotomy and stone extraction prior to laparoscopic cholecystectomy. A rational approach would be selective endoscopic retrograde cholangiopancreatography (see *Table 12.12*). On the other hand, if stones are found in the bile duct by cholangiography during laparoscopic cholecystectomy, postsurgical endoscopic stone removal could be undertaken.

Intraoperative ultrasonography

The detection of bile duct stones using a high-frequency (7.5 MHz) scanner with a hand-held probe can produce accurate detection of extrahepatic stones quickly and with cost savings compared to perioperative cholangiography. In a series of 449 patients, intraoperative ultrasound was 97.5% accurate compared to 94.4% for perioperative cholangiography.[75] The main disadvantage is the difficulty in locating intrahepatic stones using the usual hand probes, but this is a minor consideration.

INVASIVE NON-SURGICAL APPROACHES

The approach is either percutaneous[101] or retrograde using a nasobiliary catheter inserted during endoscopic retrograde cholangiopancreatography.[21] The advantage of the percutaneous approach is that the access tract may be dilated to allow mechanical extraction as well as the instillation of solvents. The endoscopic route is disadvantageous in so far as only a minority of patients have a cystic duct which is wide enough and straight enough to allow the introduction of a nasobiliary catheter. Moreover, only direct gallstone dissolution is practical for the cystic duct route.

The gallbladder may be accessed percutaneously either transhepatically or transperitoneally. The former has the advantage of minimizing bile leakage from the gallbladder but may pose problems for access. The transperitoneal route is more easily obtained but there is a small risk of puncturing bowel, the colon in particular.

Percutaneous transhepatic access in chronic cholecystitis performed in more than 100 patients has not been associated with any complications.[172] There is a high success rate with methyl-tert-butyl ether although the follow-up rate remains relatively short (see p. 1726).[173]

Mechanical methods of stone extraction remain more attractive because of speed of treatment and certainty of extraction. Large gallstones may be shattered using ultrasonic lithotripsy,[57] a rotational mechanical lithotriptor[187] or neodymium–yttrium aluminium garnet (Nd–YAG) laser lithotripsy.[74]

Completeness of extraction may be determined either by fluoroscopy or endoscopy using an adapted urological rigid endoscope or, alternatively, by a flexible fibre-optic cholecystoscope (normally used for choledochoscopy).

The appropriate place for these techniques is in those patients who do not wish to have a general anaesthetic or, alternatively, in those who are at high risk from more invasive procedures.

ACUTE GALLSTONE CHOLECYSTITIS

Aetiology

Obstruction of the cystic duct or Hartmann's pouch by a stone is the usual cause of inflammation but, rarely, occlusion is by carcinoma. In the initial 12–24 hours a chemical cholecystitis becomes established. Bacterial infection is probably a secondary event in most situations. *Emphysematous acute cholecystitis* is a particularly serious variation. Although rare, it usually occurs in patients with diabetes mellitus and is due to gas-forming organisms.[105]

Pathology

The gallbladder is distended and the gallbladder oedematous and hypervascular. The oedema and inflammation spread into Calot's triangle and the hepatoduodenal ligament. Other structures, in particular the greater omentum, hepatic colonic flexure and duodenum, may become attached to it by inflammatory adhesions. The gallbladder wall often shows patchy areas of gangrene and infected bile may exude out of the gallbladder at the site.

Microscopy reveals mucosal ulceration and the wall is oedematous with an inflammatory and fibroblastic reaction. The inflammatory reaction increases with bacterial infection. Lymphocytes are concentrated around areas of mucosal necrosis. Venous thrombosis is common and in the later stages there may be thrombosis of the cystic artery or its branches and the main arterial supply is then provided by branches from the hepatic bed. Resolution occurs spontaneously in around 85% of patients. Acute cholecystitis may progress to empyema of the gallbladder or extensive gangrene of the wall with localized perforation.

Clinical features

Pain develops in the epigastrium and right upper quadrant. There is usually fever of 37.5°C or more with a slight tachycardia and leukocystosis. These features become more marked with severe inflammation although they may be absent in the elderly who may instead present with apparent senile confusion.[34] Nausea and anorexia are present but vomiting is unusual.

Murphy's sign is usually positive: on palpating the right hypochondrium, there is mid-inspiratory arrest due to tenderness as the gallbladder moves caudally to meet the palpating fingertips. In contrast, this does not occur when palpating the left hypochondrium. There may be hyperaesthesia over the right hypochondrium (Boa's sign) and, in advanced cases, cutaneous oedema (Leeke's sign) on the right upper abdomen. In up to 25% of patients there is the suggestion of a mass in the right hypochondrium.

Mild clinical jaundice is present in 10–25% of patients, usually indicating bile duct compression from the distended gallbladder (Mirizzi's syndrome) because in icteric patients the incidence of bile duct stones is no more than the normal prevalence.[167]

Investigations

Plain radiography

An erect chest radiograph is required to exclude free air under the diaphragm which follows from a perforated viscus, which is an alternative diagnosis. An erect plain abdominal radiograph may reveal acute emphysematous cholecystitis with a fluid–gas level in the gallbladder lumen and a concentric air shadow in the gallbladder wall. Calcified stones are evident in 10–30% of patients but is not diagnostic for acute cholecystitis.

Ultrasonography

This is the investigation of choice but ultrasonography findings must be interpreted in conjunction with the clinical features. An ultrasonic Murphy's sign (tenderness when the probe is directly over the ultrasonography-located gallbladder) is positive in 63% with a specificity of 63%.[143] A thickened gallbladder wall, pericholecystic fluid collections, fine intraluminal echoes from empyema or debris, a distended gallbladder and adjacent liver abscesses are additional diagnostic features. Failure to identify the gallbladder is almost always because of a contracted gallbladder full of calculi; agenesis of the gallbladder is rare (0.03%).

Computed tomography

The sensitivity for gallstones in acute cholecystitis is similar to that for ultrasonography but there is difficulty in identifying the smallest gallstones; ultrasonography remains superior in this respect.[103]

^{99m}Tc iminodiacetic acid (^{99m}Tc-HIDA) scan

A variety of iminodiacetic acid derivatives which are readily labelled with ^{99m}Tc are available for radionuclide bilary scanning. These are constituted as high-molecular-weight organic anionic dimers with substituted side-chains, producing agents with increased lipophilicity. They are rapidly and almost exclusively taken up by the liver and excreted into the biliary tree. Although they are of limited use in diagnosing bile leaks and the patency of biliary–enteric anastamosis, their main use is in assessing cystic duct patency. Because the cystic duct is invariably blocked in acute cholecystitis, it is highly diagnostic in this situation, but, as with ultrasonography, the results must be taken in conjunction with the overall clinical picture.

The patient is fasted for at least 4 hours. The investigation may be performed in the presence of jaundice. ^{99m}Tc-HIDA is given intravenously (185 MBq; total dose to patient about 20 mGy) and the liver area is scanned with a γ camera. The biliary system is imaged within 10–15 minutes (*Figures 12.48* and *12.49*) and the gallbladder and duodenum are outlined by 30 minutes. The test is positive if the gallbladder is not demonstrated within 1 hour; occasionally, delayed scans may subsequently image the gallbladder.

The sensitivity of HIDA scanning for acute cholecystitis is 98–100%.[114,195] Although the specificity is often quoted at about 80%,[195] this is questionable because the contrasting group is usually chronic cholecystitis. Up to 82% of patients with biliary colic also have a positive scan,[114] but this is of little practical importance because the distinction between acute cholecystitis and biliary colic is often blurred.

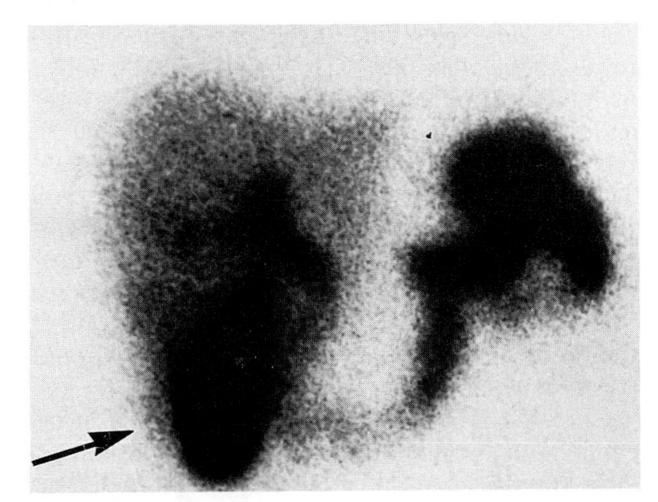

Figure 12.48 HIDA scintigram in left anterior oblique position at 1 hour after injection of radionuclide, showing take-up of the radionuclide in a normal gallbladder (arrow).

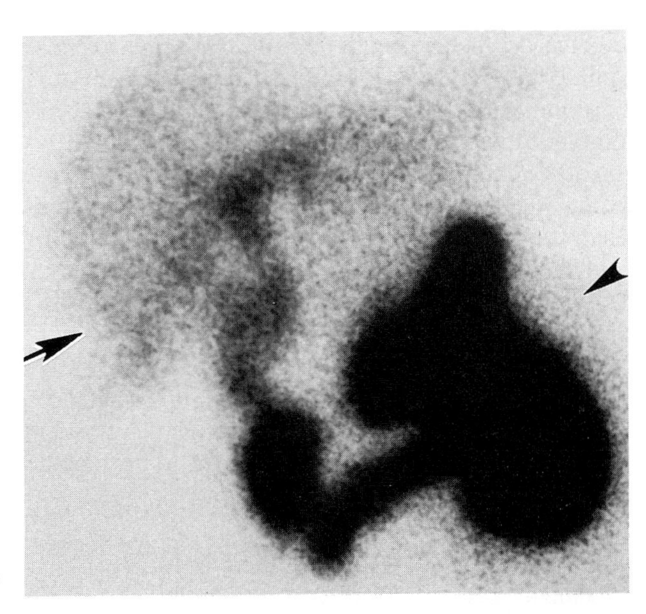

Figure 12.49 HIDA scintigram in left anterior oblique position at 1 hour after injection of the radionuclide, showing no uptake in the gallbladder (arrow). Most of the radionuclide is in the small intestine (arrowhead). This appearance is consistent with an obstructed cystic duct and a diseased gallbladder.

True false positives may occur in patients who have had prolonged oral fasting such as those on intravenous nutrition or in the postoperative period. Contrary to some opinions, it is of no value in distinguishing between gallstone and non-gallstone pancreatitis; up to 30% of patients with alcohol-induced pancreatitis have a positive scan.[103,114,115,195]

Radionuclide biliary scanning is often mentioned as the investigation of choice for acute cholecystitis but, in practice, ultrasonography is much quicker to perform. The tests are complementary.[195]

Intravenous cholangiography

The principle of this technique (see p. 1748) for diagnosing acute cholecystitis is similar to radionuclide biliary scanning, namely failure to identify the gallbladder because of a blocked cystic duct. An intravenous infusion of the soluble contrast agent, e.g. 100 ml of 10.3% iodipamide meglumine, is given over 20 minutes. Radiographs are taken at 20-minute intervals with tomographs at 40 or 60 minutes, depending on duct visualization. Unfortunately, a high proportion of the investigations (as much as 40–60%) prove not to be useful because the biliary system is not visualized.[158]

Infusion tomography of the gallbladder

The patient is given an infusion of a soluble contrast agent after a control radiograph of the gallbladder area has been performed; 300 ml of 30% methylglucamine diatrizoate (Urograffin) in 5% dextrose over 20 minutes is commonly used. Anteroposterior tomographs centred over the 12th rib are taken at 1-cm intervals and the examination is usually complete within 30 minutes. The test is interpreted as positive when the gallbladder wall is shown to be thickened, being greater than 1 mm in one or more of the cuts. A diagnostic accuracy as high as 96% for acute cholecystitis has been reported, but is only 64% for chronic cholecystitis.[108] On the other hand, misdiagnosis or technical failure may occur in up to 26% of patients and is particularly poor at diagnosing gangrenous cholecystitis because of non-perfusion of the gallbladder wall.[79]

Treatment

Initial measures include pain relief (see p. 1735) and intravenous fluids, and the patient must take nothing orally. A nasogastric tube is not usually necessary. Antibiotics should be given intravenously (see p. 1757). Patients with acute emphysematous cholecystitis must receive a bacteriocide directed against clostridia.

The type of intervention, whether surgical or by invasive percutanenous techniques (see *Table 12.10*), will depend upon associated co-morbidity (see p. 1735). The timing of intervention will be dependent upon the severity of the attack. The indications for urgent intervention include: (1) general deterioration in the patient's condition; (2) evidence of spreading or generalized peritonitis; (3) empyema of the gallbladder or abscess formation; (4) acute emphysematous cholecystitis.

Surgical treatment

The conventional treatment is a cholecystectomy through a right subcostal (Kocher's) incision. In technically difficult situations, a partial cholecystectomy may be performed and the cystic duct ligated and the anterior part of the gallbladder removed, leaving behind that part which is firmly adherent to the liver. Finally, the mucosa is destroyed by fulguration.

Provided the gallbladder is close to the anterior abdominal wall (which it often is in acute cholecystitis), a cholecystostomy can be performed under local anaesthetic. In general, operative cholecystostomy should be avoided because it is associated with a much higher mortality than cholecystectomy (see *Table 12.11*). In a collected series of 556 elderly patients undergoing cholecystostomy for acute cholecystitis, the postoperative mortality was 18%.[101] Winkler *et al.*, however, were able to report a mortality of only 5% in a recent series of 60 patients.[189]

In patients with a severe attack of acute cholecystitis who are not responding to initial measures, urgent surgery is required. Most patients, however, will respond. In this group, cholecystectomy during the same admission is to be preferred, because delaying surgery until the second elective admission will result in 10–20% having a repeat attack. Early cholecystectomy also appears to be associated with a lower incidence of postoperative biliary fistulas and lower mortality.[181]

It is likely that laparoscopic cholecystectomy will also prove to be an effective treatment for acute cholecystitis although experience is currently limited.

Invasive non-surgical approaches

Mortality in the elderly is still appreciable (10–20%),[61,70,101] although early surgical intervention undoubtedly reduces mortality even in these patients.[50] In elderly patients at high risk from surgery, primary consideration should be given to percutaneous gallbladder decompression techniques. In a collected series of 114 patients at high risk from surgery, the procedure-related morbidity was 4.4% and no immediate mortality; the 30-day mortality was 9.6%, which compares favourably with similar cases treated by surgical cholecystostomy (mortality 18%).[101]

It is important that these patients also receive full supportive measures, including intravenous fluids and antibiotics. All the infected bile and pus must be aspirated; local instillation of an antibiotic such as gentamicin is also recommended. The antibiotic regimen can be modified as a consequence of the results of the bile culture. The catheter should not be withdrawn for at least 10 days to allow a tract to form and the use of Gelfoam can reduce bile leakage. A recent survey of 250 cases revealed bile leaks in only 3.2% with only two patients (0.8%) who required surgery.[101] Patients with acute cholecystitis or gallbladder empyema are at risk of developing a pronounced vasovagal attack, especially if there is preexisting ischaemic heart disease. Attention must, therefore, be given to adequate analgesia and sedation along with atropine.[183]

Once the attack has settled, the stones must be eliminated. A number of techniques are available, including mechanical lithotripsy,[59] piezoelectric lithotripsy,[57] electrohydraulic lithotripsy[114] and laser lithotripsy.[74] Direct gallstone dissolution is an alternative (see p. 1724).[173]

EMPYEMA OF THE GALLBLADDER

Empyema of the gallbladder occurs in elderly females more often than in elderly men who present with features typical of acute cholecystitis. A palpable mass is noted in 40% of patients.[55,75] A preoperative diagnosis, however, is suspected in less than half the patients. Alternative presentations include overwhelming septicaemia,[54] mental disability, particularly in the elderly[34] or as an incidental finding of cholecystectomy for chronic cholecystitis.[55,175] Early intervention is mandatory. The mortality is 15–25%, but is increased because of delay in diagnosis.

CHOLECYSTODUODENAL FISTULA AND GALLSTONE ILEUS

A stone eroding into the duodenum from the gallbladder may give rise to intestinal obstruction.[182] Cholecystoduodenal fistulas comprise 70% of all biliary enteric fistulas. The sites of obstruction are the terminal ileum (70%), jejunum (15%), duodenal bulb (causing Bouveret's syndrome) (10%) and, rarely, the sigmoid colon (usually in association with a stricture due to diverticular disease). The diagnosis is suggested by a large calcified stone (30%) which moves on repeat radiographs, causing a change in the site of obstruction (tumbling obstruction). The diagnosis can be made with a plain radiograph which demonstrates air in the biliary tree (pneumobilia) in 30–50% of patients, but is missed all too often. A barium meal showing contrast reflux into the gallbladder or a CT scan showing pneumobilia will make the diagnosis. Treatment requires surgical intervention. The simplest operative procedure (enterotomy) should be performed because the patients are usually elderly and frail. It is important to exclude other stones in the intestines and gallbladder, which will be responsible for a recurrence in about 5% of patients. Cholecystectomy is usually unnecessary and will increase the morbidity; bile duct stones are frequent in such patients. Endoscopic retrograde cholangiopancreatography should therefore be performed if, in the postoperative period, the patient shows little sign of improvement. The mortality is as high as to 30%.[2]

CHOLECYSTOCOLIC FISTULA

Cholecystocolic fistula accounts for 15% of all biliary fistulas. They cause profuse diarrhoea from bile acid irritation of the colon, and malabsorption syndrome from interruption of the enterohepatic circulation of bile acids.[146] If the fistula is narrow there may be additional features of acute cholangitis (see p. 1746).[93] Air is present on a plain radiography in about 50% of patients. The diagnosis may be made by barium enema, radionuclide biliary scanning (see p. 1739) or endoscopic retrograde cholangiopancreatography.

Treatment

Cholecystectomy and primary closure of the colonic fistula is the treatment of choice. If the patient is unfit for surgery, endoscopic sphincterotomy may be successful.[141]

MIRIZZI'S SYNDROME AND CHOLECYSTOCHOLEDOCHAL FISTULA

Compression of the main bile duct by a distended gallbladder in acute cholecystitis or fibrotic contraction in chronic cholecystitis (Mirizzi's syndrome) may result in erosion of the bile duct wall, creating a fistula (see *Figure 12.50*).[40] Cholecystocholedochal

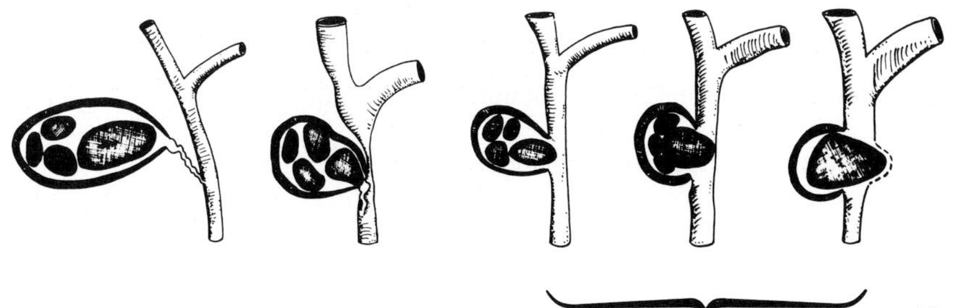

Figure 12.50 The Csendes classification of Mirizzi's syndrome and cholecystobiliary fistulas: I, external compression of the extrahepatic bile duct; II, fistula involving less than one-third of bile duct circumference; III, fistula involving one-third to two-thirds of bile duct circumference; IV, fistula with complete loss of bile duct circumference.

fistula accounts for about 1% of all biliary–enteric fistulas. Type I disease from acute cholecystitis often resolves spontaneously; otherwise, cholecystectomy is the treatment of choice.[40] Non-operative techniques are also available. Insertion of an endoscopic endoprosthesis to relieve the jaundice (see p. 1751) may be followed by percutaneous electrohydraulic lithotripsy.[27] Alternatively, the gallbladder may be decompressed endoscopically via the cystic duct and the stones shattered by extracorporeal shock wave lithotripsy (see p. 1728).[102]

Type III and some type II lesions are treated by cholecystectomy, or choledochoplasty using part of the gallbladder wall, and insertion of a T tube in the lower bile duct. Type IV lesions require a Roux-en-Y biliary–enteric anastomosis. For types I and II the mortality is 1.8%, whilst for types III and IV the mortality is 12.3%.[40]

ACALCULOUS CHOLECYSTITIS

Cholecystitis, either chronic or acute, may be primary because, in only about half the cases, a predisposing cause is identified (*Table 12.13*).[60]

The incidence of chronic acalculous cholecystitis relative to calculous cholecystitis may be as high as 6–13%.[142,145] Recent evidence suggests that acute acalculous cholecystitis may be increasing, with estimates varying from 2%[135] to 10%[62] of all cases of acute cholecystitis.

Chronic acalculous cholecystitis

There may be non-specific features of mild chronic cholecystitis or specific pathological states.

Cholesterolosis

This is a relatively common condition, being present in up to 11% of all cholecystectomy specimens.[136,153] It is characterized by an accumulation of lipid esters in macrophage foam cells of the lamina propria. The mucosal villi become oedematous. There is a macroscopic reticular appearance and the translucency of the lipids through the polypoid mucosa gives the typical strawberry gallbladder appearance. The development of cholesterolosis is associated with altered hepatic cholesterol metabolism; in the gallbladder there is altered uptake of

Table 12.13 Associated conditions in acalculous cholecystitis

Primary[60]
  No predisposing factor
Specific infections
  Typhoid,[60] leptospirosis,[192] staphylococcol septicaemia,[174] brucellosis, actinomycosis,[43] clonorchiasis, giardiasis,[64] *Toruslopsis galabrata* infection,[107] ascariasis
Major sepsis[60]
Atherosclerosis[155]
  Myocardial infarction, congestive cardiac failure, hypertension
Trauma
  Blunt trauma,[60] burns,[60] surgery (orthopaedic, abdominal, 'general surgical', urological, vascular, cardiac, neurosurgical)[46]
Cholesterolosis[153]
Adenomyomatosis[188]
Xanthogranulomatous cholecystitis[15]
Metabolic disorders
  Diabetes mellitus,[155] alcoholism,[72] acute pancreatitis,[60] total parenteral nutrition,[138] multiple blood transfusions[92]
Connective tissue disorders
  Rheumatoid arthritis,[72] systemic lupus erythematosis,[168] polyarteritis nodosa,[91] systemic sclerosis[36]
Haemobilia[72]
Pernicious anaemia[111]
Malignant disease[72]
Crohn's disease[96]
Sarcoidosis[94]
Kawasaki syndrome[163]
Sjögren's syndrome[169]
Sclerosing cholangitis[176]
Intraportal chemotherapy[37]
Porcelain gallbladder[16]
Torsion of the gallbladder[26]

biliary free sterols, mucosal esterification of sterols and accumulation of triglycerides of unknown origin.[177] Gallstones may or may not be present.

Adenomyomatosis
This is characterized by the formation of Rokitansky–Aschoff sinuses and hyperplasia of the muscularis, causing prominent diverticula or crypts. The aetiological mechanisms include muscular dysfunction and cystic duct stenosis.[188] This condition may occur in up to 10% of cholecystectomy specimens. (See also page 1817.)

Xanthogranulomatous cholecystitis
Penetration of bile pigments as well as lipid into the connective tissue gives rise to marked inflammation. Oxidation of lipids may occur to form chromolipids. The incidence of xanthogranulomatous cholecystis varies from 0.7 to 1.8% of all cholecystectomy specimens. It is associated with an increased risk of carcinoma of the gallbladder.[15] (See also page 1797.)

Symptoms and diagnosis

The symptoms are often those of biliary colic and the diagnosis may be difficult. Confirmatory investigations can be obtained by ultrasonography or CT if specific features are apparent but the sensitivity is low.[135,159,188] Radionuclide biliary scanning,[159] oral cholecystography or intravenous cholangiography may show non-gallbladder filling.

Reproducing the typical pain by intravenous cholecystokinin–pancreozymin has been promoted as an important diagnostic tool[151] but has not been generally accepted. Dynamic assessment of the gallbladder function either by cholecystography, ultrasonography or radionuclide biliary scanning following intravenous cholecystokinin–pancreozymin appears to be more valuable. In addition, the presence of duodenal bile cholesterol crystals will be evidence for microliathiasis in the presence of a normal ultrasonogram.[25,190]

Treatment

Symptomatic patients do well following a cholecystectomy,[25,151,190] and this should also be performed in patients with cholesterolosis because of a 30% risk of acute pancreatitis.[136]

Premaligant conditions

There is an increased risk of malignancy in patients with xanthogranulomatous cholecystitis[15] and a porcelain gallbladder.[16] Cholecystitis must be performed in these patients irrespective of symptoms. There may also be a risk with typhoid disease in relation to chronic cholecystitis.[8]

Acute acalculous cholecystitis

Ischaemia of the gallbladder from a variety of causes (hypertension, atherosclerosis, vasculitis etc.) is probably the single most important initiating event.[155] This is likely to predispose the mucosa to damage by potentially noxious bile constituents such as lysolecithin.[161] Activation of factor XII may be an important final pathway in causing microvascular injury to the gallbladder.[62] The incidence of secondary bacterial infection is similar to that of acute acalculous cholecystitis (63 versus 59%).[46]

Patients with acute acalculous cholecystitis have a higher mortality (10–20%) than those with the calculous type.[46,62] There is also a greater incidence of gangrenous cholecystitis, empyema of the gallbladder and free biliary perforation.[46]

Clinical features

The symptoms are usually those of severe acute cholecystitis (see p. 1738). Savoca *et al.*, recently reported that 77% of 47 patients developed acute acalculous cholecystitis at home without any preexisting evidence of illness or acute cholecystitis.[155]

INVESTIGATIONS

Radionuclide biliary scanning has a high diagnostic usefulness (97%),[155] free perforation may be indicated by peritoneal leakage of HIDA, which is superior to CT scanning (75%). Ultrasonography may show gallbladder distention and wall thickening, sludge and the halo sign of subserosal oedema; but the diagnostic accuracy is low (28%).[155] ^{111}In-labelled leukocyte imaging may be useful in some circumstances.[41]

Treatment

The main aim of treatment is the underlying condition in those patients with specific infections (see *Table 12.13*). Following recovery, typhoid carriers should undergo cholecystectomy. The desirability of undertaking cholecystectomy in patients with acute acalculous cholecystitis will to some extent be dependent upon the underlying condition. In principle, however, urgent cholecystectomy is advised. Johnson reported a perforation rate of 40% in those in whom surgery was delayed beyond 48 hours compared to only 8% in those who had a cholecystectomy within this time.[78]

GALLSTONE-RELATED DISEASES OF THE BILE DUCTS

CHOLEDOCHOLITHIASIS

Stones in the main bile duct pose distinct problems in several clinical situations:

1. Bile duct stones found during routine cholecystectomy.
2. Jaundice in patients with the gallbladder in situ.
3. Acute cholangitis – Western variety.
4. Recurrent pyogenic cholangitis – Oriental variety.
5. Acute pancreatitis – sometimes associated with acute cholangitis.
6. Retained bile duct stones detected in the early postcholecystectomy period.
7. Symptoms of retained or recurrent bile duct stones (jaundice, cholangitis and pancreatitis) following remote cholecystectomy.

The approaches to such patients include surgical, endoscopic or percutaneous stone extraction techniques or a combination of these. Adjuncts to these methods include extracorporeal shock wave lithotripsy and direct dissolution (*Table 12.14*). Which of these is appropriate for a particular patient is dependent on the clinical scenario, the fitness of the

Table 12.14 Methods of improving the success rates of non-surgical forms of treating bile duct stones

Duodenoscopic route		*Percutaneous routes*
	Gaining access	
Sphincter relaxation 'Pre-cut' papillotomy Combined percutaneous technique		Ultrasonography Computed tomography
	Widening the extraction route	
Sphincterotomy Sphincter dilatation Sphincter relaxation		Sphincterotomy Sphincter dilatation Sphincter relaxation Percutaneous tract dilatation
	Lithotripsy	
Mechanical (basket) Electrohydraulic Ultrasonic Laser ESWL		Mechanical (basket and rotational) Electrohydraulic Ultrasonic Laser ESWL
	Stone extraction	
Balloon Dormia basket		Balloon Dormia basket Steerable basket
	Biliary endoscopy	
'Mother and baby' endoscopy		Choledochoscopy Cholangioscopy
	Biliary drainage	
Nasobiliary catheter Internal stent		External drainage Internal stent Internal–external stent
	Stone dissolution	
Via nasobiliary catheter		Via percutaneous catheter

ESWL, extracorporeal shock wave lithotripsy.

patient for surgery (low, moderate or high risk) and the desirability of removing the gallbladder if such is present.[113]

Aetiology

Stones in the biliary tree found at the same time as cholecystectomy are usually of the same variety. In Westernized patients, these are either cholesterol or black pigment stones,[116] which nearly always form in the gallbladder and enter the biliary tree via the cystic duct.

Primary (or recurrent) bile duct stones are usually formed by calcium bilirubinate (or brown pigment) following the precipitation of unconjugated bilirubin secondary to increased bacterial β-glucuronidase activity. Their formation is rapid and usually results in a soft stone sometimes taking the shape of that part of the biliary tree within which they formed. Up to 30% of recurrent bile duct stones following surgery contain non-absorbent suture material which serves to promote secondary bacterial infection as well as to act as a nidus for the precipitation of bilirubinate crystals.

Acute (Western) cholangitis is associated with bacterial infection in 80–100% of patients (see p. 1738) and is generally considered to be secondary to bile duct stone disease. In contrast, patients with recurrent pyogenic (Oriental) cholangitis have a primary infection with secondary gallstone formation. Both *Escherichia coli* and *Clonorchis sinensis* have been implicated either individually or in combination.[112] Such stones are almost invariably of the brown pigment variety and are found in the bile ducts in about 80% of cases; less than 30% of patients have stones in the gallbladder.[131] Acute pancreatitis is associated with the passage of small bile duct stones through the ampulla of Vater.[1,112]

Pathology of bile duct obstruction and cholangitis

Within 48 hours of the onset of bile duct obstruction, proliferation of the dilated canaliculi occurs. There is a blunting and a reduction in the number of canalicular microvilli, a decrease of the smooth and rough endoplasmic reticulum as well as the Golgi apparatus and mitochondria. The tight junctional complexes between the hepatocytes become leaky and intracellular vacuoles may develop.[144] Bile pigment thrombi occur in the canaliculi and adjacent hepatocytes with an inflammatory cell infiltrate. Around the portal tracts there is intracytoplasmic hyaline deposition proceeding to feathery degeneration and biliary piecemeal necrosis. Unless relieved, the obstruction will lead to perilobular fibrosis. Progression of this to secondary biliary cirrhosis will ultimately lead to loss of the normal architecture. Secondary portal hypertension will also develop.

Additional features of bacterial infection may become superimposed on this picture if acute cholangitis develops. There is then portal oedema and a predominantly neutrophil infiltration extending outwards from the ductules, ultimately forming micro-abscesses. Patchy areas of necrosis may follow, resulting in multiple small abscesses communicating with the biliary tree throughout the liver. These may be observed by direct cholangiography (endoscopic retrograde cholangiopancreatography and percutaneous transhepatic cholangiography).

The extrahepatic ducts are also affected. With obstruction, there is at first mucosal atrophy and squamous metaplasia. With infection, there is a marked inflammatory infiltrate of the mucosa and submucosa, which becomes friable, followed by fibrosis.

Clinical features

Patients with bile duct stones may be asymptomatic. Vague or marked epigastric pain may occur intermittently even in the absence of jaundice and this can pose particular diagnostic problems in patients with previous cholecystectomy (see p. 1754). The only clue to diagnosis in elderly patients may be the sudden and unexplained development of mental and physical disability.[34]

Jaundice

This may be associated with abdominal discomfort in about 60% of patients. Bloating, steatorrhoea and malabsorption will follow, but patients usually present before these symptoms become marked. Prolonged biliary obstruction may result in secondary biliary cirrhosis, portal hypertension and bleeding oesophageal varices. Failure to absorb lipid-soluble vitamin K causes a marked bleeding tendency following failure of the liver to produce clotting factors. The clotting factors produced by the liver are factors I (fibrinogen), II (prothrombin), V, VII, IX and X. Vitamin K is necessary for the conversion of the precursors of factors II, V, VII, IX and X to the active coagulation factors. The liver also has two other important functions in haemostasis: the synthesis and degradation of fibrinolytic factors (plasminogen and plasminogen activators); and the clearance of activated coagulation factors. In obstructive jaundice, there is also decreased clearance by the Kupffer cells of endotoxins from the gut which may be important in the development of acute renal failure (hepatorenal syndrome).

Acute cholangitis
This is characterized by obstructive jaundice, a swinging pyrexia of 38°C or greater (Charcot's fever), chills and pain and tenderness over the liver (Charcot's triad). Jaundice may be absent in up to 2% of patients.[112] Acute cholangitis may be graded as acute non-suppurative cholangitis, acute suppurative cholangitis with incomplete obstruction, acute suppurative cholangitis with complete obstruction, and acute suppurative cholangitis with multiple liver abscesses. In the severer types there is a 'pentad' of features which also includes shock, mental confusion and lethargy.[150]

Recurrent pyogenic cholangitis[112,131]
Acute attacks of cholangitis are often superimposed on subclinical symptoms of vague discomfort and malaise. Despite jaundice and the presence of bile duct stones with infected bile, patients may be asymptomatic. These patients frequently have intrahepatic bile duct strictures with sludge and stones forming upstream. There is often extensive destruction of liver parenchyma from chronic pyogenic liver abscess formation. Patients may also present with the overwhelming features of septicaemia.

Acute pancreatitis
Most patients with acute pancreatitis (see p. 1598) do not have jaundice and, if present, it is usually transient. Patients with severe gallstone pancreatitis, however, are more prone to 'persisting' bile duct stones.[121] Acute cholangitis (Charcot's triad) may occur in association with acute pancreatitis; this applies equally to Western[118] and Oriental cholangitis.[132]

Retained postoperative stones
These are usually asymptomatic in the early postoperative period and are diagnosed on the postoperative T-tube cholangiogram. Acute cholangitis, acute pancreatitis and an internal biliary fistula (bile leak) may occur, especially if there has been primary closure of the bile duct, the limbs of the T tube are excessively long or the T tube has been inappropriately removed.

Spectrum of clinical features
There may only be the features of obstruction in uncomplicated jaundice: steatorrhoea, dark urine, scratch marks from itching (usually a feature of marked jaundice from malignant disease) and a bleeding diathesis. The gallbladder is usually neither palpable nor tender unless there is also either acute cholecystitis, or empyema of the gallbladder or Mirizzi's syndrome. A non-tender palpable gallbladder usually suggests malignant disease rather than a mucocoele. An enlarged, tender liver may indicate a liver abscess while a tender epigastric mass with features of peritonitis suggests acute pancreatitis. Tachycardia, pyrexia, hypotension and a warm periphery indicate septicaemia secondary to acute cholangitis. Mental confusion or coma indicates advanced suppurative cholangitis. There may be profound hypovolaemia and acute renal failure in patients with sepsis.

Investigations

The following tests are mandatory in the jaundiced patients: HB_sAg (to exclude hepatitis), full blood count, electrolytes and urea, plasma proteins and albumin (often low), serum bilirubin, liver transaminases and the prothrombin time. An obstructive picture is suggested by a several-fold increase in the alkaline phosphatase level relative to the liver transaminase level. There will be a mixed picture of hepatic and posthepatic cholestasis if secondary biliary cirrhosis has supervened.

The primary radiological investigation is ultrasonography to confirm an obstructed biliary tree but a full diagnosis may be obtained with this alone. More precise diagnostic information is often required, however, usually by endoscopic retrograde cholangiopancreatography, although percutaneous hepatic cholangiography, intravenous cholangiography and CT may be required occasionally.

Ultrasonography
Ultrasonography may detect a dilated extrahepatic biliary tree in early obstruction before there is dilatation of the intrahepatic bile ducts. In healthy adults the upper limit of normal or the extrahepatic bile ducts is 6 mm.[126] There is no doubt, however, that the diameter increases with age and following cholecystectomy.[125,126] The level of obstruction can be detected in no more than 50% of patients. Bile duct stones are detected in only 19–55% of patients,[39] this being less in patients with normal-sized ducts. Ultrasonography is able to detect air in the biliary tree (high echogenicity with little shadowing) and ascariasis (linear, non-shadowing structures). Liver abscesses are demonstrated as irregular hypoechogenic areas with variable echoes from debris and gas; at an early stage there may be irregular hyper- echogenicity. The distinction from a necrotic tumour may be difficult.

Endoscopic retrograde cholangiopancreatography

This technique is performed with a side-viewing flexible duodenoscope under radiographic screening, using local pharyngeal spray analgesia (1% lignocaine) and intravenous sedation (5–20 mg of midazolam in divided doses).[38] The patient lies on his or her left side with the left arm at his or her back. Once the duodenoscope has entered the second part of the duodenum, the small wheel is turned and locked full right; as the instrument is withdrawn to the 60–70 cm mark, the major papilla appears. During this later procedure, the patient is turned semi-prone and hyoscine hydrobromide (20–40 mg) is given to relax the duodenum. The ampulla is cannulated and contrast medium is slowly injected under screening control. Opacification of the pancreatic parenchyma should be avoided. As the ducts are filled with contrast medium, serial radiographs should be taken and developed immediately because stones and other lesions will be more clearly visualized. The whole of the biliary tree including the gallbladder should be outlined with contrast medium. The normal extrahepatic bile duct diameter is twice that measured by ultrasonography;[127] indeed, the correlation between the diameters measured by ultrasonography and endoscopic retrograde cholangiopancreatography is poor. At the end of the procedure the patient lies supine and further radiographs are taken to outline the gallbladder. An erect radiograph may show layering of small gallbladder stones (*Figure 12.51*).

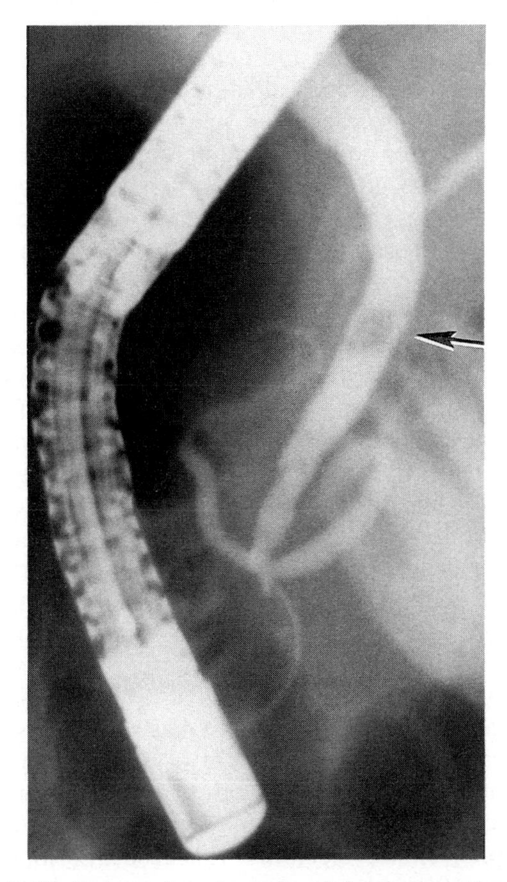

Figure 12.51 Endoscopic retrograde cholangiopancreatogram showing contrast in the bilary system and pancreatic duct. A radiolucent stone is demonstrated in the common bile duct (arrow).

The success rate of endoscopic retrograde cholangiography is around 90–98%.[38,180] This may be helped by relaxing the sphincter of Oddi with glycerol trinitrate sprayed sublingually, the use of a 'precut' papillotomy or a combined percutaneous radiological endoscopic procedure.[38,180] The complication rate is 0.8% and the mortality is 0.08%.[148] The commonest complication is acute pancreatitis, but this is rarely severe. Bacteraemia and septicaemia may occur, especially in an obstructed biliary tree; intravenous fluids, prophylactic intravenous antibiotics (see p. 1757) and adequate biliary drainage will minimize this.

Computed tomography

Although superior to ultrasonography, stones are detected at best in only 76% of patients with dilated bile ducts and recognition is much worse in the 20% of patients with normal-sized ducts.[11] The normal extrahepatic bile duct diameter is 3–6 mm as measured by CT. CT is helpful in assessing liver abscesses associated with acute cholangitis.

Percutaneous transhepatic cholangiography

Haemostasis should be as close to normal as possible; if there is prolongation of the prothrombin time or bleeding time, 2 units of fresh frozen plasma must be given half an hour before the procedure; platelets are given if the count is less than 6×10^{10}/litre.

The procedure is undertaken using a 'skinny' (Chiba) needle (15 cm long, 0.7 mm outer diameter) with prophylactic intravenous antibiotics (see p. 1757), intravenous sedation (midazolam 5–10 mg) and local anaesthesia (1% lignocaine). The patient lies supine and the needle is inserted in the mid-axillary line just below the costophrenic angle. Using screening, the needle is advanced horizontally and slightly cranially to within 2–3 cm of the vertebral column. The stylet is removed and the needle is slowly withdrawn, whilst injecting contrast material, until a biliary radical is visualized. Several passes may be necessary. The success rate is 98% in those patients with dilated ducts and 70% when the ducts are non-dilated.[68] The size of normal extrahepatic bile ducts is 6.5–7.6 mm by percutaneous transhepatic cholangiography (*Figure 12.52*).

The incidence of serious or fatal complications was 3.5% in a US national survey of 2006 patients: sepsis 1.4%, bile leakage 1.5%, bleeding 0.4% and

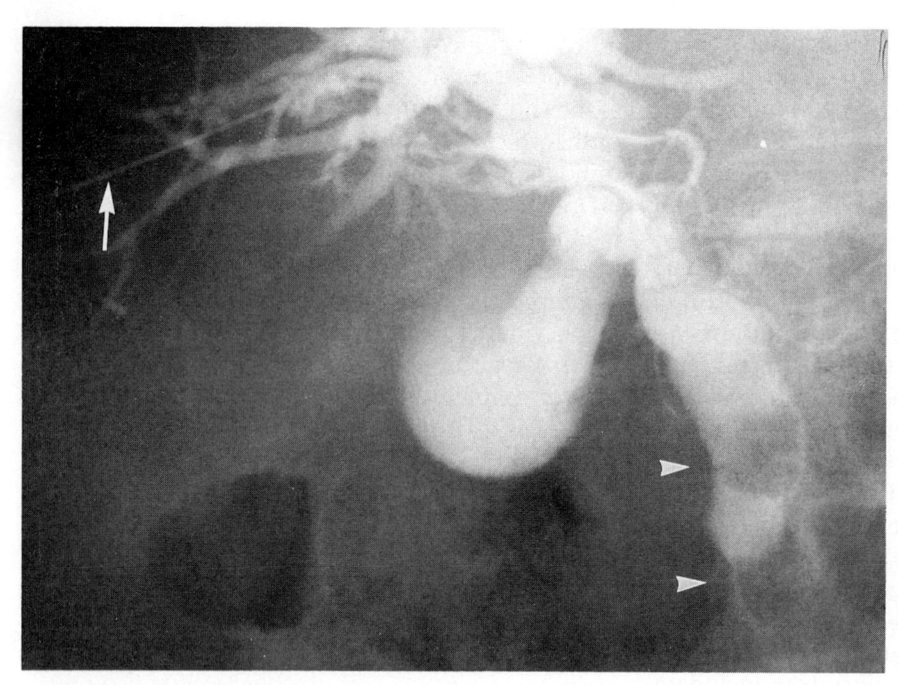

Figure 12.52 Percutaneous transhepatic cholangiogram performed with a 23 gauge needle (arrow). Contrast medium introduced into the dilated intrahepatic ducts has opacified the gallbladder and common bile duct. Two large stones are shown in the common bile duct (arrowheads).

death 0.2%.[68] Percutaneous transhepatic cholangiography should be done at a time when operating theatres and the surgical team are available if the patient is fit for surgery. If the patient is unsuitable for surgery, interventional radiological techniques should be available as well as other supportive measures to deal with complications.

Percutaneous transhepatic cholangiography may need to be used if endoscopic retrograde cholangiopancreatography has been unsuccessful or proved impossible because of a previous biliary–enteric anastomosis or a Polya gastrectomy. Percutaneous transhepatic cholangiography may be particularly useful in recurrent pyogenic cholangitis when the stones are mainly intrahepatic or there is suspicion by ultrasonography that there is a hilar cholangiocarcinoma, which is a recognized association in the Far East.[30]

Intravenous cholangiography

The patient should be fasted and the large bowel cleared of faeces. The patient must be well hydrated. An intravenous infusion of 100 ml of contrast medium (meglumine iotroxate or meglumine iodoxamate) is given over 30–45 minutes and tomographs of the bile ducts are taken at the end of the infusion. Delayed films are required to demonstrate the gallbladder (1–3 hours; 24 hours to show layering of stones).

The complications reported by Ansell in 1970[5] (death 1:5000, intermediate reactions 1:700, severe reactions 1:1600) are much less with the newer contrast materials. Absolute contradictions to intravenous cholangiography are combined liver and renal disease, sensitivity to iodine and Waldenström's macroglobulinaemia. Relative contraindications include allergy to drugs or contrast media, pregnancy, asthma and ischaemic heart disease because hypotension is still a frequent complication of the procedure. Severe reactions are more likely if two doses of contrast medium are given within 48 hours; thus, at least 1 week must elapse between intravenous cholangiography and, for example, oral cholecystography. Dehydration also increases the risk of toxicity.

Visualization of the bile ducts varies from 90% in those with a normal serum bilirubin level (<17 μmol/l) to 10% if the bilirubin concentration is over 68 μmol/l. Intravenous cholangiography fails to detect gallbladder stones in 30–50% of patients diagnosed by oral cholecystography. The detection rate for bile duct stones is less than by direct cholangiography even if the bile ducts are visualized.

Intravenous cholangiography is particularly indicated in the postcholecystectomy patient in whom endoscopic retrograde cholangiopancreatography has failed and percutaneous transhepatic cholangiography is undesirable or has also failed. Although intravenous cholangiography has several disadvantages, it is used routinely by a number of units to identify bile duct stones prior to elective cholecystectomy. This practice may increase with laparoscopic cholecystectomy because perioperative cholangiography is technically more demanding with this procedure than with conventional cholecystectomy.

Treatment

Supportive measures

While jaundice per se is not an 'emergency' condition, patients with choledocholithiasis require suitable preparation before any interventional procedure, whether surgical, endoscopic or radiological. Parenteral vitamin K (10 mg intravenously or 20 mg intramuscularly) is necessary, irrespective of the results of the clotting studies. Intravenous human albumin may be needed if the serum albumin level is less than 30 g/l, and a blood transfusion if the haemoglobin level is less than 10 g/dl. Prior to intervention the patient requires adequate hydration and a good urine output. It is wise to give intravenous fluids for 24 hours prior to intervention. If necessary, intravenous mannitol (100 ml of 20% solution) is administered to achieve a urine output of over 50 ml/h. Prophylactic antibiotics are mandatory (see p. 1757). Oral lactulose will lessen the endotoxin burden on the liver and lessen the risk of postprocedure renal failure.[134]

Surgical approaches

Overall, the results of operative choledocholithotomy appear acceptable at less than 2%, but this increases appreciably in high-risk groups, especially the elderly (9–30%).[113,119] The risks of biliary surgery in patients with acute cholangitis and severe gallstone pancreatitis are even greater.[112,113] Multivariate analysis has demonstrated that the most important risk factors for surgical morbidity are the preoperative bilirubin level and associated comorbidity.[123] Thus, surgery should be avoided in high-risk patients in preference to other techniques. Laparoscopic cholecystectomy apart, low- and moderate-risk cases do at least as well with surgery alone as with a combination of endoscopic sphincterotomy and surgery.[117]

The indications for surgical bile duct stone removal are:

1. Bile duct stones detected during elective conventional cholecystectomy (low- or moderate-risk patients).
2. Bile duct stones present during emergency cholecystectomy for complicated gallbladder stone disease including cholecystocholedochal fistula.
3. Resolving mild acute cholangitis initially treated conservatively (low or moderate risk).
4. Resolving acute pancreatitis initially treated conservatively (low or moderate risk).
5. Complicated hepatolithiasis in patients with recurrent pyogenic cholangitis (low to high risk).
6. Failed non-operative methods of bile duct stone removal or internal stenting (low to high risk).

The surgical approaches to the extrahepatic bile ducts include supraduodenal exploration, transduodenal sphincteroplasty and choledochoduodenostomy.[77] The preferred approach is through a right subcostal incision. The choice of operation is shown in the algorithm in *Figure 12.53*. Following bile duct exploration, choledochoscopy is mandatory because this has led to a reduction in retained bile duct stones from 3.5–15.5% to 1.4–6.0%.[191]

Whilst primary bile duct closure can be undertaken, successful insertion of a T tube is to be preferred. In order to avoid the complication of intraperitoneal abscess and bile leakage, the T tube

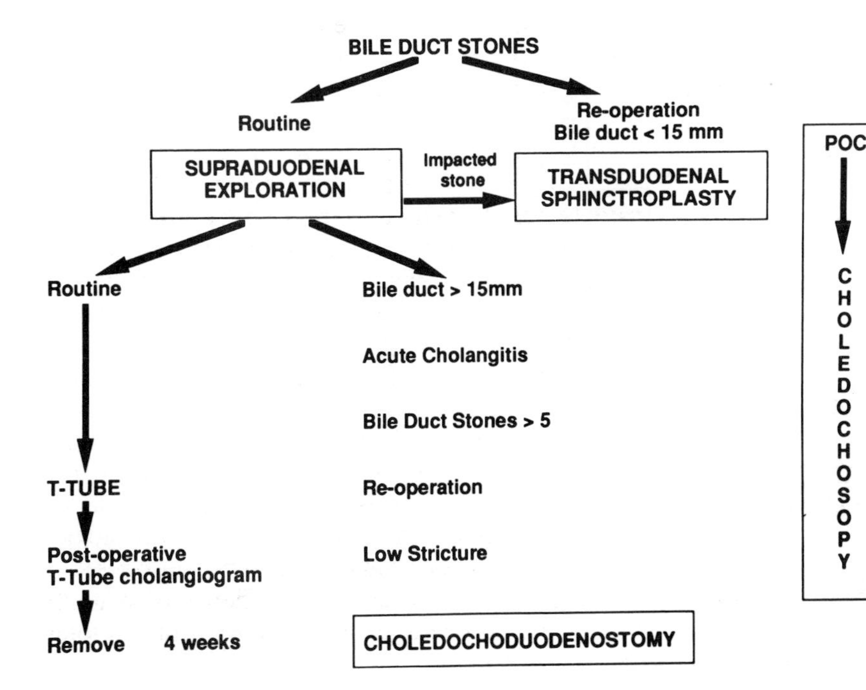

Figure 12.53 Algorithm for the surgical treatment of bile duct stones.

should be removed after several weeks. The patient may be sent home after a few days to return later for T-tube removal. The medium- and long-term results of surgical choledocholithotomy are comparable to those achieved endoscopically.[10,113]

The clinical picture is more complex in patients with *recurrent pyogenic cholangitis*: good results are obtained in 75–80% who have had transduodenal sphincteroplasty or hepaticojejunostomy.[112] Patients with intrahepatic strictures and stones require additional procedures of hepatotomy, transhepatic intubation, hepaticojejunostomy or partial hepatectomy. The mortality varies from 4.3 to 11.2%, depending upon the severity of the disease. Recurrent disease occurs in 4% following resection, 38% for transhepatic intubation and 75% for hepatotomy.[32]

Non-surgical approaches

The main choice lies between endoscopic sphincterotomy and stone extraction versus the percutaneous transhepatic route (*Figure 12.54*). The former is to be preferred but this will be dependent on the availability of local expertise. Patients with stones found on the postoperative T-tube cholangiograph may be treated by the Burhenne technique following T-tube tract dilatation. The indications for non-surgical treatment of bile duct stones are:

1. Postcholecystectomy (low- to high-risk cases).[58,157,180,191]
2. Prior to laparoscopic cholecystectomy (low to moderate risk).
3. Moderate-to-severe acute cholangitis, Western variety (irrespective of co-morbidity).[87,118]
4. Moderate-to-severe recurrent pyogenic cholangitis with stones largely in the extrahepatic biliary tree (irrespective of co-morbidity).[58,86,89]
5. Acute cholangitis secondary to ascariasis (irrespective of co-morbidity).[81]
6. Acute gallstone pancreatitis: prognostically or clinically severe cases, patients who fail to progress or patients requiring pancreatic surgery (irrespective of co-morbidity) (see p. 1602).[112,121,122]
7. Patients with the gallbladder in situ (high risk).[42,58,73,160]
8. Patients with a T tube in situ (all cases).[24,58,165]
9. Patients with an access hepaticojejunostomy; usually those with recurrent pyogenic cholangitis.[33,58,194]
10. Sump syndrome following choledochoduonostomy (all cases).[9]
11. Mirizzi's syndrome (all cases) (see p. 1741).

A variety of adjunctive measures are available which enhance the success rates of non-operative forms of treatment (see *Table 12.14*).

Endoscopic treatment

Endoscopic sphincterotomy and bile duct stone clearance can be undertaken in 85–99% of patients.[191] The success rate of sphincterotomy can be increased by needle knife papillotomy[47] or a combined percutaneous endoscopic technique.[48] The complication rate is 5–10%; the procedural mortality is 0.4–1.4% although the 30-day mortality varies from 1 to 3.5%.[191] Elderly patients and those with concomitant medical problems fare better with endoscopic than surgical treatment.[123,191] Although

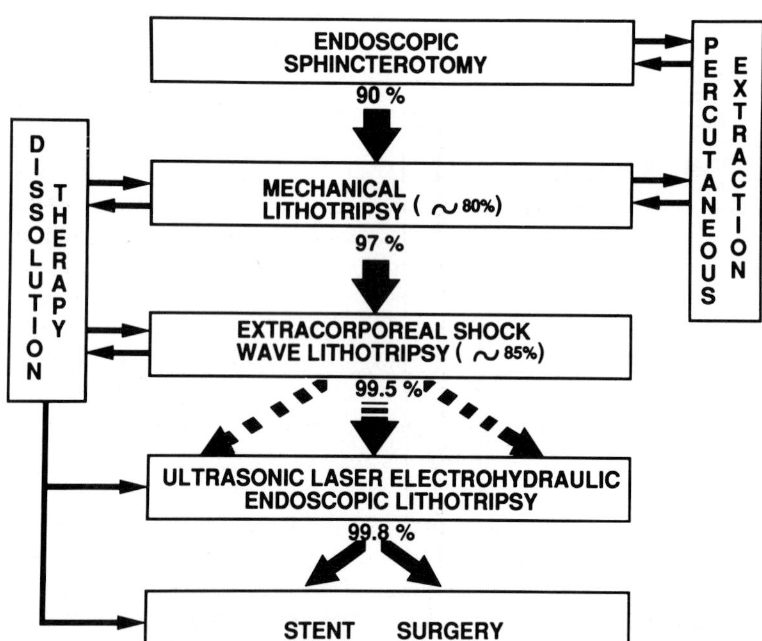

Figure 12.54 Algorithm for the non-surgical treatment of bile duct stones. The success rates of the main individual techniques are shown in parentheses and the estimated cumulative success rates are shown below the boxes.

the success rate of endoscopic sphincterotomy in patients with a duodenal diverticulum is slightly less (95 versus 98%) and the complication rate slightly higher (4.0 versus 5.2%), this is of little practical consequence.[179] Newer sphincterotomes (reverse push type or Sohma type) can also increase the success rate (up to 95%) in patients with a Polya gastrectomy.[128] A combined radiological and endoscopic technique using a paediatric colonoscope can be used to achieve stone extraction in patients with a Roux-en-Y reconstruction.[65]

ADJUNCTS TO ENDOSCOPIC SPHINCTEROTOMY

An algorithm for the use of the many techniques available is shown in *Figure 12.54*.

1. Mechanical lithotripsy

This is the most valuable adjunctive technique; the success rate is inversely proportional to the stone size.[156]

2. Extracorporeal shock wave lithotripsy (see p. 1728)

The shock waves are directed from the posterior aspect of the patient and a nasobiliary catheter is necessary. The success rate varies from 75 to 100% in collected series.[185] The initial success rate is 75%, which may be improved with further treatment sessions.[154] Adjunctive endoscopic extraction is necessary in 70%.[154] The complication rate is 30% and includes procedural pain, cutaneous petechiae, pyrexia, haematuria, haemobilia, gallbladder empyema, haematomas of the liver and kidney, ruptured duodenal diverticulum, biliary colic and acute pancreatitis. These complications are usually mild and transient; the mortality is less than 1%.[154, 185]

3. Intracorporeal lithotripsy

Ultrasonic,[45] electrohydraulic[90] and laser[51] lithotripsy devices are available. The tip of the instrument should be close to the target stones. Although it is possible to achieve this by fluoroscopy, direct endoscopic vision is preferred.[88]

4. Nasobiliary catheter and internal stenting

Temporary drainage must be provided if a sphincterotomy cannot be adequately performed or the biliary tree is not completely cleared. A nasobiliary catheter will allow this and permit repeat contrast studies to be undertaken as some stones will pass spontaneously; it buys time to enable further endoscopic attempts at removal or for consideration of alternative forms of treatment. A nasobiliary catheter is necessary for direct dissolution treatment or for extracorporeal shock wave lithotripsy. An internal stent is effective treatment when all else fails and the bile duct stones still remain.[28]

5. Direct dissolution therapy (see p. 1724)

The results are suboptimal because of the type of dissolution agents available, stone composition and physicochemical considerations.[116]

Monooctanoin Monooctanoin cleared the bile duct of stones in 26% of 343 patients; some stone reduction was achieved in a further 29%, allowing extraction by repeat mechanical methods.[135] Side-effects were common, requiring cessation of treatment in 9%. Treatment may be prolonged (mean 7.2 days).

Methyl tert-butyl ether (see p. 1726) This agent has proved disappointing for treating bile duct stones. In a collected series of 74 patients, success occurred in 55%, of whom 80% required additional intervention. Complications were common (79%), including pain, anorexia, nausea, hypotension, drowsiness and headaches.[125]

Bile acid–EDTA–modified monooctanoin solutions These have been promoted as being more successful for the brown pigment stones (found in 24–70% of bile ducts) than the cholesterol dissolution agents mentioned above. The evidence for this is limited.[116]

COMPLICATIONS OF ENDOSCOPIC TREATMENT

Immediate complications include bleeding (2.5%), perforation (1.1%) and an impacted basket (0.2%). Bleeding can usually be managed conservatively although 17.1% of patients will require surgery.[133,191] Adjunctive measures to control bleeding include the use of pressor agents, sclerosants and embolization. The overall mortality from significant bleeding is 8.9%. Retroperitoneal perforation requires surgery in 41% of patients. The overall mortality is 12%. The diagnosis can usually be made with a supine plain radiograph which shows air in the retroperitoneal tissues. Basket impaction has been associated with an operation rate of 67% and a mortality of 11%. Extracorporeal shock wave lithotripsy may help to minimize the use of surgery.[14]

Intermediate complications develop within the first 24 hours postsphincterotomy. Acute pancreatitis (2%) requires surgery in 7% of patients; the mortality is 11%.[133,191] Acute cholangitis (1.3%) is usually associated with incomplete clearance or drainage and the need for surgery is high (34%) with an overall mortality of 9%. Acute cholecystitis or empyema of the gallbladder occurs in 5–10% of patients with the gallbladder in situ and patients with pre-existing cholangitis are particularly predisposed to this complication.[42]

Late complications: long-term follow-up shows that about 3% of patients develop restenosis of the ampulla of Vater and 6% develop recurrent stones.[157]

Percutaneous techniques

The transhepatic route is used to access the biliary tree for stone dissolution or extraction and emergency decompression for cholangitis. The T-tube route is used for retained stones.

Percutaneous transhepatic techniques

These are based on percutaneous transhepatic cholangiography (see p. 1747). A guide wire is introduced following removal of the needle stylet and opacification of the biliary tree to confirm positioning. The tract is dilated to an appropriate size. A tract of at least 8 Fr is necessary and larger tract sizes may be developed at several separate sessions. Stone extraction can be achieved in 78–93% of patients but with a significant complication rate (13–38% including pain, bleeding and biliary leaks) and a mortality of about 2%.[76,166] Adjunct techniques include sphincterotomy,[35] Gruntzig balloon dilatation,[66] and electrohydraulic,[76] ultrasonic,[12] laser[83] and mechanical lithotripsy.[187] Direct dissolution may also be used.[184] Direct percutaneous endoscopic visualization of the biliary tree may be preferred in complex situations.[76]

T-tube tract techniques

Usually the tract is allowed to mature for 5–6 weeks[24,58] while repeat cholangiography is performed under antibiotic cover. If the T tube is less than 14 Fr, the T tube can be removed and the tract dilated to be replaced by a working sheath. A 13 Fr Burhenne steerable catheter is introduced and the stone grasped with the Dormia basket and extracted. Sphincter relaxation (using, for example, intravenous glucagon) can be used to relax the sphincter in order to push the stone out through the ampulla of Vater. The stone may be crushed with the Dormia basket, or Mazzariello–Caprini forceps. The success rates vary from 80 to 97%.[58] Complications occur in about 5% of patients, and include sinus tract perforation, cholangitis, pancreatitis, biliary peritonitis and vasovagal reactions, and there is a very low mortality (about 0.1%).[58]

Non-surgical treatment of choledocholithiasis – choice of treatment

Acute cholangitis

Endoscopic sphincterotomy is the preferred method of treatment in patients who do not settle with conservative measures. There is a lower complication rate (30 versus 60%) and mortality (<5 versus 20–40%) compared to surgery.[82,87,112,180] If endoscopic sphincterotomy is not possible or is not available, percutaneous biliary decompression is valuable prior to definite surgery.[137]

Recurrent pyogenic cholangitis

Endoscopic sphincterotomy is preferred in patients with predominantly extrahepatic biliary stone disease.[86,89] Success is possible in 90–97% of patients with a low complication rate (10%) and mortality (2–5%). This approach may be combined with interventional radiological procedures in those with hepatolithiasis. The use of cholangioscopy with modern forms of lithotripsy can provide high success rates (78–95%) with an acceptable complication rate (up to 38%) and a low mortality (2%).[76,194] If surgery is necessary, a large T tube can be inserted or an access hepaticojujunostomy established to allow subsequent percutaneous dilatation and extraction of retained or recurrent stones.[33,194]

Choledocholithiasis in patients with the gallbladder in situ

Endoscopic sphincterotomy is the preferred method of treatment in high-risk patients. About 10–15% of patients will develop gallbladder complications; empyema of the gallbladder may be particularly difficult to recognize in the elderly.[42,73,160] Antibiotics are given to these patients for 5–7 days. Although it has been suggested that non-filling of the gallbladder during endoscopic retrograde cholangiopancreatography indicates a high predisposition to gallbladder sepsis, the weight of evidence is against this.[191] Complications developing with the gallbladder should be treated non-operatively in the first instance (see p. 1724).

Patients with the T tube in situ

The majority of stones (60% or so) can be treated by flushing with normal saline if the stone lies below the T tube. A relaxant of the sphincter of Oddi is given (sublingual glyceryl trinitrate, intravenous glucagon or intravenous cerulatide) to assist passage.[116] The choice lies between the Burhenne technique and endoscopic sphincterotomy. The former has marginally lower complication rates but the latter can be performed immediately without the need to wait several weeks for the tract to mature.[140] Direct dissolution is a poor option at present because of poor efficacy, complications and length of treatment required (see p. 1751).[116]

Sump syndrome

This occurs in 3.3% of patients with choledochoduodenostomy; an equivalent syndrome occurs in about

4% of patients with a surgical sphincteroplasty.[10] This is usually due to narrowing of the stoma allowing accumulation of food debris and bacterial overgrowth. The symptoms are intermittent and include abdominal pain or discomfort, malaise, pyrexia and jaundice. Acute cholangitis occurs in a minority.[9] Endoscopic sphincterotomy is the treatment of choice.[9,191] If this is not possible, direct widening of the stoma using a duodenoscopic cutting diathermy needle is an alternative.[19]

BILIARY FISTULAS

Biliary fistulas may be internal, intraperitoneal or external. The former is usually due to gallstone disease and the latter usually due to trauma (mostly iatrogenic).

Internal biliary fistulas

If all the causes of biliary fistulas are considered, gallstones are responsible for 90%, peptic ulcer 6% and the remaining 4% follow cancer, trauma, parasitic infestation and congenital anomalies.[139] The incidence is about 1% in Western gallstone disease[63] compared to 13–18% in the Far East where primary bile duct stone disease predominates.[178]

Investigations

PLAIN RADIOGRAPHY

Plain radiographs may show pneumobilia (30–50%), a 'moving' calcified stone (10–30%) and 'tumbling' obstruction (see p. 1741).

BARIUM STUDIES

A barium meal may reveal a cholecystoduodenal fistula (40%) or choledochoduodenal fistula (75%); a barium enema will reveal a cholecystocolic fistula (95%).

CT SCANNING

CT is useful for showing air in the biliary tree in uncertain cases and may suggest the cause of the lesion (gallstones versus malignant disease).

CHOLANGIOGRAPHY

Endoscopic retrograde cholangiopancreatography is preferred but percutaneous transhepatic cholangiography may prove complementary at times. These techniques are particularly indicated for diagnosing complicated fistulas (e.g. cholecystocholedochal and bronchobiliary fistulas).

RADIONUCLIDE BILIARY SCAN

This technique is useful for demonstrating very small fistulas, or fistulas which allow abnormal flow of bile only intermittently (e.g. to the colon or bronchial tree), using delayed imaging.

ULTRASONOGRAPHY

Assessment of residual gallbladder stone size relative to fistula size in a patient with a cholecystoduodenal fistula may be difficult at laparotomy and ultrasonography can be useful in deciding whether to perform cholecystectomy in a patient with gallstone ileus.

Specific types of internal biliary fistula

CHOLECYSTODUODENAL FISTULA AND GALLSTONE ILEUS (see p. 1741)

CHOLECYSTOCHOLEDOCHAL FISTULA (see p. 1741)

CHOLECYSTOCOLIC FISTULA (see p. 1741)

PERIAMPULLARY CHOLEDOCHODUODENAL FISTULA

The diagnosis requires investigation by endoscopic retrograde cholangiopancreatography. The fistulas are usually caused by iatrogenic trauma or by choledocholithiasis. Symptoms may occur either because of remaining bile duct stones which give rise to jaundice or because of a variant of the 'stump' syndrome (see p. 1755). Such primary fistulas occur in patients from the Far East.

Clinical features include a history of symptoms for more than 10 years (46%), pain (88%), jaundice (69%), choleliathiasis (71%), choledocholithiasis (38%) and a demonstrable fistula by a plain radiograph or barium meal (41%).[170] Treatment is only necessary if the patient has symptoms: either endoscopic sphincterotomy or 'fistulotomy' is suitable.

CHOLEDOCHODUODENAL FISTULA DUE TO PEPTIC ULCER DISEASE

This may be noticed incidentally because of pneumobilia (15–60%). The symptoms are those of chronic peptic ulcer disease; biliary symptoms such as jaundice or cholangitis are rare. Treatment is aimed at the peptic ulcer; if surgery is performed, direct repair of the fistula is probably best avoided.[152]

BRONCHOBILIARY AND PLEUROBILIARY FISTULAS

Congenital bronchobiliary fistulas may present in the neonate or at 3–33 months of age.[29] The diagnosis is made by bronchography, bronchoscopy or radionuclide biliary scanning. Treatment is surgical. Acquired bronchobiliary and pleurobiliary fistulas are due to liver trauma, iatrogenic injury, complicated gallstone disease and parasitic infestation (e.g. echinococcosis and amoebiasis). Endoscopic sphincterotomy and biliary stenting have a high success rate for treating the fistulas.[141] Additional measures (medical, interventional, radiological and surgical) may also be necessary to deal with the underlying cause or other complications such as abscess.

External biliary fistulas

These are usually iatrogenic (surgical, radiological or endoscopic intervention) but may follow inflammation due to complicated gallstone disease. Continued major bile loss (1 l/day or more) results in the *choledochostomy acidotic syndrome*, in which sodium loss exceeds chloride loss. There is also hypokalaemia but, if renal failure supervenes, hyperkalaemia is present.

The precise site of leakage must be identified and this may be achieved by one or more of the following investigations: T-tube cholangiography (if the T tube is still present), fistulography, endoscopic retrograde cholangiopancreatography, radionuclide biliary scanning or percutaneous transhepatic cholangiography.

Treatment involves fluid and electrolyte replacement and effective biliary drainage – usually by endoscopic sphincterotomy and/or use of a nasobiliary catheter or biliary stent.[141] If this is not initially successful, endoscopic selective embolization of the biliary tree may be tried[85] before resorting to surgery.

BILIARY STRICTURE

The usual cause of biliary strictures is iatrogenic, most frequently following cholecystectomy (0.3%) but also because of inflammation from gallstone disease.[4] Intrahepatic biliary strictures in recurrent pyogenic cholangitis are common (see p. 1745).[32,131]

Surgical treatment (usually a Roux-en-Y hepaticojejunostomy) provides good long-term results in about 85% of patients.[186] Repeat operations are often required and the long-term mortality for this is about 10%. Percutaneous dilatation (especially for anastamotic strictures) and endoscopic dilatation and stenting are emerging as important alternative approaches but follow-up results are limited.[18,140]

POSTCHOLECYSTECTOMY SYNDROME

Up to 43% of patients develop some symptoms following cholecystectomy but these are severe in probably no more than 5%.[20]

The postcholecystectomy syndrome describes a clinical situation in which the patient believes that the original symptoms prior to cholecystectomy have returned to a lesser or greater extent. The symptoms vary, therefore, from vague biliary 'dyspepsia' to classical biliary colic. Gallbladder disease may not have been the cause of the original symptoms, although at least mild histopathological changes are found in nearly all gallbladders removed. Removal of the gallbladder may reveal another set of symptoms previously overshadowed by genuine biliary colic. Alternatively, the operation itself may have resulted in a complication which manifests itself months or years later. Finally, unrelated disease may arise which the patient interprets as a return of the original symptoms. The appearance of jaundice should not be included in the definition of the postcholecystectomy syndrome because it indicates a clear reason for the return of symptoms.

Aetiology

The cause of the symptoms may be pre-existing, consequent (iatrogenic or natural) or subsequent to cholecystectomy.

The causes (*Table 12.15*) may be classified into:

1. Organic: non-biliary or biliary.
2. Dysfunctional: gastrointestinal tract or biliary.
3. Psychosomatic.

Important causes include retained or recurrent bile duct stones (30%), sphincter of Oddi dysfunction (9%) (see p. 1785), peptic ulcers (5%), tumours of the pancreas or biliary tree (4%), chronic pancreatitis (3%) and bile duct stricture (2%).[120] A non-biliary (or pancreatic cause) is evident in at least 30% of cases.[120]

Investigations

The most important part of the diagnostic evaluation is a careful history and a review of precholecystectomy symptoms. This usually provides an important clue to the underlying cause, and should direct subsequent investigations. It is helpful to know if the patient has had only a cholecystectomy, if a perioperative cholangiogram has been performed and if there has been exploration of the bile ducts. If an obvious cause is not immediately apparent, upper gastrointestinal endoscopy and ultrasonography are often rewarding. Failing these, endoscopic retrograde cholangiopancreatography is warranted.[120] Patients may suffer debilitating symptoms of pain and weight loss associated with a retained or recurrent bile duct stone years after cholecystectomy and yet have a normal ultrasound examination and normal 'liver function tests'.

Table 12.15 Causes of the postcholecystectomy syndrome

Extrabiliary	*Biliary*
Reflux oesophagitis	Retained bile duct stone
Oesophageal dysmotility	Recurrent bile duct stone
Peptic dysmotility	Bile duct stricture
Irritable bowel syndrome	Internal biliary fistula
Idiopathic chronic constipation	Biliary or periampullary tumour
Diverticular disease	Sclerosing cholangitis
Chronic pancreatitis	Sphincter of Oddi dysfunction
Pancreatic carcinoma	Stenosis
Chronic active hepatitis	Dysmotility
Vertebral column osteoarthrosis	Long cyst duct stump[a]
Psychosomatic	Cystic duct sump neuroma[a]
Postoperative adhesions[a]	

[a] Questionable causes.

Recourse is often to a CT examination. Laparotomy is best avoided because a cause is rarely found and the problem is then compounded by the surgical intervention. Dynamic HIDA scanning may be a useful screening (or diagnostic) procedure[56] for sphincter of Oddi dysfunction although the patient may ultimately require manometric assessment (see p. 1785).[120]

Treatment

This depends on establishing the cause. If none is found, symptomatic relief may be obtained with simple measures such as reassurance, antacids or antispasmodics. Mild analgesics may prove useful but narcotics should be avoided. In selected patients a psychiatric referral is required.

INFECTION AND THE BILIARY SYSTEM

Bacteria are infrequently found in the normal biliary tree. Bacterial overgrowth which may lead to infection is consequent upon biliary tract disease or iatrogenic interference (percutaneous, endoscopic or surgical intervention); the exceptions are recurrent pyogenic cholangitis (see p. 1745) and specific infections or infestations (see *Table 12.13*).

ROUTES OF INFECTION

Bacteria usually reach the biliary system from the lower gastrointestinal tract via the hepatic–portal circulation. They are normally cleared by the hepatic Kupffer cells but some may escape to enter the bile canaliculi.

Those patients who have had a biliary enteric procedure will usually have bacteria present in the bile, in which event the bacteria probably reach the biliary tree from the gut lumen via the anastomosis. These patients are usually without symptoms unless biliary drainage through the anastomosis is obstructed. Common procedures in which this situation occurs are choledochoduodenostomy and transduodenal sphincteroplasty. It is important to ensure that, in patients undergoing hepaticojejunostomy for biliary stricture, the Roux-en-Y limb up to the biliary enteric anastomosis is 60–75 cm long to prevent reflux of intestinal contents, which can cause intermittent attacks of acute cholangitis.

Bacteria may also reach the biliary system via the systemic arterial supply and retrogressively via the lymphatics. These routes may be important in the aetiology of acute cholecystitis.

Bacteriology

The frequency of positive bile cultures varies considerably according to the type of biliary disease (*Table 12.16*). Factors which predispose to bacterobilia are gallstones, iatrogenic interference, obstructive jaundice (see *Table 12.16*) and increasing age (*Table 12.17*). Given the main routes of spread, it is not surprising that the bacteria commonly isolated are similar to those found in the gastrointestinal tract (*Table 12.18*). Aerobic organisms were only isolated in 41% of 371 patients studied by Bourgault *et al.*;[23] 26% had mixed aerobic and anaerobic organisms and only 0.5% had anaerobic organisms only. Anaerobes are particularly associated with increasing age, more severe sepsis, complications, and previous interference with the biliary tree.[53]

Table 12.16 Frequency of bacteria in bile according to type of biliary disease

Type of biliary disease	*Positive bile culture* (%)
Uncomplicated gallbladder stones	14
Mucocoele of the gallbladder	29
Empyema of the gallbladder	34
Acute cholecystitis	84
Resolving acute cholecystitis	48
Bile duct stones	84
Benign bile duct stricture	90
Jaundice due to cancer	29

Based on 423 patients; after Keighley and Blankharn.[80]

Table 12.17 Frequency of bacterobilia according to type of gallstone disease and patient age

	Positive bile culture by age in decades (%)								
Type of gallstone	*<20 years*	*21–30*	*31–40*	*41–50*	*51–60*	*61–70*	*71–80*	*>80*	*All*
Uncomplicated	18	10	0	7	14	17	33	50	11
Acute cholecystitis	0	0	—	23	36	70	33	100	40
Bile duct stones; no jaundice	—	66	60	25	80	55	0	66	55
Bile duct stones; jaundice	—	0	0	20	50	—	100	100	53

Based on 532 patients; after Elliott.[52]

Table 12.18 Types of bacteria found in bile in patients with gallstone disease

Aerobic		*Anaerobic*	
Common[a]	*Uncommon*	*Common*[a]	*Uncommon*
Escherichia coli[b,c]	*Staphylococcus aureus*[c]	*Bacteroides* spp.[b,c]	Microaerophilic streptococci[c]
Streptococcus faecalis[b,c]	*Staphylococcus epidermidis*[c]	*Clostridium* spp.[b,c]	Anaerobic streptococci[c]
Klebsiella spp.[b,c]	*Enterobacter* spp.	*Fusobacterium* spp.	*Bifidobacterium* spp.
Pseudomonas spp.[c]	*Corynebacterium* spp.		*Eubacterium* spp.
Streptococcus viridans[c]	*Citrobacter* spp.		*Actinomycosis* spp.
Proteus spp.[c]	*Lactobacillus*		*Proprionibacterium* spp.
	Haemophilus influenza		
	Serratia spp.		
	Morganella morganii		

[a]Usually found in at least 5% of bile samples,
[b]Found in at least 15% of bile samples,
[c]Often isolated from blood cultures in patients with acute cholangitis.

BILE DUCT OBSTRUCTION AND INFECTION

Obstructive jaundice will affect a number of hepatocyte functions, including glucose, protein and lipid metabolism. Of direct relevance to the development of sepsis are the effects on Kupffer cell activity and the luminal bile duct pressure. In the presence of jaundice, impaired clearance of bacteria and endotoxins occurs, leading to 'spill over' into the general circulation. Increased bacterial trapping occurs in the pulmonary circulation whilst endotoxins may be particularly damaging to the kidneys. In health, some bacteria normally enter the biliary canaliculi, but with normal bile flow they are ejected into the duodenum. In the presence of obstruction, bacteria will multiply, giving rise to overt sepsis (acute cholangitis).

The normal resting pressure in the intraluminal biliary tree is 10–12 cmH_2O, whilst the maximum secretory pressure of hepatocytes is 30 cmH_2O. As the biliary pressure rises above normal, there is cholangiovenous reflux of bacteria, perhaps via intracellular vacuoles,[144] resulting in bacteraemia or septicaemia. Ninety per cent of patients with a bile duct pressure over 25 cmH_2O had bacteraemia and a 30% mortality in one study; in contrast, those with a lower pressure had a 40% incidence of bacteraemia and a 10% mortality.[95]

ANTIBIOTICS

All patients undergoing routine uncomplicated biliary surgery should receive a single-dose antibiotic with appropriate cover against the main organisms found in bile (see *Table 12.18*). A meta-analysis has shown that this should apply to low-risk as well as high-risk patients and that first or subsequent generation cephalosporins are equally appropriate.[104] Single-agent cover is also recommended for prophylaxis in patients undergoing endoscopic retrograde cholangiopancreatography or percutaneous transhepatic cholangiography. In patients who are at high risk of anaerobic infection, appropriate cover should also be given.

Although a single-agent regimen is usually all that is required for most cases of acute cholecystitis, treatment aimed also at anaerobes is recommended for elderly patients and those with severe cholecystitis. A regimen which will cover microaerophilic streptococci and peptostreptococci as well as the commoner anaerobes and aerobes is required in patients with cholangitis. The ureidopenicillins (e.g. mezlocillin and piperacillin) have an appropriate wide spectrum of activity against Gram-negative bacilli, streptococci and anaerobes but they are susceptible to some β-lactamase inactivation. The broad-spectum antipseudomonal cephalosporins (cefoperazone and ceftazidime) also have useful applications in severe biliary sepsis. Although both the ureidopenicillins and cefoperazone have high biliary excretion rates, this is largely irrelevant in acute cholangitis as there is little or no penetration of antibiotics into the bile of patients with obstruction.

In general, therefore, an agent such as cefuroxime is recommended for routine prophylaxis in patients undergoing surgery, endoscopic retrograde cholangiopancreatography or percutaneous transhepatic cholangiography with uncomplicated biliary disease. In addition, metronidazole should be added for patients at particular risk of anaerobic infection such as elderly or diabetic patients with acute cholecystitis. For severe acute cholangitis, ceftazadime (or gentamicin) along with ampicillin and metronidazole is suggested.

REFERENCES

1. Acosta, J.M. and Ledema, C.L. (1974) Gallstone migration as a cause of acute pancreatitis. *New England Journal of Medicine*, **290**, 484–485.
2. Anderson, A. and Zederfeldt, B. (1969) Gallstone ileus. *Acta Chirurgica Scandinavica*, **135**, 713–717.
3. Anderson, A., Bergdahl, L. and Boquist, L. (1971) Acalculous cholecystitis. *American Journal of Surgery*, **122**, 3–7.
4. Andren-Sandberg, A., Alinder, G. and Bengmark, S. (1985) Accidental lesions of the common bile duct at cholecystectomy. Pre and perioperative factors of importance. *Annals of Surgery*, **201**, 328–332.
5. Ansell, G. (1970) Adverse reactions to contrast agents. Scope of problem. *Investigative Radiology*, **5**, 374.
6. Aranha, G.V., Sdntag, S.J. and Greenlee, H.B. (1982) Cholecystectomy in cirrhotic patients: a formidable operation. *American Journal of Surgery*, **143**, 55–59.
7. Asfar, S., Al-Refah, F.I., Al-Mokhtar, N.Y. and Baraka A. (1989) Percutaneous sclerosis of the gallbladder, *The Lancet*, **ii**, 387.
8. Axelrod, L., Munster, A.M. and O'Brien T.F. (1971) Typhoid cholecystitis and gallbladder carcinoma after interval of 67 years. *Journal of the American Medical Association*, **217**, 83.
9. Baker, A.R., Neoptolemos, J.P., Carr-Locke, D.L. and Fossard, D.P. (1985) Sump syndrome following choledocho-duodenostomy and its endoscopic treatment. *British Journal of Surgery*, **72**, 433–435.
10. Baker, A.R., Neoptolemos, J.P., Leese, T., James, D.C. and Fossard D.P. (1987) Longterm follow-up of patients with side to side choledochoduodenostomy and transduodenal

sphincteroplasty. *Annals of the Royal College of Surgeons of England*, **68**, 253–257.
11. Baron, R.L. (1987) Common bile duct stones: reassessment of criteria for CT diagnosis. *Radiology*, **162**, 419–424.
12. Bean, W.J., Daughtry, J.D., Rodan, B.A. and Mullin, D. (1985) Ultrasonic lithotripsy of retained common bile duct stone. *American Journal of Roentgenology*, **144**, 1275–1276.
13. Becker, C.D., Quenville, N.F. and Burhenne, H.J. (1988) Longterm occlusion of the porcine cystic duct by means of endoluminal radio-frequency electrocoagulation. *Radiology*, **g167**, 63–68.
14. Becker, C.D., Gibney R.G., Fache J.S., Rowley A., McLoughlin M.G. and Burhenne, H.J. (1989) Fragmentation grosser und impaktierter. Gallenblasenkankremente mittels Ultraschall. *Rontgenpraxis*, **42**, 40–44.
15. Benbow, E.W. (1990) Xanthogranulomatous cholecystitis. *British Journal of Surgery*, **77**, 255–256.
16. Berk, R.N., Armburster, T.G. and Saltzstein, S.L. (1973) Carcinoma in the porcelain gallbladder. *Radiology*, **106**, 29–31.
17. Berk, R.N., Ferrucci, J.T. and Leopold, G.R. (1983) *Radiology of the Gallbladder and Bile Ducts; Diagnosis and Intervention*. Philadelphia: W.B. Saunders.
18. Berkelhammer, C.H., Kortan, P., Hapner, G.B. (1989) Endoscopic biliary prostheses as treatment for benign postoperative bile duct strictures. *Gastrointestinal Endoscopy*, **35**, 95–101.
19. Blair, A.J., Leung, J.W.C. and Cotton, P.B. (1985) Endoscopic treatment of stomal stenosis after choledochoduodenostomy: preliminary report. *Surgery*, **97**, 487–489.
20. Bodvall, B. (1973) The postcholecystectomy syndrome. *Clinics in Gastroenterology*, **2**, 103–126.
21. Bonardi, L., Gandini, G., Gabasio, S., Fascetti, E., Gremo, L., Righi, D., Asnaghi, R., Volterrani, U. and Verme, G. (1986) Methyl-tet-butyl ether (MTBE) and endoscopic sphincterotomy. A possible dissolution for dissolving gallstones. *Endoscopy*, **18**, 238–239.
22. Bouchier, I.A.D. (1984) Imaging procedures to diagnose gall bladder disease. *British Medical Journal*, **288**, 1632–1633.
23. Bourgault, A.M., England, D.M., Rosenblatt, J.E., Forgacs, P. and Bieger, R.C. (1979) Clinical characteristics of anaerobic bactibilia. *Archives of Internal Medicine*, **139**, 1346–1349.
24. Burhenne, H.J. (1980) Percutaneous extraction of retained biliary stones: 661 patients. *American Journal of Roentgenology*, **134**, 888–898.
25. Burnstein, M.J., Vassal, K.P. and Strasberg, S.M. (1982) Results of combined biliary drainage and cholecystokinin cholecystography in 81 patients with oral cholecystograms. *Annals of Surgery*, **196**, 627–632.
26. Butsch, J.L. and Luchette, F. (1985) Torsion of the gallbladder. *Archives of Surgery*, **120**, 1323.
27. Cairns, S.R., Watson, G.N., Lees, W.R. and Salmon, P.R. (1987) Percutaneous lithotripsy and endoprosthesis: a new treatment for obstructive jaundice in Mirizzi's syndrome. *British Medical Journal*, **295**, 1448.
28. Cairns, S.R., Diaj, L., Cotton, P.B., Salmon, P.R. and Russell, R.C.G. (1989) Additional endoscopic procedures instead of urgent surgery for retained common bile duct stones. *Gut*, **30**, 335–340.
29. Chan, Y.T., Ng, W.D., Mak, W.P., Kong, M.L. and Chow, C.B. (1984) Congenital bronchobiliary fistula associated with biliary atresia. *British Journal of Surgery*, **71**, 240–241.
30. Chen, P.H., Lo, H.W. and Wang, C.S. (1984) Cholangiocarcinoma in hepatolithiasis. *Journal of Clinical Gastroenterology*, **6**, 539–547.
31. Chiverton, S.G., Inglis, J.A., Hudd, C., Kellett, M., Russell, R.C.G. and Wickham, J.E.A. (1990) Percutaneous cholecystolithotomy: the first 60 patients. *British Medical Journal*, **300**, 1310–1312.
32. Choi, T.K., Wong, J. and Ong, G.B. (1982) The surgical management of primary intrahepatic stones. *British Journal of Surgery*, **69**, 86–90.
33. Choi, T.K., Lee, M.J.R., Lui, R., Fok, M. and Wong, J. (1986) Postoperative flexible choledoschoscopy for residual primary intrahepatic stones. *Annals of Surgery*, **203**, 260–265.
34. Cobden, I., Lendrum, R., Venables, C.W. and James, O.F.W. (1984) Gallstones presenting as mental and physical debility in the elderly. *The Lancet*, **i**, 1062–1064.
35. Cobourn, C., Makowka, L., Ho, C.S., Taylor B. and Langer, B. (1986) Percutaneous transhepatic sphincterotomy in the management of biliary tract disease. *Gastrointestinal Radiology*, **17**, 273–276.
36. Copeman, P.M.W. and Medd, W.E. (1967) Diffuse systemic sclerosis with abnormal liver and gall bladder. *British Medical Journal*, **iii**, 353–354.
37. Corrasco, C.H., Freeny, P.C., Chuang, V.P. and Wallace, S. (1983) Chemical cholecystitis associated with hepatic artery infusion chemotherapy. *American Journal of Roentgenology*, **141**, 703–706.
38. Cotton, P.B. and Williams, C.B. (1990) *Practical Gastrointestinal Endoscopy*, 3rd edn. Boston: Blackwell.
39. Cronan, J.J. (1989) Ultrasound diagnosis of choledocholithiasis: a reappraisal. *Radiology*, **161**, 133–134.
40. Csendes, A., Diaz, J.C., Burdiles, P., Maluenda, F. and Nava, O. (1989) Mirizzi's syndrome and cholecystobiliary fistula: a unifying classification. *British Journal of Surgery*, **76**, 1139–1143.
41. Datz, F.L. (1986) Utility of indium^{III}-labelled leukocyte imaging in acute acalculous cholecystitis. *American Journal of Roentgenology*, **147**, 813–814.
42. Davidson, B.R., Neoptolemos, J.P. and Carr-Locke, D.L. (1988) Endoscopic sphincterotomy

for common bile duct calculi in patients with gallbladder in-situ considered unfit for surgery. *Gut*, **29**, 114–120.
43. Davies, M. and Keddie, N.C. (1973) Abdominal actinomycosis. *British Journal of Surgery*, **60**, 18–22.
44. De Lacey, G., Gajjar, B., Thromey, B., Levi, J. and Cox, A.G. (1984) Should cholecystography or ultrasound be the primary investigation for gall bladder disease. *The Lancet*, **i**, 205–207.
45. Deming, L., Ermeert, H., Riemann, J.F., Schmolke, G. and Heyder, N. (1984) Lithotripsy in the common bile duct using ultrasound. *Endoscopy*, **10**, 226–228.
46. Devine, R.M., Farvell, M.B. and Mucha, P. (1984) Acute cholecystitis as a complication in surgical patients. *Archives of Surgery*, **119**, 1389–1393.
47. Dowsett, J.F., Vaira, D. and Hatfield, A.R.W. (1989) Endoscopic biliary therapy using the combined percutaneous and endoscopic technique. *Gastroenterology*, **96**, 180–186.
48. Dowsett, J.F., Polydoron, A.A., Vaira, D. *et al.* (1990) Needle knife papillotomy: how safe and how effective? *Gut*, **31**, 905–908.
49. Dubois, F., Icard, P., Berthelot, G. and Levard, H. (1990) Coelioscopic cholecystectomy. *Annals of Surgery*, **211**, 60–62.
50. Edlund, G. and Ljungdahl, M. (1990) Acute cholecystitis in the elderly. *American Journal of Surgery*, **159**, 414–416.
51. Ell, C., Lux, G., Hochberger, J., Muller, D. and Demling, L. (1988) Laserlithotripsy of common bile duct stones. *Gut*, **29**, 746–751.
52. Elliott, D. (1980) Prevention of sepsis in biliary surgery. In *Controversies in Surgical Sepsis* (Ed.) Kuman, S. pp. 285–301. Sussex: Praeger.
53. Endland, D.M. and Rosenblatt, J.E. (1977) Anaerobes in human biliary tracts. *Journal of Clinical Microbiology*, **6**, 494–498.
54. Faber, R.G., Ibrahim, S.Z., Thomas, D.M., Beynon, G.P.Y. and Le Quesne, L.P. (1978) Gallstone disease presenting as septicaemia shock. *British Journal of Surgery*, **65**, 101–105.
55. Fry, D.E., Major, R.A.C. and Harbrecht, P.J. (1981) Empyema of the gallbladder: a complication in the natural history of acute cholecystitis. *American Journal of Surgery*, **141**, 366–369.
56. Fullarton, G.M., Hilditch, T., Campbell, A. and Murray, W.R. (1990) Clinical and scintigraphic assessment of the role of endoscopic sphincterotomy in the treatment of sphincter of Oddi dysfunction. *Gut*, **31**, 231–235.
57. Gacetta, D.J., Cohen, M.J., Crummy, H.B., Joseph, D.A., Kuglitsh, M. and Mack, E. (1984) Ultrasonic lithotripsy of gallstones after cholecystectomy. *American Journal of Roentgenology*, **143**, 1088–1089.
58. Geisenger, M.A., Owens, D.B. and Meaney, T.F. (1989) Radiologic methods of bile duct stone extraction. *American Journal of Surgery*, **158**, 222–227.
59. Gibney, R.G., Fache, J.S., Becker, C.D. *et al.* (1987) Combined surgical and radiologic intervention for complicated cholelithiasis in high risk patients. *Radiology*, **165**, 715–719.
60. Glenn, F. (1979) Acute acalculous cholecystitis. *Annals of Surgery*, **189**, 458–465.
61. Glenn, F. (1981) Surgical management of acute cholecystitis in patients 65 years of age and older. *Annals of Surgery*, **193**, 56–69.
62. Glenn, F. and Becker, C.G. (1982) Acute acalculous cholecystitis. *Annals of Surgery*, **195**, 131–136.
63. Glenn, F., Reed, C. and Graff, W.R. (1981) Biliary enteric fistula. *Surgery, Gynecology and Obstetrics*, **153**, 527–531.
64. Goldstein, F., Thornton, J.J. and Szydlowski, T. (1978) Biliary tract dysfunction in giardiasis. *American Journal of Digestive Diseases*, **23**, 559–560.
65. Gostout, C.J. and Bender, C.E. (1988) Cholangiopancreatography, sphincterotomy and common bile duct stone removal via Roux-en-Y limb enteroscopy. *Gastroenterology*, **95**, 156–163.
66. Graziani, L., Fabrizzi, G., Manfrini, E., Galeazzi, R. and Freddara, U. (1989) Percutaneous transhepatic Oddi–sphincter dilatation for bile duct stone removal. *American Journal of Roentgenology*, **152**, 73–75.
67. Harbin, W.P., Ferrucci, J.T., Wittenburg, J. and Kirkpatrick, R.H. (1979) Non-visualised gallbladder by cholecystosonography. *American Journal of Roentgenology*, **132**, 727–729.
68. Harbin, W.P., Mueller, P.R. and Ferrucci, J.T. (1980) Transhepatic cholangiography: complications and use patterns of the fine needle technique. A multi-institutional survey. *Radiology*, **135**, 15–22.
69. Hickman, M.S., Schwedinger, W.H. and Page, C.P. (1988) Acute cholecystitis in the diabetic: a case control study of outcome. *Archives of Surgery*, **123**, 409–411.
70. Houghton P.W., Jenkinson, J.L.R. and Donaldson, L.A. (1985) Cholecystectomy in the elderly: a prospective study. *British Journal of Surgery*, **72**, 220–222.
71. Houssin, D., Castain, G.D., Lemoine, J. and Bismuth, H. (1983) Microlithiasis of the gallbladder. *Surgery, Gynecology and Obstetrics*, **157**, 20–24.
72. Howard, R.J. (1981) Acute acalculous cholecystitis. *American Journal of Surgery*, **141**, 194–198.
73. Ingoldby, C.J.H., El-Saadi, J., Hall, R.I. and Denyer, M.E. (1989) Late results of endoscopic sphincterotomy for bile duct stones in elderly patients with gall bladders *in situ*. *Gut*, **30**, 1129–1131.
74. Inui, K., Nakazawa, S., Naito, Y., Kimoto, E. and Yamao, K. (1988) Non surgical treatment of

cholecystolithiasis with percutaneous transhepatic cholecystoscopy. *American Journal of Gastroenterology*, **83**, 1124–1127.

75. Jakimowicz, J.J., Rutten, H., Jurgens, P.J. and Carol, E.J. (1987) Comparison of operative ultrasonography and radiography in screening of the common bile duct for calculi. *World Journal of Surgery*, **11**, 628–634.
76. Jeng, K.S., Chiang, H.J. and Shih, S.C. (1989) Limitations of percutaneous transhepatic cholangioscopy in the removal of complicated biliary calculi. *World Journal of Surgery*, **13**, 603–610.
77. Johnson, A.G. and Hosking, S.W. (1987) Appraisal of the management of bile duct stones. *British Journal of Surgery*, **74**, 555–560.
78. Johnson, L.B. (1987) The importance of early diagnosis of acute acalculous cholecystitis. *Surgery, Gynecology and Obstetrics*, **164**, 197–203.
79. Karp, W., Herlin, P., Holmin, T. and Owman, T. (1979) Infusion tomography and ultrasonography of the gallbladder in the diagnosis of acute cholecystitis. *Gastrointestinal Radiology*, **4**, 253–261.
80. Keighley, M.R.B. and Blankharn, J.I. (1988) Infection and the biliary tree. In *Surgery of the Liver and Biliary Tract*, Vol. 1 (Ed.) Blumgart, L.H. pp. 121–132. London: Churchill Livingstone.
81. Khuroo, M.S., Zargar, S.A. and Mahajan, R. (1989) Hepatobiliary and pancreatic ascariasis in India. *The Lancet*, **335**, 1503–1506.
82. Kill, J., Kruse, A. and Rokkjaer, M. (1989) Large bile duct stones treated by endoscopic biliary drainage surgery. *Annals of Surgery*, **105**, 51–56.
83. Kozarek, R.A., Low, D.E. and Ball, T.J. (1988) Tunable dye based lithotripsy: in-vitro studies and in-vivo treatment of choledocholithiasis. *Gastrointestinal Endoscopy*, **34**, 418–420.
84. Kozoll, D.D., Dwyer, G. and Meyer, K.A. (1959) Pathological correlation of gallstones. *Archives of Surgery*, **79**, 514–536.
85. Krige, J.E.J., Bornman, P.C., Beningfield, S.J., Nieuwoudt, J.H.M. and Terblanche, J. (1990) Endoscopic embolization of external biliary fistulae. *British Journal of Surgery*, **77**, 581–583.
86. Lam, S.K. (1984) A study of endoscopic sphincterotomy in recurrent pyogenic cholangitis. *British Journal of Surgery*, **71**, 262–266.
87. Leese, T., Neoptolemos, J.P., Baker, A.R. and Carr-Locke, D.L. (1986) Management of acute cholangitis and the impact of endoscopic sphincterotomy. *British Journal of Surgery*, **73**, 988–992.
88. Leung, J.W.C. and Chung, S.S.C. (1989) Electrohydraulic lithotripsy with peroral choledochoscopy. *British Medical Journal*, **299**, 575–578.
89. Leung, J.W.C., Chung, S.C.S., Sung, J.J.Y., Banez, V.P. and Li, A.K.C. (1989) Urgent endoscopic drainage of acute suppurative cholangitis. *The Lancet*, **ii**, 1307–1309.
90. Liguory, C.L., Bonnel, D., Canard, J.M., Cornud, F. and Dumont, J.L. (1987) Intracorporeal electrohydraulic shockwave lithotripsy of common bile duct stones: preliminary results in 7 cases. *Endoscopy*, **19**, 237–240.
91. Livolsi, V.A., Perzin, K.H. and Porter, M. (1973) Polyarteritis nodosa of the gallbladder presenting as acute cholecystitis. *Gastroenterology*, **65**, 115–123.
92. Long, T.N., Heimbach, D.M. and Carrico, C.J. (1978) Acalculous cholecystitis in critically ill patients. *American Journal of Surgery*, **136**, 31–36.
93. Lygidakis, N.J. (1981) Spontaneous internal biliary fistulae: early surgery for prevention, radical surgery for cure. A report of 75 cases. *Medica Chirurgica Digestive*, **10**, 695–699.
94. Lygidakis, N.J. (1981) Surgery for acalculous cholecystitis. *American Journal of Gastroenterology*, **76**, 27–31.
95. Lygidakis, N.J. and Brummelkemp, W.H. (1985) The significance of intrabiliary pressure in acute cholangitis. *Surgery, Gynecology and Obstetrics*, **161**, 465–469.
96. McClure, J., Banerjee, S.S. and Schofield, P.S. (1984) Crohn's disease of the gallbladder. *Journal of Clinical Pathology*, **37**, 516–518.
97. McIntosh, D.M.F. and Penney, H.F. (1980) Grayscale ultrasonography as a screening procedure in the detection of gallbladder disease. *Radiology*, **136**, 725–727.
98. McSherry, C.K. (1989) Cholecystectomy. The gold standard. *American Journal of Surgery*, **158**, 174–178.
99. McSherry, C.K. (1989) Advantages of elective surgical treatment of gallstones. *Hepato-Gastroenterology*, **36**, 330–332.
100. McSherry, C.K., Ferstenberg, H., Calhoun, W.F., Lahman, E. and Virshup, M. (1985) The natural history of diagnosed gallstone disease in symptomatic and asymptomatic patients. *Annals of Surgery*, **202**, 59–63.
101. Malone, D.E. and Burhenne, H.J. (1989) Advantages and disadvantages of the newer 'interventional' procedures for the treatment of cholecystolithiasis. *Hepato-Gastroenterology*, **36**, 317–326.
102. Martin, D.F., Tweedle, D.E.F. and Rao, P.N. (1988) Endoscopic gallbladder catheterisation and extracorporeal shockwave lithotripsy in the management of Mirizzi's syndrome. *Endoscopy*, **20**, 321–322.
103. Matolo, N.M., Stadalnik, R.C. and McGahan, J.P. (1982) Comparison of ultrasonography, computerised tomography and radionuclide imaging in the diagnosis of acute and chronic cholecystitis. *American Journal of Surgery*, **144**, 676–681.
104. Meijer, W.S., Schmitz, P.I.M. and Jeekel, J. (1990) Meta-analysis of randomised, controlled clinical trials of antibiotic prophylaxis in biliary

tract surgery. *British Journal of Surgery*, **77**, 283–290.

105. Mentzer, R.M., Golden, G.T. and Chandler, J.G. (1975) A comparative appraisal of emphysematous cholecystitis. *American Journal of Surgery*, **129**, 10–15.
106. Millbourn, E. (1941) Klinische Studies uber die Choledocholithiasis. *Acta Chirurgica Scandinavica*, **65**, 1–310.
107. Miller, D.D. (1976) Post operative cholecystitis due to *Torulopsis galabrata. Archives of Surgery*, **111**, 1404–1405.
108. Moncada, R., Carduso, M., Danley, R. *et al.* (1977) Acute cholecystitis: 137 patients studied by infusion tomography of the gallbladder. *American Journal of Roentgenology*, **129**, 583–585.
109. Mujaheid, Z., Evans, J.A. and Whalen, J.P. (1974) The nonpacified gallbladder on oral cholecystography. *Radiology*, **112**, 1–3.
110. Mundith, E.D. (1962) Cholecystitis and diabetes mellitus. *New England Journal of Medicine*, **267**, 642–646.
111. Munster, A.M. and Brown, J.R. (1967) Acalculous cholecystitis. *American Journal of Surgery*, **113**, 730–734.
112. Neoptolemos, J.P. and Carr-Locke, D.L. (1989) ERCP in acute cholangitis and pancreatitis. In *ERCP: Diagnostic and Therapeutic Applications* (Ed.) Jacobson, I.M. pp. 91–126. New York: Elsevier.
113. Neoptolemos, J.P. and Rowley, S. (1989) Advantages in non-surgical treatment of bile duct stones. *Hepato-Gastroenterology*, **36**, 313–316.
114. Neoptolemos, J.P., Fossard, D.P. and Berry, J.M. (1983) A prospective study of radionuclide biliary scanning in acute pancreatitis. *Annals of the Royal College of Surgeons of England*, **65**, 180–183.
115. Neoptolemos, J.P., Hall, A.W., Finlay, D.F., Berry, J.M., Carr-Locke, D.L. and Fossard, D.P. (1984) The urgent diagnosis of gallstones in acute pancreatitis: a prospective study of three methods. *British Journal of Surgery*, **71**, 230–233.
116. Neoptolemos, J.P., Hofmann, A.F. and Moossa, A.R. (1986) Chemical treatment of stones in the biliary tree. *British Journal of Surgery*, **73**, 515–524.
117. Neoptolemos, J.P., Carr-Locke, D.L. and Fossard, D.P. (1987) Prospective randomised study of preoperative endoscopic sphincterotomy versus surgery alone for common bile duct stones. *British Medical Journal*, **294**, 470–474.
118. Neoptolemos, J.P., Carr-Locke, D.L., Leese, T. and James, D. (1987) Acute cholangitis in association with acute pancreatitis: incidence, clinical features, outcome and the role of ERCP and endoscopic sphincterotomy. *British Journal of Surgery*, **74**, 1103–1106.
119. Neoptolemos, J.P., Davidson, B.R., Shaw, D.E., Lloyd, D., Carr-Locke, D.L. and Fossard, D.P. (1987) Study of common bile duct exploration and endoscopic sphincterotomy in a consecutive series of 438 patients. *British Journal of Surgery*, **74**, 916–921.
120. Neoptolemos, J.P., Bailey, I.S. and Carr-Locke, D.L. (1988) Sphincter of Oddi dysfunction: results of treatment by endoscopic sphincterotomy. *British Journal of Surgery*, **75**, 454–459.
121. Neoptolemos, J.P., Carr-Locke, D.L., London, N., Bailey, I. and Fossard, D.P. (1988) ERCP findings and the role of endoscopic sphincterotomy in acute gallstone pancreatitis. *British Journal of Surgery*, **75**, 954–960.
122. Neoptolemos, J.P., Carr-Locke, D.L., London, N.J., Bailey, I.A., James, D. and Fossard, D.P. (1988) Controlled trial of urgent endoscopic retrograde cholangiopancreatography and endoscopic sphincterotomy versus conservative treatment for acute pancreatitis due to gallstones. *The Lancet*, **ii**, 9 79–983.
123. Neoptolemos, J.P., Shaw, D.E. and Carr-Locke, D.L. (1989) A multivariate analysis of pre-operative risk factors in patients with common bile duct stones – implications for treatment. *Annals of Surgery*, **209**, 157.
124. Neoptolemos, J.P., Hall, C.H., O'Connor, H.J., Murray, W.R. and Carr-Locke, D.L. (1990) How good is methyl-tert-butyl ether for treating bile duct stones? The British Experience. *British Journal of Surgery*, **77**, 32–35.
125. Neoptolemos, J.P., Carr-Locke, D.L. and Kelly, K. (1991) Factors affecting the diameters of the common bile duct and pancreatic duct using endoscopic retrograde cholangio-pancreatography. *Hepato-Gastroenterology*, **38**, 243–247.
126. Niederau, C., Mueller, J., Sonnenberg, A. *et al.*, (1983) Extrahepatic bile ducts in healthy subjects, in patients with cholelithiasis, and in post cholecystectomy patients: a prospective ultrasonic study. *Journal of Clinical Ultrasound*, **11**, 23.
127. Niederau, C., Sonnenberg, A. and Mueller, J. (1984) Comparison of the extrahepatic bile duct measured by ultrasound and by different radiographic methods. *Gastroenterology*, **87**, 615–621.
128. Nordback, I. and Airo, I. (1988) Endoscopic retrograde cholangiopancreatography (ERCP) and sphincterotomy (EST) after BII resection. *Annals Chirurgie Gynaecology*, **95**, 156–163.
129. Normby, S. and Sohonebeck, J. (1970) Longterm results with cholecystolithotomy. *Acta Chirurgica Scandinavica*, **136**, 711–713.
130. O'Donnell, L.D.J. and Heaton, K.W. (1988) Recurrence and re-recurrence of gall stones after medical dissolution: a longterm follow up. *Gut*, **29**, 655–658.
131. Ong, G.B. (1962) A study of recurrent pyogenic cholangitis. *Archives of Surgery*, **84**, 199–225.
132. Ong, G.B., Adiseshyah, M. and Leong, C.H. (1971) Acute pancreatitis associated with recurrent pyogenic cholangitis. *British Journal of Surgery*, **58**, 891–894.
133. Ostroff, J.W. and Shapiro, H.A. (1989)

Complications of endoscopic sphincterotomy. In *ERCP: Diagnostic and Therapeutic Applications* (Ed.) Jacobsen, I. pp. 61–73. New York: Elsevier.
134. Pain, J.A., Cahill, C.J. and Bailey, M.E. (1985) Perioperative complications in obstructive jaundice: therapeutic considerations. *British Journal of Surgery*, **72**, 942–945.
135. Palmer, K.R. and Hofmann, A.F. (1986) Intraductol mono-octanoin for the direct dissolution of bile duct stones: experience in 343 patients. *Gut*, **27**, 196–202.
136. Paricio, P.P., Olmo, D.C., Franco, E.P., Gonzalez, A.P., Gonzalez, L.C. and Lopez, J.B. (1990) Gallbladder cholesterolosis: an aetiological factor in acute pancreatitis of uncertain origin. *British Journal of Surgery*, **77**, 735–736.
137. Pessa, M.E., Hawkins, I.F. and Vogel, S.B. (1987) The treatment of acute cholangitis. Percutaneous transhepatic biliary drainage before definitive therapy. *Annals of Surgery*, **205**, 389–392.
138. Peterson, S.R. and Sheldon, G.F. (1984) Acute acalculous cholecystitis: a complication of hyperalimentation. *Archives of Surgery*, **119**, 1389–1392.
139. Piedad, O.H. and Wels, P.B. (1972) Spontaneous internal biliary fistula; obstructive and non-obstructive types. 20 year review of 55 cases. *Annals of Surgery*, **175**, 72–80.
140. Pitt, H.A., Kaufman, S.L., Coleman, J., White, R.I. and Cameron, J.L. (1989) Benign postoperative biliary strictures. Operate or dilate? *Annals of Surgery*, **210**, 417–425.
141. Ponchon, T., Gallez, J.F., Valette, P.J., Chavaillon, A. and Bory, R. (1989) Endoscopic treatment of biliary tract fistulas. Gastrointestinal *Endoscopy*, **35**, 490–498.
142. Rajagoralan, A.E. and Pickleman, J. (1982) Biliary colic and functional gallbladder disease. *Archives of Surgery*, **117**, 1005–1008.
143. Ralls, P.W., Halls, J., Lapin, S.A., Quinn, M.F., Morris, U.L. and Boswell, W. (1982) Prospective evaluation of tomographic Murphy's sign in suspected acute cholecystitis. *Journal of Clinical Ultrasound*, **10**, 113.
144. Raper, S.E., Barker, M.E., Jones, A.L. and Way, L.W. (1984) Anastomic correlates of bacterial cholangiovenous reflux. *Surgery*, **105**, 352–359.
145. Raptopoulos, V., Compton, C.C., Doherty, P. *et al.* (1986) Chronic acalculous gallbladder disease: multi-imaging evaluation with clinical–pathologic correlation. *American Journal of Roentgenology*, **147**, 721–724.
146. Rau, W.S., Matern, S., Gerok, W. and Wenz, W. (1980) Spontaneous cholecystocolonic fistula: a model situation for bile acid diarrhoea and fatty acid diarrhoea as a consequence of disturbed enterohepatic circulation of bile acids. *Hepatogastroenterology*, **27**, 231–237.
147. Reddick, E.J., Olsen, D.O. (1989) Laparoscopic laser cholecystectomy. A comparison with mini-lap cholecystectomy. *Surgical Endoscopy*, **3**, 131–133.
148. Reiertsen, D., Skjoto, J., Jaconsen, C.D. and Rosseland, A.R. (1987) Complications of fibreoptic gastrointestinal endoscopy – five years experience in a control hospital. *Endoscopy*, **19**, 1–6.
149. Reiner, R.G., Lawson, M.J. and Davies, G.T. (1980) Fractionated dose of cholecystography: a comparison between iopanoic acid and sodium ipodate. *Clinical Radiology*, **31**, 667.
150. Reynolds, B.M. and Dargan, E.L. (1959) Acute obstructive cholangitis: a distinct clinical syndrome. *Annals of Surgery*, **150**, 299–303.
151. Rhodes, M., Lennard, T.W.S., Farndon, J.R. and Taylor, R.M.R. (1988). Cholecystokinin (CCK) provocation test: longterm follow-up after cholecystectomy. *British Journal of Surgery*, **75**, 951–953.
152. Saar, M.G., Shepard, A.J. and Zuidema, G.D. (1981) Choledochoduodenal fistula: an unusual complication of duodenal ulcer disease. *American Journal of Surgery*, **141**, 736–740.
153. Salmenkivi, K. (1964) Cholesterolosis of the gallbladder: a clinical study based on 269 cholecystectomies. *Acta Chirurgica Scandinavica*, 324(suppl.), 1–93.
154. Sauerbruich, T., Stern, M. and The Study Group for Shock-Wave Lithotripsy of Bile Duct Stones (1989) Fragmentation of bile duct stones by extracorporeal shock waves. *Gastroenterology*, **96**, 146–152.
155. Savoca, P.E., Longo, W.E., Zucker, K.A., McMillen, M.M. and Modlin I.M. (1990) The increasing prevalence of acalculous cholecystitis in outpatients. *Annals of Surgery*, **211**, 433–437.
156. Schneider, M.U., Matek, W., Bauer, R. and Damschke, W. (1988) Mechanical lithotripsy of bile duct stones in 209 patients – effect of technical advances. *Endoscopy*, **20**, 248–253.
157. Seifert, E., Gail, K. and Weismuller, J. (1982) Langzeitresultate nach Endoskopischer Sphinkerotomie. *Deutsche Medizinische Wochenschrift*, **107**, 610–614.
158. Sherman, M., Ralls, P.W., Quinn, M., Halls, J. and Keats, J.B. (1980) Intravenous cholangiography and sonography in acute cholecystitis: prospective evaluation. *American Journal of Roentgenology*, **135**, 311–313.
159. Shuman, W.P., Rogers, J.V., Rudd, T.G., Mack, L.A., Plumley, T. and Larson, E.B. (1984) Low sensitivity of sonography and cholescintography in acalculous cholecystitis. *American Journal of Roentgenology*, **142**, 531–534.
160. Siegel, J.N., Safrany, L., Ben-Zvi, J.S. *et al.* (1988) Duodenoscopic sphincterotomy in patients with gallbladder *in situ*: report of a series of 1272 patients. *American Journal of Gastroenterology*, **83**, 1255–1258.
161. Sjodahl, R. and Tagesson, C. (1983) On the

development of primary acute cholecystitis. *Scandinavian Journal of Gastroenterology*, **18**, 577–579.
162. Skillings, J.C., Kumak, C. and Hinshaw, J.R. (1980) Cholecystostomy: a place in modern biliary surgery? *American Journal of Surgery*, **139**, 865–869.
163. Slovis, T.L., Hight, D.W., Philipart, A. and Dubois, R.S. (1980) Sonography in the diagnosis and management of hydrops of the gallbladder in children with mucocutaneous lymph node syndrome. *Pediatrics*, **65**, 789–794.
164. Smith, R., Williams, R. and Cotton, P.B. (1976) Gallstone pancreatitis with normal biliary radiology. *British Journal of Surgery*, **63**, 861–863.
165. Soehendra, N., Kempeneeks, I., Ekhfuss, H.P. and Reynders-Frederix, V. (1989) Early post-operative endoscopy after biliary tract surgery. *Endoscopy*, **13**, 113–117.
166. Stokes, K.P., Falchuck, K.R. and Clouse, M.E. (1989) Biliary duct stones: update on 54 cases after percutaneous transhepatic removal. *Radiology*, **170**, 994–1001.
167. Stryker, S.J. and Beal, J.M. (1983) Acute cholecystitis and common bile duct calculi. *Archives of Surgery*, **118**, 1063–1064.
168. Swanepoel, C.R., Floyd, A., Allison, H., Learmonth, G.M., Cassidy, M.J. and Pascoe, M.D. (1983) Acute acalculous cholecystitis complicating systemic lupus erythematosus: case report and review. *British Medical Journal*, **286**, 251–252.
169. Tanaka, K., Shimada, M., Hattori, M., Utsunomiya, T. and Dya, N. (1985) Sjögren's syndrome with abnormal manifestations of the gallbladder and central nervous system. *Journal of Pediatric Gastroenterology and Nutrition*, **4**, 148–151.
170. Tanaka, M. and Ikeda, S. (1983) Parapapillary choledochoduodenal fistula: an analysis of 83 conservative patients. *Gastrointestinal Endoscopy*, **29**, 84–93.
171. Taylor, T.V., Armstrong, C.P., Rimmer, S., Lucas, S.B., Jeacock, J. and Gunn, A.A. (1988) Prediction of choledocholithiasis using a pocket computer. *British Journal of Surgery*, **75**, 138–140.
172. Thistle, J.L. (1989) Pros and cons of the non-surgical treatments for gallbladder stones. *Hepato-Gastroenterology*, **36**, 327–329.
173. Thistle, J.L., May, G.R. and Bender, C.E. *et al.* (1989) Dissolution of cholesterol gallbladder stones by methyl-tert-butyl ether administered by percutaneous transhepatic catheter. *New England Journal of Medicine*, **320**, 633–639.
174. Thomas, W.E.G., Thornton, J.R. and Thompson, M.H. (1981) Staphylococcal acalculous cholecystitis. *British Journal of Surgery*, **68**, 136.
175. Thornton, J.R., Heaton, K.W., Espiner, H.J., Eltringham, W.K. (1983) Empyema of the gallbladder – reappraisal of a neglected disease. *Gut*, **24**, 1183–1185.
176. Thorpe, M.E.C., Scheuer, P.J. and Sherlock, J. (1967) Primary sclerosing cholangitis, the biliary tree and ulcerative colitis. *Gut*, **8**, 435–438.
177. Tilvis, R.S., Aro, J., Strandberg, T.E., Lempinen, M. and Miettenen, T.A. (1982) Lipid composition of bile and gallbladder mucosa in patients with acalculous cholesterolosis. *Gastroenterology*, **82**, 607–615.
178. Urakami, Y. and Kishi, S. (1978) Endoscopic fistulotomy (EFT) for parapapillary choledochoduodenal fistula. *Endoscopy*, **10**, 289–294.
179. Vaira, D., Dowsett, J.F., Hatfield, A.R.W. *et al.* (1989) Is duodenal diverticulum a risk factor for sphincterotomy? *Gut*, **30**, 939–942.
180. Vaira, D., D'Anna, L., Ainley, C. *et al.* (1989) Endoscopic sphincterotomy in 1000 consecutive patients. *The Lancet*, **ii**, 431–434.
181. Van der Linden, W. and Edlund, G. (1989) Early versus delayed cholecystectomy: the effect of a change in management. *British Journal of Surgery*, **68**, 753–757.
182. Van Landingham, S.B. and Broders, C.W. (1982) Gallstone ileus. *Surgical Clinics of North America*, **62**, 241–247.
183. Van Sonnenberg E., Wing, V.W., Pollard, J.W. and Casola E. (1984) Life threatening vagal reactions associated with percutaneous cholecystostomy. *Radiology*, **151**, 377–380.
184. Van Sonnenberg, E., Casola, G. and Zakko, S.F. (1988) Gallbladder and bile duct stones: percutaneous therapy with primary MTBE dissolution and mechanical methods. *Radiology*, **169**, 505–509.
185. Vergunst, H., Terpstra, O.T., Brakel, K., Lameris, J.S., Van Blankenstein, M. and Schroder, F.H. (1989) Extra-corporeal shockwave lithotripsy of gallstones. Possibilities and limitations. *Annals of Surgery*, **210**, 565–575.
186. Warren, K.W., Christophi, C. and Armendariz, R. (1982) The evolution and current perspectives of the treatment of benign bile duct strictures: a review. *Surgical Gastroenterology*, **1**, 141–154.
187. Wholey, M.H. and Smoot, S. (1988) Choledocholithiasis: percutaneous pulverization with a high speed rotational catheter. *American Journal of Roentgenology*, **150**, 129–130.
188. Williams, I., Slavin, G., Cox, A., Simpson, P. and Delacey, G. (1986) Diverticular disease (adenomyomatosis) of the gallbladder: a radiological–pathological survey. *British Journal of Radiology*, **59**, 29–34.
189. Winkler, E., Kaplon, O., Gutman, M., Skornick, Y. and Rozin, R.R. (1989) Role of cholecystostomy in the management of critically ill patients suffering from acute cholecystitis. *British Journal of Surgery*, **76**, 693–695.
190. Winslet, M.C., Hall, C., Harding, K. and

Neoptolemos, J.P. (1990) The use of dynamic Tc99m HIDA scanning in the diagnosis of acalculous gallbladder disease. *HPB Surgery*, **2**(suppl.), 489.
191. Winslet, M.C. and Neoptolemos, J.P. (1991) The place of endoscopy in the management of gallstones. *Clinical Gastroenterology*, **1** (in press).
192. Wong, M.W., Kaplan, S., Dunkle, L.M., Stechenberg, B.W. and Feigan, R.D. (1977) Hepatospirosis: a childhood disease. *Journal of Paediatrics*, **90**, 532–537.
193. Wood, J.J., Bolton, J.P., Cannon, S.R., Allan, A., O'Connor, B.H. and Darougar, S. (1982) Biliary-type pain as a manifestation of genital tract infection: the Curtis–Fitz–Hugh syndrome. *British Journal of Surgery*, **69**, 251–253.
194. Yoshimoto, H., Ikeda, S., Tanaka, M., Matsumoto, S. and Kuroda, Y. (1989) Choledochoscopic electrohydraulic lithotripsy and lithotomy for stones in the common bile duct, intrahepatic ducts and gallbladder. *Annals of Surgery*, **210**, 576–582.
195. Zeman, R.K., Burrell, M.I., Cahow, C.E. and Caride, V. (1981) Diagnostic utility of cholscintigraphy and ultrasonography in acute cholecystitis. *American Journal of Surgery*, **141**, 446–451.

PRIMARY SCLEROSING CHOLANGITIS

R.H. Wiesner and N. LaRusso

Sclerosing cholangitis is a syndrome characterized by pain, jaundice and recurrent fever. These symptoms result from fibrosis and inflammation of the bile ducts due to primary or secondary disturbances in the biliary tree. This section deals principally with the primary variety of the syndrome.

Primary sclerosing cholangitis, sometimes abbreviated to PSC, is a chronic, cholestatic syndrome of unknown aetiology, which is characterized by diffuse inflammation and fibrosis of, most commonly, the entire biliary ductal system.[16,122] While Delbit first described the syndrome in 1924, there were only approximately 100 cases of primary sclerosing cholangitis documented in the English-speaking literature prior to 1980.[23,103,118] Thus, primary sclerosing cholangitis had been considered a rare disease prior to the increased application in the late 1970s of endoscopic retrograde and percutaneous transhepatic cholangiography.[101] The syndrome is most commonly progressive, albeit at an unpredictable and variable rate, usually advancing to biliary cirrhosis, portal hypertension and premature death from liver failure unless appropriate intervention occurs.

The diagnosis of primary sclerosing cholangitis is most commonly based on a collection of clinical, radiological, and biochemical abnormalities; in the early stages of the disease highly characteristic histological abnormalities may be seen on liver biopsy specimens.[121] Until recently, primary sclerosing cholangitis was diagnosed most commonly in its latest stages when the patient was markedly jaundiced and cachectic. However, the recent use of diagnostic tests, including endoscopic retrograde cholangiopancreatography have resulted in earlier recognition of the disease, often in the asymptomatic stage.

DEFINITIONS, DIAGNOSTIC CRITERIA AND DIFFERENTIAL DIAGNOSIS

The designation 'primary sclerosing cholangitis' is currently accepted as the most appropriate terminology for the syndrome.[58] The term *primary* indicates that this type of sclerosing cholangitis is idiopathic and distinguishes this entity from secondary sclerosing cholangitis, a syndrome with similar clinical characteristics but with identifiable causes (*Table 12.19*). The term *sclerosing* emphasizes the induration of the biliary ductal system resulting from the chronic inflammatory and fibrotic process. Finally, the term *cholangitis*, which literally means 'inflammation of the bile ducts', describes a component of the pathological process. Because the occurrence of clinical episodes of jaundice, abdominal pain and fever, also referred to as cholangitis, is uncommon in unoperated patients with primary sclerosing cholangitis, the literal meaning of cholangitis is the more appropriate.

Two final points should be made with regard to definition. First, in situations where sclerosing cholangitis occurs in association with inflammatory bowel disease, the hepatobiliary disease is not considered a secondary manifestation of the intestinal condition. While the specifics of the relationship between primary sclerosing cholangitis and inflammatory bowel disease remain obscure, the weight of evidence (see below) is against the concept that the

Table 12.19 Sclerosing cholangitis

	Primary	*Secondary*
Clinical setting	With or without inflammatory bowel disease	Choledocholithiasis Trauma Ischaemia Chemicals Infectious agents Congenital anomalies
Ducts involved	Intra- and, extrahepatic ('classic' or global) Intrahepatic (small duct) Extrahepatic (large duct)	Perihilar and extrahepatic

inflammatory bowel disease causes the hepatobiliary disease. Secondly, the term *pericholangitis* is often used by both pathologists and clinicians to designate a form of chronic hepatitis associated with chronic ulcerative colitis.[68] This term most appropriately represents a descriptive morphological designation rather than a clinical syndrome; currently, it most often represents hepatic manifestations on liver biopsy of the earliest stages of primary sclerosing cholangitis. Moreover, the morphological observation of pericholangitis can also be seen in primary biliary cirrhosis, extrahepatic obstruction, and autoimmune or idiopathic chronic active hepatitis.[68]

The diagnosis of primary sclerosing cholangitis, in the past, had been established only with laparotomy by palpation of a fibrotic common bile duct, occasionally with associated common bile duct biopsy.[99] Later, cholangiography, usually at laparotomy, demonstrated abnormalities of the intra- and extrahepatic ducts which today are recognized as characteristic features of primary sclerosing cholangitis.[29,112] However, it was not until 1964 that the first criteria for the diagnosis of primary sclerosing cholangitis were formulated.[46] With the development of endoscopic retrograde and transhepatic cholangiography in the early 1970s, the diagnostic criteria were again modified.[29] Indeed, primary sclerosing cholangitis evolved from a disease which was diagnosed only at surgery to one that could be readily recognized cholangiographically. Today, the diagnosis of primary sclerosing cholangitis is based on an appropriate clinical setting (i.e. a male with inflammatory bowel disease), a two-fold or greater elevation of the serum alkaline phosphatase level and a typical cholangiogram.[73] Although there are no unequivocally specific biochemical markers for primary sclerosing cholangitis, recent publications have described the presence of neutrophil nuclear antibodies and neutrophil cytoplasmic antibodies in the serum of some patients with primary sclerosing cholangitis.[27]

The most important diagnostic study in a patient with suspected primary sclerosing cholangitis is a cholangiogram. Radiological abnormalities commonly seen include diffusely distributed multifocal strictures of the biliary system; these abnormalities are often associated with irregularity and tortuosity of the entire biliary system (*Figure 12.55*).[29,73]

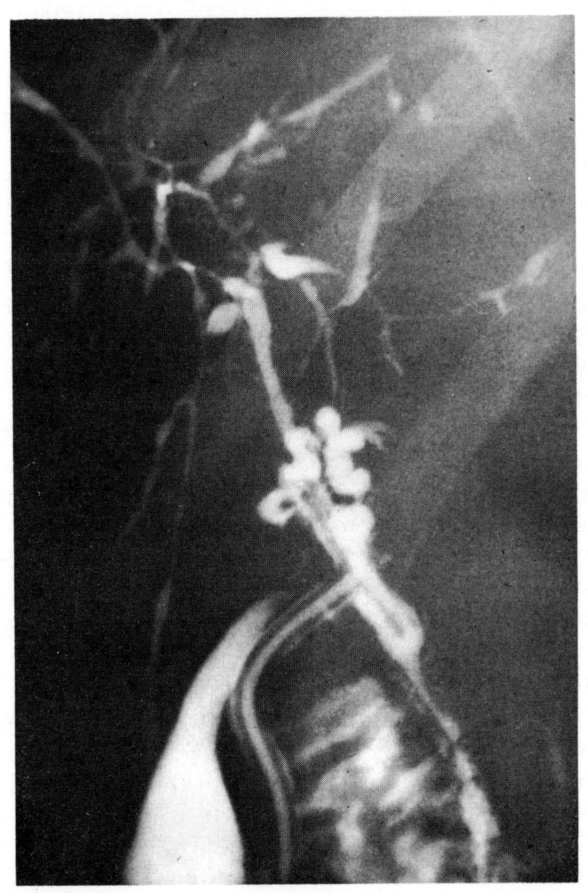

Figure 12.55 T-tube cholangiogram showing narrowing and irregularity of the common bile duct with irregularity and beading throughout the intrahepatic biliary tree.

Hepatic histological abnormalities have been previously reviewed in detail and categorized by Ludwig into four stages: stage 1, portal hepatitis or cholangitis; stage 2, periportal fibrosis or periportal hepatitis; stage 3, septal fibrosis, necrosis or both extending beyond the limiting plate; and stage 4, biliary cirrhosis.[69] Most clinicians would currently agree that a patient should not be confidently considered as having the syndrome of primary sclerosing cholangitis if that patient has had either a biliary duct reconstructive procedure (excluding simple cholecystectomy) or documented biliary tract stone disease (i.e. choledocholithiasis) prior to the diagnosis of primary sclerosing cholangitis. Conditions requiring exclusion include choledocholithiasis, congenital abnormalities of the biliary tree, cholangiopathy associated with acquired immune deficiency syndrome, biliary infection with certain organisms such as *Cryptococcus* spp., *Cryptosporidium* spp. and cytomegalovirus, toxicity related to intra-arterial infusion of floxuridine, toxicity related to caustic therapy for hydatid disease, and cholangiocarcinoma.[4,9,13,22,34,60,64,71,72,74,89,111]

Under most circumstances, the sine qua non for the diagnosis of primary sclerosing cholangitis is an abnormal cholangiogram. Indeed, most authors would now agree that abnormalities involving either the intra- or extrahepatic ducts are sufficient for the diagnosis. Finally, a form of primary sclerosing cholangitis has recently been recognized in which cholangiographic abnormalities may not be apparent but in which liver histology most often shows the finding of pericholangitis, referred to above.[68]

With this information in mind, the diagnosis of primary sclerosing cholangitis is usually not difficult assuming the clinician is aware of the syndrome. In a male with chronic cholestatic liver test abnormalities and associated inflammatory bowel disease, primary sclerosing cholangitis should be the major working diagnosis and a cholangiogram should be performed, preferably by the endoscopic rather than the transhepatic approach. Generally, a typically abnormal cholangiogram in the appropriate clinical setting is all that is required for diagnosis. A liver biopsy may be useful when the cholangiogram is equivocal or for accurate histological staging for prognosis; however, it is not essential for diagnosis. As discussed above, secondary sclerosing cholangitis can be relatively easily excluded by efforts to identify a specific causative agent. In a middle-aged female with chronic cholestasis in whom primary biliary cirrhosis would be the leading diagnosis, the most useful diagnostic test to distinguish primary biliary cirrhosis from primary sclerosing cholangitis is a cholangiogram. In general, a cholangiogram is normal in patients with primary biliary cirrhosis; indeed, the extrahepatic ducts are always normal; if radiographic abnormalities do occur in the intrahepatic ducts, they appear quite different from those seen in primary sclerosing cholangitis.[64,122] Exclusion of extrahepatic obstruction can be easily accomplished with an ultrasound scan or a cholangiogram. Some patients with chronic active hepatitis may develop a cholestatic biochemical profile; indeed, in some of these cases, a cholangiogram may show abnormalities consistent with primary sclerosing cholangitis, suggesting an overlap syndrome between chronic active hepatitis and primary sclerosing cholangitis.[64] Thus, patients with chronic active hepatitis with a cholestatic biochemical profile, particularly if the patient also has inflammatory bowel disease, should have a cholangiogram to exclude primary sclerosing cholangitis.

AETIOLOGY AND PATHOGENESIS

The cause of primary sclerosing cholangitis is unknown; genetic factors, acquired factors or both could be involved (*Table 12.20*). Several recent observations are consistent with a major role for genetic factors in the aetiopathogenesis of primary sclerosing cholangitis. Familial occurrence of primary sclerosing cholangitis has been reported in a number of studies. More recently, the frequency of selected HLA haplotypes has been shown to be higher in patients with primary sclerosing cholangitis than in control subjects. For example, several studies have shown a strong association between primary sclerosing cholangitis and the HLA haplotypes B8 and DR3, each of which is known to be associated with other autoimmune diseases.[17] Others have found that HLA haplotype DR2, in addition to B8 and DR3, may be an independent risk factor for the development of primary sclerosing cholangitis.[26] A very recent report has claimed a high association of primary sclerosing cholangitis with the newly discovered C locus (Cw7) and

Table 12.20 Potential aetiopathological factors in primary sclerosing cholangitis

1. Portal bacteraemia
2. Absorbed colon toxin
3. Toxic bile acids
4. Copper toxicity
5. Viral infection
6. Genetic predisposition
7. Immunological mechanisms
8. Ischaemic arteriole damage

DRw52A, data suggesting that the DR3 β locus may be closer to the central gene that predisposes to primary sclerosing cholangitis.[93] These findings are consistent with the hypothesis that patients with primary sclerosing cholangitis have a genetic predisposition and that primary sclerosing cholangitis may be an autoimmune disease.

In addition to genetic factors, however, important acquired factors are probably involved and could theoretically include toxins, ischaemia, or infectious agents. Regarding toxins, an elevated hepatic copper concentration was thought by some to be important in the initiation or the perpetuation of primary sclerosing cholangitis.[122] A recent negative therapeutic study, however, utilizing the cupruretic agent D-penicillimine, makes it unlikely that an elevated hepatic copper level is pathogenetically important.[59] The close association of inflammatory bowel disease, especially chronic ulcerative colitis, with primary sclerosing cholangitis has led to the hypothesis that portal bacteraemia or intestinal absorption of toxins, including toxic bile acids from an inflamed colon, may play a role in the pathogenesis of primary sclerosing cholangitis.[24,28,47,100,114] Unfortunately, studies have not supported a significant association of portal vein bacteraemia in patients undergoing surgery for chronic ulcerative colitis. Furthermore, detailed hepatic histological analysis has indicated that portal phlebitis, an important hepatic manifestation of portal vein bacteraemia, is essentially absent in most patients with primary sclerosing cholangitis.[114]

Other investigators have raised the possibility that primary sclerosing cholangitis may be caused by a reaction to toxic bile acids, such as lithocolic acid, arising in a diseased colon allowing absorption of toxin directly into the portal blood.[24,100] Unfortunately, no studies have demonstrated major abnormalities in bile acid metabolism in patients with primary sclerosing cholangitis or in patients with chronic ulcerative colitis. In a recent interesting study, it was recorded that pro-inflammatory bacterial peptides synthesized by colonic bacteria in a rat model resulted in portal inflammation and cholangitis similar to histopathological lesions seen in early primary sclerosing cholangitis.[45,88] In another study, investigators demonstrated that intestinal bacterial overgrowth in rats is associated with hepatic inflammation with some similarity to that seen in primary sclerosing cholangitis.[63] Thus, additional studies seem warranted into the potential role that pro-inflammatory peptides derived from bacteria may play in the pathogenesis of primary sclerosing cholangitis.

Recently, extrahepatic biliary tract disease closely mimicking primary sclerosing cholangitis has been described following infusion with the chemotherapeutic agent 5-fluorodeoxyuridine, a drug which causes small vessel arteriopathy probably leading to bile duct fibrosis. This syndrome, however, represents a type of secondary rather than primary sclerosing cholangitis. Indeed, there is no specific evidence of ischaemic lesions seen in patients with primary sclerosing cholangitis.

Infection of biliary epithelial cells by viral agents has also been postulated by some to be involved in the pathogenesis of primary sclerosing cholangitis. Results of several studies have excluded the hepatitis B and C viruses as potential causative agents. While cytomegalovirus may affect intrahepatic bile ducts, the histological picture generally differs from that seen in primary sclerosing cholangitis.[34] Reovirus type 3 has been associated with neonatal biliary atresia which, like primary sclerosing cholangitis, is characterized by obliterative cholangitis.[84] However, no direct evidence links reovirus infections to the development of primary sclerosing cholangitis.[82] The possibility that other viruses may be involved in the pathogenesis of primary sclerosing cholangitis remains appealing, although speculative.

Currently, the pathogenesis of primary sclerosing cholangitis is most closely linked with alterations in immune mechanisms. Like primary biliary cirrhosis, a disease thought to be a model autoimmune syndrome, primary sclerosing cholangitis is characterized by lymphocytic bile duct destruction, hypergammaglobulinaemia, and association with other diseases, such as chronic ulcerative colitis, which are thought by some to be autoimmune in origin.[14,15] Unlike primary biliary cirrhosis, however, classic autoantibodies such as antimitochondrial antibody, antinuclear antibody and anti-smooth muscle antibody are usually absent or only present in low titres in primary sclerosing cholangitis.[122] Recent studies in primary sclerosing cholangitis have found a high incidence of circulating anticolon antibodies, anti-neutrophil nuclear antibodies, and anti-neutrophil cytoplasmic antibodies.[18,104,126] Indeed, anti-neutrophil nuclear antibodies have been found to react with portal antigens and appear to correlate with disease activity in primary sclerosing cholangitis.[104]

Other lines of evidence supporting an immunological basis for the disease include the inhibition of leukocyte migration by biliary antigens, elevated IgM levels, the presence of circulating immune complexes, decreased clearance of immune complexes, and increased complement metabolism.[1,5,8,75,81] In addition, cells involved in the destruction of bile ducts in primary sclerosing cholangitis have been shown recently to be T lymphocytes, and abnormalities in peripheral blood lymphocyte subsets have also been demonstrated.[65,105,119] Also, enhanced autoreactivity of suppressor cytotoxic T lymphocytes from the peripheral blood of patients with primary sclerosing cholangitis has been reported.[66] These studies support alterations in the immune system as being pathogenetically related to the development or perpetuation of primary sclerosing cholangitis, albeit specific mechanisms are still not clearly understood. Thus, the current, most widely accepted hypothesis for the aetiopathogenesis of primary sclerosing cholangitis involves exposure of a genetically predisposed individual to an acute insult to the biliary system; for example, a transient viral infection. It is suggested that an alteration in the bile duct epithelial cell that marks them as foreign then occurs, leading to their destruction by autoimmune mechanisms.[19]

CLINICAL FEATURES

DEMOGRAPHICS

Primary sclerosing cholangitis was once considered a medical curiosity, since fewer than 100 cases had been reported in the English-speaking language prior to 1980. This situation has dramatically changed, and recent experience suggests that primary sclerosing cholangitis is among the three most common indications for liver transplantation in adults in the USA. Without question, the frequency of diagnosis of primary sclerosing cholangitis has increased dramatically in the last 10–15 years. This increase probably represents not a true increased incidence of the disease, but rather increased clinical awareness and increased utilization of diagnostic tests such as retrograde cholangiography.

The prevalence of primary sclerosing cholangitis in the USA is unknown; however, because of the frequent association of primary sclerosing cholangitis with chronic ulcerative colitis, it is possible to crudely estimate the prevalence of primary sclerosing cholangitis on the basis of studies that have been performed in patients with inflammatory bowel disease. The reported prevalence of chronic ulcerative colitis in the USA is between 40 and 100 cases per 100 000 of the population. Since approximately 4% of patients with chronic ulcerative colitis will have primary sclerosing cholangitis, one can estimate the prevalence of primary sclerosing cholangitis, to be anywhere from 1 to 4 cases per 100 000 of the population. This crude estimate has recently been supported by the results of an epidemiological study from Sweden; these data suggest the prevalence of chronic ulcerative colitis and primary sclerosing cholangitis to be 171 and 6.3 cases per 100 000 of the population, respectively.[87] These results probably underestimate the prevalence of primary sclerosing cholangitis, as this syndrome can occur in patients with normal serum levels of alkaline phosphatase (the biochemical test which, when abnormal, usually prompts suspicion of primary sclerosing cholangitis), and as much as 20% of patients with primary sclerosing cholangitis do not have associated inflammatory bowel disease.

Primary sclerosing cholangitis is predominantly a disease of young men. The average age at the time of diagnosis is 40 years, and approximately 70% of patients are male.[125] The reason for this age and sex distribution is unclear, and no major differences have yet been identified between male and female patients with primary sclerosing cholangitis.

SYMPTOMS AND SIGNS

Patients with primary sclerosing cholangitis present clinically in a number of different ways.[58] The most common mode of presentation is a cholestatic biochemical profile in an asymptomatic patient identified during a routine examination. Such individuals often have associated inflammatory bowel disease. Alternatively, a patient may develop fatigue and pruritus, a constellation of symptoms which, particularly in a young male with inflammatory bowel disease, often warrants cholangiography. Episodes of clinical cholangitis, including fever and abdominal pain with or without jaundice, occur more commonly in primary sclerosing cholangitis patients who have had previous biliary tract surgical procedures such as a choledochoenterostomy. Rarely, patients will present for the first time with complications of advanced disease such as ascites or upper gastrointestinal bleeding from gastroesophageal varices. Even less commonly in the present age of noninvasive imaging studies will be the individual in whom primary sclerosing cholangitis is discovered during a diagnostic laparotomy for obscure jaundice. Several extremely uncommon modes of presentation of primary sclerosing cholangitis are mentioned for the sake of completeness, including: (1) a patient with steatorrhoea and weight loss due to either complicating pancreatic exocrine sufficiency or associated non-tropical sprue; (2) a patient with inflammatory bowel disease and a previous diagnosis of chronic idiopathic or autoimmune chronic active hepatitis who does not respond to standard immunosuppressive therapy; (3) a patient with recurrent fever and septicaemia of unknown aetiology; and (4) a patient with a remote proctocolectomy and ileostomy for chronic ulcerative colitis who presents with peristomal variceal bleeding (see below).

It is frequently difficult to accurately determine the onset of primary sclerosing cholangitis because it usually begins insidiously. The gradual onset and progression of fatigue and pruritis followed by jaundice represents the most frequent symptom complex leading to the diagnosis of primary sclerosing cholangitis.

Approximately 75% of patients with primary sclerosing cholangitis will have an abnormality on physical examination at the time of diagnosis, most commonly hepatomegaly, icterus and/or splenomegaly.[122,124] Hyperpigmentation, xanthomas and xanthelasma occur but are found less frequently than in primary biliary cirrhosis, a syndrome with which primary sclerosing cholangitis shares many features.[122]

ASSOCIATED DISEASES

Primary sclerosing cholangitis has been found in association with a number of other diseases (*Table 12.21*). Inflammatory bowel disease is the most common and most important disease associated with primary sclerosing cholangitis. The association of primary sclerosing cholangitis and inflammatory bowel disease was first reported by Warren and Thorpe, who noted a 25–30% association of inflammatory bowel disease in patients with primary sclerosing cholangitis.[112,116] Subsequent studies have reported an association of 54–100%.[32,42] The vast majority of patients with primary sclerosing cholangitis who have associated inflammatory bowel disease have chronic ulcerative colitis. Nevertheless, Crohn's colitis has been reported to occur in up to 13% of patients with primary sclerosing cholangitis who have inflammatory bowel disease.[33,113] To the authors' knowledge, Crohn's disease isolated to the small bowel without colonic involvement has yet to be confidently documented in association with primary sclerosing cholangitis.

Table 12.21 Diseases associated with primary sclerosing cholangitis

Inflammatory bowel disease
Coeliac disease
Retroperitoneal fibrosis
Thyroiditis
Sjögren's syndrome
Autoimmune chronic active hepatitis
Lupus erythematosis
Vasculitis
Immune thrombocytopenia purpura
Histiocytosis X
Gallbladder disease
Intra-abdominal adenopathy
Chronic pancreatitis
Rheumatoid arthritis
Peyronie's disease
Bronchiectasis
Systemic sclerosis
Membranous nephropathy
Pseudotumour of orbit
Autoimmune haemolytic anaemia
Angioblastic lymphadenopathy
Cystic fibrosis
Eosinophilia

In general, the diagnosis of inflammatory bowel disease usually precedes the diagnosis of primary sclerosing cholangitis.[107] Nevertheless, inflammatory bowel disease can be diagnosed simultaneously or subsequent to the diagnosis of primary sclerosing cholangitis.[33,110] Indeed, the authors have observed the onset of inflammatory bowel disease years after liver transplantation for advanced primary sclerosing cholangitis. In addition, primary sclerosing cholangitis has been diagnosed for the first time years after proctocolectomy for chronic ulcerative colitis. Thus, inflammatory bowel disease can be diagnosed at any time during the course of primary sclerosing cholangitis and primary sclerosing cholangitis can occur at any time during the course of inflammatory bowel disease. Features of the association of chronic ulcerative colitis and primary sclerosing cholangitis include the following: (1) there appears to be no difference between patients with primary sclerosing cholangitis alone and primary sclerosing cholangitis with associated inflammatory bowel disease with respect to hepatobiliary signs and symptoms, biochemical tests, cholangiograms and hepatic histology; (2) the inflammatory bowel disease associated with primary sclerosing cholangitis is most often quiescent or mild; and (3) the rectum is commonly spared in patients with chronic ulcerative colitis associated with primary sclerosing cholangitis. Furthermore, as is the case for chronic ulcerative colitis unassociated with primary sclerosing cholangitis, patients with long-standing, extensive colitis in association with primary sclerosing cholangitis are at increased risk for colon cancer.[44] Thus, patients with primary sclerosing cholangitis who have had ulcerative colitis for 10 years or more should have annual colonoscopy with surveillance biopsies to screen for dysplasia and early colon cancer.

In addition to inflammatory bowel disease, primary sclerosing cholangitis is associated with a variety of other diseases (*see Table 12.21*). These associations may be coincidental, however. Nevertheless, many of the diseases associated with primary sclerosing cholangitis are thought to be autoimmune in nature and may be related to abnormalities in the immune system germane to the development of primary sclerosing cholangitis.

INVESTIGATIONS

Biochemical and immunological tests

Virtually all patients with primary sclerosing cholangitis will have an elevated serum alkaline phosphatase level usually greater than 3 or 4 times the upper limit of normal. Rarely, the serum alkaline phosphatase level may be normal.[3,21] Likewise, a majority of patients with primary sclerosing cholangitis will have an increase in serum aspartate and alanine transaminase levels but usually only to a very mild degree. Approximately one-half to two-thirds of patients with primary sclerosing cholangitis will have an increase in their total serum bilirubin levels at the time of diagnosis. Of importance is the fact that bilirubin levels fluctuate markedly during the course of the disease. Abnormalities in serum prothrombin and serum albumin levels at the time of diagnosis are uncommon; with progression of disease, however, the values become increasingly abnormal. The authors have reported that tests related to copper metabolism are virtually always abnormal in patients with primary sclerosing cholangitis.[38] For example, serum copper and serum ceruloplasmin levels are commonly increased, and urine copper excretion is accelerated. In addition, hepatic copper levels are increased in virtually all patients with primary sclerosing cholangitis. These abnormalities in copper metabolism are thought to be a secondary manifestation of the cholestatic nature of the syndrome.

Until recently, there were no serological markers that strongly suggested the syndrome of primary sclerosing cholangitis. Tests for antimitochondrial antibody are usually negative; if positive, the antibody is present in a very low titre. Likewise, smooth muscle antibodies and antinuclear antibodies are rarely positive. Serum levels of IgM may be increased in primary sclerosing cholangitis.[122] Recently, antibodies to as yet unidentified antigens present in the cytoplasm and the nucleus of neutrophils have been described in a large percentage of patients with primary sclerosing cholangitis.[27] Finally, unexplained eosinophilia of a mild-to-moderate degree may rarely be observed in association with primary sclerosing cholangitis.

RADIOLOGY

Direct visualization of the biliary tract cholangiographically is essential to establish the diagnosis of primary sclerosing cholangitis. Endoscopic retrograde cholangiography is currently the method of choice for diagnosis. Alternatively, under certain circumstances (for example, in a patient with previous biliary tract surgery), cholangiographic studies can be obtained via a percutaneous transhepatic approach. The radiological features most commonly seen in the syndrome of primary sclerosing cholangitis include: (1) diffusely distributed, multifocal annular strictures with intervening segments of normal or ectatic ducts; (2) short band-like strictures; and (3) diverticulum-like out-pouchings (*see Figure*

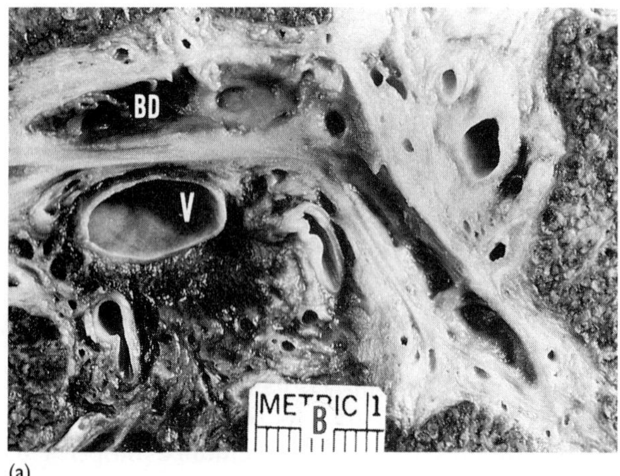

(a)

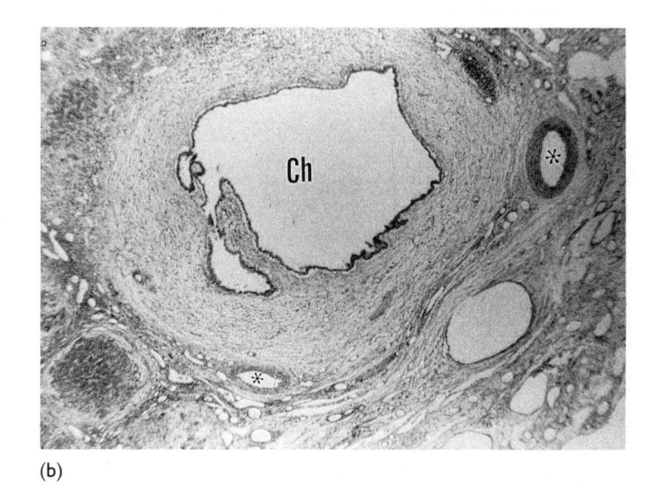

(b)

Figure 12.56 (a) Gross specimen of a primary sclerosing cholangitis liver showing biliary and peribiliary scarring of the bifurcation and the right and left hepatic ducts associated with the formation of cholangiectasis. (b) Tubulas cholangiectasisin patient with primary sclerosing cholangitis; specimen approximately 4 cm from hilum without evidence of secondary inflammation. Cholangiectasis (Ch) with prominent fibrous cholangitis of the wall (haematoxylin and eosin, × 17.5). (Reproduced, with permission, from Mosby Yearbook).

12.55).[73] These changes correspond to abnormalities detected pathologically in post-mortem liver specimens of patients with primary sclerosing cholangitis, demonstrating intrahepatic cholangiectasis and multiple stricturing (*Figure 12.56*).

Occasionally, cholangiographic abnormalities may be limited to the intrahepatic ducts, a situation that has been called 'intrahepatic sclerosing cholangitis'. Most consider this variant to represent part of the general spectrum of the syndrome of primary sclerosing cholangitis. Cholangiographic abnormalities may also be limited to the extrahepatic ducts as well.

Other diffuse liver diseases, including polycystic liver disease, metastasis, lymphoma and advanced cirrhosis, may produce narrowing and deformity of the bile ducts cholangiographically. These abnormalities, however, are rarely difficult to distinguish from the characteristic constellation of radiographic abnormalities present in primary sclerosing cholangitis. In perhaps 15% of cases with primary sclerosing cholangitis, the pancreatic duct may also be abnormal cholangiographically, demonstrating multiple short strictures and ectatic intervening segments resembling abnormalities seen in chronic pancreatitis.[6,73] Cholangiographic abnormalities may also occasionally be seen in the gallbladder and cystic duct of patients with primary sclerosing cholangitis.[7,37]

HISTOLOGY

HEPATIC HISTOLOGY

Essentially all patients with primary sclerosing cholangitis will have abnormalities apparent on liver biopsy. The most frequent abnormalities on biopsy specimens include periductal inflammation and fibrosis, bile duct proliferation alternating with bile duct obliteration, and ductopenia.[70] Ludwig has developed a staging system, shown in *Table 12.22*. Histologically (*Figure 12.57*), the abnormalities begin with enlargement of portal tracts characterized by periportal hepatitis, bile duct abnormalities or

Table 12.22 Histological staging criteria for chronic hepatitis associated with primary sclerosing cholangitis

Stage	*Criteria*
Stage 1 (portal stage)	Portal hepatitis or bile duct abnormalities or both, with little or no periportal inflammation and fibrosis. The portal tracts are not noticeably enlarged
Stage 2 (periportal stage or stage of portal enlargement)	Periportal fibrosis with or without periportal hepatitis, or prominent enlargement of portal tracts with seemingly intact, newly formed limiting plates. Both conditions may coexist. Biliary and fibrosing piecemeal necrosis may not be identifiable
	Non-essential features: portal oedema and fibrosis, proliferation of ducts and ductules, and evidence of fibrous, lymphoid, or pleomorphic cholangitis
Stage 3 (septal disease)	Septal fibrosis or bridging necrosis or both
	Non-essential features: these are the same as in the previous stages. Bridging necrosis not common. Bile ducts are often severely damaged or absent. In the parenchyma, biliary and fibrosing piecemeal necrosis and associated changes, such as prominent copper deposition, may be found
Stage 4 (cirrhotic stage)	Biliary cirrhosis
	Non-essential features: these may be the same as in the previous stages, but parenchymal changes are usually more prominent in stage 3. Bile ducts have often disappeared

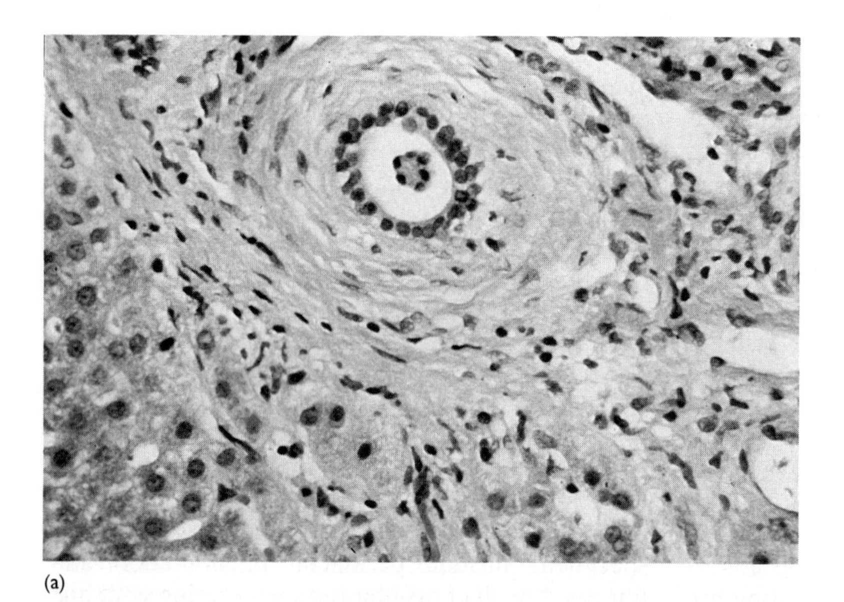

(a)

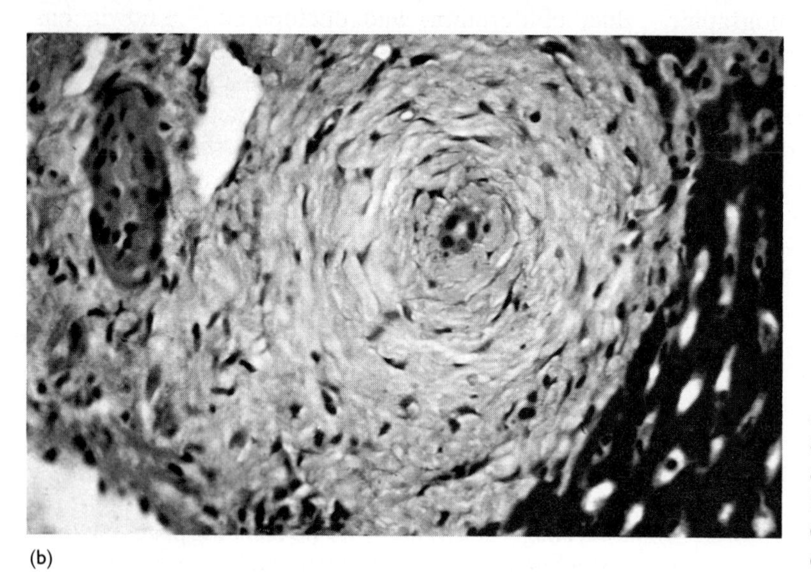

(b)

Figure 12.57 (a) Liver biopsy specimen showing an intrahepatic bile duct with abnormal epithelium and concentric periductal fibrosis surrounded by lymphocytic inflammatory cells (haematoxylin and eosin, × 170). (b) Advanced fibrous-obliterative cholangitis in primary sclerosing cholangitis.

both; oedema or fibrosis may be present but the abnormalities are confined to within the limiting plate (stage 1). With advancement, periportal fibrosis with or without inflammation extends beyond the limiting plate and may occasionally be accompanied by piecemeal necrosis (stage 2). This process progresses to septal fibrosis, bridging necrosis or both (stage 3) and, ultimately, to biliary cirrhosis (stage 4). During the early stages of the disease, most patients with primary sclerosing cholangitis will have fibrous obliterative cholangitis (chronic non-suppurative obliterative cholangitis) on biopsy. Accumulating evidence and experience suggest that this histological finding is nearly pathonomonic of the syndrome. From a histological point of view, the abnormalities seen on liver biopsy in patients with primary sclerosing cholangitis need to be differentiated from those seen in specimens from patients with primary biliary cirrhosis, prolonged extrahepatic obstruction and chronic active hepatitis. Primary biliary cirrhosis has many of the same histological features on biopsy specimens as seen in primary sclerosing cholangitis, including periportal cholestasis and copper deposition. The classic 'florid duct lesion' of primary biliary cirrhosis, however, is not seen in primary sclerosing cholangitis. Conversely, fibrous obliterative cholangitis, the histological hallmark of primary sclerosing cholangitis, is not seen in primary biliary cirrhosis. Changes showing fibrous or pleomorphic cholangitis may be present in biopsy specimens from patients with idiopathic autoimmune chronic active hepatitis. Such specimens may be difficult to distinguish from specimens of patients with primary sclerosing cholangitis and clinical information may be necessary to help the biopsy interpretation.

EXTRAHEPATIC DUCTAL HISTOLOGY

Both gross and biopsy specimens from the extrahepatic bile ducts in patients with primary sclerosing cholangitis show a thickened, fibrous wall often with mixed inflammatory infiltrates that tend to cluster around biliary glands. These changes, however, are non-specific and do not allow the pathologist to distinguish between primary sclerosing cholangitis and sclerosing cholangitis secondary to stones, strictures etc. The major value, however, of a bile duct biopsy is to exclude superimposed cholangiocarcinoma.

NATURAL HISTORY

Information regarding the natural history of primary sclerosing cholangitis continues to evolve. However, given our lack of knowledge of the pathogenesis of primary sclerosing cholangitis, the unavailability of serological markers for diagnosis, and the unpredictable nature of the syndrome, defining the natural history and prognosis of primary sclerosing cholangitis has been difficult. Nevertheless, on the basis of a number of prospective studies, there is growing evidence that primary sclerosing cholangitis is frequently a progressive disease.[120] The largest of these studies, from the Mayo Clinic, reported on 174 patients with documented primary sclerosing cholangitis who had a mean follow-up of 6.0 years.[125] The median survival from the time of diagnosis of primary sclerosing cholangitis was 11.9 years, and both symptomatic and asymptomatic patients had a shorter survival compared to a US population matched for age, sex and race (*Figure 12.58*). In this study, the authors found 31% of patients died as a result of underlying liver disease or the development of cholangiocarcinoma; an additional 10% were referred for liver transplantation. These findings have been confirmed by a number of other centres which have reported median survival from the time of diagnosis of primary sclerosing cholangitis to be between 9 and 11 years.

A subgroup of patients with primary sclerosing cholangitis without symptoms at the time of diagnosis has also been evaluated.[91] At the Mayo Clinic, 45 patients with primary sclerosing cholangitis without symptoms had a mean follow-up of 6.25 years. During this follow-up period, 76% had evidence of progression of disease on the basis of clinical and pathological findings, and 31% developed liver failure resulting in death or the need for liver transplantation. However, other institutions have found primary sclerosing cholangitis to be a more benign disease. Helzberg *et al.*, at Yale, reported a 75% 9-year survival, and studies from Norway estimated the mean survival of patients with primary sclerosing cholangitis to be 17 years from the time of diagnosis.[42] Reasons for these differences have recently been put into perspective.[92] First, primary sclerosing cholangitis progresses silently for a number of years and can be detected only by prospective follow-up of liver function tests and hepatic histology – observations which were not performed in a number of these studies. Second, early detection of the disease would be associated with prolonged survival, which seems to be the case in the Norwegian studies, in which patients with inflammatory bowel disease who had minimal abnormalities in liver function tests were aggressively evaluated with cholangiography. Third, the starting point for survival analysis is important in determining the overall

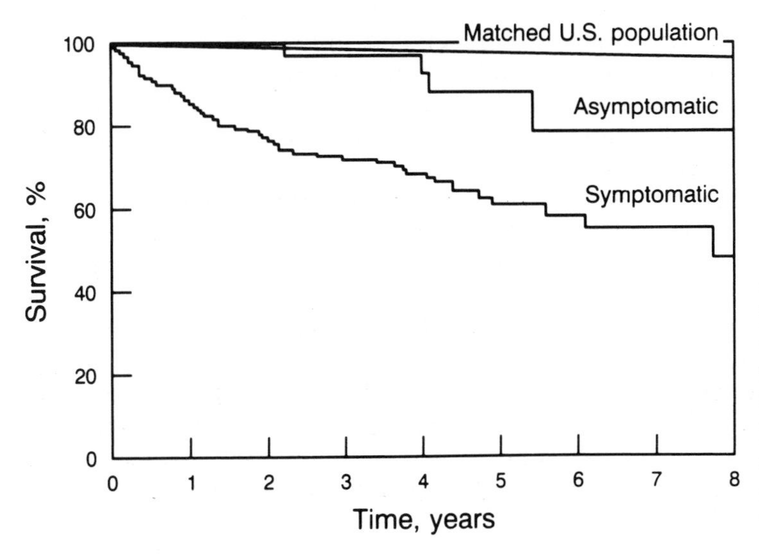

Figure 12.58 Kaplan–Meier estimated survival curves for asymptomatic and symptomatic primary sclerosing cholangitis patients. For comparison, the survival curve in the US population, matched for age, sex and race to the asymptomatic population, is also shown. Difference in survival: asymptomatic versus control ($P < 0.0001$); symptomatic versus asymptomatic ($P < 0.003$). (Reproduced, with permission, from Wiesner *et al.* (1989)[125]).

survival time. Comparing one group of patients in whom follow-up began at the time of cholangiographic diagnosis of primary sclerosing cholangitis with a second group of patients in whom a diagnosis of primary sclerosing cholangitis was backdated to the time of first onset of symptoms or biochemical abnormalities would obviously lead to differences in overall survival time. Therefore, if these differences in study design are taken into account, the authors believe the weight of evidence indicates that primary sclerosing cholangitis is indeed a progressive disease and that therapeutic intervention should be evaluated in the early as well as in the later stages of this syndrome.

PROGNOSIS

One of the main purposes of analysing the natural history of primary sclerosing cholangitis is to more accurately determine its rate of progression and to be able to estimate survival for the individual patient at any particular point in the course of his or her disease. Predicting survival based on clinical, biochemical and histological features of primary sclerosing cholangitis is also very important for the timing of liver transplantation and for monitoring therapeutic intervention. The use of sophisticated statistical approaches, most notably the Cox multivariate regression analysis, has enabled the development at the Mayo Clinic of a prognostic model based on five independent variables in which a risk score can be calculated and translated into a survival function to estimate survival for the individual patient with primary sclerosing cholangitis.[125] In the Mayo Clinic primary sclerosing cholangitis model, the important clinical variables identified are age, serum bilirubin, haemoglobin, hepatic histological stage, and the presence or absence of inflammatory bowel disease. More recently, by combining data from a number of other clinical centres interested in primary sclerosing cholangitis, a more refined model has been established in which age, bilirubin, presence or absence of splenomegaly, and histological stage represent the key prognostic clinical variables.[25]

A second primary sclerosing cholangitis model was recently developed by the Kings' College group. Multivariate analysis revealed hepatomegaly, splenomegaly, serum alkaline phosphatase level, histological stage, and age to be independent predictors of prognosis.[30] While these and other models provide some objective evidence with regard to disease progression and estimation of survival in the individual primary sclerosing cholangitis patient, additional studies are already underway to cross-validate these models and to assess the application in monitoring the effect of experimental therapy on disease progression.

PORTAL HYPERTENSION AND LIVER FAILURE

The end-stage of primary sclerosing cholangitis is associated with complications of portal hypertension, such as oesophageal variceal bleeding, ascites, and spontaneous portal systemic encephalopathy. As in other forms of chronic liver disease, oesophageal variceal bleeding is best managed by sclerotherapy. Systemic surgical shunting procedures should be avoided to keep the risk of a subsequent liver transplantation to a minimum. The recent introduction of the use of transjugular intrahepatic portasystemic shunts, which allows for the creation of an intrahepatic portacaval shunt, seems attractive in these patients. Similarly, ascites is best treated with large-volume paracentesis and diuretic therapy. In primary sclerosing cholangitis, spontaneous bacterial peritonitis is a frequent complication and is often related to biliary sepsis and cholangitis. In this situation, the use of selective bowel decontamination may be especially appropriate to prevent recurrence of this severe, life-threatening complication.[36,106]

A special complication of portal hypertension in primary sclerosing cholangitis is bleeding from peristomal varices in patients who have undergone proctocolectomy for underlying inflammatory bowel disease and who have had an ileal stoma (*Figure 12.59*).[125] Bleeding from peristomal varices can be severe; and local measures to control bleeding, including ileostomy revision, venous ligation, and injection of sclerosants, are, at best, associated with temporary relief and are generally unsuccessful long-term. Peristomal variceal bleeding can be controlled with a portosystemic shunt. However, patients with peristomal variceal bleeding generally have severe liver disease. Therefore, it is the authors' opinion that liver transplantation should be the procedure of choice because transplantation not only prevents further stomal variceal bleeding but also cures the underlying liver disease. However, in patients with primary sclerosing cholangitis who need a proctocolectomy for complications of ulcerative colitis, this troublesome complication can be prevented by performing an ileal pouch–anal anastomosis, whereby the formation of peristomal varices and associated bleeding is avoided.[53]

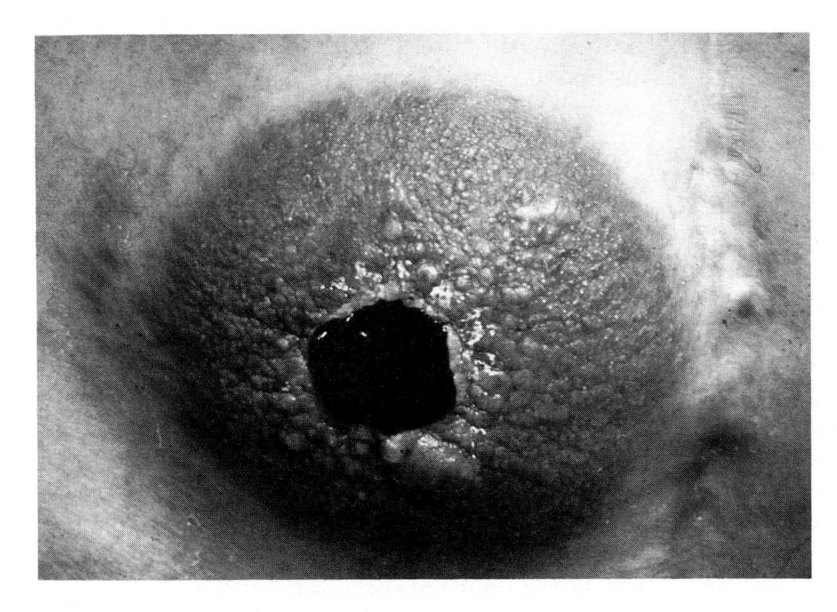

Figure 12.59 Peristomal varices occurring in a primary sclerosing cholangitis patient at the site of a Brooke ileostomy. This is a common complication in primary sclerosing cholangitis patients undergoing proctocolectomy and ileostomy who have portal hypertension. (Reproduced, with permission, from Wiesner *et al.* (1986)[124]).

COMPLICATIONS SPECIFIC FOR PRIMARY SCLEROSING CHOLANGITIS

Complications specific for primary sclerosing cholangitis include bacterial cholangitis, gallbladder and biliary stones, dominant bile duct strictures, and cholangiocarcinoma. Bacterial cholangitis is an unusual presenting symptom of primary sclerosing cholangitis but occurs frequently in patients who have undergone previous biliary surgery or in whom obstructing dominant strictures of the large bile ducts have developed.[123] These episodes of bacterial cholangitis are best treated with broad-spectrum antibiotics and, indeed, many patients appear to benefit from prophylactic antibiotic therapy to prevent recurrent bouts of cholangitis. At present, the authors use ciprofloxacin for prophylaxis of bacterial cholangitis because it achieves high biliary concentrations and has an extremely broad spectrum of action against Gram-positive and Gram-negative aerobic bacteria. However, the ability of long-term ciprofloxacin therapy to reduce the frequency and severity of bacterial cholangitis remains unstudied at this time.

Cholelithiasis and choledocholithiasis occur in 25–30% of patients with primary sclerosing cholangitis.[37] Chronic cholestasis predisposes to the formation of cholesterol gallstones, and bile stasis and bacterial cholangitis predispose to the formation of pigment stones. Indeed, if patients with primary sclerosing cholangitis, who have intact gallbladders, are surveyed by ultrasonography, gallstones will be found in approximately 25%. Because most of these patients are young men, this high incidence of gallstone disease probably represents an increased frequency of cholelithiasis in primary sclerosing cholangitis. Furthermore, the authors have shown that choledocholithiasis can cause bacterial cholangitis as a complication of primary sclerosing cholangitis. This diagnosis can be extremely difficult in patients with primary sclerosing cholangitis, because bacterial cholangitis may occur in the absence of biliary stones. A cholangiogram to exclude choledocholithiasis superimposed on primary sclerosing cholangitis should be considered, particularly in patients who have not had biliary surgery and who have recently experienced the onset of one or more episodes of bacterial cholangitis.

In primary sclerosing cholangitis, a dominant stricture of the biliary tract develops in 15–20% of patients some time during the course of the disease. These high-grade strictures most often occur at the biliary hilus but also can occur in the common bile duct and common hepatic duct. Frequently, this complication is associated with the acute onset of jaundice, pruritus, and fever. If a patient with primary sclerosing cholangitis develops these symptoms during the course of the disease, a cholangiogram should be performed. If a dominant stricture is found, cytological studies should be done to attempt to exclude cholangiocarcinoma, and balloon dilatation should be performed by either a transhepatic or endoscopic retrograde approach, depending on the location of the stricture.[39,50,78,80,102] In general, balloon dilatation of dominant strictures and removal of biliary sludge is effective in alleviating jaundice and pruritus in patients with primary sclerosing cholangitis and in decreasing the frequency and severity of bacterial cholangitis. These procedures appear to be most effective in patients whose symptoms are of recent onset and are less effective in those patients with long-standing jaundice or in those who have experienced long-standing, recurrent episodes of bacterial cholangitis. Results of dilatation of dominant strictures frequently depend on the severity of stricturing and obstruction of the intrahepatic bile ducts. The patients with primary sclerosing cholangitis and severe intrahepatic disease tend to benefit less from balloon dilatation of a dominant stricture of the common bile duct than do those who have only minimal changes of the intrahepatic biliary system. Approximately 50% of patients with primary sclerosing cholangitis having balloon dilatation of dominant strictures have improvement of symptoms for up to 2 years. Furthermore, approximately one-third require repeat balloon dilatations for recurrent strictures. In the authors' experience, stenting of the strictured area for up to 3 months has been associated with prolonged improvement.[50] However, up to one-third of patients experience episodes of bacterial cholangitis associated with the stenting procedure.

Another approach to the dominant stricture in primary sclerosing cholangitis is direct surgical intervention. Because most dominant strictures can be dilated by either a radiological or endoscopic approach, it is the authors' opinion that surgical intervention should be avoided because of the increased risk of postoperative bacterial cholangitis and the potential for causing technical difficulties if a liver transplant should be needed later (see below).

Finally, the effect of dilating biliary strictures on the long-term natural history of primary sclerosing cholangitis has been poorly defined. Further studies will be needed to evaluate dilating biliary strictures.

CHOLANGIOCARCINOMA

It is now established that cholangiocarcinoma may develop during the course of the disease in 10–15% of patients with primary sclerosing cholangitis.[31,95,96,117] The patients who appear to be at highest risk for the development of cholangiocarcinoma are those with long-standing chronic ulcerative colitis and cirrhotic stage on liver biopsy.[96] Indeed, the authors consider primary sclerosing cholangitis to be a premalignant condition of the biliary tree just as chronic ulcerative colitis is a premalignant condition of the colon. Unfortunately, bile duct carcinoma has been difficult to diagnose early in primary sclerosing cholangitis because there are no serological markers and biliary cytology has been insensitive for the early diagnosis of cholangiocarcinoma. The difficulty in making the diagnosis of cholangiocarcinoma in primary sclerosing cholangitis is supported by the recent report from the University of Pittsburgh in which 10% of patients with primary sclerosing cholangitis undergoing liver transplantation had unsuspected cholangiocarcinoma.[77] In addition, the authors' personal experience has revealed the presence of bile duct dysplasia in a number of patients with primary sclerosing cholangitis who have undergone liver transplantation. Finally, operative management, chemotherapy and radiation therapy have not been shown to be useful in this condition. Furthermore, in patients with primary sclerosing cholangitis and concomitant cholangiocarcinoma undergoing liver transplantation, recurrence of bile duct carcinoma has almost uniformly occurred.[43,108]

TREATMENT

The management of primary sclerosing cholangitis provides a real challenge to the clinician, given the array of symptoms and complications that can develop and the absence of effective, specific therapy for the underlying hepatobiliary disease. The first decision for the physician regarding management relates to whether or not any therapeutic intervention is necessary in a patient who has been newly diagnosed with primary sclerosing cholangitis. If therapeutic intervention is deemed necessary, one needs to identify the goals of such treatment. Specifically, therapy can be directed towards the relief of symptoms, the correction of complications of primary sclerosing cholangitis, or the amelioration of the underlying hepatobiliary disease. In general, management of primary sclerosing cholangitis can be divided into three categories: (1) managing complications of chronic cholestasis associated with the syndrome; (2) managing complications of portal hypertension and liver failure; and (3) specific therapy aimed at disrupting disease progression.

CHOLESTASIS

Complications associated with chronic cholestatic liver disease include fatigue, pruritus, steatorrhoea, and fat-soluble vitamin deficiency and its consequences. Fatigue, although a non-specific symptom, is a frequent complaint of patients with primary sclerosing cholangitis. Fatigue of notable severity can be present early in the course of primary sclerosing cholangitis and generally parallels the progression of the liver disease. Unfortunately, little is known about what causes fatigue in cholestatic liver diseases and, thus, no specific therapy is available for this symptom.

Pruritus, another common symptom of primary sclerosing cholangitis, can be severely debilitating, leading to severe excoriations and diminished quality of life. Although the pathogenesis of pruritus remains unknown, a recent hypothesis stated that pruritus may be related to the increased availability of endogenous opiate ligands at central opiate receptors.[51] In general, the severity of pruritus does not tend to parallel disease progression in primary sclerosing cholangitis.

A variety of therapies may help treat pruritus in patients with primary sclerosing cholangitis, including cholestyramine, activated charcoal, phenobarbitol, rifampin, plasmaphoresis, charcoal haemoperfusion and ultraviolet light therapy. While all of these therapies have been of beneficial effect in anecdotal reports, none of these therapies has been evaluated in a controlled fashion.

Steatorrhoea, associated with fat-soluble vitamin deficiency, has also been described in patients with primary sclerosing cholangitis.[85,97] As in primary biliary cirrhosis, fat malabsorption in primary sclerosing cholangitis is most probably related to diminished intestinal concentrations of bile acids.[57] However, steatorrhoea in primary sclerosing cholangitis can also be caused by chronic pancreatitis or coeliac sprue, both of which should be considered in the differential diagnosis, particularly if steatorrhoea occurs in a patient with primary sclerosing cholangitis who is not jaundiced and has early histological stage diseases.[7,40]

In the authors' experience, vitamin A deficiency occurs in about 50% of patients with primary sclerosing cholangitis and can be associated with night blindness. Similarly, deficiencies in vitamins D and E are not uncommon but, infrequently, are associated with clinical symptoms. Metabolic bone disease associated with compression fractures of trabecular bone has also been shown to occur with increased frequency in patients with primary sclerosing cholangitis.[41] Bone biopsies reveal that osteoporosis, rather than osteomalacia, is the most common form of bone disease in patients with primary sclerosing cholangitis as has previously been described in primary biliary cirrhosis. As in the latter disease, it appears that corticosteroid therapy markedly exacerbates bone disease associated with primary sclerosing cholangitis and should be avoided or used with caution in these patients.[67]

Finally, vitamin K deficiency related to malabsorption of vitamin K from the gastrointestinal tract or to severe hepatic parenchymal damage can occur in primary sclerosing cholangitis. A trial of parenteral vitamin K is reasonable to attempt to correct a prolonged prothrombin time. If the prolonged prothrombin time is related to vitamin K malabsorption, a marked improvement in prothrombin time will be noted following parenteral administration of vitamin K. If the prolonged prothrombin time is related to severe hepatic parenchymal damage, vitamin K therapy will have no effect.

TREATMENT

Primary therapy for primary sclerosing cholangitis can be categorized into medical and surgical. The diverse approach to the specific management of primary sclerosing cholangitis, however, bears witness to our lack of understanding the aetiopathogenesis to this disease (*Table 12.23*).

MEDICAL

A variety of medical therapies have been evaluated in the treatment of primary sclerosing cholangitis; however, to date, none have been proven effective.

Table 12.23 Therapy for primary sclerosing cholangitis

Medical	*Radiological*	*Surgical*
Corticosteroids	Balloon dilatation and stenting	Choledochoenterostomy
D-Penicillamine		Hepaticojejunostomy
Azathioprine		Proctocolectomy
Ursodeoxycholic acid		Liver transplantation
Methotrexate		
Biliary lavage with steroids		
Cholestyramine		
Antibiotics		

D-Penicillamine

The finding of increased hepatic copper levels in primary sclerosing cholangitis provided the major rationale for evaluating D-penicillamine in a controlled, randomized trial for this disease.[28] The authors randomized 70 patients to D-penicillamine or placebo therapy. After 36 months of follow-up, careful analysis of clinical, biochemical, radiological, histological and survival data revealed that D-penicillamine had no beneficial effect on disease progression. In addition, major side-effects, of which proteinuria was the most frequent, made it necessary to permanently discontinue this drug in 21% of patients.

Corticosteroids

Both topical and systemic corticosteroid therapy has been evaluated in primary sclerosing cholangitis. Uncontrolled observations in 10 patients with primary sclerosing cholangitis who had unusually high elevations in aminotransferase levels demonstrated a beneficial response to oral corticosteroid therapy, with early biochemical improvement.[10] However, histological assessment is not available in this study, and long-term follow-up was not performed. Other studies, including a report from the Mayo Clinic evaluating the combination of colchicine and corticosteroid therapy, have not been able to document a long-term beneficial effect of corticosteroid therapy in primary sclerosing cholangitis.[67] Furthermore, corticosteroid therapy in primary biliary cirrhosis has been shown to be associated with enhanced bone loss and, in patients treated for up to 2 years with prednisone, an increased risk of causing compression fractures of trabecular bone was noted.

Other studies have explored the use of topical corticosteroid therapy. A small, controlled trial of nasobiliary lavage with corticosteroids showed no benefit compared with the placebo group.[2] Furthermore, the treatment appeared to induce a high incidence of bacterial cholangitis. Thus, at this time, the benefits of corticosteroid therapy in primary sclerosing cholangitis remain unproven. The use of corticosteroid therapy outside of controlled clinical trials should be avoided because of the potential risk of inducing severe bone disease in patients with primary sclerosing cholangitis.

Other immunosuppressive agents

Azathioprine has been used, sporadically, to treat primary sclerosing cholangitis; in one study, two patients appeared to have clinical improvement, and in another study one patient had clinical deterioration.[49,115] Other than these two anecdotal reports, no formal studies of azathioprine treatment in primary sclerosing cholangitis have been performed. At present, the Mayo Clinic is performing a controlled clinical trial evaluating the use of cyclosporin in the treatment of primary sclerosing cholangitis. Although cyclosporin has been shown to be useful in treating primary biliary cirrhosis and chronic ulcerative colitis, preliminary evaluation of this study suggests that it apparently does not have a beneficial effect on liver disease progression in primary sclerosing cholangitis.

Methotrexate has been evaluated in the treatment of primary sclerosing cholangitis.[52,54] In a double-blind, controlled trial, methotrexate was shown to significantly reduce serum levels of alkaline phosphatase but did not have a significant effect on serum levels of bilirubin, aminotransferases and albumin. Furthermore, a subgroup of patients with primary sclerosing cholangitis who had cirrhotic stage disease apparently did not benefit from methotrexate therapy. The long-term effect of methotrexate on liver disease progression in primary sclerosing cholangitis remains unknown; therefore, further follow-up is needed to assess its efficacy. Finally, the inherent hepatotoxicity that can be associated with methotrexate therapy is of concern.[35]

Ursodeoxycholic acid therapy

Considerable enthusiasm has recently emerged for the use of ursodeoxycholic acid in the treatment of chronic cholestatic liver disease, including primary sclerosing cholangitis. The rationale for using ursodeoxycholic acid is the replacement of the bile acid pool with a bile acid that has less toxic potential than other endogenous (e.g. chenodeoxycholic or lithocholic acids), more hydrophobic bile acids. Although this hypothesis is theoretically attractive, clinical support for such therapy is lacking, and only uncontrolled data suggest that ursodeoxycholic acid is associated with improvement in pruritus and in biochemical parameters in this disease.[20,109,86] At this time, there are no data on the effect of ursodeoxycholic acid on disease progression or on survival.

Other agents

Other agents that have been used to treat primary sclerosing cholangitis include colchicine and systemic antibiotics.[83] At present, there are no controlled data on the efficacy of colchicine in the treatment of primary sclerosing cholangitis. Antibiotic trials aimed at treating or preventing portal bacteraemia have demonstrated no beneficial effect.

Although multiple medical therapies have been proposed for the treatment of primary sclerosing cholangitis, only D-penicillamine has been evaluated in a randomized, placebo, controlled clinical trial. Furthermore, none of these therapies has been shown to have a significant impact on the natural history of the disease and none has been shown to be associated with a clinical, biochemical and histological remission. Controlled studies evaluating cyclosporin and ursodeoxycholic acid remain in progress, and forthcoming reports will evaluate their efficacy.

SURGICAL

Biliary tract reconstructive surgery

Biliary tract surgery for primary sclerosing cholangitis has been advocated by a number of surgical centres.[11,90] Unfortunately, the lack of prospective, controlled data makes it impossible to totally assess the effect such surgery has had on the natural history of the disease. Because primary sclerosing cholangitis is generally a progressive disease, biliary surgery should be considered a palliative measure aimed at relieving symptoms of jaundice, pruritus, and bacterial cholangitis, and as a diagnostic approach to exclude cholangiocarcinoma. There is now agreement that biliary surgery is of little or no value in patients with primary sclerosing cholangitis who have cirrhosis or who have severe intrahepatic bile duct stricturing.[11] These patients should be considered for liver transplantation. However, patients with primary sclerosing cholangitis in whom biliary surgery may give temporary or symptomatic relief are those patients without cirrhosis who have a dominant stricture in the common bile duct, common hepatic duct or at the biliary bifurcation and who have intrahepatic disease of mild-to-moderate severity. In such cases, uncontrolled data suggest that resection of the hepatic duct bifurcation with dilatation of the intrahepatic biliary tree and placement of transhepatic biliary stents may prolong the course of the disease and postpone liver transplantation. In the authors' experience, however, dominant strictures can be readily approached radiologically and endoscopically and dilated with a balloon. Thus, the morbidity and mortality associated with a major surgical procedure and the potential surgical difficulties should the patient require liver transplantation in the future are avoided. The authors believe that, in the era of liver transplantation, biliary surgery for primary sclerosing cholangitis should be avoided, if possible, in favour of a non-operative approach.

Proctocolectomy

Because primary sclerosing cholangitis is frequently associated with chronic ulcerative colitis, the question of whether proctocolectomy has an effect on the clinical course of primary sclerosing cholangitis is intriguing. This question was recently addressed by a prospective follow-up of 45 patients with primary sclerosing cholangitis, who had chronic ulcerative colitis, of whom 20 had undergone proctocolectomy.[12] In this study, proctocolectomy had no apparent effect on clinical, biochemical, hepatic histological, or radiological features of primary sclerosing cholangitis. Additionally, proctocolectomy had no effect on overall survival.[12,77] The lack of efficacy of proctocolectomy on primary sclerosing cholangitis is further supported by reports of primary sclerosing cholangitis occurring years after proctocolectomy.[94] Therefore, the authors believe that proctocolectomy should not be performed in patients with primary sclerosing cholangitis in anticipation of having a beneficial effect on liver disease. However, as in other patients with chronic ulcerative colitis, if intractable inflammatory bowel disease symptoms, dysplasia or colon cancer develop in a patient with primary sclerosing cholangitis, proctocolectomy should be performed. In such cases, the authors believe an ileal pouch–anal anastomosis is the procedure of choice compared to an ileal stoma because it avoids the development of peristomal varices.

Liver transplantation

For patients with end-stage primary sclerosing cholangitis, liver transplantation is the only viable lifesaving therapeutic alternative. Although the initial results of liver transplantation in primary sclerosing cholangitis were poor (20% 2-year survival), more recent reports have been encouraging, noting over 85% 3-year survival.[56,79,98] Despite excellent patient survival, early surgical complications after liver transplantation have been shown to be greater in patients with primary sclerosing cholangitis than in patients with primary biliary cirrhosis.[79] Diffuse biliary strictures have been found to occur more frequently in patients with primary sclerosing cholangitis undergoing liver transplantation. Although these findings raise the question of recurrence of primary sclerosing cholangitis, other factors, such as reflux cholangitis related to the Roux-en-Y biliary anastomosis and a higher incidence of chronic rejection, represent potential causes of increased biliary stricturing in this group of patients.[48,61,62] In general, for patients with primary sclerosing cholangitis and chronic ulcerative colitis who undergo liver transplantation, symptoms related to inflammatory bowel disease usually subside or remain quiescent in the post-transplantation course. However, the development of colon cancer after liver transplantation in two patients with primary sclerosing cholangitis and chronic ulcerative colitis emphasizes the importance of continued colon cancer surveillance in this group of patients.

CONCLUSION

Primary sclerosing cholangitis is a progressive disease for which no effective medical, radiological or surgical therapy presently exists. This syndrome occurs most commonly in young men and is characterized by chronic cholestasis and a frequent association with chronic ulcerative colitis. The diagnosis is made by cholangiography, serological markers are conspicuously absent and liver histology is usually not pathognomonic. While definitive conclusions regarding the natural history of primary sclerosing cholangitis require additional study, the weight of evidence suggests the disease is slowly progressive over a 5–15-year period of time; indeed, even asymptomatic patients have a reduced life expectancy. Primary sclerosing cholangitis is complicated by cirrhosis and complications of portal hypertension, which are managed in a similar fashion to other chronic liver diseases. The disease is also complicated by a high incidence of bile duct cancer, and symptoms of pruritus and cholangitis are frequently related to the development of a dominant stricture. At this time, there is no medical therapy that is effective in the treatment of primary sclerosing cholangitis. Current medical therapies being evaluated include the use of antifibrogenic, immunosuppressive and choleretic agents. While biliary tract reconstructive surgery may alleviate symptoms, it appears to have no effect on the natural history of the disease and should be avoided, if possible, because it may interfere with subsequent liver transplantation, which is the only effective life-saving procedure for patients having advanced primary sclerosing cholangitis.

REFERENCES

1. Alberti-Flor, J.J., de Medina, M., Jeffers, L. and Schiff, E.R. (1983) Elevated immunoglobulins and immune complexes in the bile of patients with primary sclerosing cholangitis (abstract). *Hepatology*, **3**, 844.
2. Allison, M.C., Burroughs, A.K., Noone, P. and Summerfield, J.A. (1986) Biliary lavage with corticosteroids in primary sclerosing cholangitis: a clinical, cholangiographic and bacteriological study. *Journal of Hepatology*, **3**, 118–122.
3. Balasubramaniam, K., Wiesner, R.H., and LaRusso, N.F. (1988) Primary sclerosing cholangitis with normal serum alkaline phosphatase activity. *Gastroenterology*, **95**, 1395–1398.
4. Belghiti, J., Benhamou, J.P., Houry, S., Grenier, P., Hunguier, M. and Fekete, F. (1986) Caustic sclerosing cholangitis: A complication of the surgical treatment of hydatid disease of the liver. *Archives of Surgery*, **121**, 1162–1165.
5. Bodenheimer, H.C., Jr, LaRusso, N.F., Thayer, W.R., Charland, C., Staples, P.J. and Ludwig, J. (1983) Elevated circulating immune complexes in primary sclerosing cholangitis. *Hepatology*, **3**, 150–154.
6. Borkje, B., Vetvik, K., Odegaard, S., Schrumpf, E. and Larssen, T.B. (1985) Chronic pancreatitis in patients with sclerosing cholangitis and ulcerative colitis. *Scandinavian Journal of Gastroenterology*, **20**, 539–542.
7. Brandt, D.J., MacCarty, R.L., Charboneau, J.W., LaRusso, N.F., Wiesner, R.H. and Ludwig, J. (1988) Gallbladder disease in patients with primary sclerosing cholangitis. *American Journal of Roentgenology*, **150**, 571–574.
8. Brinch, L., Teisberg, P., Schrumpf, E. and Akesson, I. (1982) The in vivo metabolism of C3 in hepatobiliary disease associated with ulcerative colitis. *Scandinavian Journal of Gastroenterology*, **17**, 523–527.
9. Bucuvalas, J.C., Bove, K.E., Kaufman, R.A., Gilchrist, M.J.R., Oldham, K.T. and Balistreri, W.F. (1985) Cholangitis associated with *Cryptococcus neoformans*. *Gastroenterology*, **88**, 1055–1059.
10. Burgert, S.L., Brown, B.P., Kirkpatrick, R.B. and LaBrecque, D.R. (1984) Positive corticosteroid response in early primary sclerosing cholangitis (abstract). *Gastroenterology*, **86**, 1037.
11. Cameron, J.L., Pitt, H.A., Zinner, M.J. *et al.* (1988) Resection of hepatic duct bifurcation and transhepatic stenting for sclerosing cholangitis. *Annals of Surgery*, **207**, 614–620.
12. Cangemi, J.R., Wiesner, R.H., Beaver, S.J. *et al.* (1989) Effect of proctocolectomy for chronic ulcerative colitis on the natural history of primary sclerosing cholangitis. *Gastroenterology*, **96**, 790–794.
13. Cello, J.P. (1989) Acquired immunodeficiency syndrome cholangiopathy: spectrum of disease. *American Journal of Medicine*, **86**, 539–546.
14. Chapman, R.W. (1991) Role of immune factors in the pathogenesis of primary sclerosing cholangitis. *Seminars in Liver Diseases*, **11**, 1–4.

15. Chapman, R.W.G. and Jewell, D.P. (1985) Primary sclerosing cholangitis – an immunologically mediated disease? *Western Journal of Medicine*, **143**, 193–195.
16. Chapman, R.W., Marborgh, B.A., Rhodes, J.M. *et al.* (1980) Primary sclerosing cholangitis: a review of its clinical features, cholangiography, and hepatic histology. *Gut*, **21**, 870–877.
17. Chapman, R.W., Varghese, Z., Gaul, R., Patel, G., Kokinon, N. and Sherlock, S. (1983) Association of primary sclerosing cholangitis with HLA-B8. *Gut*, **24**, 38–41.
18. Chapman, R.W., Cottlone, M., Selby, W.S., Shepherd, H.A., Sherlock, S. and Jewell, D.P. (1986) Serum autoantibodies, ulcerative colitis and primary sclerosing cholangitis. *Gut*, **27**, 86–91.
19. Chapman, R.W., Kelly, P.M.A., Heryet, A., Jewell, D.P. and Fleming, K.A. (1988) Expression of HLA-DR antigens on bile duct epithelium in primary sclerosing cholangitis. *Gut*, **29**, 422–427.
20. Chazouilleres, O., Poupon, R., Capron, J.P. *et al.* (1990) Ursodeoxycholic acid for primary sclerosing cholangitis. *Journal of Hepatology*, **11**, 120–123.
21. Clements, D., Rhodes, J.M. and Elias, E. (1986) Severe bile duct lesions without biochemical evidence of cholestasis in a case of sclerosing cholangitis. *Journal of Hepatology*, **3**, 72–74.
22. Davis, J.J., Heyman, M.B., Ferrell, L., Kerner, J., Kerlan, R. Jr. and Thaler, M.M. (1987) Sclerosing cholangitis associated with chronic cryptosporidiosis in a child with a congenital immunodeficiency disorder. *American Journal of Gastroenterology*, **82**, 1196–1202.
23. Delbet, P. (1924) Retrecissement du choledoque cholecystoduodenostomie. *Bull. Mem. Soc. Chir. Paris*, **50**, 1144–1146.
24. Dew, M.J., van Berge Henegouwen, G.P., Huybregts, A.W.M. and Allan, R.N. (1980) Hepatotoxic effect of bile acids in inflammatory bowel disease. *Gastroenterology*, **78**, 1393–1401.
25. Dickson, E.R., Murtaugh, P., Malinchoc, M. *et al.* (1991) Primary sclerosing cholangitis (PSC): refinement and validation of survival models (abstract). *Gastroenterology*, **100**(part 2), A735.
26. Donaldson, P.T., Farrant, J.M., Wilkinson, M.L., Hayllar, K., Portmann, B.C. and Williams, R. (1991) Dual association of HLADR2 and DR3 with primary sclerosing cholangitis. *Hepatology*, **13**, 129–133.
27. Duerr, R.H., Targan, S.R., Landers, C.J. *et al.* (1991) Anti-neutrophil cytoplasmic antibodies: a link between primary sclerosing cholangitis and ulcerative colitis. *Gastroenterology*, **100**, 1385–1391.
28. Eade, M.N. and Brooke, B.N. (1969) Portal bactaeremia in cases of ulcerative colitis submitted to colectomy. *The Lancet*, **i**, 1008–1009.
29. Elias, E., Summerfield, J.A., Dick, R. and Sherlock, S. (1974) Endoscopic retrograde cholangiopancreatography in the diagnosis of jaundice associated with ulcerative colitis. *Gastroenterology*, **67**, 907–911.
30. Farrant, J.M., Hayllar, K.M., Wilkinson, M. *et al.* (1991) Natural history and prognostic variables in primary sclerosing cholangitis. *Gastroenterology*, **100**, 1710–1717.
31. Fausa, O. and Schrumpf, E. (1989) Cholangiocarcinoma (CH-CA) occurs with high frequency in primary sclerosing cholangitis (PSC) (abstract). *Scandinavian Journal of Gastroenterology*, **54**, 159.
32. Fausa, O., Schrumpf, E. and Elgjo, K. (1989) Inflammatory bowel disease (IBD) occurs in almost all patients with primary sclerosing cholangitis (PSC) (abstract). *Scandinavian Journal of Gastroenterology*, **24**(suppl. 159), 53.
33. Fausa, O., Schrumpf, E. and Elgjo, K. (1991) Relationship of inflammatory bowel disease and primary sclerosing cholangitis. *Seminars in Liver Diseases*, **11**, 31–39.
34. Finegold, M.J. and Carpenter, R.J. (1982) Obliterative cholangitis due to cytomegalovirus: a possible precursor of paucity of intrahepatic bile ducts. *Human Pathology*, **13**, 662–665.
35. Gilbert, S.C., Klintmalm, G., Menter, A. and Silverman, A. (1990) Methotrexate-induced cirrhosis requiring liver transplantation in three patients with psoriasis: a word of caution in light of the expanding use of this 'steroid-sparing' agent. *Archives of Internal Medicine*, **150**, 889–891.
36. Gines, P., Rimola, A., Planas, R. *et al.* (1990) Norfloxacin prevents spontaneous bacterial peritonitis recurrence in cirrhosis: results of a double-blind placebo-controlled trial. *Hepatology*, **12**, 716–724.
37. Gluskin, L.E. and Payne, J.A. (1983) Cystic dilatation as a radiographic sign of cholangiocarcinoma complicating sclerosing cholangitis. *American Journal of Gastroenterology*, **78**, 661–664.
38. Gross, J.B., Jr, Ludwig, J., Wiesner, R.H., McCall, J.T. and LaRusso, N.F. (1985) Abnormalities in tests of copper metabolism in primary sclerosing cholangitis. *Gastroenterology*, **89**, 272–278.
39. Hamilton, I., Soutar, J.S., Bouchier, I.A.D. and Cuschieri, A. (1987) Short-term biliary dilatation and stenting in primary sclerosing cholangitis. *Journal of Clinical Gastroenterology*, **9**, 70–75.
40. Hay, J.E., Wiesner, R.H., Shorter, R.G., LaRusso, N.F. and Baldus, W.P. (1988) Primary sclerosing cholangitis and celiac disease: a novel association. *Annals of Internal Medicine*, **109**, 713–717.
41. Hay, J.E., Lindor, K.D., Wiesner, R.H., Dickson, E.R., Krom, R.A.F. and LaRusso, N.F. (1991) Metabolic bone disease in primary sclerosing cholangitis. *Hepatology*, **14**(2), 257–261.
42. Helzberg, J.H., Petersen, J.M., Boyer and J.L. (1987) Improved survival with primary sclerosing cholangitis: a review of clinicopathologic features

and comparison of symptomatic and asymptomatic patients. *Gastroenterology*, **92**, 1869–1875.
43. Herbener, T., Zajko, A.B., Koneru, B., Bron, K.M. and Campbell, W.L. (1988) Recurrent cholangiocarcinoma in the biliary tree after liver transplantation. *Radiology*, **169**, 641–642.
44. Higashi, H., Yanaga, K., Marsh, J.W., Tzakis, A., Kakizoe, S. and Starzl, T.E. (1990) Development of colon cancer after liver transplantation for primary sclerosing cholangitis associated with ulcerative colitis. *Hepatology*, **11**, 477–480.
45. Hobson, C.H., Butt, T.J., Ferry, D.M., Hunter, J., Chadwick, V.S. and Broom, M.F. (1988) Enterohepatic circulation of bacterial chemotactic peptide in rats with experimental colitis. *Gastroenterology*, **94**, 1006–1013.
46. Holubitsky, I.B. and McKenzie, A.D. (1964) Primary sclerosing cholangitis of the extrahepatic bile ducts. *Canadian Journal of Surgery*, **7**, 277–283.
47. Holzbach, R.T., Marsh, M.E., Freedman, M.R., Fazio, V.W., Lavery, I.C. and Jagelman, D.A. (1980) Portal vein bile acids in patients with severe inflammatory bowel disease. *Gut*, **21**, 428–435.
48. Hunter, E.B., Wiesner, R.H. and MacCarty, R.L. (1989) Does primary sclerosing cholangitis recur after liver transplantation? (abstract). *Gastroenterology*, **96**(part 2), A610.
49. Javett, S.L. (1971) Azathioprine in primary sclerosing cholangitis. *The Lancet*, **i**, 810.
50. Johnson, G.K., Geenen, J.E., Venu, R.P. and Ibgan, W.J. (1987) Endoscopic treatment of biliary duct strictures in sclerosing cholangitis: follow-up assessment of a new therapeutic approach. *Gastrointestinal Endoscopy*, **33**, 9–12.
51. Jones, E.A. and Bergasa, N.V. (1990) Hypothesis. The pruritus of cholestasis: from bile acids to opiate agonists. *Hepatology*, **11**, 884–887.
52. Kaplan, M.M., Arora, S. and Pincus, S.H. (1987) Primary sclerosing cholangitis and low-dose oral pulse methotrexate therapy: clinical and histologic response. *Annals of Internal Medicine*, **106**, 231–235.
53. Kartheuser, A.H., Dozois, R.R., LaRusso, N.F., Wiesner, R.H., Ilstrup, D.M. and Schleck, C.D. (1991) Peristomal variceal bleeding after proctocolectomy for ulcerative colitis in patients with primary sclerosing cholangitis can be avoided by ileal pouch–anal anastomosis (abstract). *Gastroenterology*, **100**(part 2), A220.
54. Knox, T.A. and Kaplan, M.M. (1991) Double-blind trial of methotrexate (MTX) in the treatment of primary sclerosing cholangitis (PSC) (abstract). *Gastroenterology* **100**(part 2), A761.
55. Knox, T.A. and Kaplan, M.M. (1991) Treatment of primary sclerosing cholangitis with oral methotrexate. *American Journal of Gastroenterology*, **86**, 546–552.
56. Langnas, A.N., Grazi, G.L., Stratta, R.J. *et al.* (1990) Primary sclerosing cholangitis: the emerging role for liver transplantation. *American Journal of Gastroenterology*, **85**, 1136–1141.
57. Lanspa, S.J., Chan, A.T.H., Bell, J.S. III., Go, V.L.W., Dickson, E.R. and DiMagno, E.P. (1985) Pathogenesis of steatorrhea in primary biliary cirrhosis. *Hepatology*, **5**, 837–842.
58. LaRusso, N.F., Wiesner, R.H., Ludwig, J. and MacCarty, R.L. (1984) Primary sclerosing cholangitis. *New England Journal of Medicine*, **310**, 899–903.
59. LaRusso, N.F., Wiesner, R.H., Ludwig, J., MacCarty, R.L., Beaver, S.J. and Zinsmeister, A.R. (1988) A prospective trial of penicillamine in primary sclerosing cholangitis. *Gastroenterology*, **95**, 1036–1042.
60. Lefton, H.B., Farmer, R.G., Buchwald, R. and Haselby, R. (1974) Cryptococcal hepatitis mimicking primary sclerosing cholangitis. *Gastroenterology*, **67**, 511–515.
61. Lerut, J., Demetris, A.J., Stieber, A.C. *et al.* (1988) Intrahepatic bile duct strictures after human orthotopic liver transplantation: recurrence of primary sclerosing cholangitis or unusual presentation of allograft rejection? *Transplantation International*, **1**, 127–130.
62. Letourneau, J.G., Day, D.L., Hunter, D.W. *et al.* (1988) Biliary complications after liver transplantation in patients with preexisting sclerosing cholangitis. *Radiology*, **167**, 349–351.
63. Lichtman, S.N., Sartor, R.B., Keku, J. and Schwab, J.H. (1990) Hepatic inflammation in rats with experimental small intestinal bacterial overgrowth. *Gastroenterology*, **98**, 414–423.
64. Lindor, K.D., Wiesner, R.H., LaRusso, N.F. and Dickson, E.R. (1983) Chronic active hepatitis: overlap with primary biliary cirrhosis and primary sclerosing cholangitis. In *Chronic Active Hepatitis: The Mayo Clinic Experience* (Ed.) Czaja, A.J. and Dickson, E.R. pp. 171–187. New York: Marcel Dekker.
65. Lindor, K.D., Wiesner, R.H., Katzmann, J.A., LaRusso, N.F. and Beaver, S.J. (1987) Lymphocyte subsets in primary sclerosing cholangitis. *Digestive Diseases and Sciences*, **32**, 720–725.
66. Lindor, K.D., Wiesner, R.H., LaRusso, N.F. and Homburger, H.A. (1987) Enhanced autoreactivity of T-lymphocytes in primary sclerosing cholangitis. *Hepatology*, **7**, 884–888.
67. Lindor, K.D., Wiesner, R.H., Colwell, L.J., Steiner, B., Beaver, S. and LaRusso, N.F. (1991) The combination of prednisone and colchicine in patients with primary sclerosing cholangitis. *American Journal of Gastroenterology*, **85**, 57–61.
68. Ludwig, J. (1991) Small-duct primary sclerosing cholangitis. *Seminars in Liver Diseases*, **11**, 11–17.
69. Ludwig, J., Barham, S.S., LaRusso, N.F., Elveback, L.R., Wiesner, R.H. and McCall, J.T. (1981) Morphologic features of chronic hepatitis associated with primary sclerosing cholangitis and chronic ulcerative colitis. *Hepatology*, **1**, 632–640.

70. Ludwig, J., LaRusso, N.F. and Wiesner, R.H. (1986) Primary sclerosing cholangitis. *Contemporary Issues in Surgical Pathology*, **8**, 193–213.
71. Ludwig, J., Wiesner, R.H. and LaRusso, N.F. (1988) Idiopathic adulthood ductopenia: a cause of chronic cholestatic liver disease and biliary cirrhosis. *Journal of Hepatology*, **7**, 193–199.
72. Ludwig, J., Kim, C.H., Wiesner, R.H. and Krom, R.A.F. (1989) Floxuridine-induced sclerosing cholangitis: an ischemic cholangiopathy? *Hepatology*, **9**, 215–218.
73. MacCarty, R.L., LaRusso, N.F., Wiesner, R.H. and Ludwig, J. (1983) Primary sclerosing cholangitis: Findings on cholangiography and pancreatography. *Radiology*, **149**, 39–44.
74. McEntee, G., Wiesner, R.H., Rosen, C., Cooper, J. and Wahlstrom, H.E. (1991) A comparative study of patients undergoing liver transplantation for primary sclerosing cholangitis and primary biliary cirrhosis. *Transplantation Proceedings*, **23**, 1563–1564.
75. McFarlane, I.G., Wojcicka, B.M., Tsantoulas, D.C., Portmann, B.C., Eddleston, A.L.W.F. and Williams, R. (1979) Leukocyte migration inhibition in response to biliary antigens in primary biliary cirrhosis, sclerosing cholangitis, and other chronic liver diseases. *Gastroenterology*, **76**, 1333–1340.
76. Margulis, S.J., Honig, C.L., Soave, R., Govoni, A.F., Mouradian, J.A. and Jacobson, I.M. (1986) Biliary tract obstruction in the acquired immunodeficiency syndrome. *Annals of Internal Medicine*, **105**, 207–210.
77. Marsh, J.W. Jr, Shunzaburo, I., Makowka, L. *et al.* (1988) Orthotopic liver transplantation for primary sclerosing cholangitis. *Annals of Surgery*, **207**, 21–25.
78. Martin, E.C., Fankuchen, E.I., Schultz, R.W. and Casarella, W.J. (1981) Percutaneous dilatation in primary sclerosing cholangitis: two experiences. *American Journal of Roentgenology*, **137**, 603–605.
79. Martin, F.M., Rossi, R.L., Nugent, F.W. *et al.* (1990) Surgical aspects of sclerosing cholangitis: results in 178 patients. *Annals of Surgery*, **212**, 551–556.
80. May, G.R., Bender, C.E., LaRusso, N.F. and Wiesner, R.H. (1985) Nonoperative dilatation of dominant strictures in primary sclerosing cholangitis. *American Journal of Roentgenology*, **145**, 1061–1064.
81. Minuk, G.Y., Angus, M., Brickman, C.M. *et al.* (1985) Abnormal clearance of immune complexes from the circulation of patients with primary sclerosing cholangitis. *Gastroenterology*, **88**, 166–170.
82. Minuk, G.Y., Rascanin, N., Paul, R.W., Lee, P.W.K., Buchan, K. and Kelly, J.K. (1987) Reovirus type 3 infection in patients with primary biliary cirrhosis and primary sclerosing cholangitis. *Journal of Hepatology*, **5**, 8–13.
83. Mistilis, S.P., Skyring, A.P. and Goulston, S.J.M. (1965) Effect of long-term tetracycline therapy, steroid therapy and colectomy in pericholangitis associated with ulcerative colitis. *Australian Annals of Medicine*, **14**, 286–294.
84. Morecki, R., Glaser, J.H., Cho, S., Balistreri, W.F. and Horwitz, M.S. (1982) Biliary atresia and reovirus type 3 infection. *New England Journal of Medicine*, **307**, 481–484.
85. Munoz, S.J., Heubi, J., Deems, R., Ross, R. and Maddrey, W.C. (1991) Vitamins D and E deficiency in primary sclerosing cholangitis: mechanism, frequency and relation to deficiency in other lipid soluble vitamins (abstract). *Gastroenterology*, **100**(part 2), A539.
86. O'Brien, C.B., Senior, J.R., Aroya-Mirchandani, R. *et al.* (1991) Ursodeoxycholic acid for the treatment of primary sclerosing cholangitis: a 30-month pilot study. *Hepatology*, **14**, 838–847.
87. Olsson, R., Danielsson, A., Jarnerot, G. *et al.* (1991) Prevalence of primary sclerosing cholangitis in patients with ulcerative colitis. *Gastroenterology*, **100**, 1319–1323.
88. Palmer, K.R., Duerden, B.I. and Holdsworth, C.D. (1980) Bacteriological and endotoxin studies in cases of ulcerative colitis submitted to surgery. *Gut*, **21**, 851–854.
89. Patel, S.A., Borges, M.C., Batt, M.D. and Rosenblate, H.J. (1990) *Trichosporon* cholangitis associated with hyperbilirubemia and findings suggesting primary sclerosing cholangitis on endoscopic retrograde cholangiopancreatography. *American Journal of Gastroenterology*, **85**, 84–87.
90. Pitt, H.A., Thompson, H.H., Tompkins, R.K. and Longmire, W.P. Jr (1982) Primary sclerosing cholangitis: results of an aggressive surgical approach. *Annals of Surgery*, **196**, 259–268.
91. Porayko, M.K., Wiesner, R.H., LaRusso, N.F. *et al.* (1990) Patients with asymptomatic primary sclerosing cholangitis frequently have progressive disease. *Gastroenterology*, **98**, 1594–1602.
92. Porayko, M.K., LaRusso, N.F. and Wiesner, R.H. (1991) Primary sclerosing cholangitis: a progressive disease? *Seminars in Liver Diseases*, **11**, 18–25.
93. Prochazka, E.J., Terasaki, P.I., Park, M.S., Goldstein, L.I. and Busuttil, R.W. (1990) Association of primary sclerosing cholangitis with HLA-DRw 52a. *New England Journal of Medicine*, **322**, 1842–1844.
94. Rabinovitz, M., Gavaler, J.S., Schade, R.R., Dindzans, V.J., Chien, M.-C. and Van Thiel, D.H. (1990) Does primary sclerosing cholangitis occurring in association with inflammatory bowel disease differ from that occurring in the absence of inflammatory bowel disease? A study of sixty-six subjects. *Hepatology*, **11**, 7–11.
95. Rosen, C.B. and Nagorney, D.M. (1991) Cholangiocarcinoma complicating primary sclerosing cholangitis. *Seminars in Liver Diseases*, **11**, 26–29.

96. Rosen, C.B., Nagorney, D.M., Wiesner, R.H., Coffey, R.J. Jr and LaRusso, N.F. (1991) Cholangiocarcinoma complicating primary sclerosing cholangitis. *Annals of Surgery*, **213**, 21–25.
97. Sartin, J.S., Wiesner, R.H. and LaRusso, N.F. (1987) Fat-soluble vitamin deficiencies in primary sclerosing cholangitis (abstract). *Gastroenterology*, **92**, 1615.
98. Scharschmidt, B.F. (1984) Human liver transplantation: analysis of data on 540 patients from four centers. *Hepatology*, **4**(suppl. 1), 95–101.
99. Schwartz, S.I. and Dale, W.A. (1958) Primary sclerosing cholangitis: review and report of six cases. *Archives of Surgery*, **77**, 439–451.
100. Siegel, J.H., Barnes, S. and Morris, J.S. (1977) Bile acids in liver disease associated with inflammatory bowel disease. *Digestion*, **15**, 469–481.
101. Sivak, M.V. Jr, Farmer, R.G. and Lalli, A.F. (1981) Sclerosing cholangitis: its increasing frequency of recognition and association with inflammatory bowel disease. *Journal of Clinical Gastroenterology*, **3**, 261–266.
102. Skolkin, M.D., Alspaugh, J.P., Casarella, W.J., Chuang, V.P. and Galambos, J.T. (1989) Sclerosing cholangitis: palliation with percutaneous cholangioplasty. *Radiology*, **170**(part 1), 199–206.
103. Smith, M.P. and Loe, R.H. (1965) Sclerosing cholangitis: review of recent case reports and associated diseases and four new cases. *American Journal of Surgery*, **110**, 239–246.
104. Snook, J.A., Chapman, R.W., Fleming, K. and Jewell, D.P. (1989) Anti-neutrophil nuclear antibody in ulcerative colitis, Crohn's disease and primary sclerosing cholangitis. *Clinical and Experimental Immunology*, **76**, 30–33.
105. Snook, J.A., Chapman, R.W., Sachdeve, G.K. *et al.* (1989) Peripheral blood and portal tract lymphocyte populations in primary sclerosing cholangitis. *Journal of Hepatology*, **9**, 36–41.
106. Soriano, G., Guarner, C., Teixido, M. *et al.* (1991) Selective intestinal decontamination prevents spontaneous bacterial peritonitis. *Gastroenterology*, **100**, 477–481.
107. Steckman, M., Drossman, D.A. and Lesesne, H.R. (1984) Hepatobiliary disease that precedes ulcerative colitis. *Journal of Clinical Gastroenterology*, **6**, 425–428.
108. Stieber, A.C., Marino, I.R., Iwatsuki, S. and Starzl, T.E. (1989) Cholangiocarcinoma complicating primary sclerosing cholangitis: the role of liver transplantation. *International Surgery*, **74**, 1–3.
109. Stiehl, A., Raedsch, R., Theilmann, L. and Galle, P. (1989) The effect of ursodeoxycholic acid (UDCA) in primary sclerosing cholangitis (PSC) (abstract). *Gastroenterology*, **96**(part 2), A664.
110. Stockbrugger, R.W., Olsson, R., Jaup, B. and Jensen, J. (1988) Forty-six patients with primary sclerosing cholangitis: radiological bile duct changes in relationship to clinical course and concomitant inflammatory bowel disease. *Hepatogastroenterology*, **35**, 289–294.
111. Sullivan, W.G. and Koep, L.J. (1980) Common bile duct obstruction and cholangiohepatitis in clonorchiasis. *Journal of the American Medical Association*, **243**, 2060–2061.
112. Thorpe, M.E.C., Scheuer, P.J. and Sherlock, S. (1967) Primary sclerosing cholangitis, the biliary tree, and ulcerative colitis. *Gut*, **8**, 435–448.
113. Tobias, R., Wright, J.P., Kottler, R.E. *et al.* (1983) Primary sclerosing cholangitis associated with inflammatory bowel disease in Cape Town 1975–1981. *South African Medical Journal*, **63**, 229–235.
114. Vinnik, I.E., Kern, F. Jr, Struthers, J.E. Jr, Hill, R.B. and Guzak, S. (1964) Experimental chronic portal vein bacteremia. *Proceedings of the Society for Experimental Biology and Medicine*, **115**, 311–314.
115. Wagner, A. (1971) Azathioprine treatment in primary sclerosing cholangitis. *The Lancet*, **ii**, 663–664.
116. Warren, K.W., Athanassiades, S. and Monge, J.I. (1966) Primary sclerosing cholangitis. A study of forty-two cases. *American Journal of Surgery*, **111**, 23–38.
117. Wee, A., Ludwig, J., Coffey, R.J. Jr, LaRusso, N.F. and Wiesner, R.H. (1985) Hepatobiliary carcinoma associated with primary sclerosing cholangitis and chronic ulcerative colitis. *Human Pathology*, **16**, 719–726.
118. White, T.T. and Hart, M.J. (1987) Primary sclerosing cholangitis. *American Journal of Surgery*, **153**, 439–443.
119. Whiteside, T.L., Lasky, S., Si, L. and Van Thiel, D.H. (1985) Immunologic analysis of mononuclear cells in liver tissues and blood of patients with primary sclerosing cholangitis. *Hepatology*, **5**, 468–474.
120. Wiesner, R.H., Grambsch, P., LaRusso, N.F. and Dickson, E.R. (1988) Is primary sclerosing cholangitis a progressive disease or not? *Hepatology*, **8**, 970–972.
121. Wiesner, R.H. and LaRusso, N.F. (1980) Clinicopathologic features of the syndrome of primary sclerosing cholangitis. *Gastroenterology*, **79**, 200–206.
122. Wiesner, R.H., LaRusso, N.F., Ludwig, J. and Dickson, E.R. (1985) Comparison of the clinicopathologic features of primary sclerosing cholangitis and primary biliary cirrhosis. *Gastroenterology*, **88**, 108–114.
123. Wiesner, R.H., Ludwig, J., LaRusso, N.F. and MacCarty, R.L. (1985) Diagnosis and treatment of primary sclerosing cholangitis. *Seminars in Liver Diseases*, **5**, 241–253.
124. Wiesner, R.H., LaRusso, N.F., Dozois, R.R. and

Beaver, S.J. (1986) Peristomal varices after proctocolectomy in patients with primary sclerosing cholangitis. *Gastroenterology*, **90**, 316–322.
125. Wiesner, R.H., Grambsch, P.M., Dickson, E.R. *et al.* (1989) Primary sclerosing cholangitis: Natural history, prognostic factors and survival analysis. *Hepatology*, **10**, 430–436.
126. Zauli, D., Schrumpf, E., Crespi, C., Cassani, F., Fausa, O. and Aadland, E. (1987) An autoantibody profile in primary sclerosing cholangitis. *Journal of Hepatology*, **5**, 14–18.

BILIARY MOTOR DISORDERS

J. Toouli

The clinical relevance of motility disorders of the biliary tract has been the subject of debate for many years.[43] Similar to motility disorders in other areas of the gastrointestinal tract, they occur intermittently and are difficult to diagnose clinically. In particular, the diagnosis of biliary tract motility disorders has posed problems because of the relative inaccessibility of the biliary tract to direct investigation.[37] However, developments in methodology for the study of motility in the past decade have allowed better study of the motility of the biliary tract and, as a result, improved understanding of normal physiology has arisen. In addition, the techniques have allowed identification of motility abnormalities in patients with biliary-like symptoms, and specific treatment has led to relief of these symptoms. Undoubtedly, biliary motility disorders are well recognized and account for the cause of biliary-like symptoms in a small percentage of patients presenting clinically with recurrent upper abdominal pain.

CLINICAL FEATURES

Dyskinetic disorders of the biliary tract arise from either the gallbladder or the sphincter of Oddi.[48] These disorders are most common in middle-aged females although they are well described in men, and patients of all ages.

Gallbladder motility disorders may mistakenly be labelled as acalculous cholecystitis. The disorders present as clinically similar to calculous disease of the gallbladder. Patients complain of recurrent epigastric to right upper quadrant abdominal pain. The pain may be initiated by a fatty meal and may be associated with a degree of nausea or vomiting. Occasionally the pain may awake the patient in the early hours of the morning. There usually are no associated colonic symptoms, no increase in eructation or flatus and no relief following defaecation. Patients are normally investigated initially for gallstone disease by ultrasound or oral cholecystography. These investigations are normal. However, in some patients it may be noted that on cholecystography the gallbladder does not empty fully after oral ingestion of a radiological fatty meal. This sign is not diagnostic of a gallbladder abnormality; however, it may suggest a gallbladder motility disorder.

Sphincter of Oddi dysfunction usually presents clinically 5–10 years following cholecystectomy for either calculous or non-calculous gallbladder disease,[22] although it is theoretically possible for sphincter of Oddi dysfunction to be present at the time of gallbladder disease, and indeed account for the symptoms experienced. However, at our current state of knowledge it is difficult to make a clinical diagnosis of sphincter of Oddi dysfunction in the presence of an intact biliary tract.

Patients with sphincter of Oddi dysfunction present with recurrent episodes of epigastric to right upper quadrant abdominal pain. The pain is described as similar to that experienced previously with episodes of gallbladder pain. It is usual that patients have had a long asymptomatic period following cholecystectomy performed for stone disease of the gallbladder. The pain may follow ingestion of a fatty meal and may awake the patient in the early hours of the morning. In some patients, there is a strong association with administration of opiate-containing medications such as cough mixtures, or the pain may be experienced after parenteral administration of opiate premedication prior to an anaesthetic.

Biochemical investigation of the serum may show abnormally elevated liver transaminase levels in association with an episode of pain. Biliary ultrasound and endoscopic retrograde cholangiopancreatography are often normal. However, in a group of these patients the bile duct may be moderately dilated[25,26] and there is delayed emptying (*Figure 12.60*) of contrast medium from the duct into the duodenum.[18]

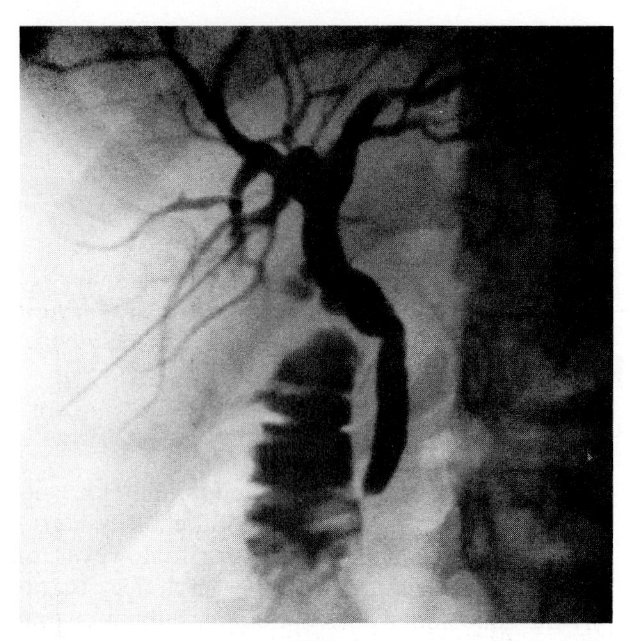

Figure 12.60 Cholangiogram illustrating a moderately dilated bile duct with a fixed stenosis of the sphincter of Oddi. The stenosis required operative division and histology revealed fibrosis.

INVESTIGATION OF BILIARY TRACT MOTILITY

A number of investigations have evolved for the study of biliary tract motility. Their relative strengths and weaknesses are discussed below. Generally, it is aimed to exclude structural abnormalities at initial investigation and then proceed with the most specific investigation which will provide the diagnosis. However, on occasion the full range of investigations may be required on these patients before either a diagnosis is made or no cause found for the symptoms.

CONTRAST RADIOLOGY

The presence or absence of stones or structural anomalies of the biliary tract are evaluated by cholecystography and choledochography. In addition, contrast studies may give valuable clues to the possibility of biliary tract motility disorders. However, most techniques which involve contrast radiography do not provide the necessary accuracy for evaluating subtle changes in motility, and are only diagnostic where there are gross changes.

The gallbladder may be imaged by radiographs after the ingestion of oral Biloptin.[19] Ingestion of a standard 'fatty meal' determines whether the gallbladder empties its contents. The test provides a subjective assessment of gallbladder emptying. Reduced emptying suggests a hypokinetic gallbladder. Unfortunately, this test is not accurate for motility abnormalities and further evaluation should be undertaken using radionuclide techniques.

Endoscopic retrograde cholangiography[38] provides an accurate image of the biliary tract and often detects any structural abnormalities. The presence of a dilated bile duct suggests that a motility abnormality of the sphincter of Oddi may exist which produces a relative resistance to outflow resulting in bile duct dilatation.

ULTRASONOGRAPHY

The gallbladder volume, bile duct and pancreatic duct diameter can be measured by non-invasive methods using ultrasonography. Following the ingestion of food or hormone infusion, changes in these measurements are determined, thus providing a means of evaluating the motility of the gallbladder biliary and pancreatic ducts.

The volume of the human gallbladder is determined by measuring the maximal length and corresponding maximal transverse diameter of the gallbladder. The volume is then calculated from the ultrasound images as the sum of a series of cylinders.[16] Serial measurement of volume changes determines the effect of various stimuli such as food or hormone infusion on gallbladder volume.

Using ultrasonography, the maximal diameter of the bile duct is measured at a fixed point adjacent to where the right hepatic artery crosses the common hepatic duct. Following the ingestion of a fatty meal, it is expected that normal changes in sphincter of Oddi motility will enhance bile flow into the duodenum, hence the diameter of the common hepatic duct should decrease. An increase in ductal diameter reflects a resistance to outflow which may reflect dysfunction of the sphincter of Oddi.[14]

Using a similar ultrasonographic method, the diameter of the pancreatic duct in normal individuals measures less than 1 mm. Following infusion of secretin 1 unit/kg, there is an increase in ductal diameter followed by a rapid return to normal size within 30 minutes. If the ductal diameter remains in excess of 1.5 mm at 30 minutes, this suggests an increase in resistance to the outflow of pancreatic juice consistent with dysfunction of the sphincter of Oddi.[6]

These ultrasonographic techniques for evaluating biliary motility have been developed as non-invasive methods for evaluating sphincter of Oddi motility.

Their specificity, sensitivity and usefulness as diagnostic tools are presently under scrutiny. Whereas it is apparent that for relatively gross abnormalities these techniques provide a positive diagnosis of abnormality, the more subtle abnormalities detected by manometry are not as readily detected via ultrasonography.

ISOTOPE STUDIES

A variety of ^{99m}Tc IDA (iminodiacetic acid) compounds are cleared through the liver into bile after intravenous administration. ^{99m}Tc produces 140 KeV γ photons that are ideally suited for imaging and counting by a γ camera. These properties of the ^{99m}Tc IDA compounds have been used to image the gallbladder[36] and the biliary tract. Temporal profiles of gallbladder emptying and flow across the bile duct in postcholecystectomy subjects can be determined by sequential monitoring of the isotope images.

The degree of gallbladder emptying can be evaluated by calculating the gallbladder ejection fraction. Following the concentration of ^{99m}Tc DIDA (diamino-diacetic acid) in the gallbladder, cholecystokinin octapeptide is infused intravenously over 45 minutes. Gallbladder emptying of the ^{99m}Tc DIDA is monitored during the infusion period and for 15 minutes after cessation of infusion.[24] The gallbladder ejection fraction is determined by use of the following formula

$$\frac{\text{counts at specified time}}{\text{maximal counts prior to infusion}} \times 100$$

The mean gallbladder ejection fraction at 15 minutes after infusion is normally 70%. Values less than 40% represent abnormalities in the gallbladder ejection fraction which reflect disorders in gallbladder motility.[53]

A similar evaluation of flow through the bile duct has been done in patients after cholecystectomy in order to determine the characteristics of flow across the sphincter of Oddi.[33] Following the injection of ^{99m}Tc DIDA, the subject is positioned under a γ camera and continuous recordings are made from the liver, biliary tract and duodenum. In order to analyse flow, areas of interest are outlined and the counts per second within those areas is determined and graphically displayed. The shape and slope of the curve of counts from the bile duct reflect flow through the biliary tree (*Figure 12.61*). Delay in outflow may represent a raised resistance to flow across the sphincter of Oddi which is due to sphincter of Oddi dysfunction (*Figure 12.62*). Similar to the ultrasonographic methods for evaluating sphincter of Oddi function, this technique appears useful in detecting major stenosis of the sphincter; but its sensitivity for the more subtle manometric changes is low.

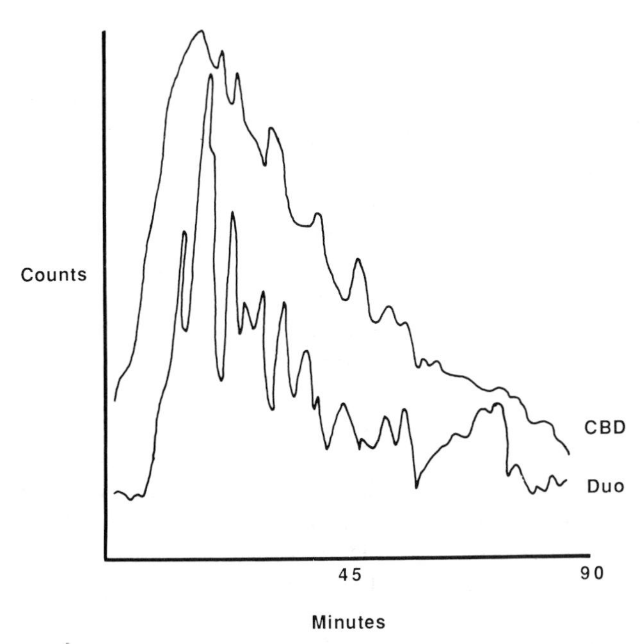

Figure 12.61 Biliary scintigram illustrating the counts in the bile duct and duodenum over 90 minutes. There is a rapid increase in counts initially, followed by a quick fall as bile flows through the bile duct. Rapid entry of bile into the duodenum is illustrated by the duodenal counts.

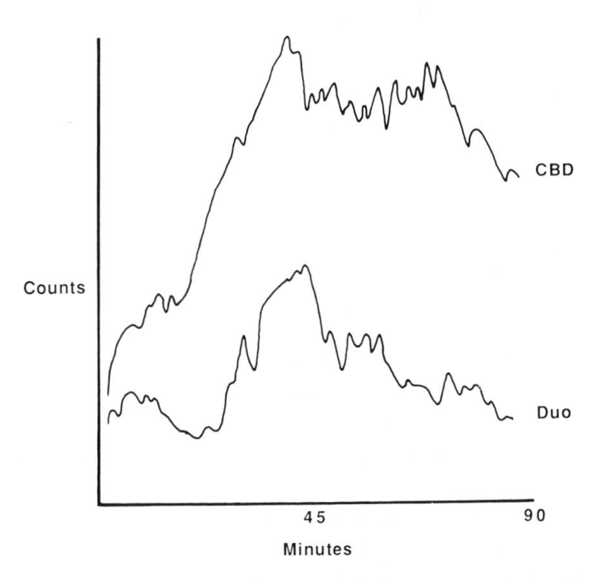

Figure 12.62 Biliary scintigram of the bile duct and duodenum in a patient with sphincter of Oddi stenosis. The bile duct curve shows a delayed outflow which is reflected by the delay in counts appearing in the duodenum.

MANOMETRY

Pressure measurement has been used for the evaluation of resistance to flow across the sphincter of Oddi at operation.[22] In some series the pressure changes have been read from fluid-filled manometers inserted into the bile duct and recorded by a transducer linked to a polygraph.[20] Using these techniques the opening, passage and closing pressures of the sphincter have been determined.[11] An increase in the opening pressure of the sphincter of Oddi is thought to represent stenosis of the opening of the sphincter of Oddi either due to an intraluminal stone or idiopathic stenosis.

Direct pressure measurements from the sphincter of Oddi became possible by miniaturization of manometry catheters and the development of fluid perfusion systems of low compliance.[1] Triple-lumen catheters made of polyethylene or Teflon are used to record sphincter of Oddi pressures. Each lumen of the catheter has an internal diameter of 0.5 mm and the whole catheter has an outer diameter of 1.7 mm. Three side holes are fashioned at 2 mm intervals starting at 10 mm from its distal tip. Therefore, the three lumens record across a length of 5 mm from within the sphincter of Oddi. The catheter is 200 cm long and is perfused with deionized bubble-free water via a pneumohydraulic capillary system at a pressure of 750 mmHg. The volume of water perfused through the catheter is 0.125 ml/min and the whole system is capable of recording accurately pressure changes up to 300 mmHg/s. Recording from three lumens allows an evaluation of the sequencing of sphincter contractions as well as determination of basal pressure, amplitude and frequency of contractions.[45]

Recordings of human sphincter of Oddi motility using the above system may be done via three different approaches. The catheter may be introduced through an endoscope (*Figure 12.63*), as in endoscopic retrograde cholangiopancreatography.[17] The patient is mildly sedated and the oropharynx anaesthetized to assist the passage of the endoscope. The manometry catheter is introduced via the biopsy channel of the duodenoscope through the papilla and into either the bile duct or pancreatic duct. The catheter is then withdrawn so that all three recording ports are situated within the sphincter of Oddi segment. In order to assist in the positioning of the catheter across the sphincter, circular markings are placed on the catheter at 2 mm intervals from the most proximal hole for a total length of 12 mm. Recordings are made for approximately 3–10 minutes. It is difficult to record for much longer via the endoscopic technique because the patient becomes intolerant of prolonged intubation via the endoscope.

During elective operation for gallstones, recordings from the sphincter of Oddi may be made by introducing the triple-lumen catheter through the cystic duct, into the bile duct and through the sphincter into the duodenum.[34] The catheter is then withdrawn so that the three lumens are recording from the sphincter. The duration of recording may be greater than that obtained at endoscopy but a major disadvantage is the fact that the patient is anaesthetized, and the effect of anaesthetic agents on biliary motility is unknown. However, in studies where manometry of the sphincter was obtained in both anaesthetized and awake patients, sphincter motility did not differ significantly when non-opiate anaesthetics were used.[49]

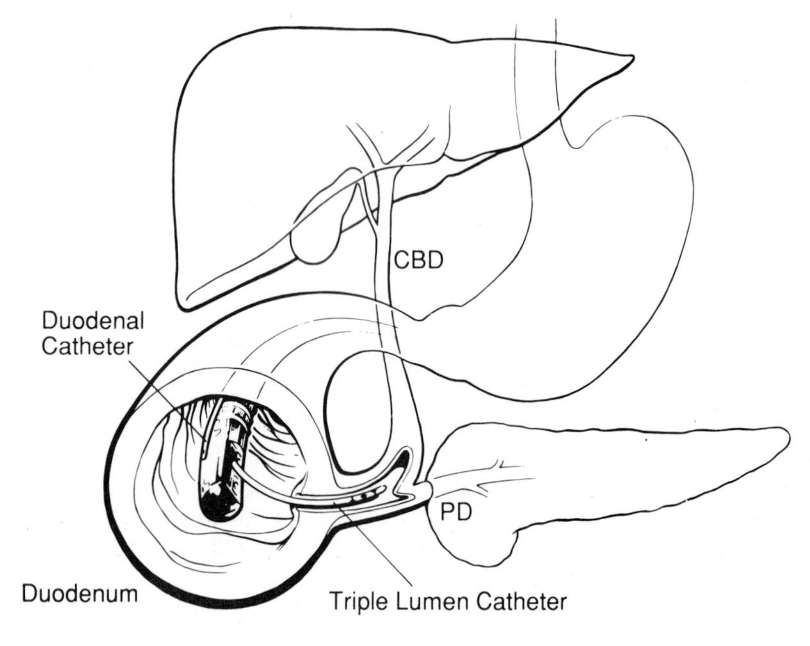

Figure 12.63 Endoscopic sphincter of Oddi manometry. The triple-lumen manometric catheter is introduced into either the bile duct (CBD) or pancreatic duct (PD) and withdrawn so that all three lumens record from the sphincter. A separate catheter records duodenal pressure.

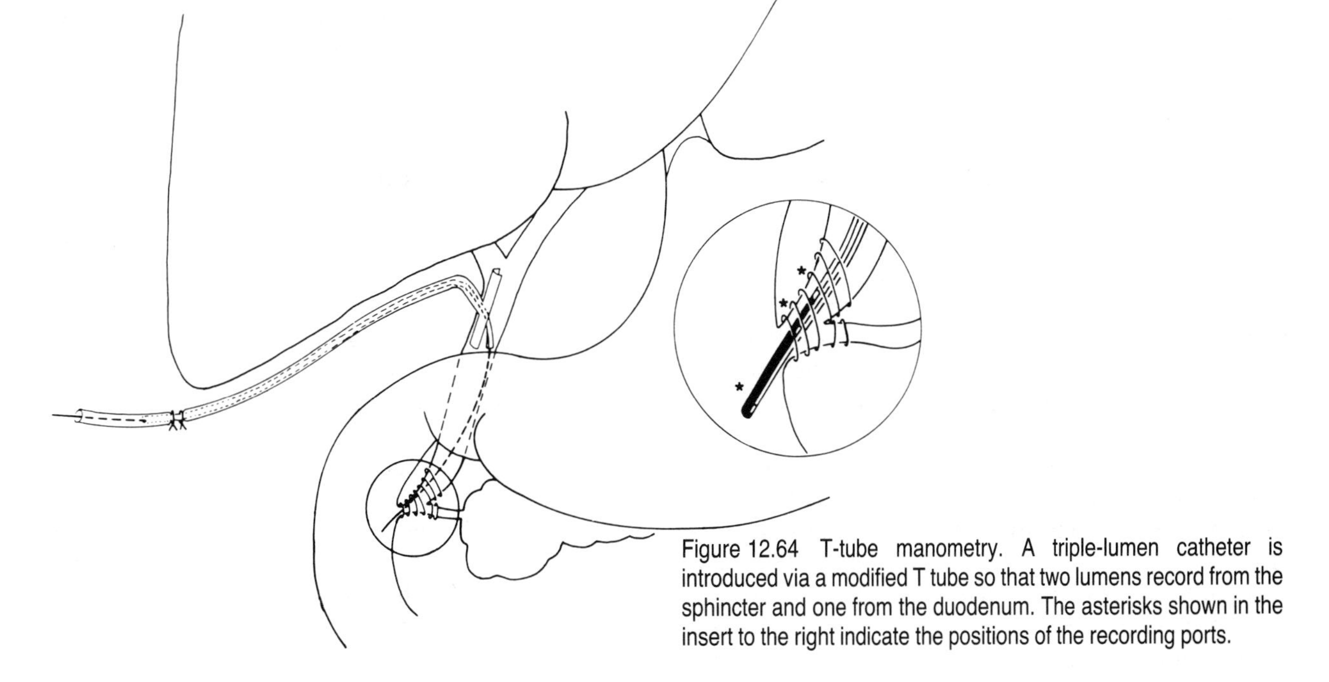

Figure 12.64 T-tube manometry. A triple-lumen catheter is introduced via a modified T tube so that two lumens record from the sphincter and one from the duodenum. The asterisks shown in the insert to the right indicate the positions of the recording ports.

In order to conduct prolonged studies of sphincter of Oddi motility, the catheter may be introduced through the T tube in patients who have undergone exploration of the bile duct for stones.[52] The manometry catheter is passed into the bile duct, through the sphincter and into the duodenum. It is then withdrawn so that two of the recording ports are situated within the sphincter and the third in the duodenum (*Figure 12.64*). The position of the catheter within the sphincter of Oddi may be confirmed fluoroscopically. Recordings of up to 8 hours may be made with this technique. The disadvantage is that, by necessity, only those patients who have had stones in the bile duct can be studied. The technique of nasobiliary intubation of the biliary tract may, in future, provide an avenue for introducing catheters for the long-term study of biliary motility in patients who have not undergone operations.

PROVOCATION STUDIES

Patients with suspected biliary motility disorder present clinically with pain which is consistent with a biliary origin. Occasionally there may be associated abnormalities in liver enzymes detected in blood taken at the time of the pain episode.

In patients presenting with suspected gallbladder dyskinesia, tests have evolved which attempt to demonstrate reproduction of the pain following the administration of standard-dose cholecystokinin octapeptide.[31] The specificity and sensitivity of these tests in selecting patients for treatment have not been reproduced by studies conducted in different institutions, thus limiting their effectiveness. One difficulty is that the investigation is dependent on a subjective assessment by the patient regarding the reproduction of the pain.[15]

The *morphine–neostigmine test* is a provocation test which aims to evaluate sphincter of Oddi motor function.[32] In a subgroup of patients who present with biliary-type pain following cholecystectomy, it is well described that administration of opiates reproduces the pain. The morphine–neostigmine test is aimed at identifying such patients following the administration of a standard dose of morphine and neostigmine. The patient records the presence of any pain and blood is taken at hourly intervals for determination of serum liver enzymes and amylase. A positive test comprises reproduction of pain associated with an abnormal rise in liver enzymes and or amylase. Although this provocation test proves useful in the selection of patients with possible sphincter of Oddi dysfunction, it does not appear to be specific for selection of patients who will respond to treatment by division of the sphincter of Oddi.[18]

NORMAL MOTILITY OF THE BILIARY TRACT

GALLBLADDER

Ultrasound studies have shown that the resting gallbladder volume is approximately 17 ml but the volume does not remain static during the interdigestive period. Studies in humans and experimental animals have demonstrated that the gallbladder contracts by up to 40% of its maximum contractile capacity during the interdigestive period. These gallbladder contractions occurred at the end of phase II of the duodenal interdigestive cycle just prior to phase III.[39,50]

The factors which control gallbladder volume changes during the interdigestive cycle are unknown. Neuronal mechanisms may be involved,[23] and, in addition, the enteric hormone motilin may have an important role. Serum motilin levels peak just prior to duodenal phase III activity, and animal studies have shown that motilin at physiological concentrations produces gallbladder contraction.[40]

Following a meal the gallbladder empties by a steady contraction which delivers bile into the duodenum. This steady contraction generates a low intraluminal pressure which is only just above that registered in the bile ducts. This type of contraction is very similar to that generated by the fundus of the stomach during gastric emptying.

Gallbladder emptying following a meal is related to the release of endogenous cholecystokinin from the mucosa of proximal small intestine. The cholecystokinin is released by fat and protein entering the duodenum whilst carbohydrates have little or no effect.[51]

SPHINCTER OF ODDI

Manometric recording and radiographic screening of the sphincter of Oddi shows that the sphincter exhibits prominent phasic contractions (*Figure 12.65*) which are superimposed on a low basal pressure (tone). Most of the phasic contractions are oriented in an antegrade direction; however, a significant percentage are either simultaneous or oriented retrogradely (*Table 12.24*).[7,44]

Table 12.24 Sphincter of Oddi manometry

	Normal[a]	*Abnormal*
Basal pressure (mmHg)	15 (5–35)	>40
Amplitude (mmHg)	135 (95–195)	>300
Frequency (contractions/min)	4 (2–6)	>7
Sequences		
Antegrade (%)	80 (12–100)	
Simultaneous (%)	13 (0–50)	
Retrograde (%)	9 (0–50)	≥50
Cholecystokinin octapeptide 20 ng/kg	Inhibits	Contracts

[a]Median (range).

During the interdigestive cycle the frequency of the sphincter of Oddi contractions relates to the duodenal interdigestive phases. However, unlike the duodenum the sphincter of Oddi does not demonstrate a quiescent period of no activity.[47] The frequency of sphincter of Oddi contractions increases towards the end of duodenal phase II activity and throughout phase III of duodenal contractions.[52]

Flow of bile across the sphincter mostly occurs across a passive pressure gradient from the bile duct to the duodenum. Most of the flow occurs between the phasic contractions; however, the contractions also expel small boluses into the duodenum.

After a meal the amplitude of the phasic contractions decreases and the sphincter of Oddi basal

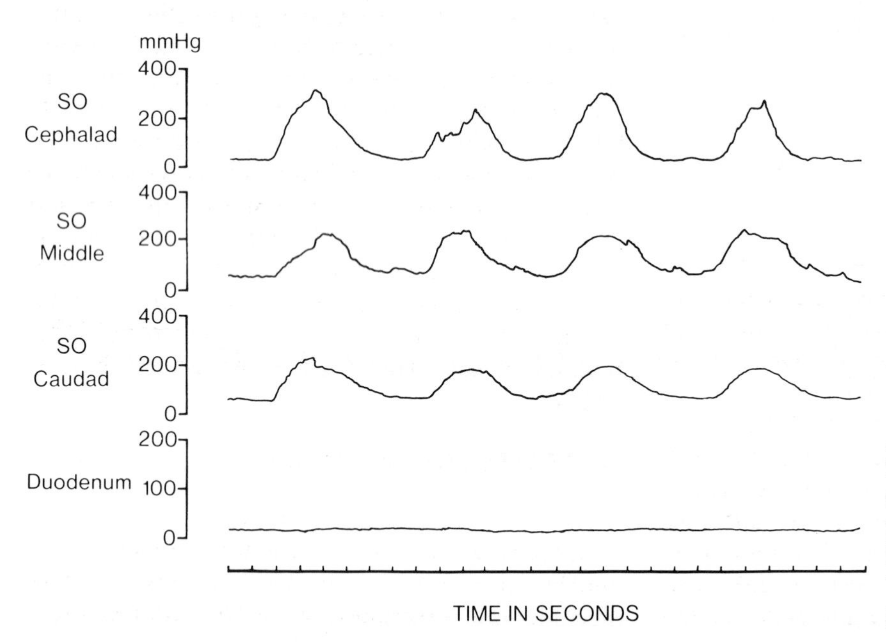

Figure 12.65 Manometric recording from the sphincter of Oddi (SO) and duodenum. The sphincter demonstrates phasic contractions which are superimposed on a modest basal pressure. This activity is independent of duodenal pressure changes.

pressure falls.[52] This effect enhances the passive flow of bile across the sphincter by decreasing the resistance to flow.

Control of these motility events of the sphincter of Oddi is via an interplay of neuronal[5,41,42] and hormonal mechanisms.[4,46] Numerous nerves and ganglia have been demonstrated in the wall of the bile duct and sphincter of Oddi.[8,9,29,30] A neural reflex has been described between the gallbladder and sphincter of Oddi[42] and such a reflex is thought to be important in coordinating the contractile events between the gallbladder and sphincter of Oddi.

A variety of gastrointestinal hormones have been shown to influence sphincter of Oddi motility. Cholecystokinin produces inhibition of the phasic contractions and a decrease in basal pressure.[46] The mechanism of its action appears to be via a stimulation of non-adrenergic non-cholinergic inhibitory neurons.[3,4] Secretin, glucagon, histamine, gastrin, vasoactive intestinal polypeptide and substance P all alter sphincter of Oddi contractions in doses that may apply in the physiological state.[10,12,13]

MOTILITY DISORDERS OF THE BILIARY TRACT

Disordered motility has been described separately to involve the gallbladder,[31] cystic duct[35] or sphincter of Oddi.[29] Evidence suggests that the gallbladder and sphincter of Oddi develop abnormalities in motility which are associated with clinical symptoms. However, isolated cystic duct motility disorders have not been convincingly described and suggest that gallbladder and cystic duct disorders may coexist.

GALLBLADDER MOTILITY DISORDERS

Acalculous gallbladder disease due to disorder of gallbladder motility presents clinically with recurrent upper abdominal pain. Both decreased contraction (hypokinesia) and excessive contraction (hyperkinesia) have been postulated to give rise to pain syndromes. Most of the current evidence supports the presence of hypokinetic disorders as demonstrated by delayed gallbladder emptying. Objective support for hyperkinetic disorders is lacking.

The cholecystokinin provocation test has been used to diagnose the hyperkinetic disorders of the gallbladder.[31] A series of prospective and retrospective studies aimed at evaluating its efficacy in selecting patients for treatment by cholecystectomy has shown variable results.[15]

The gallbladder hypokinetic disorders are supported by objective tests such as the radionuclide gallbladder ejection fraction[24,53] and ultrasound determination of gallbladder volume changes. Recently the author showed that patients undergoing cholecystectomy with an abnormal gallbladder ejection fraction showed histological evidence in the gallbladder consistent with chronic cholecystitis. The gallbladder wall was thickened and the cystic duct was narrow, suggesting an obstruction to outflow from the gallbladder.[53] In a separate study, Marzio *et al.*[27] identified evidence of decreased gallbladder emptying in response to a meal by use of ultrasound techniques in patients with symptoms consistent with acalculous gallbladder disease. However, in this study there was no histological confirmation of gallbladder disease as the patients were treated with prokinetic drugs.

SPHINCTER OF ODDI DYSFUNCTION

Motility dysfunction of the sphincter of Oddi results in recurrent biliary-type pain which presents for management several years following cholecystectomy for either calculous or non-calculous gallbladder disease.[2] The pain may be associated with an abnormal elevation of serum liver enzymes or an abnormally elevated serum amylase. Investigations normally exclude common causes of recurrent biliary pain after cholecystectomy such as stones, stricture or pancreatitis and the investigations focus on the motor activity of the sphincter of Oddi as a possible causative factor.

In order to make the diagnosis of sphincter of Oddi dysfunction, the following investigations are undertaken to evaluate sphincter of Oddi activity. Investigations include; morphine–neostigmine test, fatty meal sonography of the bile duct, radionuclide bile flow studies, secretin-stimulated estimation of pancreatic duct diameter[1] and endoscopic sphincter of Oddi manometry. The role of each investigation in identifying patients with sphincter of Oddi dysfunction has not been fully elucidated. However, endoscopic sphincter of Oddi manometry provides the most objective evaluation of sphincter of Oddi motility; hence, it is used to categorize sphincter of Oddi motility disorders as described below.

Stenosis of the sphincter of Oddi

Manometrically, patients with an abnormally elevated sphincter of Oddi basal pressure above 40 mmHg have sphincter of Oddi stenosis (*Figure 12.66*). The stenosis may be due to fibrotic changes

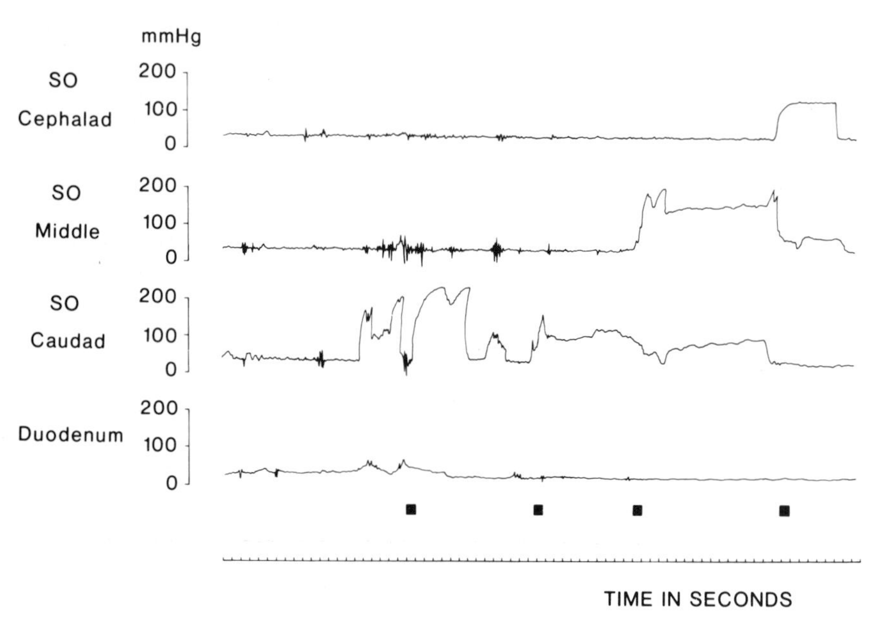

Figure 12.66 Manometric recording from the sphincter of Oddi (SO) and duodenum illustrating an abnormally elevated basal pressure. The triple-lumen catheter is withdrawn across the sphincter in stages illustrated by the black squares. Hence, the elevated basal pressure is first shown in the most caudad lumen, then the middle lumen and, finally, the most cephalad lumen. This recording illustrates sphincter of Oddi stenosis.

in the sphincter or smooth muscle hyperplasia. Pathological correlation with the manometric findings has not been described but isolated case studies support this association.

Sphincter of Oddi dyskinesia

This group of patients has a variety of findings on manometry which, at this stage, have been grouped under the heading of dyskinesia. With further understanding of sphincter of Oddi motility disorders, the groupings may become inappropriate.

Rapid phasic contraction frequency

Spontaneously occurring bursts of rapid contraction may be recorded and possibly reflect an irritable sphincter. The rapid contractions may produce transient obstruction to flow. A frequency in excess of seven contractions per minute is considered abnormal.

Intermittent episodes of elevated basal pressure

This group of patients is similar to the group described above and the abnormality may be an associated finding. This manometric pattern may also reflect an irritable sphincter which goes into spasm intermittently.

Excessive retrograde contractions

In normal subjects the majority of sphincter of Oddi contractions are oriented in an antegrade direction. However, in some patients a majority of retrograde contractions are found. A percentage of retrograde contractions in excess of 50% is considered abnormal. This finding is also seen in patients with gallbladder and common bile duct stones and it may reflect a relative retardation in flow through the sphincter.

Paradoxical response to cholecystokinin

The administration of a bolus dose of cholecystokinin octapeptide normally results in inhibition of phasic contractions of the sphincter of Oddi (*Figure 12.67*). This action is thought to be mediated through an effect on non-adrenergic non-cholinergic nerves to the sphincter of Oddi. A paradoxical response consists of sphincter contraction in place of inhibition (*Figure 12.68*) and it may be due to a direct effect of the hormone on the sphincter.[50] The finding may reflect damage to the intrinsic neurons of the sphincter of Oddi and it may be a condition that is pathogenetically similar to achalasia of the oesophagus.

TREATMENT

The most common clinical presentation of patients with biliary motility disorders, whether from the gallbladder or sphincter of Oddi, is that of recurrent upper abdominal pain. The pain has the clinical characteristics of either biliary- or pancreatic-type pain and occurs intermittently. Treatment by a variety of pharmacotherapeutic substances often fails to relieve the symptoms. However, recent studies indicate that either operative or endoscopic surgical techniques provide effective therapy for objectively identified biliary tract motor disorders.

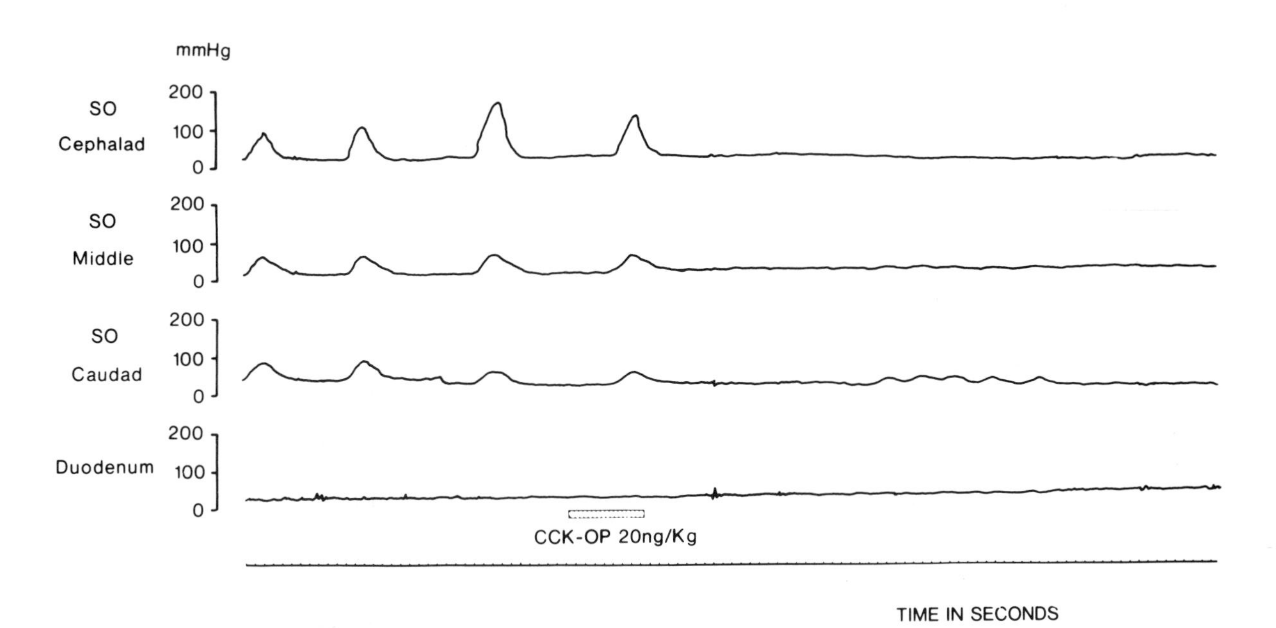

Figure 12.67 Action of cholecystokinin octapeptide (CCK-OP) on sphincter of Oddi (SO) motility. The phasic contractions are inhibited and there is a fall in basal pressure.

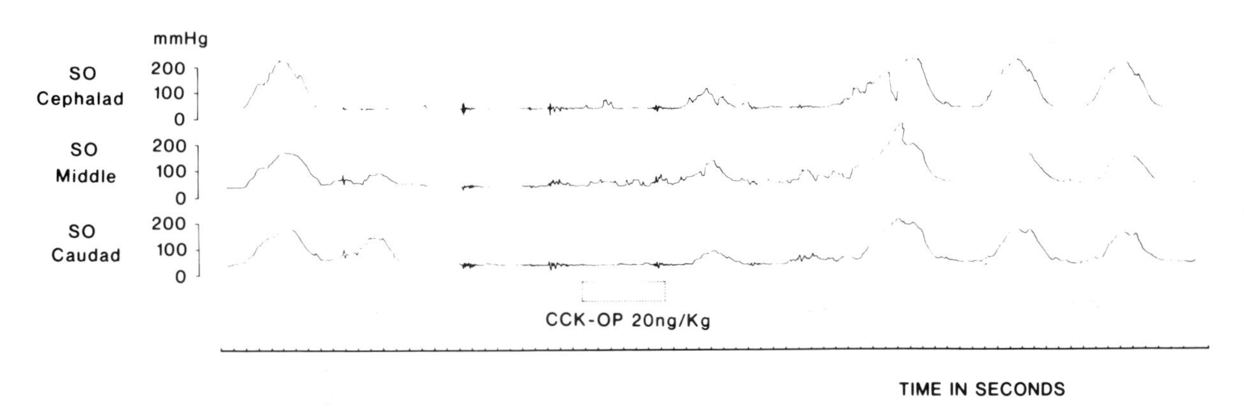

Figure 12.68 Paradoxical response of the sphincter of Oddi (SO) to cholecystokinin octapeptide (CCK-OP). An increase of the sphincter contraction frequency occurs, instead of the normal inhibition.

GALLBLADDER DYSKINESIA

Cholecystectomy has been used for the treatment of gallbladder motor dysfunction and results vary depending on the investigation used to identify the disorder. Clinical history, although often convincing, cannot be relied upon to discriminate gallbladder causes of upper abdominal pain from other origins for the pain.

One recent study has re-evaluated the role of cholecystokinin provocation tests for reproduction of the pain and selecting patients for cholecystectomy. The study has shown excellent long-term results in resolution of symptoms.[31] However, there are a number of concerns about the method used for selecting patients for this treatment. First, the selection relies on a subjective reproduction of pain. Other studies have shown that cholecystokinin induces colonic spasm as well as gallbladder contractions.[21] Hence the pain may not always originate from the biliary tract. Secondly, other studies which have evaluated this technique do not confirm the same degree of accuracy for selection[15] and, thirdly, histological examination of the gallbladders removed in this study showed little or no pathological changes when they were examined histologically.

In a separate study the gallbladder ejection fraction was used to select patients for cholecystectomy. Patients with recurrent biliary-like pain and an abnormal gallbladder ejection fraction (<40%) were randomized into either cholecystectomy or no operation. Those patients who underwent cholecystectomy were cured of their symptoms, and histology of the gallbladder revealed increased gallbladder wall thickness and evidence of chronic cholecystitis.[53] These pathological findings support the conclusions of this study that the gallbladder ejection fraction is a useful objective investigation which selects patients with gallbladder dysfunction who will benefit from cholecystectomy. Interestingly, unlike the previous study, administration of cholecystokinin via infusion did not reproduce the pain in patients with an abnormal gallbladder ejection fraction.

Recently, Marzio *et al.*[27] have reported their experience with the use of the prokinetic substance cisapride in treating patients with gallbladder hypokinesia. A group of patients presenting with dyspeptic symptoms was shown by ultrasound techniques to have abnormalities in gallbladder emptying following a meal. Long-term treatment with cisapride reversed this abnormality and produced relief of symptoms.

The results of the above two studies suggest that gallbladder hypokinetic disorders may be identified in patients presenting with clinical symptoms consistent with acalculous gallbladder disease. Treatment via cholecystectomy or prokinetic agents will provide relief of symptoms. It is too early to conclude a preference for either form of therapy as long-term follow-up is necessary in order to determine the long-term effectiveness of the two treatments.

SPHINCTER OF ODDI DYSFUNCTION

One of the uncommon causes of postcholecystectomy recurrent abdominal pain is sphincter of Oddi dysfunction. Patients present with either recurrent biliary-like pain or symptoms and signs of idiopathic recurrent pancreatitis. Endoscopic sphincter of Oddi manometry provides the most accurate guide to therapy for both of these conditions.

In a prospective study,[18] patients with biliary-like pain plus one or more of the following signs – dilated bile duct, delay in emptying of contrast from the bile duct or elevated liver enzymes during an episode of pain – were treated by endoscopic sphincterotomy or a sham procedure. Manometry was performed but not used to determine therapy. After a 4-year follow-up period it was found that patients with sphincter of Oddi stenosis diagnosed by manometry were significantly improved after division of the sphincter, when compared to patients who had the sham procedure. However, patients with dyskinesia on manometry did not have the same result and only showed a trend towards improvement when compared to the sham group. The results from this study suggest that patients with significant sphincter of Oddi dysfunction as diagnosed by manometry obtain relief of symptoms by division of the sphincter of Oddi.

Manometry of the sphincter of Oddi in patients with idiopathic recurrent pancreatitis demonstrates that a group of these patients have abnormally elevated sphincter of Oddi basal pressure. This finding may be present only when the manometry catheter is directed into the pancreatic duct and not the bile duct. Division of the biliary sphincter of Oddi by endoscopic sphincterotomy does not alter the basal pressure in the pancreatic duct and does not produce relief of symptoms. However, preliminary studies have shown that division of the pancreatic duct sphincter by operative sphincteroplasty and pancreatic duct septectomy[28] results in a significant relief of symptoms.

REFERENCES

1. Arndorfer, R.C., Steff, J.J., Dodds, W.J., Linethan, J.H. and Hogan, W.J. (1977) Improved infusion system for intraluminal oesophageal manometry. *Gastroenterology*, **73**, 23–27.
2. Bar-Meir, S. (1984) Frequency of papillary dysfunction among cholecystectomized patients. *Hepatology*, **4**, 328–330.
3. Bauer, A.J., Go, V.L.W., Koch, R.T. and Szurszewski, J. (1987) Non-adrenergic, non-cholinergic (NANC) inhibitory innervation of the canine and opossum sphincter of Oddi. *Gastroenterology*, **92**(Part 2), 1311.
4. Behar, J. and Biancani, P. (1980) Effect of cholecystokinin and the octapeptide of cholecystokinin on the feline sphincter of Oddi and gallbladder. Mechanisms of action. *Journal of Clinical Investigation*, **66**, 1231–1239.
5. Benevantano, T.C. and Rosen, R.G. (1969) The physiological effect of acute vagal section on canine biliary dynamics. *Journal of Surgical Research*, **9**, 331–334.
6. Bolondi, L., Gaiani, S., Gullo, L. and Labo, G. (1984) Secretin administration induces a dilatation of the main pancreatic duct. *Digestive Diseases and Sciences*, **29**, 802–808.
7. Bortolotti, M., Caletti, G.C., Brocchi, E., Bersani, G., Guizzardi, G. and Labo, G. (1985) Endoscopic electromyography and manometry of the human sphincter of Oddi. *Hepatology and Gastroenterology*, **32**, 250–252.
8. Cai, W.Q. and Gabella, G. (1983) Innervation of the gall bladder and biliary pathways in the guinea-pig. *Journal of Anatomy*, **136**, 97–109.
9. Cai, W.Q., Gu, J., Huang, W. *et al.* (1983) Peptide immunoreactive nerves and cells of the guinea-pig gallbladder and biliary pathways. *Gut*, **24**, 1186–1193.
10. Carr-Locke, D.L., Gregg, J.A. and Auki, T. (1983) Effects of exogenous glucagon on pancreatic and biliary ductal and sphincteric pressures in man

demonstrated by endoscopic manometry and correlation with plasma glucagon. *Digestive Disease and Sciences*, **28**, 312–320.
11. Cuschieri, A., Hughes, J.H. and Cohen, M. (1972) Biliary pressure studies during cholecystectomy. *British Journal of Surgery*, **59**, 267–273.
12. Dahlstrand, C., Bjorck, S., Edin, R., Dahlstom, A. and Ahlman, H. (1988) Substance P in the control of extrahepatic biliary motility in the cat. *Regulatory Peptides*, **20**, 11–24.
13. Dahlstrand, C., Dahlstom, A. and Ahlman, H. (1989) Adrenergic and VIPergic relaxatory mechanisms of the feline extrahepatic biliary tree. *Journal of Autonomous Nervous System*, **26**, 97–106.
14. Darweesh, R.M.A., Dodds, W.J., Hogan, W.J. *et al.* (1988) Efficacy of quantitative hepatobiliary scintigraphy and fatty meal sonography for evaluating patients with suspected partial common bile duct obstruction. *Gastroenterology*, **94**, 779–786.
15. Dunn, F.H., Christensen, E.C., Reynold, J. *et al.* (1974) Cholecystokinin cholecystectomy. *Journal of the American Medical Association*, **22**, 89–97.
16. Everson, G.T., Braverman, D.Z., Johnson, M.L. and Kern, F. Jr (1980) A critical evaluation of real-time ultrasonography for the study of gallbladder volume and contraction. *Gastroenterology*, **79**, 40–46.
17. Geenen, J.E., Hogan, W.J., Dodds, W.J., Steward, E.T. and Arndorfer, R.C. (1980) Intraluminal pressure recording from the human sphincter of Oddi. *Gastroenterology*, **78**, 317–324.
18. Geenen, J.E., Hogan, W.J., Doods, W.J., Toouli, J. and Venu, R.P. (1989) The efficacy of endoscopic sphincterotomy in post-cholecystectomy patients with sphincter of Oddi dysfunction. *New England Journal of Medicine*, **320**, 82–87.
19. Graham, E.A., Cole, W.H. and Copter, G.H. (1924) Visualisation of the gallbladder by the salt of tetrobromophthalein. *Journal of the American Medical Association*, **82**, 1777–1778.
20. Hallenbeck, G.A. (1967) Biliary and pancreatic intraductal pressures. In *The Handbook of Physiology. The Alimentary Canal*, Section 6. *Secretion*, Vol. 2 (Ed.) Code, C.F. pp. 1007–1025. Washington DC: American Physiological Society.
21. Harvey, R.F. and Read, A.E. (1973) Effects of cholecystectomy on colonic motility and symptoms in patients with the irritable bowel syndrome. *The Lancet*, **i**, 1–3.
22. Hess, W. (1979) Physiology of the sphincter of Oddi. In *The Papilla Vateri and its Diseases. Proceedings of the International Workshop of the World Congress of Gastroenterology held in Madrid 1978* (Ed.) Classen, M., Geenen, J. and Kawai, K. pp. 14–21. Kohn: Gerhard Witzshock.
23. Keast, J.R., Furness, J.B. and Costa, M. (1985) Distribution of certain peptides containing nerve fibres and endocrine cells in the gastrointestinal mucosa in five mammalian species. *Journal of Comparative Neurology*, **236**, 413–422.
24. Krishnamurthy, G.T., Bobba, V.R. and Kingston, E. (1981) Radionuclide ejection fraction: a technique for the quantitative analysis of motor function of the human gallbladder. *Gastroenterology*, **80**, 482–490.
25. LeQuesne, L.P., Whiteside, C.G. and Hand, B.T. (1959) The common bile duct after cholecystectomy. *British Medical Journal*, **i**, 329–332.
26. Mahour, G.H., Wakin, K.G., Ferris, D.O. and Soule, E.H. (1967) The common bile duct after cholecystectomy. *Annals of Surgery*, **166**, 964–967.
27. Marzio, L., Difelice, F., Laico, M.G., Celiberti, W., Grossi, L. and DelBianco, R. (1990) Gallbladder hypokinesia and normal gastric emptying of liquids in patients with dyspeptic symptoms: a double blind placebo controlled trial with cisapride. *Gastroenterology*, A255.
28. Moody, F.G., Becker, J.M. and Potts, J.R. (1983) Transduodenal sphincteroplasty and transampullary septectomy for post-cholecystectomy pain. *Annals of Surgery*, **197**, 627–636.
29. Padbury, R.T.A. (1990) The innervation of the biliary tract with catecholamine and peptide-containing nerves. Ph.D. Thesis. Flinders University of South Australia.
30. Padbury, R.T.A., Furness, J.B. and Toouli, J. (1989) Intrinsic catecholamine containing neurons in the sphincter of Oddi and duodenum of the Australian possum. *Gastroenterology*, **96**(part 2), 381.
31. Rhodes, M., Lennard, T.W.J., Farndon, J.R. and Taylor, R.M.R. (1988) Cholecystokinin (CCK) provocation test: longterm follow-up after cholecystectomy. *British Journal of Surgery*, **75**, 951–953.
32. Roberts-Thomson, I.C. and Toouli, J. (1985) Abnormal responses to morphine neostigmine in patients with undefined biliary type pain. *Gut*, **26**, 1367–1372.
33. Roberts-Thomson, I.C., Toouli, J., Blanchett, W., Lichtenstein, M. and Andrews, J.T. (1986) Assessment of bile flow by radioscintigraphy in patients with biliary type pain after cholecystectomy. *Australian and New Zealand Journal of Medicine*, **16**, 788–793.
34. Saccone, G.T.P., Toouli, J., Iannos, J. *et al.* (1988) The effect of catheter diameter on sphincter of Oddi motility. *Surgical Research Communications*, **2**, 315–321.
35. Scott, G.W. and Otto, W.J. (1979) Resistance and sphincter-like properties of the cystic duct. *Surgery, Gynaecology and Obstetrics*, **149**, 177–182.
36. Shaffer, E.A., McOrmond, P. and Duggan, H. (1980) Quantitative cholescintigraphy: assessment of gallbladder filling and emptying and duodenogastric reflux. *Gastroenterology*, **79**, 899–906.
37. Smadja, C. and Blumgart, L.H. (1988) The biliary tract and anatomy of biliary exposure. In *Surgery of the Liver and Biliary Tract* (Ed.) Blumgart, L.H., pp. 11–22. Edinburgh: Churchill Livingstone.

38. Stewart, E.T., Vennes, J.A. and Geenen, J.E. (1977) *Altas of Endoscopic Retrograde Cholangio Pancreatography*. Saint Louis: C.V. Mosby.
39. Takahashi, I., Nakaya, M., Suzuki, T. and Itoh, Z. (1982) Postprandial changes in contractile activity and bile concentration in gallbladder of the dog. *American Journal of Physiology*, **6**, G365–G371.
40. Takahashi, I., Suzuki, T., Aizawa, I. and Itoh, Z. (1982) Comparison of gallbladder contractions induced by motilin and cholecystokinin in dogs. *Gastroenterology*, **82**, 419–424.
41. Tansy, M.F., Innes, D.L., Martin, J.S. and Kendall, F.M. (1974) An evaluation of neural influences on the SO in the dog. *Digestive Diseases and Sciences*, **19**, 423–437.
42. Thune, B.A., Thornell, E. and Svanvik, J. (1986) Reflex regulation of flow resistance in the feline sphincter of Oddi by hydrostatic pressure in the biliary tree. *Gastroenterology*, **91**, 1364–1369.
43. Tondelli, P., Gyr, K., Stalder, G.A. and Allgower, M.N. (1979) The biliary tract and cholecystectomy. *Clinics in Gastroenterology*, **8**, 487–505.
44. Toouli, J. (1984) Sphincter of Oddi motility. *British Journal of Surgery*, **71**, 251–256.
45. Toouli, J., Geenen, J.E., Hogan, W.J., Dodds, W.J. and Arndorfer, R.C. (1982) Sphincter of Oddi motor activity: a comparison between patients with common bile duct stones and controls. *Gastroenterology*, **82**, 111–117.
46. Toouli, J., Hogan, W.J., Geenen, J.E., Dodds, W.J. and Arndorfer, R.C. (1982) Action of cholecystokinin octapeptide on sphincter of Oddi basal pressure and phasic wave activity in humans. *Surgery*, **92**, 497–503.
47. Toouli, J., Dodds, W.J., Honda, R. *et al.* (1983) Motor function of the opossum sphincter of Oddi. *Journal of Clinical Investigation*, **71**, 208–220.
48. Toouli, J., Roberts-Thomson, I.C., Dent, J. and Lee. J. (1985) Manometric disorders in patients with suspected sphincter of Oddi dysfunction. *Gastroenterology*, **88**, 1243–1250.
49. Toouli, J., Bushell, M., Iannos, J., Collinson, T., Wearne, J. and Kitchen, D. (1986) Peroperative sphincter of Oddi manometry: motility disorders in patients with cholelithiasis. *Australian and New Zealand Journal of Surgery*, **56**, 625–629.
50. Toouli, J., Bushell, M., Stevenson, G., Dent, J., Wycherley, A. and Iannos, J. (1986) Gallbladder emptying in man related to fasting duodenal migrating motor contractions. *Australian and New Zealand Journal of Surgery*, **56**, 147–151.
51. Weiner, I., Kazutomo, I., Fagan, C.J., Lilja, P., Watson, L.C. and Thompson, J.C. (1981) Release of cholecystokinin in man, correlation of blood levels with gallbladder contraction. *Annals of Surgery*, **194**, 321–327.
52. Worthley, C.S., Baker, R.A., Iannos, J., Saccone, G.T.P. and Toouli, J. (1989) Human fasting and post-prandial sphincter of Oddi motility. *British Journal of Surgery*, **76**, 709–714.
53. Yap, L., McGee, M.A., McKenzie, J., Wycherley, A. and Toouli, J. (1989) Acalculous biliary pain: diagnostic use of cholecystokinin cholescintography in the selection of patients for cholecystectomy. *Gastroenterology*, **96**, A558.

TUMOURS

I.S. Benjamin

Tumours of the biliary tree are not common but are important because they pose particular problems both in diagnosis and therapy. Most clinicians will encounter but few of such patients in their working lifetime, and a strong argument can be made for their referral to specialist centres for treatment. This is especially so because in the last decade there have been major advances in diagnostic and therapeutic approaches to these conditions, many of which may rely on techniques beyond the scope of the average non-specialist physician or surgeon.

EPIDEMIOLOGY

INCIDENCE

Cancer of the gallbladder constitutes 3–4% of all gastrointestinal malignancies.[79] Cancer of the extrahepatic biliary tree is uncommon. In 1983 there were an estimated 400 deaths from hilar cholangiocarcinoma diagnosed in England and Wales, and the estimated annual incidence in the USA is 3000 cases;[22] this is similar to that for cancer of the tongue. Renard *et al.*[100] reported the age-standardized incidence for gallbladder cancer in the Cote d'Or (France) as 2.7 per 100 000 of the population in women and 0.9 per 100 000 in men: corresponding rates for extrahepatic bile duct cancers were 0.5 and 1.7. Tumours of the ampulla of Vater have a similar incidence (0.3 per 100 000 for men or for women in the French review). These tumours pose a particular problem, because they have been frequently misdiagnosed and misclassified in the past as tumours of the head of the pancreas (see below). There appears to be a general increase in the incidence of these tumours, especially in younger patients.[102] In Japan the corrected age-adjusted mortality rate for intrahepatic biliary tumours rose 2.0-fold in men and 1.67-fold in women over one decade, with a more modest increase (1.2–1.4) in cancers of the gallbladder, extrahepatic bile ducts and pancreas.[61] Some regional differences have been observed in Japan and in Chile, suggestive of environmental factors.[61,102]

PATHOLOGY

Tumours of the whole biliary tract have a similar pathology but regional differences are important. This section will therefore consider tumours of the gallbladder, extrahepatic bile ducts and periampullary region separately.

All the tumours are adenocarcinomas arising from the epithelium of the biliary tract. They are to a greater or lesser extent mucus-secreting tumours.

TUMOURS OF THE GALLBLADDER

These are mucus-secreting adenocarcinomas which arise in the gallbladder mucosa of patients in late middle-age onwards, almost invariably in association with gallstones. There appears to be an unusually high incidence of an anomalous junction between the distal common bile duct and the pancreatic duct in patients with gallbladder cancer: this may be an aetiological factor, similar to that reported for malignancy in choledochal cysts.[89] A few gallbladder tumours are of the squamous variety, presumably arising in areas of squamous metaplasia in the gallbladder mucosa. The staging and grading system adopted for these tumours is that of Nevin.[84] Stage 1 tumours are confined to the mucosa of the gallbladder; stage 2 tumours are those which have breached the muscularis mucosa; stage 3 tumours have extended through the muscularis propria into surrounding tissues, frequently to invade the bed of the gallbladder. Stages 2 and 3 are almost invariably associated with lymphatic spread, which involves the hilar and periductal lymph nodes. These pathological stages are important because they have a major influence on prognosis and significantly affect decisions on surgical therapy.

TUMOURS OF THE BILE DUCTS

Cholangiocarcinoma of the extrahepatic biliary tree is morphologically similar to intrahepatic cholangiocellular carcinoma. This mucus-secreting adenocarcinoma may arise anywhere within the biliary tree. The gross morphology of the tumours has been noted to vary with different anatomical sites in the biliary tree.[115] Those in the periampullary region are generally papillary in configuration, and form a spectrum with the more common tumours of the papilla of Vater itself. Those in the mid-ductal region frequently have a nodular morphology. Tumours at the confluence of the major hepatic ducts generally have a stenosing configuration, although nodular or papillary forms at the hilus are also found.[45] For some reason this appears to be the site of predilection for these tumours: although originally described by Altemeier *et al.* in 1957,[5] major attention was first drawn to this group of tumours in a report of 13 patients by Klatskin in 1965,[63] and cholangiocarcinoma of the hilar ducts continues to bear his name.

These tumours may have an extraordinarily high degree of histological differentiation, and it may be difficult for the pathologist to distinguish between cancer and a normal or inflamed bile duct even on paraffin section; it is almost impossible on frozen section. This poses a problem for the surgeon in making decisions about surgical clearance at operation, especially as there is often severe epithelial dysplasia in adjacent mucosa. Many of these tumours express carcinoembryonic antigen on histochemical staining and this may help to delineate the extent of tumour infiltration or to identify foci of malignancy in small biopsy specimens.[28]

The tumours tend to produce a dense sclerotic reaction in the involved ducts at whatever level they occur.[6] Multicentricity is frequently described as a feature, but it is not always clear whether there is true multifocal primary disease, or intrahepatic ductal spread from retrograde seeding of tumour following biliary tract obstruction. There is certainly a tendency for tumour to spread along ducts by longitudinal subepithelial growth and it is not always possible to ascertain by gross inspection the true limits of tumour invasion. Direct spread of tumour takes place into the adjacent liver tissue and there is a strong propensity to invade adjacent vessels (portal vein and hepatic artery). There is also a strong tendency to perineural invasion.[115] Lymphatic spread is to the periductal nodes and thence to the coeliac nodes.

There is unfortunately no uniform system of staging for cholangiocarcinoma. Bismuth and Corlette[11] have published a gross descriptive staging for the primary tumours of the hepatic hilus: type I tumours are entirely below the confluence, type II tumours involve the main hepatic duct, and type III indicates invasion of second-order intrahepatic ducts. This is a practical surgical *classification* which is cited by many surgical authors. It should not, however, be mistaken for an attempt to describe *staging* of the tumours, as it is unlikely that the majority of cases follow this sequence of progression. The Japanese Surgical Society has proposed a detailed staging system which describes the lymphatic groups involved as well as the extent of ductal disease and adjacent vascular invasion. This is a complex system and has not been adopted outside Japan. The question of the influence of staging on therapy is discussed below.

TUMOURS OF THE AMPULLARY REGION

It has already been noted that many of these tumours have in the past been wrongly classified along with cancer of the head of the pancreas. This error has led to important misconceptions about the survival prospects of patients with pancreatic cancer treated without resection. Many of the 5-year survivors reported following bypass for 'pancreatic cancer' by some authors had either chronic pancreatitis (with no histological confirmation of the tumour) or tumours of the distal bile duct or papilla.[27] Tumours of the ampullary region generally have a much better prognosis than those of pancreatic origin even without surgical excision, and better prospects of cure following resection.[46]

Tumours of this region are adenocarcinomas arising in either the distal common bile duct, the papilla of Vater itself, or the adjacent duodenal mucosa. All of these tend to have a macroscopically and microscopically papillary character, and it can be very difficult to determine the true site of origin of an established tumour.[115]

Attention will be devoted for the remainder of this section to the tumours of the gallbladder and bile ducts, and only passing mention will be given to this group of distal tumours.

PATHOGENESIS

There is no known single cause for these tumours, but a number of important aetiological factors have emerged. The most important is the association between gallbladder cancer and gallstones which is very high: up to 70% of patients with gallbladder cancer have gallstones, in contrast to some 13% for other biliary cancers.[100] It is likely that the risk of cancer is related to the length of exposure of the gallbladder mucosa to the presence of stones.

A strong relationship exists between choledochal cysts and biliary tract cancer: the risk of malignancy has been shown to rise from 0.7 to 14% between cases presenting in infancy and in the third decade of life.[114] This condition is related to an anomalous junction between the pancreatic and biliary ductal systems (APBD junction). Moreover, two types of APBD junction have been defined. The type I anomaly (pancreatic duct joining the bile duct) is associated with gallbladder cancer, while the type II APBD junction (bile duct joining the pancreatic duct) is the one commonly associated with cysts of the biliary tree, and their associated malignancies. The biliary amylase level is extremely high in both types of anomaly. Ohta *et al.*[89] showed epithelial mucosal atypia with papillary or papillotubular proliferation and epithelial hyperplasia in patients with both anomalies. Kato *et al.*[62] examined the mutagenicity of the bile in type I patients, and showed positive results in 6 of 12 patients. Moreover, they also showed a high incidence of polyploid DNA in the gallbladder epithelium of 2 of 4 patients, both of whom had mutagenic bile. Suda *et al.*[104] found an APBD junction in 14.2% of patients with biliary tract carcinoma, and in 4 of 4 patients with congenital biliary dilatation. They described an experimental model of this junction constructed in puppies in which dilatation of the bile duct developed, and mucosal hyperplasia of the biliary tract was seen. Increased cell turnover was also observed on long-term follow-up.

There is a strong association of biliary tract cancers with inflammatory bowel disease and with sclerosing cholangitis. It is very difficult to establish the precise nature of this association, because it may be impossible to distinguish some cases of sclerosing cholangitis from intrahepatic or extrahepatic biliary tumours, and this remains one of the most difficult areas of differential diagnosis. The association is nevertheless a real one, and should be carefully considered in patients with ulcerative colitis who present with obstruction jaundice.[101]

Chemical carcinogens have been suggested as aetiological factors. Aflatoxin exposure in farm workers in Denmark,[90] and methylene chloride[67] and vinyl chloride monomer[18] exposure in factory workers in the USA, are amongst the substances implicated: none of these factors has been proven.

The incidence of gallbladder cancer is increased 14.7-fold 20 years after surgery for gastric ulcer, but there was no increase in the incidence of tumours in the rest of the biliary tract.[23] A single case of cholangiocarcinoma arising in biliary hamartomas (von Meyenberg complexes) has been reported.[19]

CLINICAL FEATURES

Hilar cholangiocarcinoma was first described clinically by Altemeier and colleagues in 1957.[5] Despite this, for almost two decades the diagnosis was rarely made during life, and often missed even at laparotomy for obstructive jaundice. Better understanding and recognition of the condition and improvements in diagnostic techniques have changed this situation, and it should be uncommon now to fail to recognize these tumours preoperatively. Cancers of the gallbladder are frequently diagnosed preoperatively when they present with biliary obstruction, but are still commonly reported as an incidental finding at operation for gallbladder stones.

Obstructive jaundice is the almost universal presentation for tumours of the biliary tract. However, the disease may be extensive before jaundice develops if the tumour is eccentric in origin. Tumours which arise in the left or right hepatic ducts or in segmental ducts within the liver will cause progressive obstruction of these ducts, possibly associated with lobar or segmental liver atrophy but, unless infection supervenes in the obstructed segments, this stage of the disease may be clinically silent. By the time the tumour spreads distally to involve the confluence of the hepatic ducts, there is already quite extensive liver involvement, which may significantly affect the treatment options.[9,50] This may explain why there is frequently extrahepatic tumour involvement by the time of presentation: lymph node or visceral metastases were present at diagnosis in 77% of patients with gallbladder cancers and in 83% of those with extrahepatic biliary tumours in the series reported by Renard *et al.*[100]

Fever may occur as part of the presentation of biliary tract cancers due to cholangitis in obstructed biliary segments. However, this is unusual unless there has been radiological or other intervention, because the bile is usually sterile in these patients. Some patients with gallbladder cancer present with *acute cholecystitis* or *empyema of the gallbladder*, and the diagnosis may be missed at operation. A biopsy of the gallbladder is mandatory in patients treated by cholecystostomy.[107]

Although painless obstructive jaundice is the classical presentation, many patients have had episodes of ill-defined *pain* consistent with a biliary tract origin for some time before diagnosis. This occurred in 40% of patients with biliary cancer seen at Hammersmith Hospital.[8]

The *systemic effects* of malignancy may be evident at presentation. Weight loss is common. Trousseau's syndrome of venous thromboses, a frequently reported presentation of cancers of the head of pancreas, has been reported in a patient with bile duct cancer that arose in a choledochal cyst.[97]

INVESTIGATIONS

LABORATORY TESTS

Biochemical tests of liver function are useful only in defining the degree of obstructive jaundice. An elevated alkaline phosphatase level may be the earliest sign of incomplete or segmental biliary obstruction, and should not be ignored as an isolated abnormality in a symptomatic but anicteric patient.[9]

Tumour markers are of limited value: CA19-9 and CA50 are frequently elevated in the serum of patients with jaundice, but are not specific.[91] Carcinoembryonic antigen is expressed in the cells of bile duct cancer in some patients,[28] and may be elevated in the serum.

Haematological tests should include measurement of coagulation status. Many patients are chronically anaemic on presentation and some with ampullary tumours may present with anaemia, with or without melaena, due to chronic intestinal blood loss. An elevated white cell count is a significant adverse prognostic factor.[33,95]

The nutritional status of the patient may have a major impact on prognosis and surgical risk. A low haemoglobin level may be regarded as a nutritional index in this context, but the most significant features are a low serum albumin level and the history of recent weight loss. A number of authors have attempted to construct a reliable nutritional index which is predictive of operative risk. Albumin, haemoglobin, thyroxine-binding prealbumin and anergy to recall antigen skin testing have all proved valuable. The most sensitive predictor of complications and mortality may be a reduced total body potassium level,[53] but the technology to estimate this is not widely available.

RADIOLOGY

Plain abdominal radiography

Although of limited value, this may show calcification suggestive of gallstones in patients with gallbladder cancer. The appearance of gallbladder wall calcification ('porcelain gallbladder') should raise a strong suspicion of cancer, as this is a definitely premalignant lesion.

Ultrasound

This is the most valuable screening test in patients with suspected obstructive jaundice, and it can identify the level of obstruction in practically all patients in which ultrasound examination is technically satisfactory.[41] The presence of gallbladder stones should be readily identified, and the thickness of the gallbladder wall or an obvious mass lesion may raise the suspicion of cancer of the gallbladder. Ultrasound can identify a mass lesion in the majority of patients with cancer of the bile ducts, and may be more sensitive than computed tomography (CT).[120] Hilar nodes may also frequently be identified. Masses within the liver may indicate secondaries, but multiple small deposits in the presence of biliary tract obstruction are less easy to define, and may also represent micro-abscesses when there is clinical evidence of cholangitis.

Ultrasound is valuable in assessing vascular invasion in biliary tumours. In the author's experience the specificity for portal venous invasion by tumour is at least as great as that for angiography. Duplex Doppler scanning has added further precision to this tool.

It must be emphasized that, although ultrasound has improved greatly, it is still a mistake to operate on the evidence of ultrasound *alone* in patients with obstructive jaundice.

Computed tomography

Much of the information which can be obtained from CT scanning is similar to that for ultrasound. CT is of specific value in defining lobar or segmental hepatic atrophy. The degree of extrahepatic spread may also be defined by CT, both in lymph nodes and other intraperitoneal sites, and lymphadenopathy was demonstrated in almost three-quarters of patients with gallbladder or bile duct cancer at presentation,[35] though this has not been the author's experience.

Cholangiography

In patients referred to specialist centres, some form of cholangiography will often already have been performed. However, these investigations may frequently be inadequate, either because of poor facilities or because the tests have not been directed specifically at the diagnosis of bile duct or gallbladder cancer. It is therefore frequently necessary to repeat the examinations. The objective is to delineate the full extent of tumour involvement, including definition of *all* hepatic segmental ducts. Great advances have been made in this respect, and the best reports now demonstrate the precision with which delineation can be achieved.[87]

The choice of cholangiography lies between percutaneous transhepatic cholangiography and endoscopic retrograde cholangiopancreatography. There is much debate about this selection, which is frequently dictated by local availability and expertise. However, the majority of authors agree that for a suspected distally placed tumour (ampulla, distal bile duct or head of the pancreas) endoscopic retrograde cholangiography is the procedure of first choice, because this allows visualization and biopsy of the papilla of Vater or adjacent duodenum, and cytological brushings or aspiration of pancreatic juice/bile for diagnosis.[30,40,98] Conversely, for suspected upper biliary tract lesions, percutaneous transhepatic cholangiography is preferable, because in these patients it is the proximal extent of the disease which is important in staging and planning of treatment, and endoscopic retrograde cholangiography may not allow filling of all hepatic segments and definition of the upper limits of tumour involvement. There are patients in whom both procedures may be required for a complete diagnosis.

The possibility of interventional procedures, and in particular stenting of tumours, should be considered before any diagnostic manoeuvre is undertaken. The final judgement may depend on the findings at cholangiography, and the best results will be obtained if there is close consultation between radiologist or endoscopist and the clinician managing the case at the time of the procedure. Combined approaches can then be coordinated.[42]

Percutaneous transhepatic cholangiography

The use of percutaneous transhepatic cholangiography makes complete outlining of all the biliary segments more certain. However, it is important not to produce infection of any of the biliary segments at the time of this procedure, and the smallest amount of contrast medium possible should be used to avoid cholangitis and bacteraemia. A troublesome intrahepatic abscess may result if a segment becomes infected and cannot adequately be drained, and this may compromise future treatment.

Percutaneous cholangioscopy

Percutaneous cholangioscopy has been reported by some Japanese workers to be of particular diagnostic value. Irregularly dilated and tortuous vessels within biliary strictures or polyps are of significance in differentiating benign from malignant strictures, and a 96% positive diagnostic rate has been reported on cholangioscopic biopsy.[86] This approach requires a delay following percutaneous transhepatic biliary drainage while the tract is dilated to 15 FG to allow passage of the endoscope.

CYTOLOGY

The importance of making a positive diagnosis for malignancy in suspected cancers of the biliary tract cannot be emphasized too strongly. There are many lesions which 'masquerade' as biliary malignancy including localized strictures in primary sclerosing cholangitis, and benign iatrogenic biliary strictures.[48] Other rare artefacts may be seen, such as a suture granuloma following previous surgery,[80] and amputation neuroma of the cystic duct.[112] A radiotherapy stricture may also give rise to confusion, and there is a group of patients who appear to have benign idiopathic inflammatory strictures.

The author has reported on 117 patients with suspected malignant biliary stricture, in whom cytological material was obtained either by percutaneous puncture or by retrograde or prograde biliary cannulation and examination of exfoliated cells in the bile or brushings from the ducts.[30] The overall sensitivity of the procedure was 72%, and there was only one false positive result (cytology suspicious but not diagnostic of cancer) out of 206 specimens. The sensitivity of the technique is directly related to the precision with which targeting of the lesion can be obtained. This is best done at the time of percutaneous transhepatic cholangiography, aiming for the stricture or, if a stent has been placed, directed towards the stent as it passes through the tumour. The highest sensitivity (80%) was observed for material aspirated under direct vision intraoperatively.[30]

ANGIOGRAPHY

This is performed at a late stage in the investigation of bile duct cancers. It may be of some diagnostic value because benign lesions rarely cause encasement of the arteries or portal vein, but its main use is in staging the tumour and making decisions regarding surgery. Angiographic criteria have been defined for irresectability.[113,117] A tumour of the middle part of the common hepatic duct or common bile duct may cause compression and subsequently encasement of the main stem of the portal vein. The right or left portal vein may be similarly involved by tumours which lie at or above the confluence of the right and left hepatic ducts. Occlusion of the right or left portal vein will give rise to atrophy of the ipsilateral liver, commonly associated with dilatation of the hepatic ducts on that side. The result is a fibrotic and atrophic liver lobe which may be of such long-standing before the patient's symptoms present that there may be irrecoverable loss of function of that mass of liver tissue.[49] This may be seen particularly well on CT scans. Involvement of the main stem of the portal vein will cause portal hypertension, but segmental obstruction with the atrophy–hyperplasia complex is also commonly associated with portal hypertension.[50] Involvement of the hepatic artery may not preclude resectability in the presence of a patent portal vein, but this is generally a sign of advanced disease, and most such cases prove to be irresectable.

TREATMENT

The general philosophy in dealing with tumours of the biliary tract is first to establish the diagnosis accurately using all the available modalities, including cytology, and, secondly, concurrently with the first, to determine the suitability of the case for surgical resection. Complete removal of the tumour gives the only prospect of long-term cure but, because there are now many non-operative treatments available, it is important to try to establish resectability or irresectability before undertaking possibly unnecessary or futile surgery. Therapy must be aimed at obtaining drainage to the gastrointestinal tract of the maximum amount of functioning liver tissue when complete removal of the tumour is not possible. This may be achieved by endoscopic, percutaneous radiological or surgical means. In order to determine the best approach, a combination of scanning and cholangiography is important, and a complete map of the biliary tree should be obtained. Decisions regarding palliative intubation should be made concomitantly with diagnostic cholangiography when appropriate. Finally, angiography is only required for patients in whom other tests do not preclude surgical resection.

INTUBATION AND STENTING

Types of stent

Biliary drainage can be achieved by means of intubation from above (percutaneous) or from below (endoscopic). While occasionally intubation with external or external/internal drainage may be the definitive treatment, generally speaking the endpoint of these methods is the insertion of some form of stent within the biliary tree, passing through the tumour to act as a permanent conduit for bile. A variety of designs of such stents has been developed, mostly made of a range of plastic materials. They have in common some form of device to prevent dislodgement, either in the form of barbs protruding from the plastic material, mushroom-shaped expansions at one or both ends, 'pigtail' curls at the ends, or a spiral configuration to the whole stent.[118] All of these materials suffer the same problems, in that a surface of foreign material is presented to bile and there is inevitably a degree of biliary stasis. This combination results in formation of a biofilm of bacteria inside the stent which is followed by precipitation and deposition of bile salts and pigments within the lumen. This gradually accumulates to occlude the lumen and, in combination with the bacterial contamination of the obstructed biliary tree, gives rise to further attacks of cholangitis and jaundice. Many attempts have been made to overcome these problems, including the use of various agents bonded to the stent material, but the most significant factor is the calibre of the stent, because the rate of occlusion is inversely proportional to the rate of flow, which is related to the internal diameter of the stent. Unfortunately, placement of large stents is limited both endoscopically (by the calibre of the endoscope channel) and percutaneously (by the need to dilate the percutaneous transhepatic tract and push the prosthesis across the liver).

All of these factors have led to the development of expandable metallic stents.[2] These stents can be inserted endoscopically or percutaneously over a guide wire or through a fine-bore catheter, after which they are dilated or allowed to expand within the tumour, following careful placement during screening (*Figure 12.69*). Once in place these stents are not readily dislodged and are usually irremovable. However, they can be expanded to a much larger calibre than is possible with plastic material (up to 10 mm), and also present a negligible surface for deposition of sludge; they may therefore retain their patency for a much longer period, but this remains to be proven by controlled trial. These stents are very much more expensive than the more common plastic ones. The additional advantage of expanding metal stents over wide-bore plastic stents for percutaneous insertion is that they can be placed in a single stage without the need for prolonged

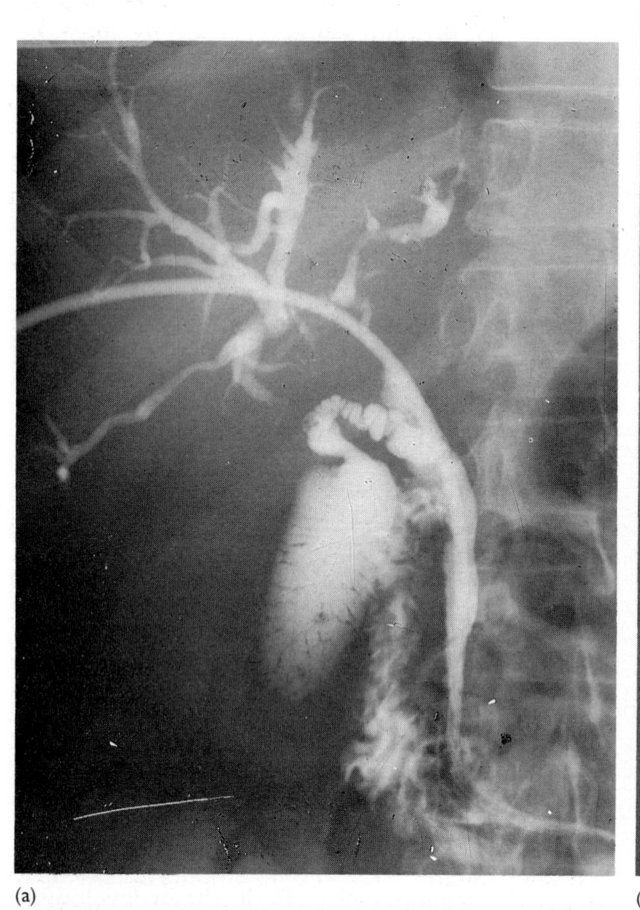

(a)

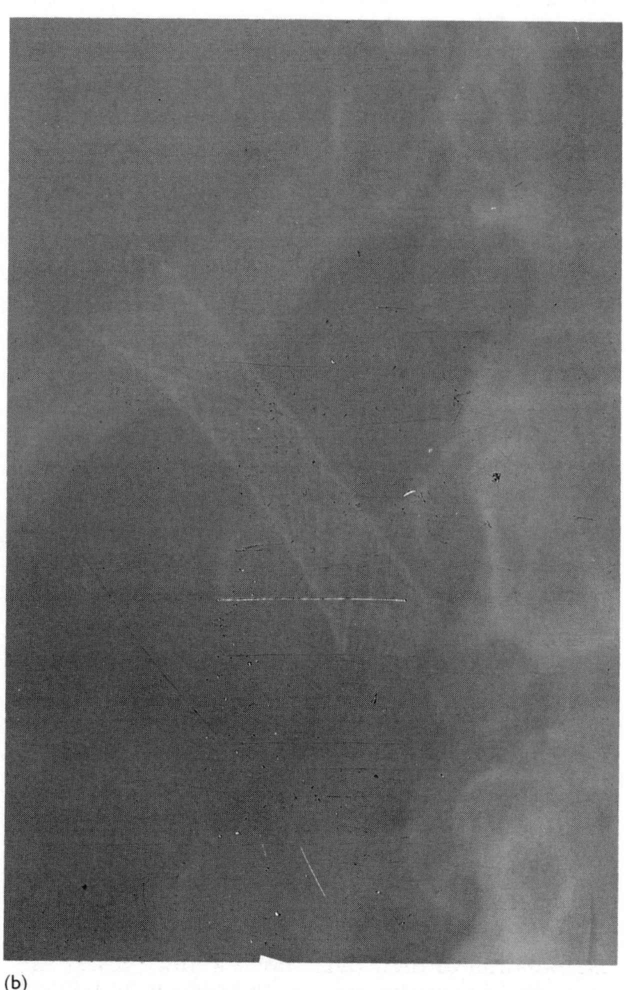

(b)

Figure 12.69 (a) A percutaneous transhepatic tube has been placed across the main stricture in a patient with extensive hilar cholangiocarcinoma. The tube passes down the common bile duct and enters the duodenum. (b) The percutaneous tube has been replaced by a self-expanding metal stent, which can be seen in this plain abdominal radiograph. Note that there is practically no 'waist' in the cylindrical stent, indicating that the tumour has been dilated to about 10 mm.

external biliary drainage and dilatation of a percutaneous transhepatic track.

Tumour ingrowth has been reported through the walls of metal stents in 2 of 5 patients followed for over 4 months.[26] This has not been the experience of the author's group and, in the author's experience, when stents have become occluded by tumour advancement there has been growth of the tumour above the highest level of the stent or below its distal end.[3] This can largely be overcome by placing the longest stents available. If stents do become occluded they can be cleared by 'diathermic cleaning',[26] or further stents can be inserted down the lumen of the original obstructed stent, or even from another segmental duct, passing through the wall of the stent.

Plastic stents which become occluded can often be cleared or removed. Endoscopically placed stents which project through the papilla of Vater can be removed endoscopically and replaced with another similar stent. Percutaneously placed stents which lie entirely within the biliary tree can be removed by a variety of techniques.[1,119] Metal stents cannot, for practical purposes, be removed once they have been placed.

An alternative configuration for the metal stent has been designed, the Gianturco stent, which has a zig-zag spring configuration (see *Figure 12.71b*). This has been used for both benign and malignant biliary strictures in a small number of patients, and has the advantage of exerting an even stronger centrifugal force than the mesh stents described above.[59] In practice, this stent has been mostly reserved for benign strictures.

Choice of technique

The choice of technique for stenting remains controversial. In many centres the selection of the percutaneous or endoscopic route will depend upon the availability of local expertise because the techniques required for effective intubation of these tumours may be quite exacting. There are no entirely satisfactory trials available. One trial from the Middlesex Hospital in London[103] appeared to show an advantage in 30-day mortality with no survival disadvantage for endoscopically placed stents. However, there was a very high complication rate for percutaneous stent placement, in comparison with other reports. Lameris *et al.*[66] compared two groups, but examination of their data shows a much lower success rate in accurate placement of stents endoscopically for hilar lesions. The endoscopic route has major advantages for distal tumours, but the author generally prefers percutaneous transhepatic intubation for tumours of the proximal hepatic ducts.

External drainage tubes

Rarely it is necessary to rely on external or external/internal biliary drainage as definitive treatment for patients with malignant bile duct obstruction. Even if the tube cannot be passed across the tumour at the first attempt, a short period of external biliary drainage will usually allow oedema to settle and a guide wire to be passed for the placement of a suitable stent. The major risk of all these procedures is cholangitis, which is especially troublesome when there are multiple segmental intrahepatic biliary obstructions.[7] It is important to avoid external contamination of biliary drainage tubes[75] and special sealed drainage systems have been designed to minimize this risk.[13]

SURGERY

Surgical treatment of biliary tumours may be internal biliary–enteric bypass, operative intubation of the tumours, or resection. The last category may consist of local resection, resection of the tumour including hepatic resection, or total hepatectomy with liver transplantation. Careful preoperative assessment should allow definition of those patients who are completely unsuitable for surgical treatment. However, decisions regarding the selection of patients for surgery and the choice of operation in individual cases may be extremely subtle and, because of the infrequency of these tumours, only clinicians working in specialist centres have the opportunity to gain experience in this decision process.

Surgical bypass

This has long been the standard palliative technique for the treatment of pancreatic cancer, and it is equally applicable to tumours of the distal bile duct. However, the use of bypass surgery for proximal biliary cancer is less widespread, largely because the procedure may be very difficult for tumours high in the hepatic ducts, or when a tumour of the gallbladder involves the common hepatic duct. Until the last decade, understanding of the biliary anatomy was relatively poor, despite the work of French surgeons and anatomists in the 1950s,[55] who demonstrated that the left hepatic duct is invariably an extrahepatic structure, and potentially accessible to the surgeon with well-directed dissection beneath the left liver. It is then possible to carry out a hepaticojejunostomy, anastomosing the left hepatic duct to a long Roux-en-Y loop of jejunum.[16] Often an anastomosis 1–2 cm in length can be achieved which will adequately drain the whole of the left liver. The right liver may be drained by this procedure if the confluence of the right and left ducts has not been disconnected by the tumour. When the left duct is not available for anastomosis because of tumour extension, it is possible to gain access to an intrahepatic duct in the left liver. The earliest method of achieving this was the Longmire procedure,[72] in which part of the left lateral segment of the liver was resected to gain access to an intrahepatic duct. This procedure has now been superseded by a bypass to the duct of Segment III, access to which can be obtained by splitting the liver just to the left of the umbilical fissure (*Figure 12.70*). This approach was described by Bismuth and Corlette,[11] who performed palliative bypass to the left duct or the segment III duct in 96 patients with an operative mortality of 7%. No internal or external tube is necessary, and the duration of palliation may be excellent.[12] These techniques are ideally suited to patients in whom there is communication between the right and left ducts. However, even in the absence of such a communication, effective palliation may still be obtained provided there is no sepsis within the right liver. For this reason it is of paramount importance to avoid introducing infection into the liver during the percutaneous cholangiography or external drainage procedures.

Similar techniques for biliary–enteric bypass have been described to the duct of segment V in the right liver, although these techniques are more difficult.[14]

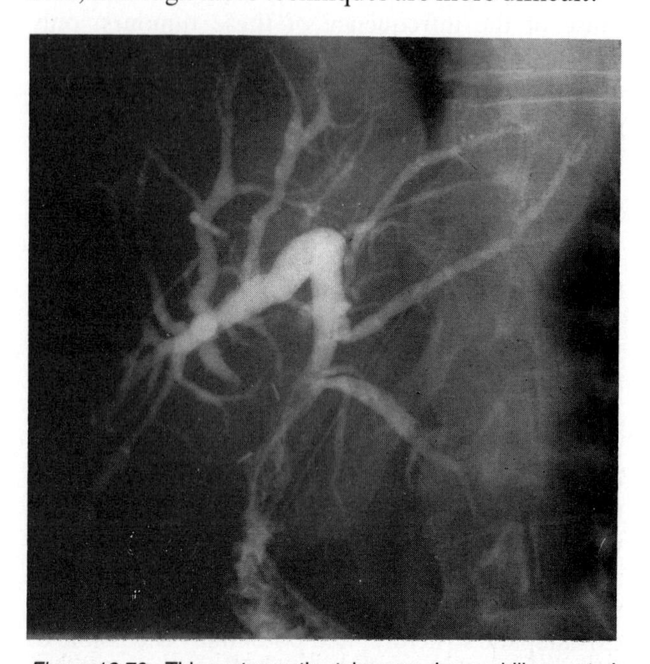

Figure 12.70 This postoperative tubogram shows a biliary–enteric bypass to the segment III duct of the right liver in a patient with irresectable carcinoma of the gallbladder. Note that the anastomosis is a long way from the hilum of the liver, and drains a large volume of liver tissue.

Intubation

Operative intubation has been largely supplanted by the use of endoscopic or radiological methods (see above). Insertion of a stent through an obstructing tumour at operation may not be easy, requiring opening of the bile duct below the tumour, operative dilatation using graduated bougies, and the insertion of a suitable stent, which may be either entirely intraductal or may exit through the common duct with or without the use of a jejunal loop. The placement of a transhepatic tube, passing through the tumour and exiting via the surface of the liver, was brought to popular attention by Terblanche and colleagues,[105] though it had been described earlier by Praderi in Uruguay. A metal instrument is passed from the duct below the tumour obstruction, and an attempt is made to railroad this through the intrahepatic ducts without traversing too much liver parenchyma, and finally brought out on to the surface of the liver. A tube of silastic or other material is then drawn through the liver and holes made in such a position as to lie above and below the tumour, allowing bile to drain internally into the distal duct. Once again a Roux loop of jejunum may sometimes be used and attached over the choledochotomy. Both ends of the tube are brought out through the skin, giving the 'U' in the U tube. If satisfactory internal drainage is established, then the ends of the tube can be closed off, or if not they can be joined together outside the body to form an external conduit. If this type of tube becomes blocked it is very easy to change it without anaesthesia by simply attaching a new tube with suitably placed holes to the end of the old one, and drawing it through to replace the blocked tube. Despite the simplicity of this procedure, the U tube is not an entirely satisfactory method of palliation, as it requires a major operative intervention and patients may suffer recurrent attacks of cholangitis, bile leakage and infection around the tube exit site. Though some authors continue to favour the use of transhepatic tubes,[22] the palliation may be relatively poor compared with that of internal bypass. If such tubes are used, it is probably wise to replace them electively at intervals (perhaps 3 months), rather than waiting for the onset of cholangitis.

Resection

World-wide experience of resection for hilar cholangiocarcinoma has remained relatively small. The difficulties of the operation have meant that the procedure is largely confined to specialist units. Resectability rates reported in the literature vary

Table 12.25 Resectability rates, mortality and survival in recent series of hilar cholangiocarcinoma

Study	*Number of cases*	*Resectability*	*Mortality*	*Survival*
Longmire *et al.*[73]	34	6 (17.6%)	5/34 (14.7%)	8 >1 year Longest 15 years
Fortner *et al.*[38]	25	9 (36%)	3 (33%)	Liver res. 7 months Tx 8 months
Launois *et al.*[68]	18	11 (61.1%)	2 (18.2%)	Mean 521 days Range 12–746 days
Tsuzuki *et al.*[110]	31	16 (51.6%)	2 (12.5%)	
Blumgart *et al.*[17]	94	18 (19.1%)	2 (11.1%)	Mean 17 months
Iwasaki *et al.*[60]	46	31 (67.4%)	0	Mean 2.2 years
Mizumoto *et al.*[78]	26	24 (92.3%)	1 (3.8%)	Mean: Local res. 9.3 months Liver res. 12.2 months
Pinson and Rossi[94]	156	25 (16%)	1 (4%)	Mean: Local res. 3.6 years Liver res. 3.9 years
Pichlmayr *et al.*[93]	108	52 (48.1%)	9 (17.3%)	Mean: Local res. 22 months Liver res. 14 months Tx 16 months
Nimura *et al.*[87]	66	55 (83.3%)	4 (7.8%)	Median 3.1 years 5-year survival 37.8%

Tx, liver transplantation; res., resection.

widely (*Table 12.25*). The majority of Western series report a resectability rate of 15–20% (Pinson and Rossi,[94] 16%; Longmire *et al.*,[73] 17.6%; Blumgart *et al.*,[17] 19.1%). Some centres have adopted a more aggressive policy, including the use of liver transplantation, and these centres report higher resectability rates (Fortner *et al.*,[38] 36%; Pichlmayr *et al.*,[93] 48.1%; Launois *et al.*,[68] 61.1%). A striking feature of the literature for cholangiocarcinoma is that the resectability rate described in Japanese series, some of which contain large numbers of patients, has been consistently higher than in Western reports (Tsuzuki *et al.*,[110] 51.6%; Iwasaki *et al.*,[60] 67.4%; Nimura *et al.*,[86] 83.3%; Mizumoto *et al.*,[78] 92.3%). It is not clear how much of this is selection bias due to different referral patterns or to differences in the population or the approach adopted.

Two contrasting philosophies relate to resection for cholangiocarcinoma. Resection with no residual tumour offers the only real prospect of long-term cure. Some authors believe that resection should be confined to patients in whom this is a realistic goal. Others, however, recognize that removal of the large bulk of tumour with a good internal biliary–enteric bypass may provide excellent palliation which, although without prospect of cure, may have useful advantages over intubational methods or simple bypass. In any event, the surgery remains difficult, and carries a significant operative mortality. It is necessary to distinguish between local resection and resection involving removal of part of the liver. The tumours frequently arise eccentrically, and have involved second-order ducts in the right or left liver before producing obstructive jaundice by encroachment on the confluence of the ducts. These patients require removal of the involved side of the liver along with the confluence of the hepatic ducts, and reconstruction of the uninvolved right or left duct to a Roux-en-Y loop of jejunum (*Figure 12.71*). By contrast, patients presenting with a mid-common bile duct or common hepatic duct tumour may be amenable to resection of the extrahepatic ducts and anastomosis of the right and left ducts to a loop of jejunum (*Figure 12.72*). This procedure (local resec-

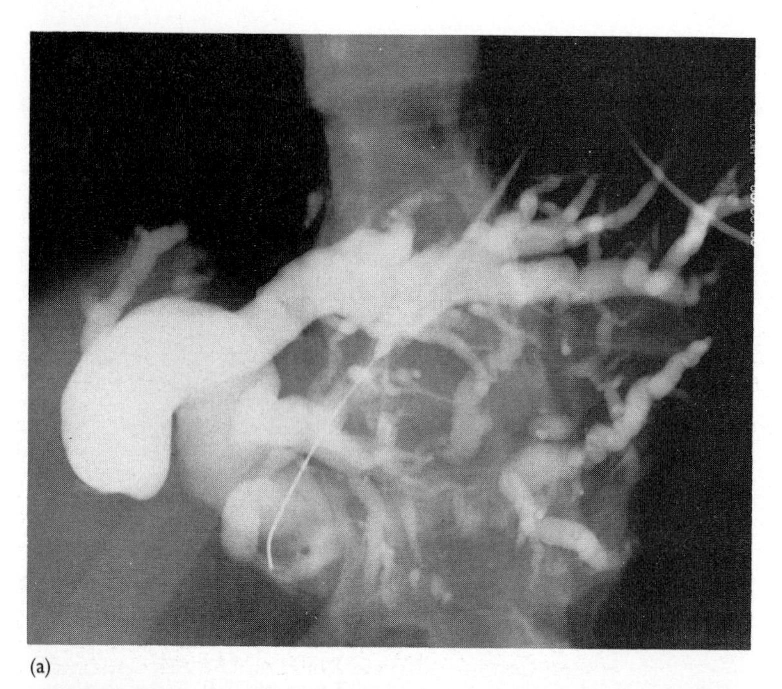

(a)

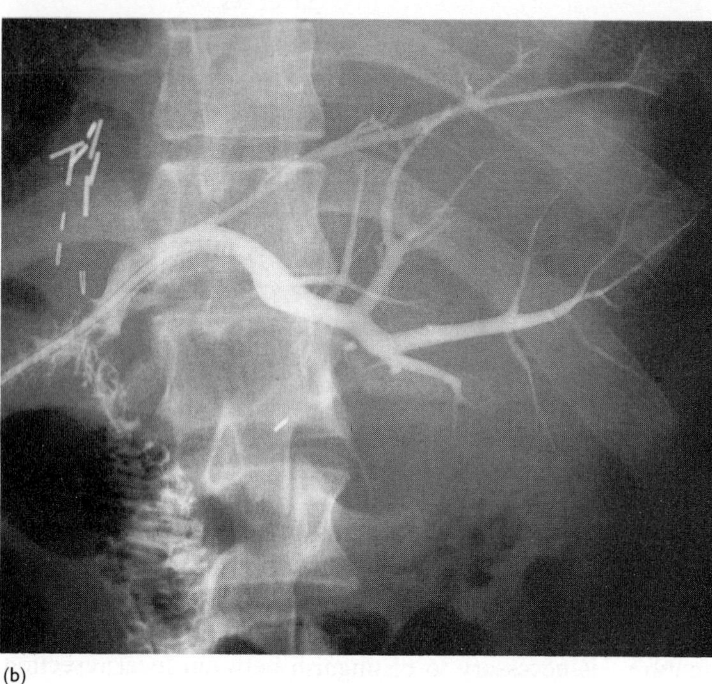

(b)

Figure 12.71 (a) A left-sided percutaneous transhepatic cholangiogram in a patient with a hilar cholangiocarcinoma. The right-sided puncture had shown extensive involvement of the right intrahepatic ducts extending to the confluence, but a good length of the main left hepatic duct is spared. (b) An extended right hepatectomy was performed, resecting the whole of the confluence, and leaving a short length of left hepatic duct: this was anastomosed to a Roux-en-Y jejunal limb, as seen on this tubogram 2 weeks postoperatively. Clips mark the cut edge of the liver, and the dilated intrahepatic ducts in the left liver have collapsed to normal size.

tion) should carry a very low mortality, but the addition of major hepatectomy raises the mortality for the operation considerably, with reports between 10 and 30% in recent series.

A further important area of controversy is whether the caudate lobe (segment I) should routinely be removed when removing bile duct cancers. This lobe drains by several short ducts, usually into the main left hepatic duct. Because of the propensity of cholangiocarcinomas to spread longitudinally along the ducts, failure to remove the caudate lobe is believed to carry the risk of leaving residual tumour.[81] The Japanese have been pioneers in this regard, and have described both the technique and the survival value of removal of the caudate lobe along with tumours of the hepatic hilum.[87] Resection of the nodes and lymphatics along the hepatoduodenal ligament may be important for survival also, though relatively few authors have undertaken major excision of the portal vein and venovenous bypass along with the resection.[77] If a short segment of the portal vein is involved by tumour, it is perfectly feasible to resect a small section of the vein and re-anastomose it end to end.[15]

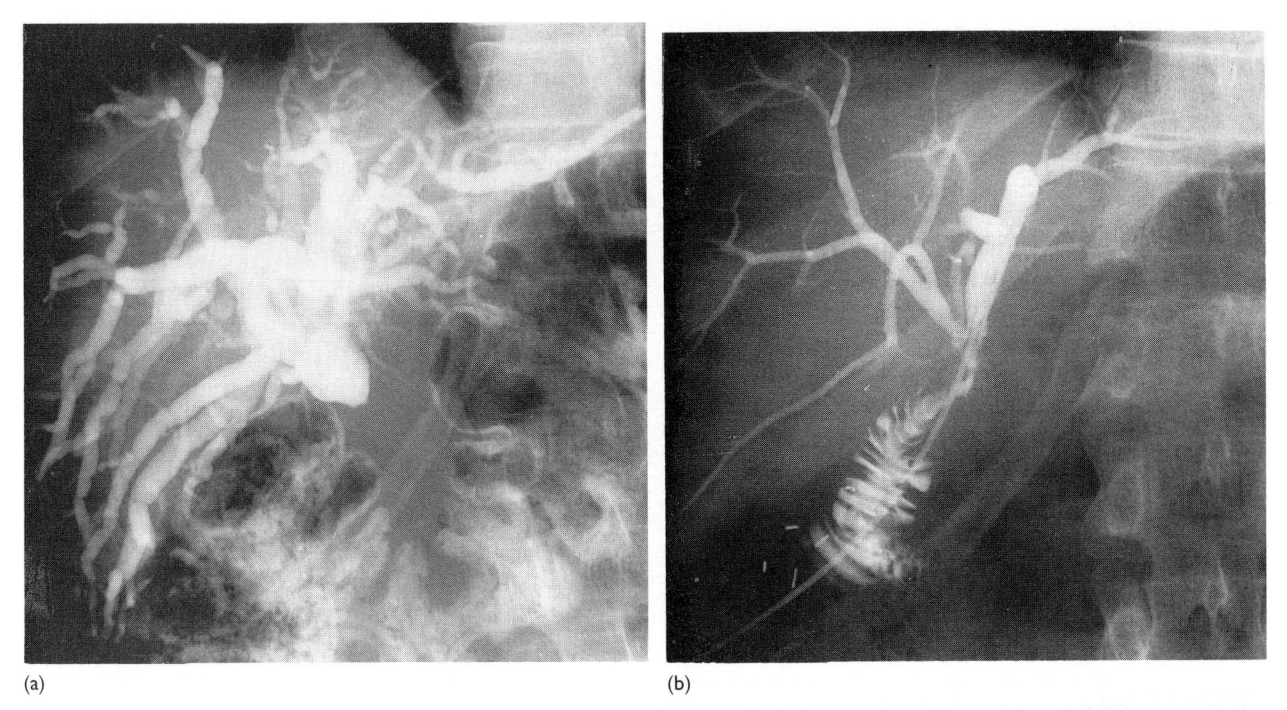

(a) (b)

Figure 12.72 (a) Percutaneous transhepatic cholangiogram in a patient with hilar cholangiocarcinoma. There is involvement of the confluence of the left and right ducts, but in this case no second order duct involvement on either side. (b) Local resection of the extrahepatic ducts was carried out, with reconstruction by means of a hepaticojejunostomy to a Roux-en-Y limb of jejunum: the postoperative tubogram shows free drainage of the whole liver.

Liver transplantation

A total hepatectomy with transplantation may be feasible for those patients in whom regional nodal metastases and other sites of extrahepatic tumour can be excluded. Pichlmayr and colleagues[93] reported 16 patients with hepatic transplantation, in whom nine were found to have extrahepatic metastases when the tissues were finally examined. Most of these patients developed tumour recurrence and the longest survival was 27 months. The seven patients without apparent residual tumour appeared to be tumour-free at 21 months. The dilemma, therefore, remains that patients with well localized tumours are the ones that are likely to survive transplantation and its associated immunosuppression, but these are also the patients likely to be amenable to conventional local resection. Few of those patients whose tumours have transgressed the boundaries of local resectability are suitable for transplantation. Current attitudes are, therefore, somewhat opposed to transplantation in this situation.

Assessment of resectability

Preoperative staging and cytological evaluation should have been performed before the operation. Conventionally, the following criteria suggest an irresectable tumour: (1) involvement of second-order intrahepatic ducts on both sides of the liver, or multifocal tumour on cholangiography; (2) involvement of the main stem of the portal vein (although some tumours may still be resectable, as described above); (3) contralateral involvement of vessels or ducts on both sides of the liver. These criteria seem logical and have been widely used. Their validity was confirmed in a series of 37 consecutive patients studied at Hammersmith Hospital.[113] All but three of these patients, who had terminal disease, underwent laparotomy, and the diagnosis and extent of the disease were confirmed. Twenty-four patients were thought to be potentially resectable before operation, and in only one of these patients was resection found to be impossible or judged futile. Sixty per cent of patients who are considered to be resectable before operation on criteria such as these are able to undergo resection. The reasons for failing to resect patients who appear to be resectable on cholangiographic, angiographic and scanning criteria are general characteristics (age and general unfitness to withstand major liver resection) or under-assessment of the extent of the disease on preoperative investigation. This is a debatable point: many tumours are technically resectable, but it has not been the author's practice to carry out major liver resection in the presence of known extrahepatic disease. Local resection can of course be undertaken quite safely for palliation, and therefore the presence of extrahepatic disease may not be a contraindication to this lesser procedure.

Techniques of resection

The following points may be made briefly. It is important to assess the patient carefully at laparotomy for extrahepatic disease, including peritoneal seedlings and lymph nodes around the porta hepatis and along the coeliac axis. Nodes can be sent for frozen section, and it is often surprising how well-differentiated the deposits of tumour from the bile ducts in adjacent lymph nodes are.[10] Even if only a palliative bypass is to be performed, there is no disadvantage in dividing the bile duct below the tumour at an early stage. The tumour can then be turned upwards off the front of the portal vein, and if it is free it can be dissected until non-cancerous dilated ducts above the tumour are encountered. Frozen section may once again be used to determine the limits of the tumour, as visual inspection may be insufficient. It is very difficult to be certain of the extent of tumour spread on frozen section, and careful definitive multiple paraffin sections of resected duct margins may reveal that the tumour has spread further than expected. This phenomenon was examined in 26 patients who underwent resection at Hammersmith Hospital, with the intent to produce cure or prolonged palliation. The involvement of the resection margins appeared to have some impact on survival, though this was not statistically significant.[43] More detailed technical accounts of the methods and results of liver resection for bile duct cancer have been given elsewhere.[15]

Gallbladder cancer

Gallbladder cancer shares many features in common with other tumours of the biliary system. However, its surgical management is worth examining separately, because it poses specific problems and the outcome may be less satisfactory. The overall 5-year survival of patients with primary gallbladder cancer is less than 5%. This is because, apart from stage 1 or 2 tumours (see above) diagnosed retrospectively after cholecystectomy for gallstones, most patients present either with advanced disease or with non-specific symptoms. Once cancer of the gallbladder has proceeded to invasion of the hilar ducts and caused obstructive jaundice, it is very rarely resectable for cure. The peak age of incidence of this tumour is 70–75 years and management must be considered in relation to the mode of presentation. When cancer of the gallbladder occurs as an incidental finding at the time of cholecystectomy (some one-third of cases) the surgeon carrying out the cholecystectomy should make a full assessment at the time of operation whenever possible and decide whether to attempt a wider excision. All gallbladders should be opened before the operation is concluded, and some surgeons believe that following the finding of a well-localized gallbladder tumour a wedge resection of the gallbladder bed or a formal excision of segments IV and V should be performed. Some have argued strongly for radical surgery of this type, or even for its extension to include formal right hepatic resection. Adson and Farnell[4] reported the Mayo Clinic experience of 12 patients out of 112 with gallbladder cancers whose tumours were resectable. Seven out of eight such patients who had simple cholecystectomy were dead within 15 months, while the four patients who underwent radical excision had a much longer survival. It is likely, however, that local invasion is the determining factor for survival even in the presence of radical excision. Evander and Ihse[36] could not demonstrate any survival advantage for radical resection in 10 out of 44 patients with gallbladder cancer who underwent such surgery. Very few will be resectable even if the diagnosis is made or suspected preoperatively.[25] Most of these patients are therefore best treated by stenting or by internal bypass, as described above. The round ligament or left duct approach may be particularly applicable to tumours of the gallbladder, because the anastomosis is at a safe distance from the tumour.

COMBINED APPROACHES

Management of tumours of the gallbladder and biliary tree should be undertaken in a cooperative manner between surgeons, endoscopists and radiologists. The therapeutic options should be considered at all stages during the assessment of these tumours. Radiologists and endoscopists may play an important part in preoperative preparation of the patients (see below). On occasions, endoscopic intubation of a tumour, particularly at the hilus, may be impossible and assistance by a percutaneous transhepatic tube or guide wire passed by the radiologist may facilitate the process.

These considerations can also be extended to surgical management when making provision at the time of operation for future access to the biliary tree, which can be achieved by fixation of the end or the side of a Roux-en-Y loop of jejunum to the parietal peritoneum, marking the loop with clips.[65] This

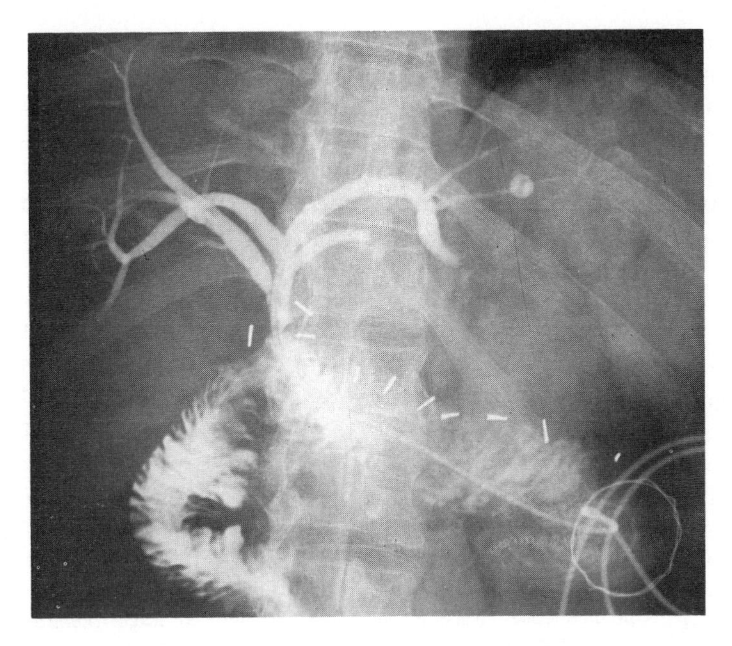

Figure 12.73 This postoperative tubogram shows the marking of the Roux loop at hepaticojejunostomy following excision of the common bile duct (in this case for a benign biliary stricture). Two metal clips mark the lateral boundaries of the anastomosis, and a row of clips on the serosa of the jejunum shows the course of the loop. At the point where the loop is attached to the peritoneum of the abdominal wall there is a circular stainless steel suture: this marks the point of percutaneous puncture for any future radiological access which may be required.

technique is much more satisfactory than creation of a cutaneous stoma in the Roux loop.[58] It is the author's practice to create an access port of this type in every case of hepaticojejunostomy, for either benign or malignant disease, by means of a circular stainless steel wire suture to mark the point of future access (*Figure 12.73*). This adds scarcely any time and no morbidity to the operation, and acts as a useful insurance policy for the future.[99]

PREOPERATIVE PREPARATION

Nutrition

Attention to nutrition is of great importance. Many patients with bile duct tumours have lost a considerable amount of weight, partly because of the general effects of the tumour and partly because of obstructive jaundice and malabsorption. An assessment of weight loss should be made preoperatively, and there is good argument for routinely instituting parenteral feeding in patients who have lost more than 10% of body weight. Moreover, patients with obstructive jaundice suffer from immune dysfunction, as shown by anergy to delayed hypersensitivity skin testing.[52,53] These patients often require several days of hospital investigation, and the need for enteral or parenteral nutrition should not be neglected during this time. A period of percutaneous transhepatic biliary drainage may allow more rapid improvement of nutrition by means of intravenous feeding,[39] but this has been disputed.[51] The role of percutaneous drainage as preoperative preparation is discussed below.

Renal function

Renal function is extremely important. It is well known that there is an increased tendency to acute renal failure in obstructive jaundice.[29] Thompson *et al.*[109] reported an 11% incidence of postoperative renal impairment following biliary surgery, and found that jaundice was an independently significant contributing factor. The mortality in established renal failure was high, but was almost always associated with other major complications; death was rarely due to renal failure alone. The hypothesis that renal failure may in large part be due to endotoxaemia has led to a number of treatments aimed at reducing the absorption of endotoxins into the portal circulation. Administration of bile salts preoperatively is of value,[21] though not all preparations are equally efficacious.[108] Preoperative bowel preparation may have a beneficial effect on electrolyte balance but not on portal endotoxaemia.[57] Preoperative lactulose reduced systemic and portal endotoxaemia, as well as mortality in jaundiced rats.[92] There is good evidence that returning bile to the gastrointestinal tract is of greater value than simple relief of biliary obstruction by means of external drainage, and there is experimental evidence to support this clinical observation.[32] Probably the most important matter for attention preoperatively is maintenance of the patient's hydration. Intravenous fluids should be administered to all patients who are deeply jaundiced, especially if they are to be fasted overnight for operation. The use of mannitol to secure a diuresis was first proposed by Dawson,[29] although it now seems possible that the effects of rehydration were as important as those of mannitol diuresis. Preoperative percutaneous drainage has also been suggested as a means of improving impaired renal function. However, in a controlled trial of percutaneous transhepatic biliary drainage it was shown that rehydration alone produced as great an improvement in renal function as rehydration combined with biliary drainage.[74]

Temporary biliary decompression

The concept of two-stage surgery for deeply jaundiced patients is not new. The first pancreatoduodenectomy described by Whipple *et al.*[116] in 1935 was performed as a two-stage procedure, the first stage being to decompress the biliary tree by means of cholecystogastrostomy. The disadvantage of a surgical bypass before attempting to undertake major resection is that the patient requires a laparotomy, in itself dangerous in the presence of jaundice, and this may prejudice the safety of future surgery. This led to the alternative treatment of percutaneous intubation. Nakayama and colleagues[83] described the use of this technique with great enthusiasm, and claimed a significant reduction in mortality, albeit in a highly selected and uncontrolled study. Since then, numerous attempts have been made to demonstrate the effectiveness of this treatment, and several controlled trials have been reported. Most of these were reviewed by Pitt *et al.*[96] That by Hatfield and colleagues in South Africa,[54] in a variety of patients with benign and malignant disease failed to show any survival advantage in patients undergoing preoperative external drainage. The trial by McPherson *et al.*[75] showed a higher mortality in patients who underwent preoperative external biliary drainage: this paper included a large number of patients with tumours of the bile ducts and gallbladder, and the increased mortality was due to introduction of infection into the biliary tree. A study by Pitt *et al.*[96] showed an identical mortality for both groups with no effective reduction in hospital costs. One trial did show a benefit.[47] These trials all relate to external percutaneous transhepatic biliary drainage and none answers the question of whether internal drainage by endoscopic stenting improves survival in patients who are to undergo major surgery.[34] The focus on endoscopic stenting as a definitive measure has considerably dampened enthusiasm for temporary biliary drainage before resection. Moreover, tumour seeding along external catheter tracks has been reported,[24] and the author has seen one such example in a patient with cholangiocarcinoma (*Figure 12.74*). The current attitude probably is that patients who are severely jaundiced, and particularly those suffering from significant acute cholangitis, are best treated by a brief period of biliary drainage. This will allow some resolution of the acute problem, though a complete return to normal liver function may take many weeks.[64]

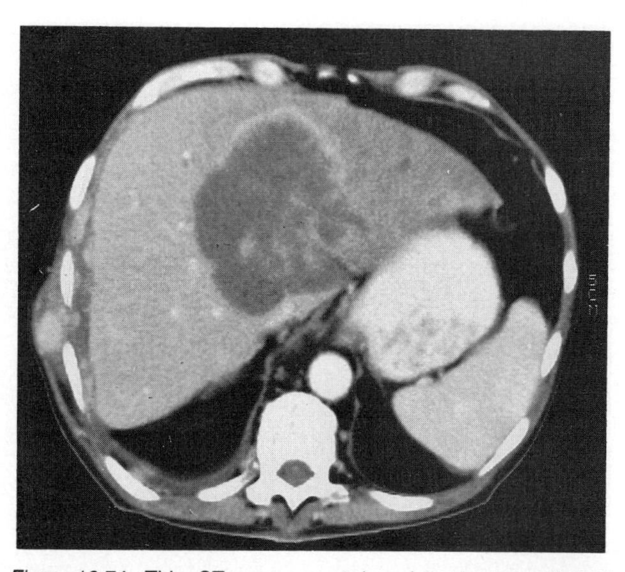

Figure 12.74 This CT scan was taken following a period of percutaneous transhepatic drainage for a large central cholangiocarcinoma. The tumour mass can be seen replacing the whole area of the central ducts. However, there is a second mass in the soft tissue of the abdominal wall, over the right ribs: this is a tumour deposit (proven on cytology) at the exit site of the transhepatic tube, and represents a complication of external drainage.

ADDITIONAL MANAGEMENT

Radiotherapy

This is another unresolved issue. While many authors have used postoperative radiotherapy for tumours of the gallbladder and biliary tree, there are no controlled studies which make it clear whether any survival advantage is conferred by these methods. Lokich and colleagues[71] reviewed nine studies which have examined radiotherapy in primary bile duct cancers. The total number of patients was only 124. Larger groups of patients have been reported in the Japanese literature. Nakama *et al.*[82] studied 122 patients treated with radiotherapy, and found that those patients who had a good local response had a longer overall survival, but it is by no means clear that there was a statistically significant effect on survival in the group as a whole. Terblanche and colleagues[106] used external beam radiotherapy in combination with transhepatic U tubes, and claimed several long survivors. However, not all of these had histologically proven tumours, and this was a study of a small number of highly selected patients seen over a number of years.

One of the problems with external beam radiotherapy (total doses used varying between 20 and 60 Gy), is the significant incidence of radiation duodenitis which may cause intractable gastrointestinal bleeding. In attempts to circumvent this problem, intracavitory therapy has been given, using a ^{192}Ir wire inserted inside the tumour, generally via a catheter passing through a stent. ^{192}Ir is a β emitter with only a few millimetres depth of penetration. It seems unlikely, therefore, that this therapy will have a major effect on large tumours. It may be that its maximum beneficial effect may be in slowing the local progression of tumours, and possibly in delaying the onset of further biliary obstruction or stent overgrowth. The delivery of ^{192}Ir has mostly been achieved by transhepatic catheterization.[37,76] The local dose of radiotherapy achieved may be 30–50 Gy, which may be supplemented by external beam irradiation, possibly with another 30–45 Gy. More recent reports have shown the possibility of delivering iridium radiotherapy via nasobiliary tubes introduced through biliary strictures using the endoscope.[69,111] Unfortunately, none of these were controlled studies, and the need for such a trial has been stressed.[22]

In the absence of any controlled trial evidence, it has been the author's practice to use radiotherapy in those patients who have irresectable tumours and are expected to live for more than a few months, as well as for adjuvant therapy in some cases following tumour resection. The technique used is usually percutaneous transhepatic insertion of iridium wire and external beam administration localized to the region of the stent. There have been no significant complications in more than 50 patients treated by this method, though it is of course impossible to evaluate the impact of this additional treatment on survival.

Intraoperative radiotherapy has been reported from a few specialised centres with little morbidity and a low mortality, though again the effects on survival are undefined.[20] Deziel *et al.*[31] reported their experience with nine patients treated with intraoperative radiotherapy and found no significant difference in mean survival between these patients (16.8 months) and those treated by external beam irradiation with or without ^{192}Ir (11 months). The 1-year survivals in these groups were 56 and 46%, respectively.

Chemotherapy

There is little evidence for the value of chemotherapy for tumours of the bile duct and gallbladder. Oberfield and Rossi[88] reported a significant local response rate to drugs such as 5FU and mitomycin, alone or in combination with doxorubicin (Adriamycin) in 29% of 97 patients. Intra-arterial therapy has also been suggested, but has yet to be widely evaluated. Finally, there remains the intriguing possibility of hormone manipulation in biliary cancer, because retardation of tumour growth by cholecystokinin was shown in 2 of 6 cancer lines from human gastrointestinal tumours xenografted in nude mice, including a metastatic cholangiocarcinoma cell line.[56]

RESULTS

The above account of tumours of the bile ducts and gallbladder may have seemed complex and confusing, but this is because we have not reached any consensus as to the optimum methods of the evaluation of treatment in difficult patients. On the one hand some authors report higher resectability rates and more adventurous and complex forms of resection, while on the other hand radiologists and endoscopists have made numerous technical advances resulting in more expeditious treatment of patients and shorter hospital stay. While philosophically it is reasonable to accept that the only prospects of cure are afforded by complete resection of the cancer, it is by no means certain that this is so, nor indeed that complete as opposed to almost complete resection confers a significant survival advantage in the majority of patients.[44] Little[70] has recently reviewed this dichotomy of views. The one thing which stands out through all these reports is the need for a unified approach to assessment of quality of survival and the extent to which we are able to palliate the patient's symptoms. Bismuth only resects some 10% of the large number of gallbladder and bile duct cancers referred to his unit, and has accepted that excellent palliation may be obtained by a left-sided biliary–enteric anastomosis.

The mortality of surgical treatment, which is not inconsiderable, must be considered. *Table 12.25*, modified from Nimura *et al.*[87] summarizes the resectability, mortality and survival figures of more than 600 patients in 10 recent series. Mortality is reasonably low for those not requiring hepatectomy, but may be as high as 70% for those in whom liver resection is required. However, as liver resection has improved so mortality has decreased. The latest of these series[87] contains only four deaths in 51 patients undergoing liver resection, including the extension of the resection in most to include the caudate lobe, a difficult surgical manoeuvre. Few authors quote 5-year survival rates following radical treatment, and the reported mean survivals vary from 9 months to 3.6 years and the median from 7 to 15 months. The author's experience[44] in almost 200 patients treated over a 10-year period was that 22% of patients were suitable for resection. Approximately half of these were amenable to local resection, and half to liver resection. There were no deaths in the patients who underwent local resection, and five (12%) in those undergoing liver resection. Of 18 patients with complete tumour clearance, 12 have died of recurrent tumour, as have 14 of 17 patients with proven involved resection margins. Five patients with clear margins are still alive and apparently tumour-free more than 5 years after resection, and two between 2 and 5 years, though there is one with recurrent disease. Of the patients not suitable for resection, the majority were treated by internal drainage, roughly equally by surgical bypass and the insertion of a stent. Overall, the percentage of patients for whom internal drainage could be achieved was 87% in the first 5 years of the author's series, and 97% in the second 5 years. This reflects both greater determination to achieve internal drainage and improvements in radiological technology. Although radiotherapy has been used for many of these patients, its results remain unproven.

REFERENCES

1. Adam, A. (1987) Use of the modified Cope introduction set for transhepatic removal of obstructed Carey-Coons biliary endoprosthesis. *Clinical Radiology*, **38**, 171–174.
2. Adam, A. (1990) Percutaneous biliary drainage for malignancy – an expanding field. *Clinical Radiology*, **41**, 225–227.
3. Adam, A., Chetty, N., Roddie, M., Yeung, E. and Benjamin, I.S. (1990) Self-expandable stainless steel endoprostheses for treatment of malignant bile duct obstruction. *American Journal of Radiology*, **156**, 321–325.
4. Adson, M.A. and Farnell, M.B. (1981) Hepatobiliary cancer – surgical considerations. *Mayo Clinic Proceedings*, **56**, 686–699.
5. Altemeier, W.A., Gall, E.A., Zinninger, M.M. and Hoxworth, P.E. (1957) Sclerosing carcinoma of the major intrahepatic bile ducts. *Archives of Surgery*, **75**, 450.
6. Al-Zuhair, A.G., Al-Adnani, M.S., Al-Bader, A.A. and Francis, I.M. (1987) Expression of connective tissue stromal elements in human cholangiocarcinomas. An immunohistochemical and ultrastructural study. *Journal of Submicroscopic Cytology*, **19**, 321–327.
7. Audisio, R.A., Bozzetti, F., Severini, A. *et al.* (1988) The occurrence of cholangitis after percutaneous biliary drainage: evaluation of some risk factors. *Surgery*, **103**, 507–512.
8. Beazley, R.N., Hadjis, N.S., Benjamin, I.S. and Blumgart, L.H. (1984) Clinicopathological aspects of high bile duct cancer: experience with resection and bypass surgical treatment. *Annals of Surgery*, **199**, 623–636.
9. Benjamin, I.S. (1983) Biliary tract obstruction. *Surgical Gastroenterology*, **2**, 105–120.
10. Benjamin, I.S. (1990) Pancreas and biliary tract. In *Treatment of Cancer* (Ed.) Sikora, K. and Halnan, K.E. pp. 455–471. London: Chapman and Hall.
11. Bismuth, H. and Corlette, M.B. (1975) Intrahepatic cholangioenteric anastomosis in carcinoma of the hilus of the liver. *Surgery, Gynecology and Obstetrics*, **140**, 170–178.
12. Bismuth, H., Castaing, D. and Traynor, O. (1988) Resection or palliation: priority of surgery in the treatment of hilar cancer. *World Journal of Surgery*, **12**, 39–47.
13. Blenkharn, J.I., McPherson, G.A.D. and Blumgart, L.H. (1981) An improved system for external biliary drainage. *Lancet*, **ii**, 781–782.
14. Blumgart, L.H. (1988) Hilar and intrahepatic biliary-enteric anastomosis. In *Surgery of the Liver and Biliary Tract*, Vol. 2 (Ed.) Blumgart, L.H. pp. 899–913. Edinburgh: Churchill Livingstone.
15. Blumgart, L.H. and Benjamin, I.S. (1989) Liver resection for bile duct cancer. *Surgical Clinics of North America*, **69**, 323–337.
16. Blumgart, L.H. and Kelly, C.J. (1984) Hepaticojejunostomy in benign and malignant high bile duct stricture: approaches to the left hepatic ducts. *British Journal of Surgery*, **71**, 257–261.
17. Blumgart, L.H., Benjamin, I.S., Hadjis, N.S. and Beazley, R.M. (1984) Surgical approaches to cholangiocarcinoma at confluence of hepatic ducts. *The Lancet*, **i**, 66–70.
18. Bond, G.G., McLaren, E.A., Sabel, F.L., Bodner, K.M., Lipps, T.E. and Cook, R.R. (1990) Liver and biliary tract cancer among chemical workers. *American Journal of Industrial Medicine*, **18**, 19–24.
19. Burns, C.D., Kuhns, J.G. and Wieman, T.J. (1990) Cholangiocarcinoma in association with multiple biliary microhamartomas. *Archives of Pathology and Laboratory Medicine*, **114**, 1287–1289.
20. Busse, P.M., Stone, M.D., Sheldon, T.A. *et al.* (1989) Intraoperative radiation therapy for biliary tract carcinoma: results of a 5-year experience. *Surgery*, **105**, 724–733.
21. Cahill, C.J. (1983) Prevention of postoperative renal failure in patients with obstructive jaundice – the role of bile salts. *British Journal of Surgery*, **70**, 590–595.
22. Cameron, J.L. (1988) Proximal cholangiocarcinomas. *British Journal of Surgery*, **75**, 1155–1156.
23. Caygill, C., Hill, M., Kirkham, J. and Northfield, T.C. (1988) Increased risk of biliary tract cancer

following gastric surgery. *British Journal of Cancer*, **57**, 434–436.
24. Chapman, W.C., Sharp, K.W., Weaver, F. and Sawyers, J.L. (1989) Tumor seeding from percutaneous biliary catheters. *Annals of Surgery*, **209**, 708–715.
25. Collier, N.A., Carr, D., Hemingway, A. and Blumgart, L.H. (1984) Preoperative diagnosis and its effect on the treatment of carcinoma of the gallbladder. *Surgery, Gynecology and Obstetrics*, **159**, 465–470.
26. Cremer, M., Deviere, J., Sugai, B. and Baize, M. (1990) Expandable biliary metal stents for malignancies: endoscopic insertion and diathermic cleaning for tumor ingrowth. *Gastrointestinal Endoscopy*, **36**, 451–457.
27. Crile, G. Jr (1970) The advantages of bypass operations over radical pancreatoduodenectomy in the treatment of pancreatic carcinoma. *Surgery, Gynecology and Obstetrics*, **130**, 1049–1053.
28. Davis, R.I., Sloan, J.M., Hood, J.M. and Maxwell, P. (1988) carcinoma of the extrahepatic biliary tract: a clinicopathological and immunohistochemical study. *Histopathology*, **12**, 623–631.
29. Dawson, J.L. (1965) The incidence of postoperative renal failure in obstructive jaundice. *British Journal of Surgery*, **52**, 663–665.
30. Desa, L.A., Akosa, A.B., Lazzara, S., Domizio, P., Krausz, T. and Benjamin, I.S. (1991) Cytodiagnosis in the management of extrahepatic biliary stricture. *Gut*, **32**, 1188–1191.
31. Deziel, D.J., Kiel, K.D., Kramer, T.S., Doolas, A. and Roseman, D.L. (1988) Intraoperative radiation therapy in biliary tract cancer. *American Surgeon*, **54**, 402–407.
32. Diamond, T., Dolan, S., Thompson, R.L.E. and Rowlands, B.J. (1990) Development and reversal of endotoxemia and endotoxin-related death in obstructive jaundice. *Surgery*, **108**, 370–375.
33. Dixon, J.M., Armstrong, C.P., Duffy, S.W. and Davies, G.C. (1983) Factors affecting morbidity and mortality after surgery for obstructive jaundice: a review of 373 patients. *Gut*, **24**, 845–852.
34. Dooley, J.S. (1985) External bile drainage – the state of the art. *Journal of Hepatology*, **1**, 681–686.
35. Engels, J.T., Balfe, D.M. and Lee, J.K. (1989) Biliary carcinoma: CT evaluation of extrahepatic spread. *Radiology*, **172**, 35–40.
36. Evander, A. and Ihse, I. (1981) Evaluation of intended radical surgery in carcinoma of the gallbladder. *British Journal of Surgery*, **68**, 158–160.
37. Fletcher, M.S., Brinkley, D., Dawson, J.L., Nunnerley, H. and Williams, R. (1983) Treatment of hilar carcinoma by bile drainage combined with internal radiotherapy using ^{192}iridium wire. *British Journal of Surgery*, **70**, 733–735.
38. Fortner, J.G., Kallum, B.O. and Kim, D.K. (1976) Surgical management of carcinoma of the junction of the main hepatic ducts. *Annals of Surgery*, **184**, 68.
39. Foschi, D., Cavagna, G., Callioni, F., Morandi, E. and Rovati, V. (1986) Hyperalimentation of jaundiced patients on percutaneous transhepatic biliary drainage. *British Journal of Surgery*, **73**, 716–719.
40. Foutch, P.G., Kerr, D.M., Harlan, J.R., Manne, R.K., Kummet, T.D. and Sanowski, R.A. (1990) Endoscopic retrograde wire-guided brush cytology for diagnosis of patients with malignant obstruction of the bile duct. *American Journal of Gastroenterology*, **85**, 791–795.
41. Gibson, R.N., Yeung, E., Thompson, J.N. *et al.* (1986) Bile duct obstruction: radiologic evaluation of level, cause and tumour resectability. *Radiology*, **160**, 43–47.
42. Gibson, R.N., Adam, A., Halevy, A. *et al.* (1987) Benign biliary strictures: a proposed combined surgical and radiological management. *Australian and New Zealand Journal of Surgery*, **57**, 361–368.
43. Gompertz, R.H., Benjamin, I.S. and Blumgart, L.H. (1988) Resection for hilar cholangiocarcinoma: does clearance matter? *Gut*, **29**, A736–A737.
44. Gompertz, R.H., Benjamin, I.S., Yip, A., O'Sullivan, R., Blumgart, L.H. and Williamson, R.C.N. (1990) Hilar cholangiocarcinoma: a 10-year experience. *Gut*, **31**, A589.
45. Gouma, D.J., Mutum, S.S., Benjamin, I.S. and Blumgart, L.H. (1984) Intrahepatic biliary papillomatosis. *British Journal of Surgery*, **71**, 72–74.
46. Grace, P.A., Pitt, H.A., Tompkins, R., den Besten, L. and Longmire, W.P. Jr (1980) Deceased morbidity–mortality after pancreatoduodenectomy. *American Journal of Surgery*, **151**, 141–149.
47. Gundry, S.R., Strodel, W.E., Knol, J.A., Eckhauser, F.E. and Thompson, N.W. (1984) Efficacy of preoperative biliary tract decompression in patients with obstructive jaundice. *Archives of Surgery*, **119**, 703–708.
48. Hadjis, N.S., Collier, N.A. and Blumgart, L.H. (1985) Malignant masquerade of the hilum of the liver. *British Journal of Surgery*, **72**, 659–661.
49. Hadjis, N.S., Adam, A., Gibson, R., Blenkharn, J.I., Benjamin, I.S. and Blumgart, L.H. (1989) Nonoperative approach to hilar cancer determined by the atrophy–hypertrophy complex. *American Journal of Surgery*, **157**, 395–399.
50. Hadjis, N.S., Blenkharn, J.I., Hatzis, G., Demianiuk, C., Guzail, M. and Benjamin, I.S. (1990) Pathologic and hemodynamic sequelae of unilobar biliary obstruction and associated liver atrophy. *Surgery*, **109**, 671–676.
51. Halliday, A.W., McPherson, G.A.D. and Benjamin, I.S. (1987) Hyperalimentation of jaundiced patients during percutaneous transhepatic biliary drainage (letter). *British Journal of Surgery*, **74**, 964.

52. Halliday, A.W., McPherson, G.A.D., Benjamin, I.S. and Blumgart, L.H. (1987) Does preoperative biliary drainage allow an improvement of nutritional status in the jaundiced patient? *Digestive Surgery*, **4**, 187–191.
53. Halliday, A.W., Benjamin, I.S. and Blumgart, L.H. (1988) Nutritional risk factors in major hepatobiliary surgery. *Journal of Parenteral and Enteral Nutrition*, **12**, 43–48.
54. Hatfield, A.R.W., Terblanche, J., Fataar, S. *et al.* (1982) Pre-operative external biliary drainage in obstructive jaundice. *The Lancet*, **ii**, 896–899.
55. Hepp, J. and Couinaud, C. (1956) L'abord et l'utilisation due canal hepatique gauche dans les reparations de la voie bilaire principale. *Presse Medicin*, **64**, 947–948.
56. Hudd, C., LaRegina, M.C., Devine, J.E. *et al.* (1989) Response to exogenous cholecystokinin of six human gastrointestinal cancers xenografted in nude mice. *American Journal of Surgery*, **157**, 386–394.
57. Hunt, D.R. and Blumgart, L.H. (1982) Sodium homeostasis with obstructive jaundice: a randomized trial of preoperative bowel preparation. *Chir. Epatobil*, **2**, 99–102.
58. Hutson, D.G., Russell, E., Schiff, E., Levi, J.J., Jeffers, L. and Zeppa, R. (1984) Balloon dilatation of biliary strictures through a choledochojejunocutaneous fistula. *Annals of Surgery*, **199**, 637–647.
59. Irving, J.D., Adam, A., Dick, R., Dondelinger, R.F., Lunderquist, A. and Roche, A. (1989) Gianturco expandable metallic biliary stents: results of a European clinical trial. *Radiology*, **172**, 321–326.
60. Iwasaki, Y., Okamura, T., Ozaki, A. *et al.* (1986) Surgical treatment of carcinoma of the confluence of the major hepatic ducts. *Surgery, Gynecology and Obstetrics*, **162**, 457.
61. Kato, I., Kuroishi, T. and Tominaga, S. (1990) Descriptive epidemiology of subsites of cancers of the liver, biliary tract and pancreas in Japan. *Japanese Journal of Clinical Oncology*, **20**, 232–237.
62. Kato, T., Matsuda, K., Kayaba, H. *et al.* (1989) Pathology of anomalous junction of the pancreaticobiliary ductal system: mutagenicity of the contents of the biliary tract and nuclear atypia of the biliary epithelium. *Keio Journal of Medicine*, **38**, 167–176.
63. Klatskin, G. (1965) Adenocarcinoma of the hepatic duct at its bifurcation within the porta hepatis: an unusual tumour with distinctive clinical and pathological features. *American Journal of Medicine*, **38**, 241–256.
64. Koyama, K., Takaqi, Y. and Hok Sato, T. (1981) Experimental and clinical studies on the effect of biliary drainage in obstructive jaundice. *American Journal of Surgery*, **142**, 293–299.
65. Krige, J.E.J., Bornman, P.C., Harries-Jones, E.P. and Terblanche, J. (1987) Modified hepaticojejunostomy for permanent biliary access. *British Journal of Surgery*, **74**, 612–613.
66. Lameris, J.S., Stoker, J., Dees, J. *et al.* (1987) Non-surgical palliative treatment of patients with malignant biliary obstruction – the place of endoscopic and percutaneous drainage. *Clinical Radiology*, **38**, 603–608.
67. Lanes, S.F., Cohen, A., Rothman, K.J., Dreyer, N.A. and Soden, K.J. (1990) Mortality of cellulose fibre production workers. *Scandinavian Journal of Work, Environment and Health*, **16**, 247–251.
68. Launois, B., Campion, J.P., Brissot, P. and Gosselin, M. (1979) Carcinoma of the hepatic hilus. Surgical management and the case for resection. *Annals of Surgery*, **190**, 151.
69. Levitt, M.D., Laurence, B.H., Cameron, F. and Klemp, P.F.B. (1988) Transpapillary iridium-192 wire in the treatment of malignant bile duct obstruction. *Gut*, **29**, 149–152.
70. Little J.M. (1989) Hilar biliary cancer – are we getting it right? (Editorial comment.) *HPB Surgery*, **1**, 93–96.
71. Lokich, J.J., Kane, R.A., Harrison, D.A. and McDermott, W.V. (1987) Biliary tract obstruction secondary to cancer: management guidelines and selected literature review. *Journal of Clinical Oncology*, **5**, 969–981.
72. Longmire, W.P. Jr and Lippman, H.N. (1956) Intra-hepatic cholangiojejunostomy – an operation for biliary obstruction. *Surgical Clinics of North America*, **36**, 849–862.
73. Longmire, W.P., McArthur, M.S. and Bastounis, E.A. (1973) Carcinoma of the extrahepatic biliary tract. *Annals of Surgery*, **178**, 333.
74. McPherson, G.A.D., Benjamin, I.S. and Blumgart, L.H. (1984) Improving renal function in obstructive jaundice without preoperative drainage. *The Lancet*, **i**, 511.
75. McPherson, G.A.D., Benjamin, I.S., Hodgson, H.J.F., Bowley, N.B., Allison, D.J. and Blumgart, L.H. (1984) Pre-operative percutaneous transhepatic biliary drainage: the results of a controlled trial. *British Journal of Surgery*, **71**, 371–375.
76. Meyers, W.C. and Scott Jones, R. (1988) Internal radiation for bile duct cancer. *World Journal of Surgery*, **12**, 99–104.
77. Mimura, H., Kim, H., Ochiai, Y. *et al.* (1988) Radical block resection of hepatoduodenal ligament for carcinoma of the bile duct with double catheter bypass for portal circulation. *Surgery, Gynecology and Obstetrics*, **167**, 527–529.
78. Mizumoto, R., Kawarada, Y. and Suzuki, H. (1986) Surgical treatment of carcinoma of the bile duct. *Surgery, Gynecology and Obstetrics*, **162**, 153.
79. Morrow, C.E., Sutherland, D.E.R., Florack, G., Eisenberg, M.M. and Grage, T.B. (1983) Primary gallbladder carcinoma: significance of subserosal lesions and results of aggressive surgical treatment and adjuvant chemotherapy. *Surgery*, **94**, 709–714.

80. Murphy, J.R., Shay, S.S., Moses, F.M., Braxton, J., Jaques, D.P. and Wong, R.K. (1990) Suture granuloma masquerading as malignancy of the biliary tract. *Digestive Diseases and Sciences*, **35**, 1176–1179.
81. Nagino, M., Nimura, Y., Hayakawa, N., Kamiya, J., Kondoh, S. and Shionoya, S. (1988) Diagnostic value of computed tomography for the detection of invasion of the caudate bile duct branch in carcinoma of the hepatic hilum. *Nippon-Geka-Gakkai-Zasshi*, **89**, 889–897.
82. Nakama, M., Sugawara, T. and Ohgawara, K. (1990) Radiotherapy of carcinoma of the biliary system. *Nippon-Igaku-Hoshasen-Gakkai-Zasshi*, **50**, 398–403.
83. Nakayama, T., Ikeda, A. and Okuda, K. (1978) Percutaneous transhepatic drainage of the biliary tract. *Gastroenterology*, **74**, 554–559.
84. Nevin, J.E., Moran, T.J., Kay, S. and King, R. (1976) Carcinoma of the gallbladder. *Cancer*, **37**, 141–148.
85. Nimura, Y., Shionoya, S., Hayakawa, N., Kamiya, J., Kondo, S. and Yasui, A. (1988) Value of percutaneous transhepatic cholangioscopy (PTCS). *Surgical Endoscopy*, **2**, 213–219.
86. Nimura, Y., Kamiya, J., Hayakawa, N. and Shionoya, S. (1989) Cholangioscopic differentiation of biliary strictures and polyps. *Endoscopy*, **21**(suppl. 10), 351–356.
87. Nimura, Y., Hayakawa, N., Kamiya, J., Kondo, S. and Shionoya, S. (1990) Hepatic segmentectomy with caudate lobe resection for bile duct carcinoma of the hepatic hilus. *World Journal of Surgery*, **14**, 535–544.
88. Oberfield, R.A. and Rossi, R.L. (1988) The role of chemotherapy in the treatment of bile duct cancer. *World Journal of Surgery*, **12**, 105–108.
89. Ohta, T., Nagakawa, T., Ueno, K. *et al.* (1990) Clinical experience of biliary tract carcinoma associated with anomalous union of the pancreaticobiliary ductal system. *Japanese Journal of Surgery*, **20**, 36–43.
90. Olsen, J.H., Dragsted, L. and Autrup, H. (1988) Cancer risk and occupational exposure to aflatoxins in Denmark. *British Journal of Cancer*, **58**, 392–396.
91. Paganuzzi, M., Onetto, M., Marroni, P. *et al.* (1988) CA 19-9 and CA 50 in benign and malignant pancreatic and biliary diseases. *Cancer*, **61**, 2100–2108.
92. Pain, J.A. and Bailey, M.E. (1986) Experimental and clinical study of lactulose in obstructive jaundice. *British Journal of Surgery*, **73**, 775–778.
93. Pichlmayr, R., Ringe, B., Lauchart, W., Bechstein, W.O., Gubernatis, G. and Wagner, E. (1988) Radical resection and liver grafting as the two main components of surgical strategy in the treatment of proximal bile duct cancer. *World Journal of Surgery*, **12**, 68–77.
94. Pinson, C.W. and Rossi, R.L. (1988) Extended right hepatic lobectomy, left hepatic lobectomy, and skeletonization resection for proximal bile duct cancer. *World Journal of Surgery*, **12**, 52.
95. Pitt, H.A., Cameron, J.L., Postier, R.G. and Gadacz, T.R. (1981) Factors affecting mortality in biliary tract surgery. *American Journal of Surgery*, **141**, 66–72.
96. Pitt, H.A., Gomes, A.S., Lois, J.F., Mann, L.L., Deutsch, L.S. and Longmire, W.P. (1985) Does preoperative percutaneous biliary drainage reduce operative risk or increase hospital cost? *Annals of Surgery*, **201**, 9–16.
97. Poole, G.V. (1989) Trousseau's syndrome caused by malignant degeneration of a choledochal cyst. *Southern Medical Journal*, **82**, 1283–1284.
98. Pugliese, V., Barone, D., Saccomanno, S., Conio, M., Aste, H. and Santi, L. (1987) Tissue sampling from the common bile duct through endoscopic retrograde cholangiopancreatography, endoscopic papillo(sphinctero)tomy and drainage in juxtapapillary malignancies. *Surgical Endoscopy*, **1**, 83–87.
99. Ravindranath, K., Roddie, M., Adam, A. and Benjamin, I.S. (1990) Subparietal access loop for hepaticojejunostomy. *HPB Surgery*, **2**(suppl.), 335.
100. Renard, P., Boutron, M.C., Faivre, J. *et al.* (1987) Biliary tract cancers in Cote d'Or (France): incidence and natural history. *Journal of Epidemiology and Community Health*, **41**, 344–348.
101. Roberts-Thompson, I.C., Strickland, R.J. and MacKay, I.R. (1973) Bile duct carcinoma in chronic ulcerative colitis. *Australian and New Zealand Journal of Medicine*, **3**, 264–267.
102. Serra, I., Calvo, A., Maturana, M. and Sharp, A. (1990) Biliary tract cancer in Chile. *International Journal of Cancer*, **46**, 965–971.
103. Speer, A.G., Cotton, P.B., Russell, R.C.G. *et al.* (1987) Randomised trial of endoscopic versus percutaneous stent insertion in malignant obstructive jaundice. *The Lancet*, **ii**, 57–62.
104. Suda, K., Miyano, T., Suzuki, F. *et al.* (1987) Clinicopathologic and experimental studies on cases of abnormal pancreatico-choledocho-ductal junction. *Acta Pathologica Japonica*, **37**, 1549–1562.
105. Terblanche, J., Saunders, S.J. and Louw, J.H. (1972) Prolonged palliation in carcinoma of the main hepatic duct junction. *Surgery*, **71**, 720–731.
106. Terblanche, J., Kahn, D., Bornman, P.C. and Werner, D. (1988) The role of U-tube palliative treatment in high bile duct carcinoma. *Surgery*, **103**, 624–632.
107. Thomas, M.G., Grace, P.A., Benjamin, I.S. and Williamson, R.C.N. (1991) Carcinoma of the gallbladder, acute cholecystitis and cholecystostomy. *European Journal of Gastroenterology and Hepatology* (in press).
108. Thompson, J.N., Cohen, J., and McConnell, J.S. *et al.* (1985) A randomized controlled trial of pre-

operative oral ursodeoxycholic acid in obstructive jaundice. *British Journal of Surgery*, **72**, 1027.
109. Thompson, J.N., Edwards, W.H., Winearls, C.G., Blenkharn, J.I., Benjamin, I.S. and Blumgart, L.H. (1987) Renal impairment following biliary tract surgery. *British Journal of Surgery*, **74**, 843–847.
110. Tsuzuki, Y., Ogata, Y., Iida, S., Nakanishi, I., Takenaka, Y. and Yoshii, H. (1983) Carcinoma of the bifurcation of the hepatic ducts. *Archives of Surgery*, **118**, 1147.
111. Urban, M.S., Siegel, J.H., Pavlou, W. *et al.* (1990) Treatment of malignant biliary obstruction with a high-dose rate remote afterloading device using a 10 F nasobiliary tube. *Gastrointestinal Endoscopy*, **36**, 292–296.
112. Van Gulik, T.M., Brummelkamp, W.H. and Lygidakis, N.J. (1989) Traumatic neuroma giving rise to biliary obstruction after reconstructive surgery for iatrogenic lesions of the biliary tract – a report of three cases. *Hepatogastroenterology*, **36**, 255–257.
113. Voyles, C.R., Bowley, N.J., Allison, D.J., Benjamin, I.S. and Blumgart, L.H. (1983) Carcinoma of the proximal extrahepatic biliary tree. Radiological assessment and therapeutic alternatives. *Annals of Surgery*, **197**, 188–193.
114. Voyles, C.R., Smadja, C., Shands, C. and Blumgart, L.H. (1983) Carcinoma in choledochal cysts – age-related incidence. *Archives of Surgery*, **118**, 986–988.
115. Weinbren, K. and Mutum, S.S. (1983) Pathological aspects of cholangiocarcinoma. *Journal of Pathology*, **139**, 217–238.
116. Whipple, A.O., Parsons, W.B. and Mullins, C.R. (1935) Treatment of carcinoma of the ampulla of Vater. *Annals of Surgery*, **102**, 763–779.
117. Williamson, B.W., Blumgart, L.H. and McKellar, N.J. (1980) Management of tumours of the liver. Combined use of arteriography and venography in the assessment of resectability especially in hilar tumours. *American Journal of Surgery*, **139**, 210–215.
118. Yeung, E.Y.C., Adam, A., Gibson, R.N., Benjamin, I.S. and Allison, D.J. (1988) Spiral-shaped biliary endoprosthesis: initial study. *Radiology*, **168**, 365–369.
119. Yeung, E., O'Donnell, C., Carvalho, P. and Adam, A. (1989) A new technique for removal of double mushroom-tipped endoprostheses. *American Journal of Radiology*, **152**, 527–528.
120. Yeung, E., McCarthy, P., Gompertz, R.H. *et al.* (1989) Ultrasonic appearances of hilar cholangiocarcinoma. *British Journal of Radiology* (in press).

OTHER DISORDERS

I.A.D. Bouchier

GALLBLADDER DISEASE IN CHILDREN

Cholelithiasis and cholecystitis are rare in neonates and children[12] but present clinically in a manner similar to adults: right upper quadrant pain, nausea, vomiting and jaundice. The diagnosis can be made by plain abdominal radiography, for there is a greater possibility of the gallstones being calcified in children than in adults, and by cholecystography, ultrasonography and radionuclide scanning if necessary.

A variety of causes has been implicated in the genesis of gallbladder disease in children, including congenital abnormalities in the case of neonates, systemic infections in young children and cholelithiasis in older children. It is claimed that acalculous cholelithiasis is commoner in children than in adults. Haemolytic disease is uncommonly responsible for gallstones in children but patients with sickle cell anaemia, congenital spherocytosis, and glucose-6-phosphate dehydrogenase deficiency are at risk of developing pigment stones, and gallstone disease must be considered when patients with sickle cell disease present with an abdominal crisis.[2] There is a prominent association between cholelithiasis and early pregnancy in adolescence, disease or resection of the terminal ileum and long-term parenteral nutrition. Many of the children are obese and, in contrast to adults, gallstones in children occur with almost equal frequency in males and females.[7]

The management of children follows the same principles as for adults and a cholecystectomy is recommended. Intraoperative cholangiography is recommended for patients with bilirubin levels greater than 35 μmol/l, a dilated common bile duct, palpable common bile duct stones, or a history of pancreatitis.[2]

HYPERPLASTIC CHOLECYSTOSES

This term has been used to describe a variety of degenerative and non-inflammatory hyperplastic disorders involving the gallbladder mucosa and muscle. The unitary concept remains controversial and includes such conditions as adenomyomatosis, cholesterolosis, neuromatosis, lipomatosis, fibromatosis and calcified gallbladder. The lesions can be generalized, localized or segmental.[1]

ADENOMYOMATOSIS

In this disorder there is hyperplasia of the muscle and mucosa of the gallbladder. The projection of pouches of mucous membrane through weak points in the muscle coat, possibly due to raised intracystic pressure, produces the so-called Rokitansky–Aschoff sinuses or crypts. These are probably identical with intramural diverticula.[20] Muscular dysfunction, spasm and stenosis of the cystic duct have also been implicated. The diverticula (or sinuses or crypts) are usually intramural and are not recognized with the naked eye. They may contain pigmented stones. The diverticula may opacify on cholecystography and are best seen after gallbladder contraction when they appear as a 'halo' or ring of opacified beads around the gallbladder. Other appearances include hyperconcentration, hyperfunction, deformity of the body of the gallbladder or marked irregularity of outline. Localized adenomyomatosis is responsible for the appearance of a phrygian cap at the gallbladder fundus.

Ultrasonographic features of adenomyomatosis include thickening of the gallbladder wall, round anechoic areas in the thickened portion of the gallbladder wall, and echogenic areas within the gallbladder wall representing stones within diverticula.[6]

CHOLESTEROLOSIS

The question whether cholesterolosis of the gallbladder produces symptoms or is simply a pathological curiosity has been debated since the condition was first described by Virchow more than 100 years ago.

Cholesterolosis is an acalculous disease of the gallbladder characterized by the accumulation of lipids in the mucosa producing characteristic yellow, golden lipid deposits in the mucosa, called by some the 'strawberry gallbladder' appearance. Although gallstones may be present, the condition occurs independently of stone formation. The aetiology is not fully understood. The bile is frequently supersaturated with cholesterol and the mucosal changes might arise from increased cholesterol uptake from the bile. Other hypotheses are that there is increased mucosal synthesis of lipids, or that the submucosal macrophages fail to metabolize or excrete cholesterol which is absorbed from the bile.

Cholesterolosis has a prevalence of 9–26% based on surgical studies and about 12% from autopsy data. The condition is found most frequently in women aged 30–50 years. The commonest complaint (96%) is colicky right upper quadrant or epigastric pain which may be severe. Nausea and vomiting occur in 61%, dyspepsia in 60% with some degree of selective food intolerance. Obviously the symptoms can be difficult to distinguish from those of the irritable bowel syndrome.

The radiological diagnosis of cholesterolosis is difficult because oral cholecystography detects only 35% of cases (the features are small, fixed filling defects) and ultrasound is equally unrewarding. The cholecystokinin provocation test[17] has been suggested as a means of making a preoperative diagnosis. Symptomatic patients with acalculous biliary disease have their pain reproduced by an intravenous injection of cholecystokinin. Treatment is by cholecystectomy but the dilemma remains one of patient selection and how to avoid performing an unnecessary cholecystectomy on the patient with the irritable bowel syndrome.[14]

CLINICAL FEATURES

There is much disagreement over the clinical significance of the hyperplastic cholecystoses and whether or not they produce symptoms. Some authors attribute right upper quadrant pain and other digestive disorders to the condition,[9] whereas others are more cautious in ascribing a clinical syndrome to the pathology. Hyperplastic cholecystoses are probably common, one or other of the features being recognized histologically in up to 50% of resected gallbladders. Cholecystitis and cholelithiasis may be superimposed on a gallbladder with hyperplastic cholecystoses.

TREATMENT

Management is controversial and depends on whether or not there is a belief that the disorder is a cause of symptoms in which event cholecystectomy is recommended. The indication for surgery is more certain when there is, in addition, cholecystitis or cholelithiasis, which occurs in about 20% of patients.

VASCULITIS

Cholecystitis may occur as a rare complication in polyarteritis nodosa, systemic lupus erythematosus and giant cell arteritis. The gallbladder disease takes the form of an acute acalculous cholecystitis and is managed by a cholecystectomy.

EMPHYSEMATOUS CHOLECYSTITIS

In this disorder there is acute cholecystitis with the formation of gas in the wall or lumen of the gallbladder and in the biliary tract. The organisms are similar to those found in the more commonly encountered variety of cholecystitis. The condition is rare and found particularly in aged patients and those with diabetes mellitus.

The presentation is that of an acute severe cholecystitis and plain radiographs reveal gas in the biliary system. The patient requires an urgent cholecystectomy with adequate antibiotic cover particularly with penicillin and an aminoglycoside because the most common gas-forming bacteria in bile are clostridia and *Escherichia coli*.

HAEMOBILIA

Bleeding from the gallbladder is rare and the term 'haemocholecyst' has been suggested to distinguish gallbladder bleeding from bleeding into the extra- and intrahepatic ducts.[4] The causes of gallbladder bleeding include erosion of the cystic artery by a gallstone, haemorrhagic cholecystitis, cancer of the gallbladder and aberrant pancreatic tissue in the gallbladder wall. Rarely, the bleeding may produce sufficient pressure to rupture the viscus thereby inducing a haemoperitoneum.

INTRAHEPATIC LITHIASIS

Three varieties of intrahepatic gallstones have been described: (1) primary intrahepatic gallstones when stones are present only in the intrahepatic biliary radicals; (2) intrahepatic gallstones secondary to infection or biliary stasis; (3) mixed intrahepatic and extrahepatic bile duct gallstones.

Primary intrahepatic gallstones are usually found in the Far East and are related particularly to the parasitic infestations ascariasis and clonorchiasis. *Ascaris lumbricoides*, together with the liver flukes *Clonorchis sinensis* (Chinese liver fluke), *Fasciola hepatica* (sheep liver fluke) and *Opisthorchis viverrini*, may be a cause for acalculous cholecystitis of gallstones.

Mixed intra- and extrahepatic bile duct stones are a complication in 1–2.5% of patients with gallstones in the West. The presentation is with right-sided abdominal pain, fever and jaundice, and the diagnosis is established either by percutaneous, transhepatic cholangiography or endoscopic retrograde cholangiography. The management is by surgical removal of the gallstones, flushing of the biliary tree and the establishment of permanent, adequate, biliary drainage. Usually a papillotomy or choledochotomy is sufficient but occasionally it is necessary to perform a segmental hepatic resection. A Roux-en-Y hepaticojejunostomy is advised if the calibre of the biliary tree is greater than 2 cm.

Surgical drainage is not always successful and about 10% of patients suffer from recurrent bile stasis and cholangitis, and eventually they develop liver failure.

TORSION OF THE GALLBLADDER

This is a rare condition in which ageing and a distinct mesentery to the gallbladder are predisposing factors but others include weight loss, cirrhosis and kyphoscoliosis. Gallstones are not necessarily present. The patient presents with acute abdominal pain, nausea and vomiting, and the condition is difficult to diagnose preoperatively but the absence of fever and jaundice and the presence of a right upper quandrant mass are suggestive features. Management is by early cholecystectomy once the general condition of the patient has been stabilized.[8,19]

XANTHOGRANULOMATOUS CHOLECYSTITIS

This is characterized by an irregularly thickened gallbladder wall with poorly demarcated yellow nodules of varying size which on microscopy are seen to comprise foamy histiocytes and chronic inflammatory cells. The clinical features are those of chronic cholecystitis and ultrasonography reveals a thickened sonolucent gallbladder wall containing finely echogenic non-shadowing material.[18] Half the patients have gallstones, and a carcinoma complicates the condition in 15%.

ACUTE BILIARY TRACT DISEASE IN PREGNANCY

Biliary tract disease in pregnancy is rare and usually due to calculous cholecystitis. Ultrasonography, being non-invasive, is the diagnostic test of choice. The patient's complaints must be distinguished from other intra-abdominal conditions. Hyperamylasaemia seems to be common. Patients explored in the third trimester will proceed to a normal pregnancy but operations in the first trimester appear to be associated with an increased risk of the pregnancy not proceeding to full term.[11,13] Many patients can be managed conservatively without cholecystectomy until the pregnancy has been completed, or else the operation delayed where possible until the second or third trimester. Analgesia and antibiotics such as broad-spectrum β-lactam agents should be used with care.

MISCELLANEOUS CONDITIONS

Acute cholecystitis due to cytomegalovirus invasion of the gallbladder may occur in the acquired immunodeficiency syndrome. The gallbladder may become gangrenous.[5,15] Cytomegalovirus infection of the gallbladder has been recorded following liver transplantation. Acute cholecystitis occurs as a complication in sarcoidosis[10] and following hepatic arterial infusion of floxuridine.[16] Tuberculous cholecystitis may be part of a tuberculous process involving the other intra-abdominal organs, or may be limited to the gallbladder, or may occur as part of miliary tuberculosis or severe generalized tuberculosis.[3] Perforation of the gallbladder is a rare occurrence in the absence of gallstones.[22]

REFERENCES

1. Aguirre, J.R., Boher R.O. and Guraeib, S. (1969) Hyperplastic cholecystoses: a new contribution to the unitarian theory. *American Journal of Roentgenology*, **107**, 1–13.
2. Bailey, P.V., Connors, R.H., Tracy, T.F.J. *et al.* (1989) Changing spectrum of cholelithiasis and cholecystitis in infants and children. *American Journal of Surgery*, **158**, 585–588.
3. Bergdahl, L. and Boquist, L. (1972) Tuberculosis of the gall-bladder. *British Journal of Surgery*, **59**, 289–292.
4. Bismuth, H. (1973) Hemobilia. *New England Journal of Medicine*, **288**, 617–619.
5. Blumberg, R.S., Kelsey, P., Perrone, T. *et al.* (1984) Cytomegalovirus- and cryptosporidium-associated calculous gangrenous cholecystitis. *American Journal of medicine*, **76**, 1118–1123.
6. Costa-Greco, M.A. (1987) Adenomyomatosis of the gallbladder. *Journal of Clinical Ultrasound*, **15**, 198–199.
7. Crichlow, R.W., Seltzer, M.H. and Janetta, P.J. (1972) Cholecystitis in adolescents. *American Journal of Digestive Diseases*, **17**, 68–72.
8. Duari, M. (1966) Two cases of acute torsion of the gallbladder. *Gut*, **7**, 73–76.
9. Elfving, G., Lehtonen, T. and Teir, H. (1967) Clinical significance of primary hyperplasia of gallbladder mucosa. *Annals of Surgery*, **165**, 61–69.
10. Freed, J.S. and Reiner, M.A. (1983) Acute cholecystitis as a complication of sarcoidosis. *Archives of Internal Medicine*, **143**, 2188–2189.
11. Gray, J.R. and Bouchier, I.A.D. (1989) Liver disease and pregnancy. *Gastroenterology International*, **2**, 217–221.
12. Harned, R.K. and Babbit, D.P. (1975) Cholelithiasis in children. *Radiology*, **117**, 391–393.
13. Hiatt, J.R., Hiatt, J.C.G., Williams, R.A. and Klein, S.R. (1986) Biliary disease in pregnancy: strategy for surgical management. *American Journal of Surgery*, **151**, 263–265.
14. Jacyna, M.R. and Bouchier, I.A.D. (1987) Cholesterolosis: a physical cause of "functional" disorder. *British Medical Journal*, **295**, 619–620.
15. Kavin, H., Jonas, R., Chowdhury, L. and Kabins, L. (1986) Acalculous cholecystitis and cytomegalovirus infection in the acquired immunodeficiency syndrome. *Annals of Internal Medicine*, **104**, 53–54.
16. Lafon, P.C., Reed, K. and Rosenthal, D. (1984) Acute cholecystitis associated with hepatic arterial infusion of floxuridine. *American Journal of Surgery*, **150**, 687–689.
17. Lennard, T.W.J., Farndon, J.R. and Taylor, R.M.R. (1984) Acalculous biliary pain: diagnosis and selection for cholecystectomy using the cholecystokinin test. *British Journal of Surgery*, **71**, 368–370.
18. Lichtman, J.B. and Varma, V.A. (1987) Ultrasound demonstration of Xanthogranulomatous cholecystitis. *Journal of Clinical Ultrasound*, **15**, 342–345.
19. McGregor, J.R., Akyol, M. and Macpherson, S.G. (1988) Acute torsion of the gallbladder. *Scottish Medical Journal*, **33**, 277.
20. Ochsner, S.F. (1971) Intramural lesions of the gallbladder. *American Journal of Roentgenology*, **113**, 1–9.
21. Simi, M., Loriga, P., Basoli, A. *et al.* (1979) Intrahepatic lithiasis. *American Journal of Surgery*, **137**, 317–322.
22. Thornton, J.G. (1984) Spontaneous performation of the gallbladder without gallstones. *British Journal of Surgery*, **71**, 314.

CHAPTER 13

THE PERITONEUM

CONGENITAL ABNORMALITIES OF THE ANTERIOR ABDOMINAL WALL, PERITONEUM AND MESENTERY

M.H. Lyall

ANTERIOR ABDOMINAL WALL

The anterior abdominal wall contains and protects the abdominal viscera. During early intrauterine life the wall is severely deficient, permitting herniation of the midgut loop into the extra-embryonic coelom. In this way a 'physiological' umbilical hernia is produced. By the 10th week of intrauterine life the mid-gut returns to the abdominal cavity and, simultaneously, the abdominal wall develops to completely enclose the abdominal viscera. The umbilical cord is attached to the abdominal wall at the umbilical ring. Within about 10 days of birth the cord shrivels, dries and separates at its junction with the skin, and the umbilical ring closes.

Congenital abnormalities of the abdominal wall and umbilicus are common, although most are of a minor nature.

UMBILICAL HERNIA

This is caused by the umbilical ring failing to close completely. A small sac of peritoneum is forced through the gap in the linea alba and becomes attached to the overlying skin. During crying or straining, bowel or omentum bulges through the gap into the peritoneal sac. The hernia is almost always easily reducible and incarceration is rare. In most children the gap closes spontaneously and the hernia disappears. If the hernia persists after the age of three years, however, it is unlikely to close spontaneously and surgical repair should be carried out.

PARA-UMBILICAL HERNIA

In this condition the umbilical ring closes normally after birth, but there is a small defect usually just above or, less commonly, just below the umbilicus, giving rise to a para-umbilical hernia. This will not close spontaneously, so is repaired surgically.

EPIGASTRIC HERNIA

This is caused by a defect in the linea alba, usually located midway between the xiphoid process and the umbilicus. A small piece of extraperitoneal fat protrudes through the defect, causing a swelling. This will often produce pain and tenderness. The fat should be removed and the defect repaired.

DIVARICATION OF THE RECTUS MUSCLE

Occasionally the rectus muscles are separated from the midline leaving a wide, weak linea alba. This causes ventral herniation. Minor degrees do not require surgical treatment but, if the defect is large, surgical repair can be carried out.

EXOMPHALOS (OMPHALOCELE)

This is a rare, but serious, major hernia through the anterior abdominal wall at the umbilicus. The intestine is covered by a glistening, transparent membrane consisting of amniotic sac lined by peritoneum. As the membrane is avascular, it disintegrates rapidly, becoming opaque in 12 hours and rupturing by 36 hours, thus exposing the abdominal viscera. Prompt surgical intervention is essential if the life of the baby is to be saved.

The two main types are hernia into the umbilical cord (exomphalos minor) and exomphalos major.

Hernia into the umbilical cord (exomphalos minor)

In this condition the midgut loop has failed to return normally into the abdominal cavity. The neck of the sac is an abnormally wide umbilical ring but is usually less than 5 cm in diameter. The herniated loops of gut occupy the base of the cord. It is often possible to reduce the hernia by simply twisting the cord. As the umbilical defect is usually small, it is possible to excise the avascular sac and repair the abdominal wall in layers.

Exomphalos major

In this case the defect in the abdominal wall is much larger. The avascular sac contains multiple loops of small intestine and often liver as well. Because the physiological umbilical hernia of intrauterine life fails to return to the abdominal cavity, it is common to have associated malrotation of the midgut loop. Other congenital defects are common, especially cardiac and renal tract abnormalities.

Immediate treatment consists of covering the sac with a sterile plastic bag. Definitive treatment should be carried out within a few hours of delivery. The abdominal cavity is often too small, however, to allow reduction of the hernia. The aim of the operation is, therefore, to remove the avascular sac, to mobilize skin flaps from the remainder of the abdominal wall and to suture the skin over the defect. No attempt is made to repair the muscle layers. In this way skin cover is produced but with a ventral hernia. A formal repair of the abdominal musculature is performed at about 2 years of age.[1]

If skin cover is not possible, it is necessary to carry out a staged repair of the defect using silastic sheeting.[2] This method is extremely useful in dealing with very large defects. The sac is excised and the skin is undercut from the margins of the defect. Silastic sheets are then sutured to the muscle at the margins of the defect. They are then sutured to each other over the exposed viscera like the ridge of a tent. The skin is sutured to the silastic sheets as far up the side of the sheeting as possible. Every 2–3 days the abdominal contents are squeezed further into the abdominal cavity and a fresh row of sutures is placed between the silastic sheets. The length of the sheets covering the defect is thus gradually shortened and the skin and rectus muscle of each side are brought closer together. After 2 weeks it is usually possible to remove the silastic sheets and to approximate the skin.

GASTROSCHISIS

In gastroschisis there is a defect in the anterior abdominal wall, in the region of the umbilicus, allowing loops of bowel to protrude. There are, however, several important differences between this condition and exomphalos. In gastroschisis, the umbilical cord is situated in the normal position, and the defect is usually just to the right of the cord. There is no sac and the herniated viscera are completely exposed. Unlike exomphalos, associated congenital abnormalities are rare, which improves the prognosis. Treatment is similar, the aim also being to return the bowel to the abdominal cavity and to obtain skin cover in a manner such as that described for exomphalos.

PERSISTENCE OF THE VITELLOINTESTINAL DUCT

In early intrauterine life the vitellointestinal duct connects the apex of the midgut loop with the vitelline sac. It normally becomes obliterated and disappears completely. Whole or part of the vitello-intestinal duct may occasionally persist, however, giving rise to several characteristic congenital abnormalities. If the entire duct remains, there is a patent communication between the ileum and the umbilicus which may discharge faeces or flatus; if only the proximal end persists, a Meckel's diverticulum is formed. Persistence of the distal part of the duct leads to an umbilical sinus which is lined by intestinal mucosa and secretes mucus. Rarely, the proximal and distal ends of the vitellointestinal duct are closed but the middle part remains patent. Mucus is secreted into the open part causing cystic dilatation.

THE PERITONEUM AND MESENTERY

Major abnormalities of fixation of the mesentery to the posterior abdominal wall are rare and are associated with either non-rotation, incomplete rotation or malrotation of the midgut loop. Incomplete fixation of the small intestinal mesentery, which is then free to twist, gives rise to neonatal volvulus of the small intestine.

Minor abnormalities of peritoneal fixation are common, especially at the duodenojejunal junction and in the ileocaecal region. The peritoneum may be folded beneath the bowel and reflected on to the posterior abdominal wall forming a pouch. Such pouches are of clinical importance, as loops of small intestine may be trapped within them, causing internal herniation and intestinal obstruction.

Occasionally abnormal peritoneal bands are present, passing between the intestine and the posterior abdominal wall. These may cause compression of the small intestine and mechanical obstruction.

CONGENITAL CYSTS OF THE MESENTERY

Congenital cysts are occasionally found within the peritoneal cavity. They may be small and asymptomatic: an incidental finding at laparotomy; or they may become very large and present either as a painless abdominal swelling or as recurrent attacks of abdominal pain and vomiting. Acute abdominal symptoms may be precipitated by infection, torsion or rupture. The two most common congenital cysts of the mesentery are chylolymphatic and enterogenous.

The chylolymphatic cyst arises in congenitally abnormal lymphatic tissue. There is no efferent communication with the rest of the lymphatic system and cystic dilatation occurs. The commonest site is in the small-bowel mesentery. The cyst may be multilocular or unilocular and contains either clear lymph or chyle. Treatment is by surgical excision.

An enterogenous cyst arises as a result of duplication of the intestine and is usually situated on the mesenteric side of the small intestine. Its wall is similar to that of the small intestine, being lined with mucous membrane. There is no communication with the adjacent intestine but the cyst shares the same blood supply; hence enucleation is impossible and resection of the affected part of the intestine is necessary.

REFERENCES

1. Gross, R.E. (1948) A new method for surgical treatment of large omphaloceles. *Surgery*, **24**, 277.
2. Schuster, S.R. (1967) A new method for the staged repair of large omphaloceles. *Surgery, Gynaecology and Obstetrics*, **125**, 837.

ASCITES

I.A.D. Bouchier

PERITONEUM

The peritoneum is a complex serous membrane which lines the abdominal wall and is reflected over the viscera within the abdomen. The parietal and visceral layers are developed, respectively, from the somatopleural and splanchnopleural layers of the lateral plate mesoderm. The peritoneal cavity is closed in the male but communicates with the open ends of the uterine tubes in females. There are many ligaments, two omenta, a greater and a lesser mesentery, and many peritoneal recesses and folds between the organs. The total area of peritoneal surface in the adult is between 1.5 and 2.0 m^2, approximately equal to the total body surface area. The blood flow to the peritoneum is from 50–70 ml/min.

The normal peritoneum consists of a single layer of flattened mesothelial cells with round or oval nuclei and a submesothelial layer of collagen and reticular fibres. Microvilli protrude from the free mesothelial surface, which is lubricated by a small volume of serous fluid.[14] In women of reproductive age the amount of fluid varies, being greatest (20 ± 6 ml) during the luteal phase. If the ovaries are inactive, the volume is 4 ± 2 ml.[32] Peritoneal fluid in females may be derived in part from ovarian exudation.

The peritoneum participates in solute exchange and is permeable to molecules of small and intermediate molecular weight (500–5000 daltons). Transfer of substances occurs probably by both simple intercellular and transcellular movement. Diffusion of ions is quantitatively greater across the mesentery than by transfer across the parietal peritoneum. Particulate material is taken up by phagocytic cells.

There is still controversy over the mechanism of peritoneal repair. The most favoured concept is that healing occurs by the development of new mesothelial cells from metaplasia of subperitoneal fibroblasts. It is unlikely that the mechanism is by transformation of peritoneal macrophages or by the seeding of mesothelial cells from adjacent normal peritoneal surfaces. Three phases are discernible in the development of adhesions: first, from 0–7 hours after injury, degeneration and desquamation of mesothelial cells occurs; second, from 7 hours to 10 days, fibrin is deposited on the exposed basement membrane and fibrinous adhesions are formed; third, from 10–30 days, the transformation of fibrinous to fibrous adhesions occurs.[55]

Ascites is the accumulation of excess fluid in the peritoneal cavity. The causes are listed in *Table 13.1*, the commonest in the UK being malignant disease and cirrhosis of the liver. Fluid accumulates when it enters the peritoneal cavity from the mesenteries, the peritoneum and hepatic surface at a rate greater than can be returned to the circulation via the capillaries and lymphatics.

Table 13.1 Causes of ascites

Liver disease (see Table 13.2)	Cirrhosis
	Budd-Chiari syndrome
	Subacute hepatic necrosis
	Fulminant hepatic failure
	Malignant infiltration
	Veno-occlusive disease
	Hepatocellular cancer
	Cholangiocarcinoma
Cardiac	Congestive cardiac failure
	Constrictive pericarditis
	Tricuspid insufficiency
	Cardiomyopathies
Renal	Nephrotic syndrome
	Acute glomerulonephritis
	Chronic peritoneal dialysis
	Long-term haemodialysis
	Renal transplant
Pancreatic	Malignant disease
	Chronic pancreatitis
	Acute pancreatitis
	Pseudocyst
Infection/inflammation	Bacterial peritonitis
	acute
	spontaneous
	Intestinal perforation
	Tuberculosis
	Syphilis
	Pyogenic infection
	Filariasis
	Fungal (candidiasis)
Malignant disease	Metastatic cancer of:
	pancreas
	ovary
	colon
	stomach
	prostate
	uterus
	testes
	breasts
	neuroblastoma

Table 13.1 Continued

Malignant disease *Continued*	Mesothelioma Leukaemia Sarcoma Lymphoma Myeloma Pseudomyxomi peritonei
Ovarian disease (Meig's syndrome)	Ovarian tumours Struma ovarii Ovarian hyperstimulation syndrome
Venous thrombosis	Portal vein obstruction Inferior vena cava obstruction
Malnutrition/protein–energy malnutrition	Protein-losing enteropathy

Miscellaneous	Trauma
	Bile leak
	Endometriosis
	Myxoedema
	Recurrent polyserositis
	Familial Mediterranean Fever
	Whipple's disease
	Congenital dysplasia of the lymphatic system
	Vasculitis
	  systemic lupus erythematosus
	  Henoch-Schonlein purpura
	Crohn's disease
	Sarcoidosis
	Eosinophilic ascites
	Granulomatous peritonitis
	Urinary ascites of newborn (see Table 13.4)

CLINICAL FEATURES

The patient may be unaware of the presence of ascites, but sudden and marked accumulation of peritoneal fluid is accompanied by abdominal discomfort, which may be severe, and cause dyspnoea. Pain is often a feature of malignant ascites.

The classic physical sign of free fluid is shifting dullness. The demonstration of a fluid thrill is less satisfactory. However, even the clinical detection of ascites is unreliable. Clinicians are accurate in only 50% of patients in diagnosing small volumes of ascites, the error usually being to overdiagnose the presence of free fluid. At least one litre of fluid is necessary to detect shifting dullness and the sign can be mimicked by a loaded colon with a long mesentery. It is claimed that as little as 300–400 ml of fluid can be detected when the abdomen is percussed with the patient in the knee – chest position – the 'puddle' sign, but this is an inelegant and uncomfortable examination.

With greater accumulation of fluid, there is abdominal distension and bulging of the flanks, elevation of the diaphragm, eversion of the umbilicus, and scrotal and lower limb oedema, probably from pressure upon the inferior vena cava. Renal function may be compromised by compression of the renal veins and proteinuria ensues. In gross ascites, slightly elevated jugular venous pressure may be observed. A pleural effusion develops in about 10% of patients, probably from the passage of ascitic fluid through small tears in the peritoneum overlying defects in the diaphragm. The effusion is usually found in the right pleural cavity. An umbilical hernia may develop and if the ascites is very tense it may rupture,[31] but this is a rarity occurring only once in the author's experience.

Ascites must be distinguished from gaseous distension of the bowel (the abdomen is resonant and the umbilicus never becomes everted), obesity, pregnancy, large intra-abdominal tumours, and ovarian cysts. Characteristically, ovarian cysts demonstrate dullness in the centre of the abdomen and resonance in the flanks – the very opposite of the finding in ascites.

INVESTIGATIONS

The clinical diagnosis of gross ascites is generally easy but, if there is any doubt, the fluid may be demonstrated radiologically, or by diagnostic paracentesis. Paracentesis with chemical, microbiological and cytological examination of the fluid is mandatory in all patients presenting for the first time with ascites, unless there are specific contraindications.

PLAIN RADIOGRAPH OF THE ABDOMEN

In the presence of ascites, there is a generalized hazy appearance with loss of density and detail, particularly at the hepatic angle, and obliteration of the psoas shadow. Supine and lateral views show the gut to be floating on fluid: but the plain radiograph is diagnostic in less than 50% of patients.

ULTRASONIC SCAN

Longitudinal and transverse abdominal scans are performed on patients who are supine, but occasionally other positions are used to demonstrate a fluid shift. The technique is more sensitive than radiology and can detect as little as 100–300 ml of the fluid; but the technique is highly dependent on the operator.

Early features on the scan are free fluid in the superior right paracolic gutter, lateral to the liver, or in the pelvis. As fluid accumulates, it is detected around and beneath the liver and in the lesser sac, the transverse colon floats on the surface of the fluid and loops of small intestine are arranged around the mesentery. The bowel has a characteristic polycystic or arcuate appearance; it usually floats but sinks when empty. Ultrasonography can differentiate between free fluid, loculated fluid, and between fluid in the gallbladder, urinary bladder or an ovarian cyst.[17] The features of a *transudate* are homogeneous echo-free areas surrounding and interposed between the loops of bowels and the viscera in a uniform manner; the features of an *exudate* are small amorphous echoes, septa and matted loops of bowel. Upper abdominal ultrasound allows screening of the liver, spleen, pancreas and kidneys for disease. Both the portal and splenic veins can be evaluated by this technique which can be combined with Doppler sonography. Ultrasound examination of the abdomen helps in the differentiation of ascitic fluid from cystic ovarian tumours and is of particular value in the diagnosis of the Budd-Chiari syndrome.[7]

COMPUTED TOMOGRAPHY

This technique accurately detects small volumes of fluid, particularly when in the pelvic, perihepatic or perisplenic regions. It is of especial help in the diagnosis of intra-abdominal masses associated with ascites, to delineate the retroperitoneal area, and to diagnose haemoperitoneum.

PARACENTESIS

This simple and safe procedure can be undertaken for diagnostic purposes but also may be used to relieve the discomfort of massive ascites and, more recently, as a therapeutic procedure in the management of ascites. The patient should first empty the bladder. Aspiration is made under local anaesthesia using a 21 gauge needle. The usual site is in either of the iliac fossae, midway between the anterior superior iliac spine and the umbilicus. For diagnostic purposes, about 50 ml of fluid is aspirated and examined microscopically, microbiologically, chemically and cytologically. Leakage of fluid following removal of the needle is avoided by using a 'Z' track entry, applying pressure to the site of paracentesis and keeping the patient supine for a few hours after paracentesis.[5]

MACROSCOPIC APPEARANCES

The fluid in cirrhosis is generally translucent and yellow to light green in appearance, deriving some of its colour from bilirubin. Blood-stained ascites is a feature of trauma, neoplastic involvement of the peritoneum or tuberculosis. The fluid may be bile-stained or chylous which can be recognized by the white, turbid appearance. A cloudy fluid suggests infection but this appearance also occurs in one-third of patients with uninfected ascites, and in the absence of raised white-blood-cell concentrations.[3]

BIOCHEMISTRY

Proteins

The protein content is used to distinguish a transudate, which has a total protein of less than 25 g/l, from an exudate, which has a greater concentration of protein. A transudate is typical in cirrhosis of the liver, cardiac failure and in those diseases with a low serum albumin. Protein levels as high as 50 g/l have been reported in chronic liver disease, congestive cardiac failure and constrictive pericarditis, however, when the protein probably originates from the lymphatics. Of those patients with liver disease,

17% have an ascitic fluid protein greater than 30 g/l and 12% have concentrations of more than 40 g/l. An exudate suggests that the fluid is inflammatory, malignant or traumatic in origin but rarely, malignant ascites has a protein level of less than 20 g/l.

The ratio of serum ascites to albumin is an effective method for differentiating transudative from exudative ascites.[39,59] A ratio of more than 1.1 is indicative of portal hypertension. The ratio is also valuable in distinguishing the raised ascitic protein found in malignant peritonitis from the high protein ascites found in both congestive cardiac failure and hypothyroidism, where the ratio is greater than 1.1.

Glucose

Ascitic glucose concentration is generally low in bacterial infections, tuberculosis and malignant ascites, but the results are variable and the measurement does not have diagnostic value.

Enzymes

Amylase concentrations of more than 2000 u/l and elevated lipase levels occur in ascites of pancreatic origin. Lactic dehydrogenase levels greater than 500 sigma units occur in malignant disease, but this enzyme does not distinguish clearly between a transudate and an exudate.

pH

The ascitic fluid in patients with bacterial peritonitis may have a low pH, ranging from 7.12–7.31 in contrast to the normal range of 7.38–7.58,[23] but the finding is not sufficiently consistent to be a reliable sign of infected ascites. Claims that an ascitic fluid pH of 7.34 or less or an arterial blood:ascitic fluid pH gradient of 0.10 or more is of diagnostic value[60] have not been substantiated.[2,54]

CYTOLOGY

White cell count

A white cell count greater than 500/mm^3, with more than 50% polymorphonuclear cells, suggests bacterial peritonitis. Only 10% of cirrhotic patients with sterile ascites have a cell count greater than 500 cells/mm^3, and 90% of the cells in such effusions are mononuclear. If mononuclear cells predominate in a raised ascitic white cell count, tuberculosis, neoplasm and pancreatic ascites should be considered.[9] The presence of candida in the absence of peritoneal dialysis suggests intestinal perforation.

Cytodiagnosis

Cells are exfoliated from the peritoneum in the presence of ascites but they are often so grossly deformed and coated with mucus and fibrin that conventional light and electron microscopy are unhelpful. These techniques lack both specificity and sensitivity. Scanning electron microscopy holds more promise because it provides a three-dimensional view and it is possible to distinguish lymphocytes (with short microvilli), mesothelial cells (with denser microvilli), histocytes (with laminar-shaped microvilli) and adenocarcinoma (with very dense microvilli).

DIAGNOSTIC PARACENTESIS IN THE ACUTE ABDOMEN

A variety of methods has been described. A four-quadrant tap is regarded as unnecessary. Either needle aspiration under local anaesthesia is performed at the point of maximum abdominal tenderness, or a dialysis catheter is introduced in the midline below the umbilicus and manipulated into the pelvis. Aspiration of more than 1 ml of fluid is regarded as a positive indication of intraperitoneal disease. The technique is useful in assessing abdominal trauma, acute pancreatitis and in assessment of postoperative complications.[24]

OTHER INVESTIGATIONS

Other investigations which may provide diagnostic help include peritoneal biopsy (of particular value in tuberculous peritonitis rather than malignant disease), laparoscopy and serum thyroxine levels.

ASCITES IN CIRRHOSIS OF THE LIVER

The process of fluid accumulation in cirrhotic patients has been studied intensively and a number of mechanisms are recognized which operate to varying degrees in individual patients.

PORTAL HYPERTENSION

The causes of an increased portal venous pressure, that is a pressure greater than 14 mmHg, are shown in *Table 13.2*. Under normal resting conditions only one fifth of the sinusoids are perfused by portal blood; there is no increase in the portal blood pressure until the portal blood flow has increased five-fold.[12] Conversely, small increases in portal

Table 13.2 Classification of portal hypertension

Suprahepatic	Veno-occlusive disease Hepatic vein occlusion (Budd-Chiari syndrome) Constrictive pericarditis Right-sided heart failure
Intrahepatic	Cirrhosis – from any cause Hepatitis Congenital hepatic fibrosis Partial nodular transformation Idiopathic non-cirrhotic portal hypertension Sarcoidosis Schistosomiasis Reticuloendothelial system diseases Veno-occlusive disease
Extra(pre)hepatic	Portal vein thrombosis owing to pancreatic disease, sepsis, thrombotic states, trauma, malignant disease
Increased hepatic blood flow	Tropical splenomegaly syndrome Blood dyscrasias Cirrhosis with congestive splenomegaly

blood flow (which occur after meals with splenic enlargement) readily increase the portal pressure in patients with cirrhosis. Increased vascular resistance to hepatic outflow develops in cirrhotic patients for several reasons. Vascular channels in the liver may be compressed by fibrosis and regenerating nodules, and there is a decrease in hepatic outflow tracks because of a reduction in the number of central and hepatic veins in association with an increase in hepatic arterial channels. Arteriovenous shunts may develop and contribute to portal hypertension.

Portal vein occlusion is rarely accompanied by ascites, whereas the accumulation of fluid in the peritoneum is a common association of obstruction of the hepatic veins.

SODIUM AND WATER RETENTION IN CIRRHOSIS

Two major hypotheses, the 'underfill' and the 'overfill' dominate the thinking in the pathogenesis of cirrhotic ascites.[42,46]

Underfill hypothesis

This is the older 'classic' hypothesis which postulates that ascites forms when there is an imbalance in Starling's forces across the hepatic splanchnic capillary beds (increased hydrostatic pressure and low colloid osmotic pressure). Increased lymph production eventually exceeds the drainage capacity of the thoracic duct and lymph accumulates in the hepatic interstitium finally leaking into the peritoneal cavity. Fluid and electrolytes are drawn into the peritoneal cavity resulting in a contraction of plasma volume. The low effective blood volume acts as a stimulus to the sympathetic nervous system, and to the renal tubule increasing sodium and water reabsorption. Thus, according to the underfill hypothesis, renal sodium retention is secondary to ascites formation. The immersion studies of Epstein[19] support the underfill hypothesis. It is unclear to what extent the systemic arteriovenous fistulae which are known to occur in cirrhosis may contribute to sodium retention and the expanded plasma volume found in early cirrhosis. A number of inconsistencies with the hypothesis, such as the presence of an expanded plasma volume in cirrhosis, the finding that systemic haemodynamics cannot be held responsible for ascites, and the observation that decompensated cirrhotics fail to respond to plasma volume expansion with a natriuresis has led to the proposal of the 'overfill' hypothesis.

Overfill hypothesis

According to this hypothesis, the initiating event is retention of sodium by the kidneys. Plasma volume expands and fluid moves out of the splanchnic circulation ('overflow') into the peritoneal cavity. Support for the hypothesis comes from animal and human studies. The stimulus for excessive, primary, renal tubular sodium reabsorption remains unclear. It has been postulated that intrahepatic hypertension in cirrhosis causes sodium and water retention by stimulating aldosterone release and stimulating efferent renal sympathetic nerves to retain sodium in the absence of an underfilled vascular system. There are many studies in decompensated cirrhotics, however, demonstrating activation of the sympathetic nervous system as well as the renin–angiotensin–aldosterone system and the non-osmotic release of vasopressin, observations incompatible with the overflow hypothesis for, as Schrier has emphasized, this sequence of events should suppress not stimulate these hormonal systems.[57]

The failure of either the overfill or underfill hypothesis to explain adequately renal sodium and water retention, has led to the suggestion that these renal events may be stimulated by peripheral arterial vasodilatation which is known, under some circumstances, to cause sodium retention.[46,57]

Increased sympathetic activity can be demonstrated in cirrhotic patients but it is unclear whether significant systemic arteriovenous fistulae have developed sufficiently early in cirrhosis to cause sodium retention. The author's studies on hand thermography in cirrhosis support the concept of peripheral vasoconstriction at some stage of cirrhosis.[28]

RENIN–ANGIOTENSIN–ALDOSTERONE SYSTEM

This system is activated in cirrhosis, and elevated aldosterone concentrations are associated with sodium retention but the question remains why, when there is sodium overload in the cirrhotic, concentrations of renin and aldosterone are not lower than observed. Hormonal and haemodynamic measurements which have been made by the author in cirrhotics, with and without ascites, suggest that the only index that distinguishes the two groups is the plasma–renin–urinary kallikrein ratio. Cirrhotics without ascites have a low value but a sodium excretion similar to volume-expanded individuals. Cirrhotics with ascites have a high plasma renin–urinary–kallikrein ratio and low urinary sodium. This author postulates that non-ascitic cirrhotics 'normalize' sodium excretion at the expense of extracellular volume expansion which suppresses the plasma renin–urinary kallikrein ratio. There must be an, as yet undefined, anti-natriuretic influence in these patients.[29]

PLASMA ATRIAL NATRIURETIC FACTOR

This peptide suppresses the renin–aldosterone system, produces arterial hypotension, and increases glomerular filtration, sodium excretion and urinary volume. Studies on cirrhotics with ascites show basal atrial natriuretic factor values which are normal or higher. The mechanism causing the increased release and the precise role of the peptide in the genesis of ascites remains unclear.[21,33]

INCREASED LYMPH FLOW

Cirrhosis of the liver is characterized by the production of large volumes of splanchnic lymph secondary to hepatic sinusoidal hypertension. A narrow plasma : tissue oncotic gradient associated with hypoalbuminaemia and the discontinuous endothelial lining of the hepatic sinusoids allow plasma proteins to pass into the interstitial tissue, thereby further reducing the colloid osmotic gradient. Normally, infiltration occurs at a very low sinusoidal pressure, and a small increase in hydrostatic pressure will encourage the outpouring of protein-rich hepatic lymph.[63] Thoracic lymph rises from a normal level of 1–1.5 litres per day to as high as 20 litres per day when ascites is present. Ascites develops when the capacity of intra-abdominal lymphatics to remove fluid is exceeded. Hepatic lymph drainage may be impaired, not only by lymphatic obstruction from fibrous tissue and regenerating nodules, but also by obstruction at the junction of the thoracic duct and the subclavian vein.[16] In hepatic venous obstruction there is a leak of high-protein lymph from the liver itself; in portal vein obstruction the fluid tends to originate from the extensive surface of the peritoneum and is low in protein. The combination of fluid originating from these two separate sites, with differing protein content, explains the variation that is encountered in the protein content of the ascitic fluid in the cirrhosis of the liver.

HYPOALBUMINAEMIA

Hypoalbuminaemia may accompany chronic or subacute liver disease. The presence of a reduced plasma colloid oncotic pressure and an increase in the splanchnic venous hydrostatic pressure does not predict accurately the development of ascites in cirrhotic patients.

TREATMENT

Minor volumes of ascites do not require treatment and the aim of therapy should not be to remove all the ascitic fluid. Up to 15% of patients will respond to bed rest and a daily sodium intake restricted to 22 mmol. It may take up to two weeks to achieve an effective diuresis. Patients most likely to respond to sodium restriction alone are those with normal renal function, urinary sodium greater than 10 mmol per day and recent onset of ascites. When ascites is resistant to dietary means and when there is moderate to severe distension with abdominal discomfort or respiratory embarrassment, diuretic therapy is essential. If respiratory distress is marked, a preliminary paracentesis of 3–4 litres may be necessary. Spironolactone or triamterene is introduced. The initial dose of spironolactone is 100 mg daily and this may need to be increased to up to 600 mg and, rarely, 1000 mg daily in resistant patients. Occasionally spironolactone treatment may need to be supplemented with a loop diuretic such as frusemide 40–80 mg daily. The introduction of frusemide must be undertaken with careful attention to plasma electrolytes and urea. Weight loss should not exceed 1 kg daily in patients without peripheral oedema and 1.5 kg daily when peripheral oedema is present.[43] Fluid restriction to 1 litre per day is unnecessary unless the plasma sodium is below 130 mmol/l. Nonsteroidal drugs are contraindicated.

It has been traditional practice to avoid large paracenteses to treat ascites because of the fear of hypervolaemia, renal failure and encephalopathy. Recent evidence suggests that repeated large-volume paracentesis can be performed safely and effectively, so long as intravenous albumin or some other plasma expander is given which prevents the renal and electrolyte complications of fluid depletion.[22,58] Paracentesis of 4–6 litres daily is performed until the disappearance of ascites. Intravenous infusion of 40 g salt-free albumin is performed after each tap. As with diuretic therapy, patients with peripheral oedema are less likely to develop renal impairment with large-volume paracenteses, because peripheral oedema acts as a reserve extravascular compartment from which the intravascular compartment can be replenished. Patients have a shorter hospital stay than with traditional diuretic therapy which, in patients being treated with large volume paracentesis, is reserved for out-patient maintenance therapy.

It is rare for ascites to be totally unresponsive to therapy but in such an event, a peritoneovenous shunt using either the LeVeen or the Denver shunt may be inserted. Peritoneal fluid is drained via a plastic tube which passes subcutaneously between the peritoneal cavity and the internal jugular vein into the superior vena cava. There is an operative mortality of 10–15% and complications include pulmonary oedema initially and, subsequently, occlusion of the shunt, infection and disseminated intravascular coagulation. Survival in decompensated alcoholic cirrhotics is not altered by peritoneovenous shunting.[60]

SPONTANEOUS BACTERIAL PERITONITIS

This term is used when infection of pre-existing ascites occurs in the absence of any obvious intra-abdominal source. The incidence is uncertain. Early reports suggested that about 8% of cirrhotics with ascites develop spontaneous bacterial peritonitis but recent data suggest figures more in the range of 25%, probably because awareness of the syndrome has led to the frequent examination of ascitic fluid in all cirrhotic patients who develop ascites.[14,64]

PATHOGENESIS

Spontaneous bacterial peritonitis develops in cirrhotic ascites and only rarely complicates ascites secondary to heart failure, malignant disease or systemic lupus erythematosus. Decompensated alcoholic cirrhotics with portal hypertension, hypoalbuminaemia, and severe hepatic dysfunction and ascites are most prone to develop the condition but it can occur in cirrhosis with other causes as well as viral hepatitis and secondary malignant disease of the liver. Gram-negative organisms are identified in 70%, usually *Escherichia coli*. Gram-positive cocci, particularly *Diplococcus pneumoniae*, occur in 10–25% of patients and anaerobes are reported in 6–14%. *Klebsiella pneumoniae* and *Pasteurella multocida* infections are on record. The pathogenic mechanisms are almost certainly multifactorial. In most, haematogenous seeding is probably the most important factor and cultures from blood are frequently positive for the same organisms which are found in the ascitic fluid.

Another mechanism is transmural migration of bacteria, and it is noteworthy that in cirrhotics there is ileal and even jejunal contamination with Gram-negative enteric organisms while additionally there is oedema and venostasis in the intestinal villi. Alterations in lymphatic function in cirrhosis occur with leakage of intestinal lymph into the peritoneal cavity. The development of spontaneous bacterial peritonitis seems to occur more readily following a severe gastrointestinal bleed, but there is little evidence that it is a complication of invasive diagnostic or therapeutic procedures.

Of particular significance is impaired function of the reticuloendothelial system which reduces host defences in hepatic cirrhosis. Portal-systemic and intrahepatic shunting of blood from sites of reticulo endothelial cell activity such as the spleen and Kupffer cells is relevant. The neutrophils and monocytes may be less effective in cirrhosis and cirrhotic patients with spontaneous bacterial peritonitis tend to have reduced opsonic activity which may be suspected by finding a low protein concentration in ascitic fluid.[47,48]

CLINICAL FEATURES AND DIAGNOSIS

Increasing awareness of spontaneous bacterial peritonitis has demonstrated that it may be asymptomatic in up to a third of patients, but it should be suspected in cirrhotics who develop fever, diarrhoea, renal insufficiency, hypothermia, encephalopathy and who fail to respond to diuretics.[64] Fever occurs in 50–80% of patients, hypotension in 5–14% and abdominal pain in 27–72%. Nausea and vomiting are also common.

The diagnosis is established by paracentesis. Removal of 10–20 ml of fluid is necessary for good results. This should be inoculated into two blood culture bottles at the bedside[49] rather than plating ascitic material in the laboratory. A Gram stain of centrifuged ascitic fluid can demonstrate bacterial infection before culture results are available. However, because it takes 24–72 hours for cultures to become positive, and because of a high mortality from the condition, it is necessary to evaluate the features of ascitic fluid for signs of infection. The ascitic fluid is cloudy in more than 75% of patients and the most helpful procedure is measurement of the polymorphonuclear leukocyte count, which is greater than 500 mm^3,[61,64] although some authors put the volume as low as 250 mm^3.[14] Total white blood cell counts (over 300 cells) in ascitic fluid are less helpful, as are the ascitic protein (greater than 2.5 g/l) or glucose (less than 50 mg/l) levels.[50] Values vary widely and may increase during a diuresis. Raised ascitic fluid lactic dehydrogenase values (greater than 225 u/ml) are indicative of infection. The initial report that an ascitic fluid pH of less than 7.31 is diagnostic of the condition[23] was supported by Stassen *et al.*[61] but not by Attali *et al.*[2] and the diagnostic value of measuring ascitic fluid pH must remain uncertain. The consensus is that the diagnosis is made on the basis of an elevated polymorphonuclear ascitic fluid level and positive fluid culture, but the other indices may offer additional diagnostic help if the polymorphonuclear cell count is equivocal.

TREATMENT

Treatment must be prompt and effective, failing which, the mortality rate is between 80–97%. Earlier diagnosis and the institution of appropriate antibiotic treatment on clinical suspicion can reduce mortality rates to below 50% and as low as 7%. Because there will be a delay before the organisms are identified, 'best guess' antibiotic therapy should be instituted. The combination of ampicillin and an aminoglycoside is no longer recommended because of nephrotoxicity of aminoglycosides. Third-generation cephalosporins such as cefotoxin are favoured with or without metronidazole. The antibiotics are administered intravenously, adequate nutritional support is necessary and there should be careful monitoring of renal function. It is recognized that the most important determinant of survival is the severity of the underlying liver disease.[14,64]

MALIGNANT ASCITES

Those tumours responsible for malignant ascites are shown in *Table 13.1*, the most frequent being pancreas, ovary and colon, but the type of tumour will differ depending on the centre and patient referral pattern. Ascites may develop for a number of reasons; peritoneal carcinomatosis which accounts for two-thirds of patients, massive liver secondaries or chylous ascites.[52] Alteration in the vascular permeability to large molecules, and blockage of diaphragmatic lymphatics contribute to a raised protein content.[36]

Ultrasonography demonstrates that the fluid is irregularly distributed into pockets. Cytological diagnosis of malignant cells in ascites is difficult because of varying morphology and staining characteristics so that reported figures for positive morphology vary between 50–90%.[20,36,52] A blind peritoneal biopsy is safe but not sensitive. The carcinoembryonic antigen titre may be helpful because, in malignant ascites, the titre ranges from 1.6–2.6500 ng/ml and is usually greater than 10 ng/ml, whereas in only 2% of those with non-malignant ascites is the titre greater than 5 ng/ml. If the ascitic fluid titre is between 5.0 and 9.9 ng/ml, and is twice that in the plasma, a diagnosis of malignant ascites is suggested. Gastrointestinal and breast cancers often have high ascitic titres. Titres are only 34–74% sensitive but 100% specific. The addition of an estimation of human chorionic gonadotrophin in the fluid has been claimed to increase sensitivity to greater than 70% in ovarian, breast and lung cancers.[13] Another marker of human cancer cells is the CaI antibody, which reacts with the determinant present on two glycoproteins on the cell membrane. This test is very specific and is particular in distinguishing benign (reactive) mesothelial cells from a mesothelioma.[65] The diagnostic value of an ascitic fluid cholesterol greater than 1.2 mmol/l as a predictor of malignant ascites is 87.5%, and the measurement of cholesterol can be used to supplement the cytological examination.[41]

Ascites formation in patients with primary hepatocellular cancer is always secondary to portal hypertension and the hepatoma cells produce α-fetoprotein. Ascitic α-fetoprotein is 87% sensitive and 95% specific for the diagnosis of hepatocellular cancer.[53] Concentrations of fibronectin (over 75 mg/ml) and lactic acid dehydrogenase (over 150 u/l) are thus elevated in malignant ascites and, when combined with cytology and α-fetoprotein measurements, provide an accurate method of diagnosis.[44,51,56]

Pseudomyxoma peritonei is an uncommon disorder in which the peritoneum is filled with large quantities of yellow-green mucus. It arises from either a mucus-secreting ovarian cancer or, rarely, a mucus-secreting cancer of the appendix.

TREATMENT

The treatment of malignant ascites is unsatisfactory. The usual management is to perform recurrent abdominal paracentesis via a trocar with the attendant problem of fluid, electrolyte and protein depletion. The rapid loss of fluid can precipitate shock, so that drainage should be undertaken using 16-gauge catheters inserted via a 14-gauge needle, and fluid and albumin replaced by intravenous infusions. Irradiation, radioactive isotopes, sclerosing agents and alkylating drugs have all been used with limited success. The abdomen is drained to dryness and the particular agent instilled. Bleomycin has been recommended because it has low systemic toxicity and can be injected directly into the peritoneal cavity at a dose of 60–120 mg in 100 ml normal saline. Fluorouracil 2.5 mg has also been used but, as with other cytotoxic agents, it is less effective when large intra-abdominal tumour masses are present in association with ascites. Other agents used include mustine and doxorubicin. The injection of *Corynebacterium parvum* intraperitoneally, and oral spironolactone have also been tried.[36] The LeVeen or Denver peritoneovenous shunt may be used, as they may make a terminal illness more comfortable, although life is not necessarily prolonged. Problems with shunting are frequent, occurring in about 40% of patients and include febrile reactions, sepsis, thromboembolism, disseminated intravascular coagulation, ascitic fluid leakage, pulmonary oedema and occlusion. While dissemination of the primary tumour is frequently discussed, it is seldom documented. Shunts in carefully selected patients, particularly those with ovarian and breast tumours, offer effective palliation without undue morbidity.[18,29]

TUBERCULOUS ASCITES

Tuberculous peritonitis has an insidious onset and is frequently unsuspected and easily missed, particularly when the infection complicates cirrhosis of the liver. The chest radiograph is abnormal in 65% of patients. The usual presentation is with abdominal swelling and discomfort, fever and weight loss. Other complaints include anorexia, lethargy and constipation.[4] A doughy feel to the abdomen is a rare physical finding but an abdominal mass of matted bowel or omentum is felt in 25% of patients. The ascitic fluid is usually yellow and turgid and contains more than 250 white cells per mm^3, most of which are mononuclear. Rarely the ascites is haemorrhagic. The identification of organisms may be difficult but the disease is readily diagnosed by blind peritoneal biopsy, laparoscopy or laparotomy. Intermediate strength purified protein derivative (PPD) is positive in 61% of patients.[4] Measurements of adenosine deaminase activity of greater than 32.3 u/l in ascitic fluid give a sensitivity of 95% and a specificity of 98% for tuberculous peritonitis.[62] The treatment is along conventional lines for tuberculosis (see Chapter 9).

CHYLOUS ASCITES

In chylous ascites, there is an accumulation of lymph or lymph-like fluid which has a milky appearance. The triglyceride content is high (often greater than 5 g/l) and on centrifugation a clear subnatant fluid separates from a floating layer of chylomicrons. Chylous ascites is rare but may be caused by many intra-abdominal situations (*Table 13.3*) in which there is either a direct leak of lymph from traumatized or obstructed lymphatics, or transudation of lymph from the surface of the intestine, liver or

Table 13.3 Causes of chylous ascites

Infections	Tuberculosis
	Filariasis
	Dysentery
	Syphilis
Neoplastic	Lymphoma
	Leukaemia
	Cancer of the stomach, pancreas, ovary
Trauma	
Congenital	Dysplasia of the lymphatic system
Cirrhosis of the liver	
Protein-losing enteropathy	

porta hepatis. The commonest causes are inflammatory disease (35%) and neoplasms (30%); no cause is identified in 20% of patients. A patient has been described in whom chylous ascites occurred in association with intestinal lymphangiectasia and the 'yellow nail' syndrome: uniform thickening, dystrophy and yellow discoloration of the fingers and toenails.[15]

HAEMORRHAGIC ASCITES

Ascites is considered to be haemorrhagic if there are more than 50 000 red cells/mm^3. It may follow damage to large vessels, invasion of Glisson's capsule, rupture of mesenteric varices, or lymphomatous involvement of the spleen. Other causes include tuberculous peritonitis, malignant involvement of the peritoneum (usually hepatocellular cancer or peritoneal carcinomatosis), trauma, mesothelioma, mesenteric cysts, hepatic vein thrombosis, multiple myeloma, perforated viscus, lymphoma and endometriosis. Ultrasonography or computerized tomography are valuable techniques in the evaluation of haemorrhagic ascites, because if a solid peritoneal mass is identified, a guided needle biopsy can be used to establish the diagnosis.[26]

PANCREATIC ASCITES

Ascites develops in 10–20% of patients with cancer of the pancreas who have widespread peritoneal metastases. On the other hand, ascites and pleural effusions are unusual in chronic pancreatitis. About 60% of such patients have an accompanying pseudocyst of the pancreas; and about 60% of patients have chronic alcoholic pancreatitis. Ascites may also complicate acute pancreatitis.

Pancreatic ascites usually develops when there has been a rupture of the pancreatic duct and pancreatic secretions leak into the peritoneal cavity; this mechanism operates in both chronic and acute pancreatitis. The internal fistula may communicate directly with the peritoneal cavity, the peritoneum or the mediastinum. Fluid accumulation is often insidious and relatively painless, but the ascites is usually described as 'massive'.

The diagnosis is established by demonstrating a markedly elevated ascitic amylase concentration (greater than 2000 U/l) or lipase content in the fluid which has a protein concentration in the range typical of exudates. Serum amylase may be elevated. Endoscopic retrograde pancreatography is helpful in defining the anatomy prior to surgery.

The management of patients with pancreatic ascites is initially by nasogastric suction, atropine, acetazolamide (Diamox) 500 mg twice daily and repeated abdominal paracentesis to encourage spontaneous closure of the leak. If the patient is in poor nutritional condition (common in patients with alcohol abuse), parenteral hyperalimentation is recommended. Such therapy is effective in 50% of patients but, if fluid continues to re-accumulate after 4–6 weeks, surgical intervention is advisable, preceded by endoscopic retrograde cholangio pancreatography to reveal ducts, the site of any leak, and the presence of a pseudocyst. Small pseudocysts are resected; if large, drainage is required. A direct leak into the peritoneum is managed by either resection, usually distal pancreatectomy; or, if the leak cannot be defined, a cystogastrostomy. Radiotherapy in the form of a single dose of 5 Gy (500 rad) has been used in patients who are at high operative risk.[10]

BILE ASCITES

A distinction may be made between bile peritonitis, when bile in the peritoneal cavity is associated with severe pain and shock, and bile ascites, when large quantities of bile enter the peritoneal cavity without causing pain. The reason for the different presentations is unknown but bile ascites is most frequently seen as a complication of operations on the biliary tree. In this situation, the bile is sterile and the mortality rate low.[1] The free escape of bile into the peritoneal cavity is usually an acute serious event with a mortality rate from 10–80%. Bile evokes a brisk chemical peritonitis and there is severe pain, shock, dehydration and eventually sepsis and renal failure. Bile peritonitis has been reported after trauma, percutaneous transhepatic cholangiography and liver biopsy, particularly when extrahepatic bile duct obstruction is present. Other causes are typhoid fever, steroid therapy and acute pancreatitis. Spontaneous rupture of the biliary tree is a rare event which has been recorded in children. The treatment of bile peritonitis requires initial resuscitation with fluid replacement, analgesics and antibiotics, and thereafter a prompt laparotomy to repair the bile leak.

ASCITES IN RENAL DISEASE (NEPHROGENIC ASCITES)

Ascites occurs in the nephrotic syndrome as a consequence of severe hypoalbuminaemia. The fluid may become infected. However, pneumococcal peritonitis is now very rate. Acute glomerulonephritis may be complicated by ascites.

Ascites develops in a few patients with renal failure, usually after they have started haemodialysis. The condition has become less frequent as dialysis techniques have improved. The mechanism is unclear but the nephrotic syndrome, circulatory overload, infection, inferior vena cava compression or reduced lymphatic removal of fluid have all been implicated.[40] The peritoneum may have become more leaky following peritoneal dialysis. Peritonitis is a major complication of long-term peritoneal dialysis and fungi, particularly *Candida* spp. are increasingly recognized as being important. Treatment is with intraperitoneal fluorocytosine or miconazole, and oral ketoconazole should be tried with peritoneal lavage in patients with viscid peritoneal effluent. If there is no response, the catheter is removed and a temporary peritoneal dialysis catheter replaced for lavage and antifungal drugs.[6,11]

Prognosis is poor, a third of patients with ascites dying within a year. Rarely and inexplicably, ascites may develop for the first time following renal transplantation.

ASCITES IN THE NEWBORN

Neonates who develop ascites present with abdominal distension and the diagnosis of fluid can be made on plain abdominal radiograph or by ultrasound, and confirmed by an ascitic tap. The presence of calcium on a plain radiograph suggests meconium peritonitis.[25] The causes of ascites in the newborn are listed in *Table 13.4*. About 25% of neonatal ascites is urinary in nature and the common predisposing factor is posterior urethral valves with the resultant leak of urine from the kidney. Urine enters the peritoneal space by diffusion, or rarely by rupture of the overlying peritoneum. Urinary ascites is seven times more common in male than female children and carries a mortality rate of more than 70%. It is treated by prompt decompression of the urinary tract using a temporary diversion procedure, followed by relief of obstruction.

EOSINOPHILIC ASCITES

A raised concentration of eosinophilic cells in ascitic fluid is encountered in the hypereosinophilic syn-

Table 13.4 Causes of neonatal ascites

Urinary	Urethral stricture/atresia
	Renal vein thrombosis
	Congenital nephrosis
	Perforated bladder
	Posterior urethral valve
	Pelvic neuroblastoma
	Uterocele
Gastrointestinal	Perforated appendix
	Perforated Meckel's diverticulum
	Perforated ileum
	Meconium peritonitus
	Imperforate anus
Cardiac	All causes of congestive cardiac failure
Hepatobiliary	Polycystic disease of the liver
	Meckel-Gruber syndrome
	Biliary atresia
	Perforation of the biliary tract
	Cirrhosis of the liver
	Portal vein hypoplasia/obstruction
Infection	Sepsis
	Syphilis
	Toxoplasmosis
	Cytomegalovirus infection
Chylous	Constricting peritoneal band
	Thoracic duct occlusion/stenosis
Erythroblastosis fetalis	
Hydrometrocolpos	
Unknown	

drome, eosinophilic gastroenteritis, chronic peritoneal dialysis, metastatic malignant disease, abdominal lymphoma, ruptured hydatid cyst and vasculitis. The hypereosinophilic syndrome is more frequent in males and is characterized by mitral valve disease, congestive cardiac failure, segmental small bowel deformities, hepatomegaly, malabsorption and peripheral eosinophilia.

MYXOEDEMA ASCITES

Ascites is rarely encountered in myxoedema. Pleural and pericardial effusions occur much more frequently. The mechanism is not known but the fluid usually has a protein content of 40–60 g/l and responds readily to thyroid replacement.

RARE CAUSES OF ASCITES

Chronic ascites has been reported in the Fitz-Hugh-Curtis syndrome in which right upper quadrant pain and perihepatitis occur due to *Chlamydia trachomatis* and, less frequently, *Neissera gonorrhoea*.[27,38] Exudate of ascites is reported in infectious mononucleosis,[37] mastocytosis[8,45] and peritoneal lymphomatosis[51] and the syndrome of polyneuropathy, organomegaly, endocrinopathy, M-proteins and skin changes (POEMS syndrome).[34] Ascites may occur transiently in systemic sclerosis[35] and also in hepatic amyloidosis where peritoneal fluid accumulation is secondary to portal hypertension.[30]

REFERENCES

1. Ackerman, N.B., Sillin, L.F. and Suresh, K. (1985) Consequences of intraperitoneal bile: bile ascites versus bile peritonitis. *American Journal of Surgery*, **149**, 244–246.
2. Attali, P., Turner, K., Pelletier, G., Ink, O. and Etienne, J.P. (1986) pH of ascitic fluid: diagnostic and prognostic value in cirrhotic and non-cirrhotic patients. *Gastroenterology*, **90**, 1255–1260.
3. Bar-Meir, S., Lerner, E. and Conn, H.O. (1979) Analysis of ascitic fluid in cirrhosis. *Digestive Diseases and Sciences*, **24**, 136–144.
4. Bastani, B., Shariatzadeh, M.R. and De Hoashti, F. (1985) Tuberculous peritonitis – report of 30 cases and review of literature. *Quarterly Journal of Medicine*, **56**, 549–557.
5. Bateson, M.C. and Bouchier, I.A.D. (1988) *Clinical Investigations in Gastroenterology*. London: Kluwer Academic Publisher.
6. Bayer, A.S., Blumenkrantz, M.J., Montgomerie, J.A. *et al.* (1976) Candida peritonitis. Report of 22 cases and review of the English literature. *American Journal of Medicine*, **61**, 832–840.
7. Black, M. and Friedman, A.C. (1989) Ultrasound examination in patients with ascites. *Annals of Internal Medicine*, **110**, 253–255.
8. Bonnet, P., Smadja, C., Szekely, A.-M. *et al.* (1987) Intractable ascites in systemic mastocytosis treated by portal diversion. *Digestive Diseases and Sciences*, **32**, 209–213.
9. Boyer, T.D., Kahn, A.M. and Reynolds, T.B. (1978) Diagnostic value of ascitic fluid lactic dehydrogenase protein and WBC levels. *Archives of Internal Medicine*, **138**, 1103–1105.
10. Cameron, J.L. (1978) Chronic pancreatic ascites and pancreatic pleural effusions. *Gastroenterology*, **74**, 134–140.
11. Cheng, I.K.P., Fang, G.-X., Chan, T.-M., Chan, P.C.K. and Chan, M.-K. (1989) Fungal peritonitis complicating peritoneal dialysis: report of 27 cases and review of treatment. *Quarterly Journal of Medicine*, **265**, 407–416.
12. Conn, H.O. (1979) Portal hypertension and its consequences. In *Current Gastroenterology and Hepatology*, pp. 338–404. (Ed.) Gitnick, G.L. Boston, MA: Houghton and Mifflin.
13. Couch, W.D. (1981) Combined effusion fluid tumour market assay, carcinoembryonic antigen (CEA) and human chorionic gonadotrophin (hCG) in the detection of malignant tumours. *Cancer*, **48**, 1103–1105.
14. Crossley, I.R. and Williams, R. (1985) Spontaneous bacterial peritonitis. *Gut*, **26**, 325–331.
15. Duhra, P.M., Quigley, E.M.M. and Marsh, M.N. (1985) Chylous ascites, intestinal lymphangiectasia and the 'yellow nail' syndrome. *Gut*, **26**, 1266–1269.
16. Dumont, A.E. and Mulholland, J.H. (1960) Flow rate and composition of thoracic-duct lymph in patients with cirrhosis. *New England Journal of Medicine*, **263**, 471–474.
17. Edell, S.L. and Gefter, W.B. (1979) Ultrasonic differentiation of types of ascitic fluid. *American Journal of Roentgenology*, **133**, 111–114.
18. Edney, J.A., Hill, A. and Armstrong, D. (1989) Peritoneovenous shunts palliate malignant ascites. *American Journal of Surgery*, **158**, 598–601.
19. Epstein, M. (1979) Deranged sodium homeostasis in cirrhosis. *Gastroenterology*, **76**, 622–635.
20. Garrison, R.N., Kaelin, R.D. and Galloway, R.H. (1986) Malignant ascites. *Annals of Surgery*, **203**, 644–651.
21. Gines, P., Jimenez, W., Arroyo, V. *et al.* (1988) Atrial natriuretic factor in cirrhosis with ascites: plasma levels, cardiac release and splanchnic extraction. *Hepatology*, **8**, 636–642.
22. Gines, P., Tito, L., Arroyo, V. *et al.* (1988) Randomized, comparative study of therapeutic paracentesis with and without intravenous albumin in cirrhosis. *Gastroenterology*, **94**, 1493–1502.
23. Gitlin, N., Stauffer, J.L. and Silvestri, P.C. (1982) The pH of ascitic fluid in the diagnosis of

spontaneous bacterial peritonitis in alcoholic cirrhosis. *Hepatology*, **2**, 408–411.
24. Gjessing, J., Oskarsson, B.M., Tomlin, P.J. and Brock-Utne, J. (1972) Diagnostic abdominal paracentesis. *British Medical Journal*, **i**, 617–619.
25. Griscom, N.T., Colodny, A.H., Rosenberg, H.K. *et al.* (1977) Diagnostic aspects of neonatal ascites: report of 27 cases. *American Journal of Roentology*, **128**, 961–970.
26. Hacker, J.F. III, Richter, J.E., Pyatt, R.S. and Fin, M.P. (1982) Haemorrhagic ascites: an unusual presentation of splenic lymphoma. *Gastroenterology*, **83**, 470–473.
27. Haight, J.B. and Ockner, S.A. (1988) *Chlamydia trachomatis* perihepatitis with ascites. *American Journal of Gastroenterology*, **83**, 323–325.
28. Hauer, J.L., Plevris, J.N., Hayes, P.C. and Bouchier, I.A.D. (1990) Reduced hand temperature in patients with alcoholic liver disease. *European Journal of Gastroenterology and Hepatology*, **2**, 61–65.
29. Hayes, P.C., Cumming, A.D. and Bouchier, I.A.D. (1989) Haemodynamic and hormonal influences in cirrhosis with and without ascites. *Gut*, **30**, A1505.
30. Itescu, S. (1984) Hepatic amyloidosis. *Archives of Internal Medicine*, **144**, 2257–2258.
31. Kirkpatrick, S. and Schubert, T. (1988) Umbilical hernia rupture in cirrhosis with ascites. *Digestive Diseases and Sciences*, **33**, 762–765.
32. Koninckx, P.R., Renaer, M. and Brosens, I.A. (1980) Origin of peritoneal fluid in women: an ovarian exudation product. *British Journal of Obstetrics and Gynaecology*, **87**, 177–183.
33. Laffi, G., Pinzami, M., Meacci, E. *et al.* (1989) Renal hemodynamic and natriuretic effects of human atrial natriuretic factor infusion in cirrhosis with ascites. *Gastroenterology*, **96**, 167–177.
34. Loeb, J.M., Hauger, P.H., Carney, J.D. and Cooper, A.D. (1989) Refractory ascites due to POEMS syndrome. *Gastroenterology*, **96**, 247–249.
35. McAleer, J.J.A., Cunningham, S., Dickey, W., Burrows, D. and Callender, M.E. (1986) Transient ascites in progressive systemic sclerosis. *British Medical Journal*, **293**, 1211–1212.
36. Malden, L.T. and Tattesall, M.H.N. (1986) Malignant effusions. *Quarterly Journal of Medicine*, **58**, 221–239.
37. Marano, A.R., Lanse, S.B., Garsten, J.J. *et al.* (1986) Exudative ascites complicating infectious mononucleosis. *American Journal of Gastroenterology*, **81**, 808–811.
38. Marbet, U.A., Stalder, G.A., Vogtlin, J. *et al.* (1986) Diffuse peritonitis and chronic ascites due to infection with *Chlamydia trachomatis* in patients without liver disease: new presentation of the Fitz-Hugh-Curtis syndrome. *British Medical Journal*, **293**, 5–6.
39. Mauer, K. and Manzione, N.D. (1988) Usefulness of serum ascites albumin difference in separating transudative from exudative ascites. *Digestive Diseases and Sciences*, **33**, 1208–1212.
40. Mauk, P.M., Schwartz, J.T., Lowe, L.E., Smith, I.L. and Graham, D.Y. (1988) Diagnosis and course of nephrogenic ascites. *Archives of Internal Medicine*, **148**, 1577–1579.
41. Mortensen, P.B., Kristensen, S.D., Bloch, A., Jacobsen, B.A. and Rasmussen, S.N. (1988) Diagnostic value of ascitic fluid cholesterol levels in the prediction of malignancy. *Scandinavian Journal of Gastroenterology*, **23**, 1085–1088.
42. Panos, M. and Williams, R. (1988) Ascites in cirrhosis: pathophysiology and management. *British Journal of Hospital Medicine*, **40**, 256–262.
43. Pockros, P.J. and Reynolds, T.B. (1986) Rapid diuresis in patients with ascites from chronic liver disease: the importance of peripheral edema. *Gastroenterology*, **90**, 1827–1833.
44. Prieto, M., Gomez-Lechon, M.J., Hoyos, M. *et al.* (1988) Diagnosis of malignant ascites. *Digestive Diseases and Sciences*, **33**, 833–838.
45. Reisberg, I.R. and Oyakawa, S. (1987) Mastocytosis with malabsorption, myelofibrosis and massive ascites. *American Journal of Gastroenterology*, **82**, 54–60.
46. Rocco, V.K. and Ware, A.J. (1986) Cirrhotic ascites: pathophysiology, diagnosis and management. *Annals of Internal Medicine*, **105**, 573–585.
47. Runyon, B.A. (1986) Low-protein-concentration ascitic fluid is predisposed to spontaneous bacterial peritonitis. *Gastroenterology*, **91**, 1343–1346.
48. Runyon, B.A. (1988) Patients with deficient ascitic fluid opsonic activity are predisposed to spontaneous bacterial peritonitis. *Hepatology*, **8**, 632–635.
49. Runyon, B.A., Canawati, H.N. and Akriviads, E.A. (1988) Optimization of ascitic fluid culture technique. *Gastroenterology*, **95**, 1351–1355.
50. Runyon, B.A. and Hoefs, J.C. (1985) Ascitic fluid chemical analysis before, during and after spontaneous bacterial peritonitis. *Hepatology*, **5**, 257–259.
51. Runyon, B.A. and Hoefs, J.C. (1986) Peritoneal lymphomatosis with ascites. *Archives of Internal Medicine*, **146**, 887–888.
52. Runyon, B.A., Hoefs, J.C. and Morgan, T.R. (1988) Ascitic fluid analysis in malignant-related ascites. *Hepatology*, **8**, 1104–1109.
53. Salerno, F., Restelli, B., Incerti, P. *et al.* (1990) Utility of ascitic fluid analysis in patients with malignancy-related ascites. *Scandinavian Journal of Gastroenterology*, **25**, 251–256.
54. Scemama-Clergue, J., Doutrellot-Philippon, C., Metreau, J.-M. *et al.* (1985) Ascitic fluid pH in alcoholic cirrhosis: a re-evaluation of its use in the diagnosis of spontaneous bacterial peritonitis. *Gut*, **26**, 332–335.
55. Schade, D.A. and Williamson, J.R. (1968) The pathogenesis of peritoneal adhesions: an ultra-structural study. *Annals of Surgery*, **167**, 500–510.

56. Scholmerich, J., Volk, B.A., Kottgen, E., Ehlers, S. and Gerok, W. (1984) Fibronectin concentration in ascites differentiates between malignant and nonmalignant ascites. *Gastroenterology*, **87**, 1160–1164.
57. Schrier, R.W. (1988) Pathogenesis of sodium and water retention in high-output and low-output cardiac failure, nephrotic syndrome, cirrhosis and pregnancy. *New England Journal of Medicine*, **319**, 1127–1134.
58. Simon, D.M., McCain, J.R., Bonkovsky, H.L. *et al.* (1987) Effects of therapeutic paracentesis on systemic hepatic hemodynamics on renal and hormonal function. *Hepatology*, **7**, 423–429.
59. Soderlund, C. (1986) Denver peritoneovenous shunting for malignant or cirrhotic ascites. *Scandinavian Journal of Gastroenterology*, **21**, 1161–1172.
60. Stanley, M.M., Ochi, S., Lee, K.K. *et al.* (1989) Peritoneovenous shunting as compared with medical treatment in patients with alcoholic cirrhosis and massive ascites. *New England Journal of Medicine*, **321**, 1632–1638.
61. Stassen, W.N., McCullough, A.J., Bacon, B.R. *et al.* (1986) Immediate diagnostic criteria for bacterial infection of ascitic fluid. *Gastroenterology*, **90**, 1247–1254.
62. Volgt, M.D., Kalvaria, I., Trey, C. *et al.* (1989) Diagnostic value of ascites adenosine deaminase in tuberculous peritonitis. *The Lancet*, **i**, 751–754.
63. Witte, C.L., Witte, M.H. and Dumont, A.E. (1980) Lymph imbalance in the genesis and perpetuation of the ascites syndrome in hepatic cirrhosis. *Gastroenterology*, **78**, 1059–1068.
64. Wilcox, C.M., Dismukes, W.E. (1987) Spontaneous bacterial peritonitis. *Medicine*, **66**, 447–456.
65. Woods, J.C., Harris, H., Spriggs, A.I. and McGee, J.O'D. (1982) A new marker for human cancer cells. Immunocytochemical detections of malignant cells in serous fluids with the CaI antibody. *The Lancet*, **ii**, 512–515.

FAMILIAL MEDITERRANEAN FEVER (RECURRENT POLYSEROSITIS)

S.E. Goldfinger

Familial Mediterranean fever (FMF), also known as recurrent polyserositis, is a rare, inherited disorder characterized by spontaneous, irregularly occurring attacks of fever and serosal inflammation involving the peritoneum, pleura and synovia. Amyloidosis occurs frequently in some ethnic groups, but not in others.

FMF is most often found in persons of Mediterranean ancestry. Although Sephardic Jews and Armenians are regarded as the major populations at risk. FMF is prevalent in Egypt, Turkey, Lebanon, Libya, Kuwait, Italy and other Mediterranean countries. Jews in the USA who develop FMF are Ashkenazi as well as Sephardic. In addition, irrefutable instances of FMF in other ethnic groups (such as Anglo-Saxon, Japanese, American Indian) suggest that no person exhibiting typical symptoms should be excluded from diagnostic consideration on the basis of ancestry. This, together with the absence of a positive family history in many patients, has raised appropriate concern about the aptness of the term FMF to designate this disease. One suggested alternative – recurrent polyserositis – is more accurate than FMF, but has not achieved wide acceptance as yet.

AETIOLOGY AND PATHOGENESIS

The most careful genetic studies of FMF, performed in Israel, suggest that the disorder is inherited as an autosomal recessive trait carried by a gene that is located on the short arm of chromosome 16.[9] However, the precise series of events responsible for triggering an attack remain a complete mystery. There is no body of evidence to support any infectious agent, or an autoimmune or hypersensitivity basis for the disease. The separate reports of a deficiency of the inhibitor of C5 in peritoneal fluid[8] and of an increase in dopamine β-hydoxylase in the plasma[3] of FMF patients suggest that an inherited biochemical abnormality may play a fundamental role in the pathogenesis of the disease. The observation that infusion of metaraminol can reproduce components of an FMF attack in patients at baseline[2] is of uncertain significance.

CLINICAL FEATURES

Most patients with FMF report the onset of disease during childhood or adolescence, but initial attacks have been reported in infancy as well as during the sixth decade of life. Attacks vary in frequency, occurring once every 3–4 weeks in many patients, but happening as often as once a week or as seldom as once a year in others. There is no temporal regularity to the onset, and interval periods are generally characterized by robust health with complete freedom from symptoms. A typical peritoneal or pleural attack will last from 24 to 72 hours. The onset is usually abrupt with a peak in fever and pain intensity occurring within the first 12 hours. Occasionally, mild prodromal symptoms, such as fatigue or minor abdominal discomfort, may signal a full-blown attack.

FEVER

Fever either precedes or accompanies serosal manifestations of the disease. The temperature rise is usually brisk and may be accompanied by a rigor. Typical temperature elevations range between 38.5 and 40°C. At times, fever may be the sole manifestation of an attack, and patients have been reported whose serosal symptoms began only after years of recurrent episodes of unexplained fever. Conversely, serosal symptoms occur without fever in some patients.

PERITONEAL SYMPTOMS

The peritoneum is by far the most frequently involved serosal surface. Nearly all FMF patients have been stricken with peritonitis which is, for most, the principal manifestation of each attack. Pain and tenderness is usually initially localized to one sector of the abdomen; this progresses to more generalized pain and distension. Classical signs of peritonitis (guarding, rebound tenderness, board-like rigidity, absent bowel sounds) parallel the severity of the attack.

These findings, together with fever and leukocytosis, often lead to early surgical exploration if a diagnosis of FMF has not been made. Conversely, the concern that any single peritoneal attack could represent an unrelated abdominal emergency has prompted some physicians to recommend prophylactic appendectomy for the patient with FMF.

PLEURAL SYMPTOMS

Many patients experience referred chest and shoulder pain from diaphragmatic irritation during bouts of peritonitis. In addition, typical unilateral pleuritic chest pain with an accompanying pleural effusion may occur with or without peritonitis. Isolated pleuritic episodes were reported in 40% of a large group of patients seen at the Tel Hashomer Hospital in Tel Aviv.

SYNOVIAL SYMPTOMS

Approximately 75% of FMF patients seen in Israel have experienced at least one episode of acute arthritis. In contrast, inflammatory joint disease is uncommon among Armenian and Jewish FMF patients reported from the USA. The reason for this discrepancy is not known. The arthritis of FMF is usually restricted to a single joint at any one time, and has a predilection for the large joints, in particular the knee, ankle, hip and elbow, in order of frequency. Synovitis can occur independently of other manifestations of FMF, and tends to last longer than peritoneal or pleuritic attacks. Effusions are common. Radiographs and joint fluid analyses show only non-specific changes. Short attacks of arthritis, which last only 1–2 weeks, undergo complete resolution. However, protracted forms, which may last as long as a year, may result in serious consequences, including osteoporosis with periarticular fractures and aseptic necrosis of the femoral head.

SKIN MANIFESTATIONS

An erysipeloid erythema is commonly observed in FMF patients in Israel, but is rare elsewhere. Typical lesions occupy between 15 and 50 cm^2 of skin surface, are fairly sharply defined, and almost always occur below the knee.

AMYLOIDOSIS

The complication of amyloidosis, observed much more frequently in the Mediterranean region than elsewhere, has become much less of a threat to patients with FMF since the advent of colchicine therapy. Before this treatment, approximately 25% of FMF patients in Israel developed amyloidosis, and the incidence in Turkey approached 60%. The onset and progression of amyloidosis seemed to bear no consistent relationship to the number or severity of serosal attacks. The characteristic pathological features of FMF-associated amyloidosis is the deposition of serum amyloid A (SAA) protein in the intima and media of arterioles. The two organs most heavily involved are the kidneys and spleen; the liver is spared. The clinical hallmark of FMF-associated amyloidosis is nephropathy, which presents as the nephrotic syndrome before proceeding to progressive renal failure. Death due to FMF is almost always a consequence of renal amyloidosis.

OTHER MANIFESTATIONS

Rarely episodes of non-infectious, self-limited pericarditis orchitis, and meningitis occur. Intestinal obstruction owing to bowel adhesions has also been observed. The most disturbing complications of FMF observed in the USA – depression and narcotic addition – have diminished considerably since the advent of effective treatment to prevent attacks.

INVESTIGATIONS

Although typical attacks of serositis are accompanied by elevated markers of inflammation (leucocytosis, and elevated sedimentation rate, C-reactive protein, fibrinogen and haptoglobin), there are no routine laboratory findings specific for, or even particularly suggestive of, FMF. Biochemical assessment of renal and hepatic function is normal, as are lipid studies and a variety of serological tests. The finding of elevated dopamine β-hydroxylase in the plasma of patients with FMF awaits confirmation before this test can be recommended to assist in the diagnosis of the disease. Patients with associated amyloidosis show proteinuria and the biochemical abnormalities consistent with the stage of renal failure. Examination of serosal effusions typically show sterile exudates with a predominance of neutrophils and fibrin strands. Radiological studies may show the expected small pleural effusions (for pleural attacks) and non-obstructive ileus (for peritoneal attacks).[4,13]

TREATMENT

Although acute attacks of FMF are not alleviated by conventional anti-inflammatory drugs, these episodes can be prevented in most patients by the prophylactic use of colchicine, taken orally in a dose of two 0.6 mg tablets daily. Approximately 85% of patients will experience either complete cessation of their attacks or marked reduction in their frequency and severity. A few may require as many as four tablets spread over the day to achieve symptom control, whereas others manage quite well taking one tablet daily. Many describe the value of an extra tablet to abort the progression of prodromal symptoms, which may still appear during maintenance colchicine treatment.[3,5,6,12,15] Since the advent of prophylactic colchicine therapy for FMF, new cases of amyloidosis are unusual and are generally associated with failure to take colchicine as prescribed.[16] Long-term studies have shown that prophylactic colchicine treatment is safe; in particular, adverse effects upon bone marrow, liver or renal function have not been detected.[7,10] Additional medication for control of loose stools may be required by some patients. Despite the theoretical potential for colchicine to affect cell division, its continued use during conception and pregnancy has been observed to carry virtually no risk to the fetus. The previous recommendation that the drug be discontinued before planned conception and throughout pregnancy is probably unnecessary. In fact, renewal of FMF attacks occasioned by colchicine withdrawal is apt to reduce fecundity and predispose to spontaneous abortion. Wright *et al.*[14] have introduced, as an alternative to daily maintenance colchicine, a protocol for more intensive colchicine therapy to be initiated at the first premonition of an attack. This benefits most patients and is the treatment of choice for infrequent attacks. The value of prodrome-initiated therapy in patients with frequent attacks will depend on the pace of an attack following its first signal, the amount of amelioration afforded by colchicine, and the degree of bowel upset caused by the higher dose of colchicine.

REFERENCES

1. Barakat, M.H., Gumaa, K.A., El-Khawad, A.O. *et al.* (1984) Metaraminol provocation test: a specific diagnostic test for familial Mediterranean fever. *The Lancet*, **i**, 656–658.
2. Barakat, M.H., Malhas, L.N., Gumaa, K.A. *et al.* (1988) Plasma dopamine beta-hydroxylase: rapid diagnostic test for recurrent hereditary polyserositis. *The Lancet*, **ii**, 1280–1283.
3. Dinarello, C.A., Wolff, S.M., Goldfinger, S.E. *et al.* (1974) Colchicine therapy for familial Mediterranean fever. A double-blind trial. *New England Journal of Medicine*, **291**, 934–937.
4. Ehrenfield, E.N., Eliakim, M. and Rachmilewitz, M. (1961) Recurrent polyserositis (familial Mediterranean fever, periodic disease). A report of fifty-five cases. *American Journal of Medicine*, **31**, 107–123.

5. Goldfinger, S.E. (1972) Colchicine for familial Mediterranean fever. *New England Journal of Medicine*, **287**, 1302.
6. Goldfinger, S.E. (1975) Colchicine suppression of attacks of familial Mediterranean fever. *Frontiers of Internal Medicine: 12th International Congress of Internal Medicine*, Tel Aviv 1974, pp. 334–338. Basel: Karger.
7. Goldstein, R.C. and Schwabe, A.D. (1974) Prophylactic colchicine therapy in familial Mediterranean fever. A controlled double-blind study. *Annals of Internal Medicine*, **81**, 792–794.
8. Matzner, Y. and Brzezenski, A. (1984) C5a-inhibitor deficiency in peritoneal fluids from patients with familial Mediterranean fever. *New England Journal of Medicine*, **311**, 287–290.
9. Pras, E., Aksenfijevich, M.D., Gruberg, M.D. *et al.* (1992) Mapping of a gene causing Familial Mediterranean Fever to the short arm of chromosome 16. *New England Journal of Medicine*, **326**, 1510–1513.
10. Ravid, M., Robson, M. and Kedar (Keizman), I. (1977) Prolonged colchicine treatment in four patients with amyloidosis. *Annals of Internal Medicine*, **87**, 568–570.
11. Schwabe, A.D. and Peters, R.S. (1974) Familial Mediterranean fever in Armenians. Analysis of 100 cases. *Medicine (Baltimore)*, **53**, 453–462.
12. Schwabe, A.D., Terasaki, P.I., Barnett, E.V. *et al.* (1977) Familial Mediterranean fever: recent advances in pathogenesis and management. *Western Journal of Medicine*, **127**, 15–23.
13. Sohar, E., Gafni, J., Pras, M. and Heller, H. (1967) Familial Mediterranean fever. A survey of 470 cases and review of the literature. *American Journal of Medicine*, **43**, 227–253.
14. Wright, D.G., Wolff, S.M., Fauci, A.S. and Alling, D.W. (1977) Efficacy of intermittent colchicine therapy in familial Mediterranean fever. *Annals of Internal Medicine*, **86**, 162–165.
15. Zemer, D., Revach, M., Pras, M. *et al.* (1974) A controlled trial of colchicine in preventing attacks of familial Mediterranean fever. *New England Journal of Medicine*, **291**, 932–934.
16. Zemer, D., Pras, M., Sohar, E. *et al.* (1986) Colchicine in the prevention and treatment of familial Mediterranean fever. *New England Journal of Medicine*, **314**, 1001–1005.

RETROPERITONEAL FIBROSIS (ORMOND'S DISEASE)

A.E. Read

Retroperitoneal fibrosis is a rare disease of uncertain aetiology. It is characterized by the deposition of fibrous tissue in the retroperitoneal space extending from the aortic bifurcation upwards to the level of the renal arteries. The clinical picture is usually the result of compression of important retroperitoneal structures, in particular the ureters.

PATHOLOGY

The fibrous tissue deposited forms a thick rubbery plaque lying mainly over the bodies of the third and fourth lumbar vertebrae. It is in close apposition to the aorta below the renal arteries, and spreads laterally over the psoas muscles. There is no involvement of the peritoneum itself, and the mesentery is usually free of fibrosis. Extension may occur along the course of the common iliac arteries, but usually stops at the brim of the pelvis. Upward extension may occasionally lead to involvement of the mediastinum. The ureters, major veins, aorta and lumbar nerves may all be involved in the fibrotic process. Histologically dense collagen tissue is seen. In the early stages, this is cellular with a prominent lymphocytic and polymorph infiltration, and with a vascular stroma; later the fibrous tissue becomes avascular and acellular. The abdominal aorta is often the site of severe atherosclerosis, and aneurysmal changes may occur[8,2] together with vasculitis[30] in the surrounding tissue.

AETIOLOGY

In up to 10% of patients, the fibrotic process develops in relation to a malignant tumour.[27,28] It may be associated with carcinoid[21] which has a particular propensity to cause widespread fibrosis, but neoplasms of the breast[6] and stomach, and lymphoma[14] are also rare causes.

Some of the patients develop evidence of an abnormal tendency to fibrosis in other organs, and the following disorders are recorded as occurring with retroperitoneal fibrosis: scleroderma, mediastinal fibrosis, Riedel's thyroiditis, pseudotumour of the orbit,[37] retractile mesenteritis, and sclerosing cholangitis. Generally these disorders are thought to represent the effects of an abnormal immunological and fibrotic response to some unknown antigen and may pre-or postdate the retroperitoneal fibrosis.

Interest has centred around the possibility that β-blocking drugs could be a factor in the production of retroperitoneal fibrosis.[9,33,42] These reports were of interest in view of the abnormal fibrous reaction to the β-blocker practolol seen in the visceral peritoneum.[32] The other important drug association of retroperitoneal fibrosis is with the serotonin antagonist, methysergide. About 12% of cases of retroperitoneal fibrosis have been associated with this drug which is used in the treatment of migraine. The association is of practical importance since the process commonly remits on withdrawal of the methysergide. The disorder has occasionally been associated with therapy with ergotamine,[13] hydralazine, methyldopa, and some analgesics such as Distalgesic.[7] Bromocriptine,[9,12,43] a further ergot derivative and not a serotonin antagonist, when used in high doses, usually in elderly men, for the relief of Parkinson's disease, is a further drug cause of this disorder which has been recognized in recent years. Bromocriptine used for prolactinoma treatment may also be associated with this disorder.[22]

A variety of autoimmune disorders, and disorders of uncertain aetiology apart from those associated with fibrosis, may occur with retroperitoneal fibrosis. Thus Raynaud's phenomenon, arteritis, polyarthritis, sarcoidosis,[20] Crohn's disease, interstitial nephritis,[26] scleroderma[31] and systemic lupus erythematosus,[19] ankylosing spondylitis,[41] with and without radiotherapy, primary biliary cirrhosis,[38] and eosinophilic fasciitis[19] are all recorded accompaniments. It also occurs in families.[15]

The precise cause of the disease remains uncertain. The close relationship of the fibrosis to the abdominal aorta and the presence of severe aortic atheroma[18] and aneurysms has led to the suggestion that the process develops in relation to aortic disease. Some cases are caused without doubt by the inflammatory changes around abdominal aortic aneurysms.[8] It is suggested that an immunological reaction resulting in macrophage-induced fibrosis occurs as a result of antigenic material leaking from the blood stream or atheromatous aortic wall. Certainly inflammatory changes around some aneurysms are widely recognized at aortic surgery. Similarly the possibility that chronic leakage of urine from an obstructed kidney could cause a fibrous reaction has been entertained, because a granulomatous and fibrotic reaction around the renal pelvis is sometimes recorded with obstructed kidneys. Most observers, however, feel that this disease represents the effects of some immunological stimulation of collagen formation.

CLINICAL FEATURES

This is a rare disorder. Up to 1977 only about 500 cases were recorded in the world literature. The incidence is uncertain as it is probable that some examples are not associated with clinical consequences.

Characteristically, except in cases following methysergide, males are more commonly affected than females. Most patients are between 50 and 70 years of age; children can, however, be affected.[39] The symptoms are often non-specific and insidious, and are usually related primarily to obstruction of the ureters. Loin pain, lower abdominal pain or backache are early symptoms. The pain is often poorly localized, and dull and aching in character; there may also be abdominal tenderness and distension on palpation. When the ureters are completely or partially occluded the patient develops attacks of renal colic and the features of oliguric renal failure. Partial ureteric obstruction causes abdominal pain, frequency and lassitude. Obstruction of the ureters also leads to the onset of hypertension with retinopathy, dyspnoea and headaches. Occasionally generalized oedema occurs owing to the nephrotic syndrome secondary to involvement of the renal veins.

Compression of the inferior vena cava, and the iliac veins and lymphatics results in swelling of one or both legs owing to oedema and occasionally a varicocele or hydrocele or testicular retraction[11] develops in males. Involvement of the lumbar nerve roots may give rise to backache with radiation of pain into the thigh and leg, and pain on movement of the hip. Accompanying these symptoms there is often systemic upset, including lassitude, weight loss and occasionally fever.[11]

Physical signs are remarkably few and no doubt this causes the observed delay in diagnosis. A palpable mass owing to the fibrotic process is unlikely, presumably because of its deep, midline position. Nevertheless, about 30% of patients have an abdominal mass or a mass felt rectally or vaginally. Involvement of the ureters may result in one or more enlarged palpable kidneys. Hypertension is common.

Additional features in patients with other types of fibrotic disease include a hard, woody goitre with stridor (Reidel's thyroiditis), venous obstruction due to superior vena caval obstruction (mediastinal fibrosis) and proptosis (pseudotumour of the orbit).

DIFFERENTIAL DIAGNOSIS

This is extremely wide because of the common lack of physical signs and the vagueness of the symptoms. Because swelling of the ankles may occur, a diagnosis of venous insufficiency or heart failure may be made. Back and hip pain may simulate a primary orthopaedic disorder of the back or hip, whilst reference of the pain to the abdomen without physical signs may lead to a diagnosis of renal tract disease or irritable bowel syndrome.[24] The presence of hypertension, proteinuria and elevated blood urea may suggest a diagnosis of chronic renal failure of uncertain cause with secondary hypertension. There is a risk, however, that patients with this disorder will be labelled as 'functional' or 'neurotic'.

The following are rare but recognized complications of the disease which can lead to unusual abdominal manifestations.

1. A mass is sometimes felt on rectal examination owing to the fibrotic process involving the pelvis; this may simulate a rectal or pararectal tumour.
2. Portal hypertension with bleeding oesophageal varices can follow secondary involvement of the porta hepatis and the portal vein.[10,35]
3. Obstructive jaundice due to common bile duct constriction may rarely be seen.
4. Nausea, vomiting and weight loss may occur and may closely simulate gastric ulceration or neoplasia.
5. Toxic megacolon, proctitis and rectal stenosis are all rarely recorded.
6. Intermittent claudication[40] due to involvement of the iliac arteries can occur, as well as testicular retraction.

INVESTIGATION

BLOOD AND URINE TESTS

Three blood tests provide helpful but non-specific evidence of the presence of this disease: the haemoglobin, which is unexplainedly reduced so that a mild and usually normochromic anaemia results; the erythrocyte sedimentation rate, which is elevated in over 50% of patients; and the serum albumin, which is reduced.

Where there is secondary involvement of the kidneys and ureteric obstruction, proteinuria or frank evidence of renal tract infection (pyuria, proteinuria casts and organisms) can be seen on microscopy or are revealed by culture. Once renal function is deranged there is evidence of impaired creatinine clearance and later elevation of the blood urea. In two cases a raised hepatic alkaline phosphatase was the only biochemical abnormality.[4]

THE INTRAVENOUS PYELOGRAM

Until recently this was the main investigation by which a definite diagnosis could be made and it still has an important part to play in diagnosis, although its specificity has been questioned. Obstruction of the ureters may cause dilatation of the upper third, medial deviation, particularly of the middle third, owing to involvement of the ureters in the fibrotic process, which contract to produce ureteric tethering, and hydronephrosis affecting one or both kidneys. Of these radiological signs, dilatation and medial deviation are non-specific: it is well recognized that some medial deviation of the ureters may be seen in normal pyelograms. Nevertheless, these findings, particularly in the face of a compatible history and physical examination and with suggestive results from simple blood tests, make the diag-nosis probable. The value of the intravenous pyelogram diminishes with increasing evidence of secondary renal failure and on occasions can be normal.

SCANNING

These techniques have a useful part to play in diagnosis, although experience with them in this rare disease is small. Fagan, Larrieu and Amparo[16] studied three patients with retroperitoneal fibrosis in whom ultrasound showed the presence of an echogenic mass with clear margins and irregular contours enveloping but not displacing structures such as the aorta, vena cava and ureters. The kidney may be pushed anteriorly by the mass. There was a clear margin between the mass and the posterior peritoneum anteriorly. Similar features are shown on computed tomography (CT). The density of the fibrous tissue is similar to that of the muscles which it covers, and the infiltration of tissue planes between muscles is clearly shown. CT is particularly good at defining the extent of the fibrotic process and monitoring its progress.

Magnetic resonance imaging (MRI) seems to be even more helpful in delineating the extent of fibrosis.[44] Arrive *et al.*[1] showed that on MRI the fibrous tissue had ill-defined margins and heterogeneous signal intensity in 5 of 9 cases associated with malignancy.

Isotope scanning using gallium^{67}, which is taken up by macrophages, may be a useful way of detecting early retroperitoneal fibrosis.[29]

BIOPSY

A biopsy for histological examination is taken at laparotomy (see below).

TREATMENT

An accurate diagnosis must always be made where this is feasible,[25,34] which usually requires surgery and biopsy with careful histology. This is to ensure that cases caused by malignant disease are diagnosed, as the prognosis is much worse than in idiopathic cases. Even with careful scrutiny of the tissue obtained, however, malignant fibrosis may be missed and the diagnosis only becomes apparent by the subsequent clinical course. A laparotomy is necessary to expose both ureters and retroperitoneal spaces, to mobilize the ascending and descending colon and to dissect the retroperitoneal tissues.

If the ureters are involved in the fibrous tissue they are first mobilized in their upper and lower portions. The part encased in fibrous tissue is freed by blunt dissection following incision through the fibrous plaque along the course of the ureter (ureterolysis). This procedure is worthwhile even if it is known that the diagnosis is one of malignant retroperitoneal fibrosis. Once freed the ureters are placed laterally surrounded by omentum and retained by stitching the peritoneum onto the psoas muscles. Alternative approaches have been balloon dilatation of narrowed ureters, peritoneal flap ureteropexy[17] and where there is obstruction at the level of the renal pelvis, nephrostomy.

Most patients in whom this operation is performed improve, and long-term survival for 10–20 years is possible. There is argument as to whether patients in whom the diagnosis has been confirmed histologically and in whom bilateral ureterolysis has been performed should also be given steroid drugs. Reports of successful corticosteroid therapy are found in the literature, and relapse is recorded following cessation of this treatment. Furthermore, patients have been managed with corticosteroids alone[23] and this may be the best treatment at least in those who are ill or elderly and unsuitable for immediate surgery. Usually, however, as biopsy is essential ureterolysis will be carried out at the same procedure. It is important to treat any underlying disease such as an aortic aneurysm and to exclude any drugs which are possible causes.

Progesterone has been used with beneficial results[5] and, because of a presumed hormonal dependence of the fibrous tissue, it was used as intramuscular injections of medroxyprogesterone acetate 1 g, every 2 weeks for 18 months with complete disappearance of the lesion[3] in a 22-year-old female. Azathioprine may also be effective – it seems to be so by itself rather than when used merely as a corticosteroid-sparing agent.

PROGNOSIS

Patients who present with acute oliguric renal failure or renal failure which does not respond to ureterolysis alone or coupled with corticosteroids have a poor prognosis; about 10% of all patients die from these causes. The others are usually cured, and apart from the complications of hypertension, survive normally. The prognosis may be altered by the presence of another fibrosing disease.

A recent review[2] of 60 cases seen at St Bartholomew's Hospital, London, between 1965 and 1984 showed a 3:1 male sex predominance, a 2-year survival rate of 78% and death in 17 patients, usually the elderly and the uraemic. Only four were associated with malignancy and four with aneurysms.

REFERENCES

1. Arrive, L., Hricak, H., Tavares, N.J. and Miller, T.R. (1989) Malignant versus nonmalignant retroperitoneal fibrosis: differentiation with MR imaging. *Radiology*, **171**, 139–143.
2. Baker, L.R., Mallinson, W.J., Gregory, M.C. *et al.* (1987) Idiopathic retroperitoneal fibrosis. A retrospective analysis of 60 cases. *British Journal of Urology*, **60**, 497–503.
3. Barnhill, D., Hoskins, W., Burke, T., Weiser, E., Heller, P. and Park, R. (1987) The treatment of retroperitoneal fibromatosis with medroxyprogesterone acetate. *Obstetrics and Gynaecology*, **70**, 502–504.
4. Barrison, I.G., Walker, J.G., Jones, C. and Snell, M.E. (1988) Idiopathic retroperitoneal fibrosis – is serum alkaline phosphatase a marker of disease activity? *Postgraduate Medical Journal*, **64**, 239–241.
5. Bilder, C.R., Barousse, A.P. and Mazure, P.A. (1985) Progesterone as therapy for retroperitoneal fibrosis. *Medicina (Buenos Aires)*, **45**, 159–163.
6. Blairon, J., Paulet, P., Rutsaert, J. and Limbosch, J.M. (1979) Oesophageal stenosis and retroperitoneal fibrosis appearing as a late consequence of a breast carcinoma. *Acta Gastroenterologica Belgica*, **42**, 285–293.
7. Bowler, J.V., Ormerod, I.E. and Legg, N.J. (1986) Retroperitoneal fibrosis and bromocriptine (letter). *The Lancet*, **2**, 466.
8. Buchanan, L.D. and Holden, W. (1989) Inflammatory aneurysm: a cause of obstructive

nephropathy. *Journal of the American Osteopathy Association*, **89**, 1069–1072.
9. Bullimore, D.W. (1980) Retroperitoneal fibrosis associated with atenolol. *British Medical Journal*, **281**, 59–60.
10. Bullimore, D.W., Mascie Taylor, B.H., Muers, M. and Losowsky, M.S. (1987) Combined retroperitoneal and mediastinal fibrosis associated with variceal haemorrhage. *British Journal of Clinical Practice*, **41**, 1064–1065.
11. Byrd, W.E., Hunt, R.E. and Burgess, R. (1981) Retroperitoneal fibrosis as a cause of fever of undetermined origin. *Western Journal of Medicine*, **134**, 357–361.
12. Critchley, J.A., Smith, M.F. and Prescott, L.F. (1985) Distalgesic abuse and retroperitoneal fibrosis. *British Journal of Urology*, **57**, 486–487.
13. Damstrup, L. and Jensen, T.T. (1986) Retroperitoneal fibrosis after long-term daily use of ergotamine. *International Urology and Nephrology*, **18**, 299–301.
14. Diabel, P.W., Mullins, J.D. and Coltman, C.A. Jr. (1980) An unusual manifestation of non-Hodgkins lymphoma fibrosis masquerading as Ormond's disease. *Journal of the American Medical Association*, **243**, 1161–1162.
15. Doolin, E.J., Goldstein, H., Kessler, B., Vinocur, C. and Marchildon, M.B. (1987) Familial retroperitoneal fibrosis. *Journal of Paediatric Surgery*, **22**, 1092–1094.
16. Fagan, C.J., Larrieu, A.J. and Amparo, E.G. (1979) Retroperitoneal fibrosis: ultrasound and CT features. *American Journal of Roentgenology*, **133**, 239–243.
17. Fowler, J.W. (1987) Peritoneal flap ureteropexy for idiopathic retroperitoneal fibrosis. *British Journal of Urology*, **60**, 18–22.
18. Gabrielli, L. and Lorenzi, G. (1979) Arteriosclerotic obliteration of the infrarenal aorta and retroperitonel fibrosis. *Angiologia*, **31**, 105–111.
19. Garcia Morteo, O., Nitsche, A., Maldonado Cocca, J.A. and Barcelo, H.A. (1987) Eosinophilic fasciitis and retroperitoneal fibrosis in a patient with systemic lupus erythematosus (letter). *Arthritis and Rheumatism*, **30**, 1314–1315.
20. Godin, M., Fillastre, J.P., Ducastelle, T. *et al.* (1980) Sarcoidosis. Retroperitoneal fibrosis, renal arterial involvement and unilateral focal glomerulosclerosis. *Archives of Internal Medicine*, **140**, 1240–1242.
21. Gupta, A., Saibil, F., Kassim, O. and McKee, J. (1985) Retroperitoneal fibrosis caused by carcinoid tumour. *Quarterly Journal of Medicine*, **56**, 367–375.
22. Herzog, A., Minne, H. and Ziegler, R. (1989) Retroperitoneal fibrosis in a patient with macroprolactinoma treated with bromocriptine. *British Medical Journal*, **298**, 1315.
23. Higgins, P.M., Bennett Jones, D.N., Naish, P.F. and Aber, G.M. (1988) Non-operative management of retroperitoneal fibrosis. *British Journal of Surgery*, **75**, 573–577.
24. Hulnick, D.H., Chatson, G.P., Megibow, A.J., Bosniak, M.A. and Ruoff, M. (1988) Retroperitoneal fibrosis presenting as colonic dysfunction: CT diagnosis. *Journal of Computer Assisted Tomography*, **12**, 159–161.
25. Kinder, C.H. (1979) Retroperitoneal fibrosis (editorial). *Journal of the Royal Society of Medicine*, **22**, 63–67.
26. Kirschbaum, B.B., Koontz, W.W. and Olichney, M.J. (1981) Association of retroperitoneal fibrosis and interstitial nephritis. *Archives of Internal Medicine*, **141**, 1361–1363.
27. Koep, L. and Zuidema, G.D. (1977) The clinical significance of retroperitoneal fibrosis. *Surgery*, **81**, 250–257.
28. Larrieu, A.J., Weiner, I., Abston, S. and Warren, M.M. (1980) Retroperitoneal fibrosis. *Surgery, Gynaecology and Obstetrics*, **150**, 699–702.
29. Leibowich, S. and Tumeh, S.S. (1988) Gallium-67 imaging and computed tomography in early retroperitoneal fibrosis. *Clinical Nuclear Medicine*, **13**, 829–830.
30. Lindell, O.I., Sariola, H.V. and Lehtonen, T.A. (1987) The occurrence of vasculitis in perianeurysmal fibrosis. *Journal of Urology*, **138**, 727–729.
31. Mansell, M.A. and Watts, R.W. (1980) Retroperitoneal fibrosis and scleroderma. *Postgraduate Medical Journal*, **56**, 730–733.
32. Marshall, A.J., Baddeley, H., Barritt, D.W. *et al.* (1977) Practolol peritonitis. *Quarterly Journal of Medicine*, **46**, 135–149.
33. McClusky, D.R., Donaldson, R.A. and McGeown, M.G. (1980) Oxprenolol and retroperitoneal fibrosis. *British Medical Journal*, **281**, 1459–1460.
34. McComb, J.E. and Gall, E.P. (1979) Retroperitoneal fibrosis. *Arizona Medicine*, **36**, 41–44.
35. Mosimann, F. and Mange, B. (1980) Portal hypertension as a complication of idiopathic retroperitoneal fibrosis. *British Journal of Surgery*, **67**, 804.
36. Murphy, F. and Pickard, R.S. (1989) Bromocriptine-associated retroperitoneal fibrosis presenting with testicular retraction. *British Journal of Urology*, **64**, 318–319.
37. Richards, A.B., Shalka, H.W., Roberts, F.J. and Flint, A. (1980) Pseudotumour of the orbit and retroperitoneal fibrosis. A form of multifocal fibroschlerosis. *Archives of Ophthalmology*, **98**, 1617–1620.
38. Sevenet, F., Capron Chivrac, D., Delcenserie, R., Lelarge, C., Delamarre, J. and Capron, J.P. (1985) Idiopathic retroperitoneal fibrosis and primary biliary cirrhosis. A new association? *Archives of Internal Medicine*, **145**, 2124–2125.
39. Sherman, C., Winchester, P., Brill, P.W. and Mininberg, D. (1988) Childhood retroperitoneal fibrosis. *Pediatric Radiology*, **18**, 245–247.

40. Shortland, G.J., Archer, T.J. and Webster, J.H. (1986) Intermittent claudication caused by retroperitoneal fibrosis. *British Journal of Surgery*, **73**, 156–157.
41. Solomon, S.D. and Maurer, K.H. (1985) The association of retroperitonel fibrosis and ankylosing spondylitis (letter). *Journal of Rheumatology*, **12**, 818.
42. Thompson, J. and Julian D.G. (1982) Retroperitoneal fibrosis associated with metoprolol. *British Medical Journal*, **284**, 83–84.
43. Ward, C.D., Thompson, J. and Humby, M.D. (1987) Pleuropulmonary and retroperitoneal fibrosis associated with bromocriptine treatment (letter). *Journal of Neurology, Neurosurgery and Psychiatry*, **50**, 1706–1707.
44. Yuh, W.T., Barloon, T.J., Sickels, W.J., Kramolowsky, E.V. and Williams, R.D. (1989) Magnetic resonance imaging in the diagnosis and followup of idiopathic retroperitoneal fibrosis. *Journal of Urology*, **141**, 602–605.

INDEX

Note: Page references in *italics* refer to figures; those in **bold** refer to tables